Clinical Classification in Orthopaedics Trauma

图书在版编目（CIP）数据

临床骨折分型 = Clinical Classification in Orthopaedics Trauma：英文 / 张英泽主编. —北京：人民卫生出版社，2018
ISBN 978-7-117-26033-6

Ⅰ. ①临… Ⅱ. ①张… Ⅲ. ①骨折-诊疗-英文 Ⅳ. ①R683

中国版本图书馆CIP数据核字（2018）第021079号

临床骨折分型（英文版）

主　　编：张英泽
出版发行：人民卫生出版社（中继线 010-59780011）
地　　址：北京市朝阳区潘家园南里 19 号
邮　　编：100021
E - mail：pmph @ pmph.com
购书热线：010-59787592　010-59787584　010-65264830
印　　刷：北京建宏印刷有限公司
经　　销：新华书店
开　　本：889 × 1194　1/16　　**印张**：44
字　　数：1363 千字
版　　次：2018 年 2 月第 1 版　2018 年 2 月第 1 版第 1 次印刷
标准书号：ISBN 978-7-117-26033-6/R · 26034
定　　价：580.00元

Yingze Zhang
Editor

Clinical Classification in Orthopaedics Trauma

PEOPLE'S MEDICAL PUBLISHING HOUSE

Springer

人民卫生出版社
PMPH PEOPLE'S MEDICAL PUBLISHING HOUSE

Website: http://www.pmph.com/

Book Title: Clinical Classification in Orthopaedics Trauma

Contact address: No. 19, Pan Jia Yuan Nan Li, Chaoyang District, Beijing 100021, P.R. China, phone/fax: 8610 5978 7236, E-mail: pmph@pmph.com

First published: 2018
ISBN: 978-7-117-26033-6/R · 26034

Cataloguing in Publication Data:

A catalogue record for this book is available from the CIP-Database China.

ISBN 978-7-117-26033-6

9 787117 260336 >

Printed in The People's Republic of China

Contents

1 **Classifications of Shoulder Girdle Fractures** 1
Yingze Zhang and Bo Lu

2 **Classification of Humeral Fractures** 53
Yingze Zhang and Bo Lu

3 **Classifications of Radius and Ulna Fractures** 117
Yingze Zhang and Juan Wang

4 **Classifications of Hand and Wrist Fractures** 183
Yingze Zhang and Xin Xing

5 **Classification of Dislocation of Shoulder and Upper Limb** 231
Yingze Zhang and Wenjuan Wu

6 **Classifications for Spine Fractures** 265
Yingze Zhang and Wei Chen

7 **Classification of Pelvic Ring Fracture and Dislocation** 319
Yingze Zhang and Zhiyong Hou

8 **Classification of Femoral Fractures** 361
Yingze Zhang and Yanbin Zhu

9 **Classifications of Patellar Fracture** 431
Yingze Zhang and Yanbin Zhu

10 **Classification of Tibial and Fibular Fractures** 445
Yingze Zhang and Juan Wang

11 **Classification of Foot Fractures** 523
Yingze Zhang and Haotian Wu

12 **Classification of Hip Joint and Lower Extremity Dislocations** 597
Yingze Zhang and Haotian Wu

13 **Classifications of Soft-Tissue Injuries** 627
Yingze Zhang and Xin Xing

14 **Fracture and Dislocation Classification for Children** 631
Yingze Zhang and Liang Shi

Contributors

Wei Chen Department of Orthopedics, The Third Hospital of Hebei Medical University, Shijiazhuang, China

Zhiyong Hou Department of Orthopedics, The Third Hospital of Hebei Medical University, Shijiazhuang, China

Bo Lu Department of Orthopedics, The Third Hospital of Hebei Medical University, Shijiazhuang, China

Liang Shi Department of Orthopedics, The Third Hospital of Hebei Medical University, Shijiazhuang, China

Juan Wang Department of Orthopedics, The Third Hospital of Hebei Medical University, Shijiazhuang, China

Haotian Wu Department of Orthopedics, The Third Hospital of Hebei Medical University, Shijiazhuang, China

Wenjuan Wu Department of Orthopedics, The Third Hospital of Hebei Medical University, Shijiazhuang, China

Xin Xing Department of Orthopedics, The Third Hospital of Hebei Medical University, Shijiazhuang, China

Yingze Zhang Department of Orthopedics, The Third Hospital of Hebei Medical University, Shijiazhuang, China

Yanbin Zhu Department of Orthopedics, The Third Hospital of Hebei Medical University, Shijiazhuang, China

Classifications of Shoulder Girdle Fractures

1

Yingze Zhang and Bo Lu

1.1 Classification of Clavicular Fractures

Allman first proposed his classification scheme for clavicular fractures that was widely accepted in 1967. Thereafter, many classification systems involving clavicular fractures were provided. Allman's classification is still the most frequently used system, and its use became more practical when some scholars supplemented it with sub-types. According to literature over the last 5 years, other classifications of clavicular fractures also frequently used are the Craig classification, Robinson classification, etc.

Y. Zhang (✉) • B. Lu
Department of Orthopedics,
The Third Hospital of Hebei Medical University,
Shijiazhuang, China
e-mail: yzzhangdr@126.com; yzling_liu@163.com

Y. Zhang (ed.), *Clinical Classification in Orthopaedics Trauma*, https://doi.org/10.1007/978-981-10-6044-1_1

1.1.1 Craig Classification of Clavicle Fractures

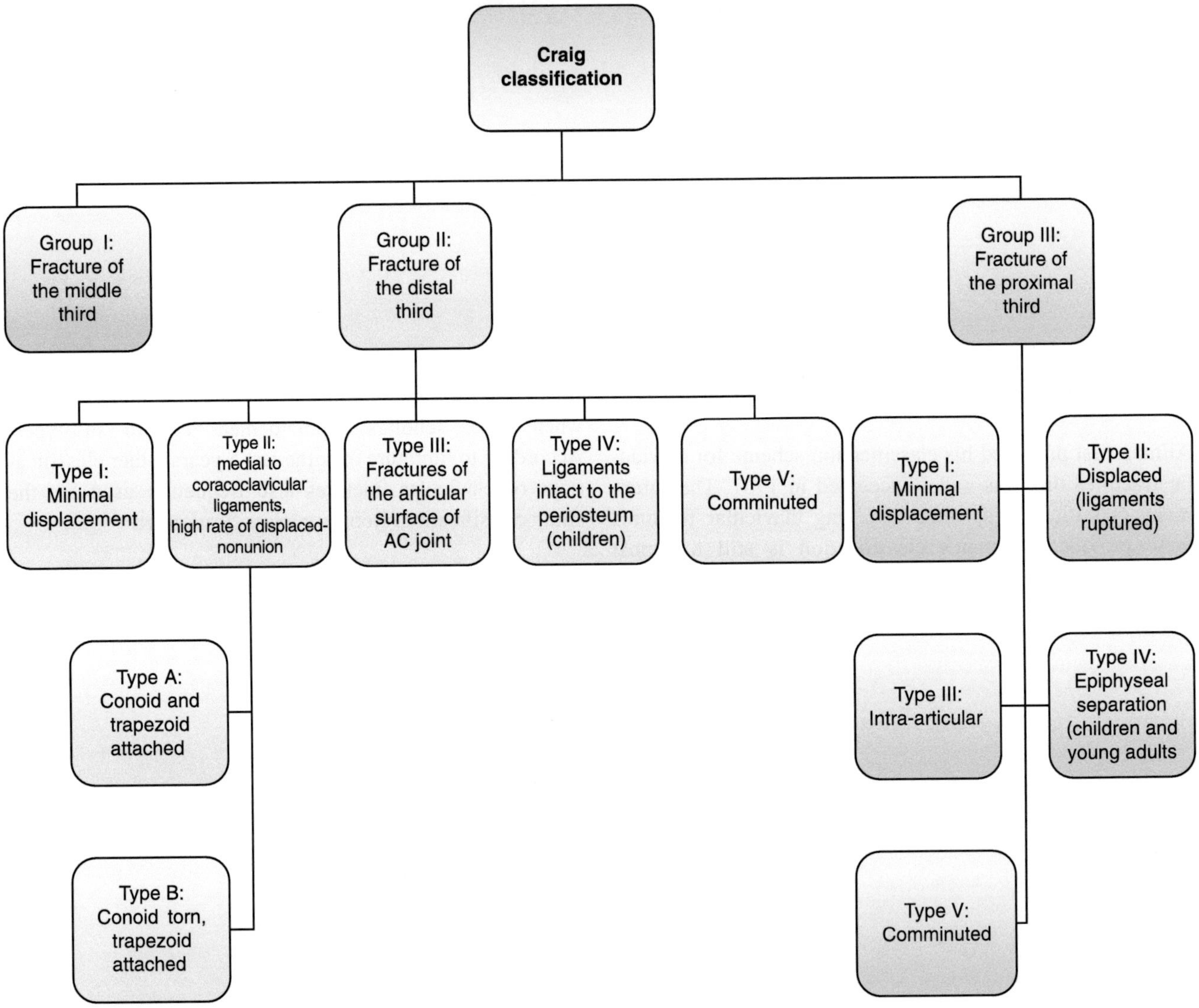

Group I: Fracture of the middle third.

Group II: Fracture of the distal third.

- Type I: Minimal displacement, an interligamentous fracture that occurs between the conoid and the trapezoid or between the coracoclavicular and acromioclavicular ligaments.
- Type II: A fracture medial to the coracoclavicular ligaments, with high rate of displaced nonunion.
  - A. Conoid and trapezoid attached.
  - B. Conoid torn, trapezoid attached.
- Type III: Fractures of the articular surface of the acromioclavicular joint, without a ligamentous injury. A type III injury may be confused with a first-degree acromioclavicular separation.
- Type IV: Ligaments intact to the periosteum (children), with displacement of the proximal fragment.
- Type V: Comminuted, with ligaments attached neither proximally nor distally, but to an inferior, comminuted fragment.

Group III: Fracture of the proximal third.

- Type I: Minimal displacement.
- Type II: Displaced (ligaments ruptured).
- Type III: Intra-articular.
- Type IV: Epiphyseal separation (children and young adults).
- Type V: Comminuted.

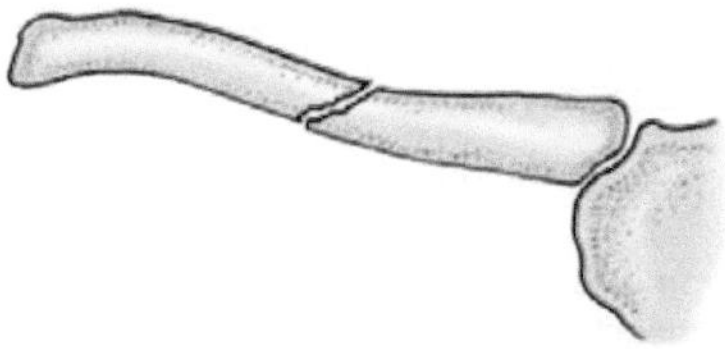

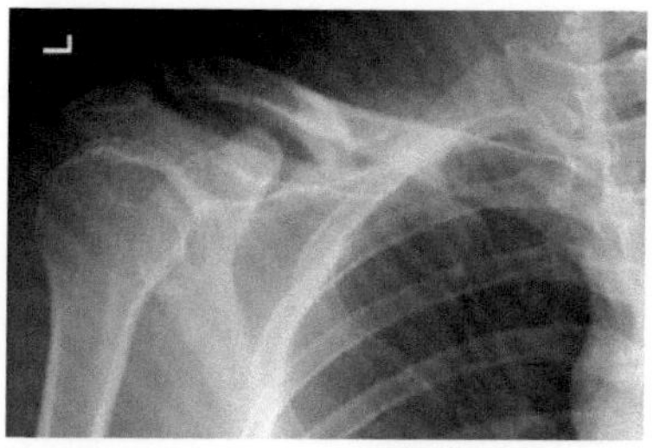

Craig Classification of Clavicle Fractures

Group I: Fracture of the middle third

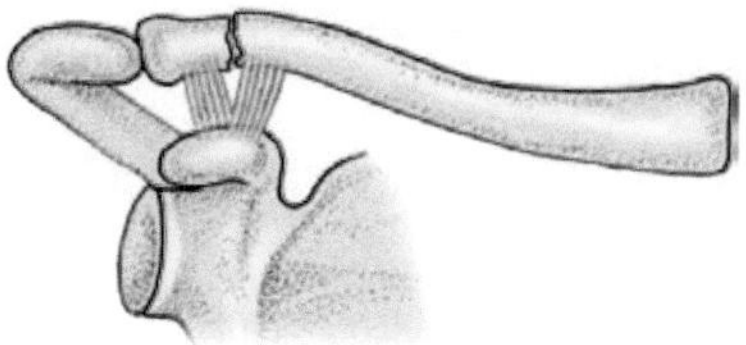

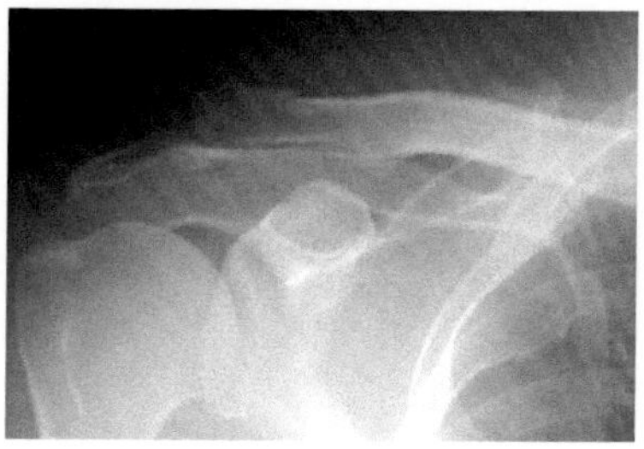

Craig Classification of Clavicle Fractures

Group II: Fracture of the distal third.

Type I: Minimal displacement, an interligamentous fracture

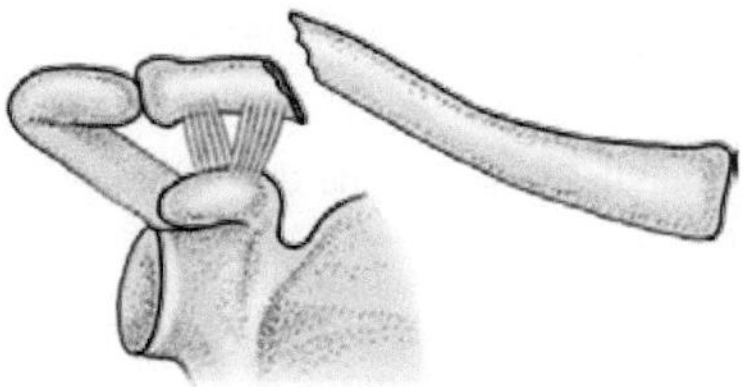

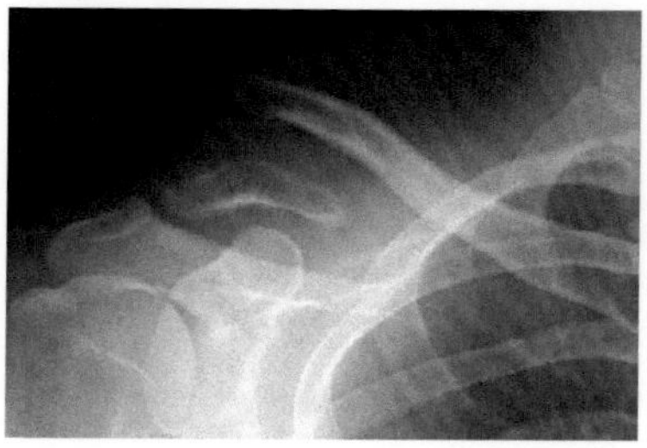

Craig Classification of Clavicle Fractures

Group II: Fracture of the distal third.

Type II: A fracture of medial to the coracoclavicular ligaments, with high rate of displaced-nonunion.

Type IIA: Conoid and trapezoid attached

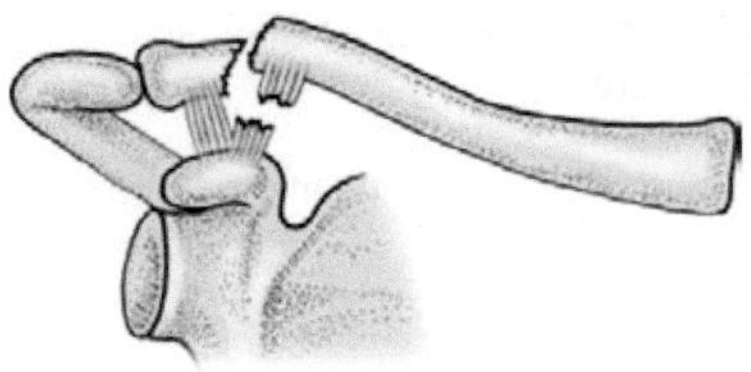

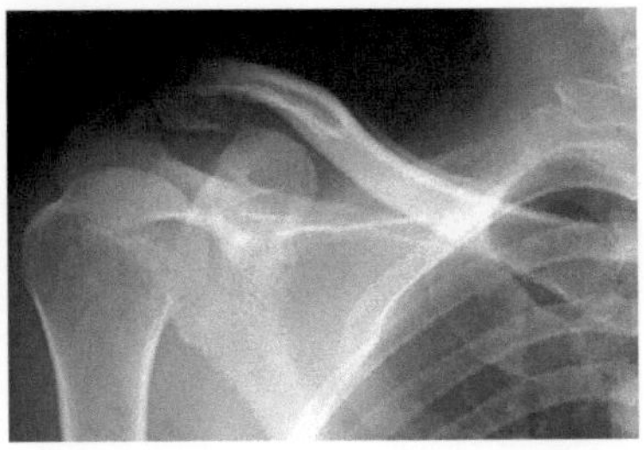

Craig Classification of Clavicle Fractures

Group II: Fracture of the distal third.

Type II: A fracture of medial to the coracoclavicular ligaments, with high rate of displaced-nonunion.

Type II B: Conoid torn, trapezoid attached

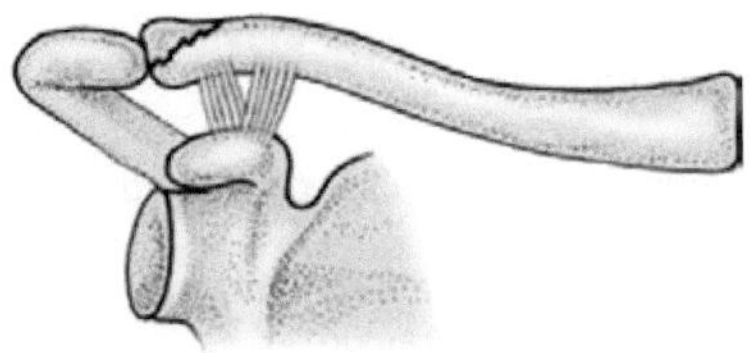

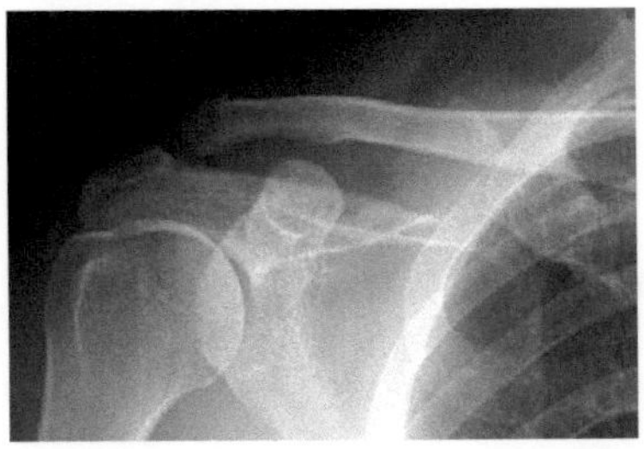

Craig Classification of Clavicle Fractures

Group II: Fracture of the distal third.

Type III: Fractures of the articular surface of the acromioclavicular joint, without a ligamentous injury

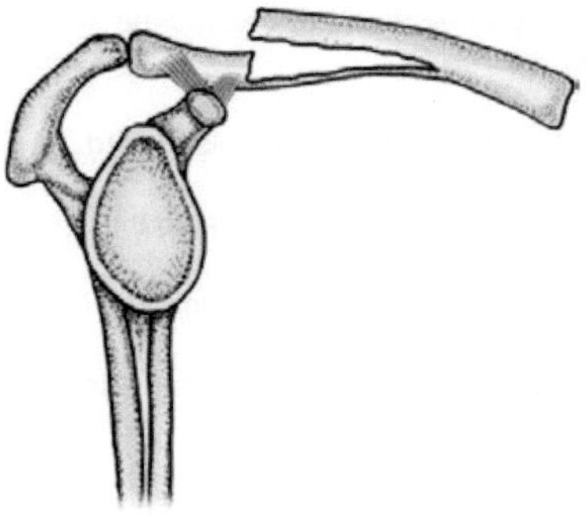

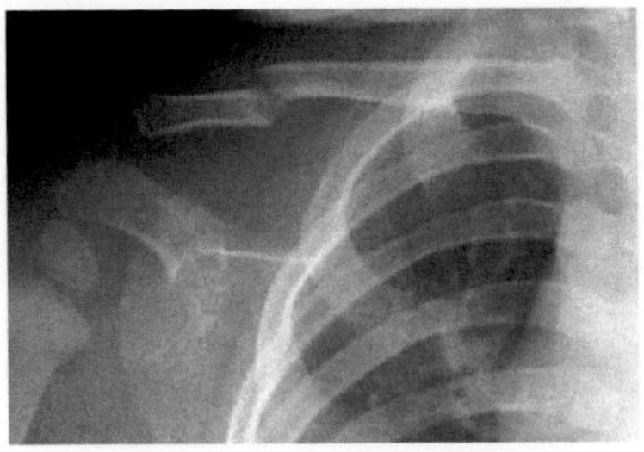

Craig Classification of Clavicle Fractures

Group II: Fracture of the distal third.

Type IV: Ligaments intact to the periosteum (children), with displacement of the proximal fragment

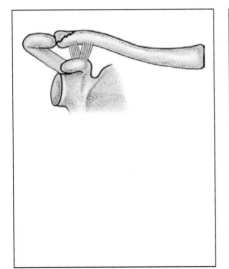

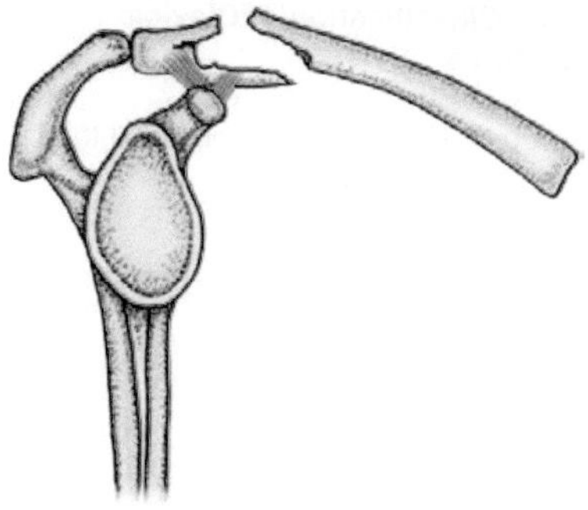

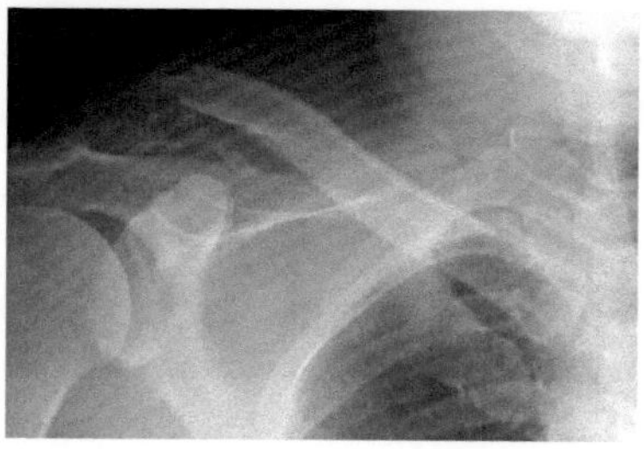

Craig Classification of Clavicle Fractures

Group II: Fracture of the distal third.

Type V: Comminuted

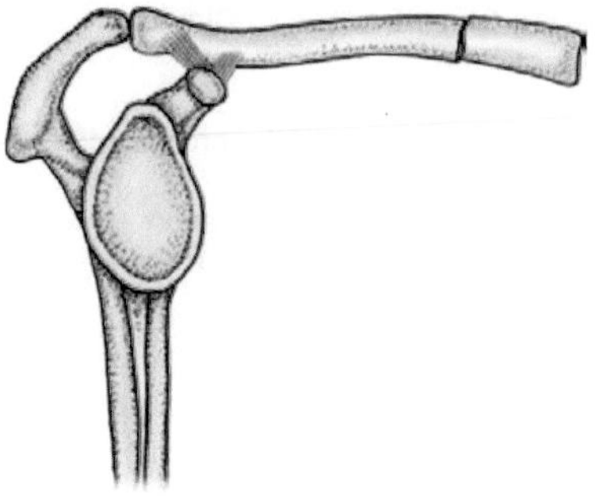

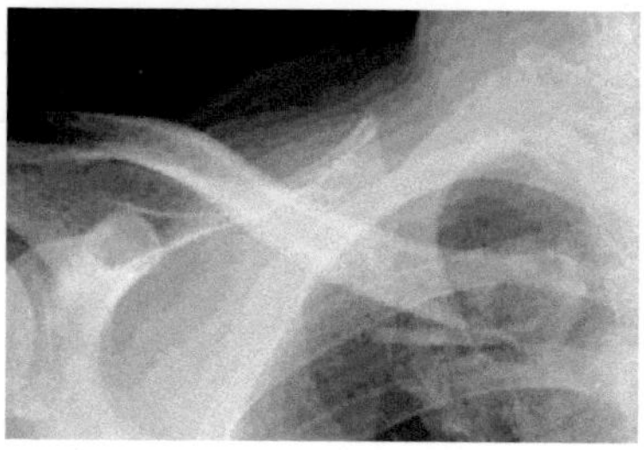

Craig Classification of Clavicle Fractures

Group III: Fracture of the proximal third.

Type I: Minimal displacement

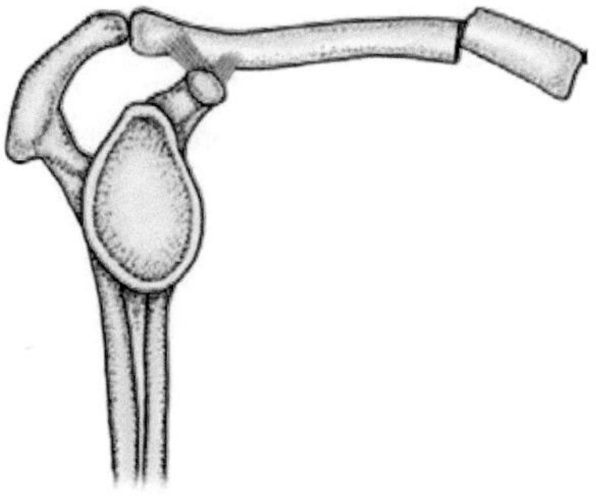

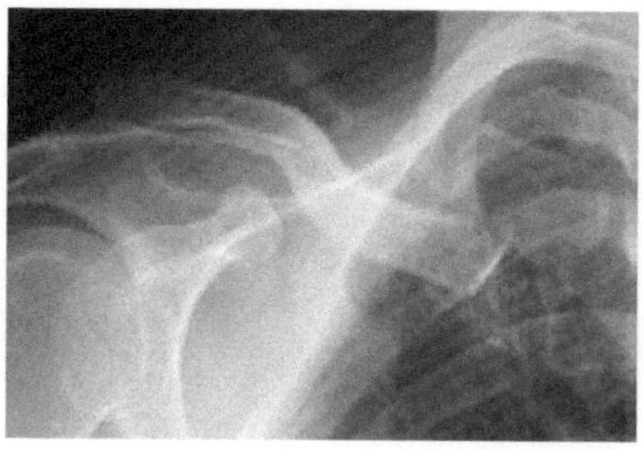

Craig Classification of Clavicle Fractures

Group III: Fracture of the proximal third.

Type II: Displaced (ligaments ruptured)

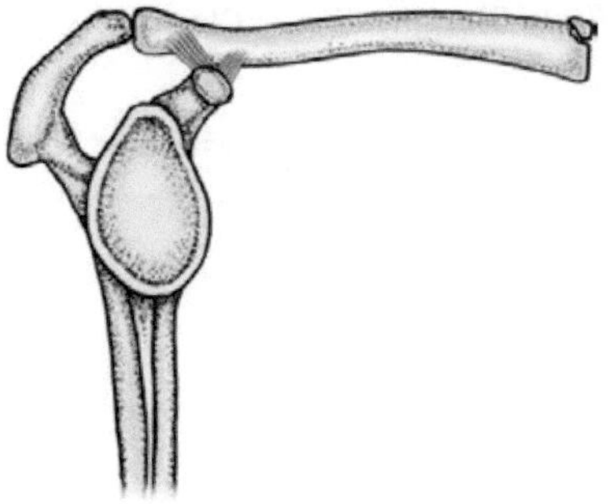

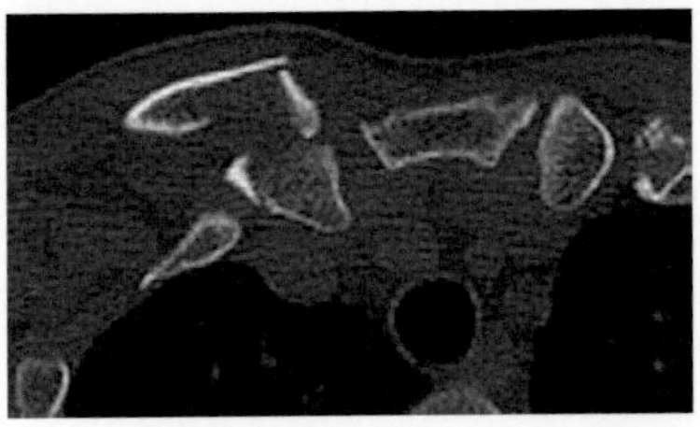

Craig Classification of Clavicle Fractures

Group III: Fracture of the proximal third.

Type III: Intra-articular

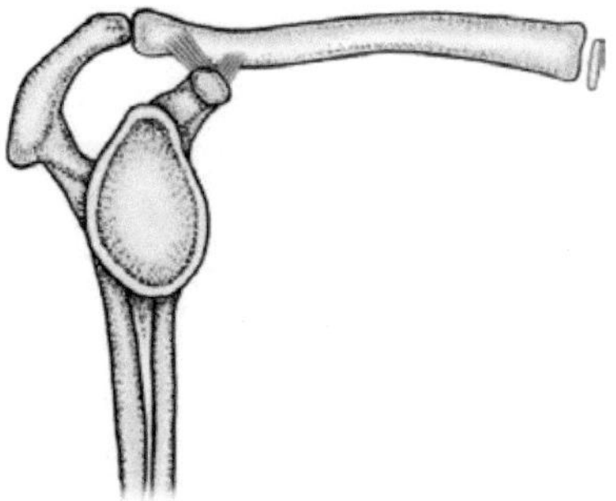

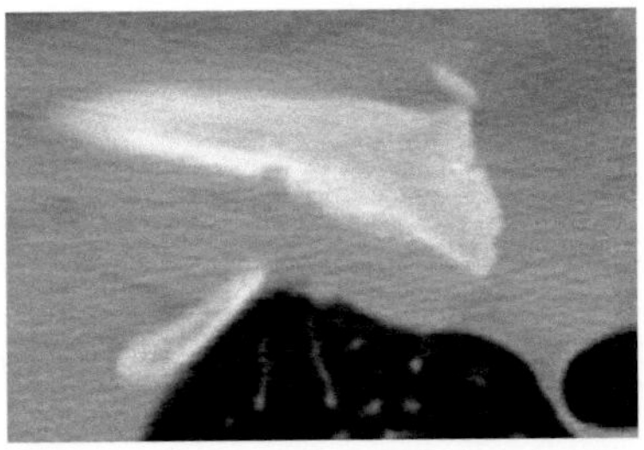

Craig Classification of Clavicle Fractures

Group III: Fracture of the proximal third.

Type IV: Epiphyseal separation (children and young adults)

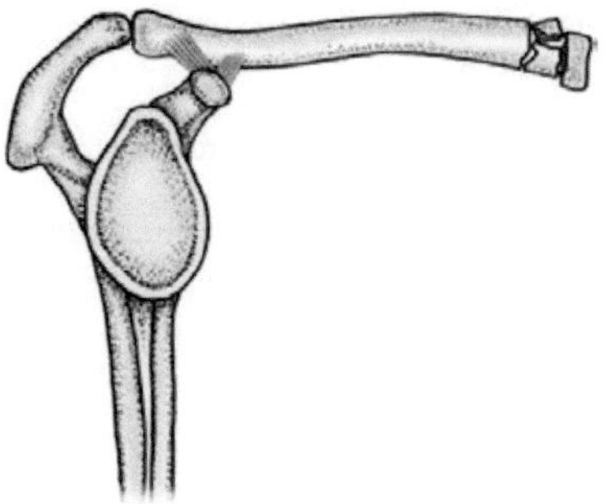

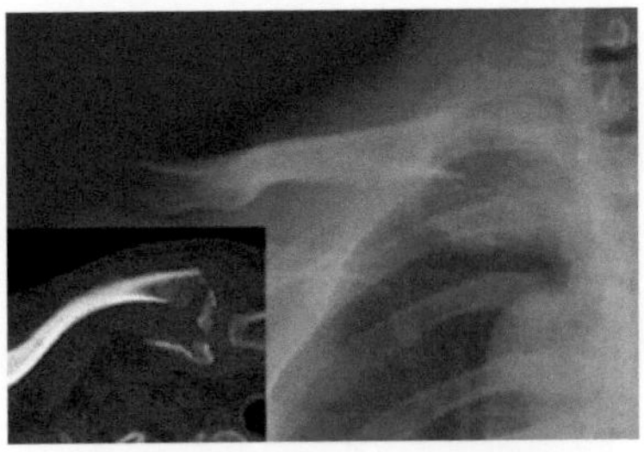

Craig Classification of Clavicle Fractures

Group III: Fracture of the proximal third.

Type V: Comminuted

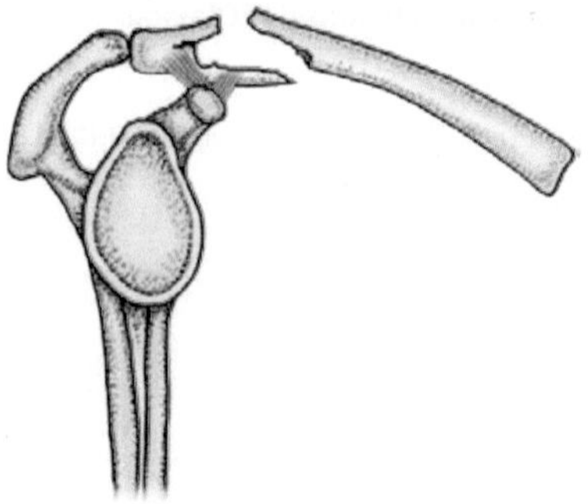

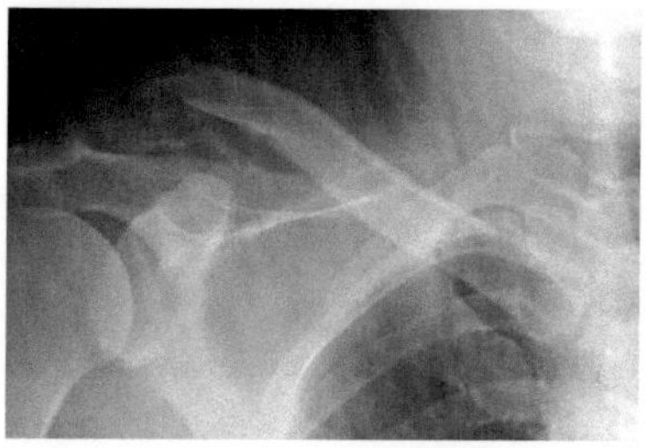

Craig Classification of Clavicle Fractures

Group II: Fracture of the distal third.

Type V: Comminuted

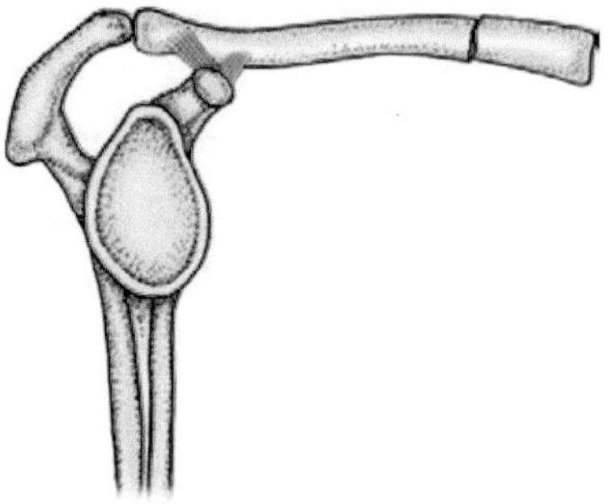

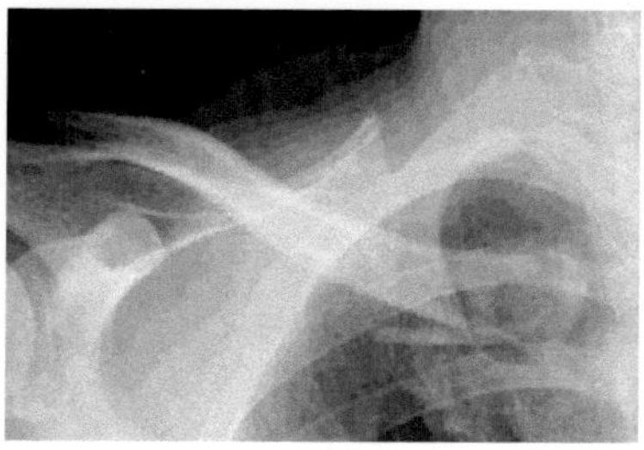

Craig Classification of Clavicle Fractures

Group III: Fracture of the proximal third.

Type I: Minimal displacement

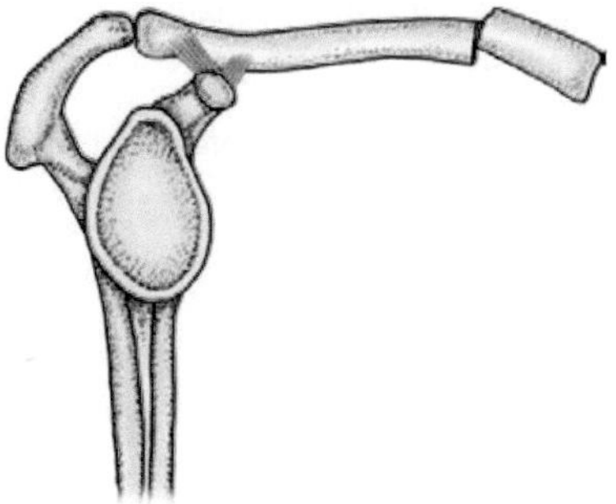

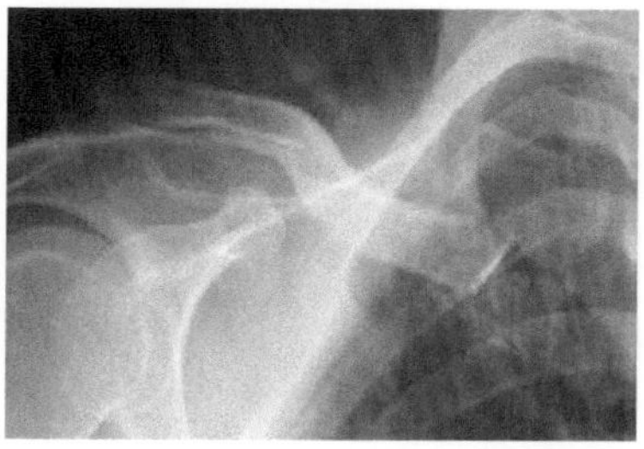

Craig Classification of Clavicle Fractures

Group III: Fracture of the proximal third.

Type II: Displaced (ligaments ruptured)

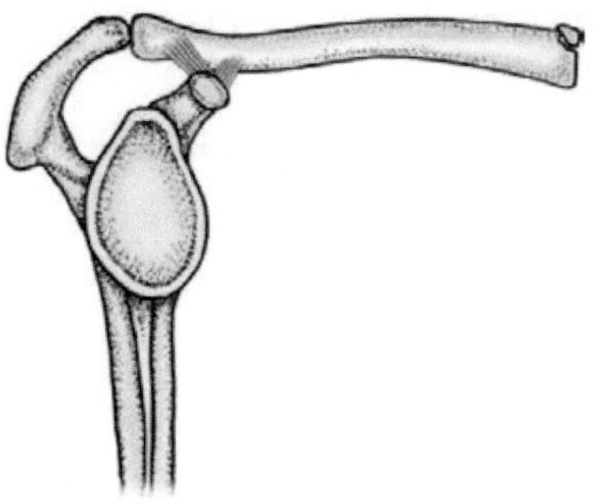

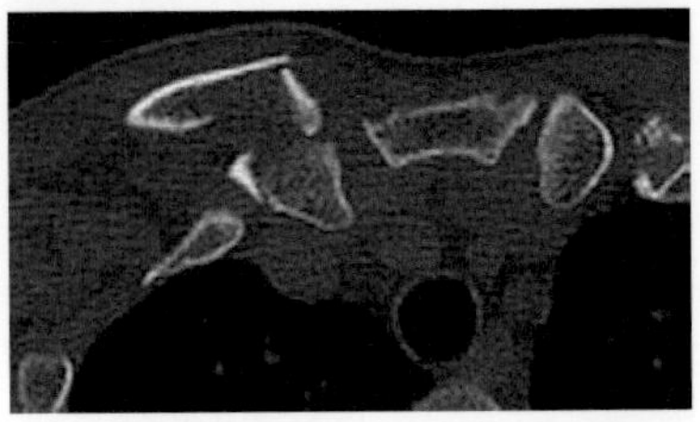

Craig Classification of Clavicle Fractures

Group III: Fracture of the proximal third.

Type III: Intra-articular

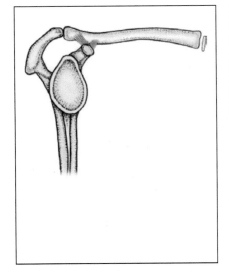

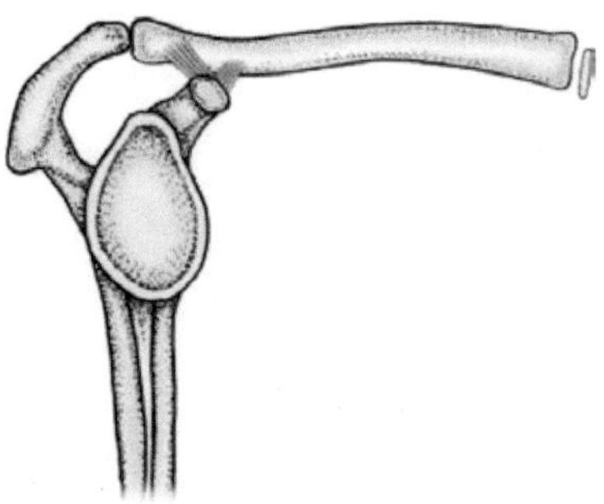

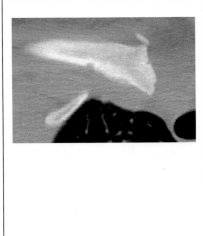

Craig Classification of Clavicle Fractures

Group III: Fracture of the proximal third.

Type IV: Epiphyseal separation (children and young adults)

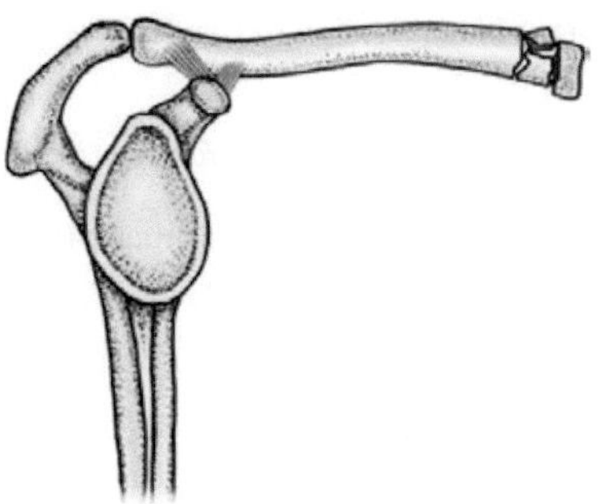

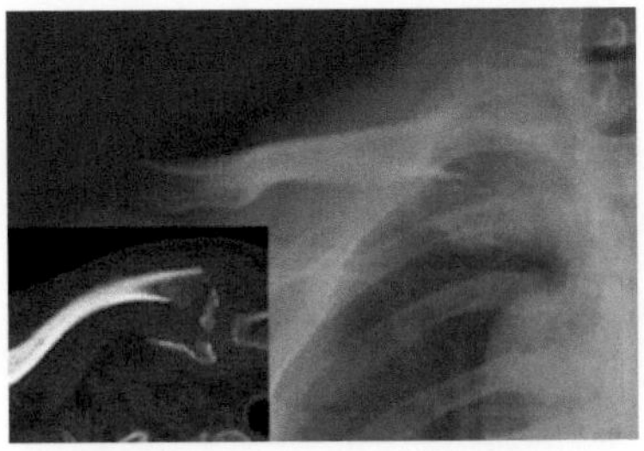

Craig Classification of Clavicle Fractures

Group III: Fracture of the proximal third.

Type V: Comminuted

1.1.2 Robinson's Classification [1]

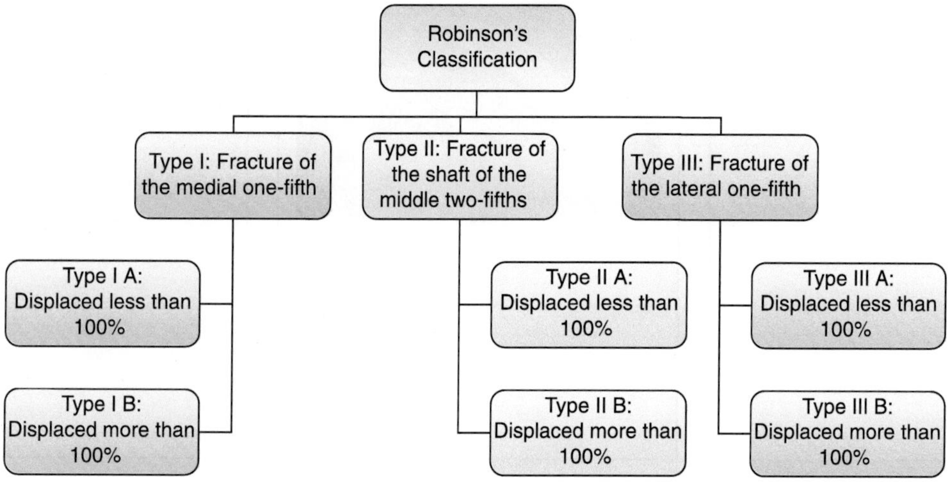

Type I: Fracture of the medial one-fifth, separated from the diaphysis by a vertical line drawn up from the centre of the first rib. Displacement further subdivides these fractures if they are displaced less than 100% (subgroup A) or more than 100% (subgroup B). These fractures are further subdivided with regard to their articular involvement, with subgroup 1 having no intra-articular involvement and subgroup 2 having intra-articular extension.

Type II: Fracture of the shaft of the middle two-fifths. Displacement further subdivides these fractures if they are displaced less than 100% (subgroup A) or more than 100% (subgroup B). These fractures are further subdivided with regard to their comminution. Simple or wedge comminution is classified into subgroup 1, and segmental or comminuted fractures are classified into subgroup 2.

Type III: Fracture of the lateral one-fifth, separated from the diaphysis by a vertical line drawn up from the centre of the base of the coracoid. Displacement further subdivides these fractures if they are displaced less than 100% (subgroup A) or more than 100% (subgroup B). These fractures are further subdivided with regard to their articular involvement, with subgroup 1 having no intra-articular involvement and subgroup 2 having intra-articular extension.

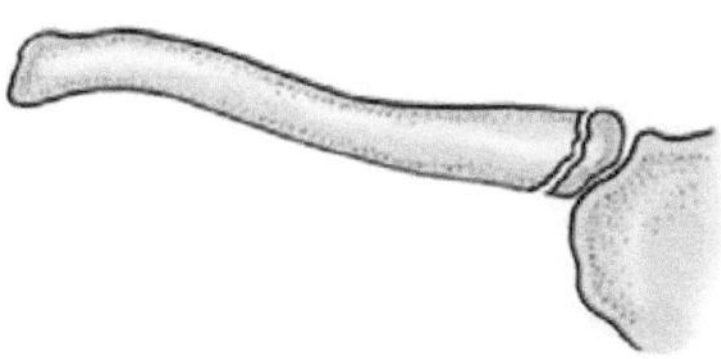

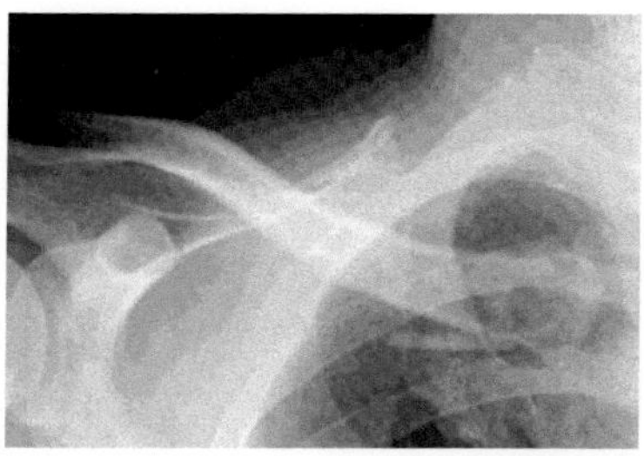

Robinson's Classification

Type I: Fracture of the medial one-fifth.

Type I A: Displaced less than 100%

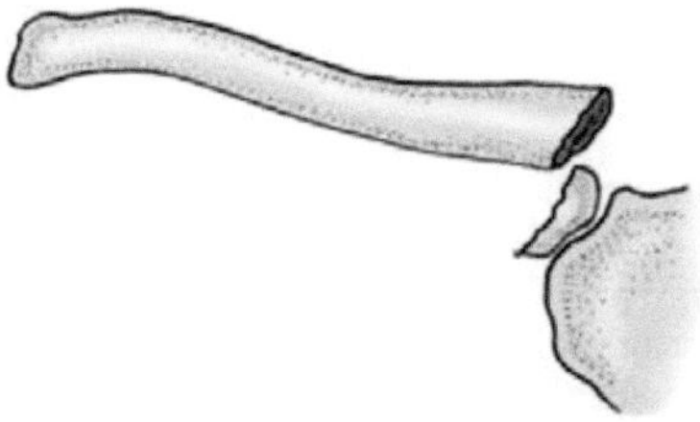

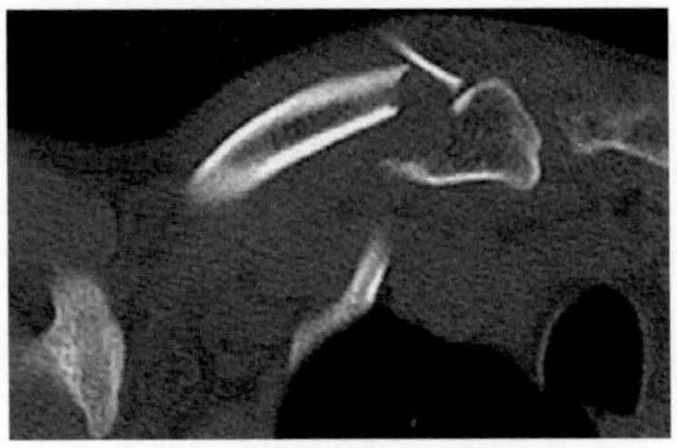

Robinson's Classification

Type I: Fracture of the medial one-fifth.

Type I B: Displaced more than 100%

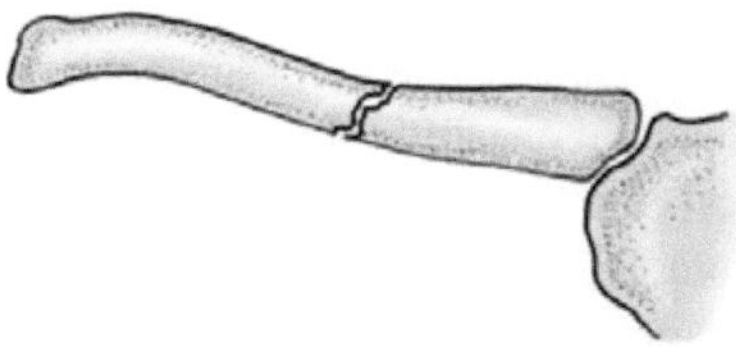

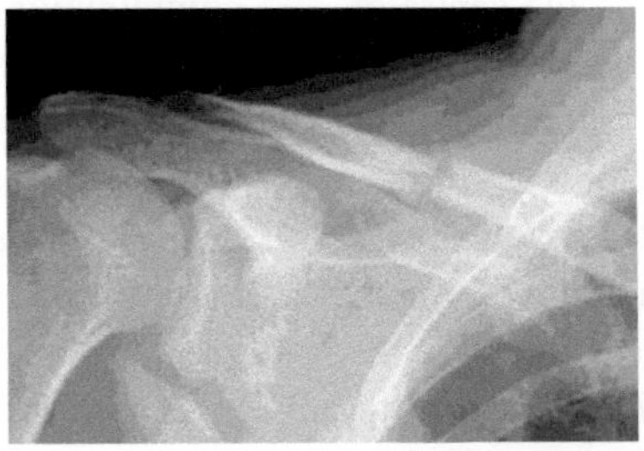

Robinson's Classification

Type II: Fracture of the shaft of
the middle two-fifths.

Type II A: Displaced less than 100%

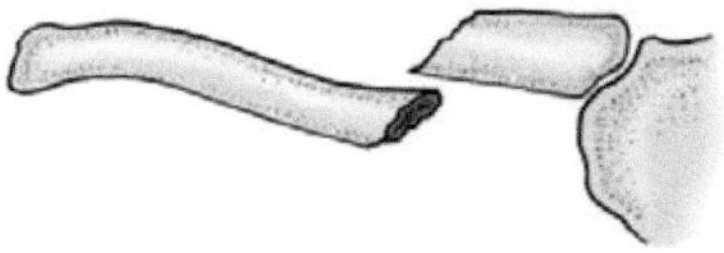

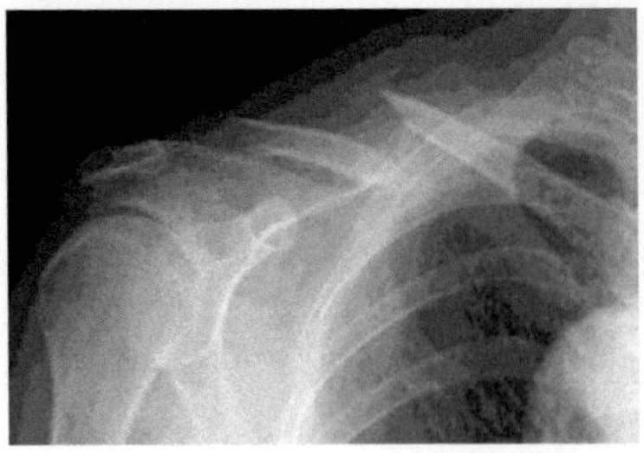

Robinson's Classification

Type II: Fracture of the shaft of the middle two-fifths.

Type II B: Displaced more than 100%

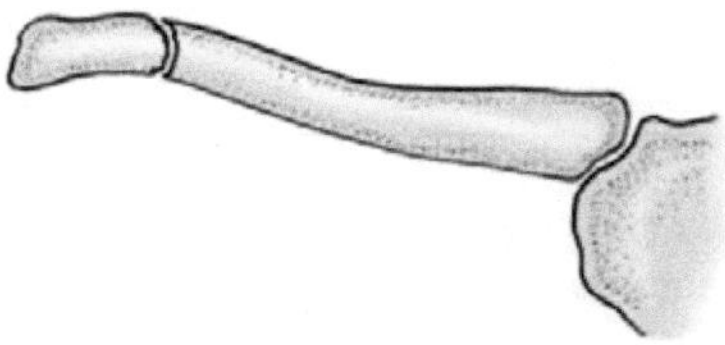

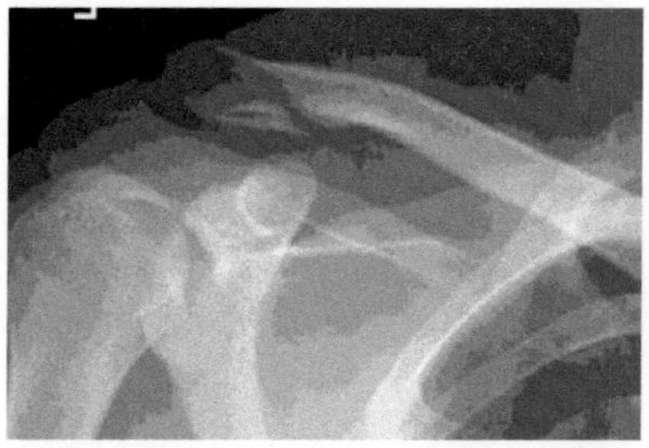

Robinson's Classification

Type III: Fracture of the lateral one-fifth.

Type III A: Displaced less than 100%

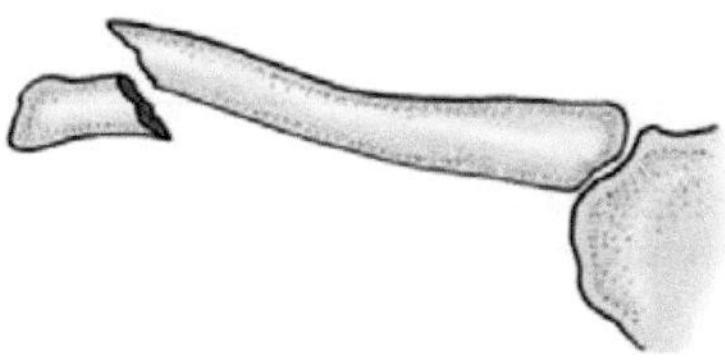

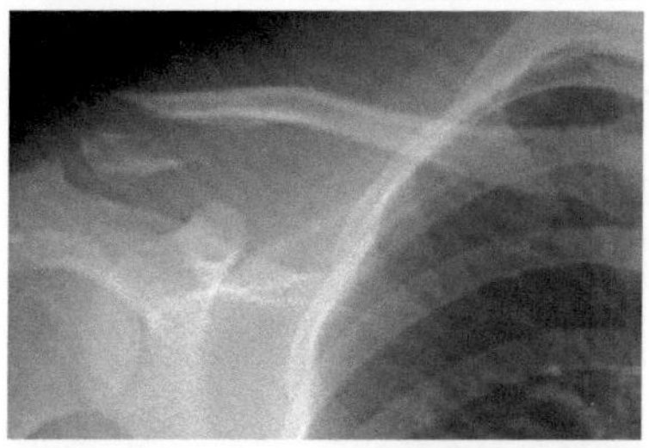

Robinson's Classification

Type III: Fracture of the lateral one-fifth.

Type III B: Displaced more than 100%

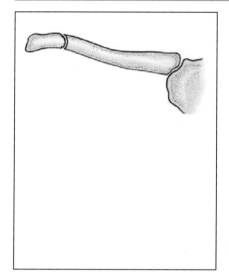

1.1.3 AO/OTA Classification of Clavicle Fractures [2]

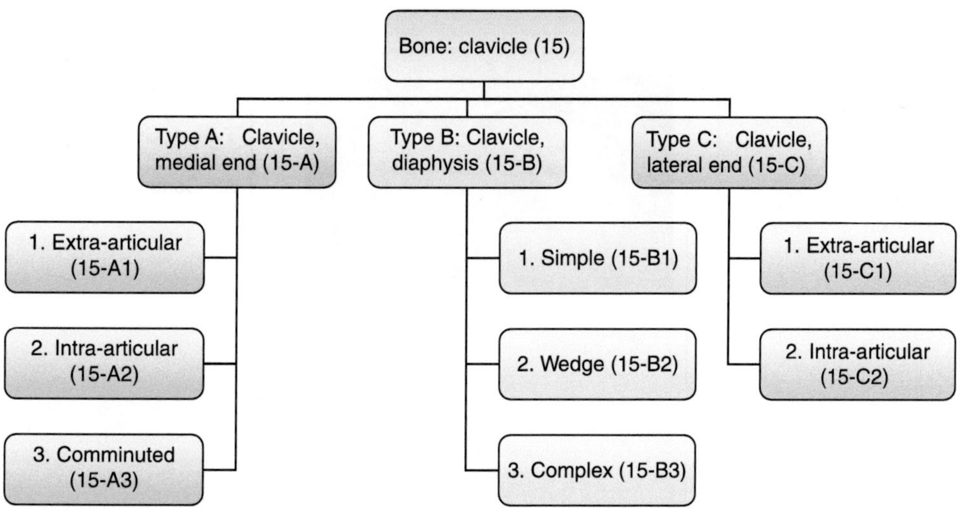

Type A: Clavicle, medial end (15-A).
A1: Extra-articular (15-A1).
A2: Intra-articular (15-A2).
A3: Comminuted (15-A3).

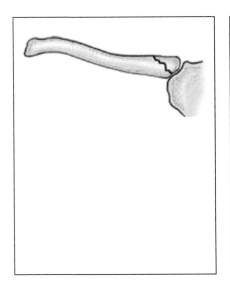

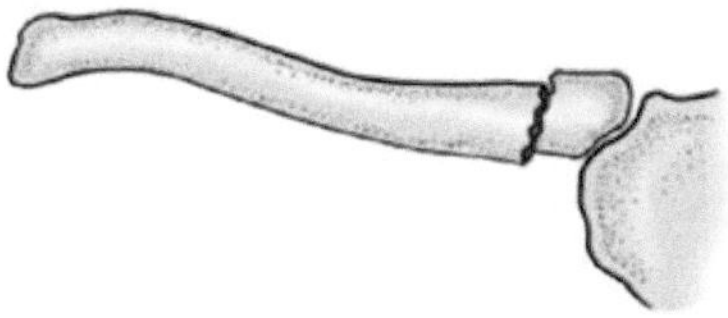

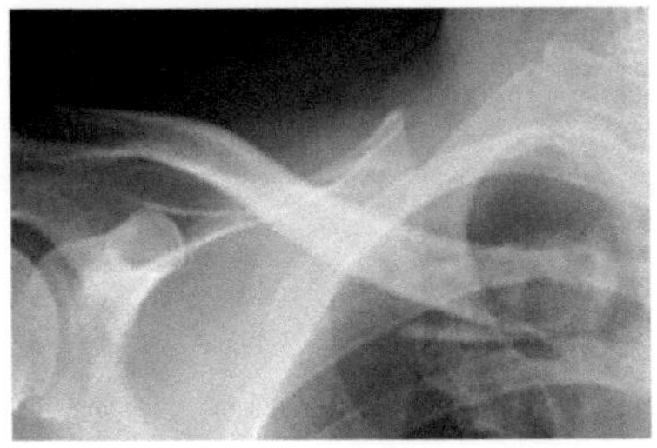

15 AO/OTA classification of clavicle fractures

Type A: Clavicle, medial end (15-A).

A1: Extra-articular (15-A1)

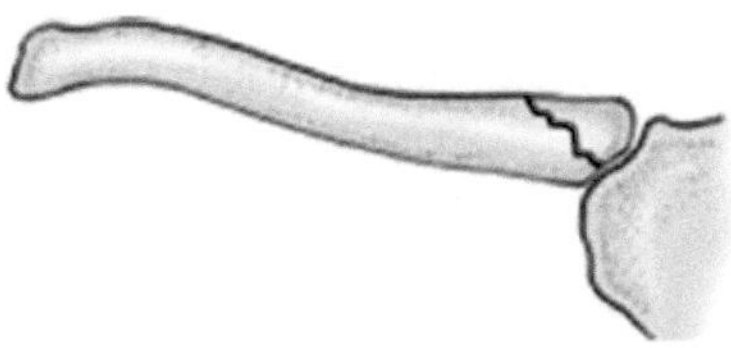

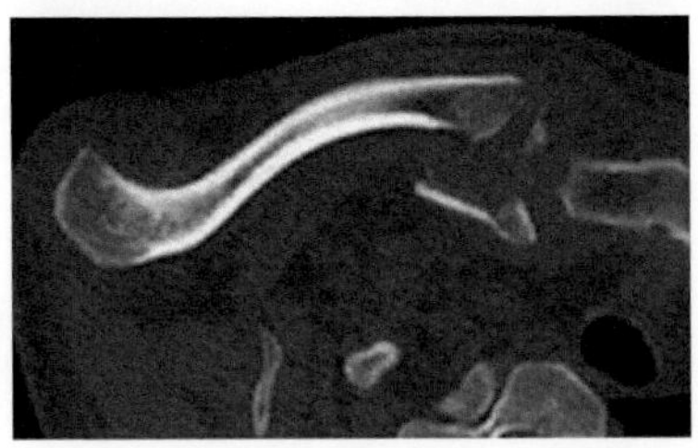

15 AO/OTA classification of clavicle fractures

Type A: Clavicle, medial end (15-A).

A2: Intra-articular (15-A2)

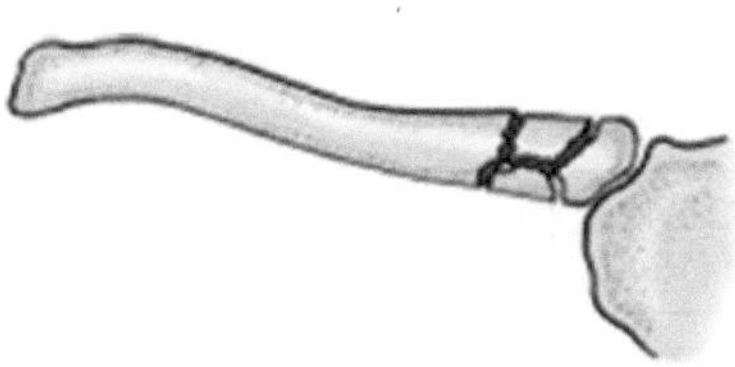

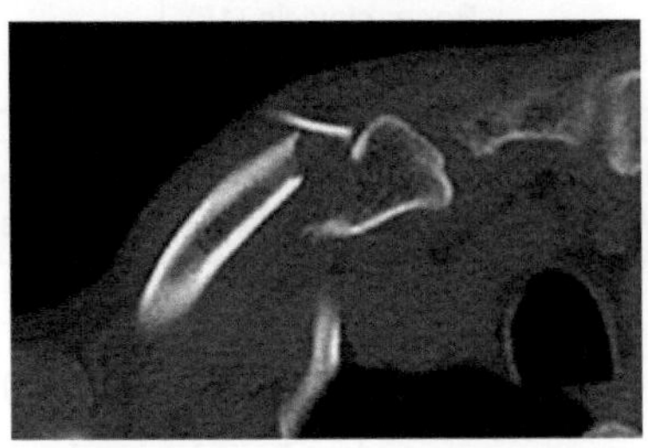

15 AO/OTA classification of clavicle fractures

Type A: Clavicle, medial end (15-A).

A3: Comminuted (15-A3)

Type B: Clavicle, diaphysis (15-B).
- B1: Simple (15-B1).
  - B1.1: Spiral (15-B1.1).
  - B1.2: Oblique (15-B1.2).
  - B1.3: Transverse (15-B1.3).
- B2: Wedge (15-B2).
  - B2.1: Spiral wedge (15-B2.1).
  - B2.2: Bending wedge (15-B2.2).
  - B2.3: Comminuted (15-B2.3).
- B3: Complex (15-B3).
  - B3.1: Spiral (15-B3.1).
  - B3.2: Transverse (15-B3.2).
  - B3.3: Complex comminuted (15-B3.3).

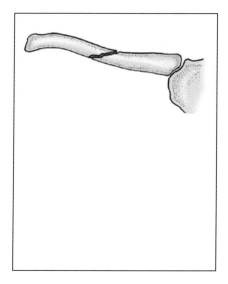

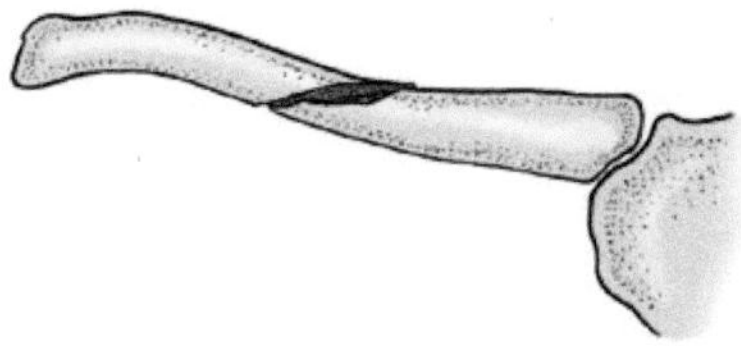

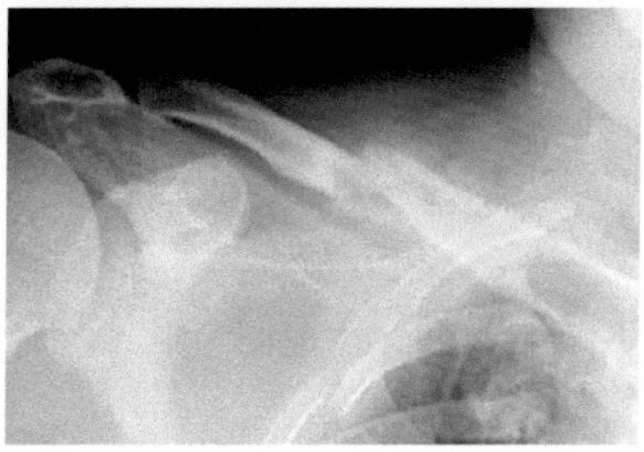

15 AO/OTA classification of clavicle fractures

Type B: Clavicle, diaphysis (15-B).

B1: Simple (15-B1)

B1.1: Spiral (15-B1.1)

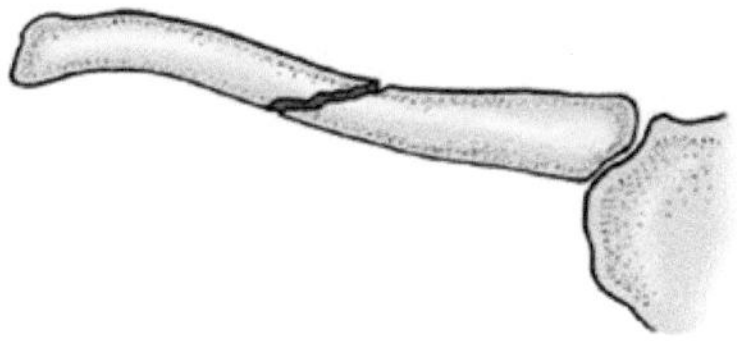

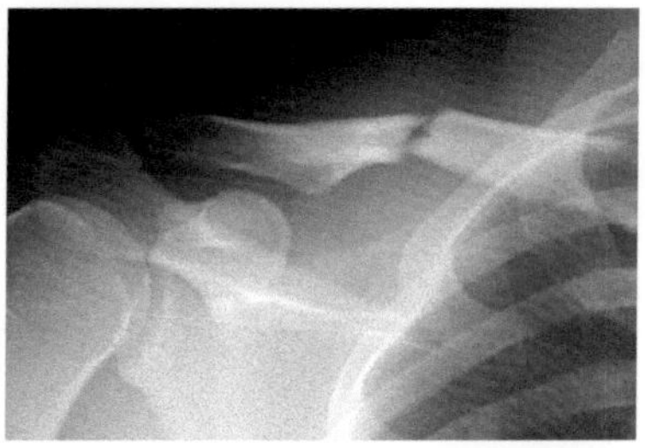

15 AO/OTA classification of clavicle fractures

Type B: Clavicle, diaphysis (15-B).

B1: Simple (15-B1).

B1.2: Oblique (15-B1.2)

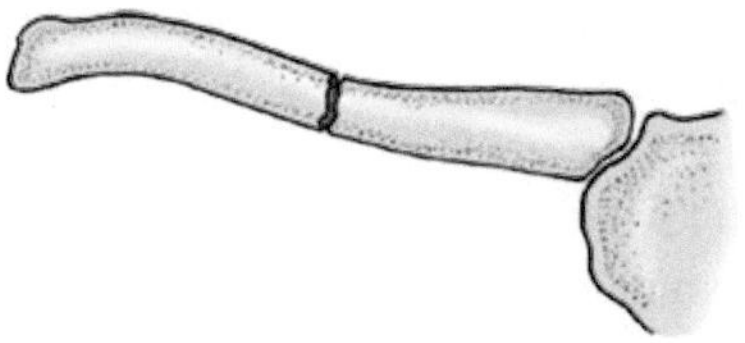

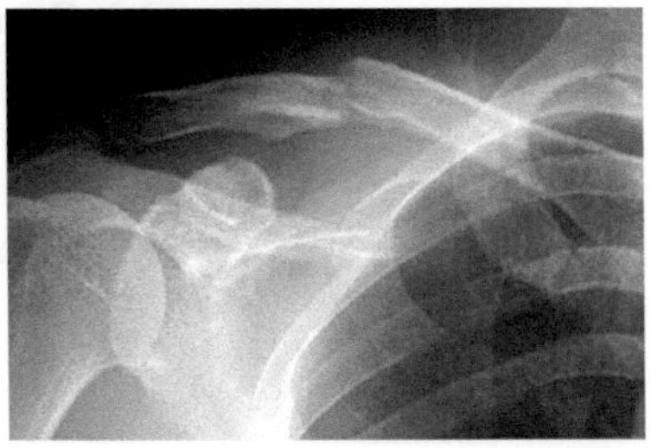

15 AO/OTA classification of clavicle fractures

Type B: Clavicle, diaphysis (15-B).

B1: Simple (15-B1).

B1.3: Transverse (15-B1.3)

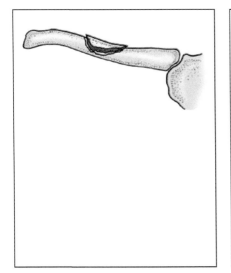

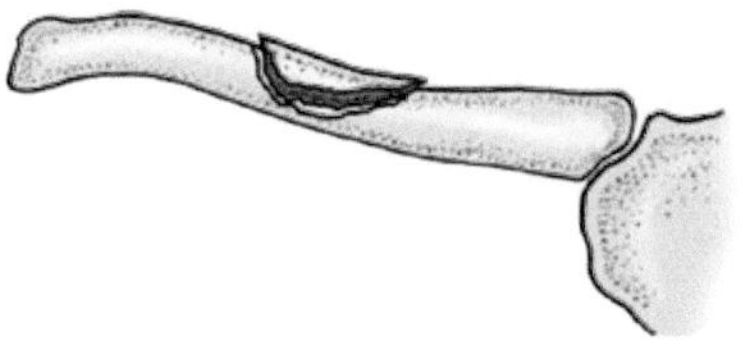

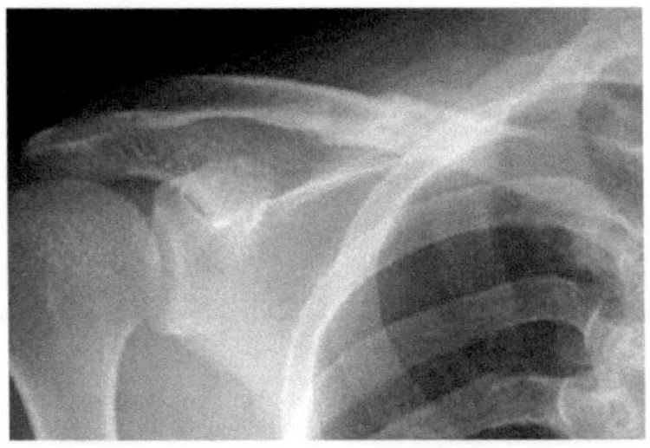

15 AO/OTA classification of clavicle fractures

Type B: Clavicle, diaphysis (15-B).

B2: Wedge (15-B2).

B2.1: Spiral wedge (15-B2.1)

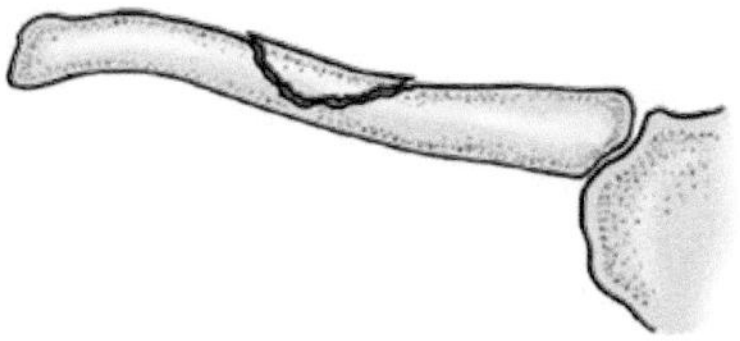

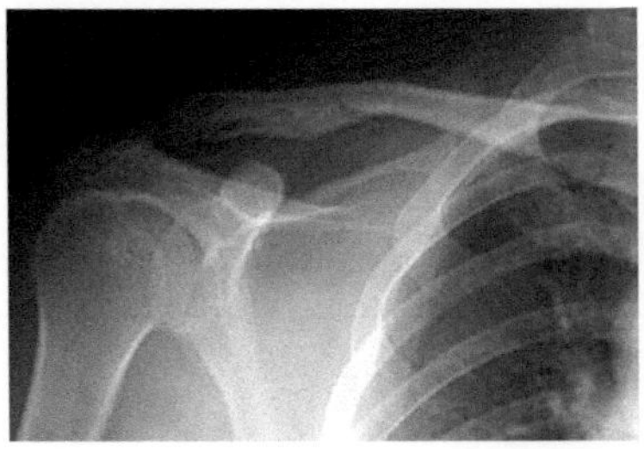

15 AO/OTA classification of clavicle fractures

Type B: Clavicle, diaphysis (15-B).

B2: Wedge (15-B2).

B2.2: Bending wedge (15-B2.2)

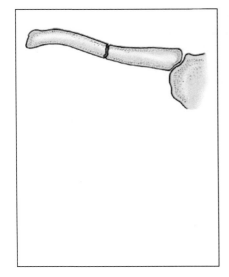

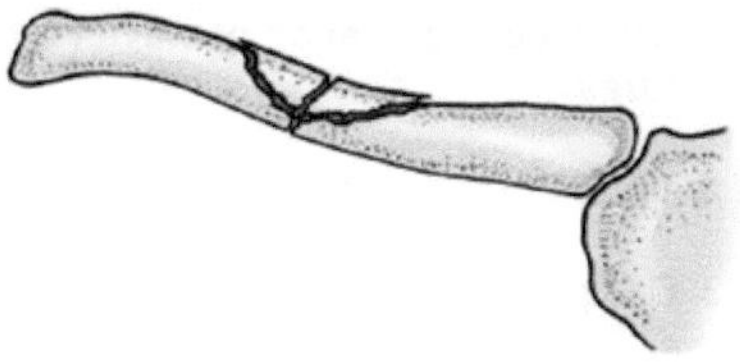

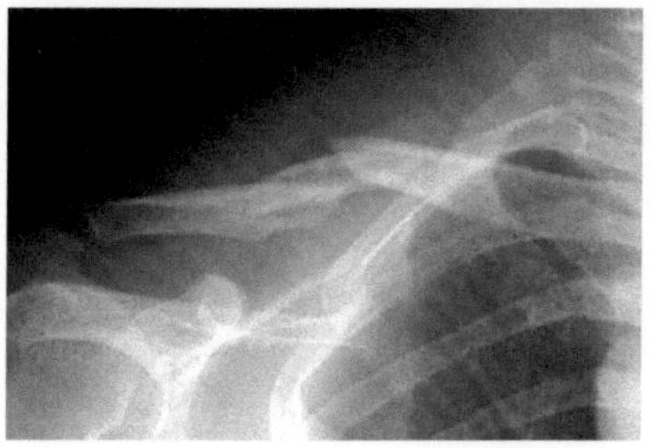

15 AO/OTA classification of clavicle fractures

Type B: Clavicle, diaphysis (15-B).

B2: Wedge (15-B2).

B2.3: Comminuted (15-B2.3)

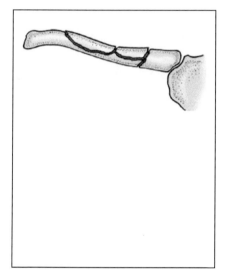

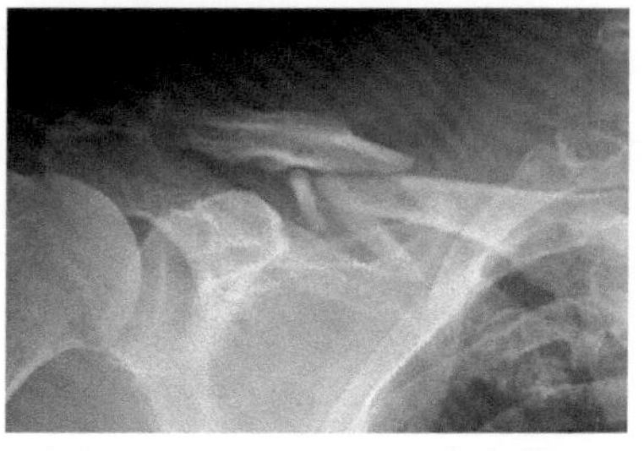

15 AO/OTA classification of clavicle fractures

Type B: Clavicle, diaphysis (15-B).

B3: Complex (15-B3).

B3.1: Spiral (15-B3.1)

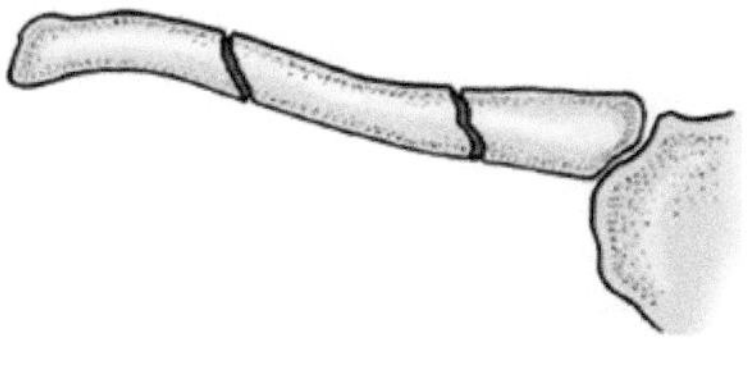

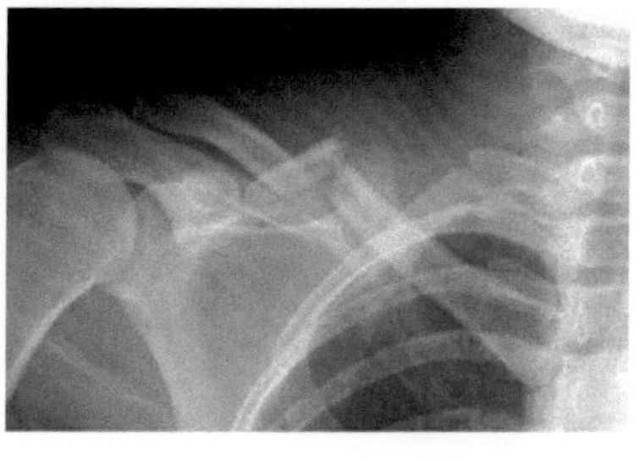

15 AO/OTA classification of clavicle fractures

Type B: Clavicle, diaphysis (15-B).

B3: Complex (15-B3).

B3.2: Transverse (15-B3.2)

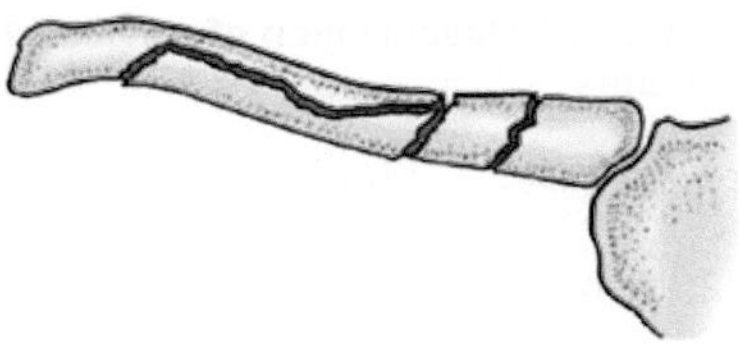

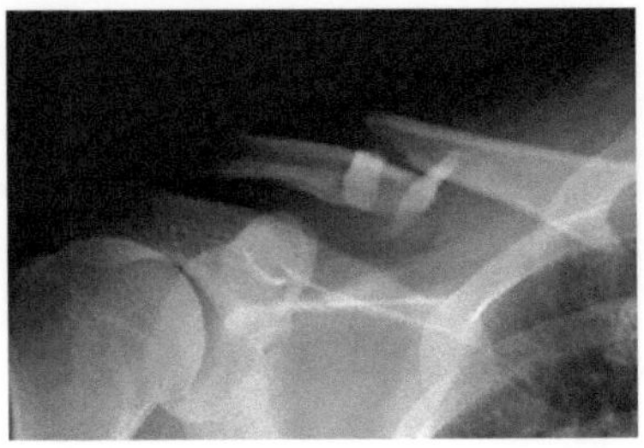

15 AO/OTA classification of clavicle fractures

Type B: Clavicle, diaphysis (15-B).

B3: Complex (15-B3).

B3.3: Complex comminuted (15-B3.3)

Type C: Clavicle, lateral end (15-C).
- C1: Extra-articular (15-C1).
  - C1.1: Impacted (C-C ligament intact) (15-C1.1).
  - C1.2: Noncomminuted (C-C ligament disrupted) (15-C1.2).
  - C1.3: Comminuted (C-C ligament disrupted) (15-C1.3).
- C2: Intra-articular (15-C2).
  - C2.1: With slight displacement (C-C ligament intact) (15-C2.1).
  - C2.2: Noncomminuted (C-C ligament disrupted) (15-C2.2).
  - C2.3: Comminuted (C-C ligament disrupted) (15-C2.3).

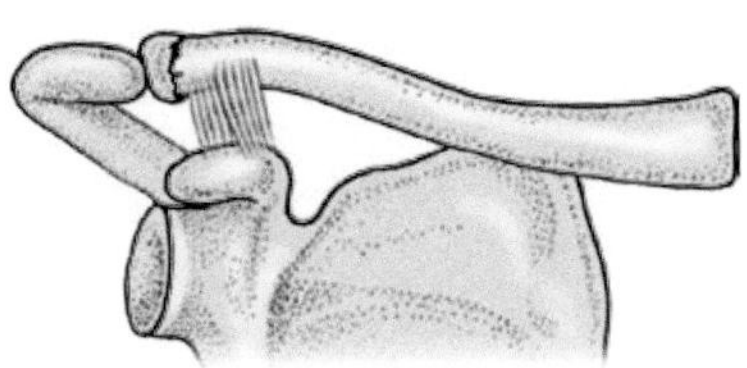

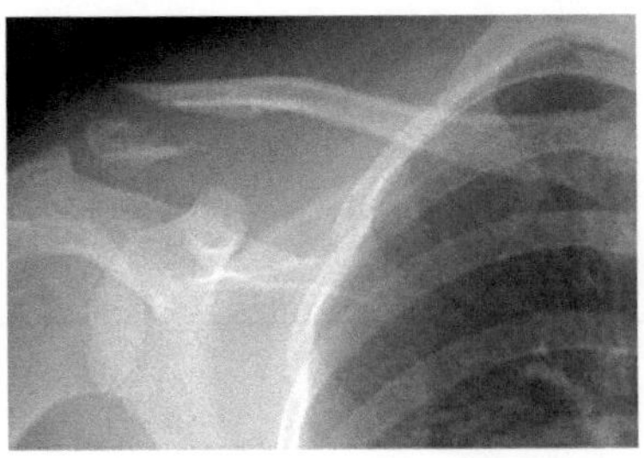

15 AO/OTA classification of clavicle fractures

Type C: Clavicle, lateral end (15-C).

C1: Extra-articular (15-C1).

C1.1: Impacted (C-C ligament intact) (15-C1.1)

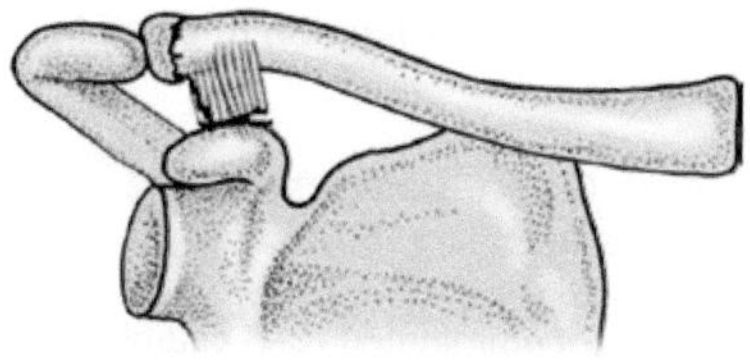

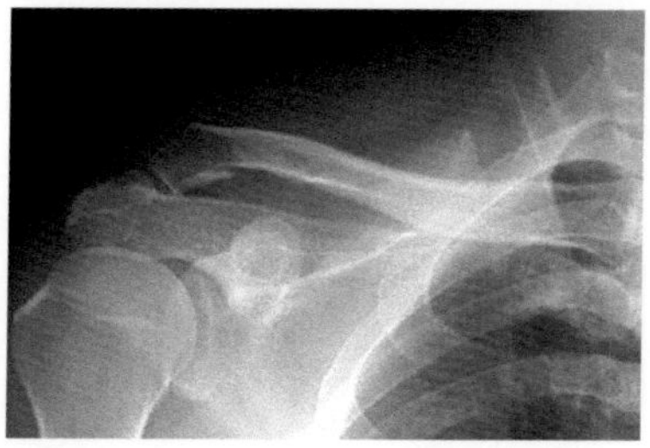

15 AO/OTA classification of clavicle fractures

Type C: Clavicle, lateral end (15-C).

C1: Extra-articular (15-C1),

C1.2: Noncomminuted (C-C ligament disrupted) (15-C1.2)

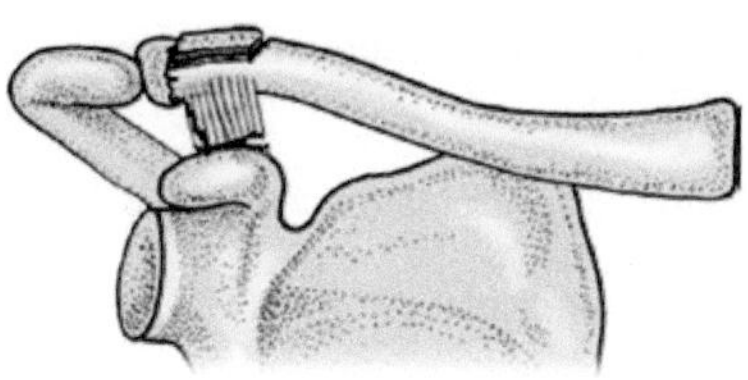

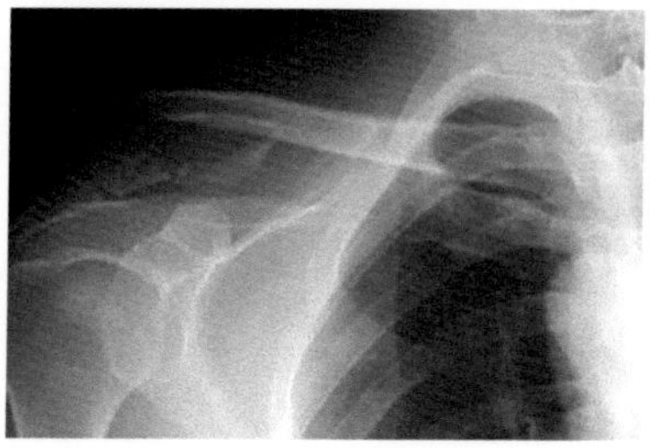

15 AO/OTA classification of clavicle fractures

Type C: Clavicle, lateral end (15-C).

C1: Extra-articular (15-C1).

C1.3: Comminuted (C-C ligament disrupted) (15-C1.3)

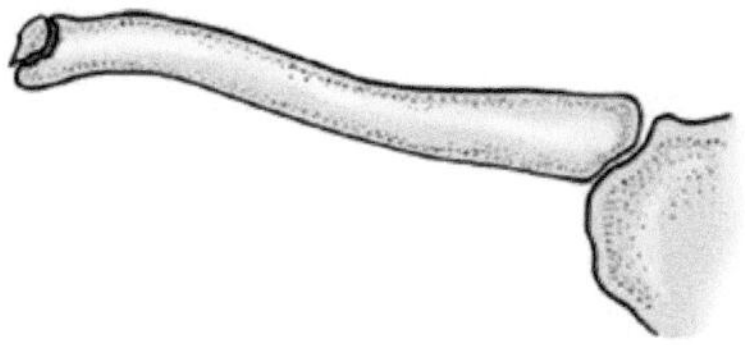

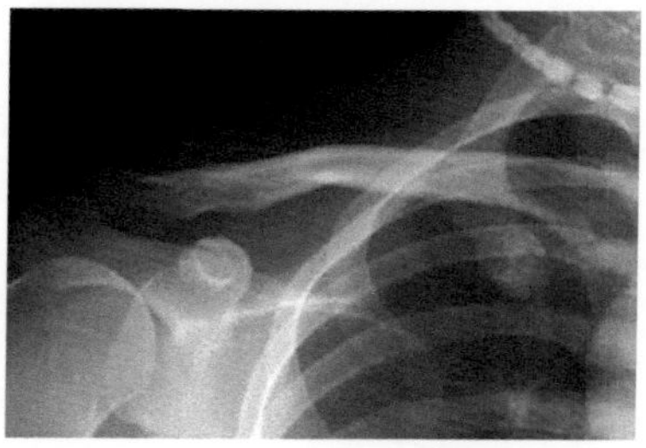

15 AO/OTA classification of clavicle fractures

Type C: Clavicle, lateral end (15-C).

C2: Intra-articular (15-C2).

C2.1: With slight displacement (C-C ligament intact) (15-C2.1)

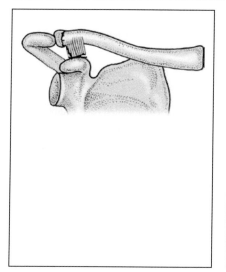

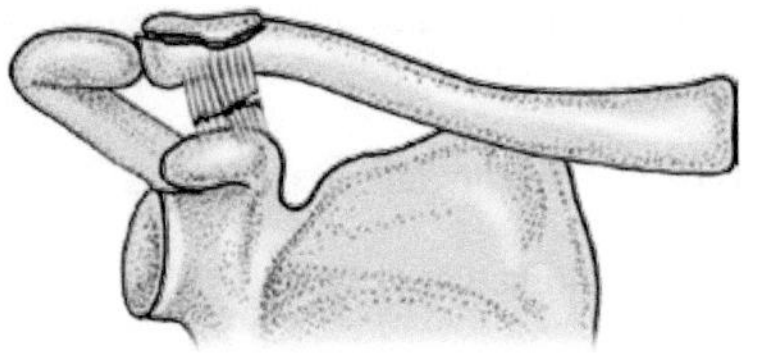

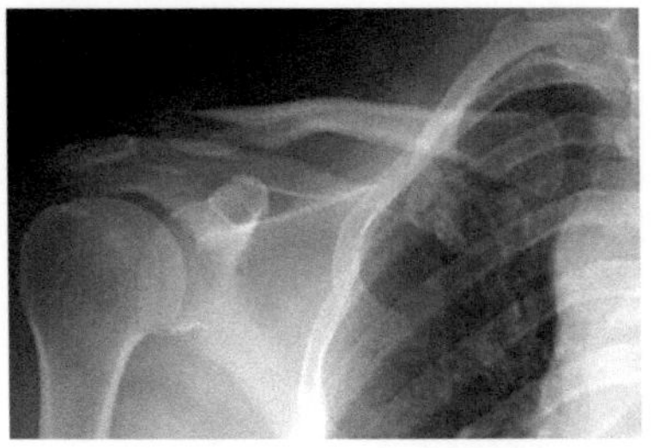

15 AO/OTA classification of clavicle fractures

Type C: Clavicle, lateral end (15-C):
C2: Intra-articular (15-C2).

C2.2: Noncomminuted (C-C ligament disrupted)(15-C2.2)

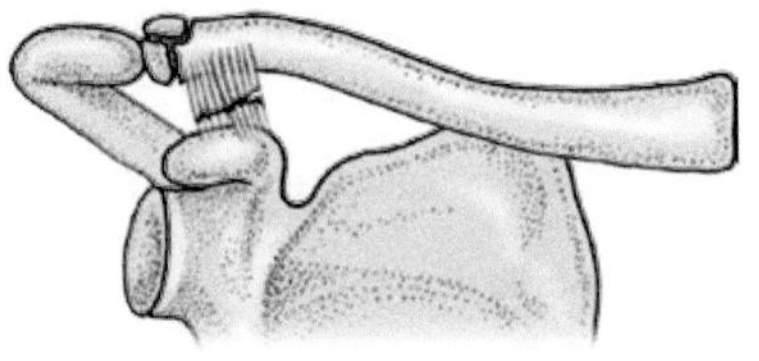

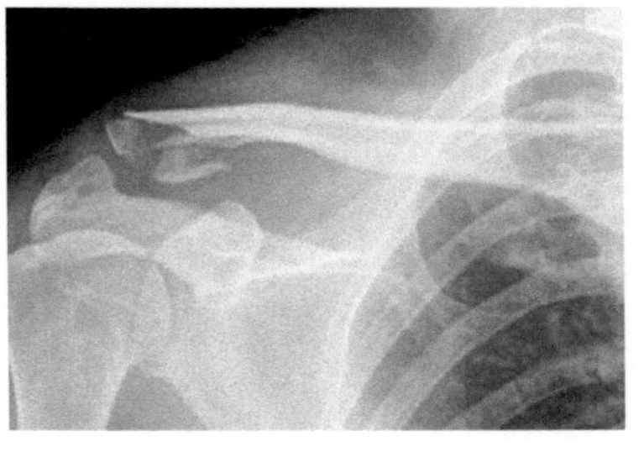

15 AO/OTA classification of clavicle fractures

Type C: Clavicle, lateral end (15-C).

C2: Intra-articular (15-C2).

C2.3: Comminuted (C-C ligament disrupted)(15-C2.3)

1.1.4 **Allman's Classification** [3]

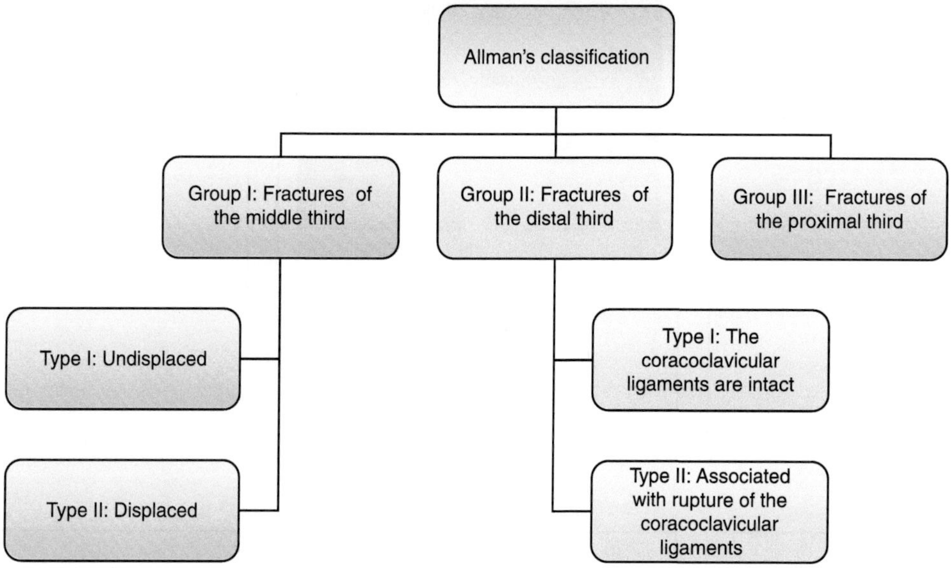

Group I: Fractures of the middle third, divided into two types.

Type I: Undisplaced.

Type II: Displaced.

Group II: Fractures of the distal third, distal to the coracoclavicular ligament. Neer classified this group into two types.

Type I: The coracoclavicular ligaments are intact.

Type II: Associated with rupture of the coracoclavicular ligaments and consequent greater posterior and superior displacement of the proximal clavicular fragment.

Group III: Fractures of the proximal third.

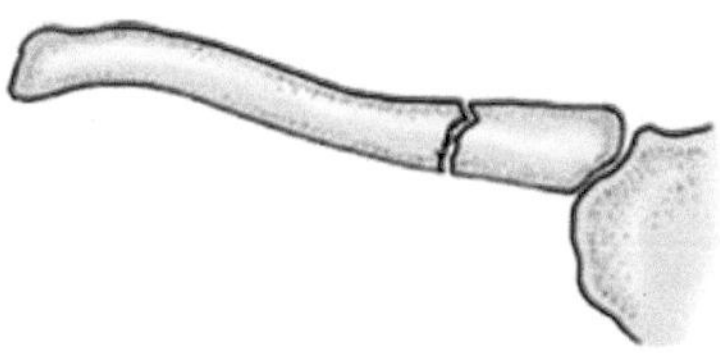

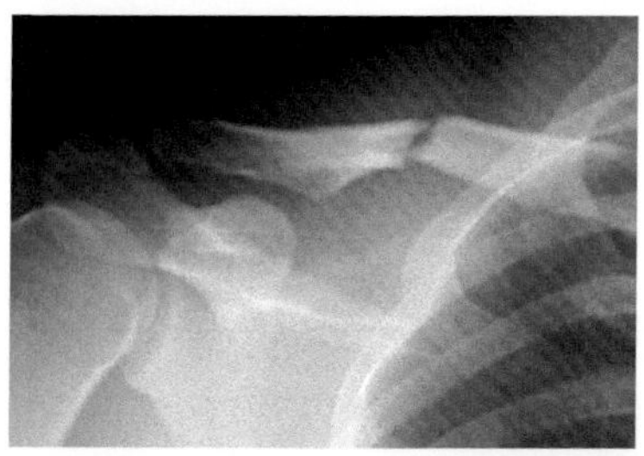

Allman's classification of clavicle fractures

Group I: Fractures of the middle third.

Type I: Undisplaced

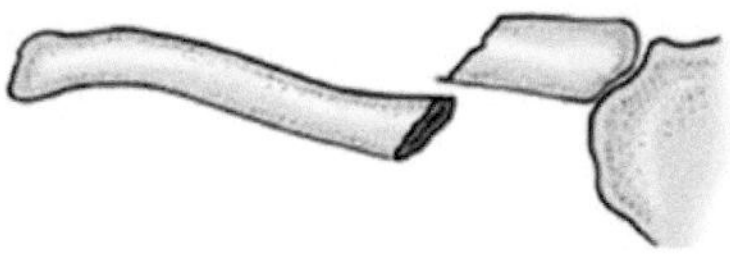

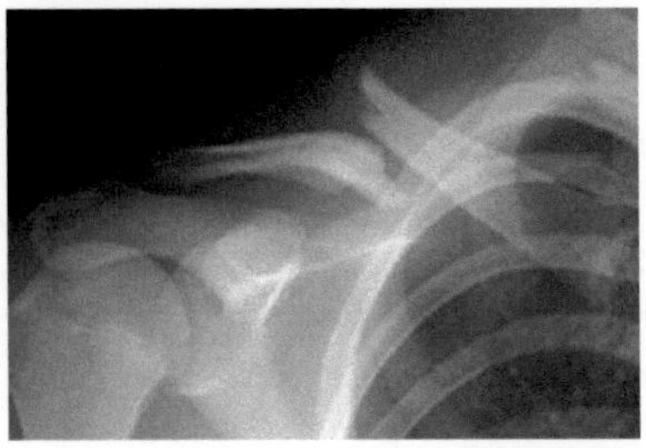

Allman's classification of clavicle fractures

Group I: Fractures of the middle third.

Type II: Displaced

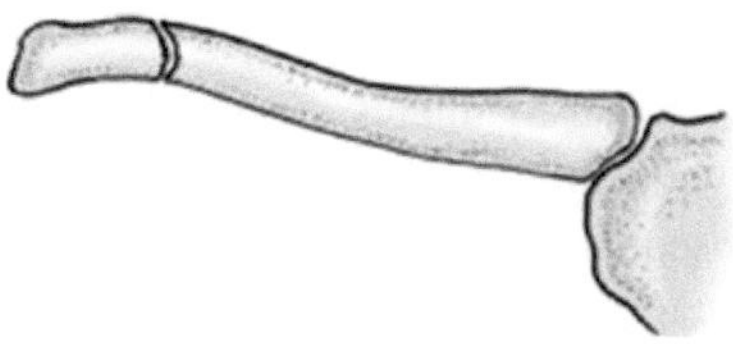

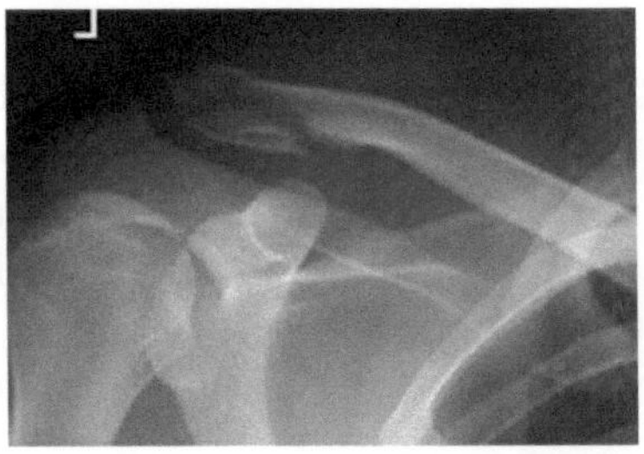

Allman's classification of clavicle fractures

Group II: Fractures of the distal third.

Type I: The coracoclavicular ligaments are intact

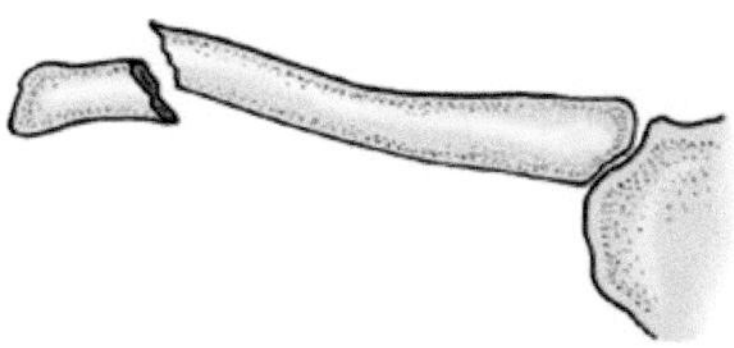

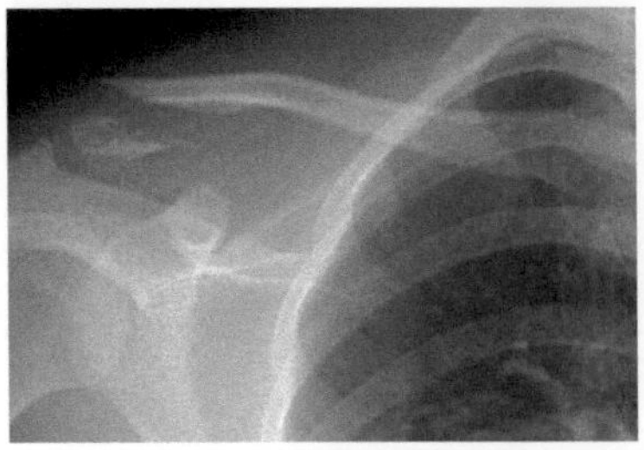

Allman's classification of clavicle fractures

Group II: Fractures of the distal third.

Type II: Associated with rupture of the coracoclavicular ligaments ,with the proximal clavicular fragment diplaced posteriorly and superiorly

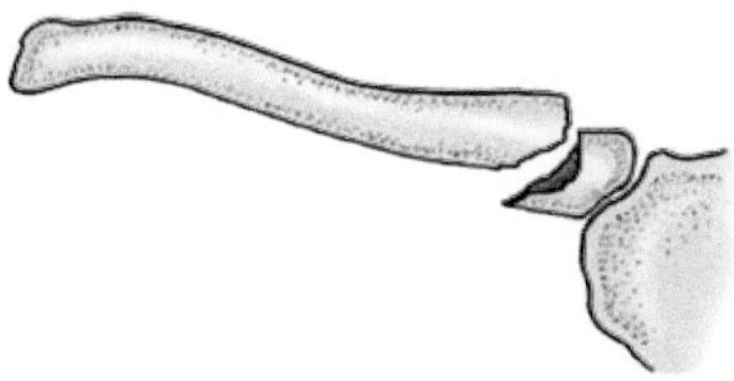

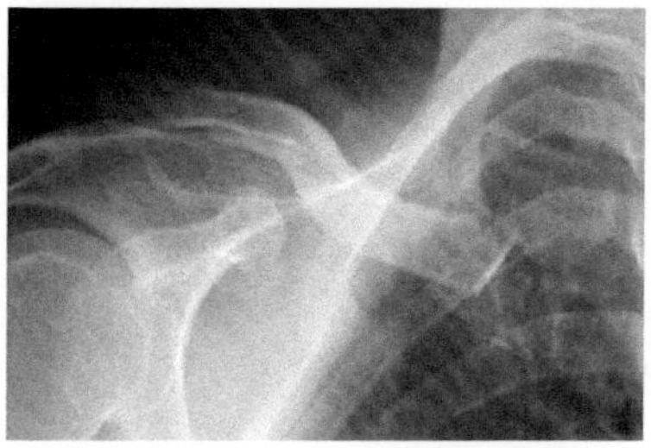

Allman's classification of clavicle fractures

Group III: Fractures of the proximal third

1.1.5 Neer's Classification [4]

Neer modified Allman's classification of clavicular fractures, with group II (distal third clavicular fractures) divided into three types based on the fracture site and ligamentous stability.

Type I: Stable; undisplaced; fracture line lying between the conoid and trapezoid.
Type II: Unstable; displaced.
IIA: Fracture medial to the CC ligaments; both the conoid and trapezoid are intact.
IIB: Fracture of the lateral end of the clavicle, with disruption of the conoid portion of the CC ligament and the trapezoid intact.
Type III: Stable; intra-articular fractures extending into the AC joint.

1.2 Classification of Scapular Fractures

To date, there are >10 scapular fracture classification systems in literature. According to literature over the last 5 years, the usage rate of these systems is in turn Hardegger classification, Ada-Miller classification, Ideberg classification, etc.

1.2.1 Classification of Scapular Fractures

1.2.1.1 Hardegger Classification [5]

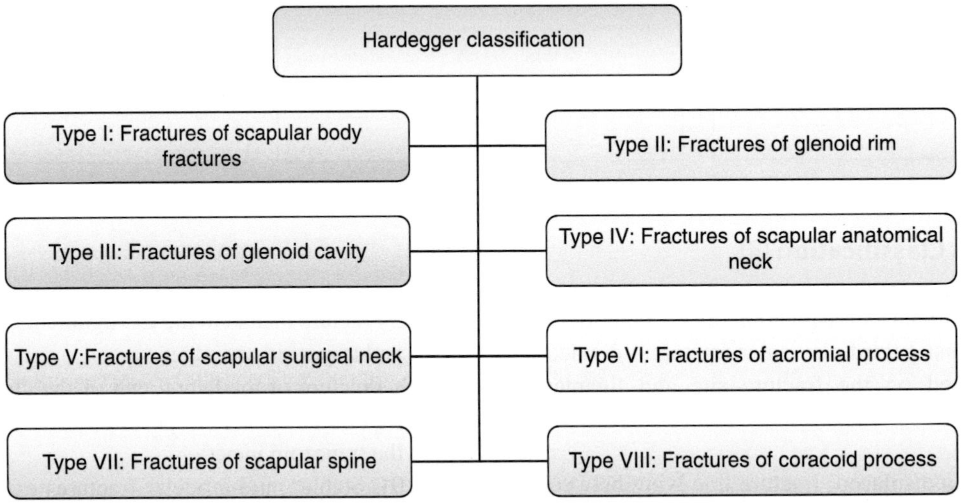

Type I: Fractures of scapular body fractures (A).
Type II: Fractures of glenoid rim (B).
Type III: Fractures of glenoid cavity (C).
Type IV: Fractures of scapular anatomical neck (D).
Type V: Fractures of scapular surgical neck (E).
Type VI: Fractures of acromial process (F).
Type VII: Fractures of scapular spine (G).
Type VII: Fractures of coracoid process (H).

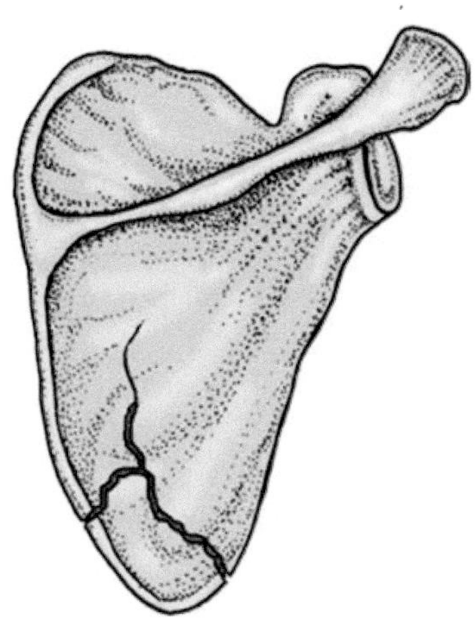

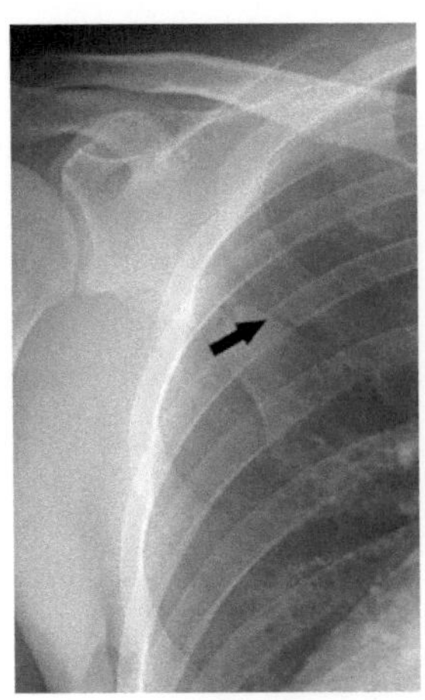

Hardegger classification

Type I: Fractures of scapular body fractures

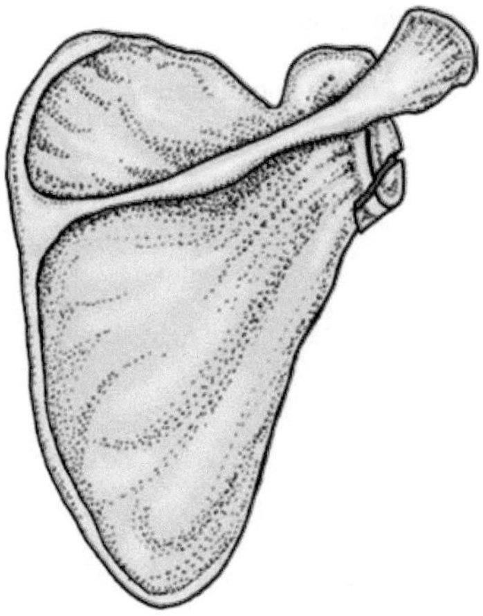

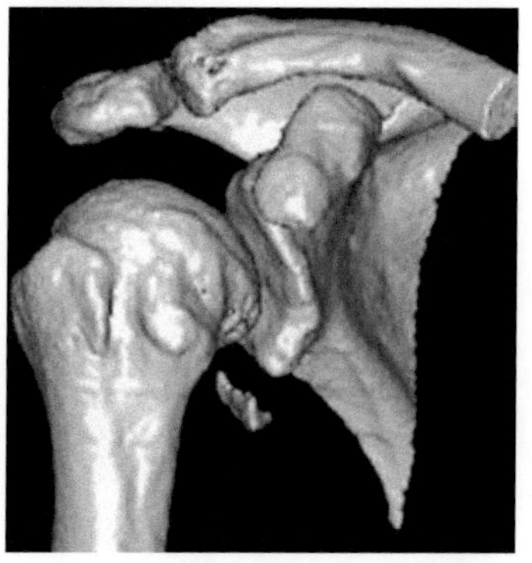

Hardegger classification

Type II: Fractures of glenoid rim

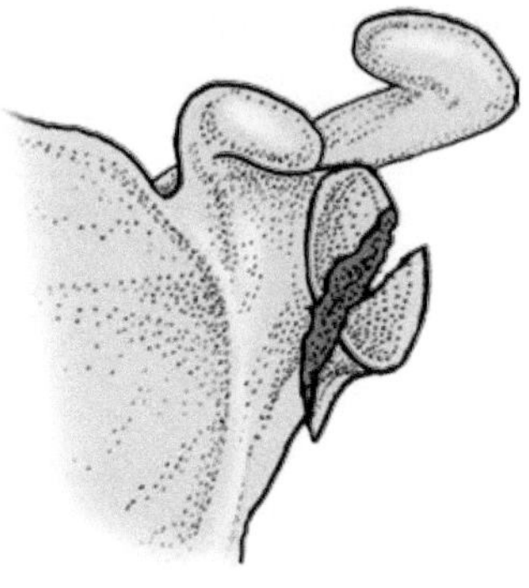

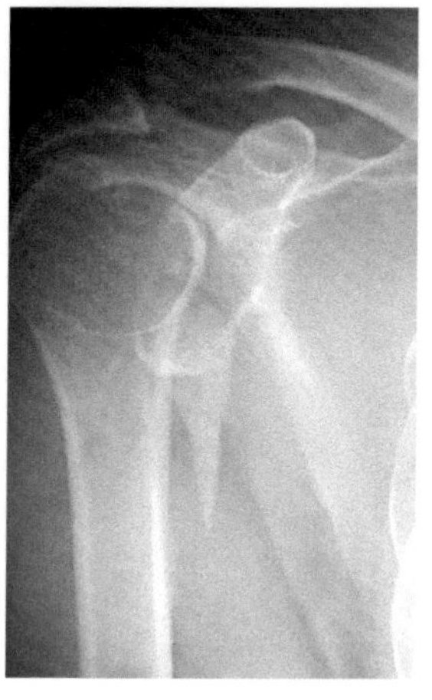

Hardegger classification

Type III: Fractures of glenoie cavity

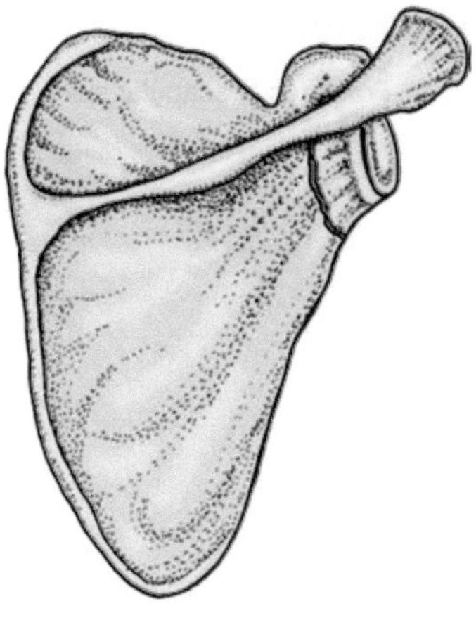

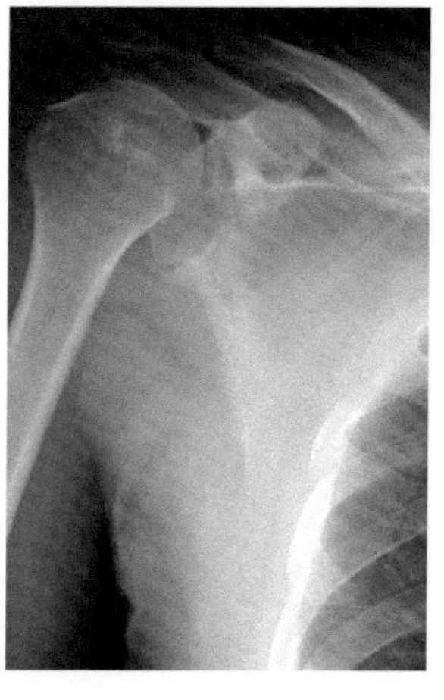

Hardegger classification

Type IV: Fractures of scapular anatomical neck

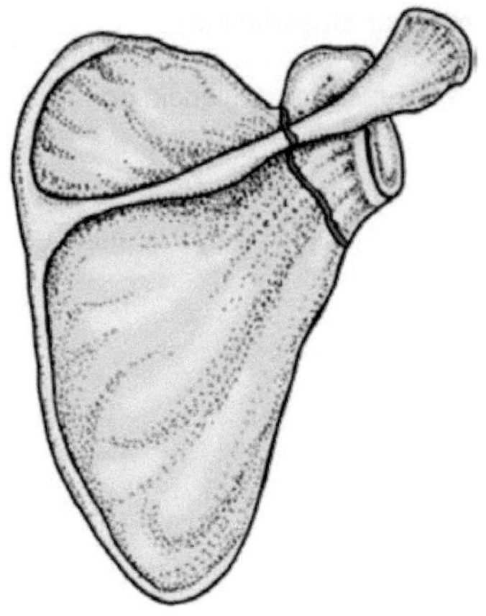

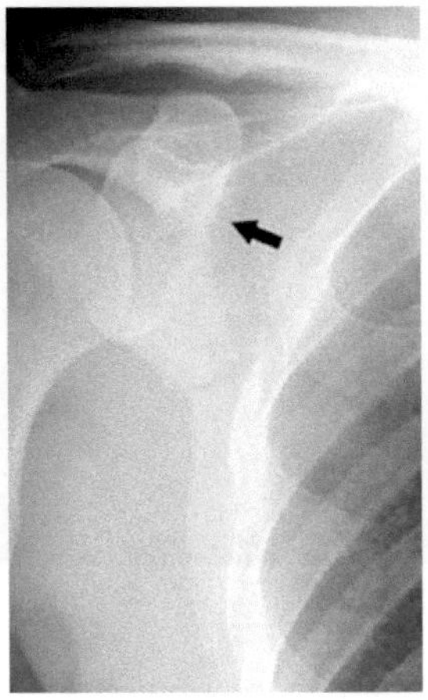

Hardegger classification

Type V: Fractures of scapular surgical neck

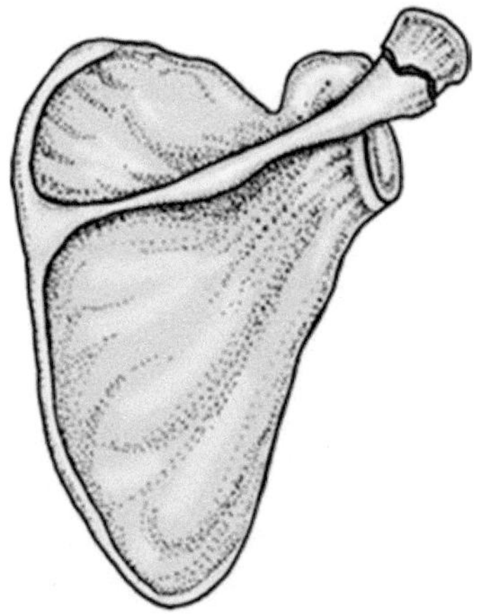

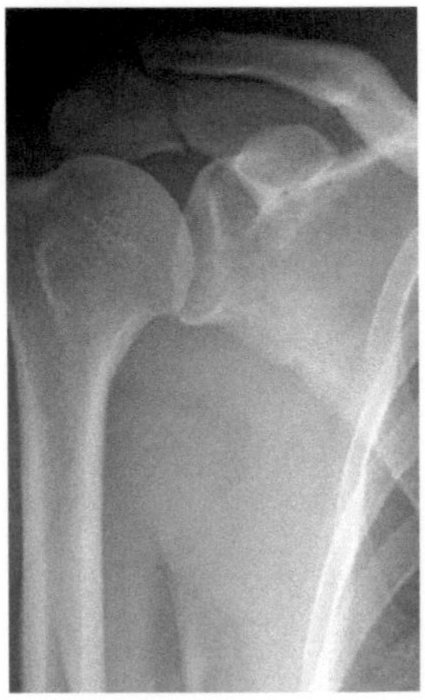

Hardegger classification

Type VI: Fractures of acromial process

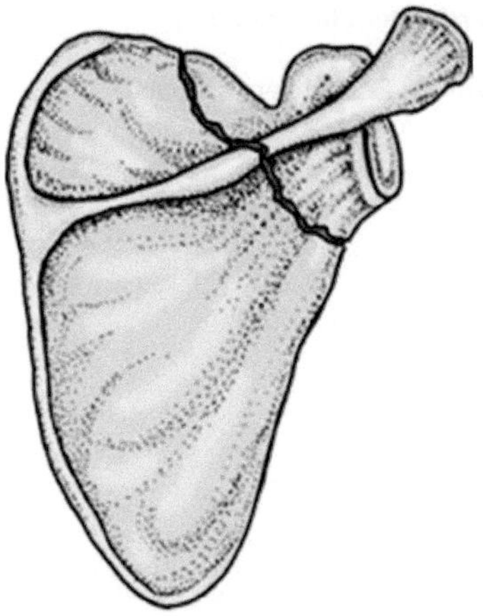

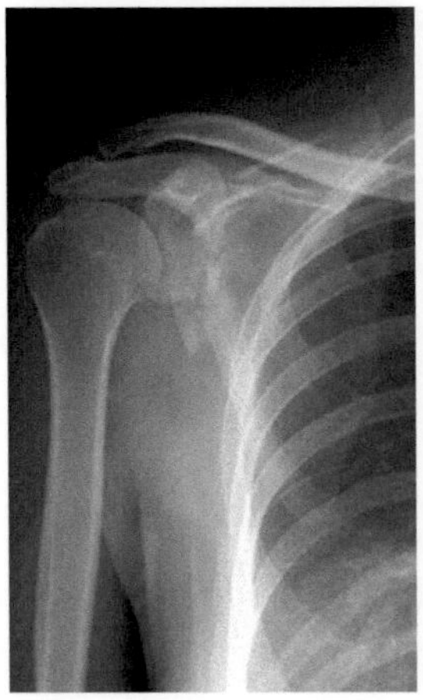

Hardegger classification

Type VII: Fractures of scapular spine

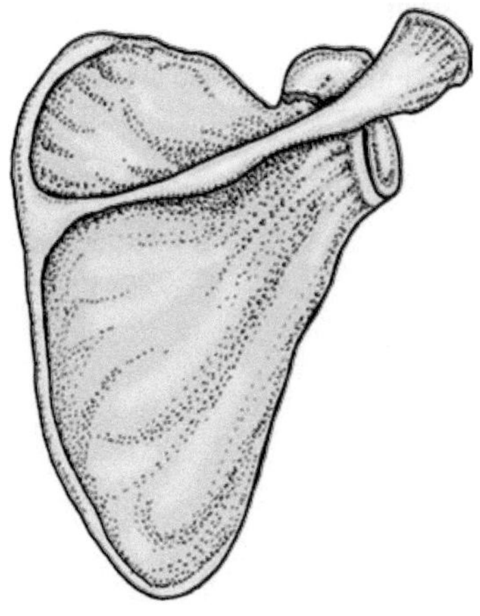

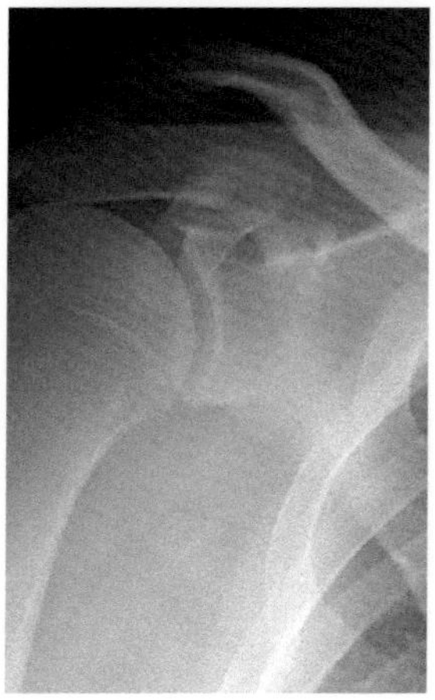

Hardegger classification

Type VIII: Fractures of coracoid process

1.2.1.2 Ada-Miller Classification [6]

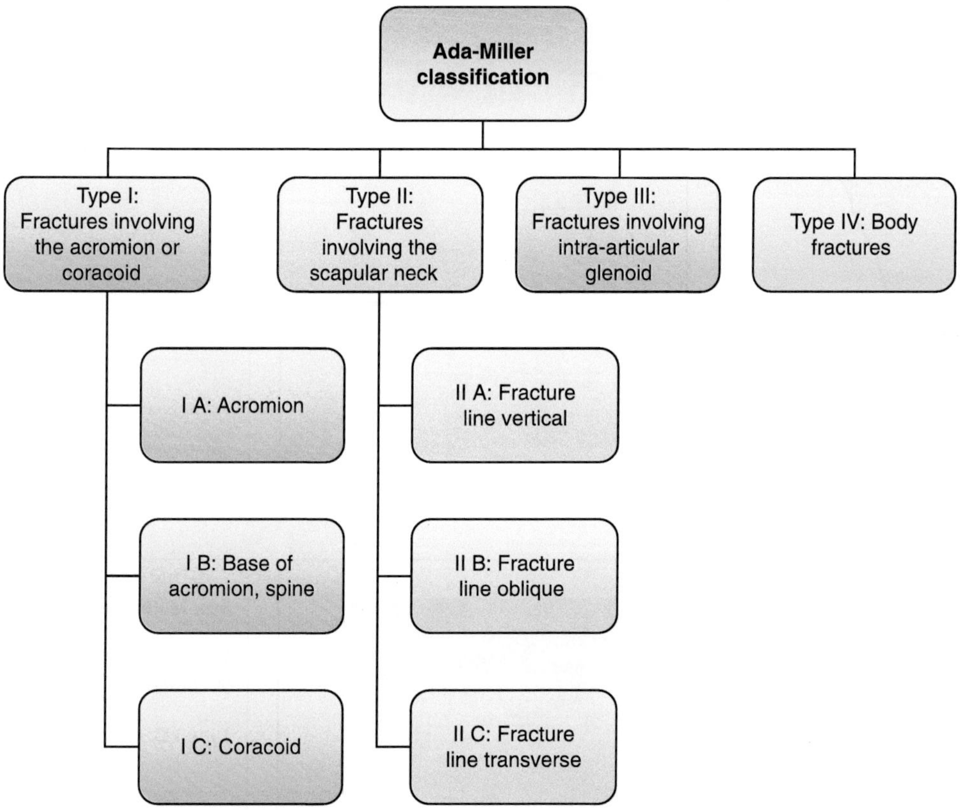

Type I: Fractures involving the acromion or coracoids.
- IA: Acromion.
- IB: Base of acromion, spine.
- IC: Coracoid.

Type II: Fractures involving the scapular neck.
- IIA: Fracture line vertical, within scapular neck, lateral to base of acromion-spine.
- IIB: Fracture line oblique, extending to base of acromion or spine
- IIC: Fracture line transverse.

Type III: Fractures involving intra-articular glenoid.

Type IV: Body fractures.

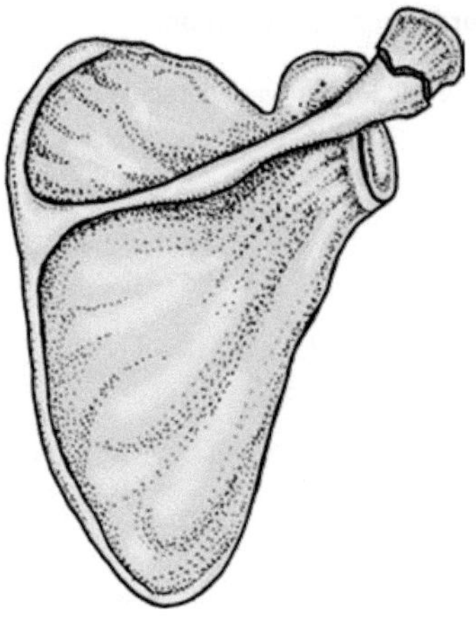

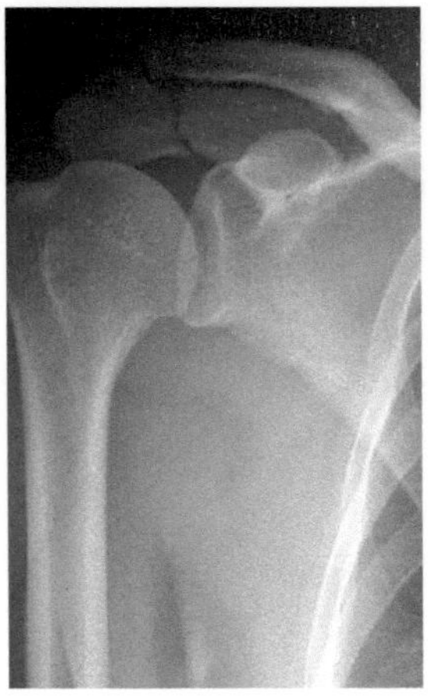

Ada-Miller classification

Type I: Fractures involving the acromion or coracoids.

Type I A: Acromion

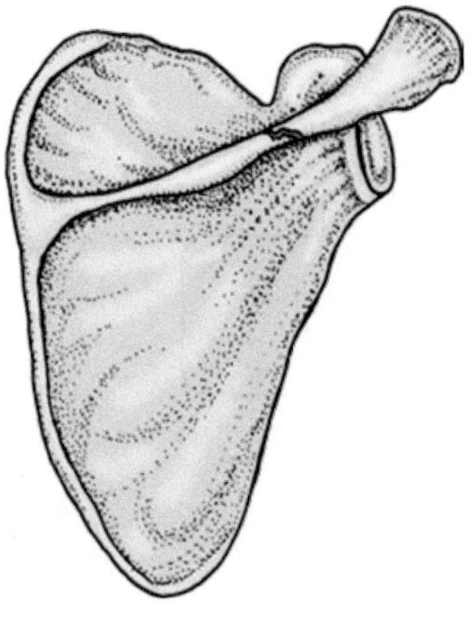

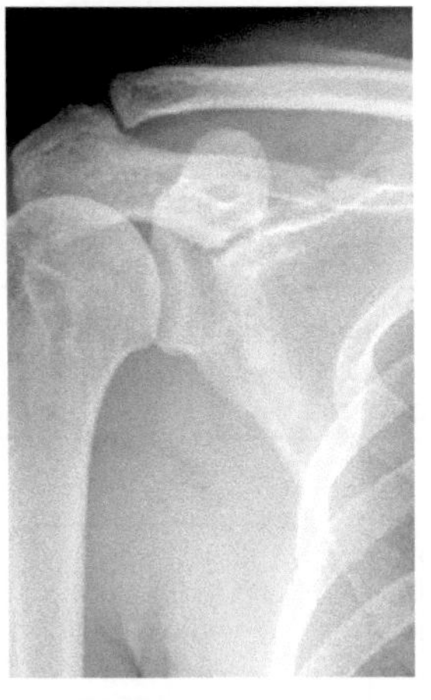

Ada-Miller classification

Type I: Fractures involving the acromion or coracoids.

Type I B: Base of acromion, spine

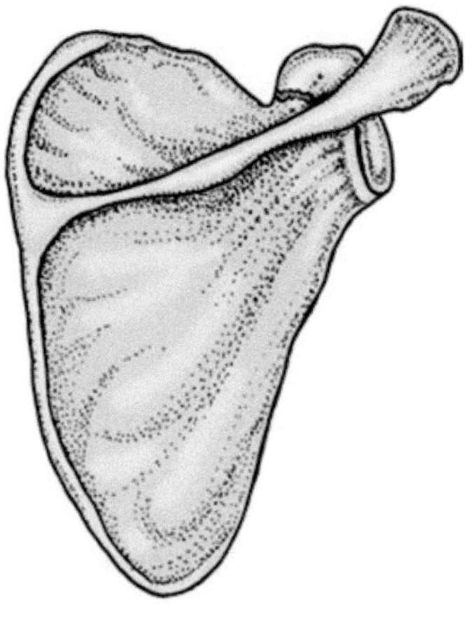

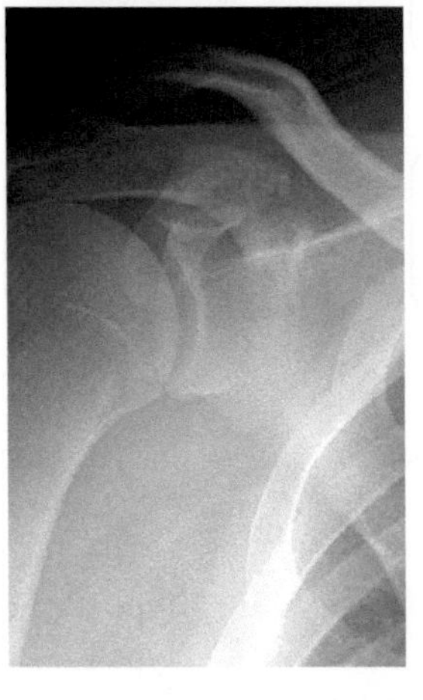

Ada-Miller classification

Type I: Fractures involving the acromion or coracoids.

Type I C: Coracoid

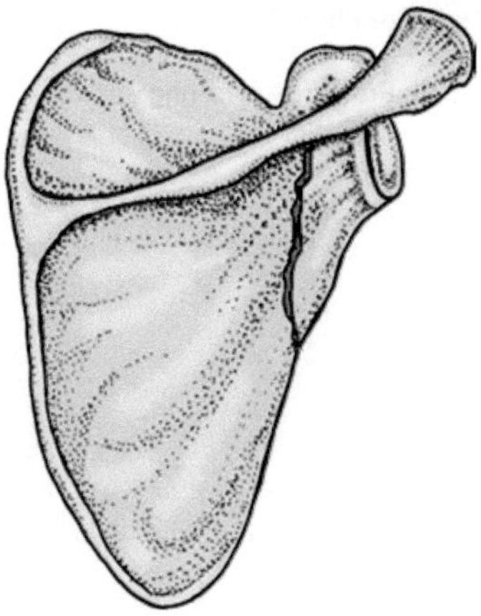

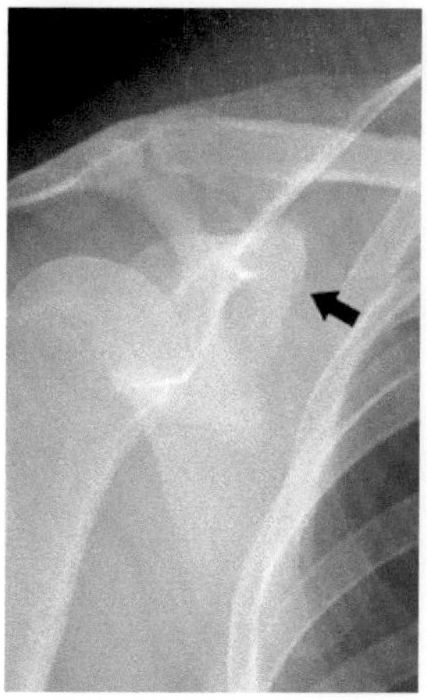

Ada-Miller classification

Type II: Fractures involving the scapular neck.

Type II A: Fracture line vertical, within scapular neck, lateral to base of acromion-spine

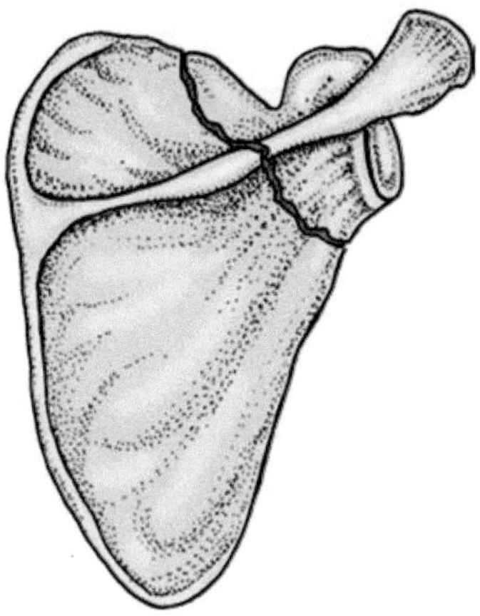

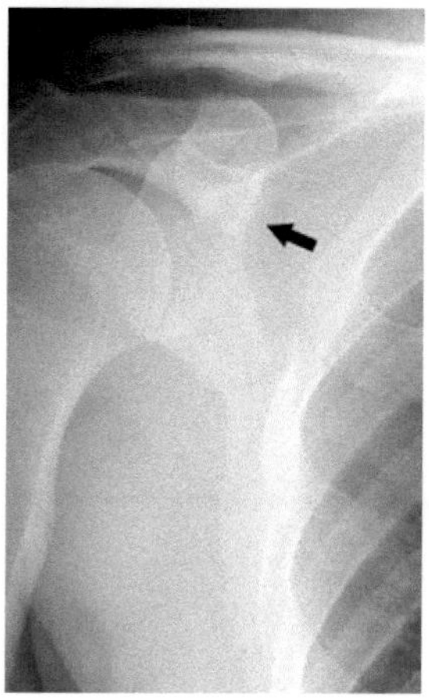

Ada-Miller classification

Type II: Fractures involving the scapular neck.

Type II B: Fracture line oblique, extending to base of acromion or spine

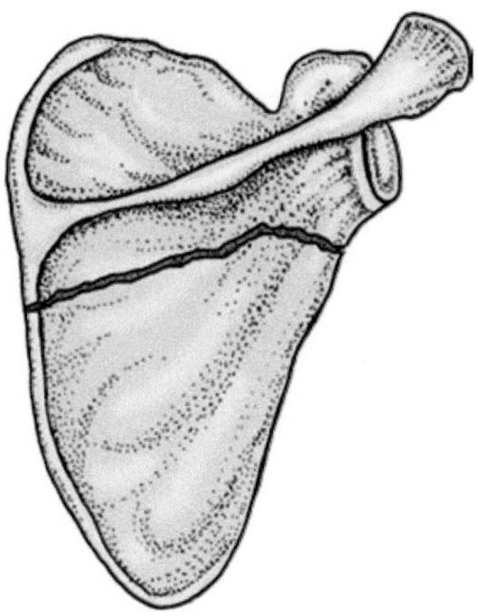

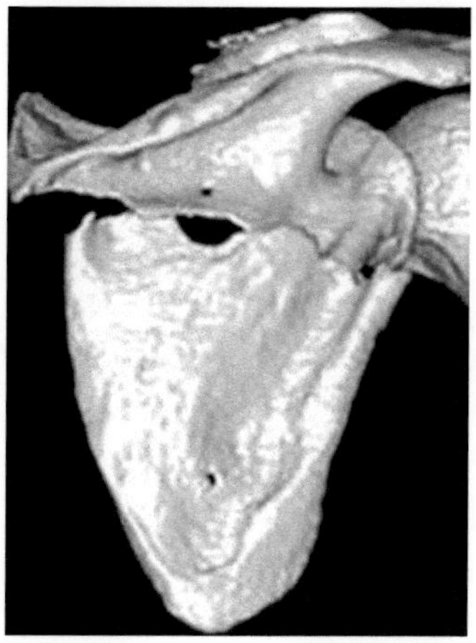

Ada-Miller classification

Type II: Fractures involving the scapular neck.

Type II C: Fracture line transverse

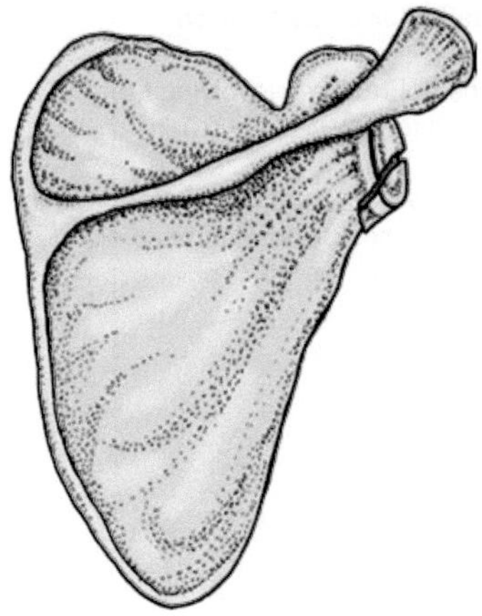

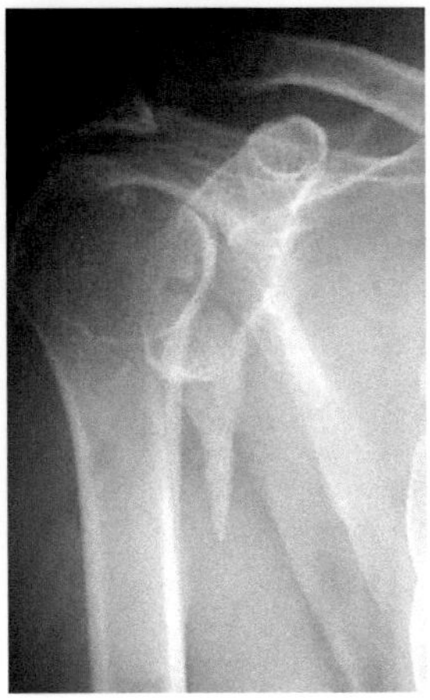

Ada-Miller classification

Type III: Fractures involving intra-articular glenoid

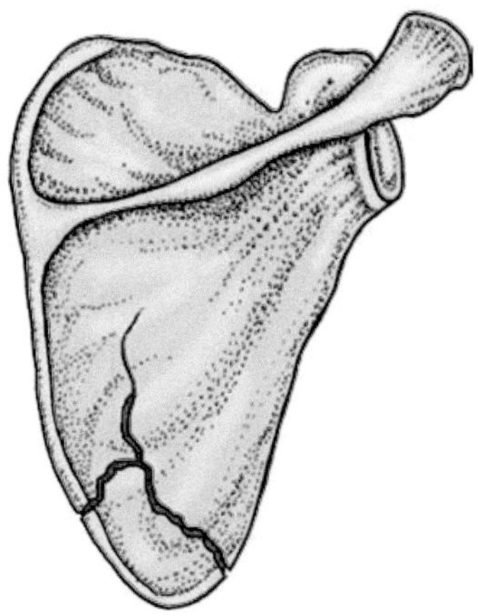

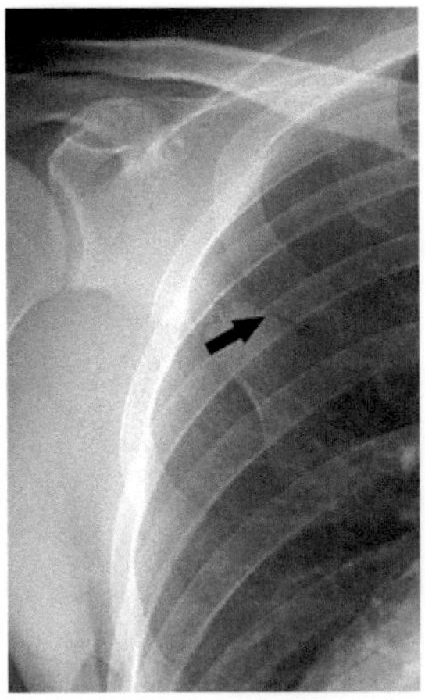

Ada-Miller classification

Type IV: Body fractures

1.2.1.3 AO/OTA Classification of Scapular Fractures [2]

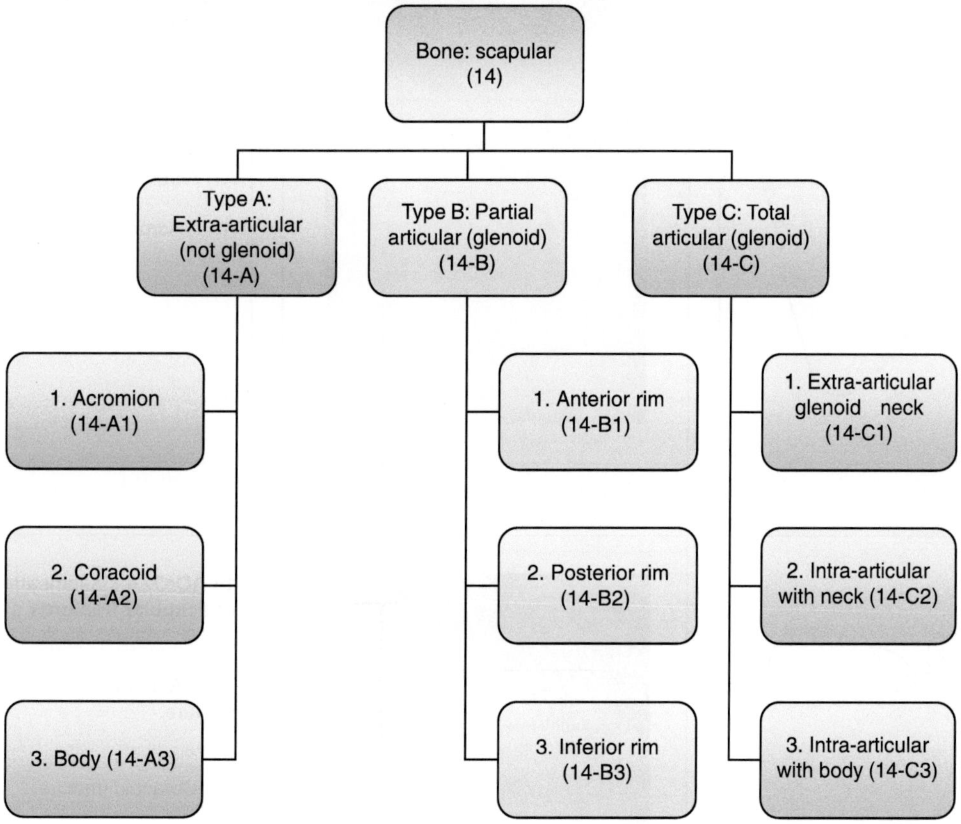

Type A: Extra-articular (not glenoid) fracture.
- A1: Acromion fracture.
  - A1.1: Acromion noncomminuted.
  - A1.2: Acromion comminuted.
- A2: Coracoid fracture.
  - A2.1: Coracoid noncomminuted.
  - A2.2: Coracoid comminuted.
- A3: Scapular body fracture.
  - A3.1: Scapular body noncomminuted.
  - A3.2: Scapular body comminuted.

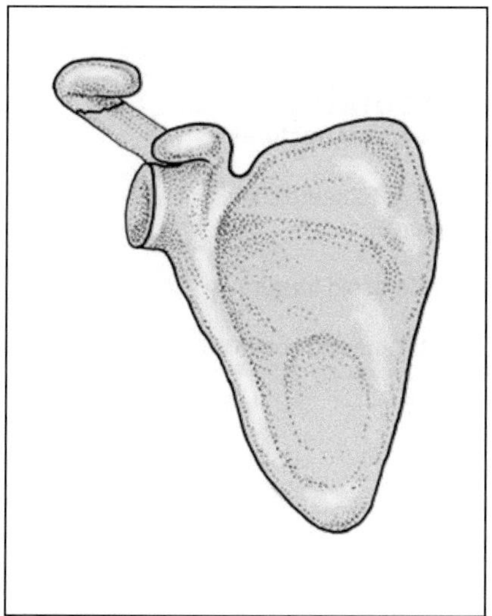

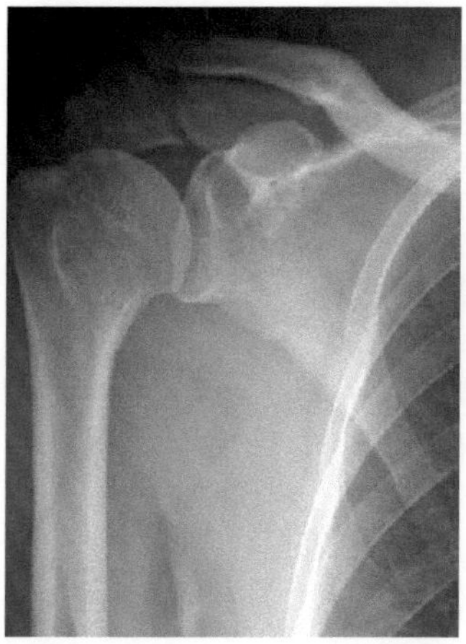

14 AO/OTA classification of scapular fractures

Type A: Extra-articular (not glenoid) fracture.

A1: Acromion fracture.

A1.1: Acromion non-comminuted

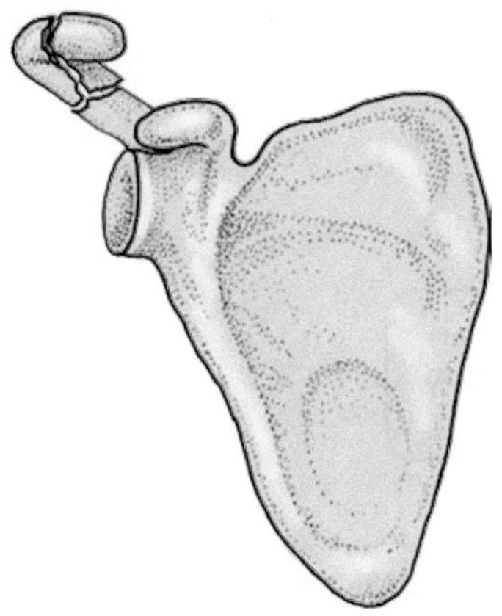

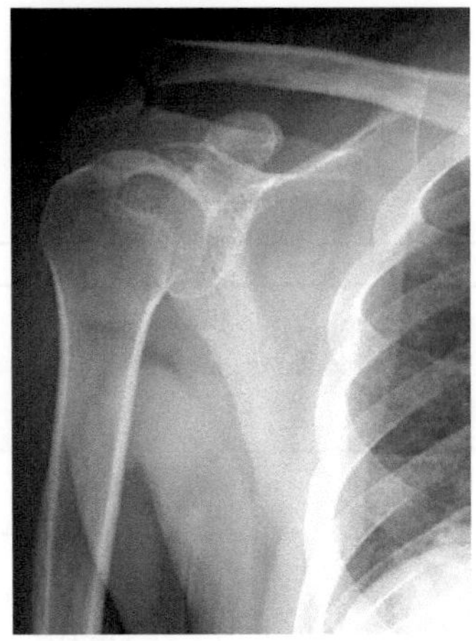

14 AO/OTA classification of scapular fractures

Type A: Extra-articular (not glenoid) fracture.

A1: Acromion fracture.

A1.2: Acromion comminuted

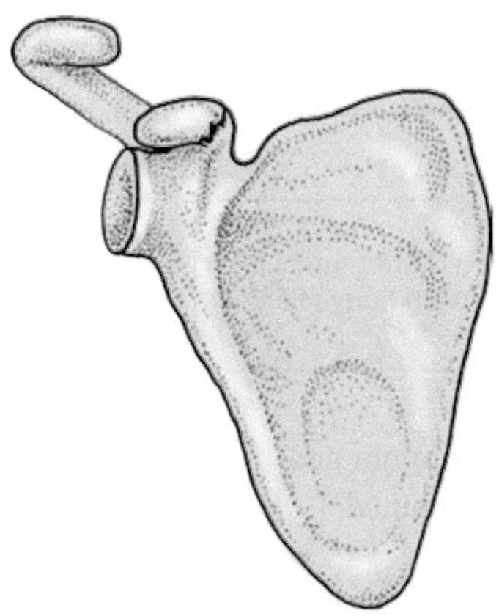

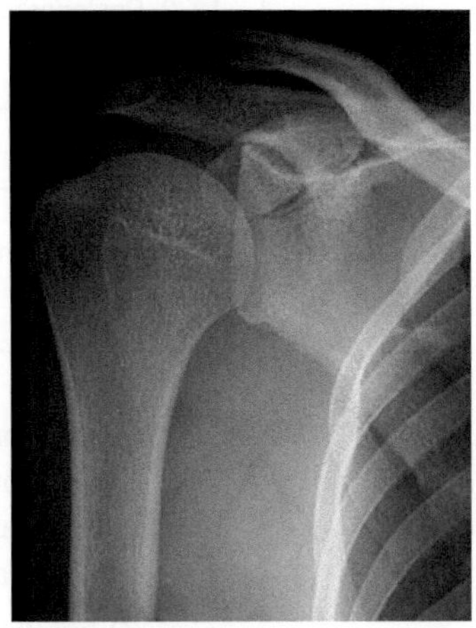

14 AO/OTA classification of scapular fractures

Type A: Extra-articular (not glenoid) fracture.

A2: Coracoid fracture.

A2.1: Coracoid non-comminuted

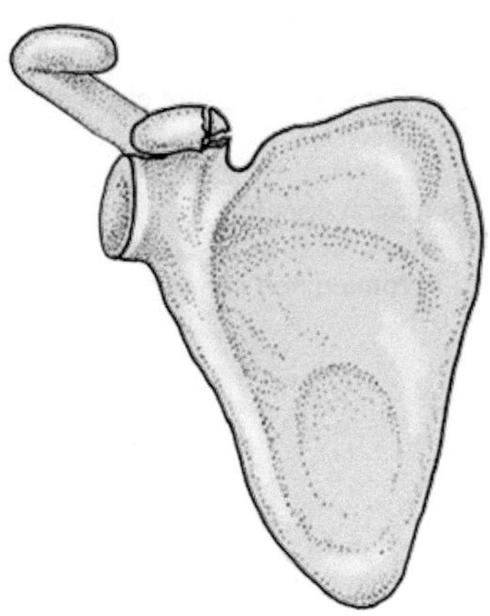

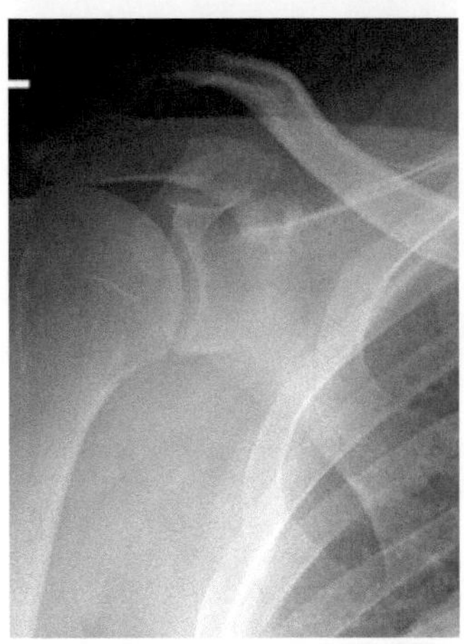

14 AO/OTA classification of scapular fractures

Type A: Extra-articular (not glenoid) fracture.

A2: Coracoid fracture.

A2.2: Coracoid comminuted

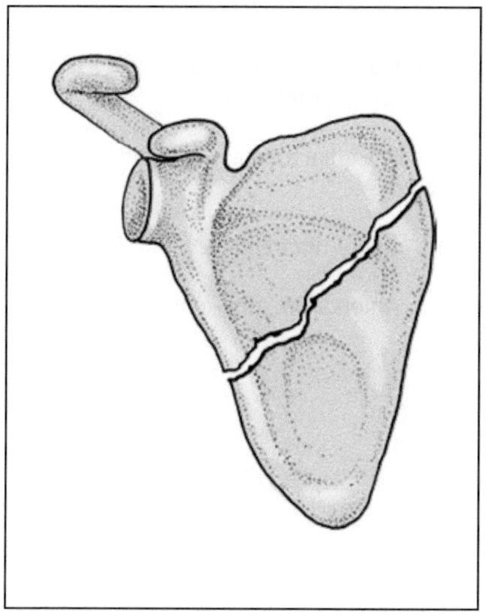

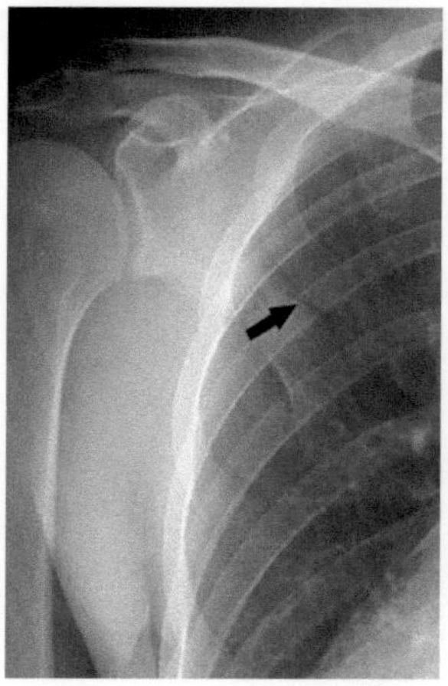

14 AO/OTA classification of scapular fractures

Type A: Extra-articular (not glenoid) fracture.

A3: Scapular body fracture.

A3.1: Scapular body non-comminuted

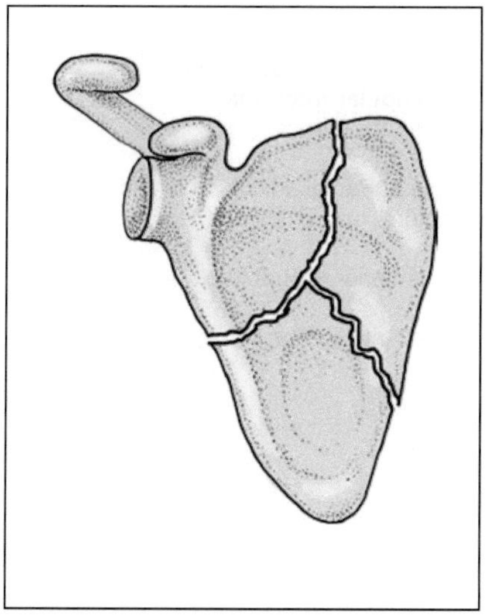

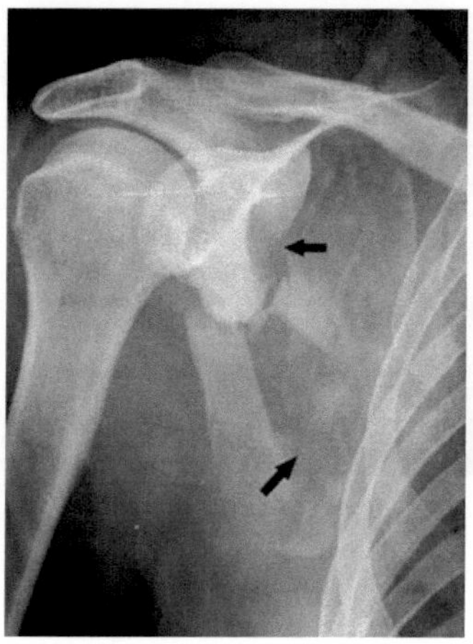

14 AO/OTA classification of scapular fractures

Type A: Extra-articular (not glenoid) fracture.

A3: Scapular body fracture.

A3.2: Scapular body comminuted

Type B: Partial articular (glenoid) fracture.
- B1: Anterior rim fracture.
  - B1.1: Anterior rim, noncomminuted.
  - B1.2: Anterior rim, comminuted.
- B2: Posterior rim fracture.
  - B2.1: Posterior rim, noncomminuted.
  - B2.2: Posterior rim, comminuted.
- B3: Inferior rim fracture.
  - B3.1: Inferior rim, noncomminuted.
  - B3.2: Inferior rim, comminuted.

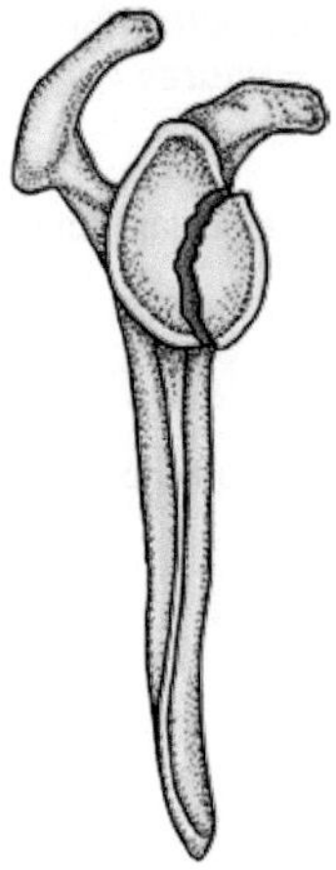

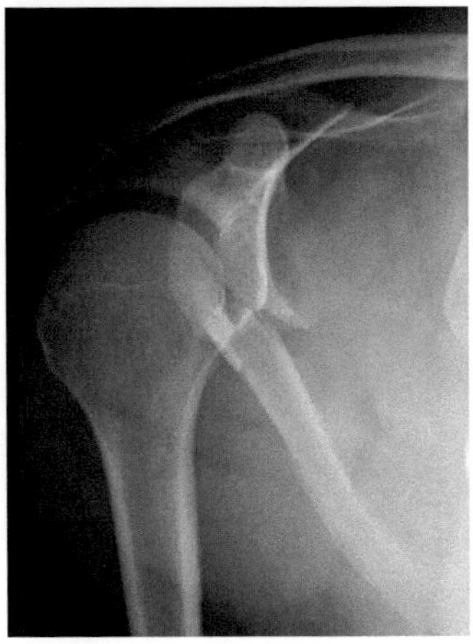

14 AO/OTA classification of scapular fractures

Type B: Partial articular (glenoid) fracture.

B1: Anterior rim fracture.

B1.1: Anterior rim, non-comminuted

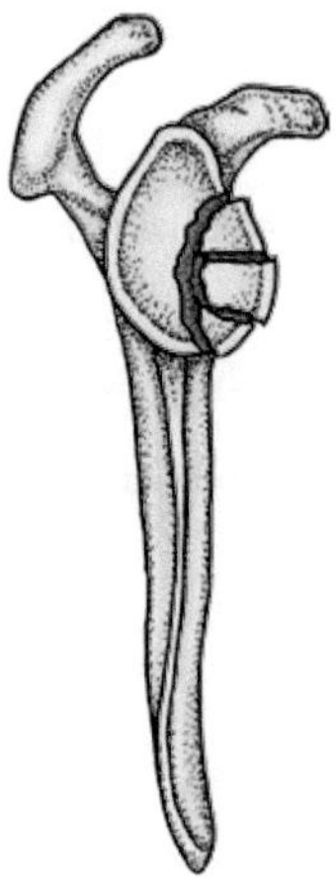

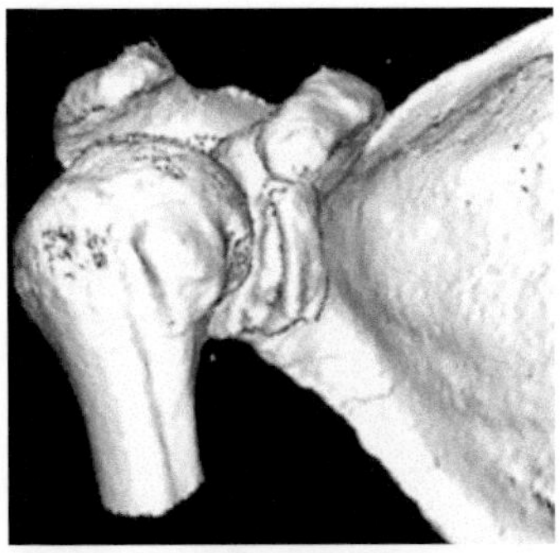

14 AO/OTA classification of scapular fractures

Type B: Partial articular (glenoid) fracture.

B1: Anterior rim fracture.

B1.2: Anterior rim, comminuted

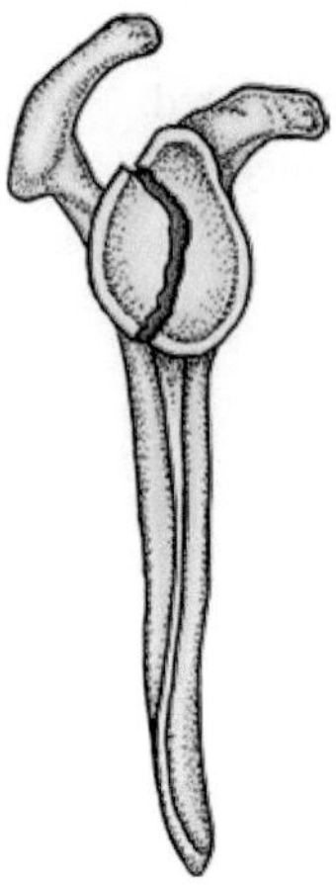

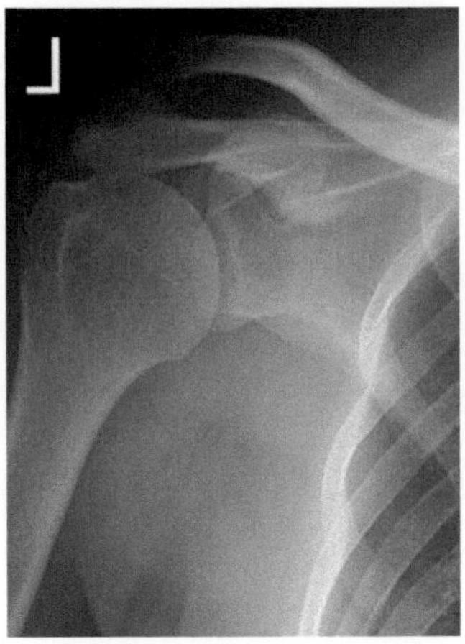

14 AO/OTA classification of scapular fractures

Type B: Partial articular (glenoid) fracture.

B2: Posterior rim fracture.

B2.1: Posterior rim, non-comminuted

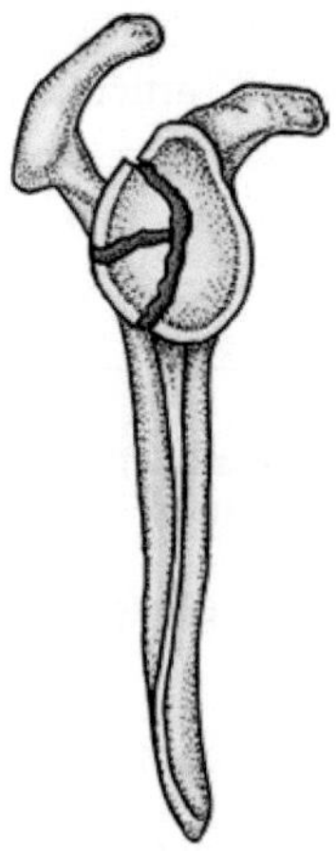

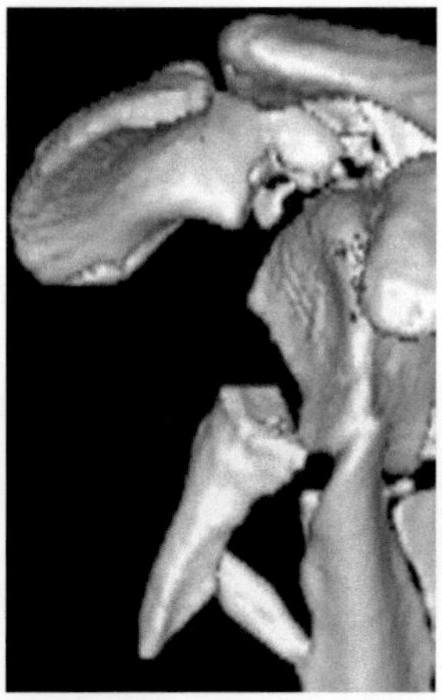

14 AO/OTA classification of scapular fractures

Type B: Partial articular (glenoid) fracture.

B2: Posterior rim fracture.

B2.2: Posterior rim, comminuted

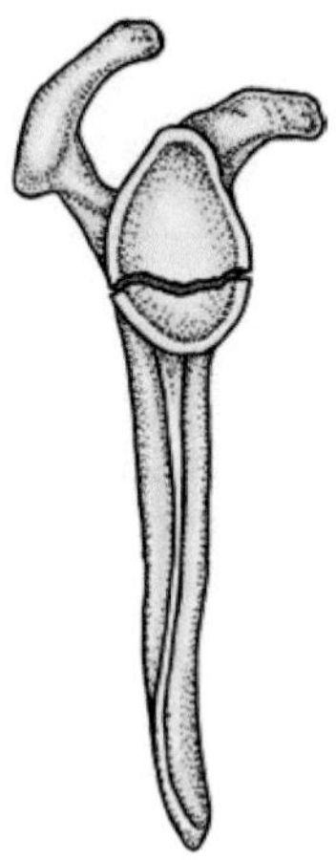

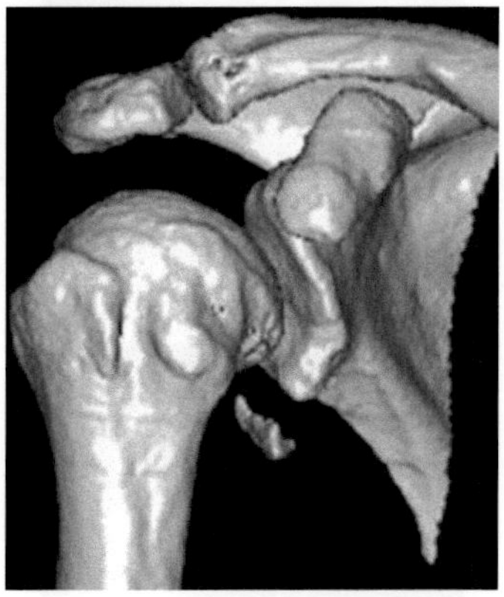

14 AO/OTA classification of scapular fractures

Type B: Partial articular (glenoid) fracture.

B3: Inferior rim fracture.

B3.1: Inferior rim, non-comminuted

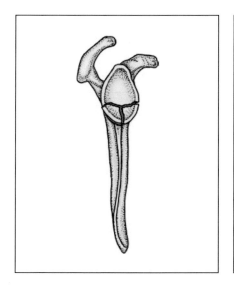

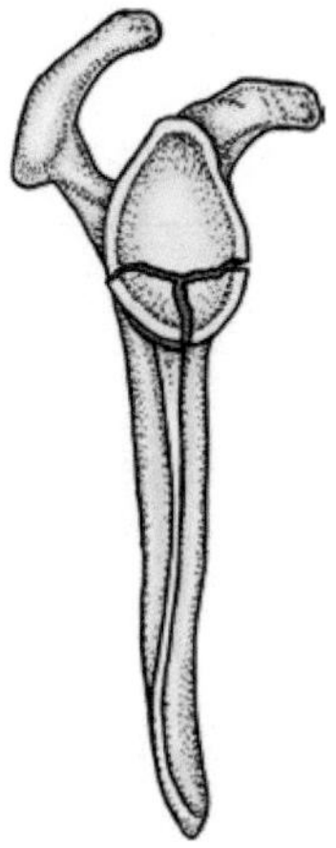

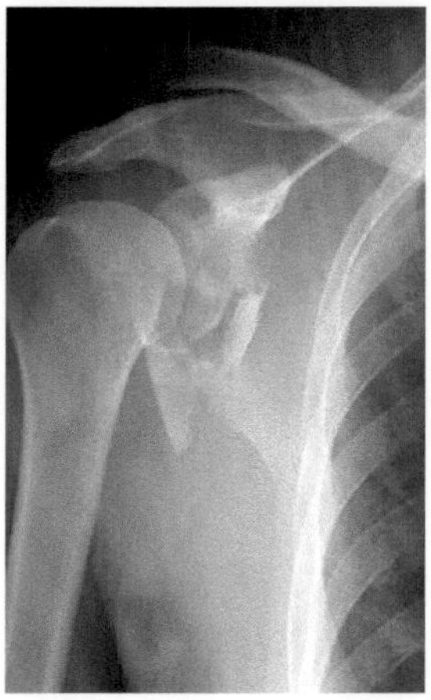

14 AO/OTA classification of scapular fractures

Type B: Partial articular (glenoid) fracture.

B3: Inferior rim fracture

B3.2: Inferior rim, comminuted

Type C: Total articular (glenoid) fracture.
- C1: Extra-articular glenoid neck fracture.
  - C1.1: Extra-articular glenoid neck, noncomminuted.
  - C1.2: Extra-articular glenoid neck, comminuted.
- C2: Intra-articular with neck.
  - C2.1: Intra-articular with neck, articular noncomminuted, neck noncomminuted.
  - C2.2: Intra-articular with neck, articular noncomminuted, neck comminuted.
  - C2.3: Intra-articular with neck, articular comminuted.
- C3: Intra-articular with body.

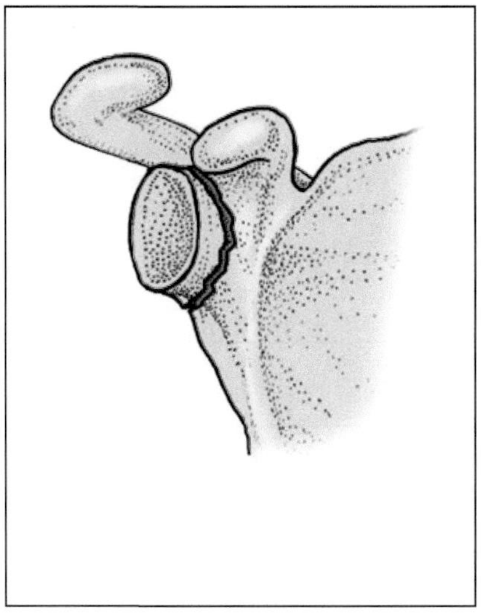

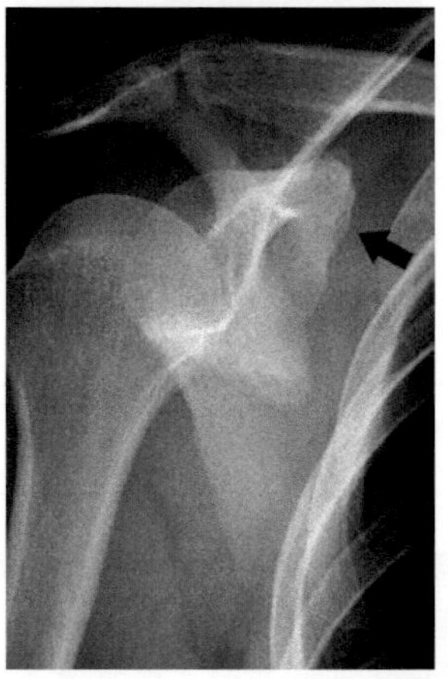

14 AO/OTA classification of scapular fractures

Type C: Total articular (glenoid) fracture.

C1: Extra-articular glenoid neck fracture.

C1.1: Extra-articular glenoid neck, non-comminuted

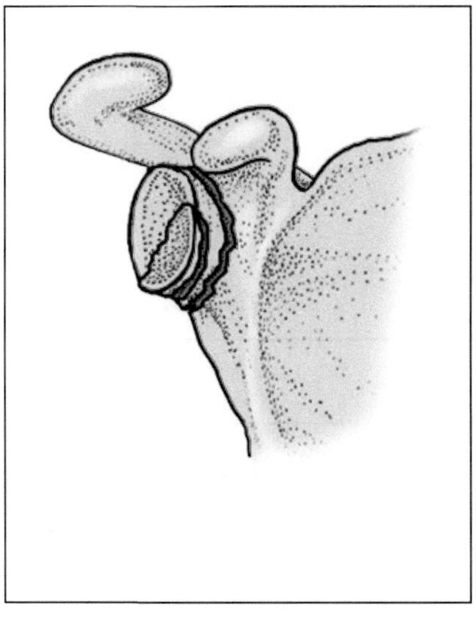

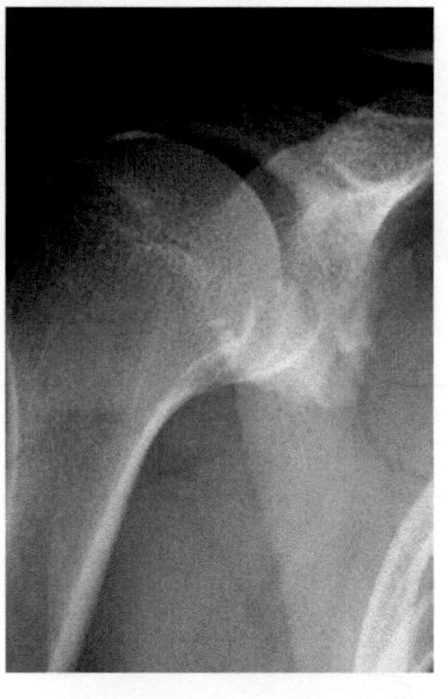

14 AO/OTA classification of scapular fractures

Type C: Total articular (glenoid) fracture.

C1: Extra-articular glenoid neck fracture.

C1.2: Extra-articular glenoid neck, comminuted

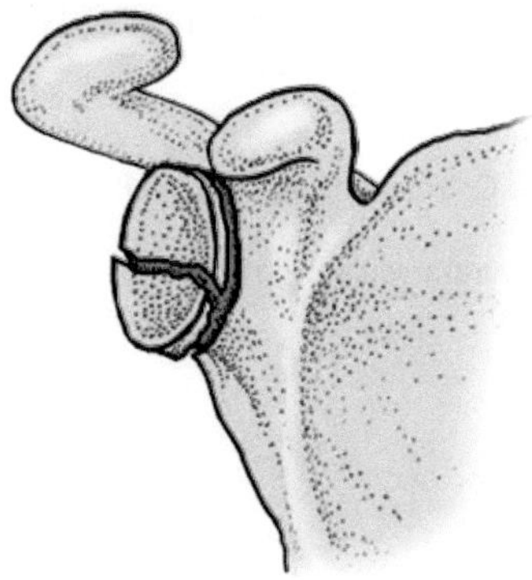

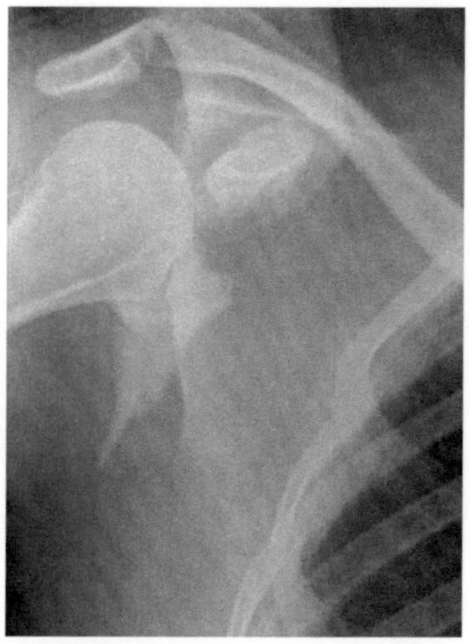

14 AO/OTA classification of scapular fractures

Type C: Total articular (glenoid) fracture.

C2: Intra-articular with neck.

C2.1: Intra-articular with neck, articular non-comminuted, neck non-comminuted

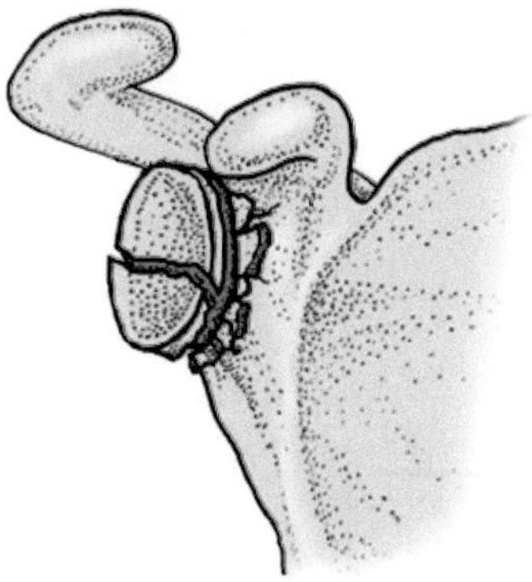

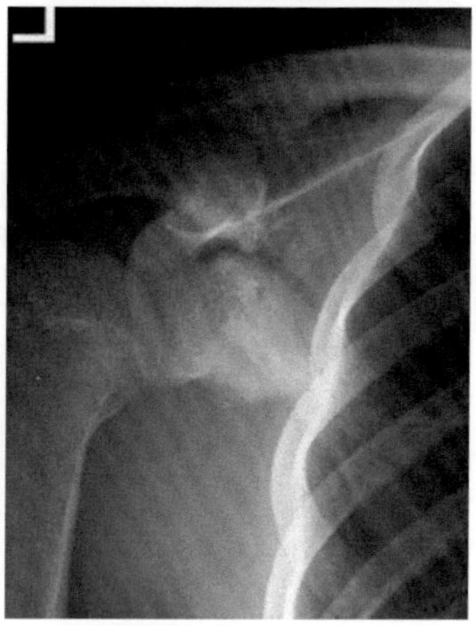

14 AO/OTA classification of scapular fractures

Type C: Total articular (glenoid) fracture.

C2: Intra-articular with neck.

C2.2: Intra-articular with neck, articular non-comminuted, neck comminuted

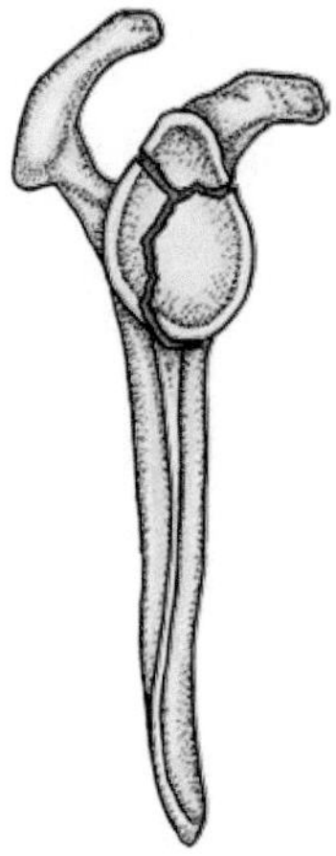

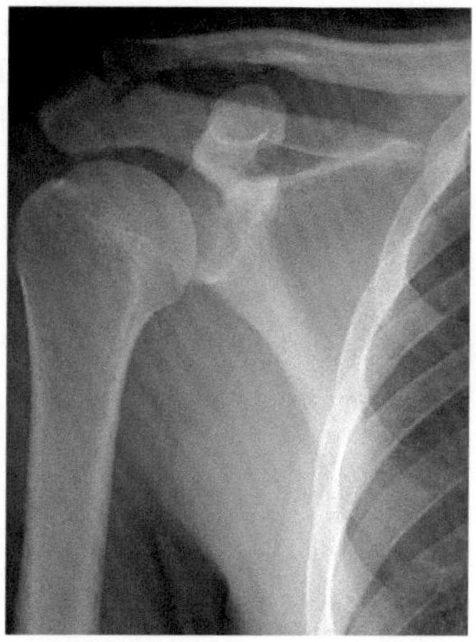

14 AO/OTA classification of scapular fractures

Type C: Total articular (glenoid) fracture.

C2: Intra-articular with neck.

C2.3: Intra-articular with neck, articular comminuted

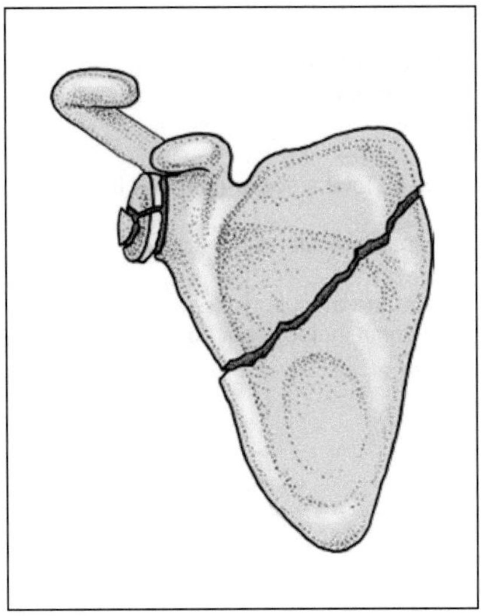

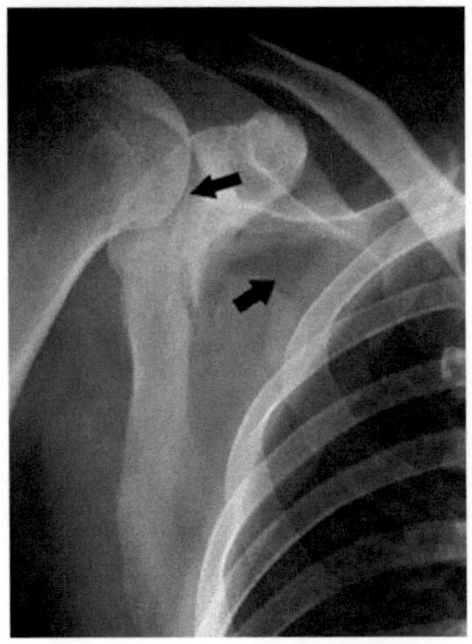

14 AO/OTA classification of scapular fractures

Type C: Total articular (glenoid) fracture.

C3: Intra-articular with body

1.2.1.4 Zdravkovic-Damholt Classification

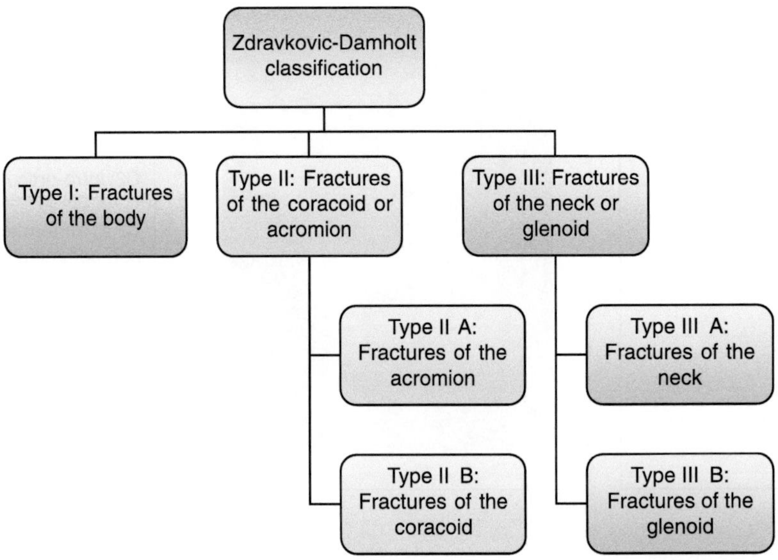

Type I: Fractures of the body.
Type II: Fractures of the coracoid or acromion.
  Type IIA: Fractures of the acromion.
  Type IIB: Fractures of the coracoids.
Type III: Fractures of the neck or glenoid.
  Type IIIA: Fractures of the neck.
  Type IIIB: Fractures of the glenoid.

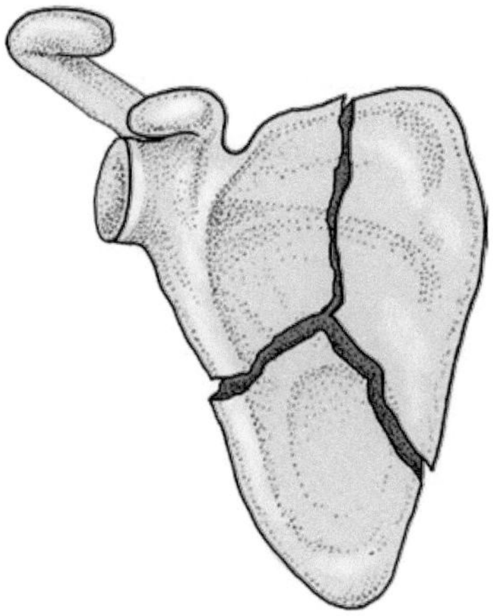

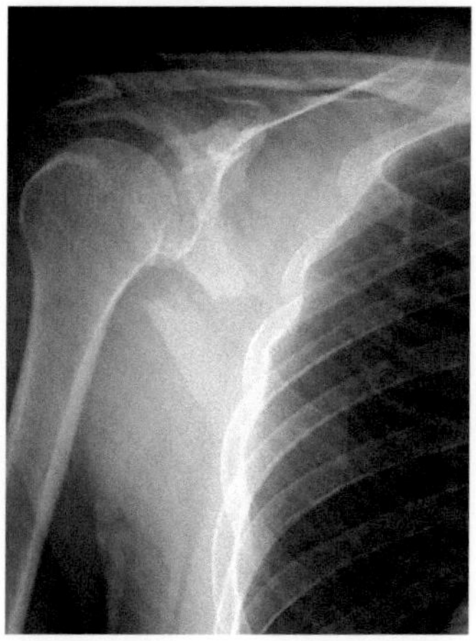

Zdravkovic-Damholtclass ification

Type I: Fractures of the body

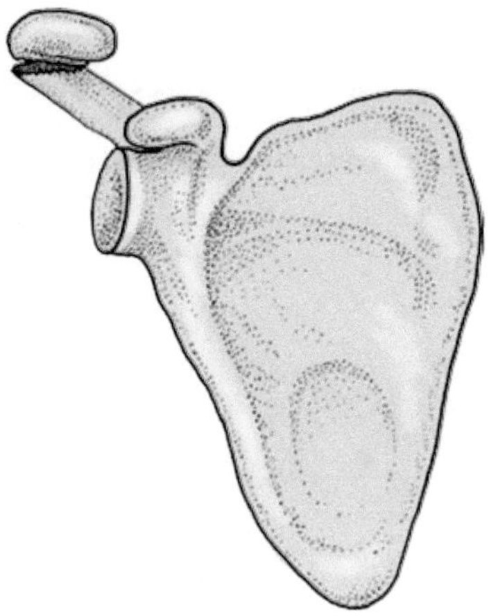

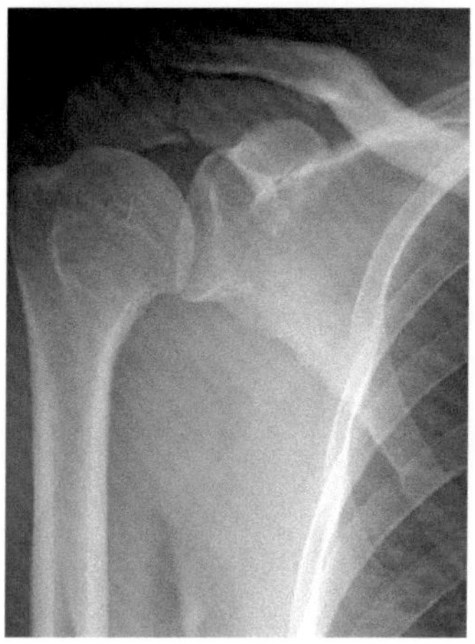

Zdravkovic-Damholtclass ification

Type II: Fractures of the coracoid or acromion.

Type II A: Fractures of the acromion

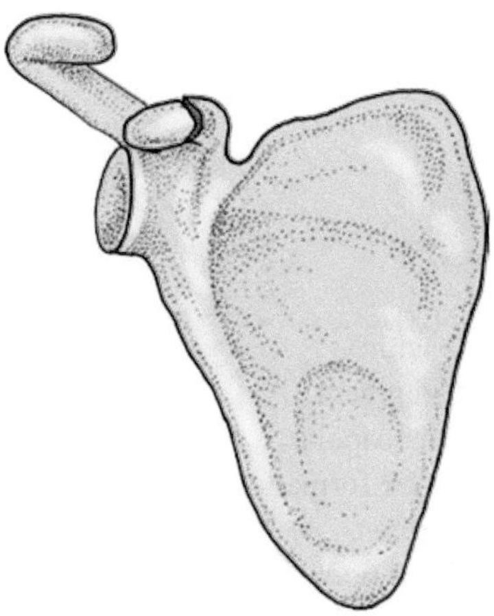

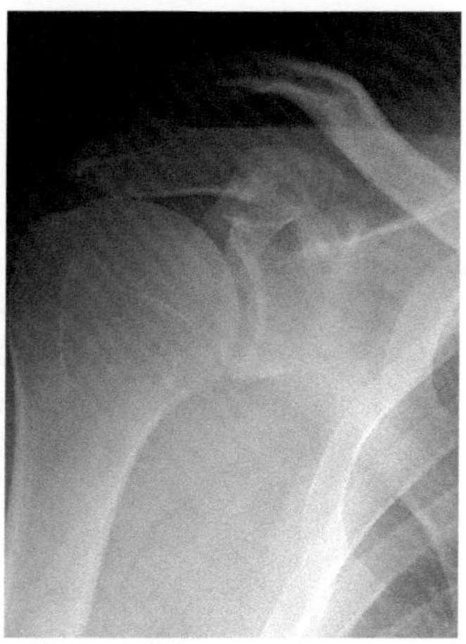

Zdravkovic-Damholtclass ification

Type II: Fractures of the coracoid or acromion.

Type II B: Fractures of the coracoid

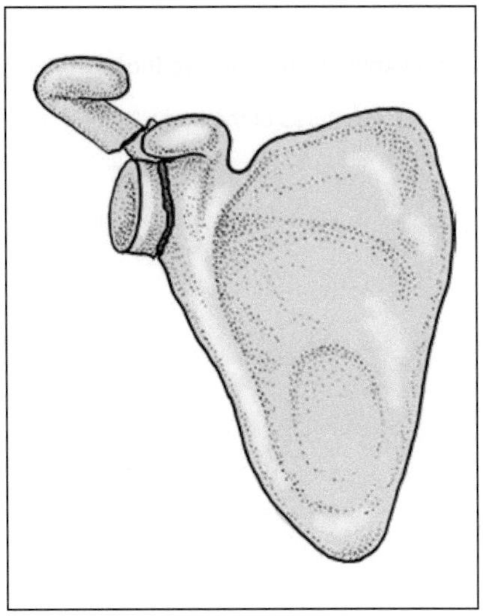

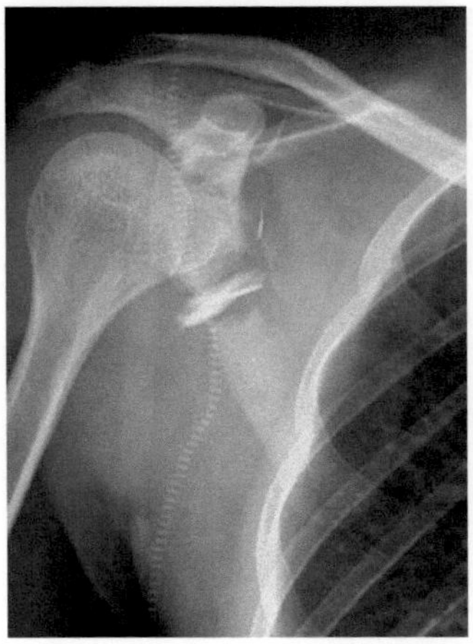

Zdravkovic-Damholtclass ification

Type III: Fractures of the neck or glenoid.

Type IIIA: Fractures of the neck.

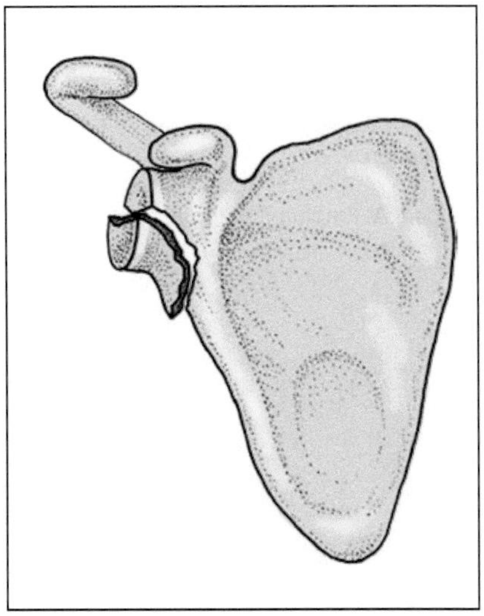

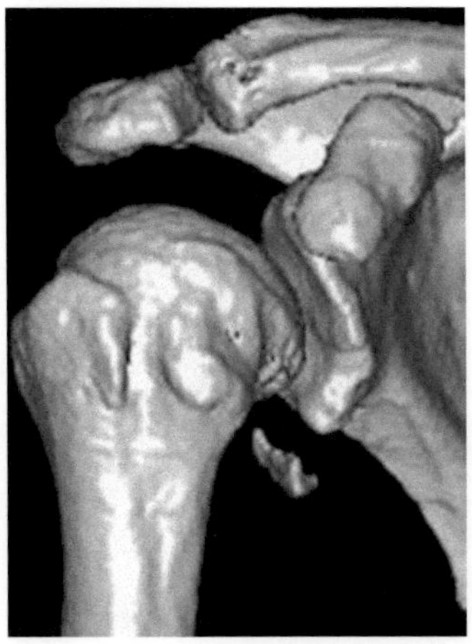

Zdravkovic-Damholtclass ification

Type III: Fractures of the neck or glenoid.

Type IIIB: Fractures of the glenoid.

1.2.1.5 Thompson Classification [7]

Type I: Coracoid and acromion fractures.

Type II: Glenoid and neck fractures.

Type III: Major body fractures.

1.2.1.6 Euler-Ruedi Classification [8]

Type A, type B, and type C are extra-articular, and type D is intra-articular.

Type A: Fractures of the body of scapula, isolated or multifragmentary.

Type B: Fractures of the process.
- Type B1: Spine.
- Type B2: Coracoids.
- Type B3: Acromion.

Type C: Fractures of scapular neck.
- Type C1: Anatomical neck.
- Type C2: Surgical neck.
- Type C3: Surgical neck with:
  - (a) Fractures of clavicle and acromion.
  - (b) Torn CC and CA ligaments.

Type D: Articular fractures.
- Type D1: Glenoid rim.
- Type D2: Glenoid fossa with:
  - (a) Inferior glenoid fragment.
  - (b) Horizontal split of scapula.
  - (c) Coracoglenoid block formation.
  - (d) Comminuted fractures.
- Type D3: Scapula neck and body fracture.

Type E: Fracture combination with humeral head fractures.

1.2.1.7 Goss Classification: Types of Traumatic Superior Shoulder Suspensory Complex (SSSC) Disruptions [9]

Goss introduced the concept of the SSSC. The "SSSC" is an osseous and ligamentous ring supported by the superior and inferior osseous struts that serve as a suspension for the upper extremities. It includes the glenoid, coracoid, acromion, distal clavicle, and connecting ligaments.

SSSC single disruptions
- Type A: Single disruption by a break
- Type B: Single disruption by a ligament disruption

SSSC double disruptions
- Type C: Double-ligament disruption
- Type D: Double break
- Type E: Combined bone and ligament disruption
- Type F: Disruption of both struts
- Type G: One strut and one ring disruption

Traumatic SSSC single disruptions, e.g., grade II acromial-clavicular separation, are more frequent than SSSC double disruptions, with no obvious influence to stability. SSSC double or more disruptions are potentially unstable and can result in delayed union, nonunion, malunion, decreased strength, and long-term problems. SSSC single disruptions combined with clavicular shaft fracture, scapular body fracture, or scapular spine fracture yield the same clinical result as SSSC double or more disruptions, such as glenoid neck fracture combined with acromial-clavicular separation or clavicular fracture, which often need open reduction and internal fixation.

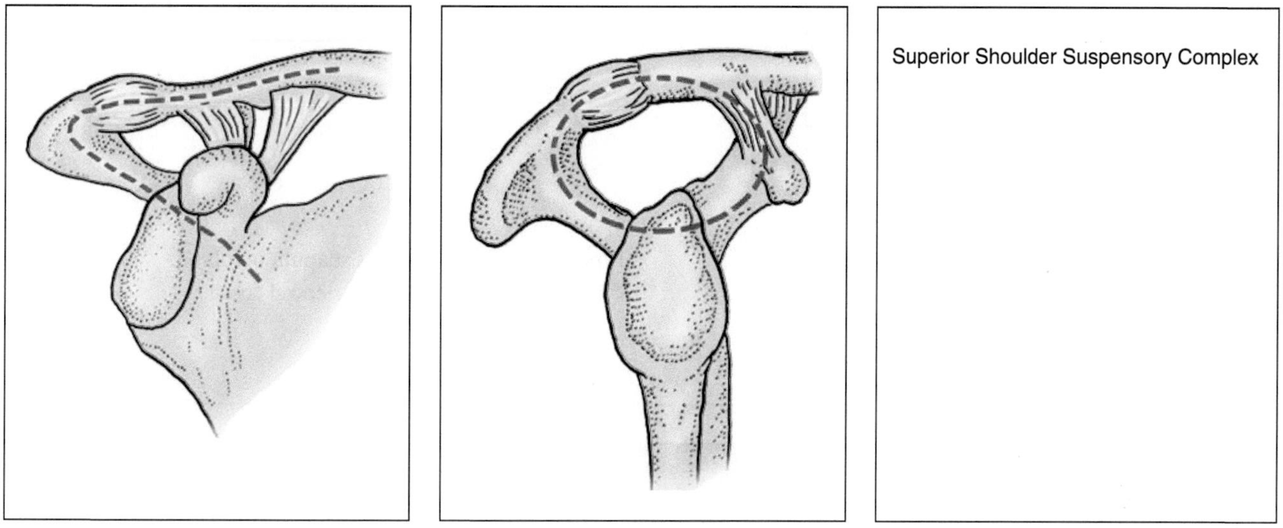

1.2.2 Classification of Fractures of the Coracoid Process

1.2.2.1 Eyres Classification [10]

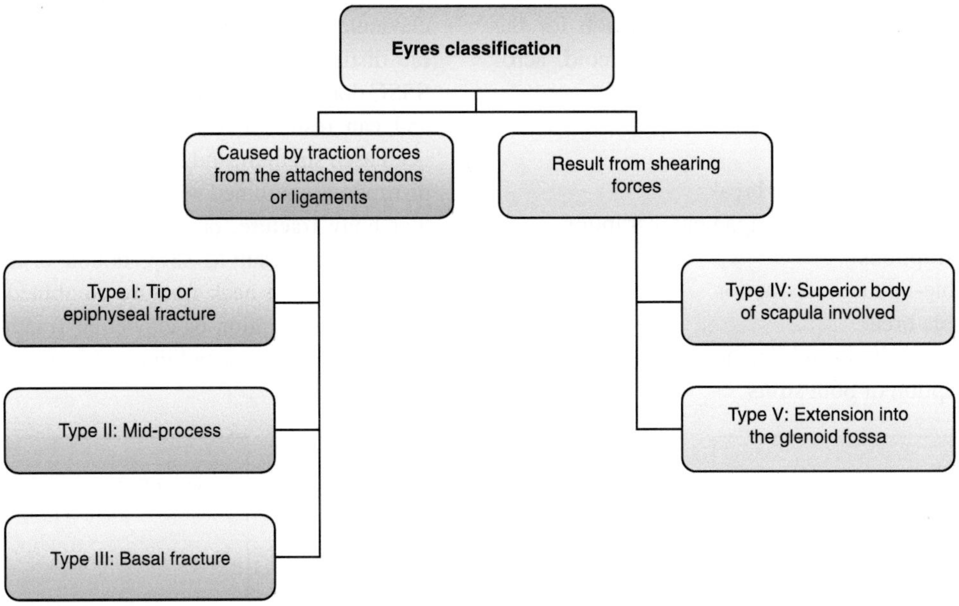

Type I: Tip or epiphyseal fracture.
Type II: Mid-process.
Type III: Basal fracture.

Type IV: Superior body of scapula involved.
Type V: Extension into the glenoid fossa.

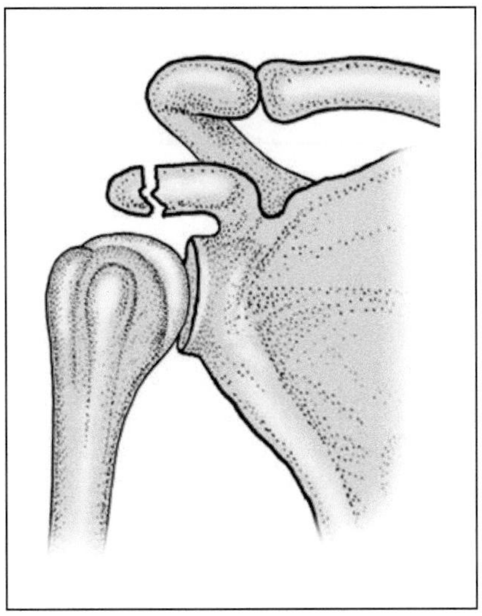

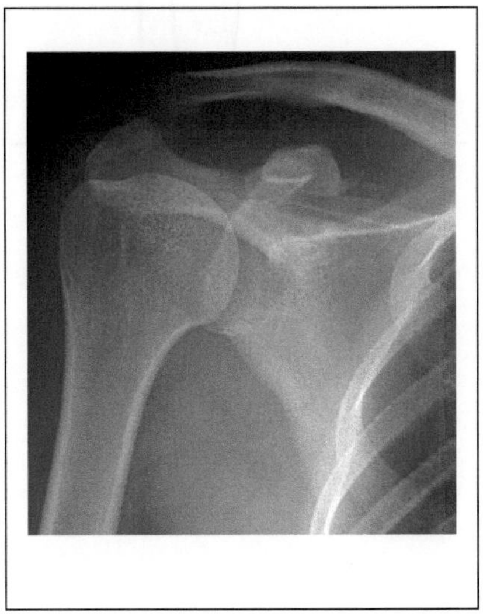

Eyres Classification of fractures of the coracoid process

Type I: Tip or epiphyseal fracture

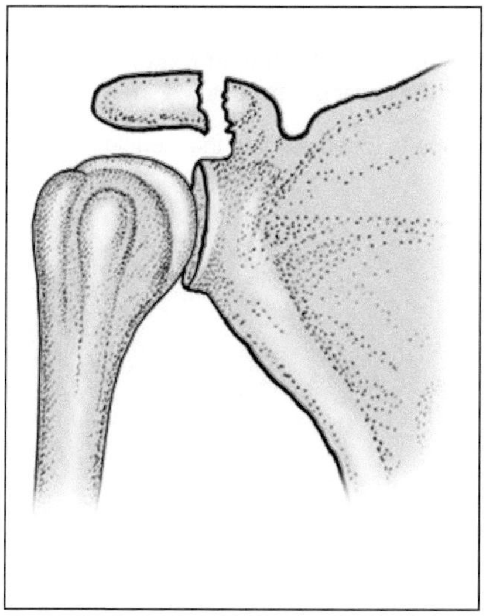

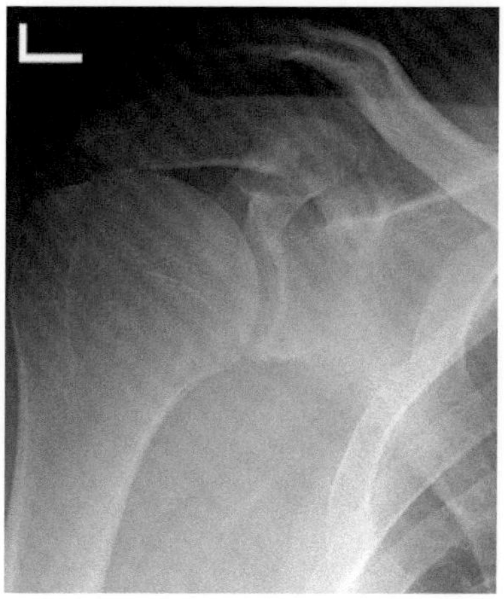

Eyres Classification of fractures of the coracoid process

Type II: Mid-process

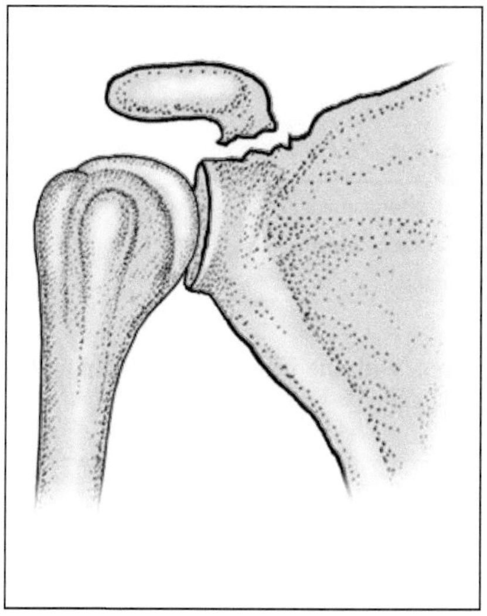

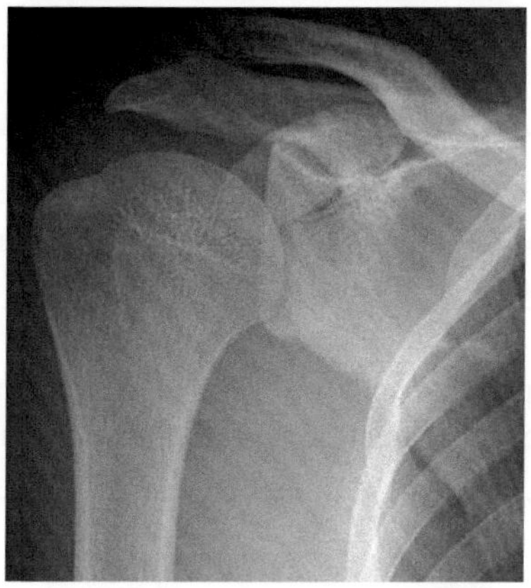

Eyres Classification of fractures of the coracoid process

Type III: Basal fracture

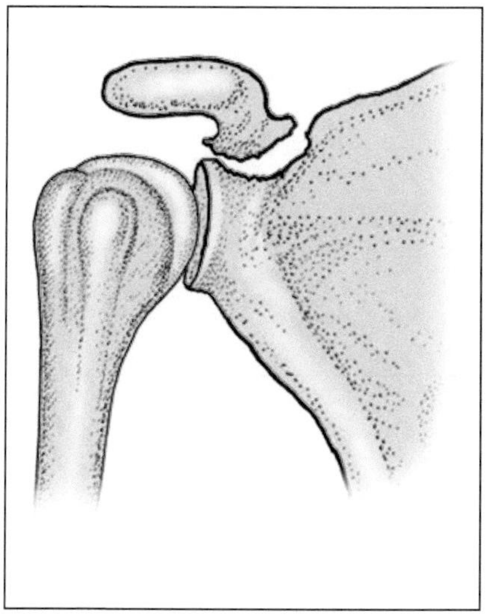

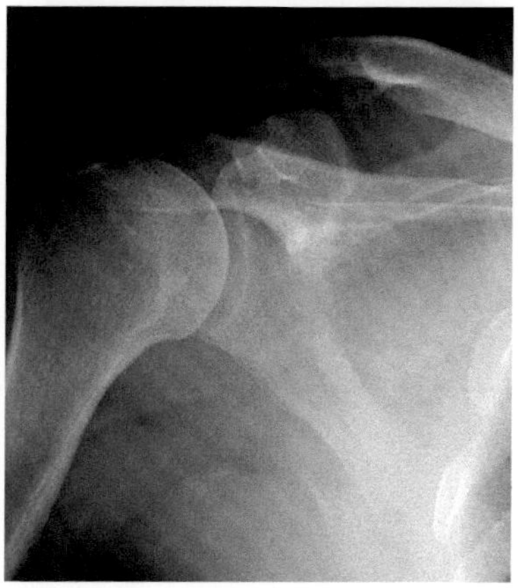

Eyres Classification of fractures of the coracoid process

Type IV: Superior body of scapula involved

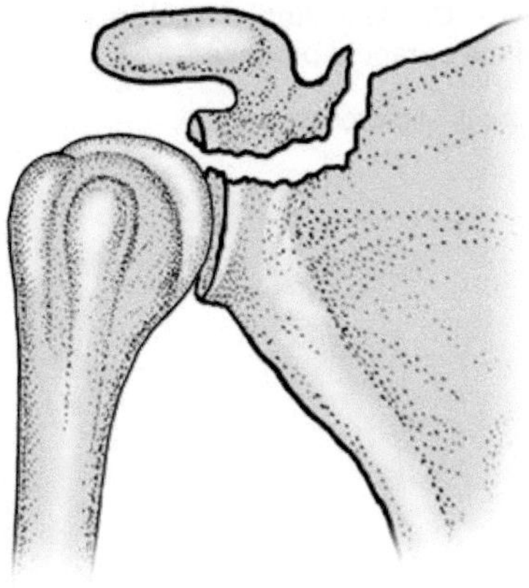

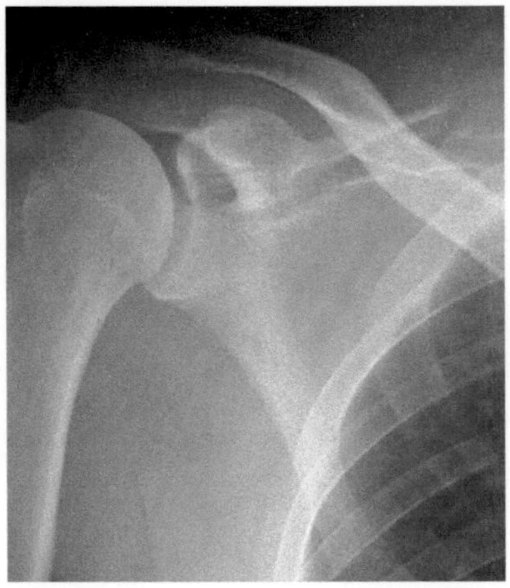

Eyres Classification of fractures of the coracoid process

Type V: Extension into the glenoid fossa

1.2.2.2 Ogawa Classification [11]

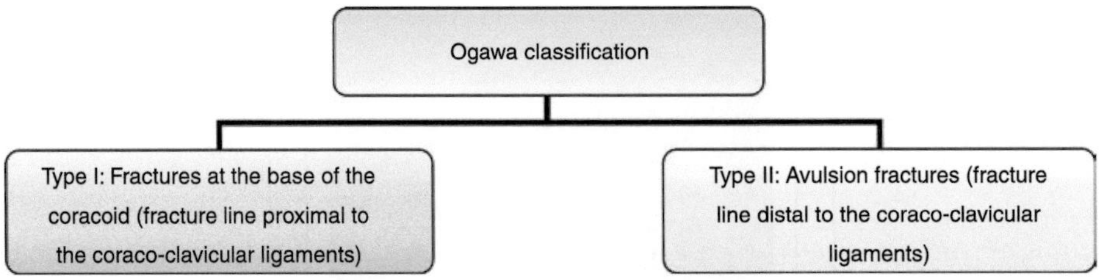

Type I: Fractures at the base of the coracoid process, with the fracture line proximal to the coracoclavicular ligaments.

Type II: Avulsion fractures, with the fracture line distal to the coracoclavicular ligaments.

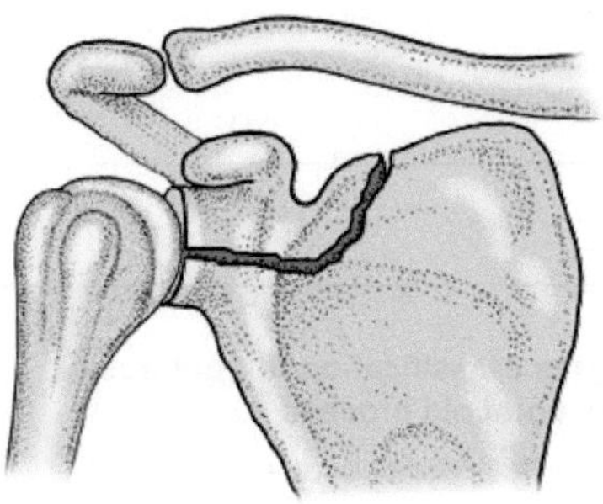

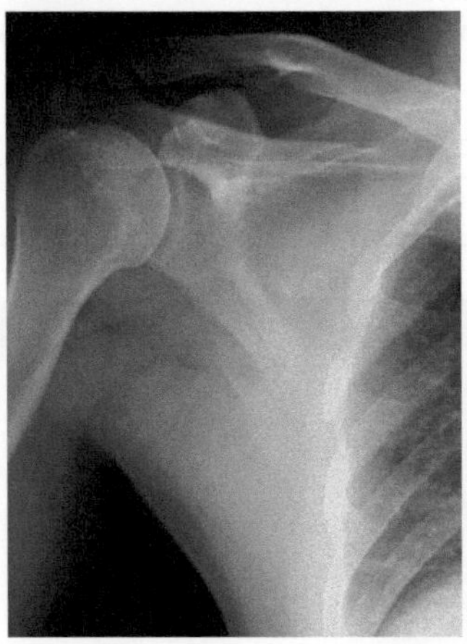

Ogawa Classification of fractures of the coracoid process

Type I: Fractures at the base of the coracoid (fracture line proximal to the coraco-clavicular ligaments)

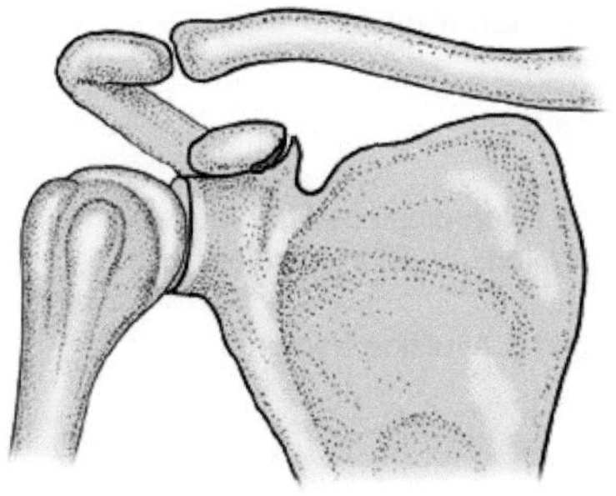

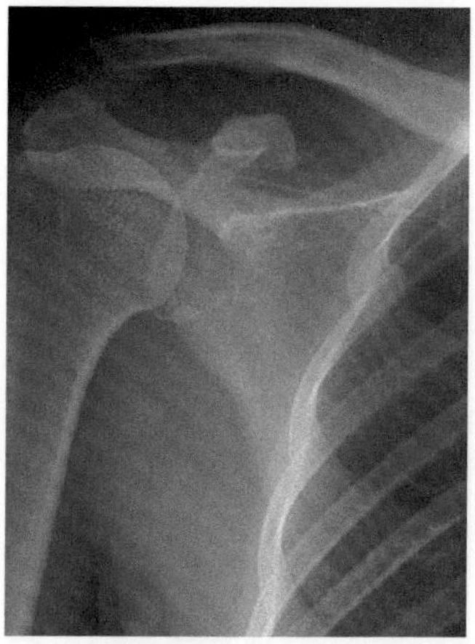

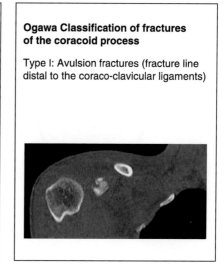

Ogawa Classification of fractures of the coracoid process

Type I: Avulsion fractures (fracture line distal to the coraco-clavicular ligaments)

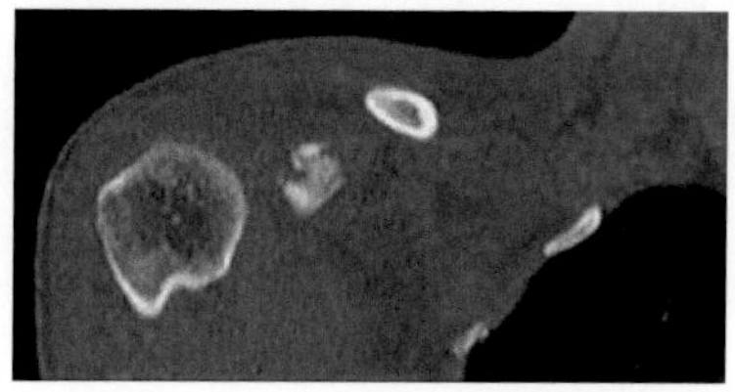

1.2.3 Classification System of Acromion Fractures

1.2.3.1 Area Classification

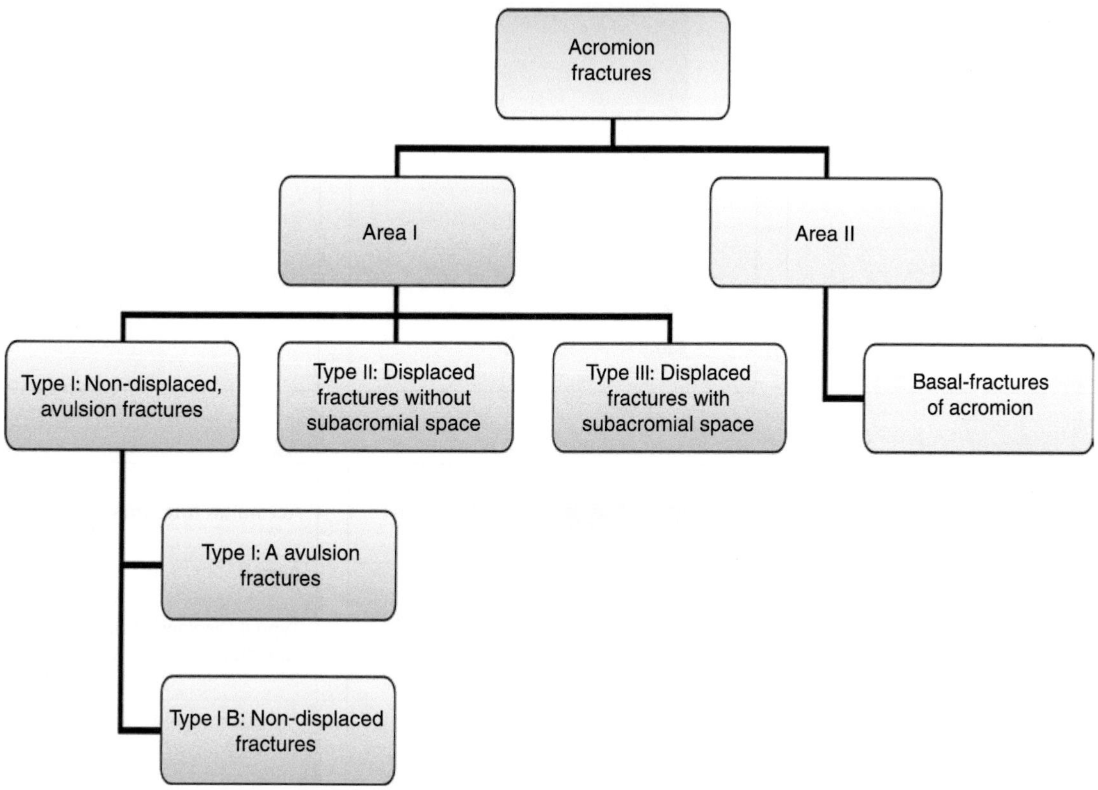

Area I

Type I: Non-displaced fractures of the acromion, avulsion fractures

Type IA: Avulsion fractures.

Type IB: Non-displaced fractures.

Type II: Displaced fractures without subacromial space reducing

Type III: Displaced fractures with subacromial space reducing

Area II

Basal fractures of acromion

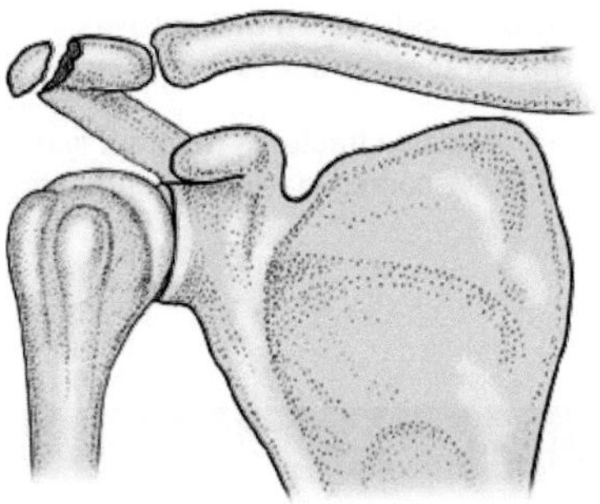

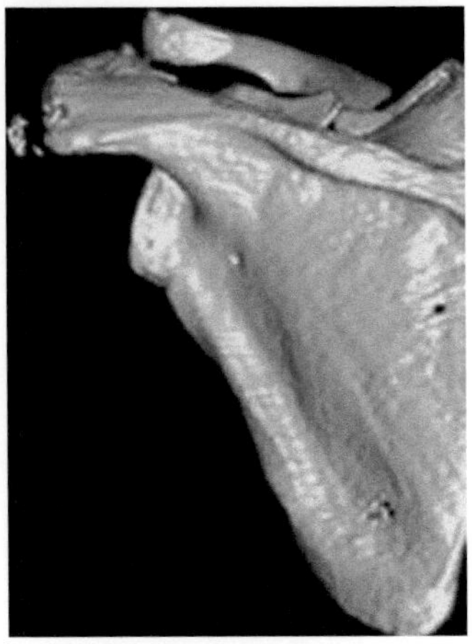

Acromion fractures

Area I:

Type I Non-displaced fractures of the acromion, avulsion fractures:

Type I A Avulsion fractures

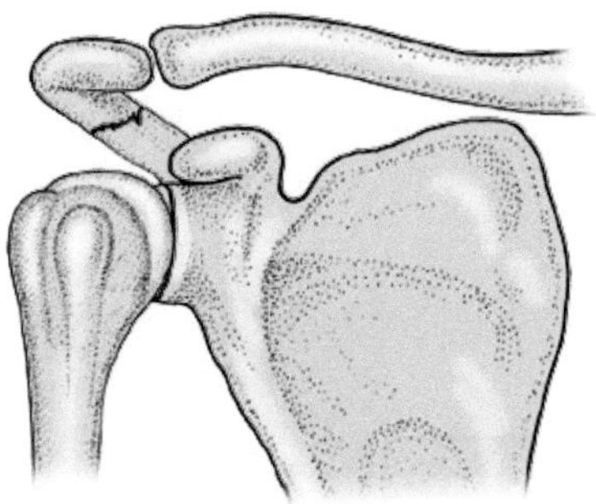

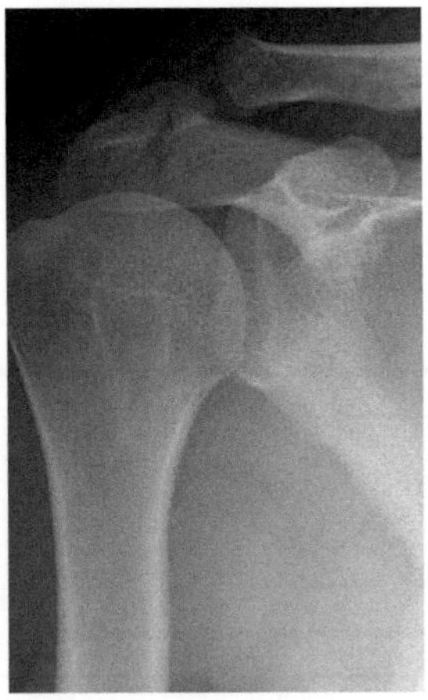

Acromion fractures

Area I:

Type I Non-displaced fractures of the acromion, avulsion fractures:

Type I B Non-displaced fractures

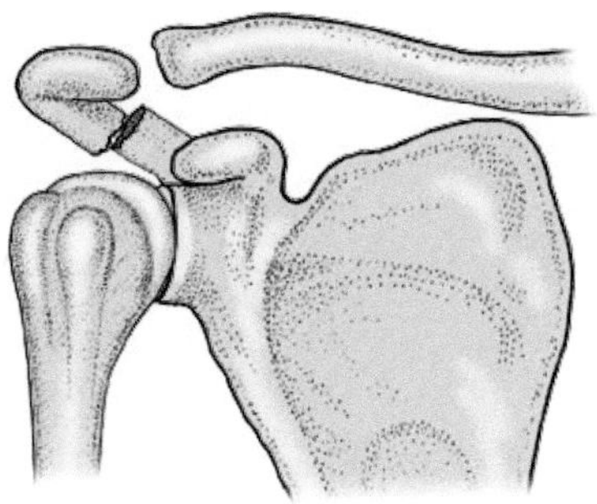

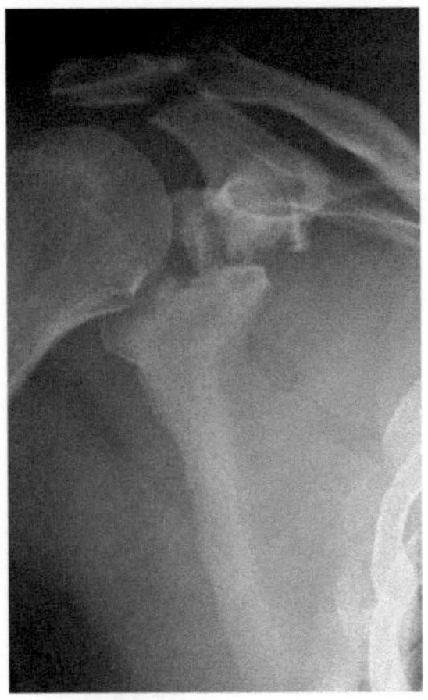

Acromion fractures

Area I:

Type II Displaced fractures without subacromial space reducing

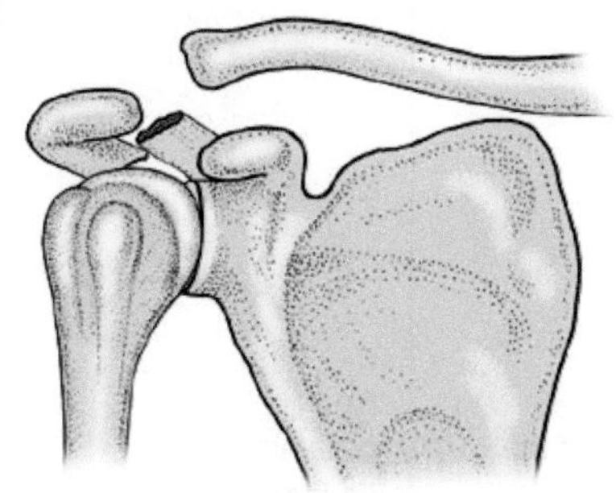

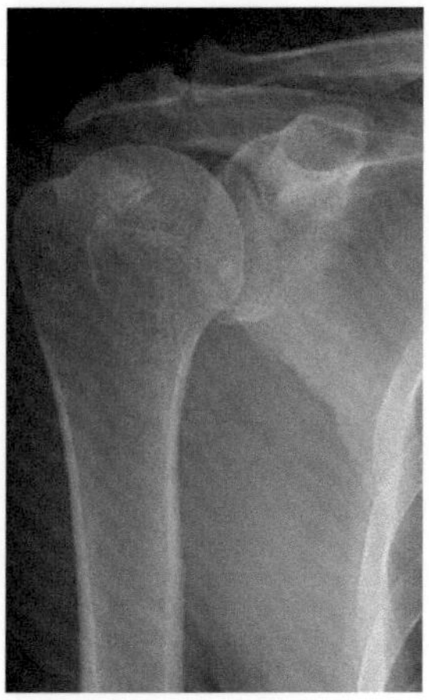

Acromion fractures

Area I:

Type III Displaced fractures with subacromial space reducing

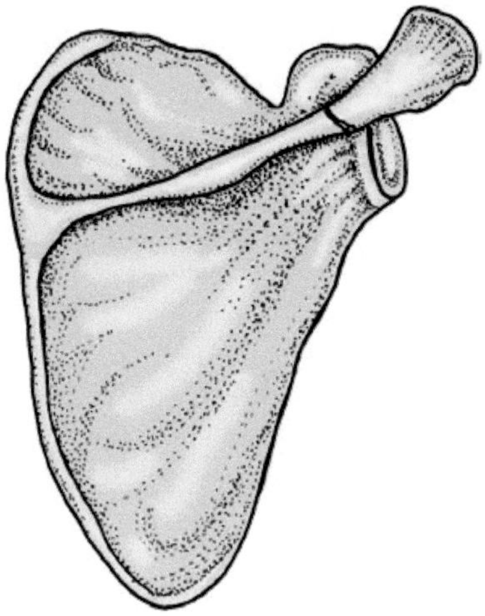

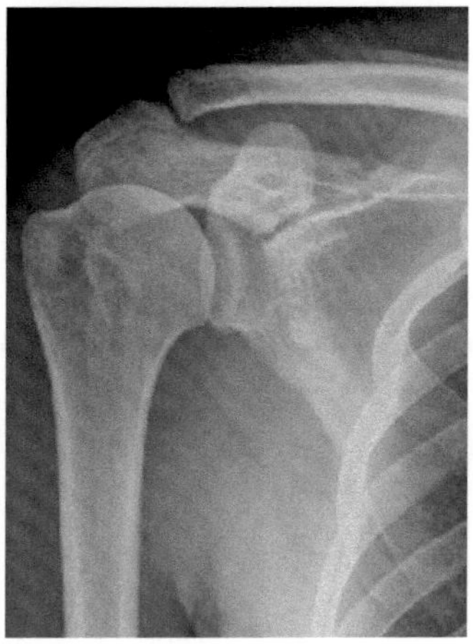

Acromion fractures

Area II:

Basal fractures of acromion

1.2.3.2 Classification According to Kuhn [12]

Type I: Non-displaced fractures of the acromion.
- Type Ia: Avulsion fracture.
- Type Ib: Complete fracture.

Type II: Displaced fractures of the acromion, but not reducing the subacromial space.

Type III: Displaced fractures of the acromion with reduction of the subacromial space.
- Type IIIa: Inferior displacement of the acromion.
- Type IIIb: With ipsilateral superiorly displaced glenoid neck fracture.

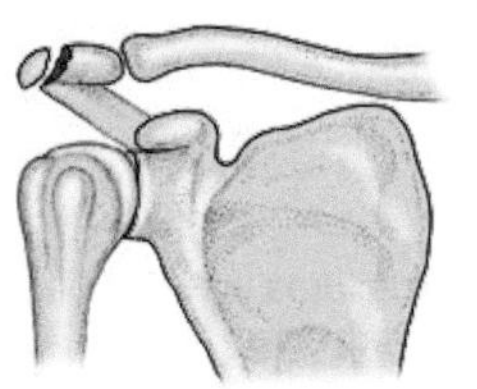	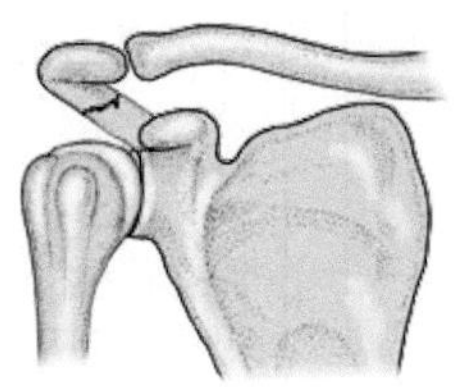	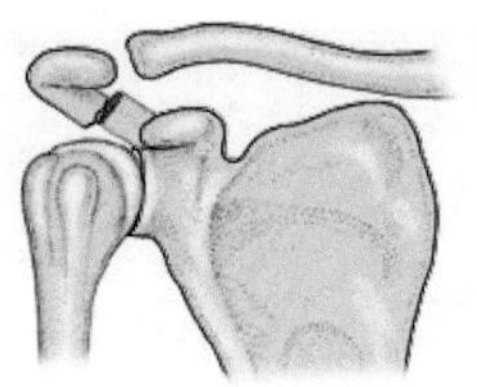	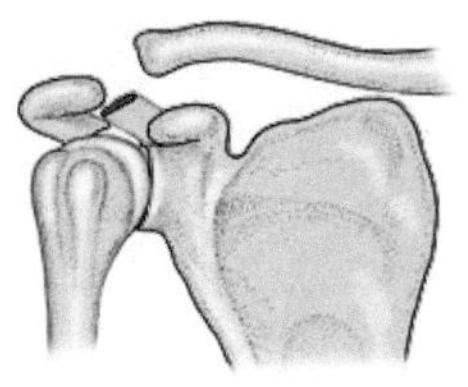	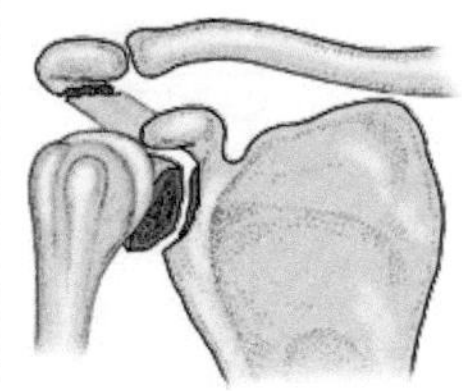
Type Ⅰa: Non-displaced fractures of the acromion, avulsion fracture	Type Ⅰb: Non-displaced fractures of the acromion, complete fracture	Type Ⅱ: Displaced fractures of the acromion, but not reducing the subacromial space	Type Ⅲa: Inferior displacement of the acromion	Type Ⅲb: With ipsilateral superiorly-displaced glenoid neck fracture

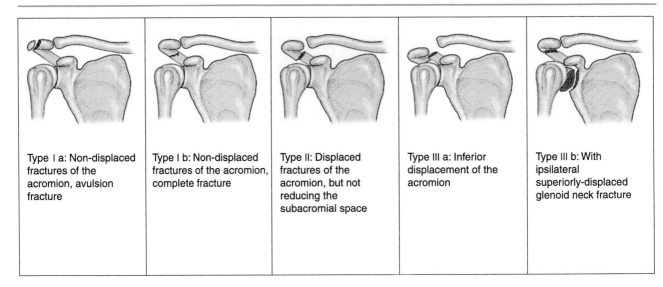

1.2.4 Classification of Fractures of the Glenoid Neck

1.2.4.1 Miller Classification

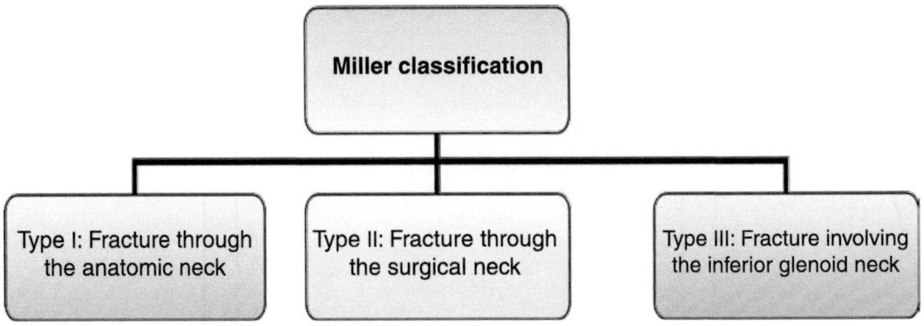

Type I: Fracture through the anatomic neck.
Type II: Fracture through the surgical neck.
Type III: Fracture involving the inferior glenoid neck that then courses medially to exit through the medial border of the scapular body.
Type IV: Fracture involving the inferior glenoid neck that then exits through the superior border of the scapular body via the scapular spine.

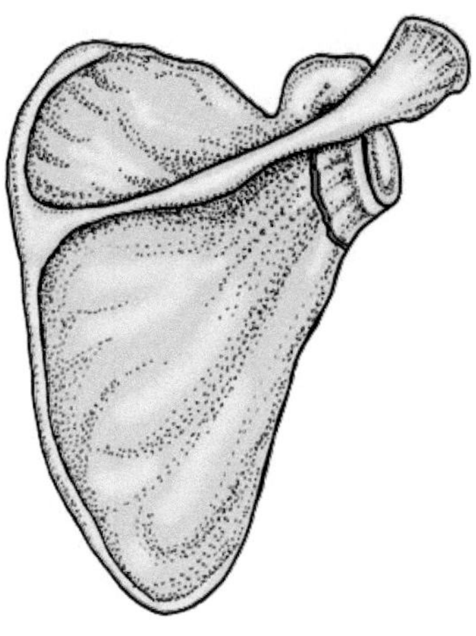	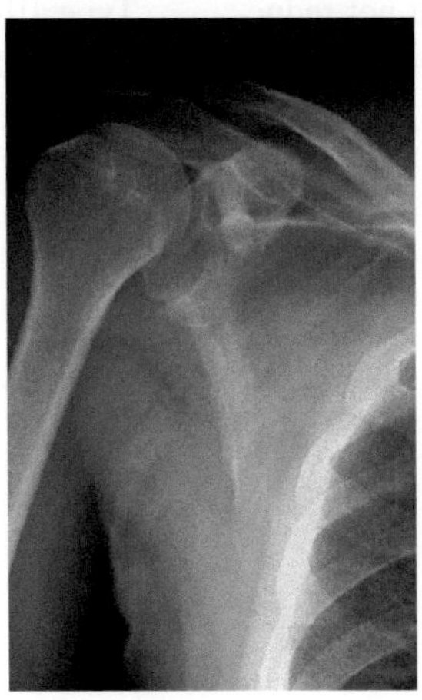	**Miller Classification of fractures of the glenoid neck** Type I: Fracture through the anatomic neck

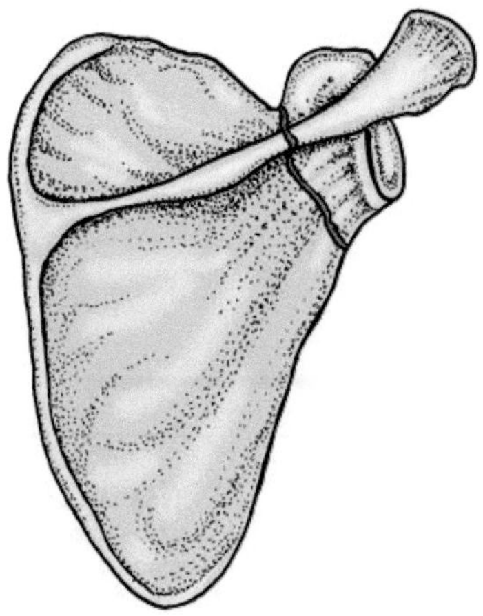

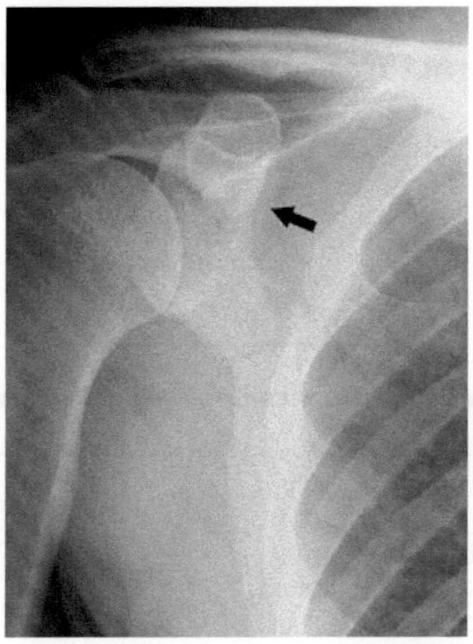

Miller Classification of fractures of the glenoid neck

Type II: Fracture through the surgical neck

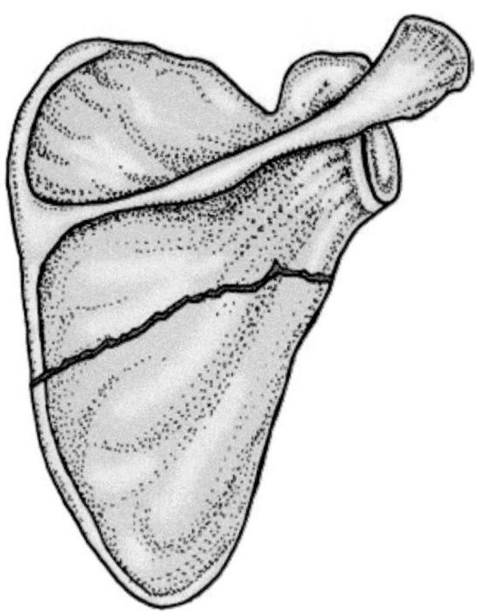

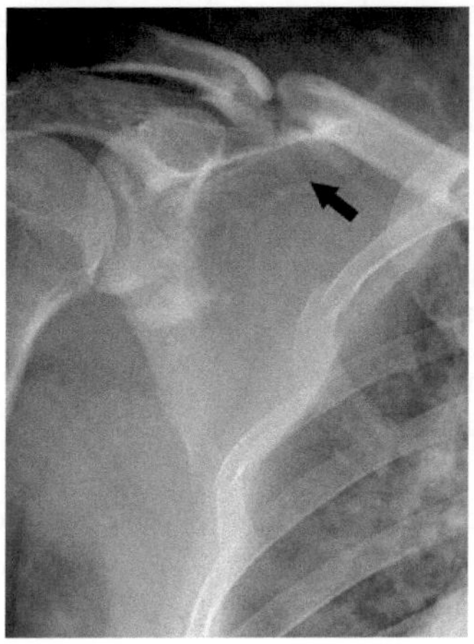

Miller Classification of fractures of the glenoid neck

Type III: Fracture involving the inferior glenoid neck that then courses medially to exit through the medial border of the scapular body

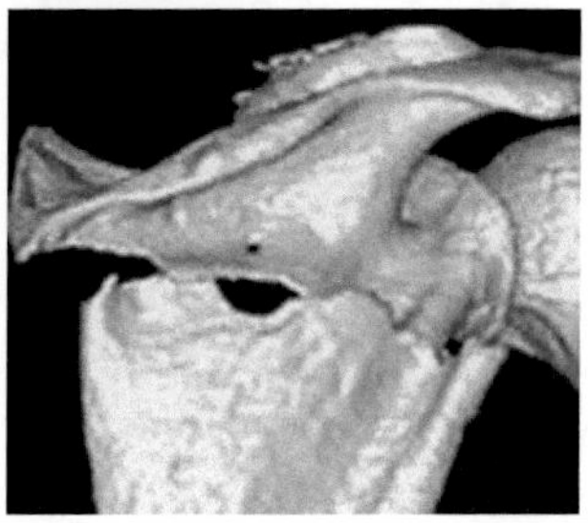

1.2.4.2 Goss Classification [13]

Type I: Fractures are non-displaced and minimally displaced (<10 mm).

Type II: Fractures of which the translational displacement >10 mm or angular displacement >40 in the sagittal or coronal plane.

1.2.5 Classification of Fractures of the Glenoid Cavity

1.2.5.1 Goss-Ideberg Classification for Fractures of the Glenoid Cavity [14]

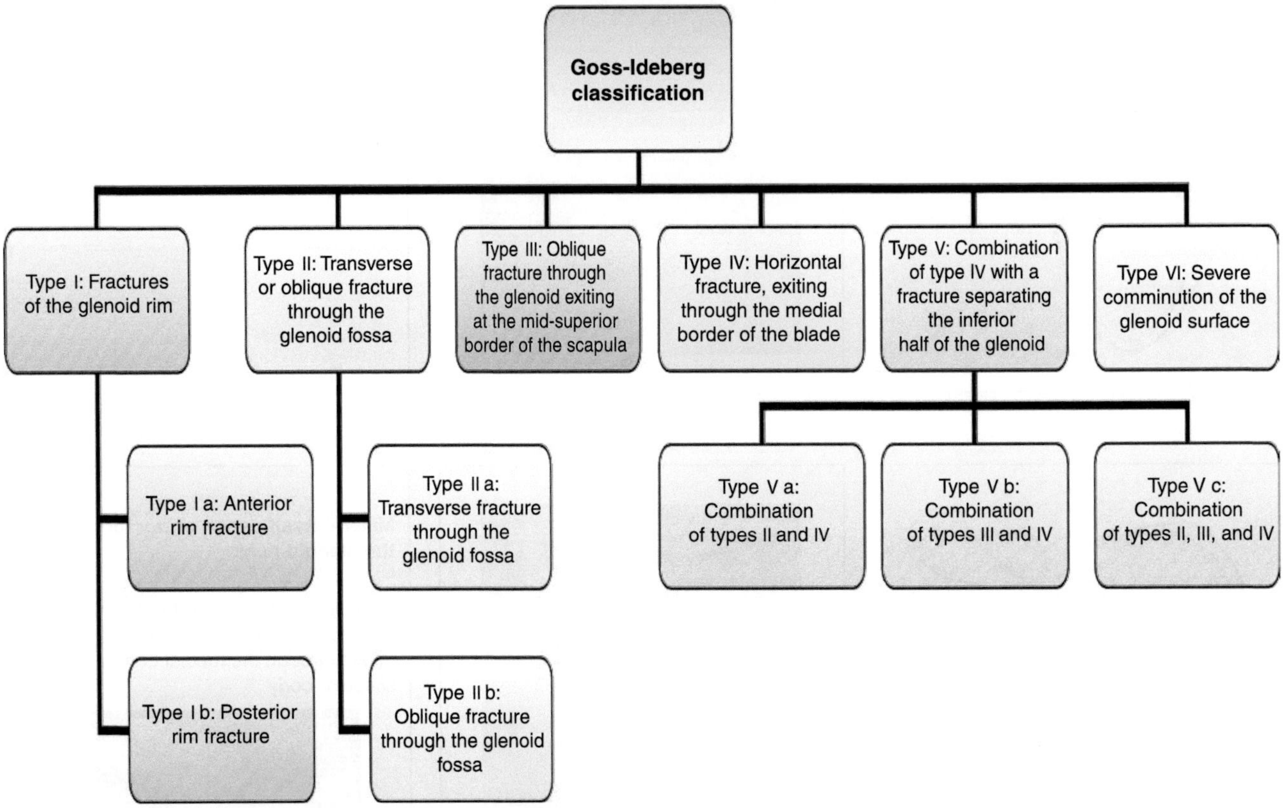

Type I: Fractures of the glenoid rim, further divided into Ia (anterior) and Ib (posterior).

Type Ia: Anterior rim fracture.

Type Ib: Posterior rim fracture.

Type II: Transverse or oblique fracture through the glenoid fossa.

Type IIa: Transverse fracture through the glenoid fossa, with an inferior triangular fragment displaced with the subluxated humeral head.

Type IIb: Oblique fracture through the glenoid fossa, with an inferior triangular fragment displaced with the subluxated humeral head.

Type III: Oblique fracture through the glenoid exiting at the mid-superior border of the scapula.

Type IV: Horizontal fracture, exiting through the medial border of the blade.

Type V: Combination of type IV with a fracture separating the inferior half of the glenoid.

Type Va: Combination of types II and IV.

Type Vb: Combination of types III and IV.

Type Vc: Combination of types II, III, and IV.

Type VI: Severe comminution of the glenoid surface.

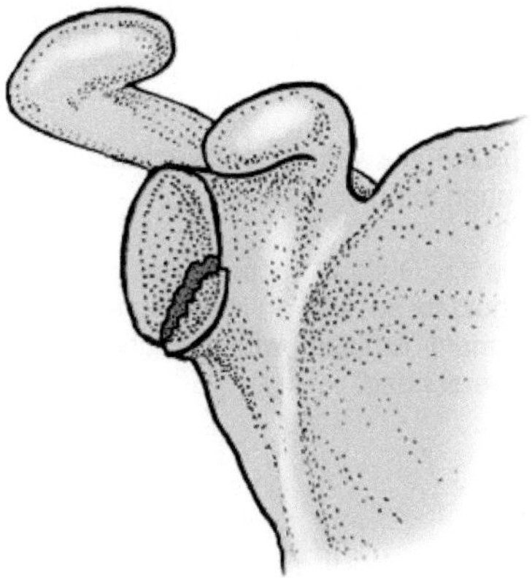

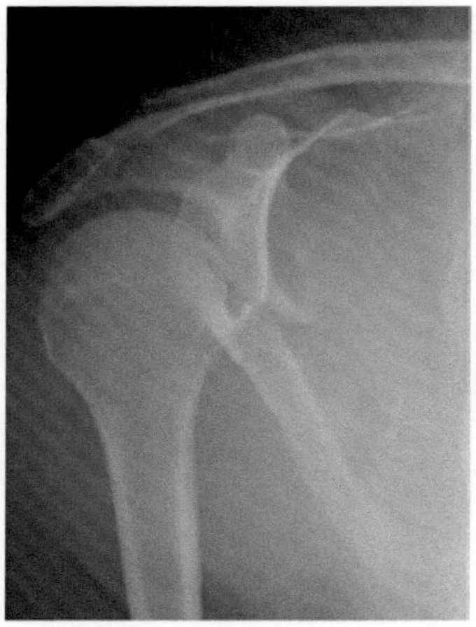

Goss-Ideberg classification of the glenoid cavity

Type I: Fractures of the glenoid rim.

Type I a: Anterior rim fracture

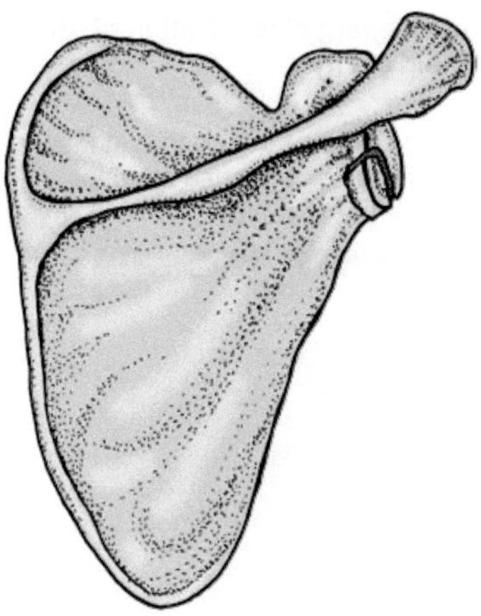

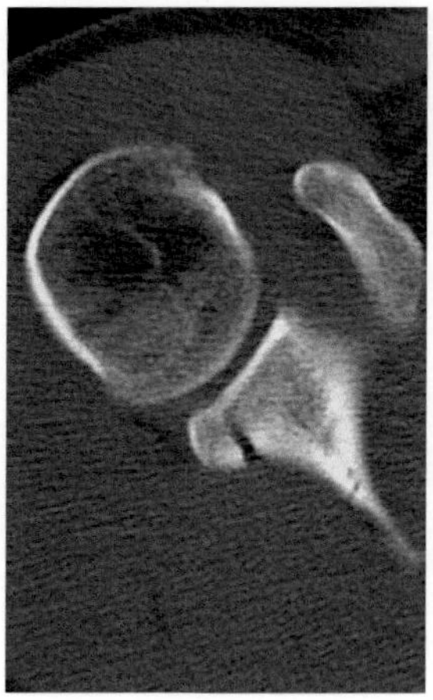

Goss-Ideberg classification of the glenoid cavity

Type I: Fractures of the glenoid rim.

Type I b: Posterior rim fracture

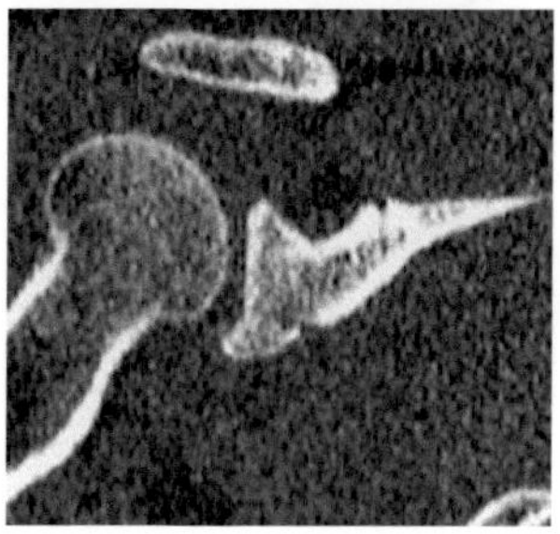

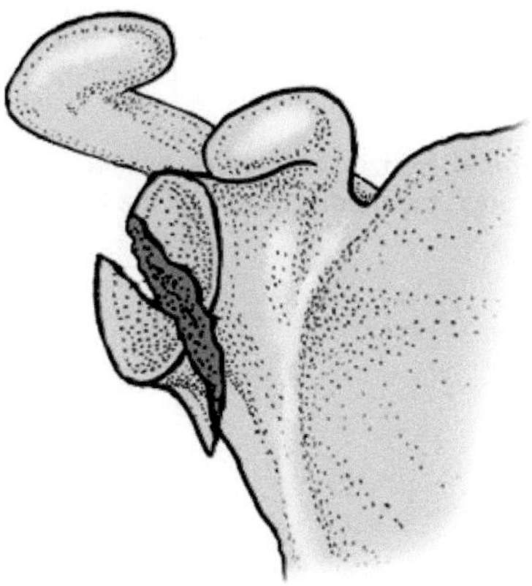

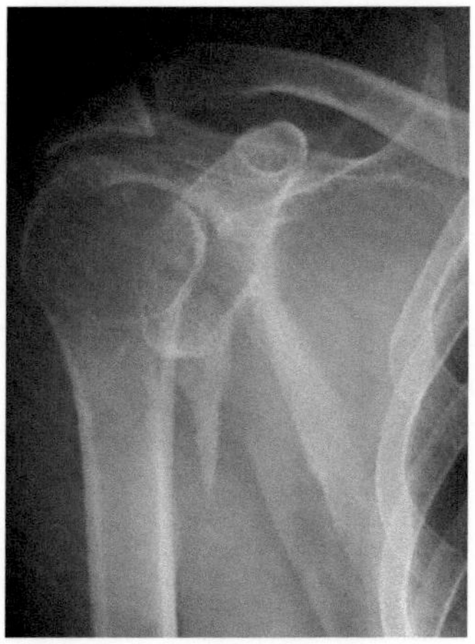

Goss-Ideberg classification of the glenoid cavity

Type II: Transverse or oblique fracture through the glenoid fossa.

Type II a: Transverse fracture through the glenoid fossa, with an inferior triangular fragment displaced with the subluxated humeral head

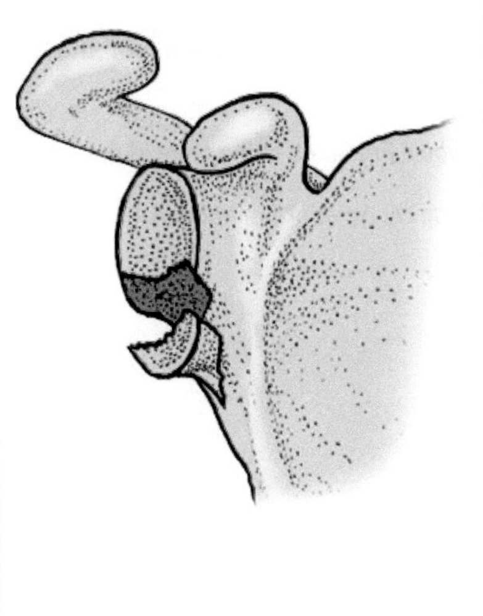

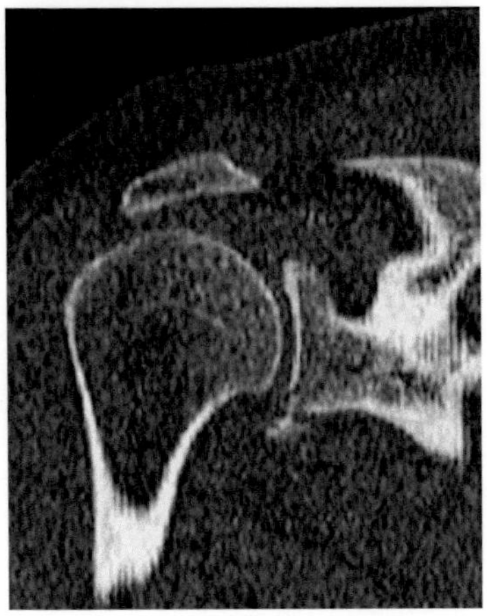

Goss-Ideberg classification of the glenoid cavity

Type II: Transverse or oblique fracture through the glenoid fossa.

Type II b: Oblique fracture through the glenoid fossa, with an inferior triangular fragment displaced with the subluxated humeral head

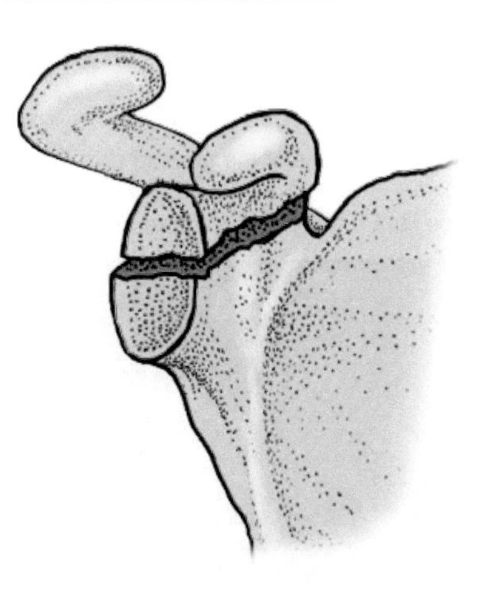

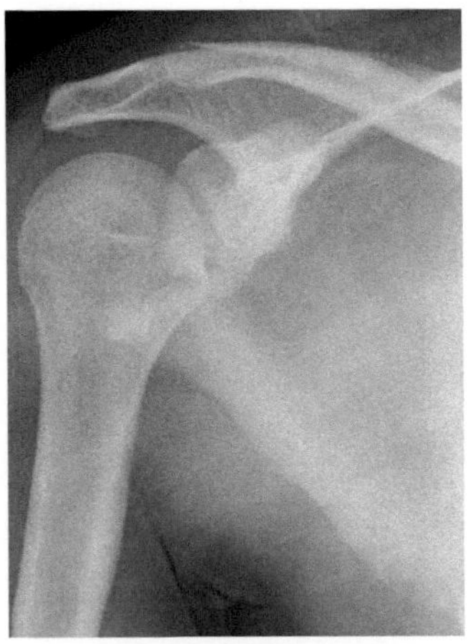

Goss-Ideberg classification of the glenoid cavity

Type III: Oblique fracture through the glenoid exiting at the mid-superior border of the scapula

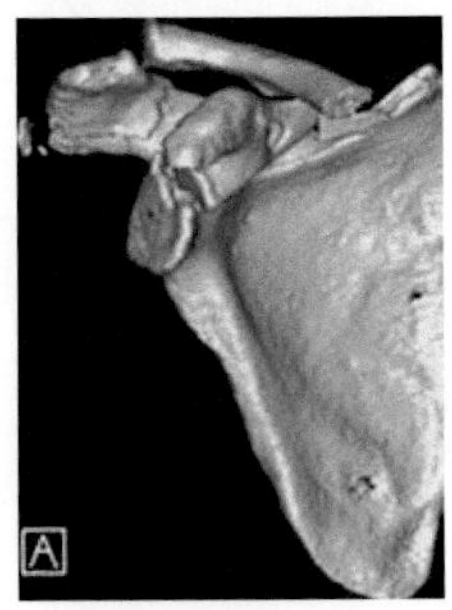

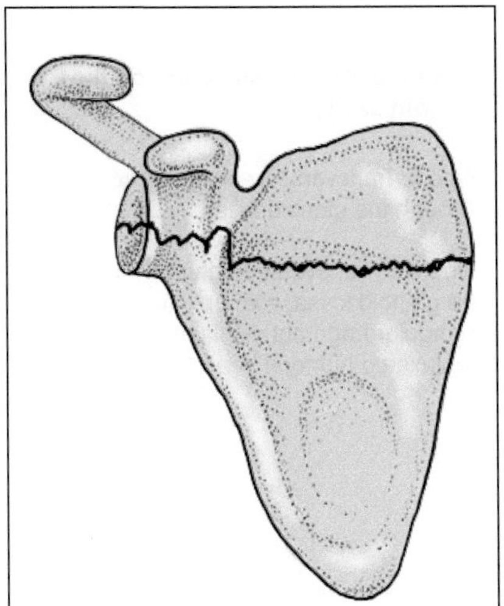

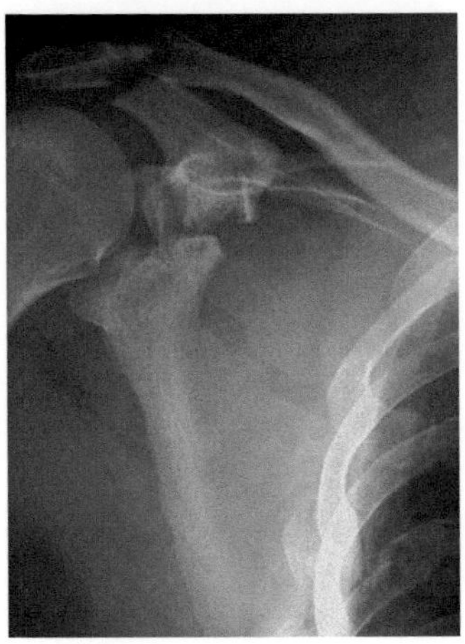

Goss-Ideberg classification of the glenoid cavity

Type IV: Horizontal fracture, exiting through the medial border of the blade

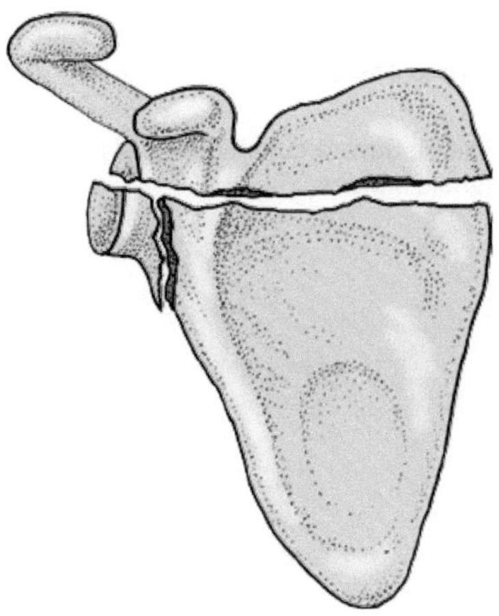

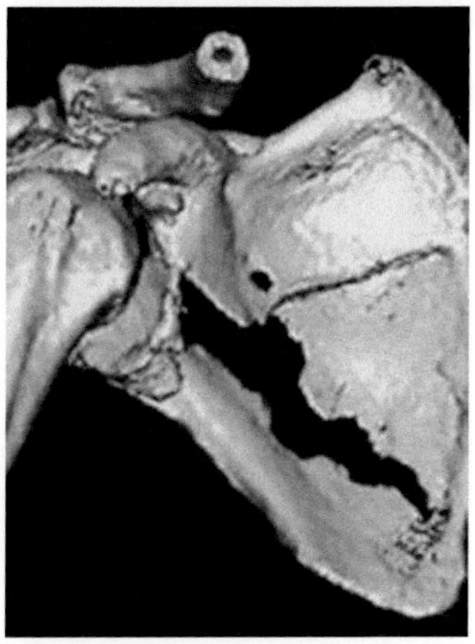

Goss-Ideberg classification of the glenoid cavity

Type V: Combination of type IV with a fracture separating the inferior half of the glenoid.

Type V a: Combination of types II and IV

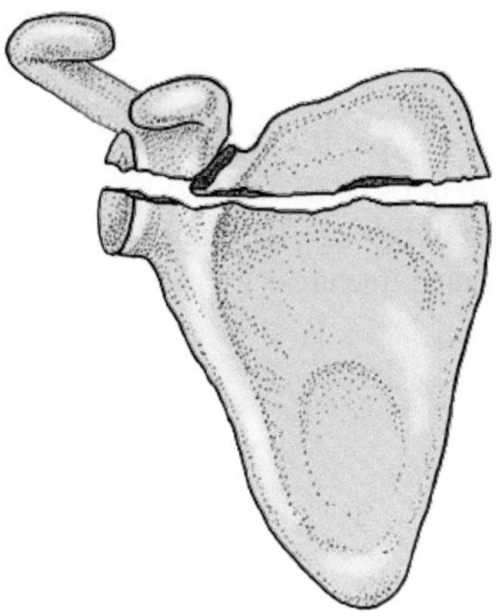

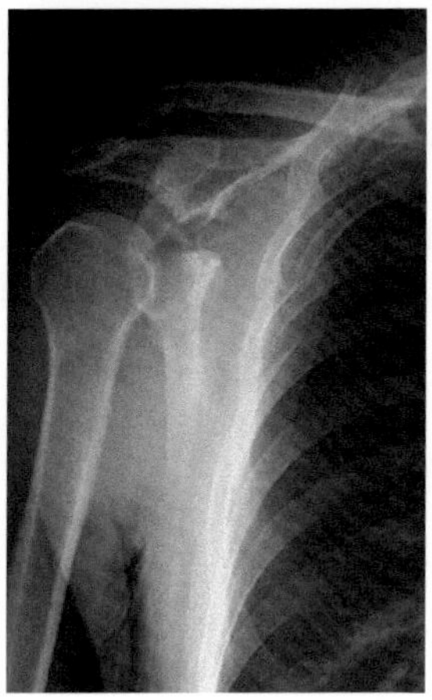

Goss-Ideberg classification of the glenoid cavity

Type V: Combination of type IV with a fracture separating the inferior half of the glenoid

Type V b: Combination of types III and IV

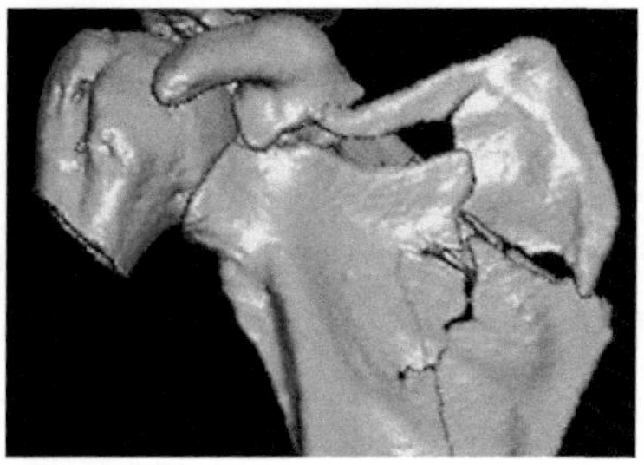

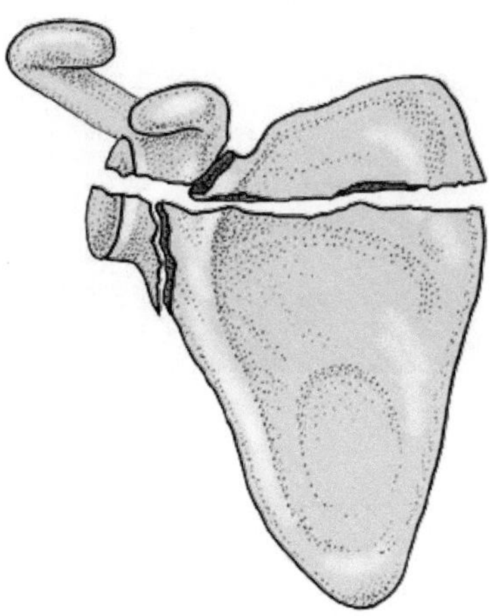

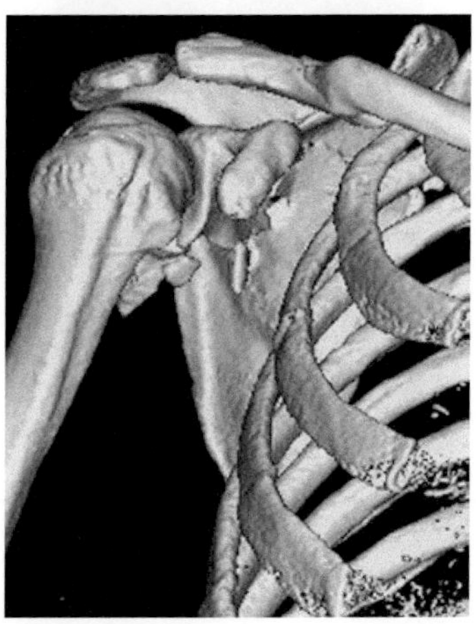

Goss-Ideberg classification of the glenoid cavity

Type V: Combination of type IV with a fracture separating the inferior half of the glenoid.

Type V c: Combination of types II, III, and IV

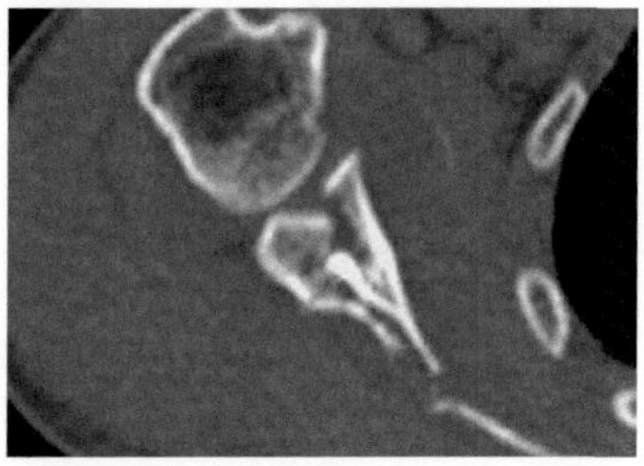

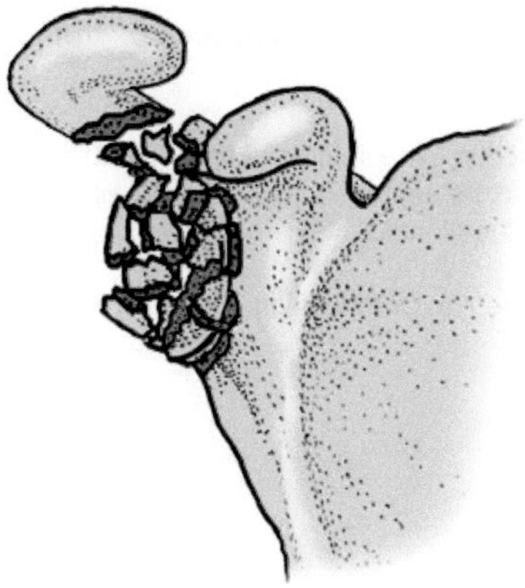

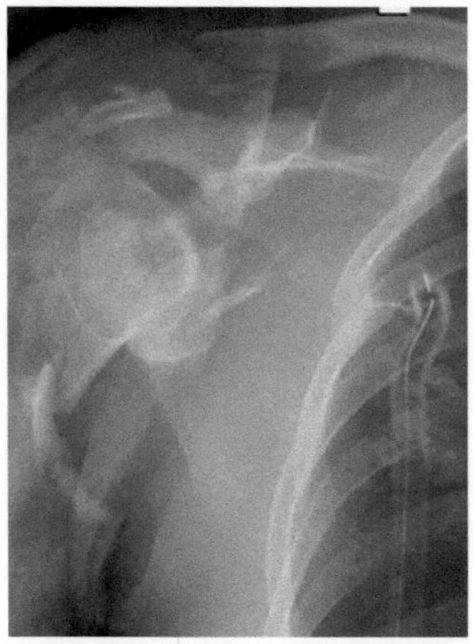

Goss-Ideberg classification of the glenoid cavity

Type VI: Severe comminution of the glenoid surface

1.2.5.2 Goss Classification [9]

Type I: Fractures of the glenoid rim.
  Type Ia: Anterior rim fracture.
  Type Ib: Posterior rim fracture.

Type II: Fracture through the glenoid fossa and lateral border of the scapula.

Type III: Fracture through the glenoid fossa and superior border of the scapula.

Type IV: Fracture through the glenoid fossa and medial border of the scapula.

Type V:
  Type Va: Combination of types II and IV.
  Type Vb: Combination of types III and IV.
  Type Vc: Combination of types II, III, and IV.

Type VI: Severe comminuted fractures.

1.2.6 Bankart Fracture

Fractures of the anterior-inferior glenoid rim, with or without anterior shoulder dislocation.

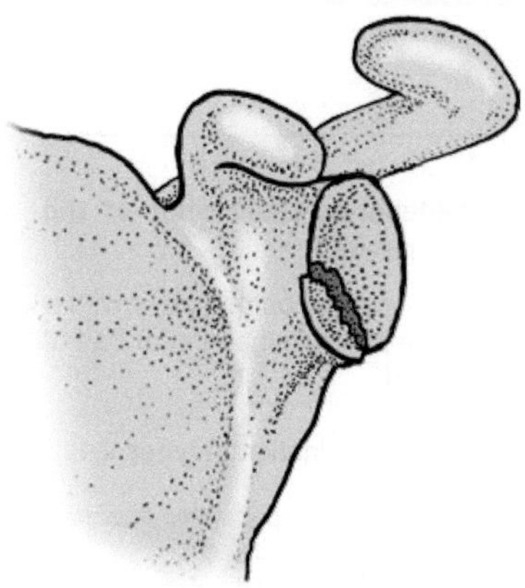

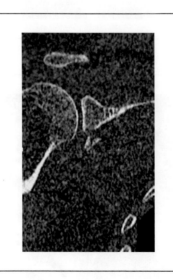

Bankart fracture

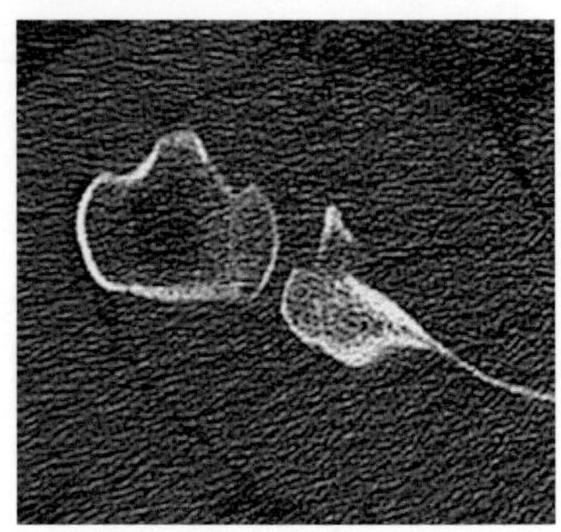

References

1. Robinson CM. Fractures of the clavicle in the adult. Epidemiology and classification. J Bone Joint Surg Br. 1998;80(3):476–84.
2. Marsh JL, Slongo TF, Agel J, Broderick JS, Creevey W, DeCoster TA, Prokuski L, Sirkin MS, Ziran B, Henley B, et al. Fracture and dislocation classification compendium - 2007: orthopaedic trauma association classification, database and outcomes committee. J Orthop Trauma. 2007;21(10 Suppl):S1–133.
3. Allman FL Jr. Fractures and ligamentous injuries of the clavicle and its articulation. J Bone Joint Surg Am. 1967;49(4):774–84.
4. Neer CS 2nd. Fractures of the distal third of the clavicle. Clin Orthop Relat Res. 1968;58:43–50.
5. Hardegger FH, Simpson LA, Weber BG. The operative treatment of scapular fractures. J Bone Joint Surg Br. 1984;66(5):725–31.
6. Ada JR, Miller ME. Scapular fractures. Analysis of 113 cases. Clin Orthop Relat Res. 1991;269:174–80.
7. Thompson DA, Flynn TC, Miller PW, Fischer RP. The significance of scapular fractures. J Trauma. 1985;25(10):974–7.
8. Euler E, Rüedi T. Scapulafraktur. Schulterchirurgie Urban und Schwarzenberg, München. 1996:261–72.
9. Goss TP. Double disruptions of the superior shoulder suspensory complex. J Orthop Trauma. 1993;7(2):99–106.
10. Eyres KS, Brooks A, Stanley D. Fractures of the coracoid process. J Bone Joint Surg Br. 1995;77(3):425–8.
11. Ogawa K, Yoshida A, Takahashi M, Ui M. Fractures of the coracoid process. J Bone Joint Surg Br. 1997;79(1):17–9.
12. Kuhn JE, Blasier RB, Carpenter JE. Fractures of the acromion process: a proposed classification system. J Orthop Trauma. 1994;8(1):6–13.
13. Goss TP. Fractures of the glenoid neck. J Shoulder Elbow Surg. 1994;3(1):42–52.
14. Goss TP. Fractures of the glenoid cavity. J Bone Joint Surg Am. 1992;74(2):299–305.

2 Classification of Humeral Fractures

Yingze Zhang and Bo Lu

2.1 Classification of Proximal Humeral Fractures

Kocher first proposed his classification of proximal humeral fractures based on anatomic location in 1896; to date, there are >5 classification systems of proximal humeral fractures in literature. According to the literature over the last 5 years, the most commonly used system is the Neer's classification, followed by the AO/OTA classification.

2.1.1 Neer's Classification [1]

This system is based on the anatomic relations of the four major anatomic segments: articular segment, greater tuberosity, lesser tuberosity, and proximal shaft. For a segment to be considered displaced, it must be either displaced >1 cm or angulated >45° from its anatomic position.

1. One-part fractures or minimally displaced fractures: The most common type.
2. Two-part fractures: Characterized by displacement of one of the four segments, with the remaining three segments either not fractured or not fulfilling the criteria for displacement. Four types of two-part fractures can be encountered (greater tuberosity, lesser tuberosity, anatomic neck, and surgical neck).
3. Three-part fractures: Characterized by displacement of two of the segments from the remaining two nondisplaced segments. Two types of three-part fracture patterns can be encountered. The more common pattern is characterized by displacement of the greater tuberosity and the shaft, with the lesser tuberosity remaining with the articular segment. The less commonly encountered pattern is characterized by displacement of the lesser tuberosity and shaft, with the greater tuberosity remaining with the articular segment.
4. Four-part fractures: Characterized by displacement of all four segments.
5. Fracture dislocations: Displaced proximal humeral fractures: Two-part, three-part, or four-part fractures associated with either anterior or posterior dislocation of the articular segment.
6. Articular surface fractures: Two types: Impression fractures or head-splitting fractures.
7. Impression fractures: Most often occur in association with chronic dislocations. As such, they can be either anterior or posterior and involve variable amounts of articular surface.
8. Head-splitting fractures: Usually associated with other displaced fractures of the proximal humerus, in which the disruption or "splitting" of the articular surface is the most significant component.

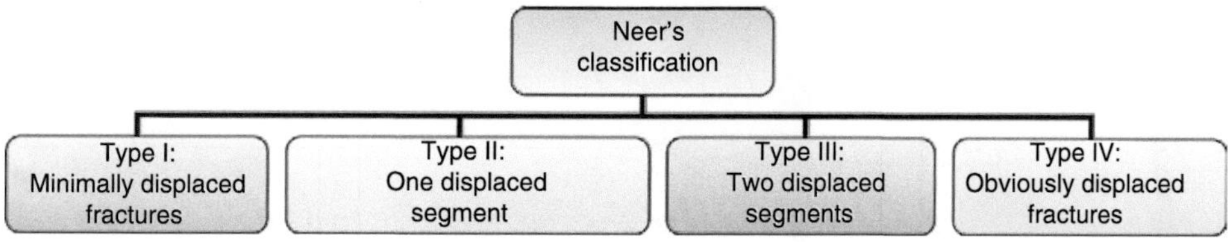

Y. Zhang (✉) • B. Lu
Department of Orthopedics,
The Third Hospital of Hebei Medical University,
Shijiazhuang, China
e-mail: yzzhangdr@126.com, yzling_liu@163.com

Y. Zhang (ed.), *Clinical Classification in Orthopaedics Trauma*, https://doi.org/10.1007/978-981-10-6044-1_2

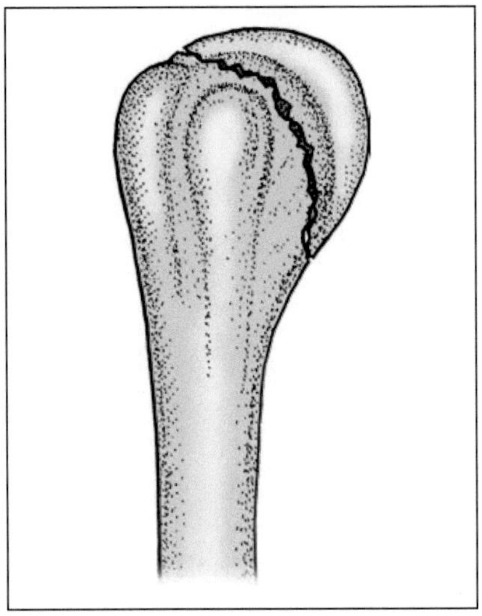

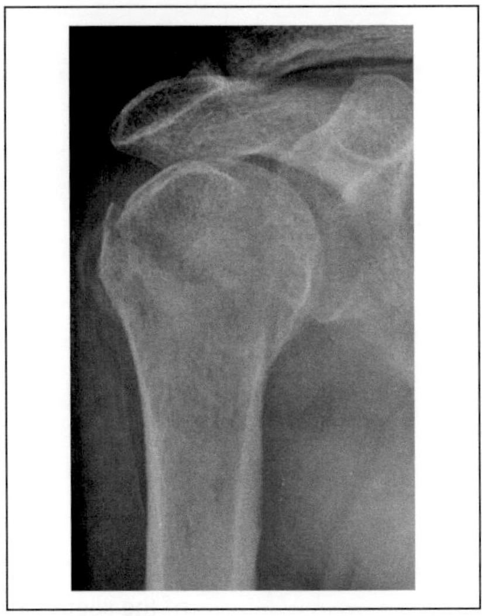

Neer's classification

One-part fractures: Minimally displaced fractures, segments neither displaced more than 1 cm nor angulated more than 45 °

Anatomic neck fracture

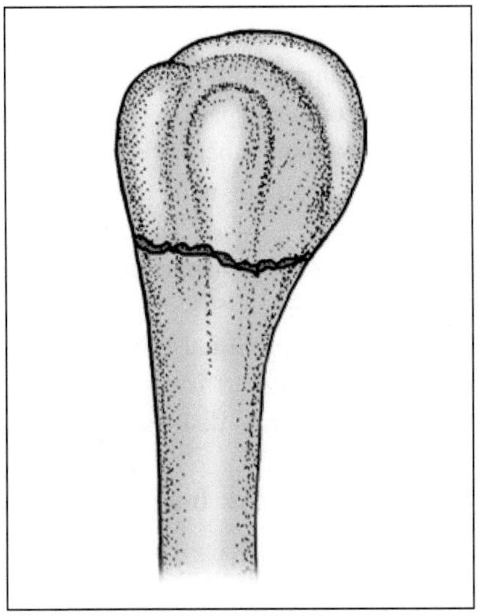

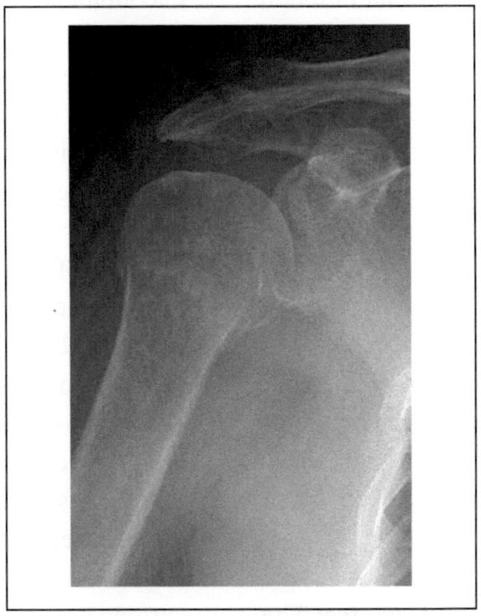

Neer's classification

One-part fractures: Minimally displaced fractures, segments neither displaced more than 1 cm nor angulated more than 45 °

Femoral neck fracture

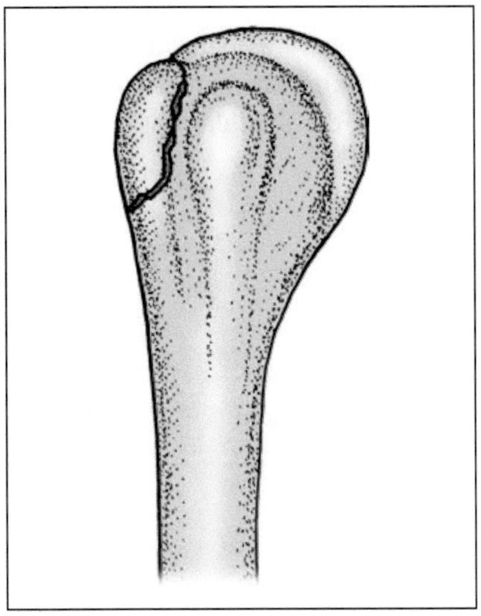

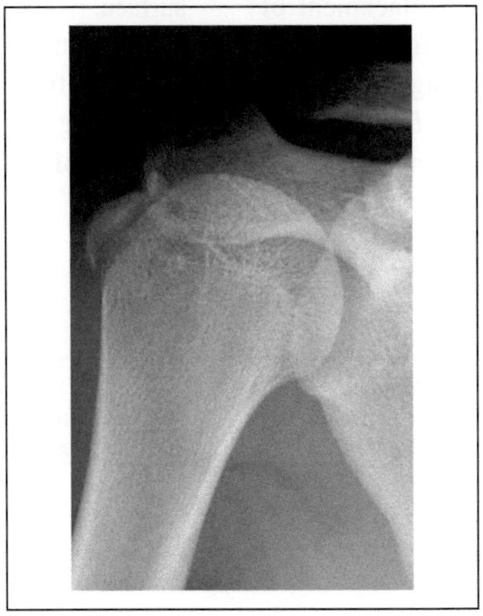

Neer's classification

One-part fractures: Minimally displaced fractures, segments neither displaced more than 1 cm nor angulated more than 45 °

Greater trochanter fracture

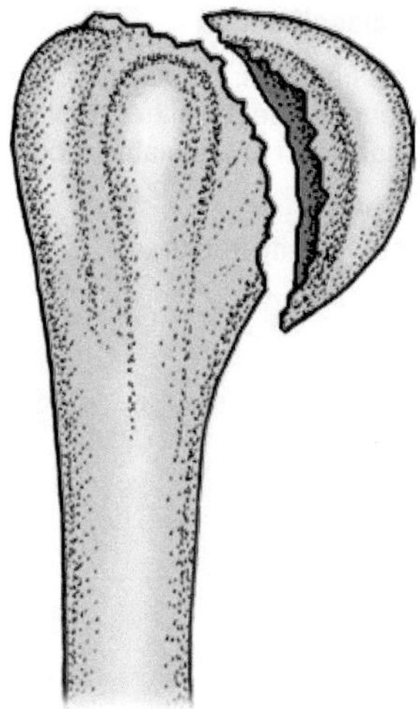

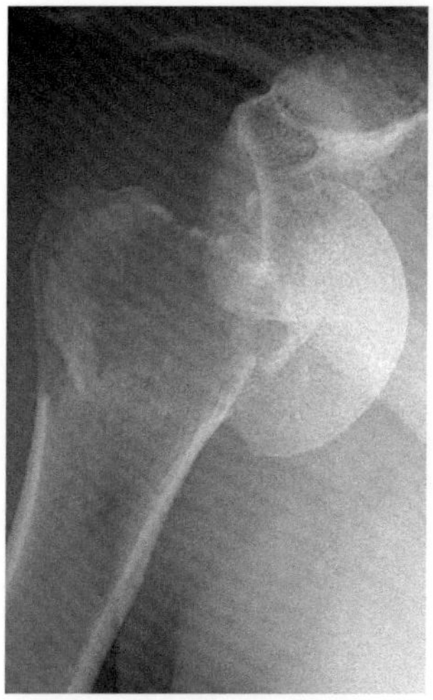

Neer's classification

Two-part fractures: Displacement of one of the four segments, either displaced more than 1 cm or angulated more than 45 °

Anatomic neck fracture

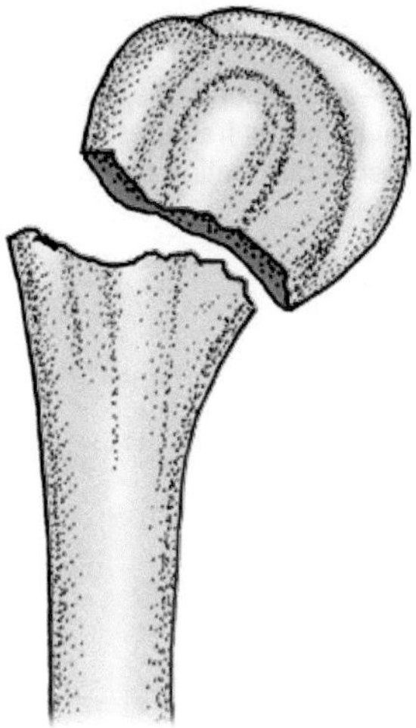

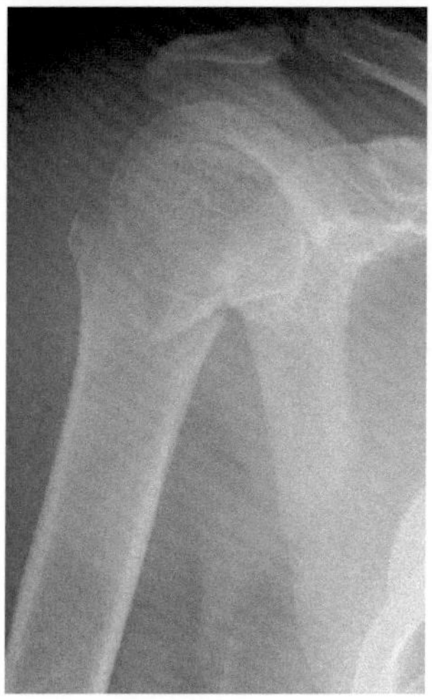

Neer's classification

Two-part fractures: Displacement of one of the four segments, either displaced more than 1 cm or angulated more than 45 °

Surgical neck fracture

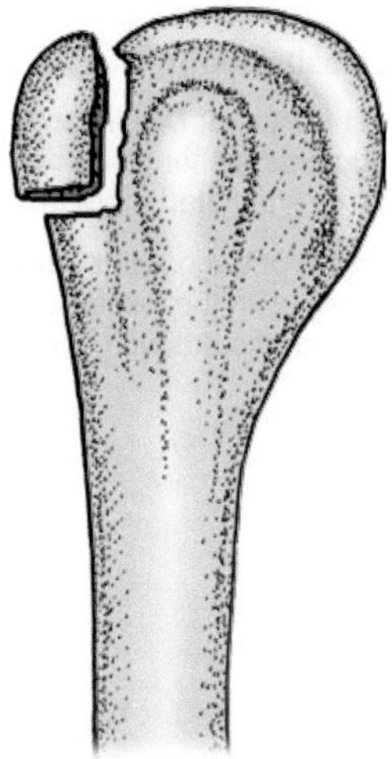

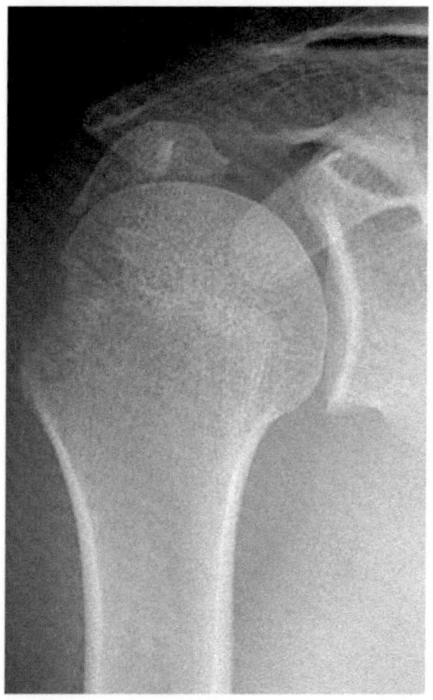

Neer's classification

Two-part fractures: Displacement of one of the four segments, either displaced more than 1 cm or angulated more than 45 °

Greater tuberosity fracture

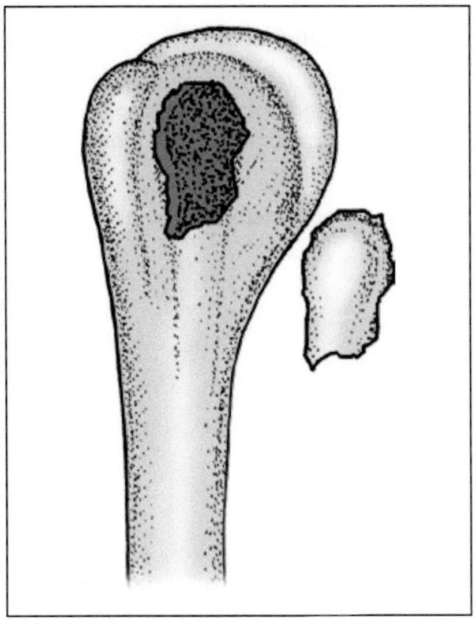

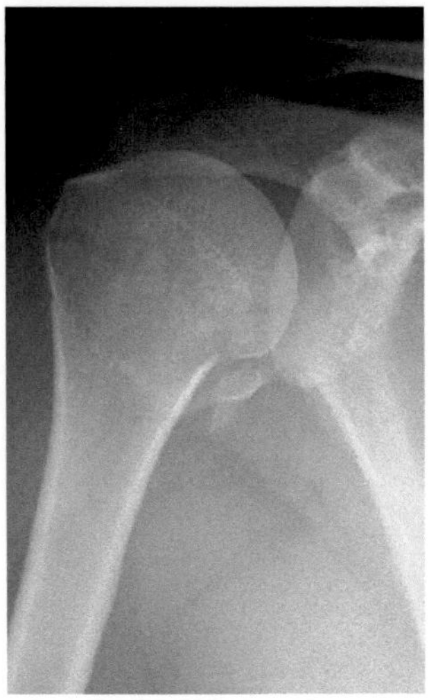

Neer's classification

Two-part fractures: Displacement of one of the four segments, either displaced more than 1 cm or angulated more than 45 °

Lesser tuberosity fracture

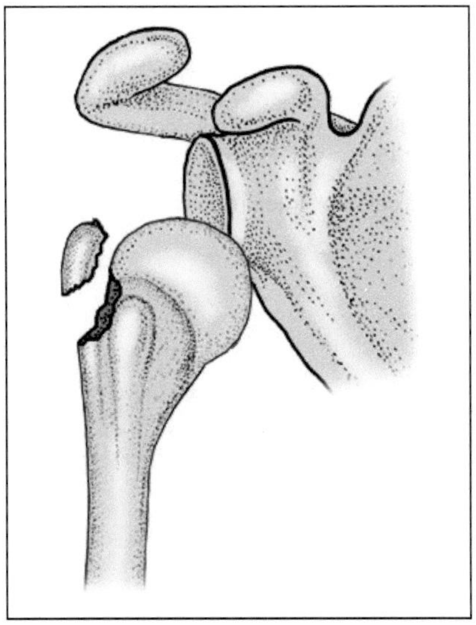

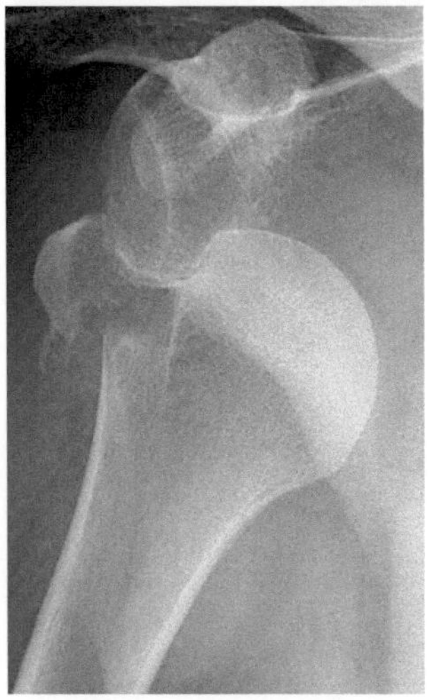

Neer's classification

Fracture–dislocations: Displaced two-part proximal humerus fractures, associated with anterior dislocation of the articular segment

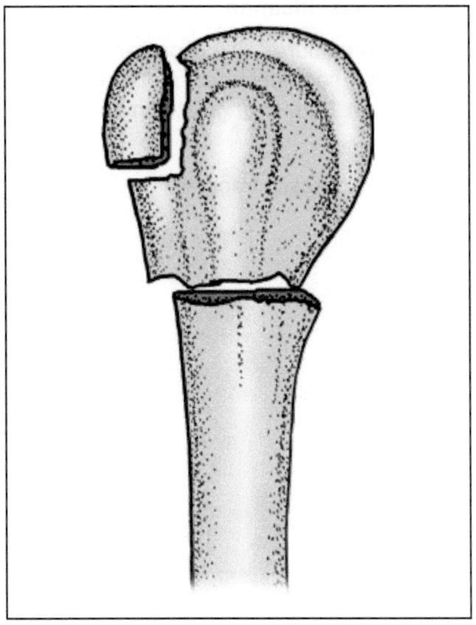

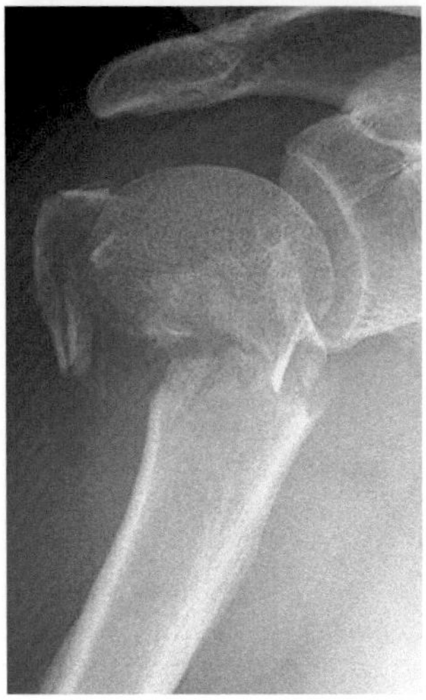

Neer's classification

Three-part fractures: Displacement of two of the segments, either displaced more than 1 cm or angulated more than 45 °

Displacement of the greater tuberosity and the shaft, with the lesser tuberosity remaining with the articular segment

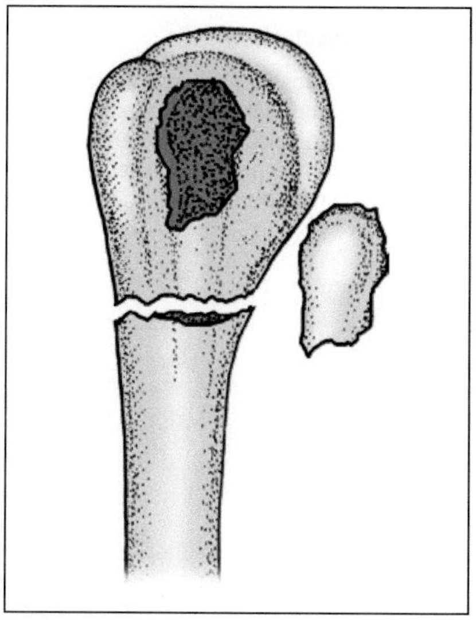

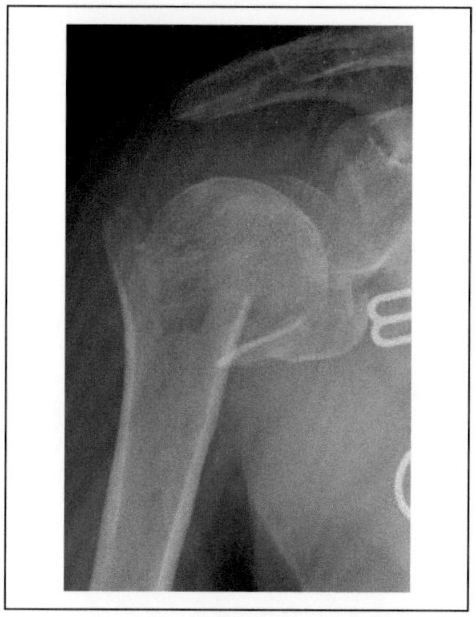

Neer's classification

Three-part fractures: Displacement of two of the segments, either displaced more than 1 cm or angulated more than 45 °

Displacement of the lesser tuberosity and shaft, with the greater tuberosity remaining with the articular segment

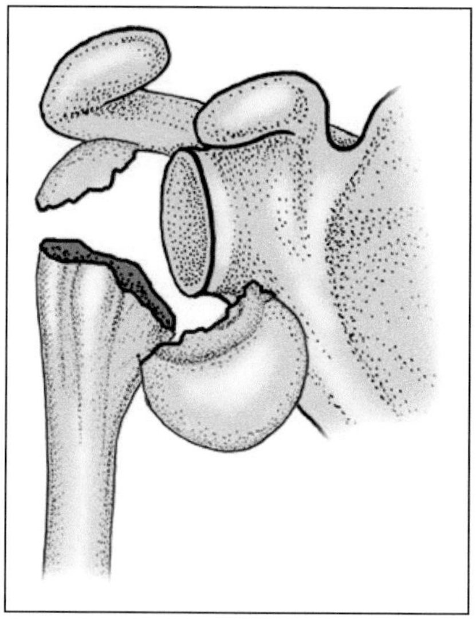

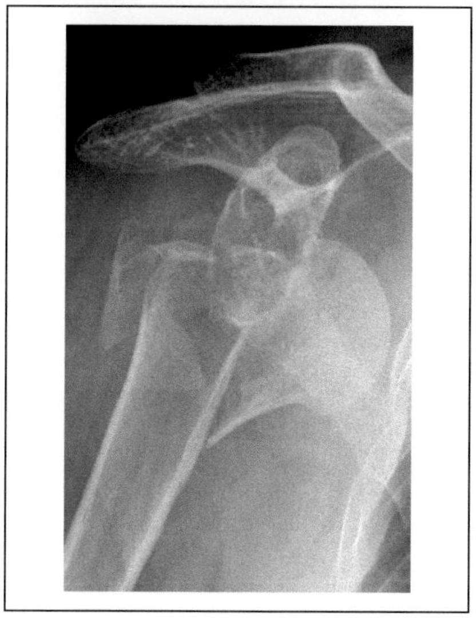

Neer's classification

Fracture–dislocations: Displaced three-part proximal humerus fractures, associated with anterior dislocation of the articular segment

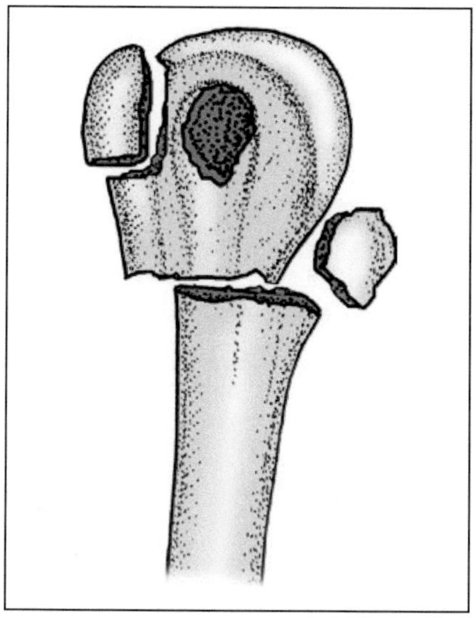

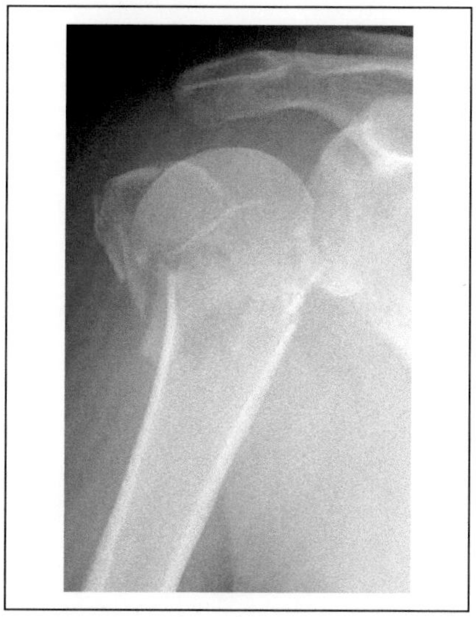

Neer's classification

Four-part fractures: Displacement of all four segments, either displaced more than 1 cm or angulated more than 45 °

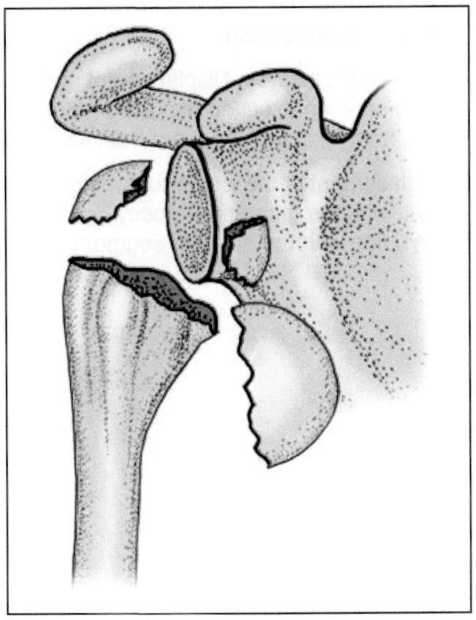

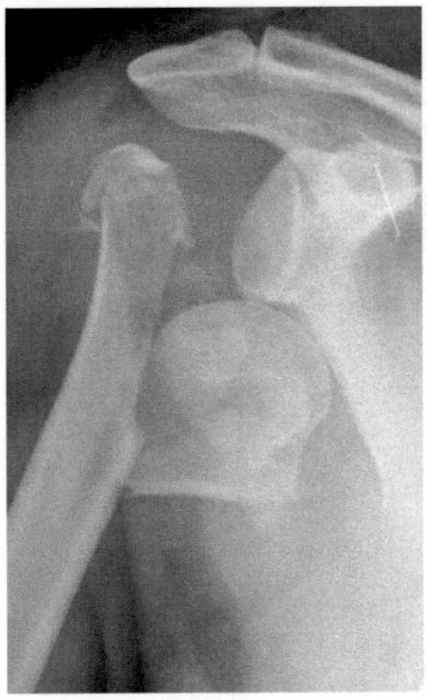

Neer's classification

Fracture–dislocations: Displaced four-part proximal humerus fractures, associated with anterior dislocation of the articular segment, the humeral head is isolated and lost main blood supply

2.1.2 AO/OTA Classification [2]

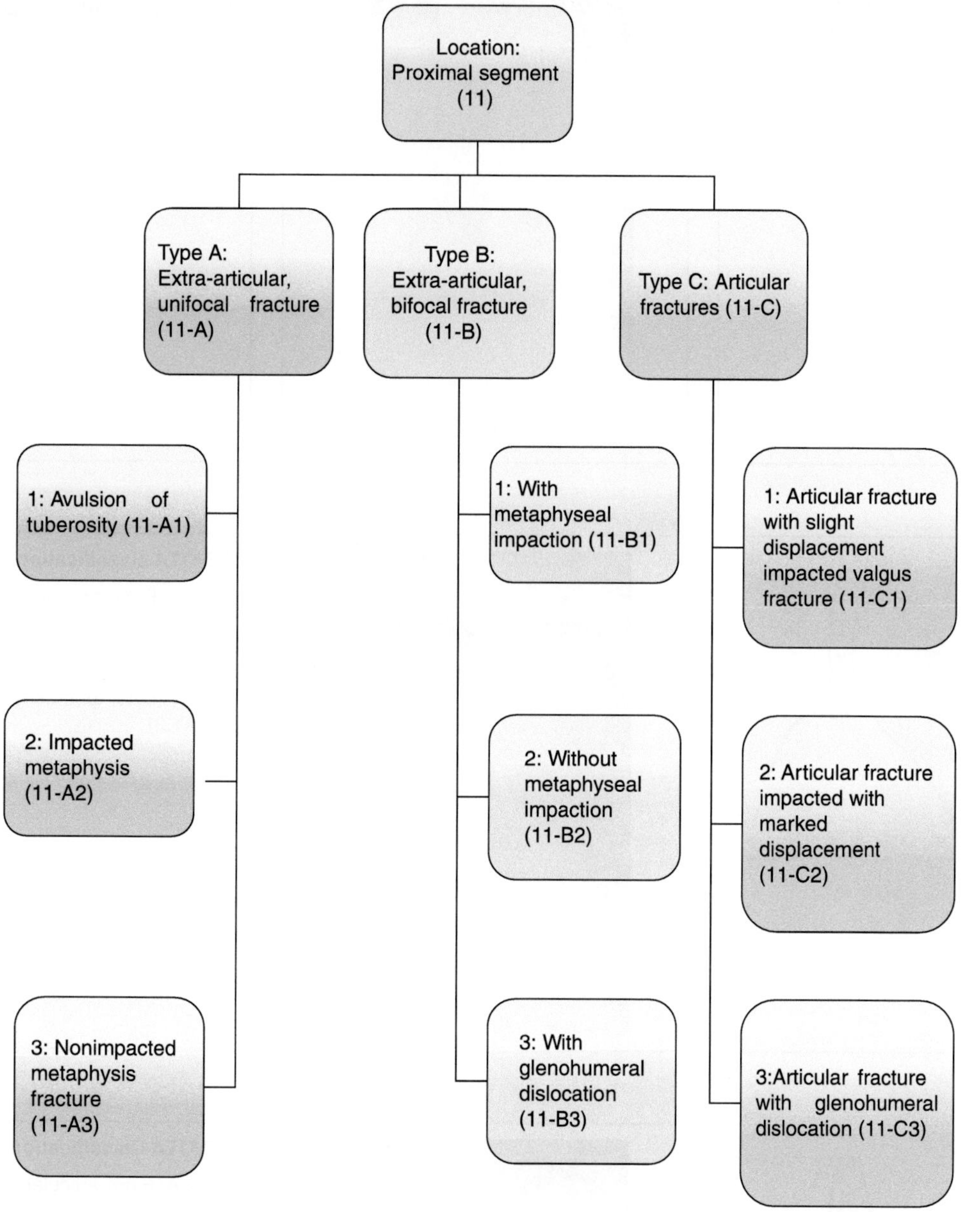

Type A: Extra-articular, unifocal fracture (11-A).
- A1: Avulsion of tuberosity (11-A1).
  - A1.1: Greater tuberosity not displaced (11-A1.1).
  - A1.2: Greater tuberosity displaced (11-A1.2).
  - A1.3: With glenohumeral dislocation (11-A1.3).
- A2: Impacted metaphysis (11-A2).
  - A2.1 Without frontal malalignment (11-A2.1).
  - A2.2 With varus malalignment (11-A2.2).
  - A2.3 With valgus malalignment (11-A2.3).
- A3: Non-impacted metaphysis fracture (11-A3).
  - A3.1: Simple with angulation (11-A3.1).
  - A3.2: Simple with translation (11-A3.2).
  - A3.3: Multifragmentary (11-A3.3).

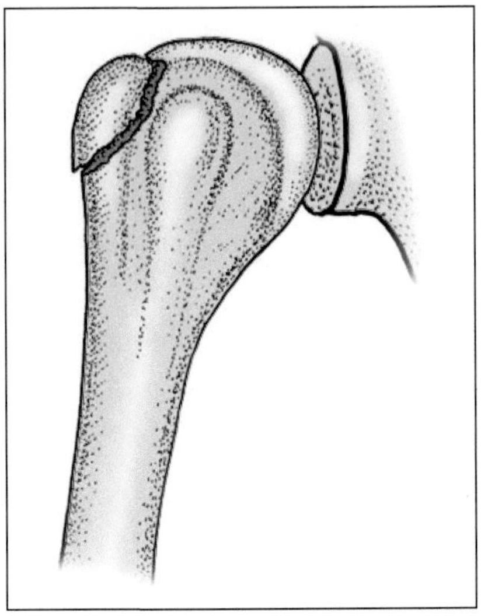

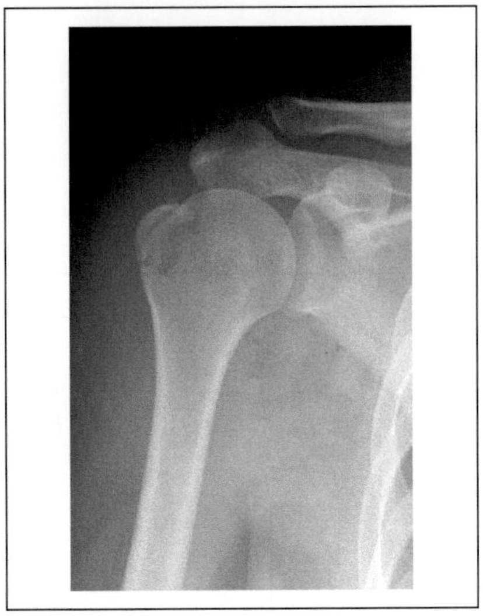

AO/OTA classification

Type A: Extra-articular, unifocal fracture (11-A)

A1: Avulsion of tuberosity (11-A1)

A1.1: Greater tuberosity not displaced (11-A1.1)

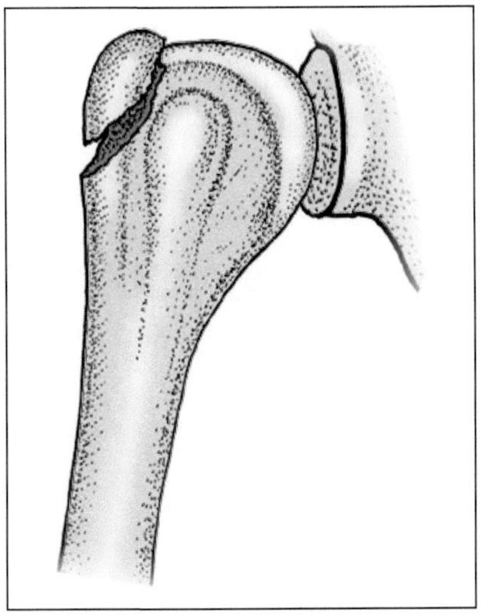

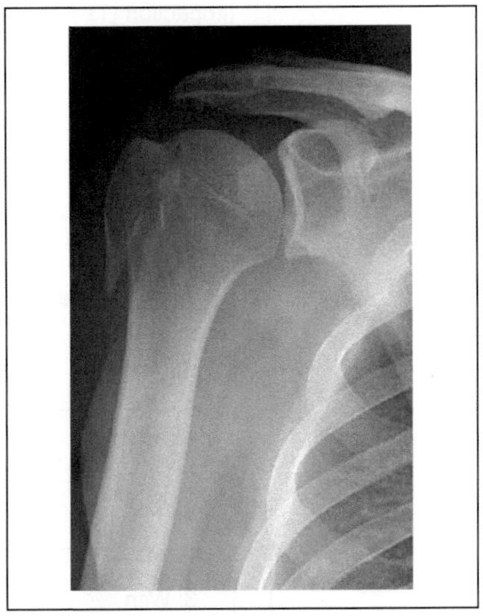

AO/OTA classification

Type A: Extra-articular, unifocal fracture (11-A)

A1: Avulsion of tuberosity (11-A1)

A1.2: Greater tuberosity displaced (11-A1.2)

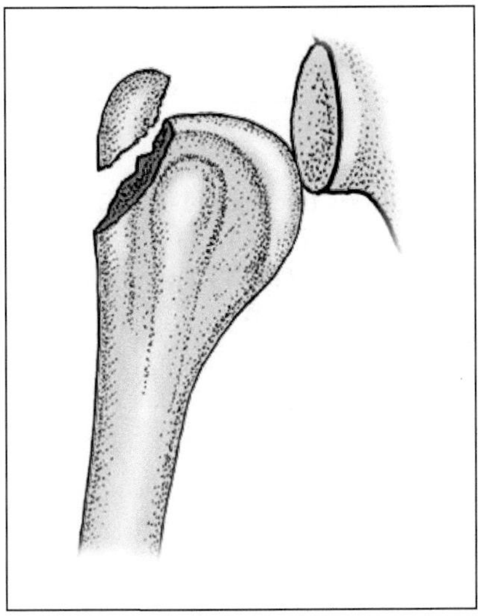

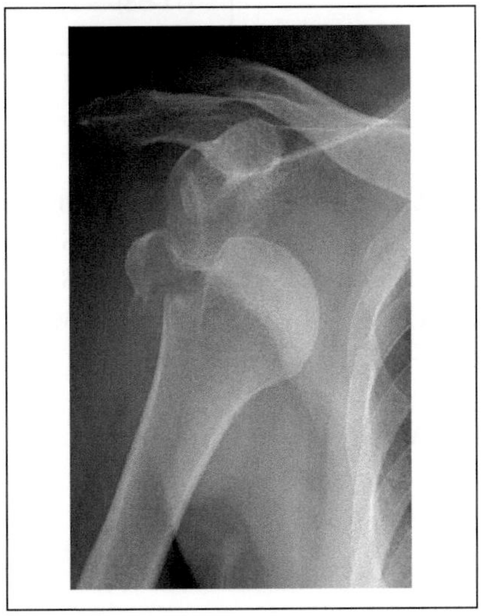

AO/OTA Classification

Type A: Extra-articular, unifocal fracture (11-A)

A1: Avulsion of tuberosity (11-A1)

A1.3: With glenohumeral dislocation (11-A1.3)

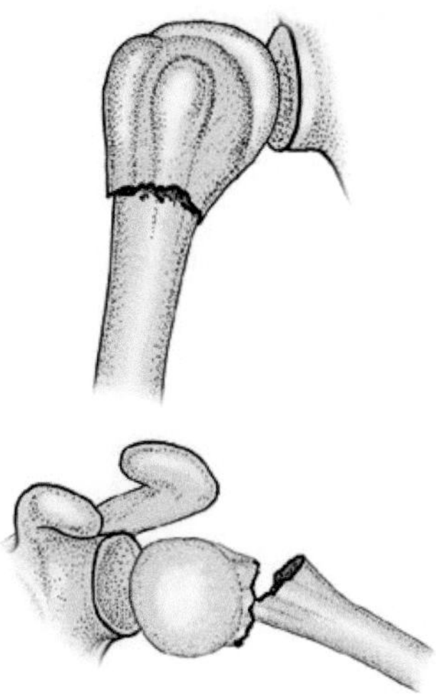

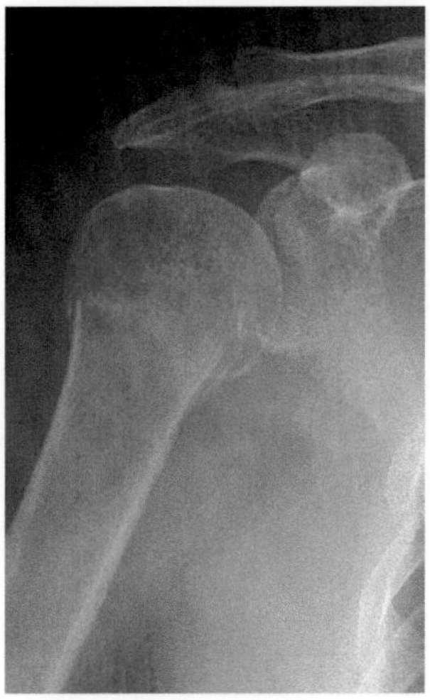

AO/OTA classification

Type A: Extra-articular, unifocal fracture (11-A)

A2: Impacted metaphysis (11-A2)

A2.1: Without frontal malalignment (11-A2.1)

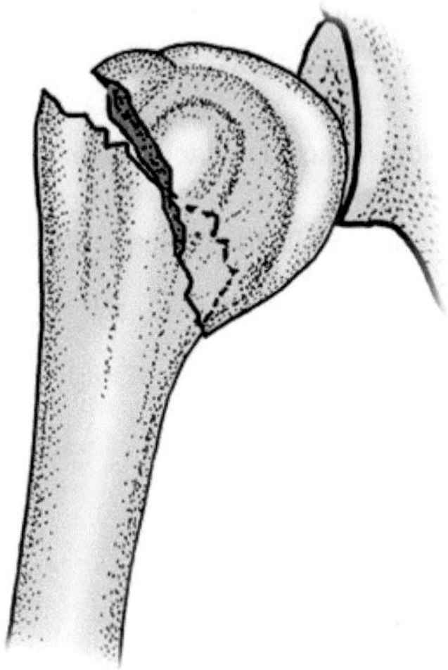

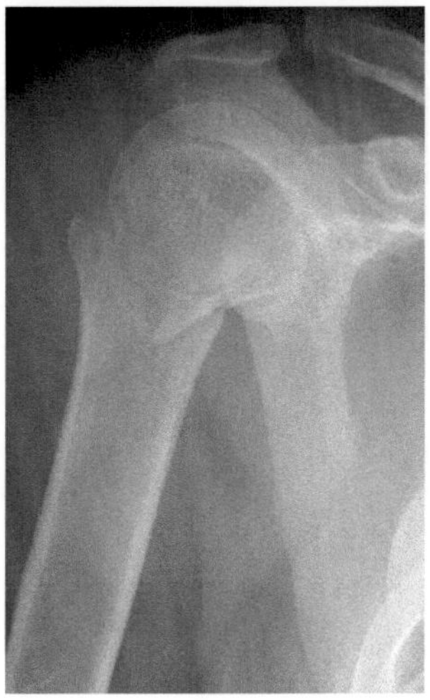

AO/OTA classification

Type A: Extra-articular, unifocal fracture (11-A)

A2: Impacted metaphysis (11-A2)

A2.2: With varus malalignment (11-A2.2)

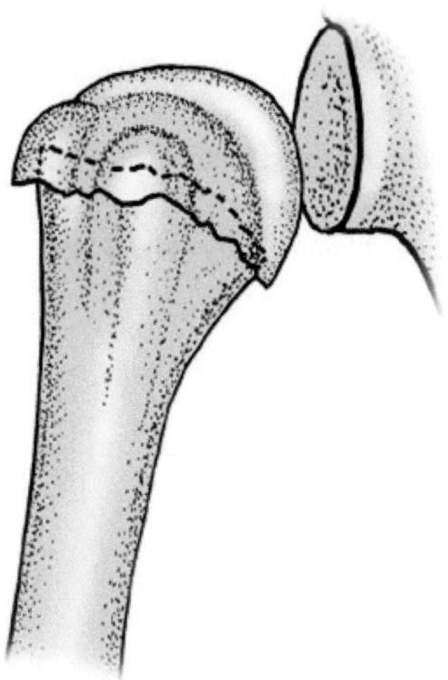

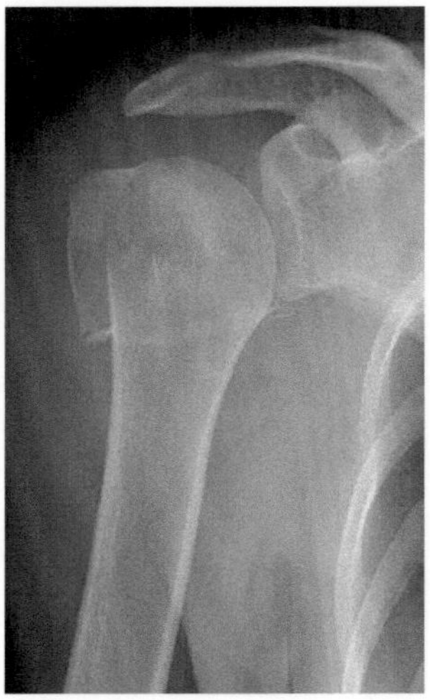

AO/OTA classification

Type A: Extra-articular, unifocal fracture (11-A)

A2: Impacted metaphysis (11-A2)

A2.3: With valgus malalignment (11-A2.3)

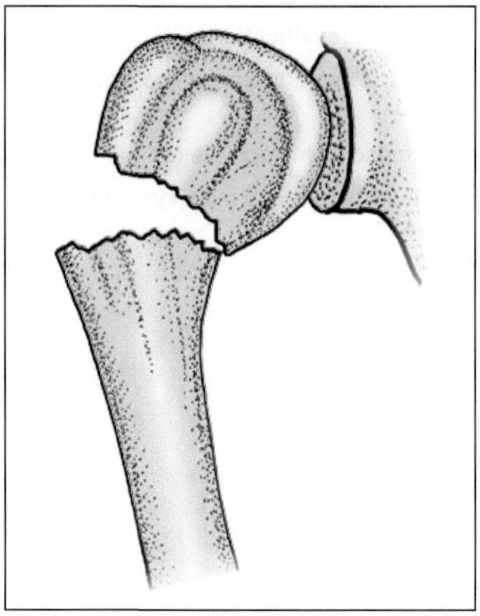

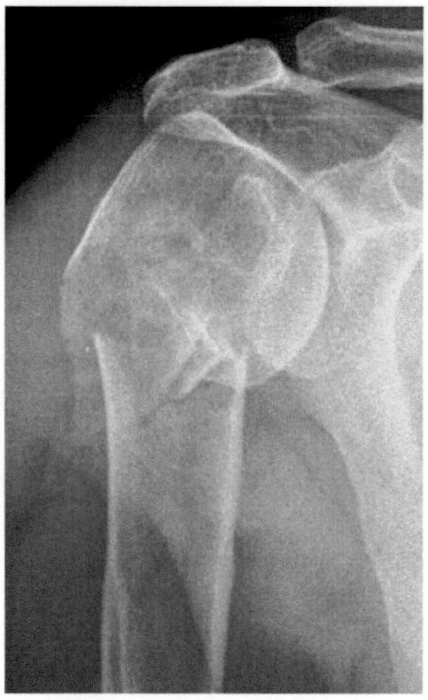

AO/OTA classification

Type A: Extra-articular, unifocal fracture (11-A)

A3: Non-impacted metaphysis fracture (11-A3)

A3.1: Simple with angulation (11-A3.1)

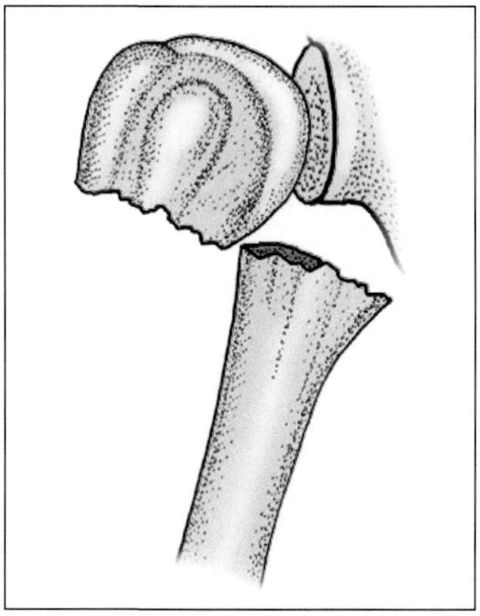

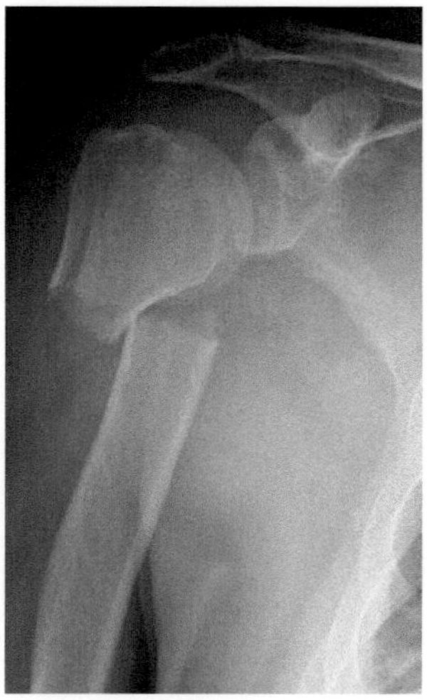

AO/OTA classification

Type A: Extra-articular, unifocal fracture (11-A)

A3: Non-impacted metaphysis fracture (11-A3)

A3.2: Simple with translation (11-A3.2)

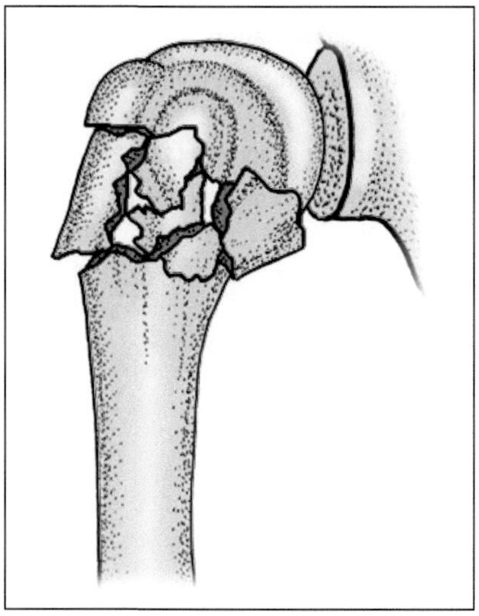

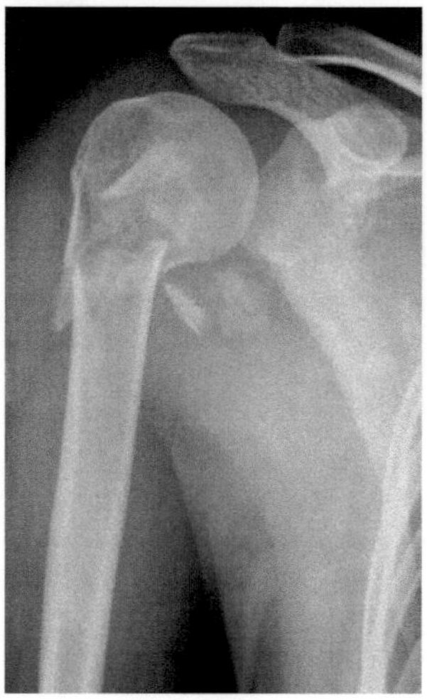

AO/OTA classification

Type A: Extra-articular, unifocal fracture (11-A)

A3: Non-impacted metaphysis fracture (11-A3)

A3.3: Multifragmentary (11-A3.3)

Type B: Extra-articular, bifocal fracture (11-B).
- B1: With metaphyseal impaction (11-B1).
  - B1.1: Lateral plus greater tuberosity (11-B1.1).
  - B1.2: Medial plus lesser tuberosity (11-B1.2).
  - B1.3: Posterior plus greater tuberosity (11-B1.3).
- B2: Without metaphyseal impaction (11-B2).
  - B2.1: Without rotatory displacement of the epiphyseal fracture fragment (11-B2.1).
  - B2.2: With rotatory displacement of the epiphyseal fragment (11-B2.2).
  - B2.3: Multifragmentary metaphysis plus one of the tuberosities (11-B2.3).
- B3: With glenohumeral dislocation (11-B3).
  - B3.1: "Vertical" cervical line plus greater tuberosity intact plus anterior medial dislocation (11-B3.1).
  - B3.2: "Vertical" cervical line plus greater tuberosity fracture plus anterior medial dislocation (11-B3.2).
  - B3.3: Lesser tuberosity fracture plus posterior dislocation (11-B3.3).

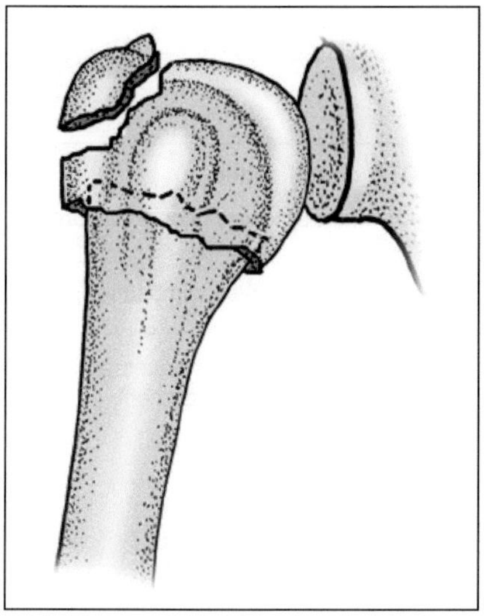
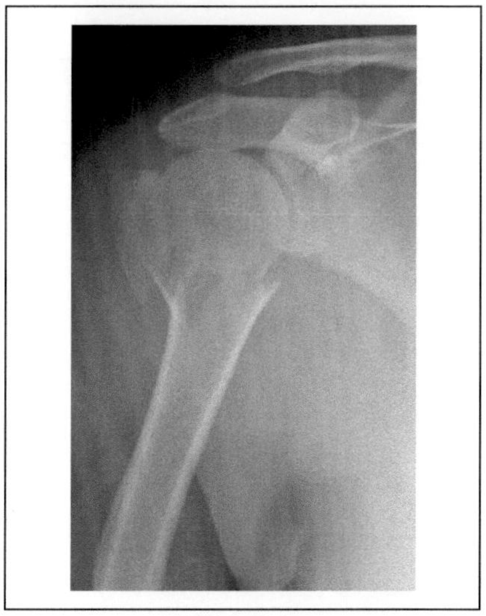

AO/OTA classification

Type B: Extra-articular, bifocal fracture (11-B)

B1: With metaphyseal impaction (11-B1)

B1.1: Lateral plus greater tuberosity (11-B1.1)

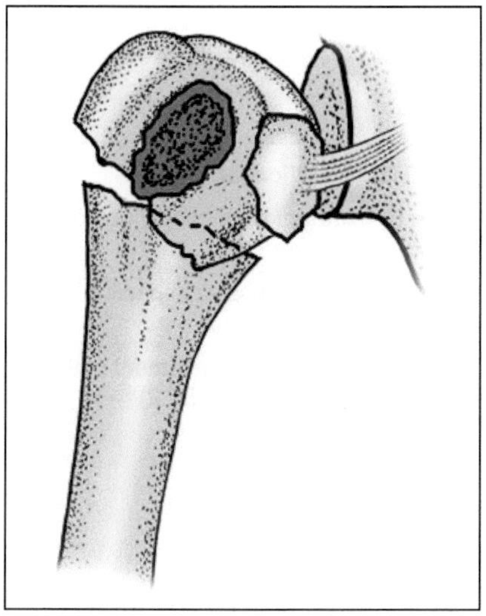
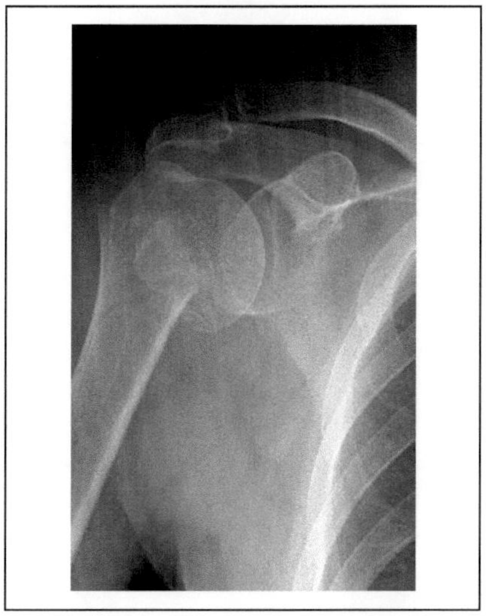

AO/OTA classification

Type B: Extra-articular, bifocal fracture (11-B)

B1: With metaphyseal impaction (11-B1)

B1.2: Medial plus lesser tuberosity (11-B1.2)

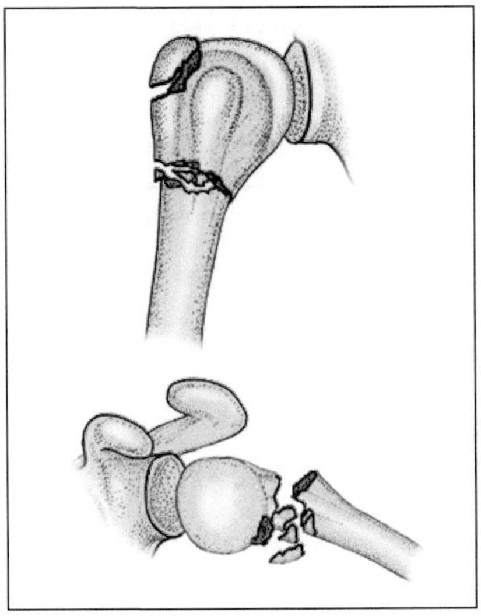

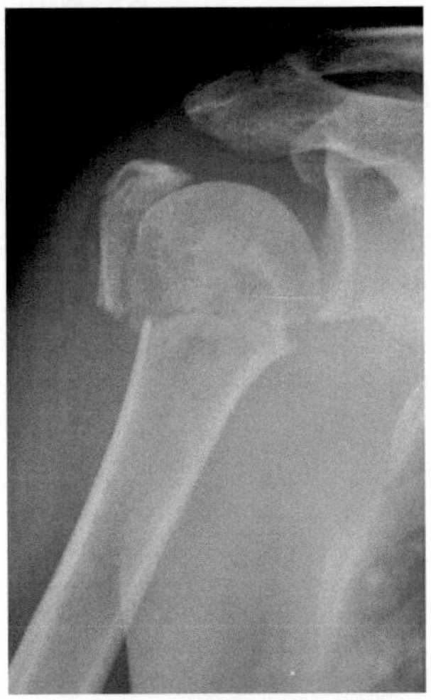

AO/OTA classification

Type B: Extra-articular, bifocal fracture (11-B)

B1: With metaphyseal impaction (11-B1)

B1.3: Posterior plus greater tuberosity (11-B1.3)

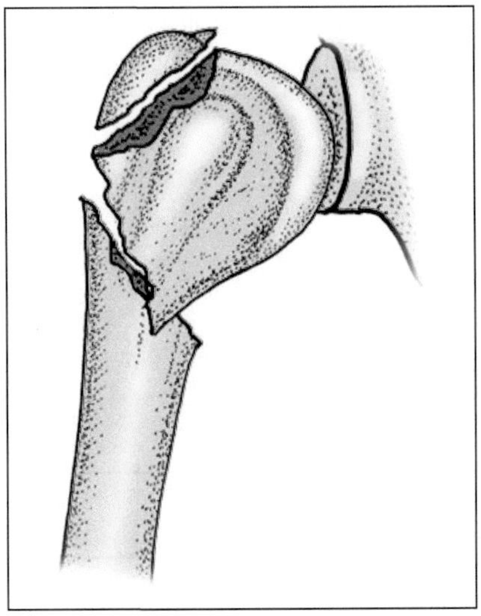

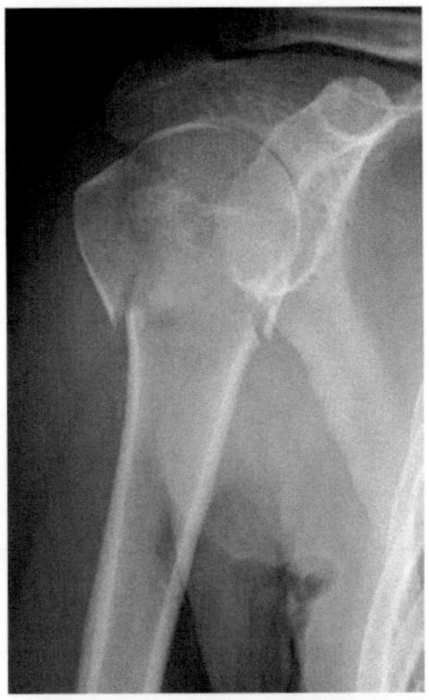

AO/OTA classification

Type B: Extra-articular, bifocal fracture (11-B)

B2: Without metaphyseal impaction (11-B2)

B2.1: Without rotatory displacement of the epiphyseal fracture fragment (11-B2.1)

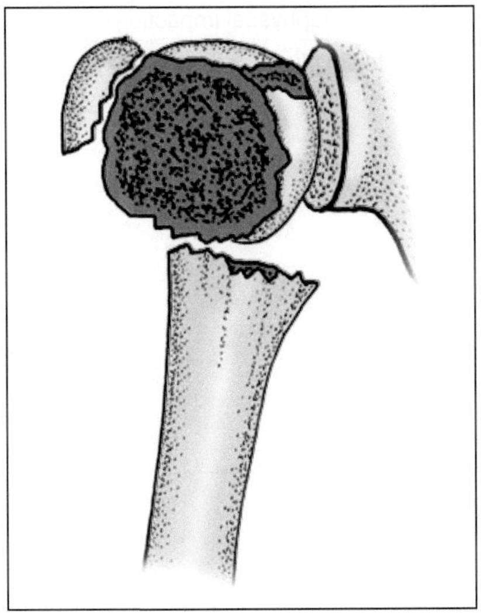

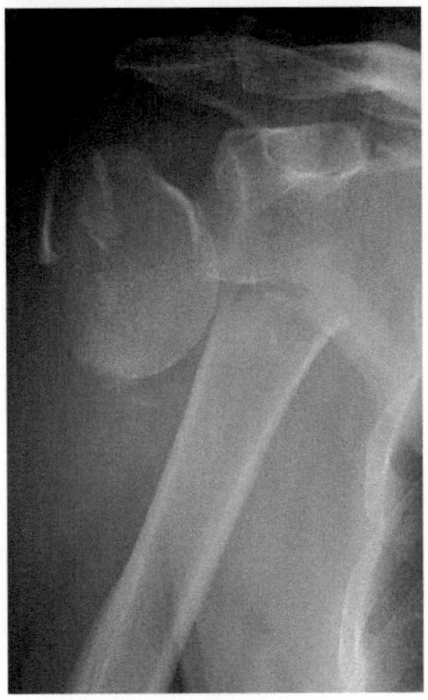

AO/OTA classification

Type B: Extra-articular, bifocal fracture (11-B)

B2: Without metaphyseal impaction (11-B2)

B2.2: With rotatory displacement of the epiphyseal fragment (11-B2.2)

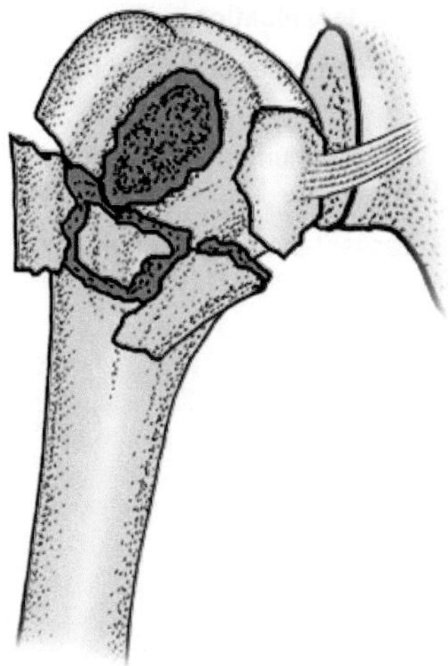

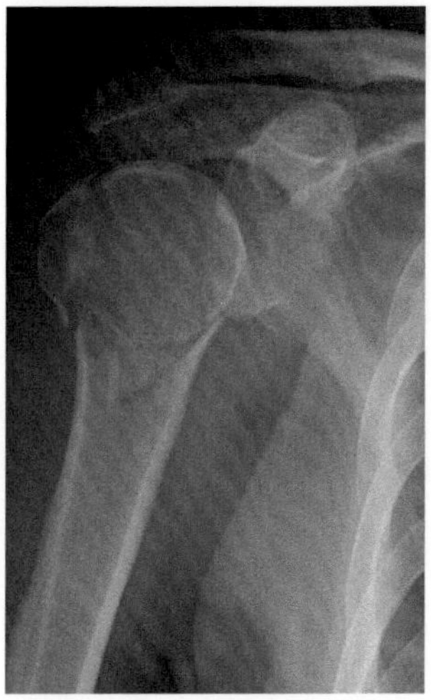

AO/OTA classification

Type B: Extra-articular, bifocal fracture (11-B)

B2: Without metaphyseal impaction (11-B2)

B2.3: Multifragmentary metaphysis plus one of the tuberosities (11-B2.3)

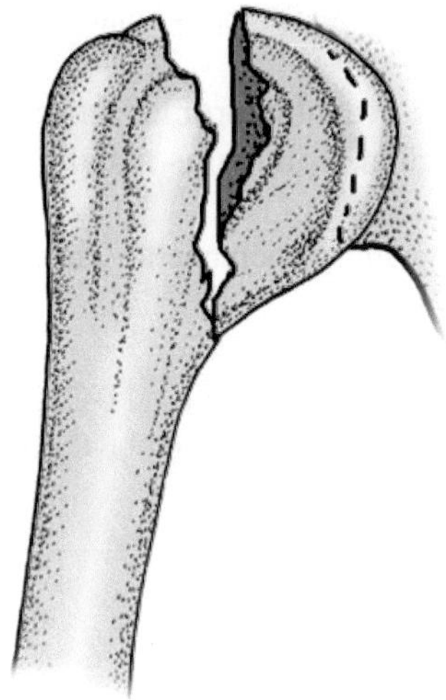

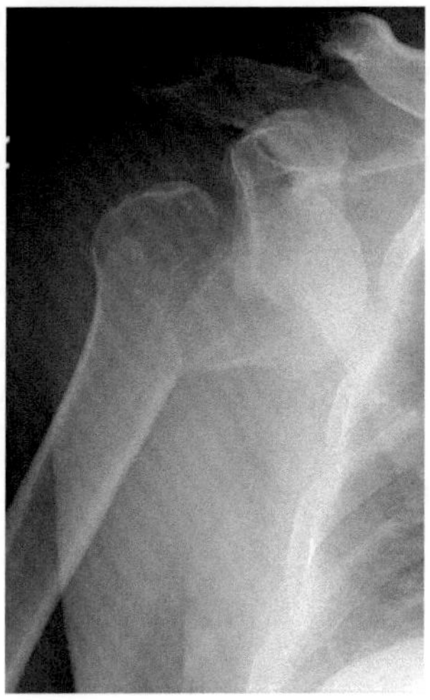

AO/OTA classification

Type B: Extra-articular, bifocal fracture (11-B)

B3: With glenohumeral dislocation (11-B3)

B3.1: "Vertical" cervical line plus greater tuberosity intact plus anterior medial dislocation (11-B3.1)

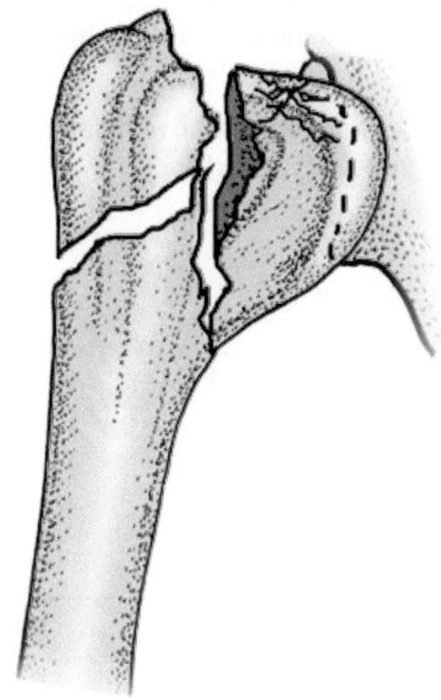

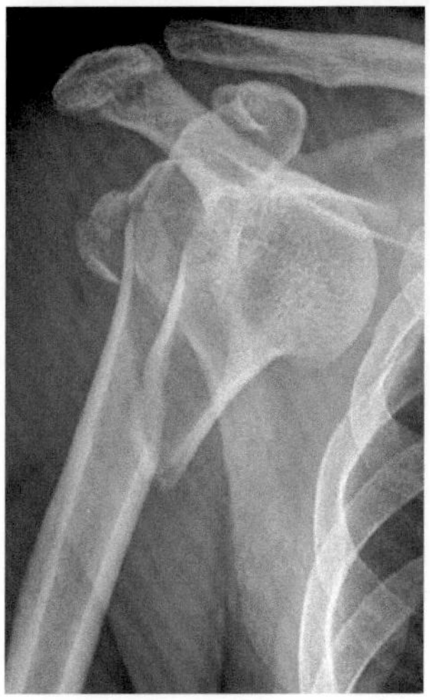

AO/OTA classification

Type B: Extra-articular, bifocal fracture (11-B)

B3: With glenohumeral dislocation (11-B3)

B3.2: "Vertical" cervical line plus greater tuberosity fracture plus anterior medial dislocation (11-B3.2)

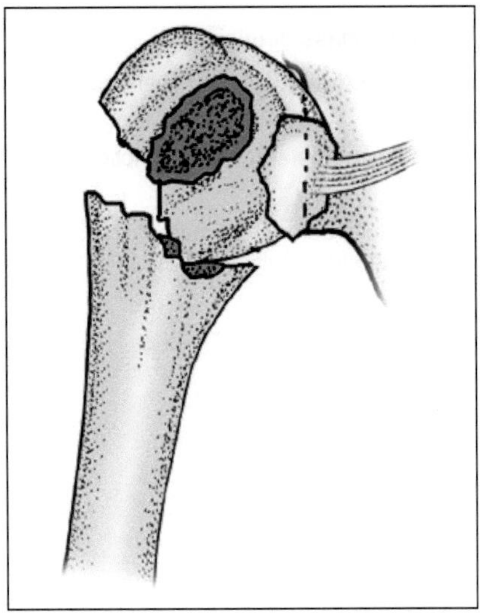

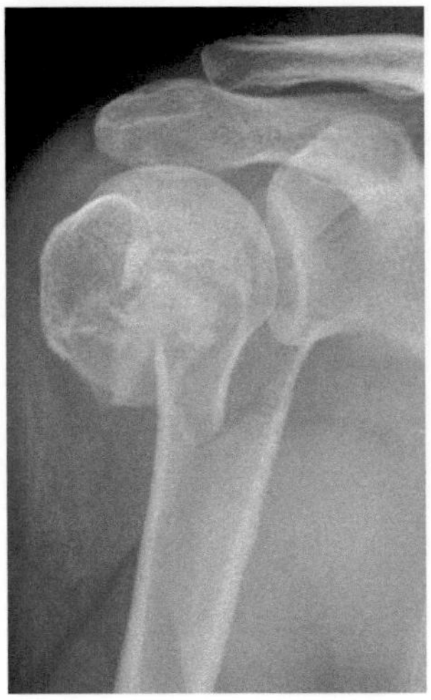

AO/OTA classification

Type B: Extra-articular, bifocal fracture (11-B)

B3: With glenohumeral dislocation (11-B3)

B3.3: Lesser tuberosity fracture plus posterior dislocation (11-B3.3)

Type C: Articular fractures (11-C).

- C1: Articular fracture with slight displacement impacted valgus fracture (11-C1).
  - C1.1: Cephalotubercular with valgus malalignment (11-C1.1).
  - C1.2: Cephalotubercular with varus malalignment (11-C1.2).
  - C1.3: Anatomical neck (11-C1.3).
- C2: Articular fracture impacted with marked displacement (11-C2).
  - C2.1: Cephalotubercular with valgus malalignment (11-C2.1).
  - C2.2: Cephalotubercular with varus malalignment (11-C2.2).
  - C2.3: Transcephalic (double-profile image on X-ray) and tubercular, with varus malalignment (11-C2.3).
- C3: Articular fracture with glenohumeral dislocation (11-C3).
  - C3.1: Anatomical neck (11-C3.1).
  - C3.2: Anatomical neck and tuberosities (11-C3.2).
  - C3.3: Cephalotubercular fragmentation (11-C3.3).

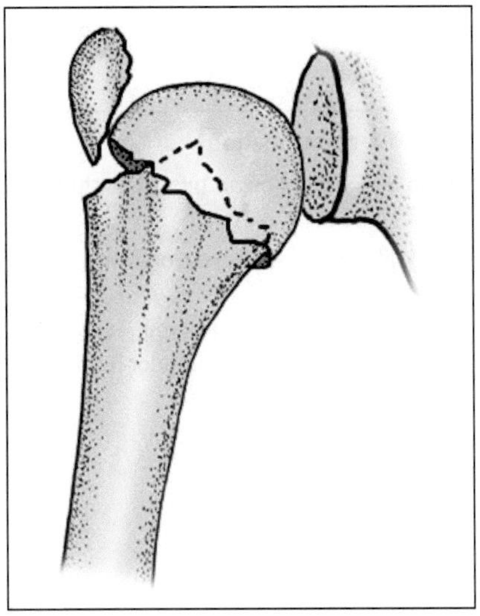

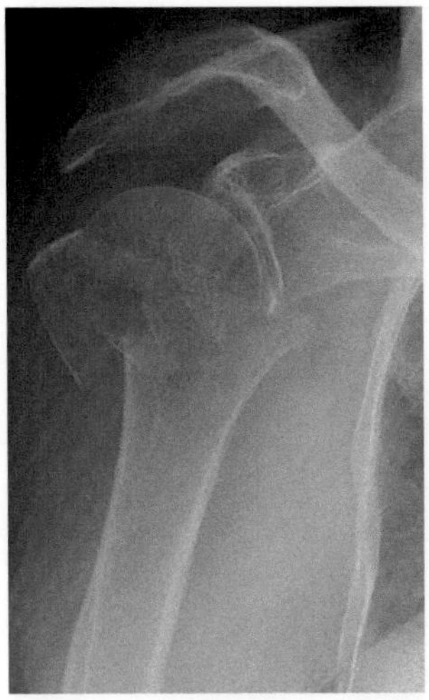

AO/OTA classification

Type C: Articular fractures (11-C)

C1: Articular fracture with slight displacement impacted valgus fracture (11-C1)

C1.1: Cephalotubercular with valgus malalignment (11-C1.1)

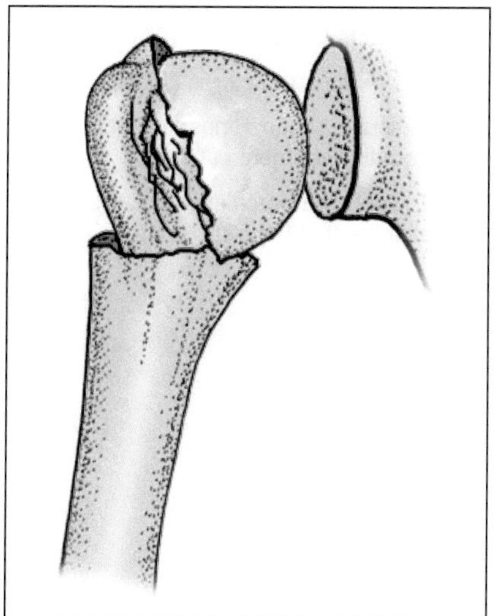

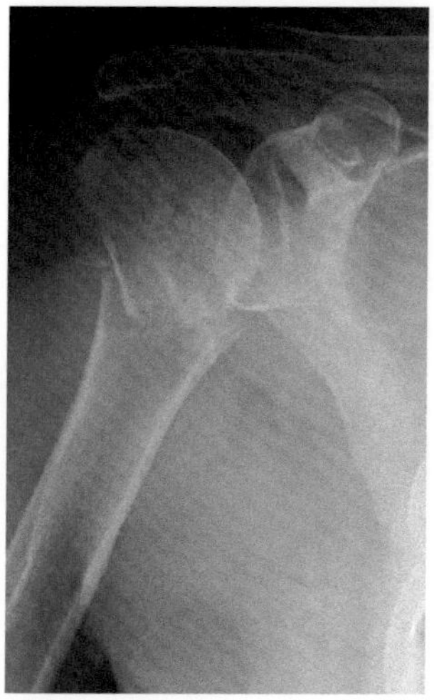

AO/OTA classification

Type C: Articular fractures (11-C)

C1: Articular fracture with slight displacement impacted valgus fracture (11-C1)

C1.2: Cephalotubercular with varus malalignment (11-C1.2)

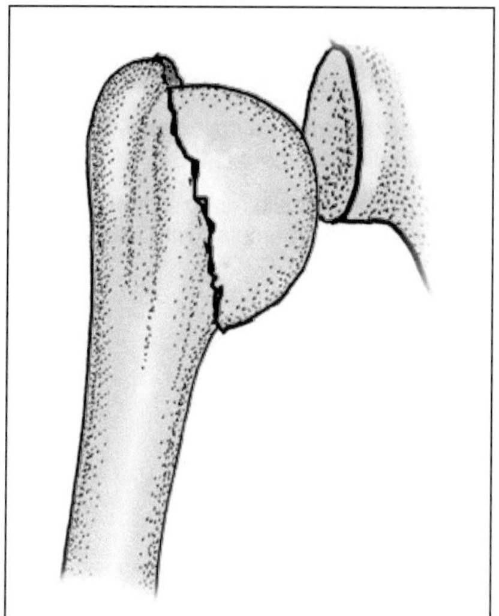

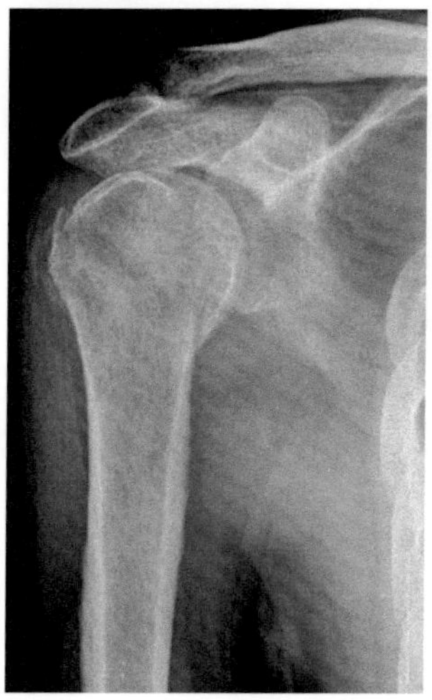

AO/OTA classification

Type C: Articular fractures (11-C)

C1: Articular fracture with slight displacement impacted valgus fracture (11-C1)

C1.3: Anatomical neck (11-C1.3)

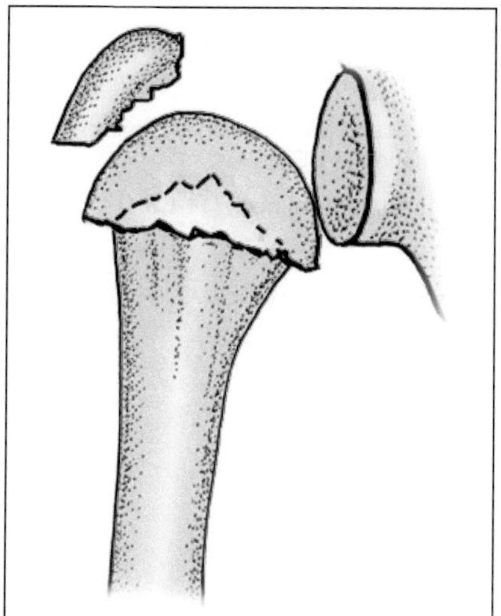

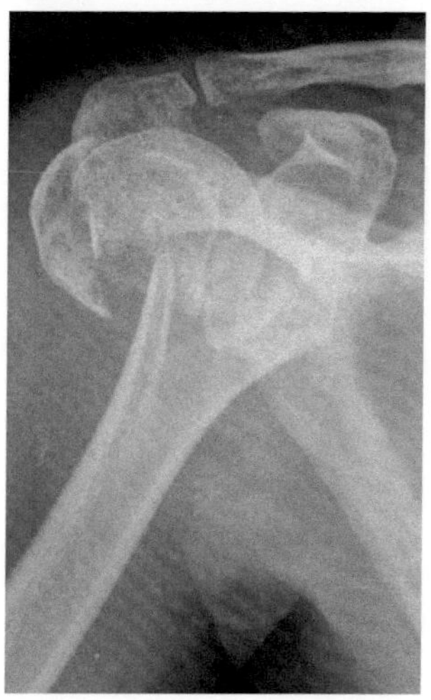

AO/OTA classification

Type C: Articular fractures (11-C)

C2: Articular fracture impacted with marked displacement (11-C2)

C2.1: Cephalotubercular with valgus malalignment (11-C2.1)

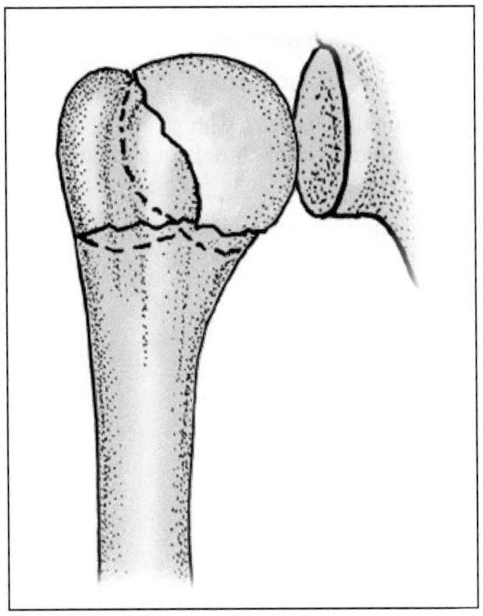

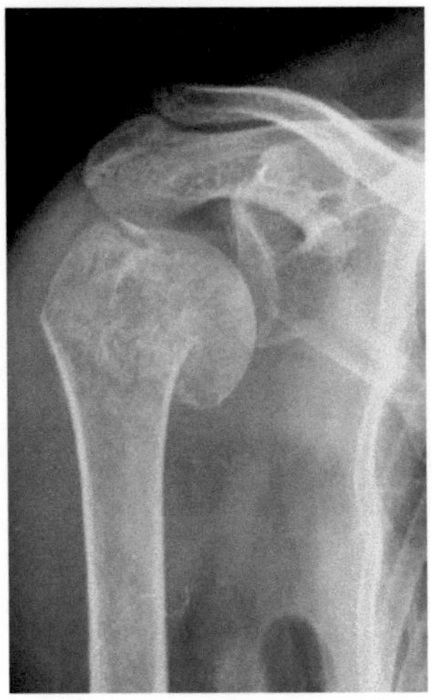

AO/OTA classification

Type C: Articular fractures (11-C)

C2: Articular fracture impacted with marked displacement (11-C2)

C2.2: Cephalotubercular with varus malalignment (11-C2.2)

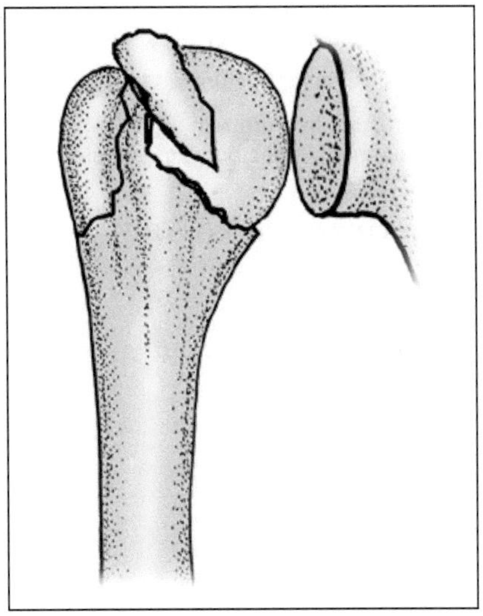

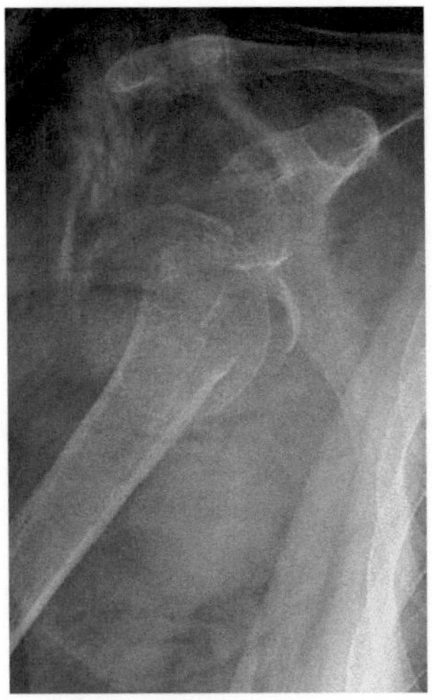

AO/OTA classification

Type C: Articular fractures (11-C)

C2: Articular fracture impacted with marked displacement (11-C2)

C2.3: Transcephalic (double-profile image on X-ray) and tubercular, with varus malalignment (11-C2.3)

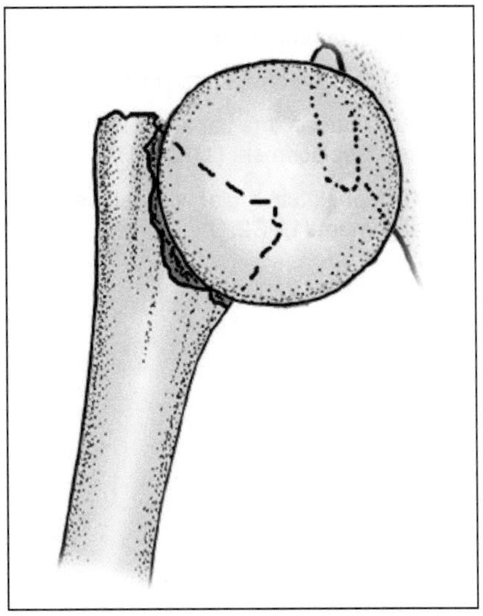

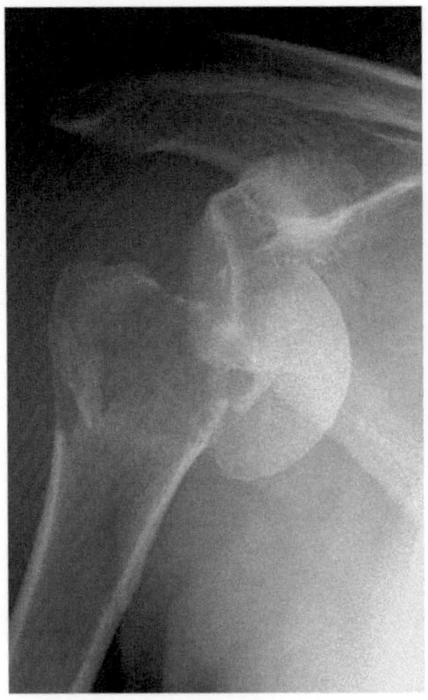

AO/OTA classification

Type C: Articular fractures (11-C)

C3: Articular fracture with glenohumeral dislocation (11-C3)

C3.1: Anatomical neck (11-C3.1)

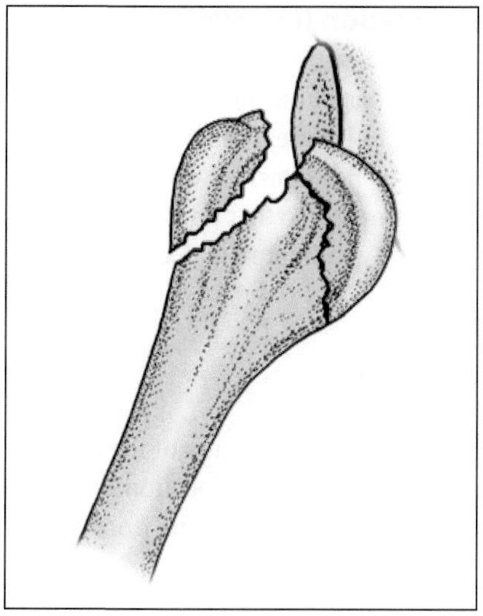

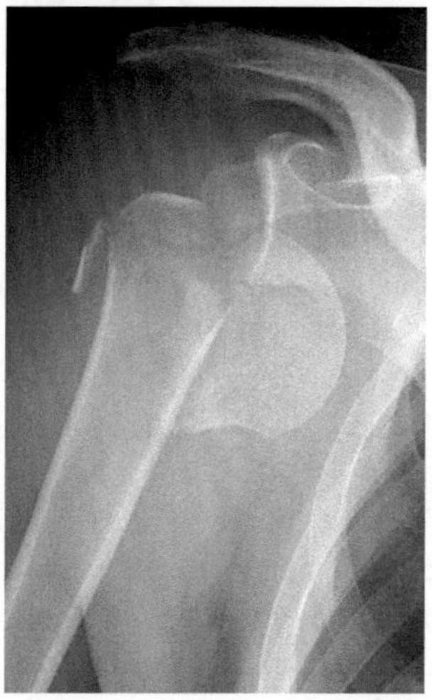

AO/OTA classification

Type C: Articular fractures (11-C)

C3: Articular fracture with glenohumeral dislocation (11-C3)

C3.2: Anatomical neck and tuberosities (11-C3.2)

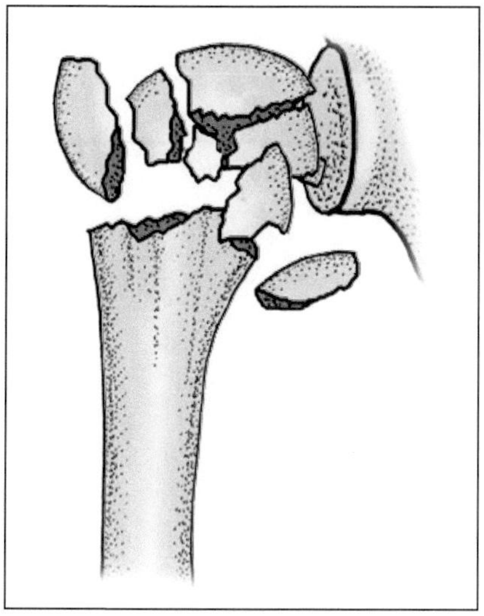

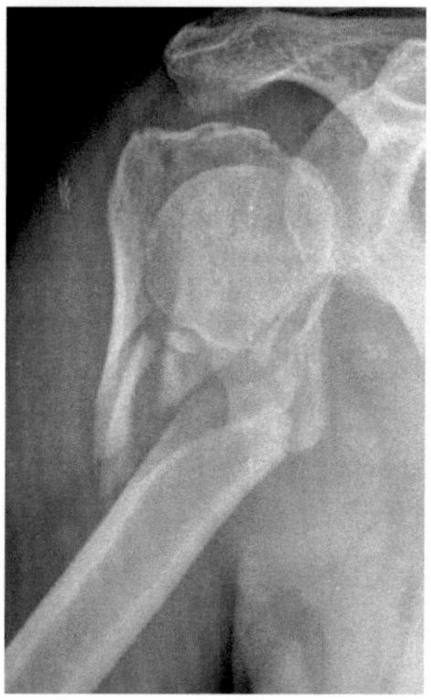

AO/OTA classification

Type C: Articular fractures (11-C)

C3: Articular fracture with glenohumeral dislocation (11-C3)

C3.3: Cephalotubercular fragmentation (11-C3.3)

2.1.3 Codman Classification [3]

Codman divided the proximal end of the humerus into four distinct fragments according to anatomic lines of epiphyseal union: *a*, greater tuberosity; *b*, lesser tuberosity; *c*, head; and *d*, shaft. All those different types of fractures are variable combinations of the four major fragments mentioned above.

2.1.4 Watson-Jones Classification (in 1955)

Watson-Jones divided the proximal humeral fractures into abduction fracture and adduction fracture according to injury mechanism. The apex of angulation of the proximal humerus usually is directed anteriorly, and anterior angulation can produce in X-rays either the abduction fracture or the adduction fracture, depending on the position of humerus rotation. Therefore, this classification can mislead the therapy as classifying criteria is not strict or accurate.

2.1.5 Kocher Classification (in 1896)

The Kocher classification is based on three anatomic levels of fractures: anatomic neck, epiphyseal region, and surgical neck. This classification does not consider displacement of fractures and amount of fragments, so that it results in confusion of diagnosis and difficulty in treatment decision.

2.1.6 Hill-Sachs Fracture

A bony trough in the posterior-superior region of the humeral head which occurs during the anterior dislocation of shoulder as the humeral head impacts against the front of the glenoid.

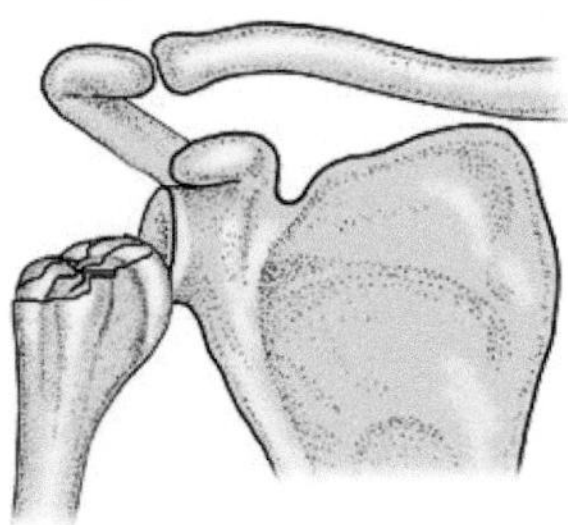

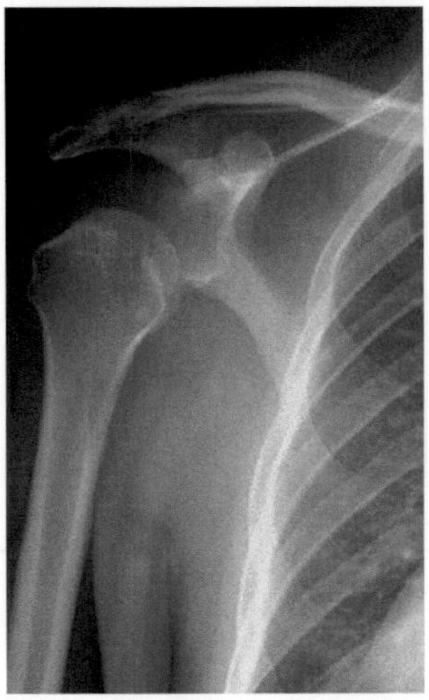

Hill-Sachs fracture

2.2 Classification Systems of Humeral Shaft Fractures

To date, there are five classification systems of humeral shaft fractures in literature. According to the literature over the last 5 years, the most frequently used system is the AO/OTA classification.

2.2.1 AO/OTA Classification [2]

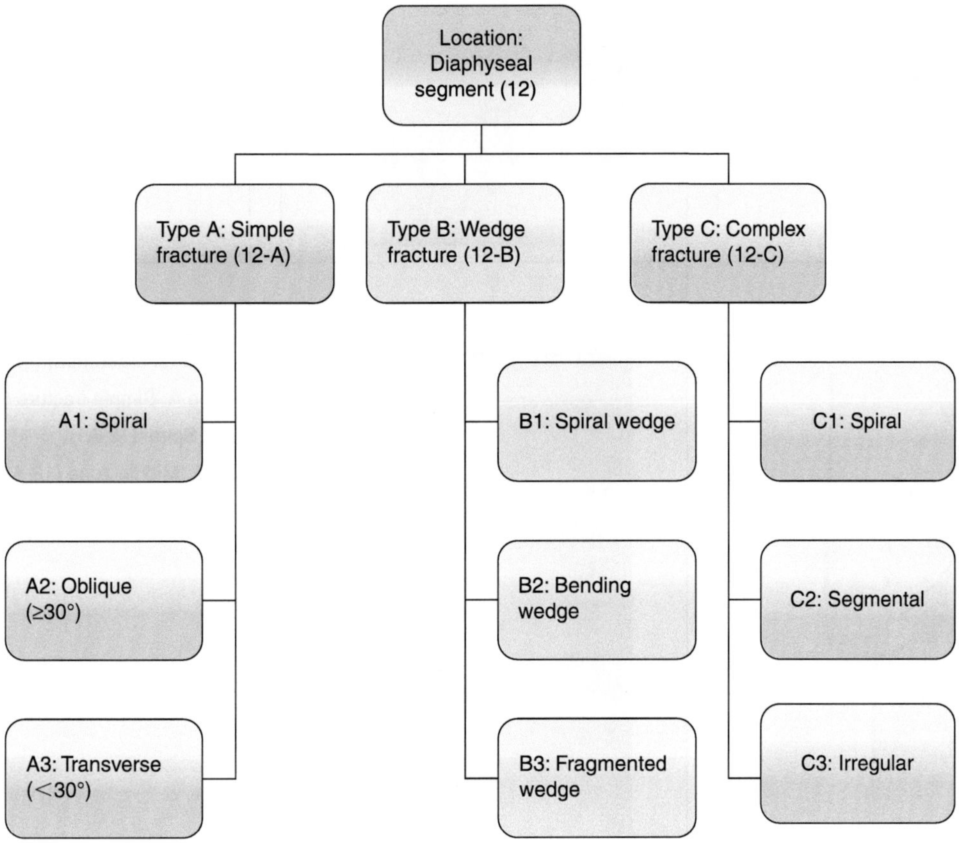

Type A: Simple fracture (12-A).
- A1: Spiral (12-A1).
  - A1.1: Proximal zone (12-A1.1).
  - A1.2: Middle zone (12-A1.2).
  - A1.3: Distal zone (12-A1.3).
- A2: Oblique (≥30°) (12-A2).
  - A2.1: Proximal zone (12-A2.1).
  - A2.2: Middle zone (12-A2.2).
  - A2.3: Distal zone (12-A2.3).
- A3: Transverse (<30°) (12-A3).
  - A3.1: Proximal zone (12-A3.1).
  - A3.2: Middle zone (12-A3.2).
  - A3.3: Distal zone (12-A3.3).

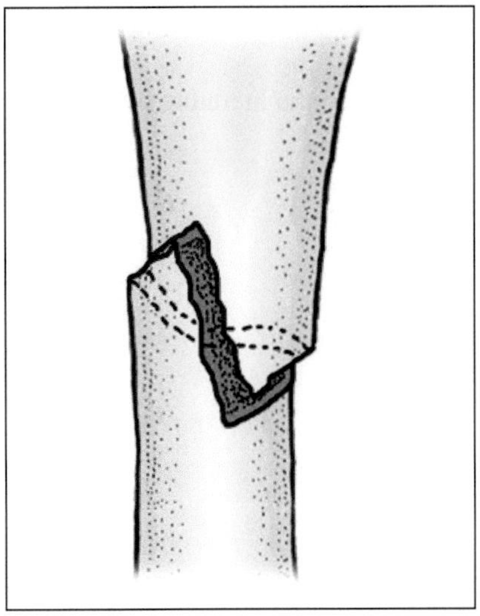

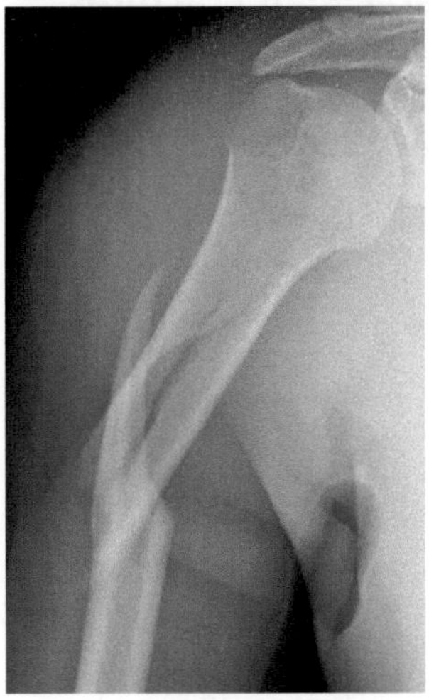

AO/OTA classification

Type A: Simple fracture (12-A)

A1: Spiral (12-A1)

A1.1: Proximal zone (12-A1.1)

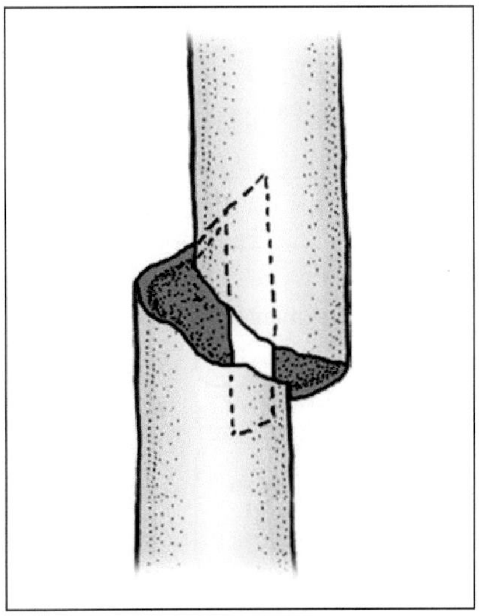

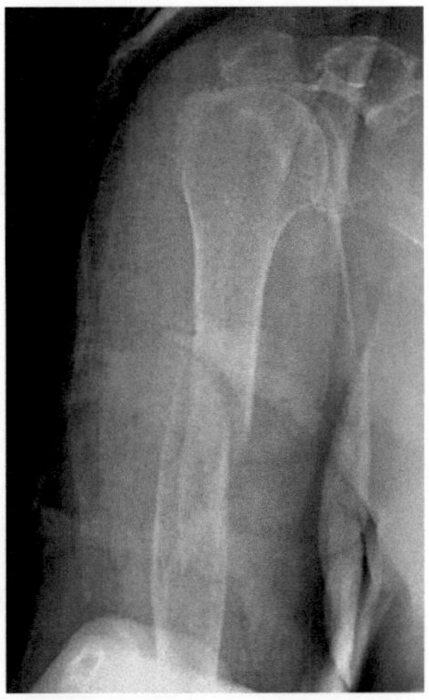

AO/OTA classification

Type A: Simple fracture (12-A)

A:1 Spiral (12-A1)

A1.2: Middle zone (12-A1.2)

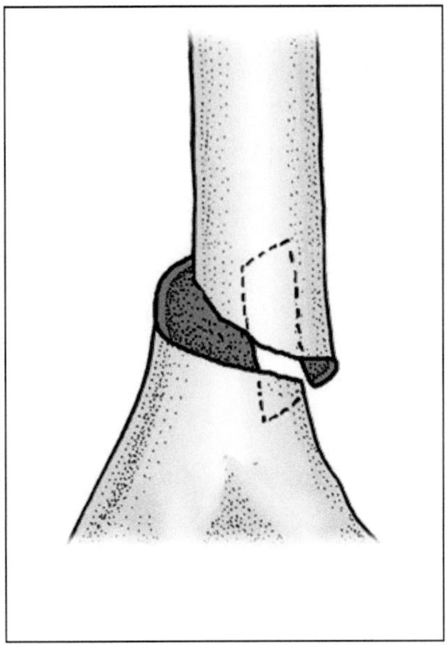

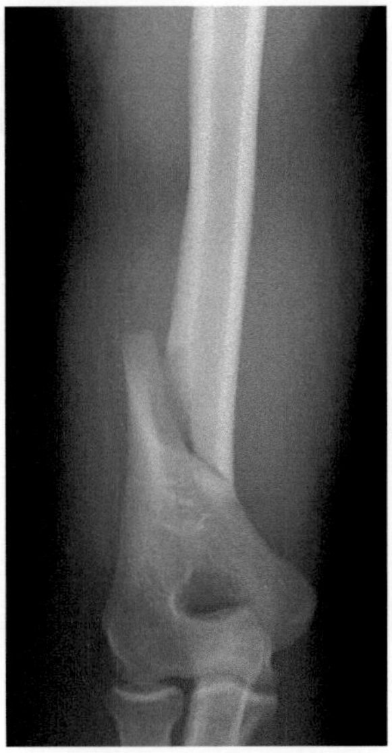

AO/OTA classification

Type A: Simple fracture (12-A)

A1: Spiral (12-A1)

A1.3: Distal zone (12-A1.3)

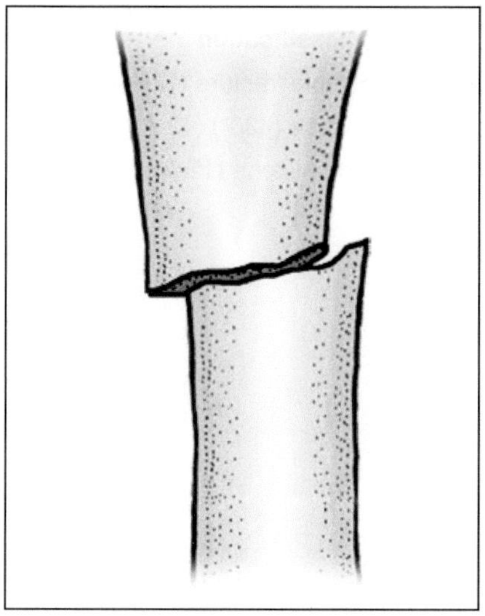

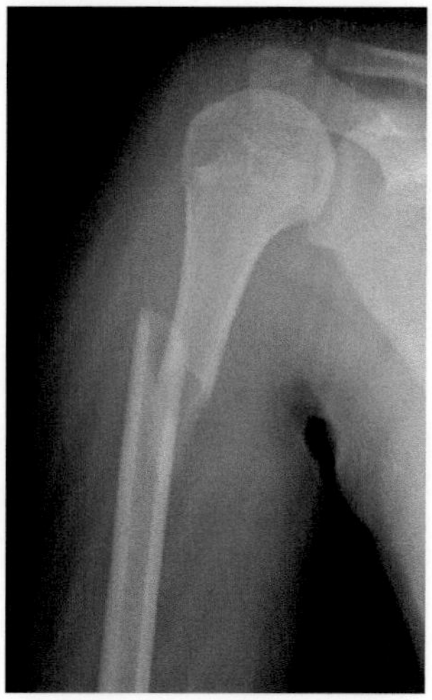

AO/OTA classification

Type A: Simple fracture (12-A)

A2: Oblique (≥30°) (12-A2)

A2.1: Proximal zone (12-A2.1)

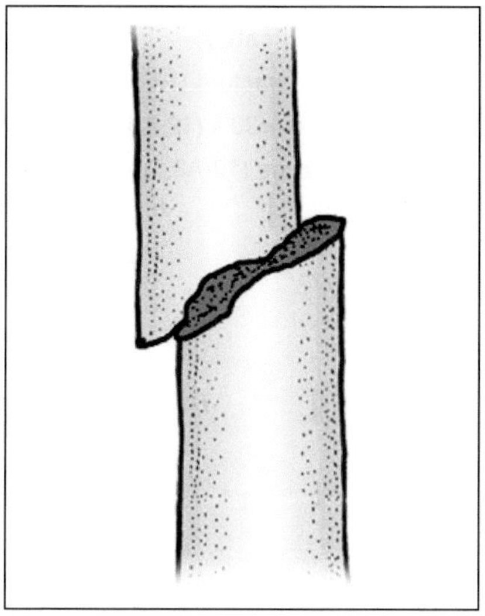

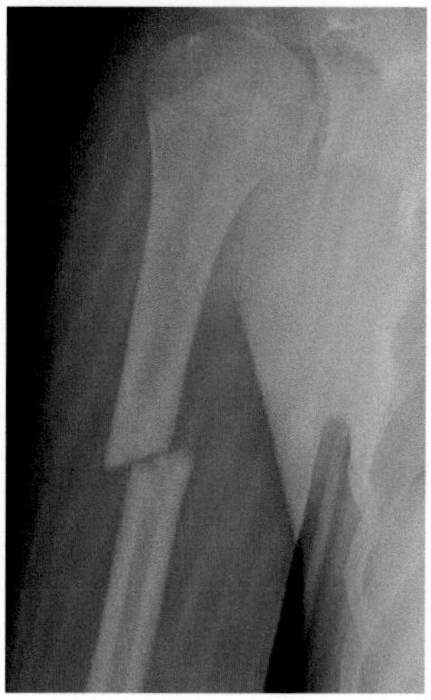

AO/OTA classification

Type A: Simple fracture (12-A)

A2: Oblique (≥30°) (12-A2)

A2.2: Middle zone (12-A2.2)

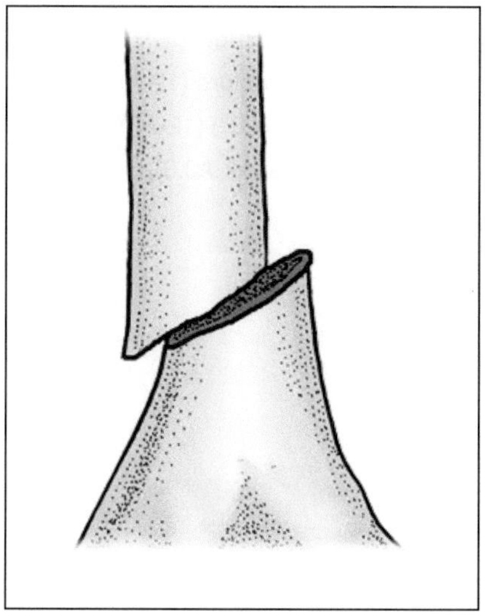

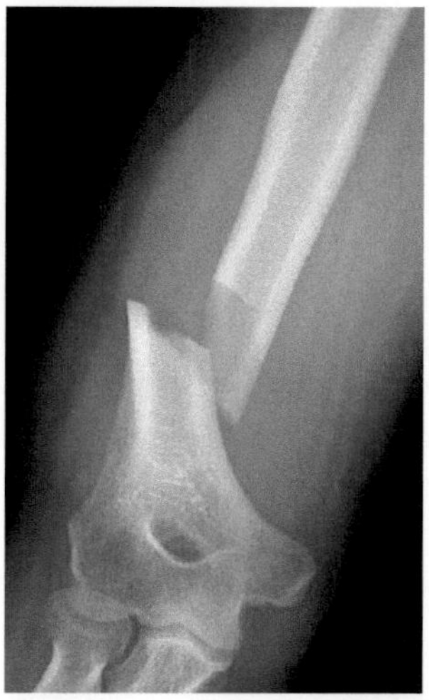

AO/OTA classification

Type A: Simple fracture (12-A)

A2: Oblique (≥30°) (12-A2)

A2.3: Distal zone (12-A2.3)

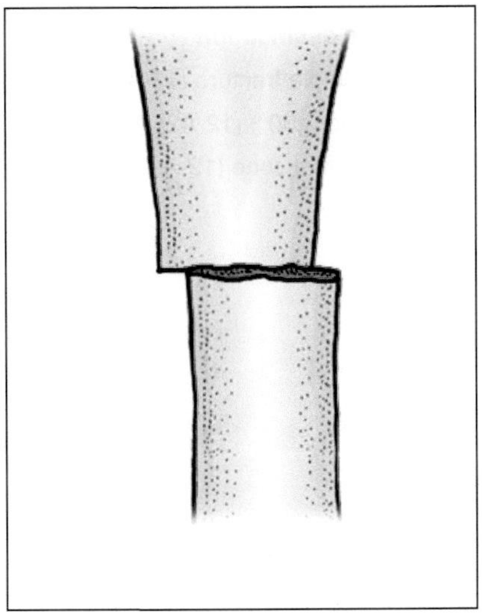

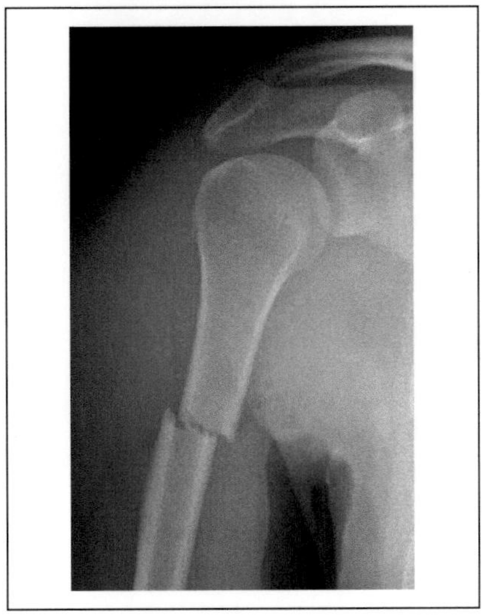

AO/OTA classification

Type A: Simple fracture (12-A)

A3: Transverse (<30°) (12-A3)

A3.1: Proximal zone (12-A3.1)

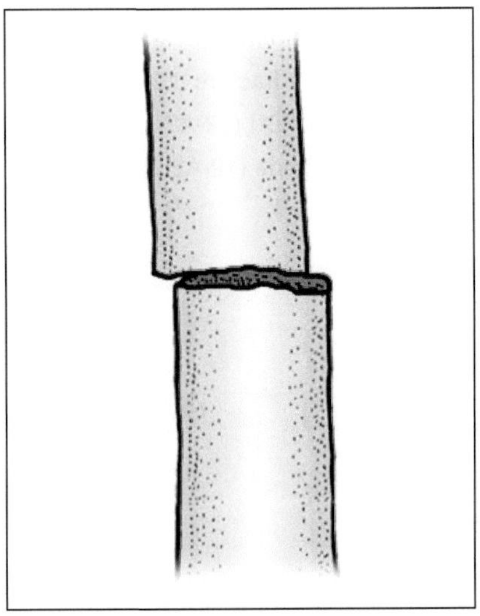

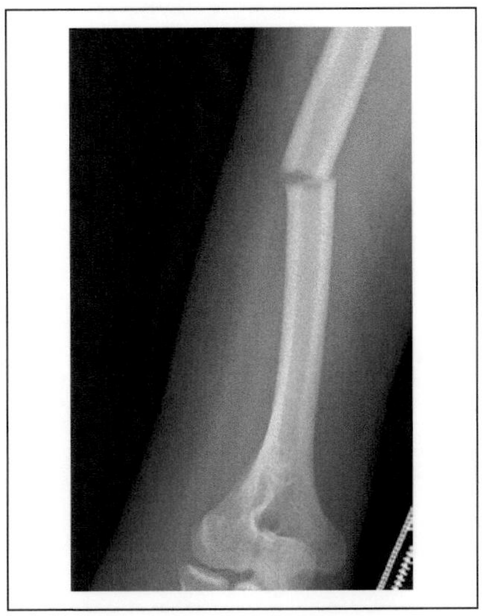

AO/OTA classification

Type A: Simple fracture (12-A)

A3: Transverse (<30°) (12-A3)

A3.2: Middle zone (12-A3.2)

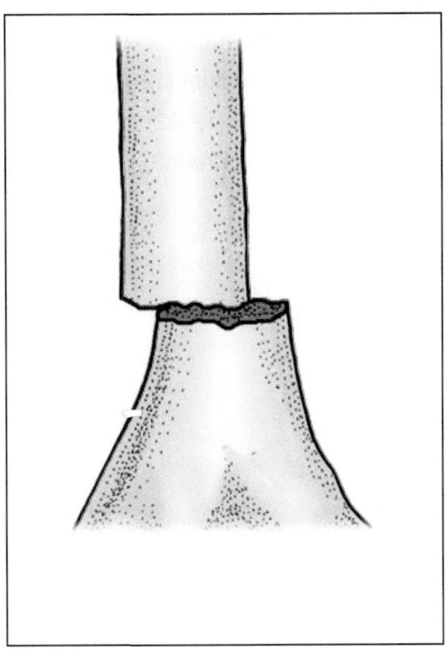

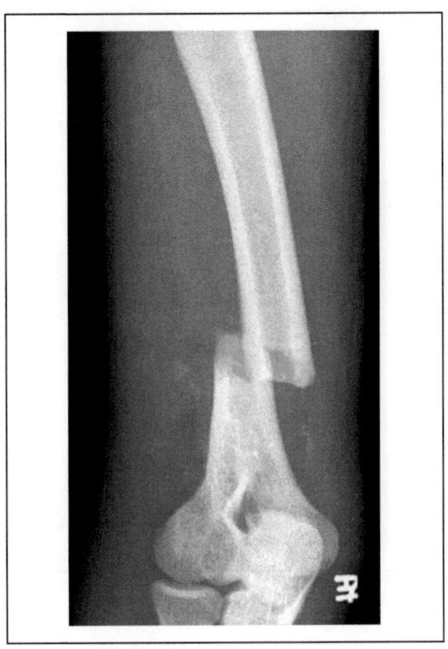

AO/OTA classification

Type A: Simple fracture (12-A)

A3: Transverse (<30°) (12-A3)

A3.3: Distal zone (12-A3.3)

Type B: Wedge fracture (12-B)
- B1: Spiral wedge (12-B1).
  - B1.1: Proximal zone (12-B1.1).
  - B1.2: Middle zone (12-B1.2).
  - B1.3: Distal zone (12-B1.3).
- B2: Bending wedge (12-B2).
  - B2.1: Proximal zone (12-B2.1).
  - B2.2: Middle zone (12-B2.2).
  - B2.3: Distal zone (12-B2.3).
- B3: Fragmented wedge (12-B3).
  - B3.1: Proximal zone (12-B3.1).
  - B3.2: Middle zone (12-B3.2).
  - B3.3: Distal zone (12-B3.3).

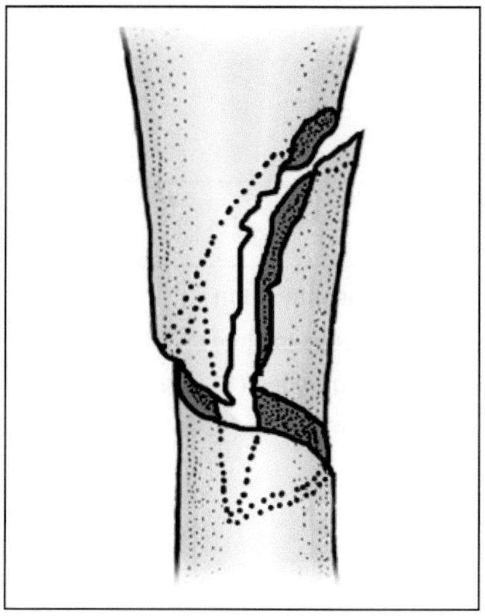

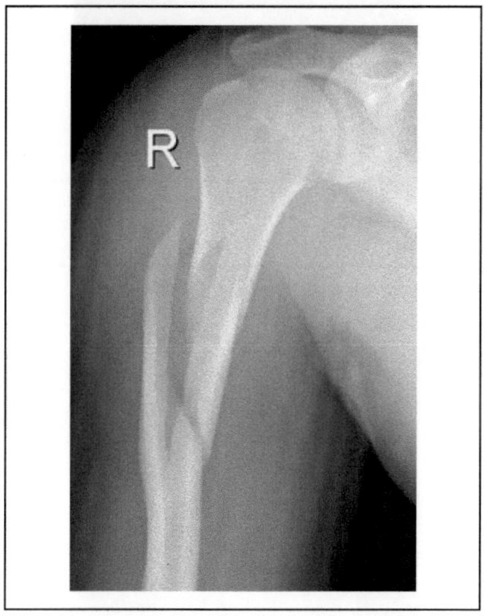

AO/OTA classification

Type B: Wedge fracture (12-B)

B1: Spiral wedge (12-B1)

B1.1: Proximal zone (12-B1.1)

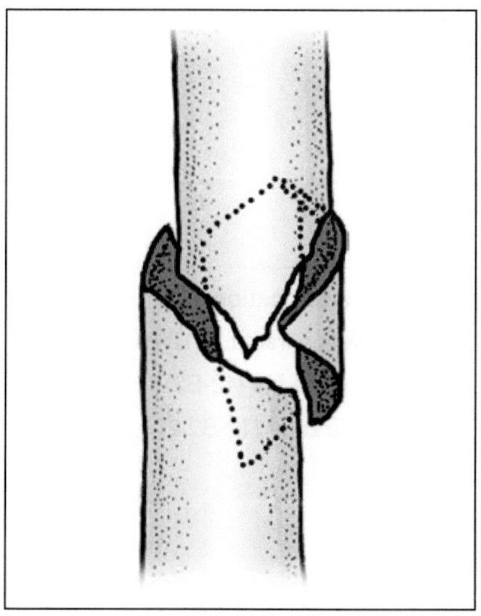

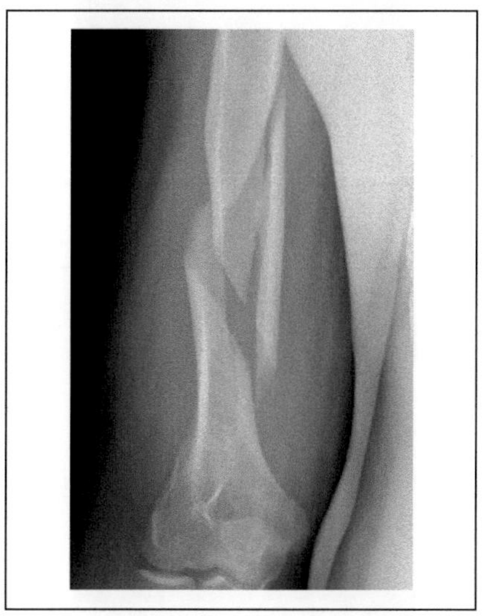

AO/OTA classification

Type B: Wedge fracture (12-B)

B1: Spiral wedge (12-B1)

B1.2: Middle zone (12-B1.2)

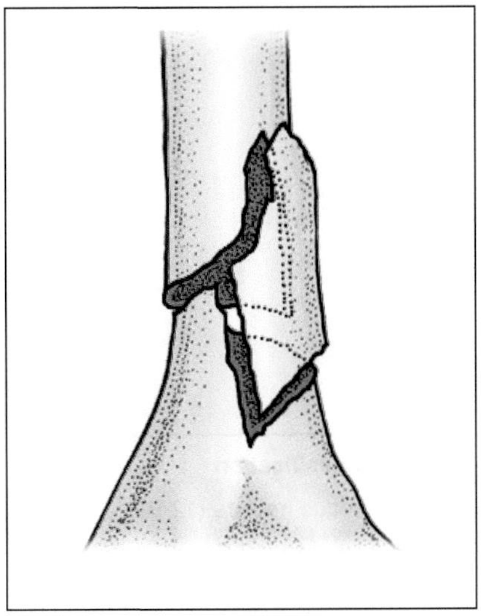

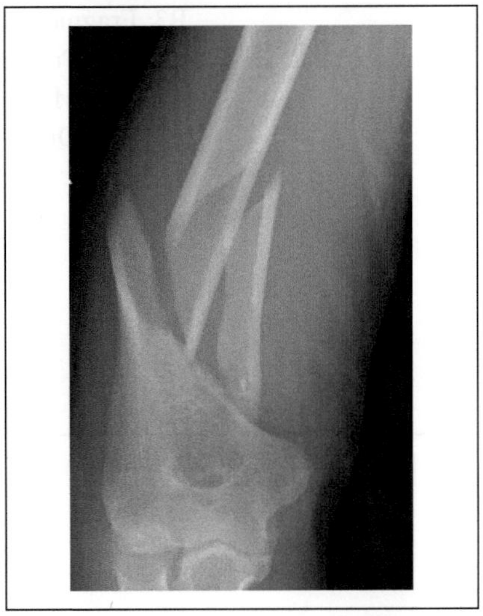

AO/OTA classification

Type B: Wedge fracture (12-B)

B1: Spiral wedge (12-B1)

B1.3: Distal zone (12-B1.3)

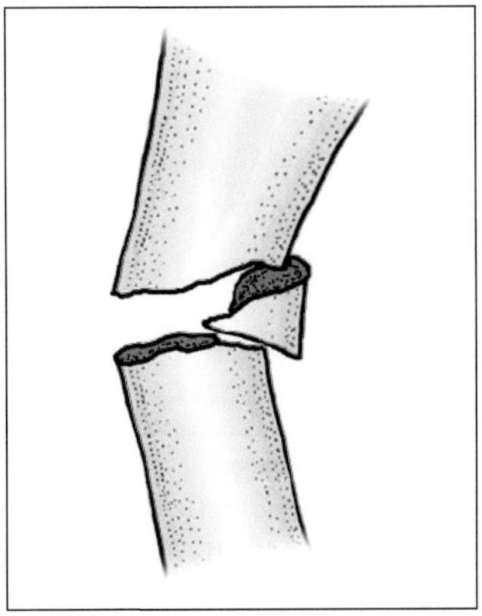

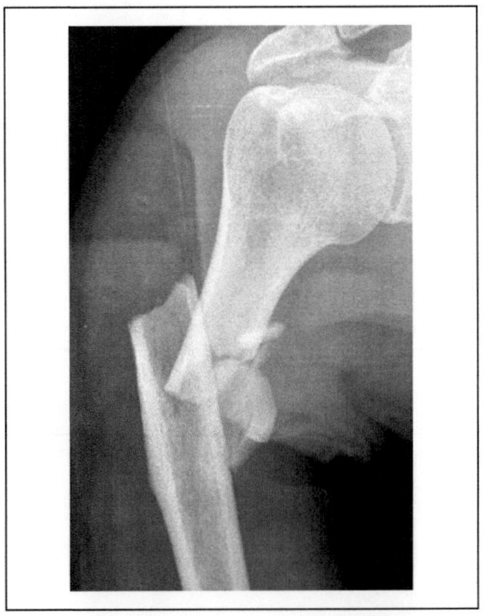

AO/OTA classification

Type B: Wedge fracture (12-B)

B2: Bending wedge (12-B2)

B2.1: Proximal zone (12-B2.1)

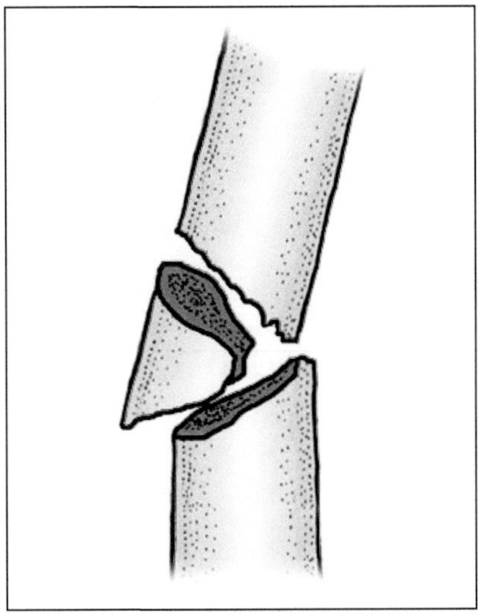

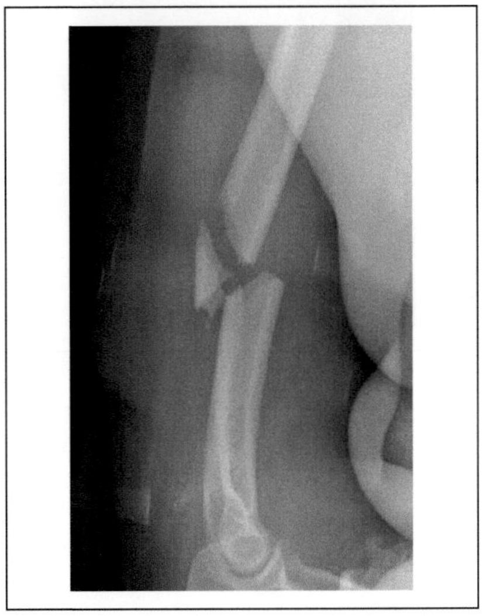

AO/OTA classification

Type B: Wedge fracture (12-B)

B2: Bending wedge (12-B2)

B2.2: Middle zone (12-B2.2)

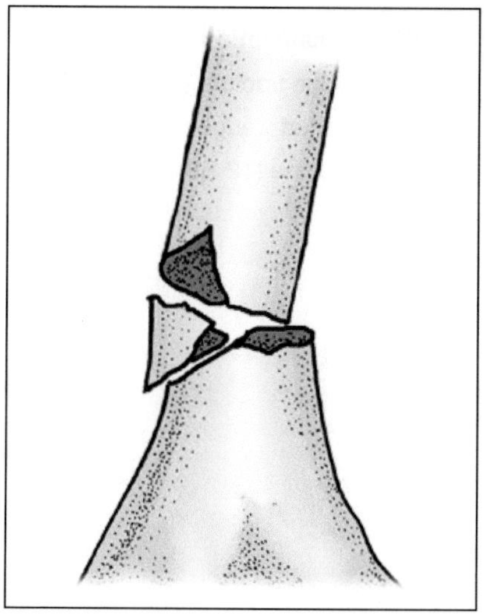

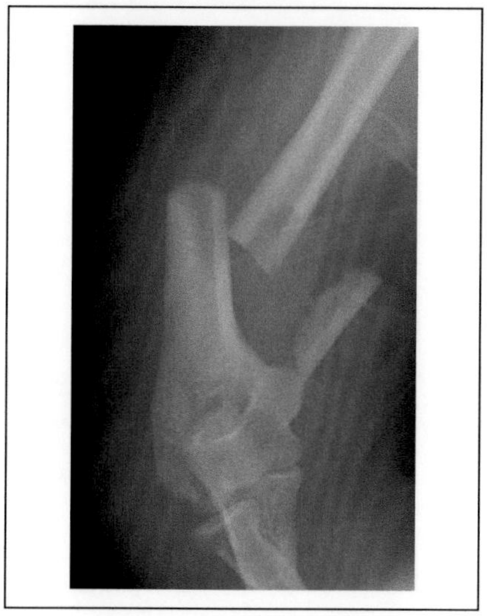

AO/OTA classification

Type B: Wedge fracture (12-B)

B2: Bending wedge (12-B2)

B2.3: Distal zone (12-B2.3)

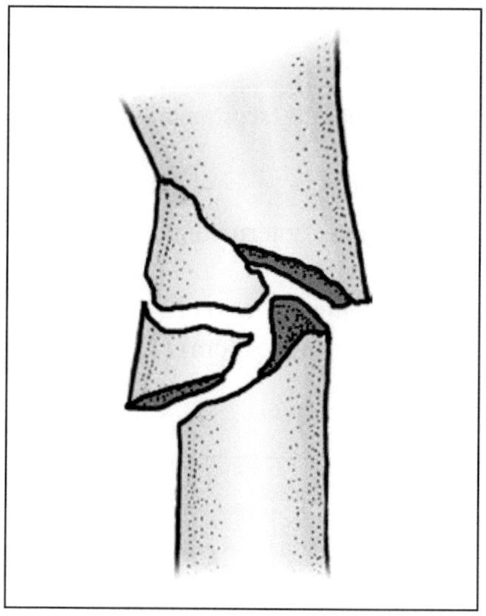

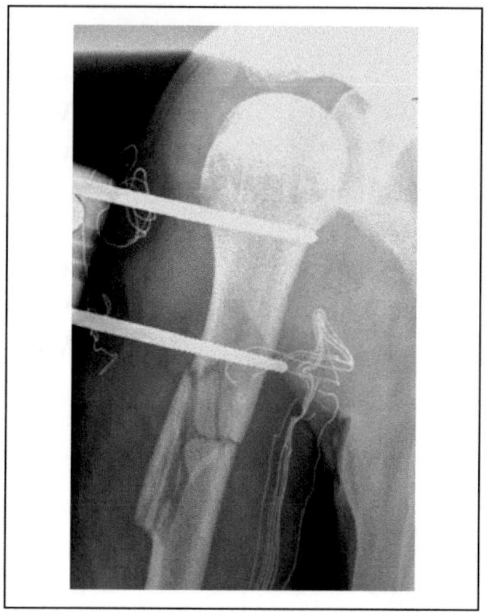

AO/OTA classification

Type B: Wedge fracture (12-B)

B3: Fragmented wedge (12-B3)

B3.1: Proximal zone (12-B3.1)

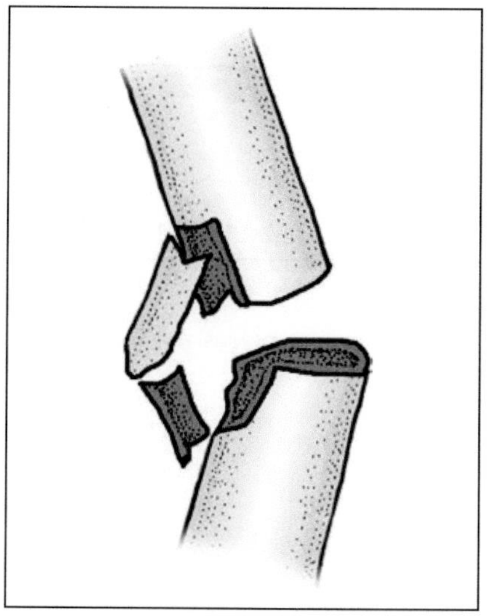

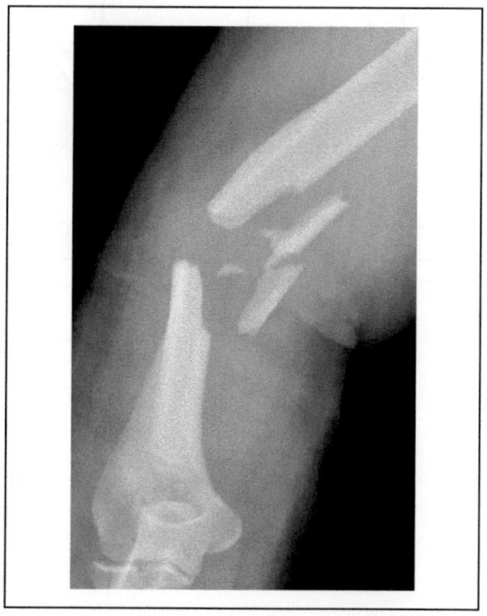

AO/OTA classification

Type B: Wedge fracture (12-B)

B3: Fragmented wedge (12-B3)

B3.2: Middle zone (12-B3.2)

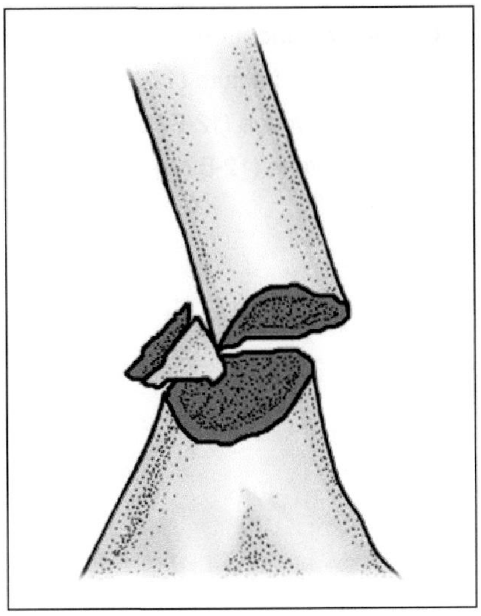

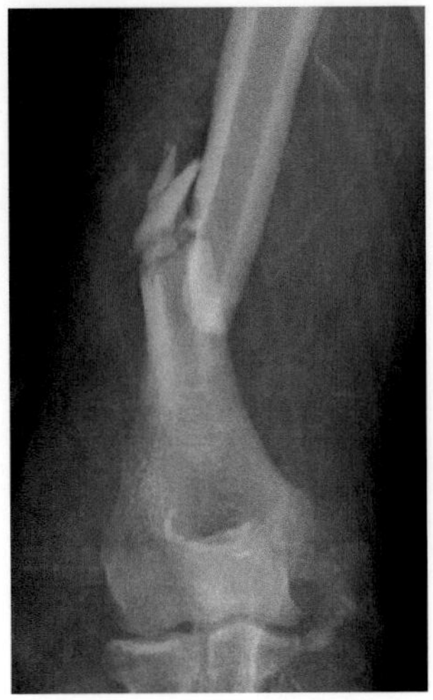

AO/OTA classification

Type B: Wedge fracture (12-B)

B3: Fragmented wedge (12-B3)

B3.3: Distal zone (12-B3.3)

Type C: Complex fracture (12-C).

- C1: Spiral (12-C1):
  - C1.1: With two intermediate fragments (12-C1.1).
  - C1.2: With three intermediate fragments (12-C1.2).
  - C1.3: With more than three intermediate fragments (12-C1.3).
- C2: Segmental (12-C2):
  - C2.1: With one intermediate segmental fragment (12-C2.1).
  - C2.2: With one intermediate segmental and additional wedge fragments (12-C2.2).
  - C2.3: With two intermediate segmental fragments (12-C2.3).
- C3: Irregular (12-C3):
  - C3.1: With two or three intermediate fragments (12-C3.1).
  - C3.2: With limited shattering (<4 cm) (12-C3.2).
  - C3.3: With extensive shattering (>4 cm) (12-C3.3).

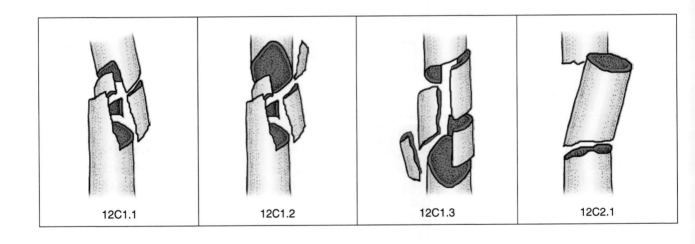

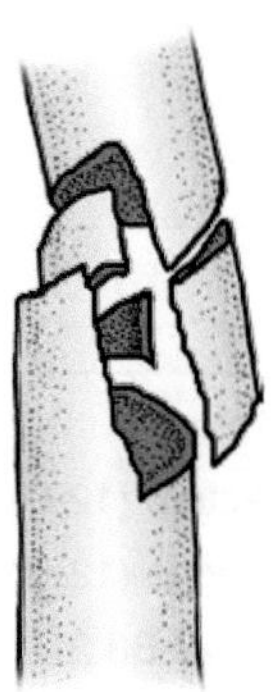

12C1.1

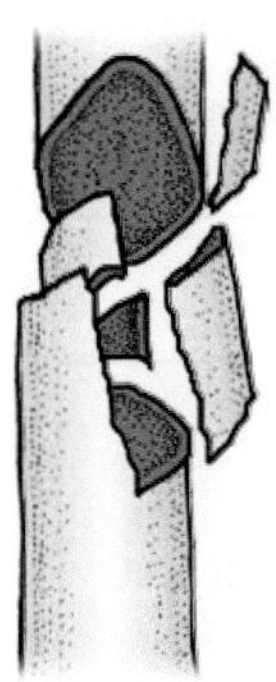

12C1.2

12C1.3

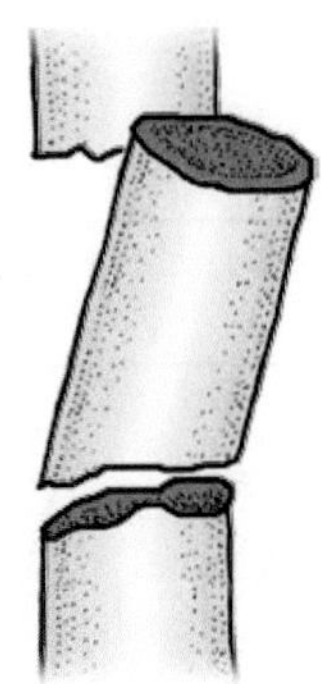

12C2.1

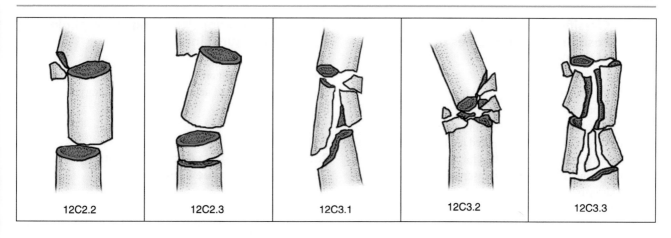

12C2.2

12C2.3

12C3.1

12C3.2

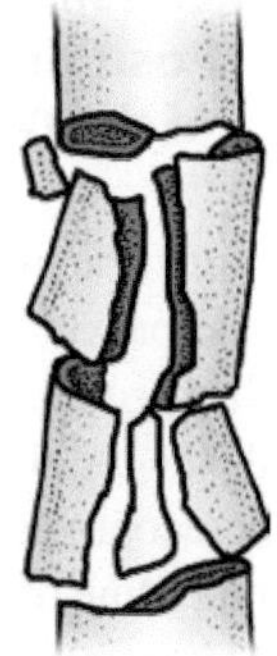
12C3.3

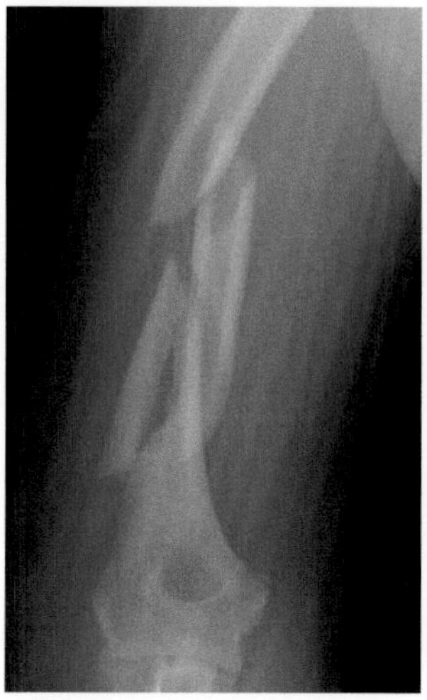
C1.1: With two intermediate fragments (12-C1.1)

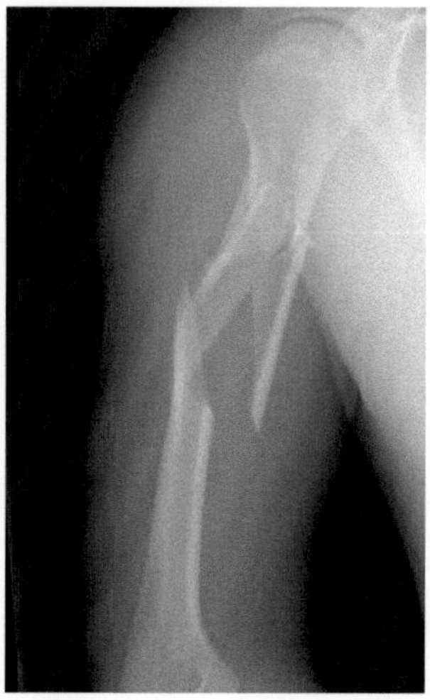
C1.2: With three intermediate fragments (12-C1.2)

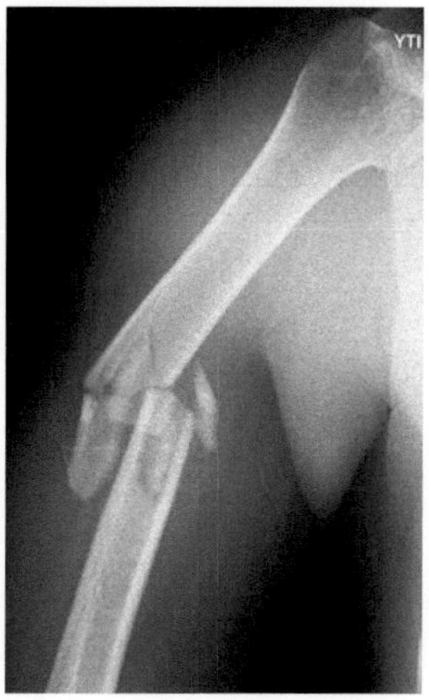

C1.3: With more than three intermediate fragments (12-C1.3)

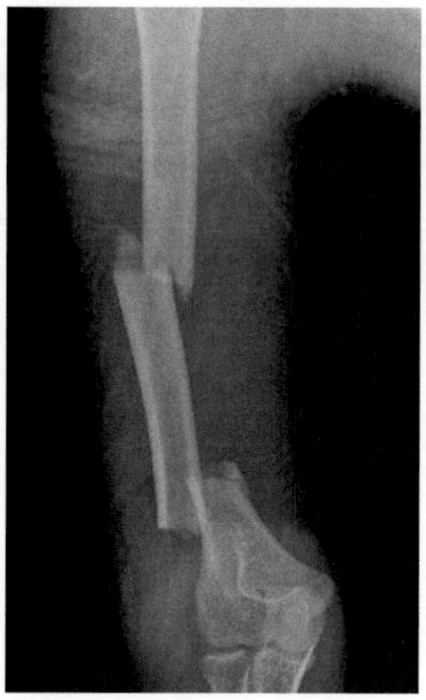
C2.1: With one intermediate segmental fragment (12-C2.1)

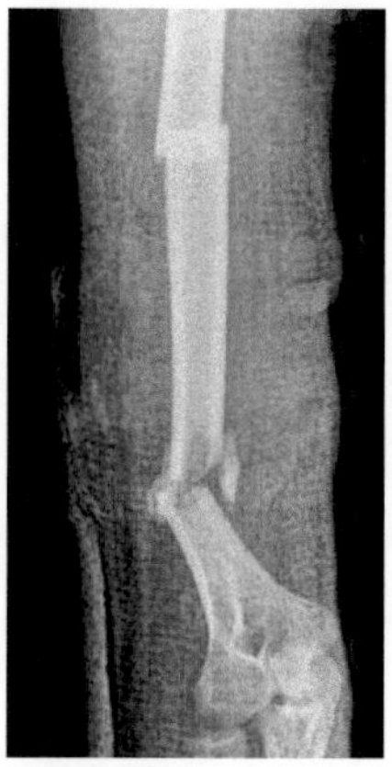
C2.2: With one intermediate segmental and additional wedge fragments (12-C2.2)

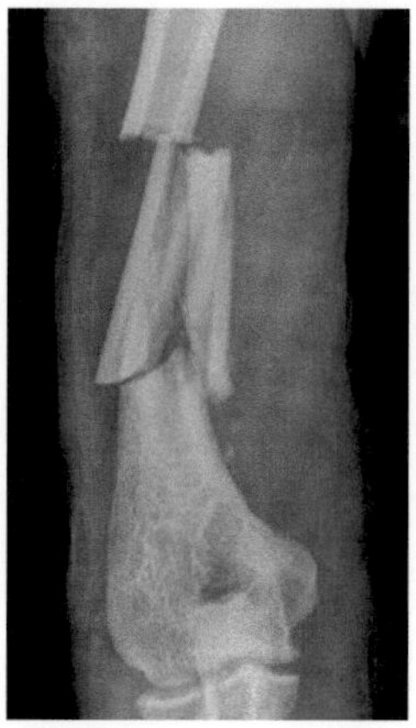
C2.3: With two intermediate segmental fragments (12-C2.3)

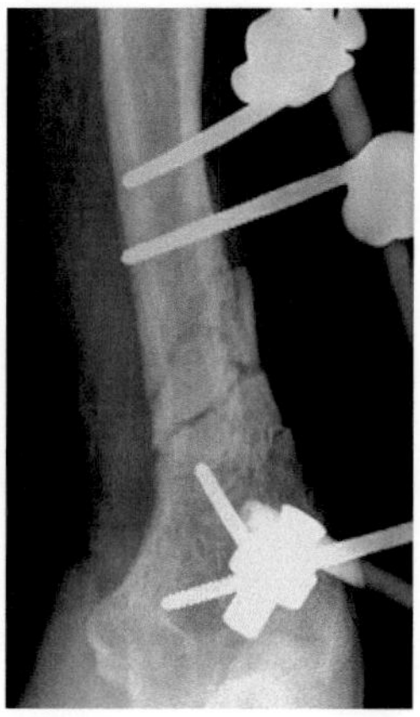
C3.2: With limited shattering (<4 cm) (12-C3.2)

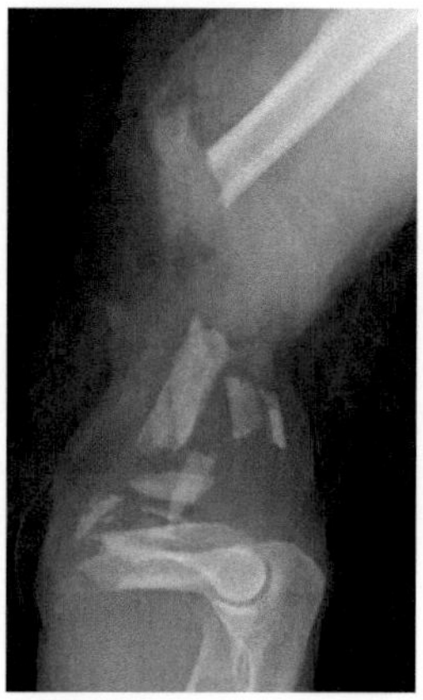
C3.3: With extensive shattering (>4 cm) (12-C3.3)

2.2.2 Classification According to Relative Position of Fracture Lines to Insertion of the Deltoid

1. Fracture line proximal to deltoid insertion of humerus:
   The proximal fragment is pulled medially and anteriorly by pectoralis major, latissimus dorsi, and teres major, while the distal fragment is pulled laterally and proximally by coracobrachialis, biceps brachii, and triceps brachii.
2. Fracture line distal to deltoid insertion of humerus:
   The proximal fragment is pulled laterally and anteriorly by the deltoid, while the distal fragment is pulled proximally by biceps brachii and triceps brachii.

2.2.3 Classification According to Anatomic Location of Fractures

Depending on the anatomic location of the fracture lines, fractures of the humeral shaft can be divided into proximal third, mid-third, and distal third.

2.2.4 Classification According to Morphology of Fracture Lines

Fractures of the humeral shaft can be transverse, oblique, spiral, or comminuted according to morphology of the fracture lines.

2.2.5 Classification According to Integrity of Soft-Tissue Envelope

Depending on whether the soft-tissue envelope at fracture site is integrated or not, there are two types: closed fracture and open fracture.

2.3 Classification of Distal Humeral Fractures

Distal humeral fractures are traditionally classified in accordance with the anatomic location. Reich first proposed the "T" shape and "Y" shape fractures in his classification of intercondylar fractures of the humerus in 1936. There have been >10 classification systems of distal humeral fractures to date in the literature. According to the literature over the last 5 years, the most commonly used system is the Jupiter classification, followed by the AO/OTA classification and that according to the anatomic location.

2.3.1 Jupiter Classification of Distal Humeral Fractures [4, 5]

The distal humerus consists of medial and lateral bony columns with an intervening trochlea.

The medial column ends ~1 cm proximal to the distal end of the trochlea, consisting of the medial cortex bone of the metaphysis and its extension, i.e., medial epicondyle. The lateral column extends to the level of the distal aspect of the trochlea, consisting of the lateral cortex bone of the metaphysis, lateral epicondyle, and capitellum. The trochlea, olecranon fossa, and coronoid fossa compose the inter-column triangle.

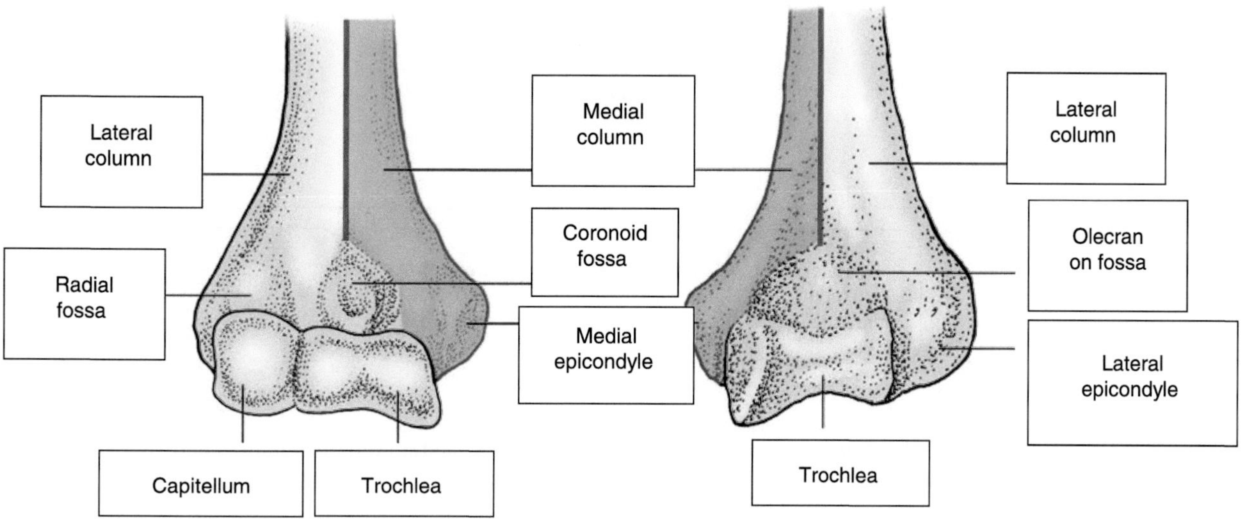

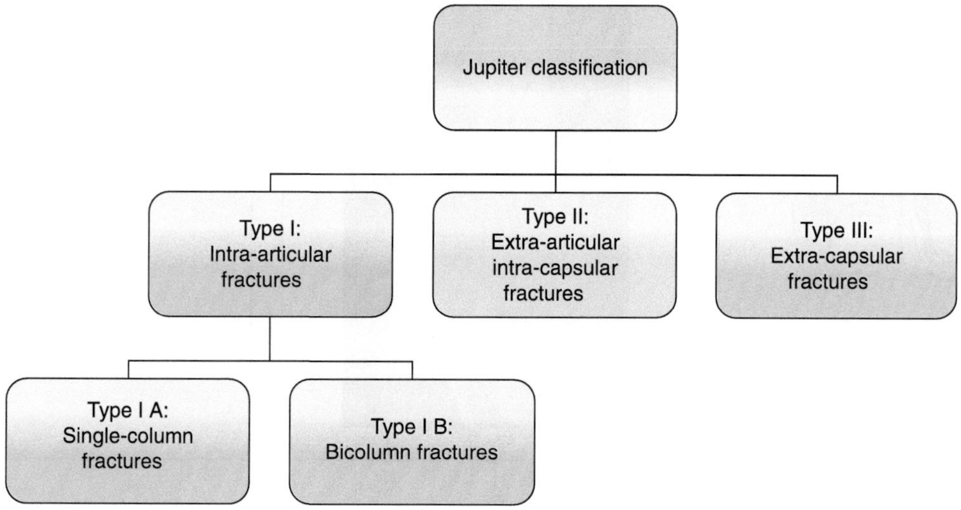

Type I: Intra-articular fractures:

Intra-articular fractures are divided into four groups, including single-column injury, bicolumn injury, capitellar fractures, and trochlea fractures.

- Type IA: Single-column fractures. Single-columnar injuries are divided into medial or lateral column fractures and subdivided into high and low fractures.
- Type IB: Bicolumn fractures. Subdivided into high "T", low "T", "Y", "H", and medial lambda, lateral lambda patterns.

Type II: Extra-articular intra-capsular fractures:

Transcolumn fractures, subdivided into high-extension fracture, high-flexion fracture, low-extension fracture, low-flexion fracture, abduction fracture, and adduction fracture.

Type III: Extracapsular fractures:

- Type IIIA: Medial epicondyle.
- Type IIIB: Lateral epicondyle.

2.3.1.1 Type I A: Intra-articular Fracture, Single-Column Fracture

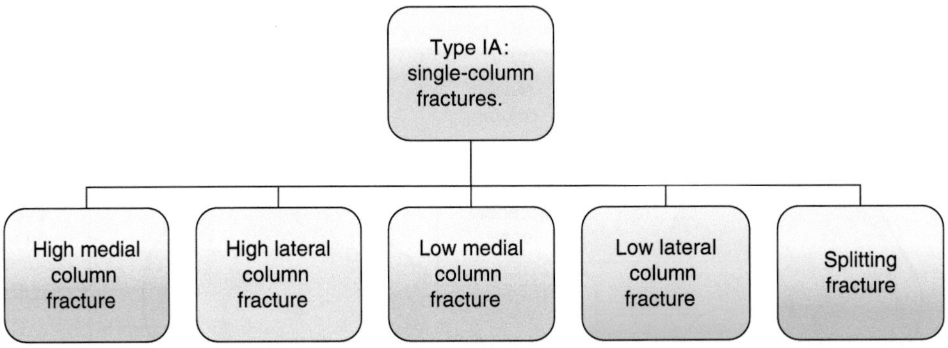

Single-column fractures: Single- columnar injuries are divided into medial or lateral column fractures and subdivided into high and low fractures, and splitting fractures.

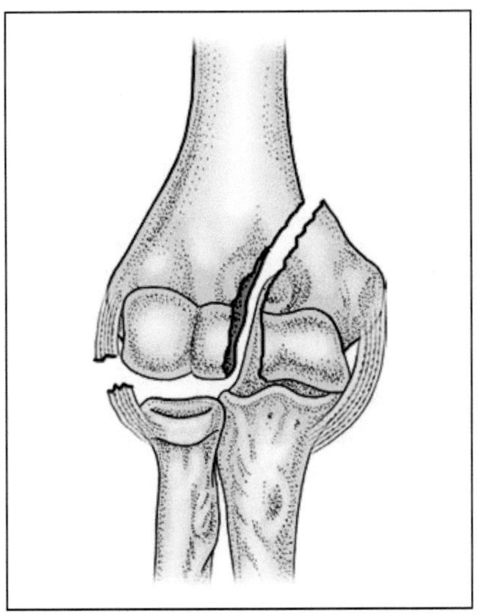

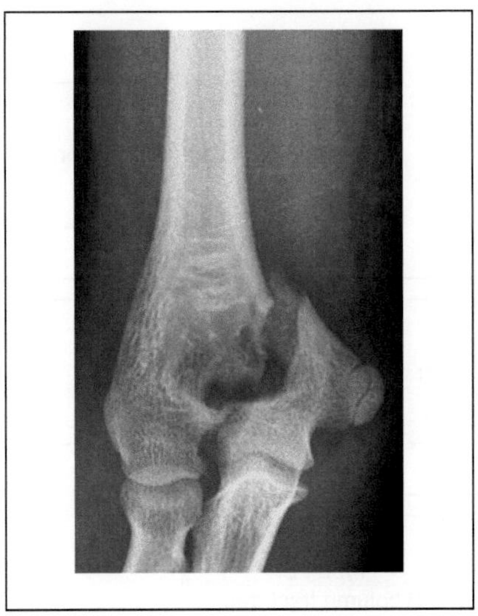

Jupiter classification

Type I A: Intra-articular fracture

Single-column fracture

High medial column fracture

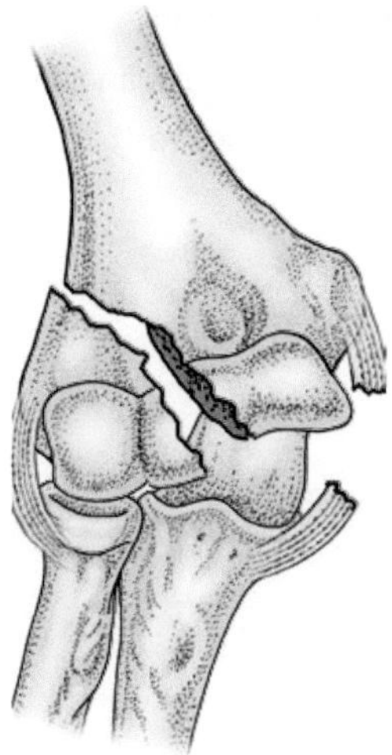

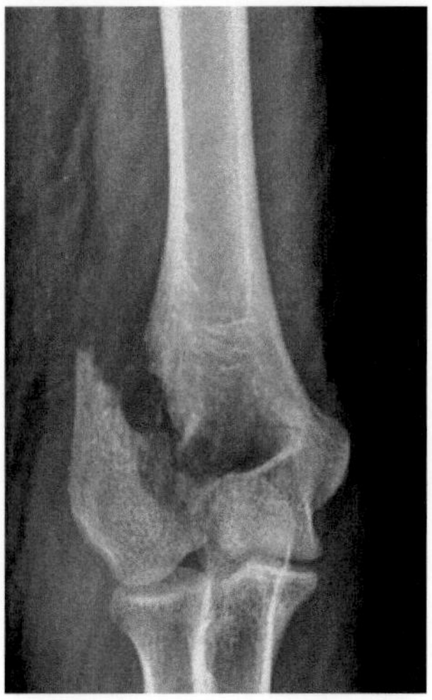

Jupiter classification

Type I A: Intra-articular fracture

Single-column fracture

High lateral column fracture

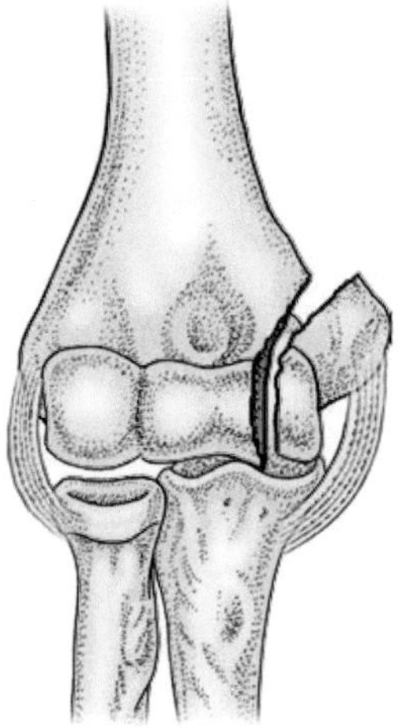

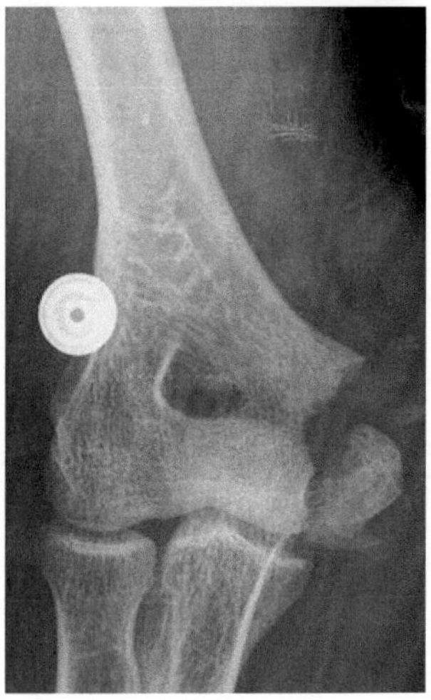

Jupiter classification

Type I A: Intra-articular fracture

Single-column fracture

Low medial column fracture

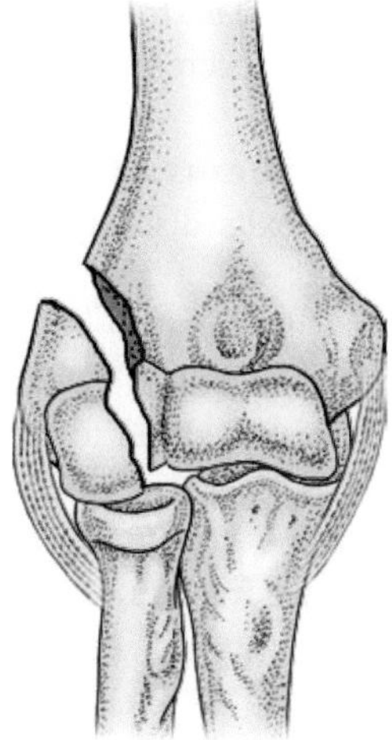

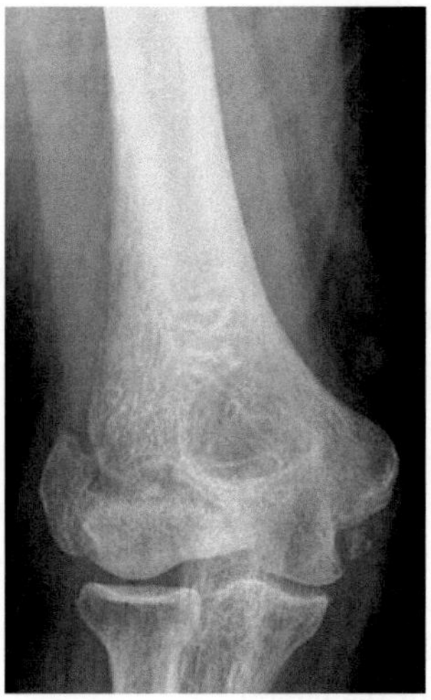

Jupiter classification

Type I A: Intra-articular fracture

Single-column fracture

Low lateral column fracture

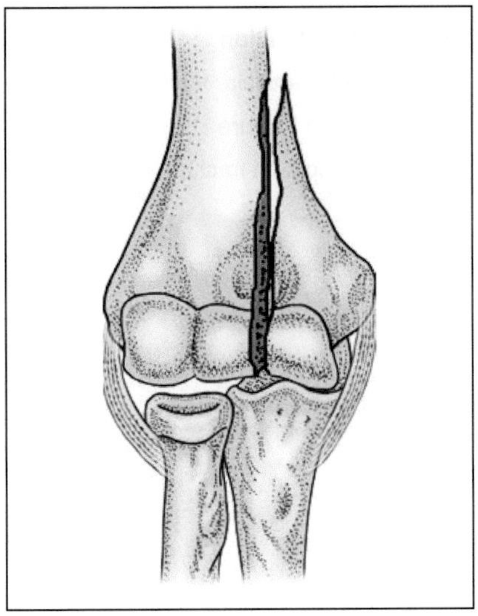

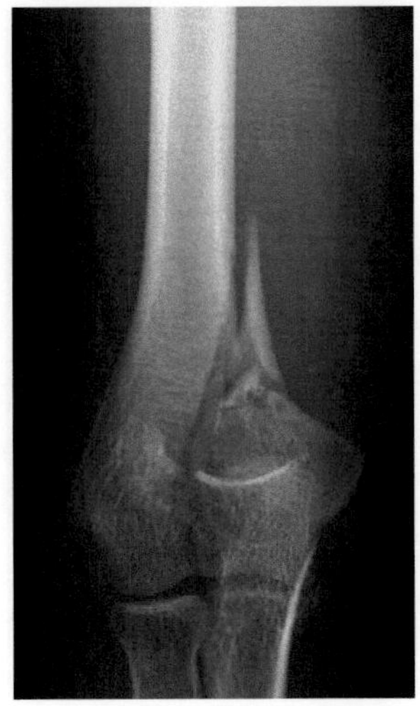

Jupiter classification

Type I A: Intra-articular fracture

Single-column fracture

Splitting fracture

2.3.1.2 Type I B: Intra-articular Fractures, Bicolumn Fractures

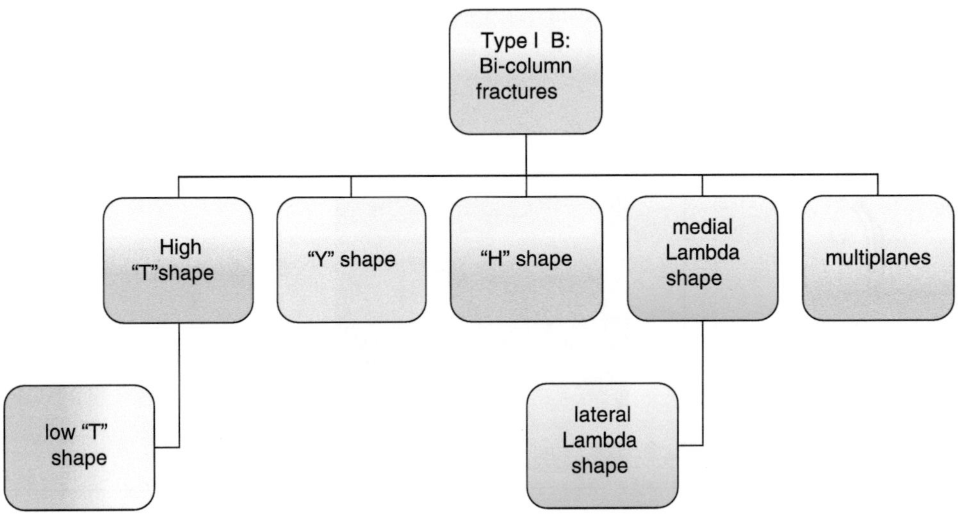

1. High "T" shape
   The fracture lines are T shape. A transverse fracture line divides both columns proximal to or at the upper limits of the olecranon fossa.
2. Low "T" shape
   The fracture lines are T shape. A transverse fracture line crosses the olecranon fossa, usually just proximal to the trochlea, leaving relatively small distal fragments.
3. "Y" shape
   The fracture lines are Y shape. Oblique fracture lines cross each column, joining into the olecranon fossa, extending distally as a vertical line.
4. "H" shape
   Fracture lines of the medial column are above and below the medial epicondyle. Fracture lines of the lateral column are in a T or Y pattern. The trochlea is a free fragment and at risk for avascular necrosis.
5. Medial lambda shape
   The most proximal fracture line exits at the medial column. The lateral fracture line exits distal to the lateral epicondyle.
6. Lateral lambda shape
   The most proximal fracture line exits at the lateral column. The medial fracture line exits distal to the medial epicondyle.
7. Multiplanes: Standard T-shape fractures of distal humerus, combined with another fracture of which fracture lines, are in coronal plane.

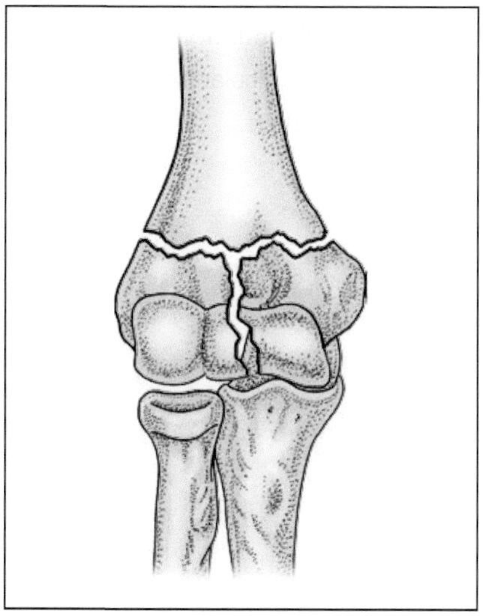

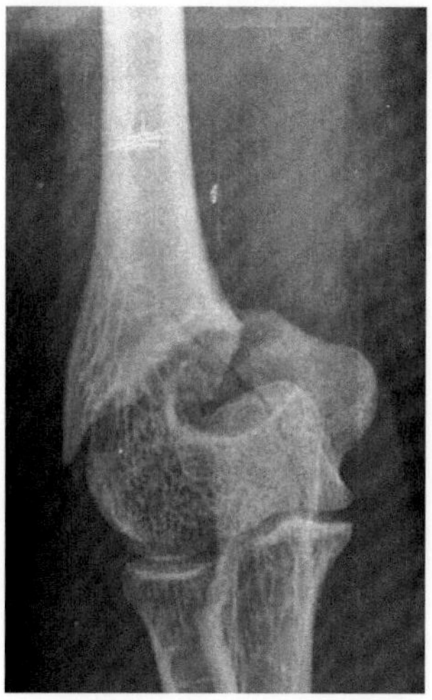

Jupiter classification

Type I B: Intra-articular fractures

Bicolumn fractures

High "T" shape

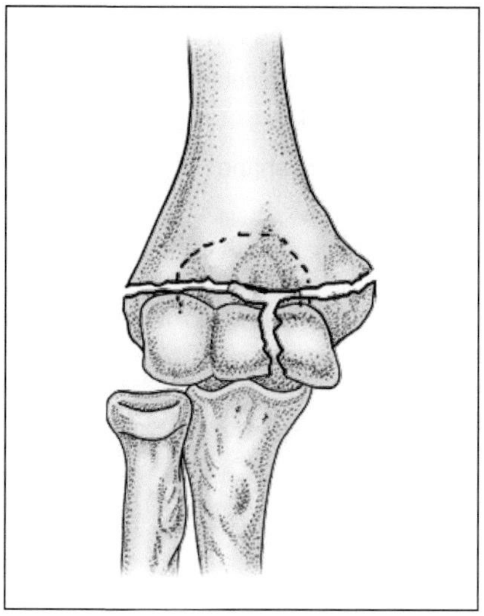

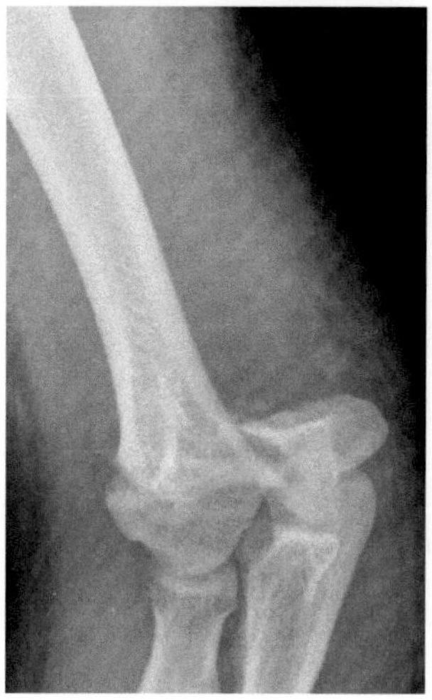

Jupiter classification

Type I B: Intra-articular fractures

Bicolumn fractures

Low "T" shape

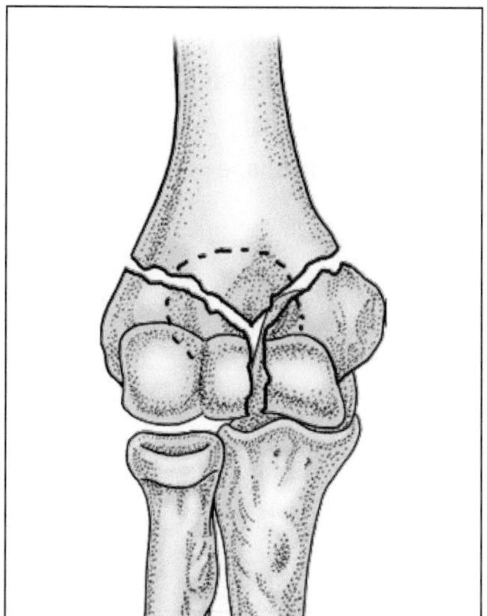

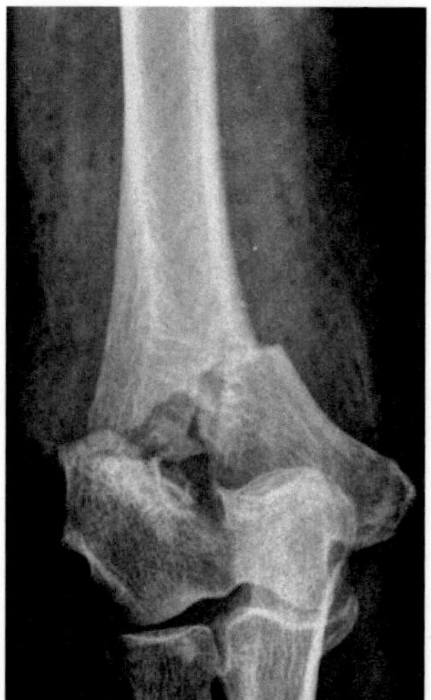

Jupiter classification

Type I B: Intra-articular fractures

Bicolumn fractures

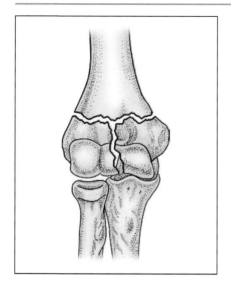

"Y" shape

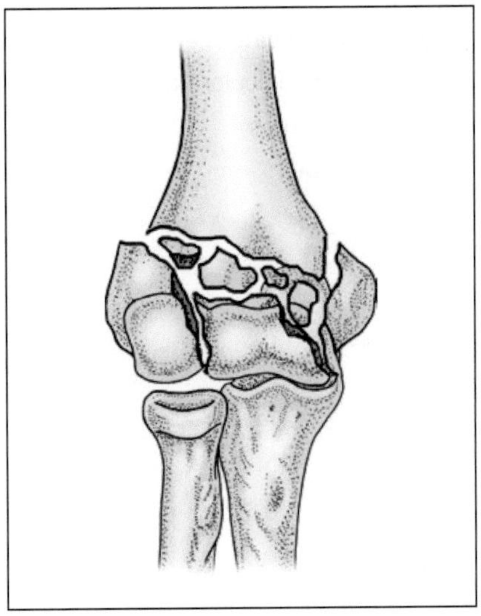

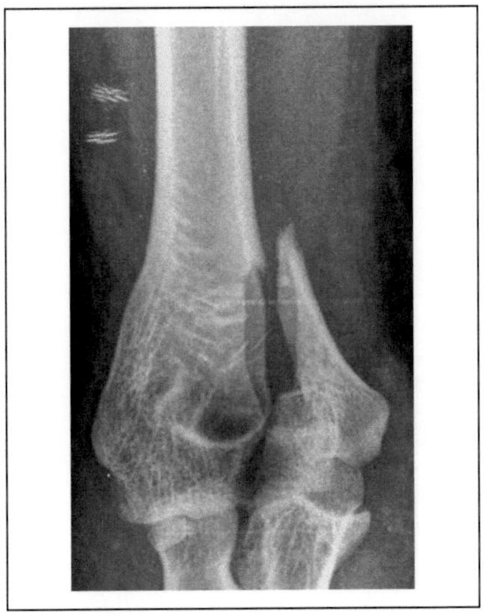

Jupiter classification

Type I B: Intra-articular fractures

Bicolumn fractures

"H" shape

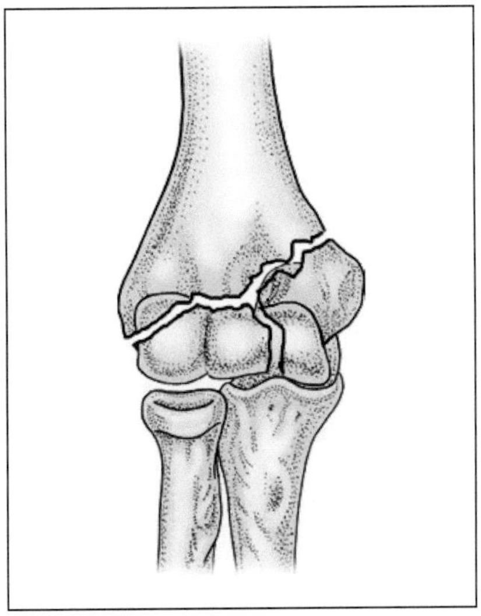

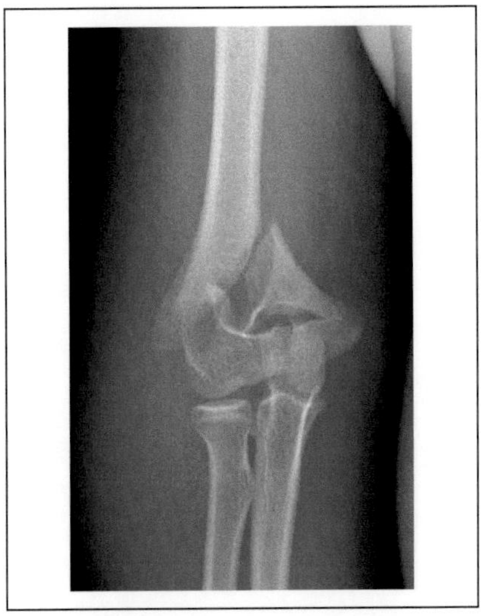

Jupiter classification

Type I B: Intra-articular fractures

Bicolumn fractures

Medial lambda shape

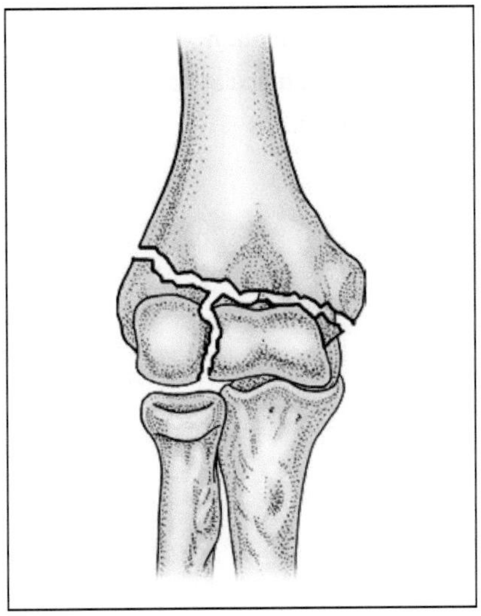

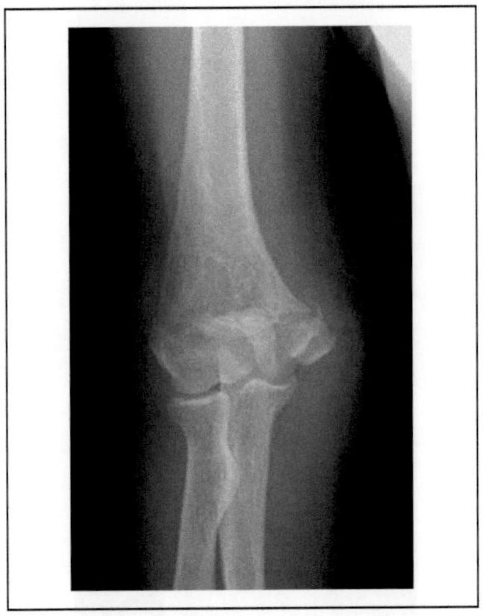

Jupiter classification

Type I B: Intra-articular fractures

Bicolumn fractures

Lateral lambda shape

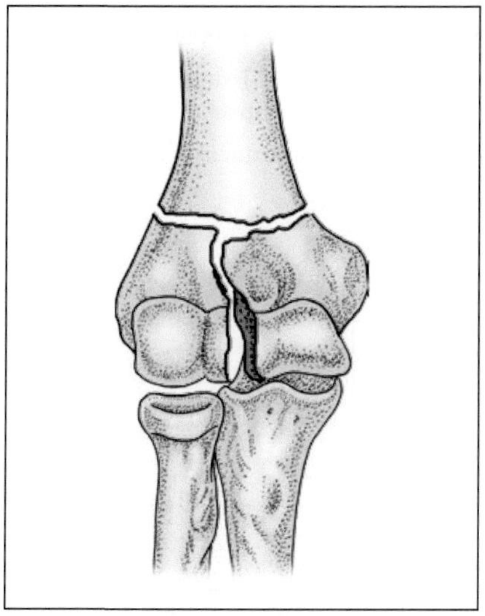

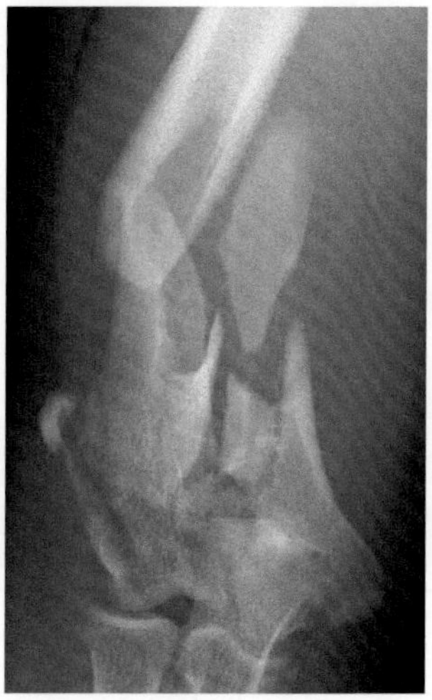

Jupiter classification

Type I B: Intra-articular fractures

Bicolumn fractures

Multiplanes

2.3.1.3 Type II: Extra-Articular Intra-capsular Fractures, Transcolumn Fractures

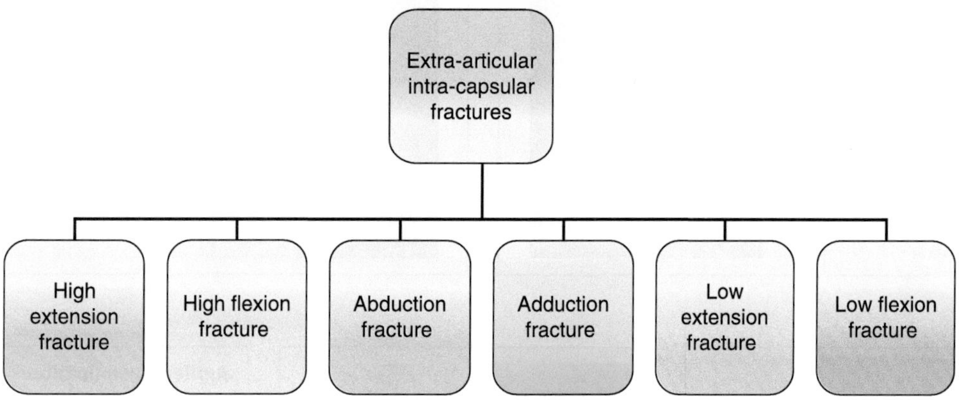

1. **High-extension fracture**: The oblique fracture line extends from a posterior proximal position to a low anterior position, and the distal fragment is displaced posteriorly (the same with the extension-type supracondylar fractures).
2. **High-flexion fracture**: The oblique fracture line extends from an anterior proximal position to a low posterior position, and the distal fragment is displaced anteriorly (the same with the flexion-type supracondylar fractures).
3. **Abduction fracture**: The oblique fracture line extends from a lateral proximal position to a distal medial position, and the distal fragment is displaced laterally.
4. **Adduction fracture**: The oblique fracture line extends from a medial proximal position to a distal lateral position, and the distal fragment is displaced medially.
5. **Low-extension fracture**: The fracture line is transverse or slightly oblique, and the distal fragment is displaced posteriorly.
6. **Low-flexion fracture**: The fracture line is transverse or slightly oblique, and the distal fragment is displaced anteriorly.

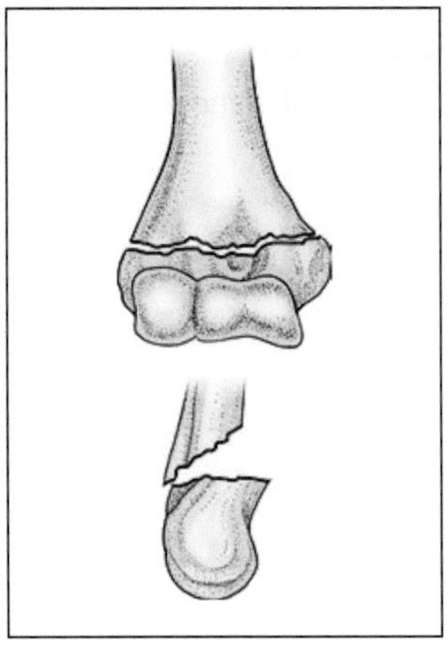
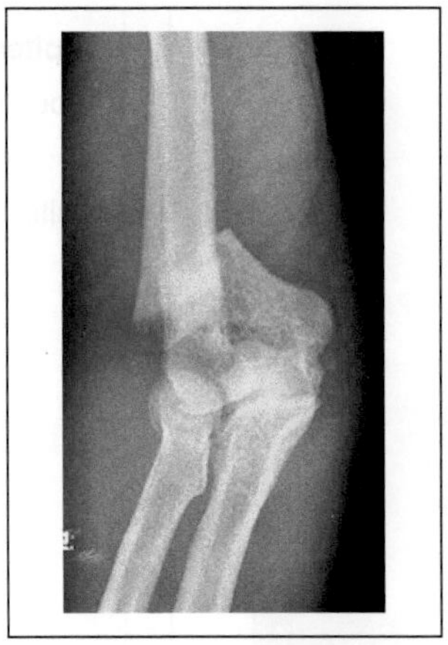
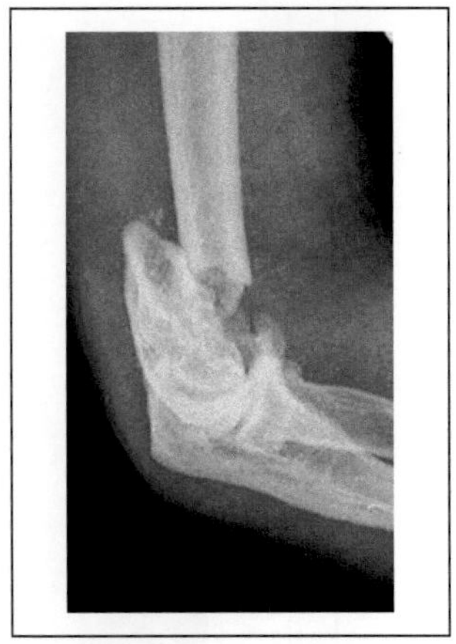

Jupiter classification

Type II: Extra-articular intra-capsular fractures.

High-extension fracture

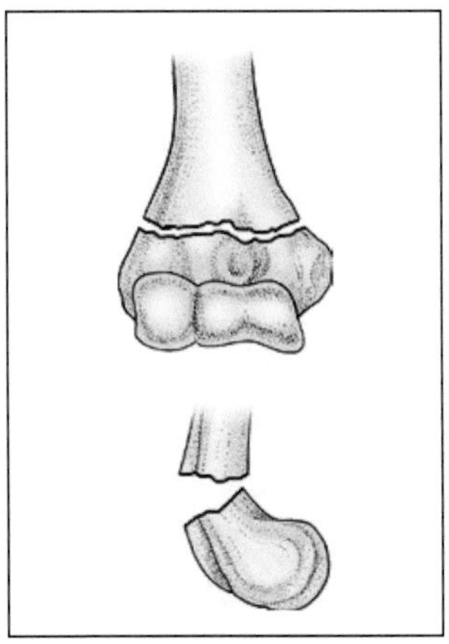
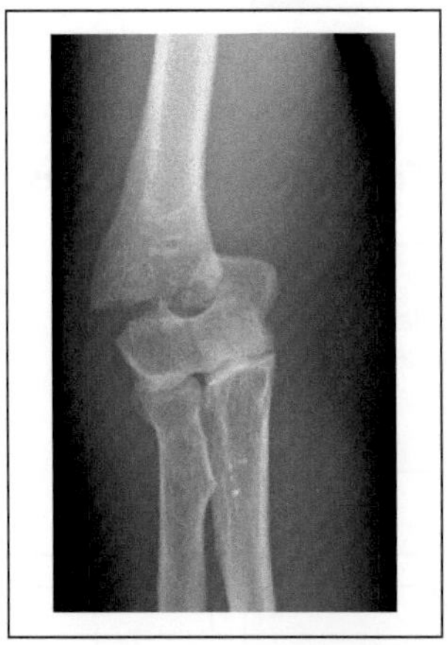
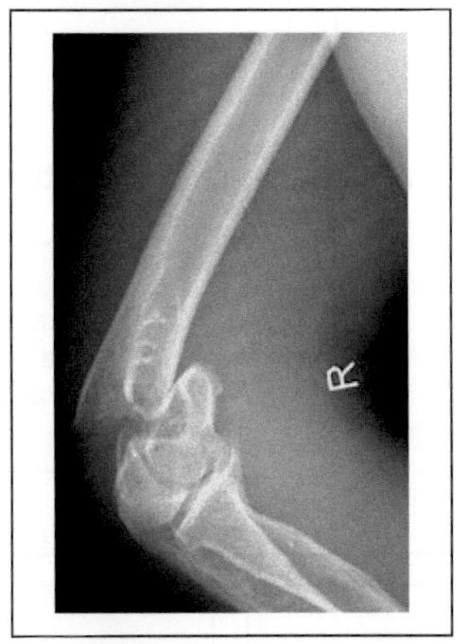

Jupiter classification

Type II: Extra-articular intra-capsular fractures.

High-flexion fracture

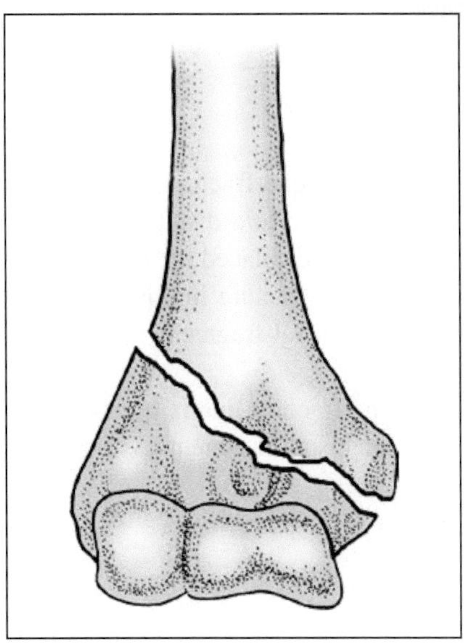
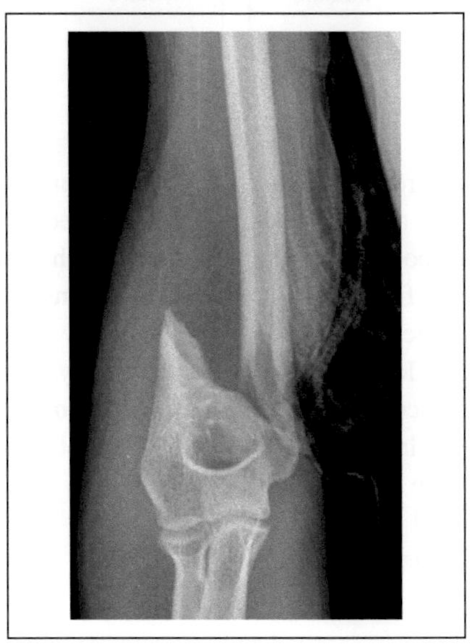

Jupiter classification

Type II: Extra-articular intra-capsular fractures.

Abduction fracture

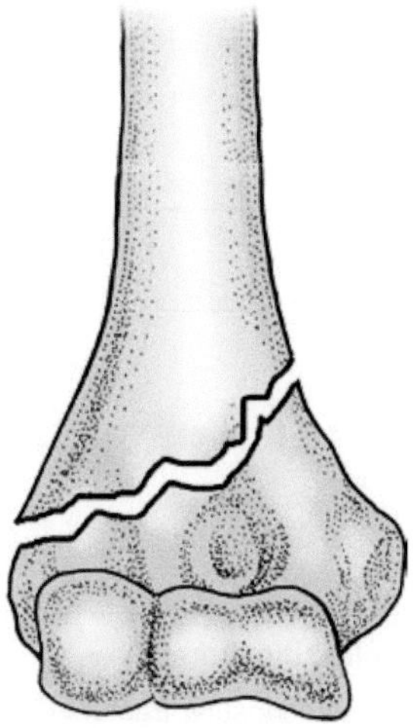

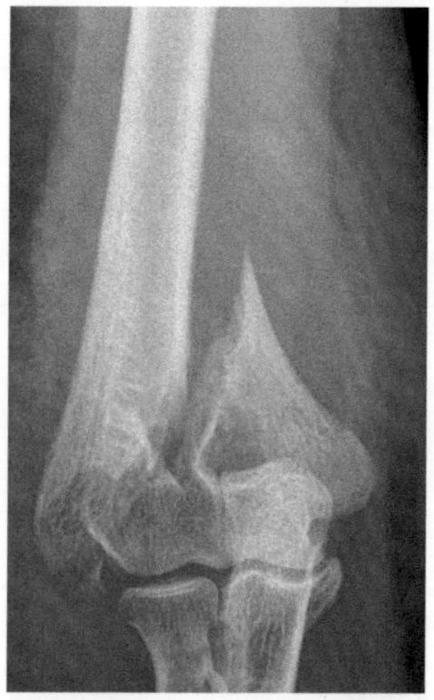

Jupiter classification

Type II: Extra-articular intra-capsular fractures.

Adduction fracture

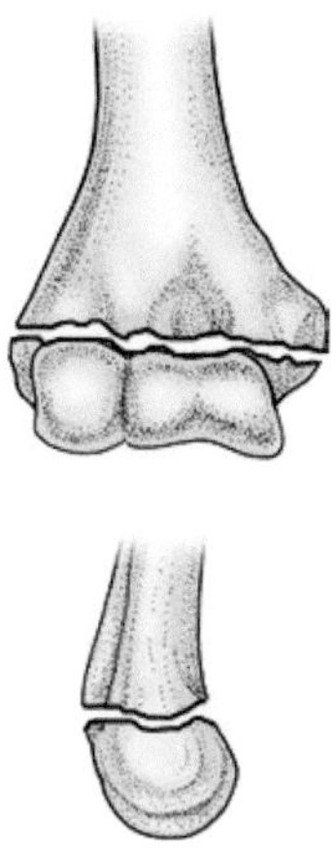

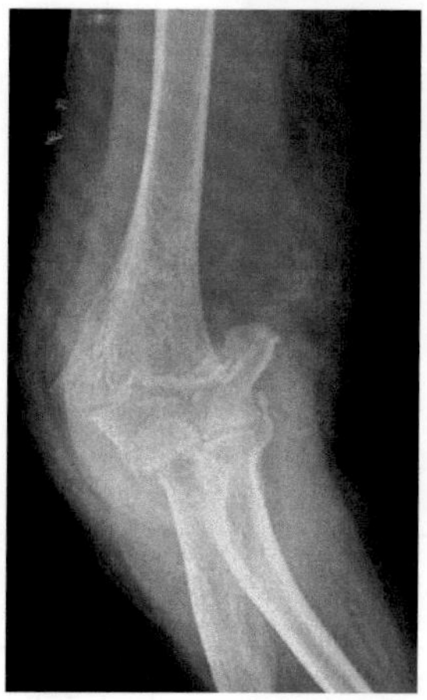

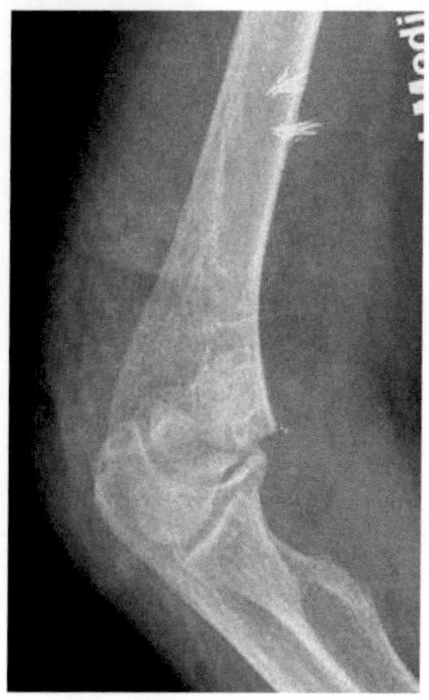

Jupiter classification

Type II: Extra-articular intra-capsular fractures.

Low-extension fracture

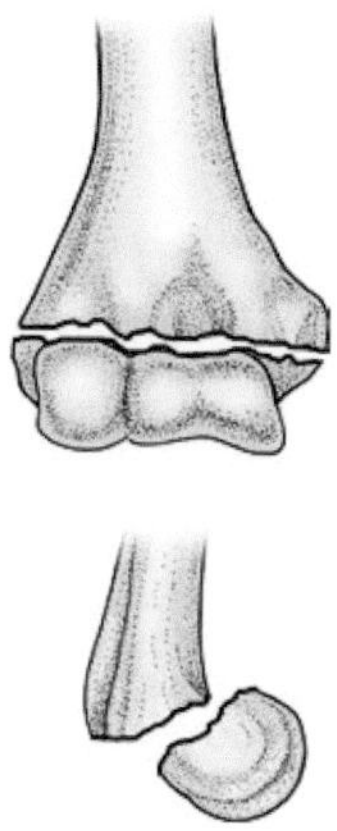

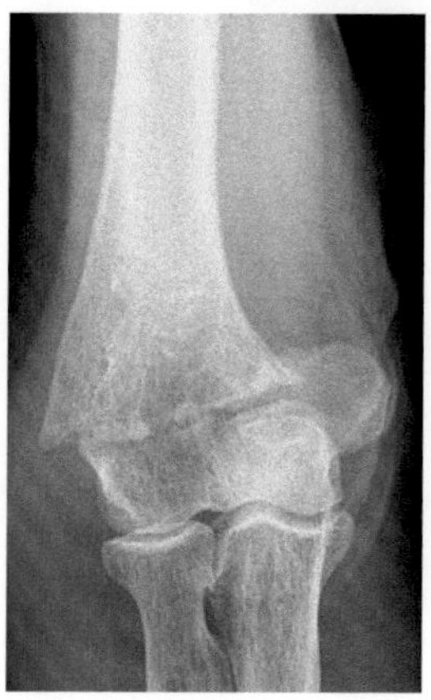

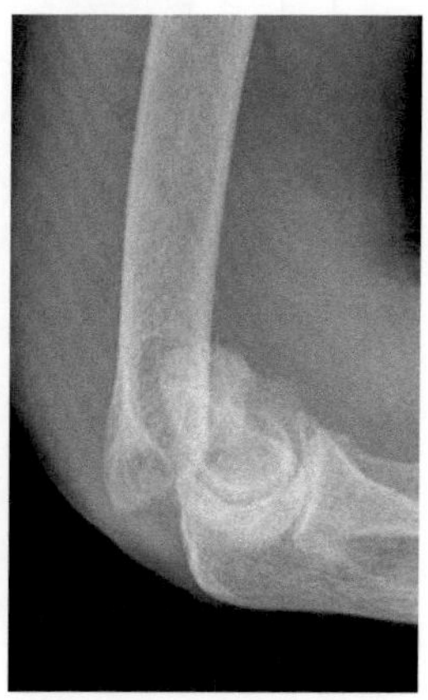

Jupiter classification

Type II: Extra-articular intra-capsular fractures.

Low-flexion fracture

2.3.1.4 Type III: Extracapsular Fractures

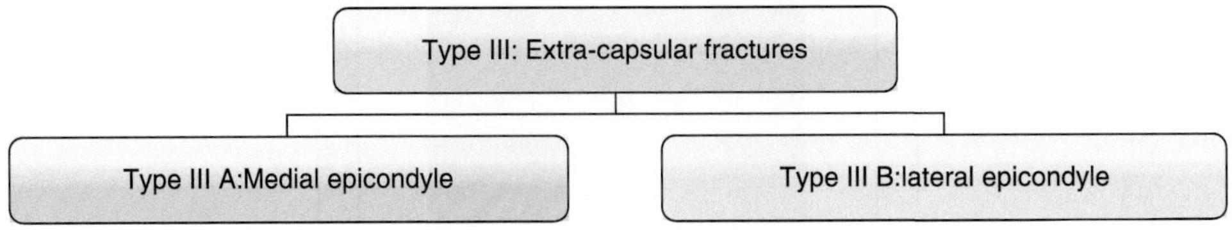

Type III A: Medial epicondyle.
Type III B: Lateral epicondyle.

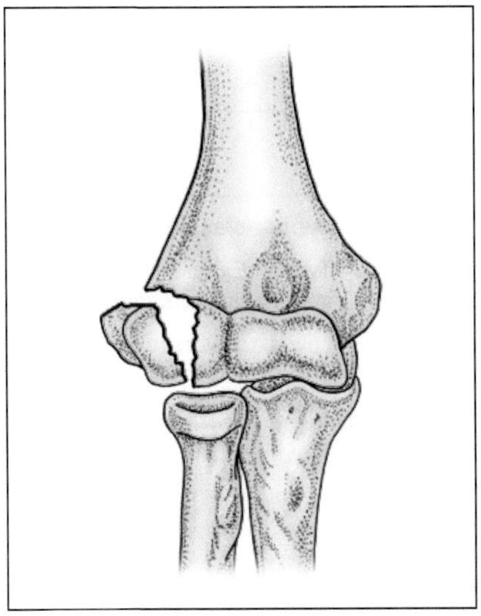

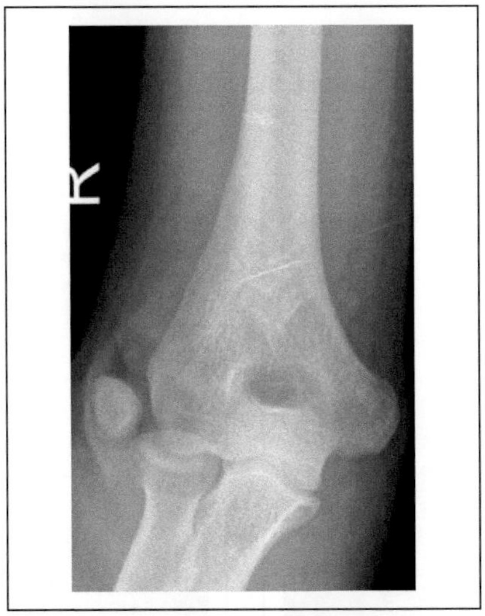

Jupiter classification

Type III: Extracapsular fractures.

Type III B: Lateral epicondyle

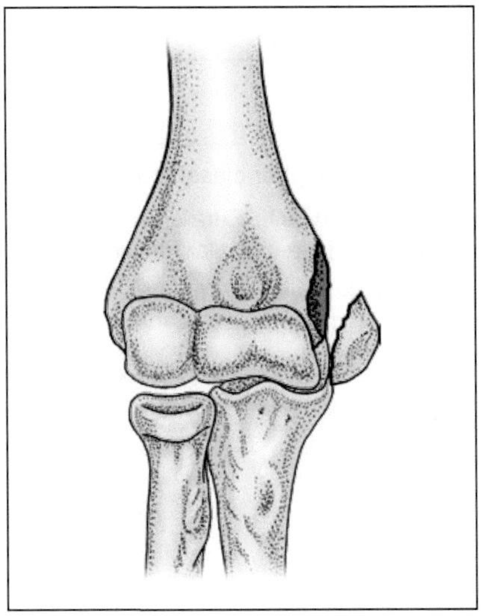

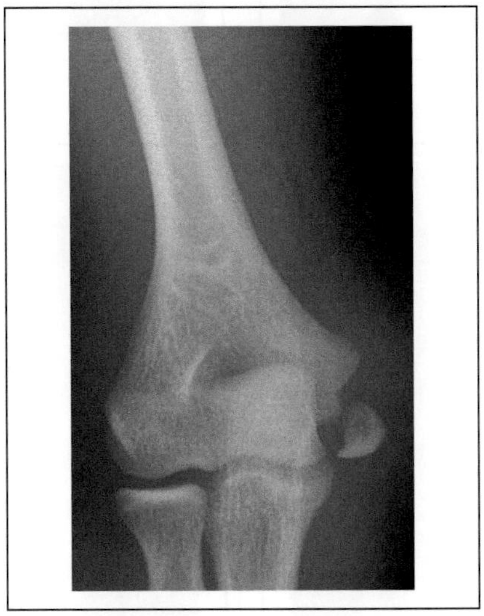

Jupiter classification

Type III: Extracapsular fractures.

Type III A: Medial epicondyle

2.3.2 AO/OTA Classification [2]

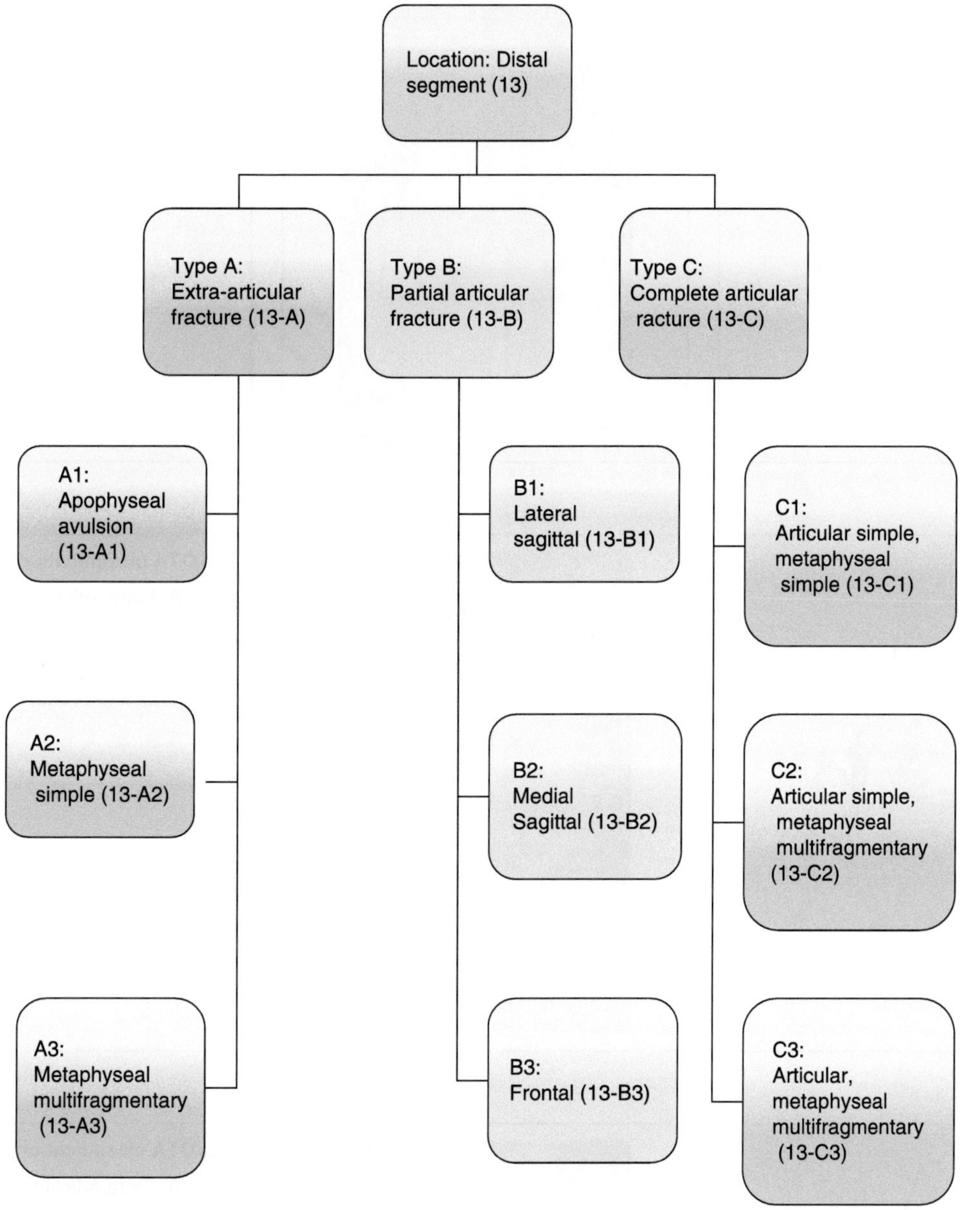

Type A: Extra-articular fracture (13-A).
- A1: Apophyseal avulsion (13-A1):
  - A1.1: Lateral epicondyle (13-A1.1).
  - A1.2: Medial epicondyle, non-incarcerated (13-A1.2).
  - A1.3: Medial epicondyle, incarcerated (13-A1.3).
- A2: Metaphyseal simple (13-A2):
  - A2.1: Oblique downwards and inwards (13-A2.1).
  - A2.2: Oblique downwards and outwards (13-A2.2).
  - A2.3: Transverse (13-A2.3).
- A3: Metaphyseal multifragmentary (13-A3):
  - A3.1: With intact wedge (13-A3.1).
  - A3.2: With fragmented wedge (13-A3.2).
  - A3.3: Complex (13-A3.3).

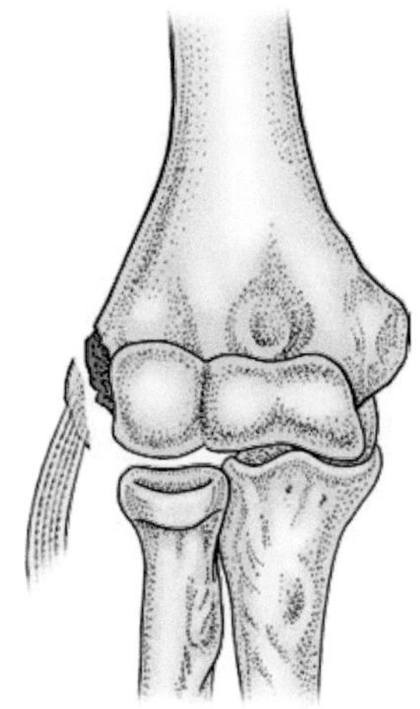

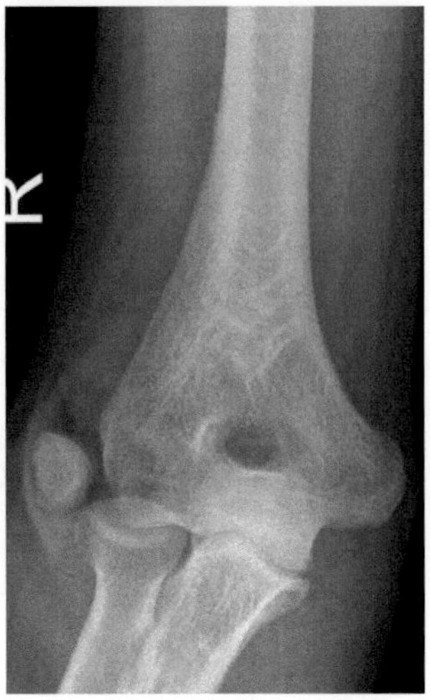

AO/OTA classification

Type A: Extra-articular fracture (13-A)

A1: Apophyseal avulsion (13-A1)

A1.1: Lateral epicondyle (13-A1.1)

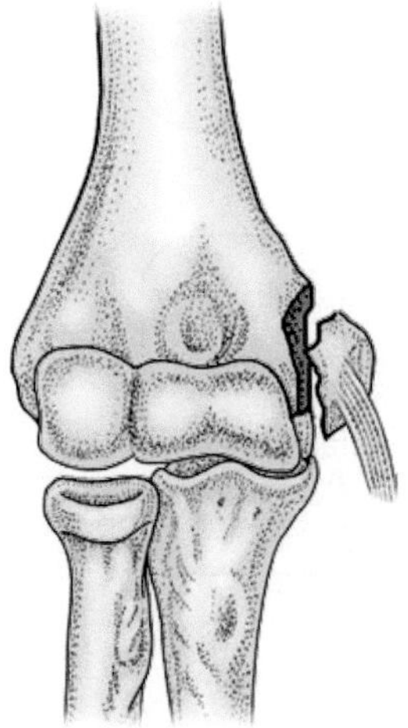

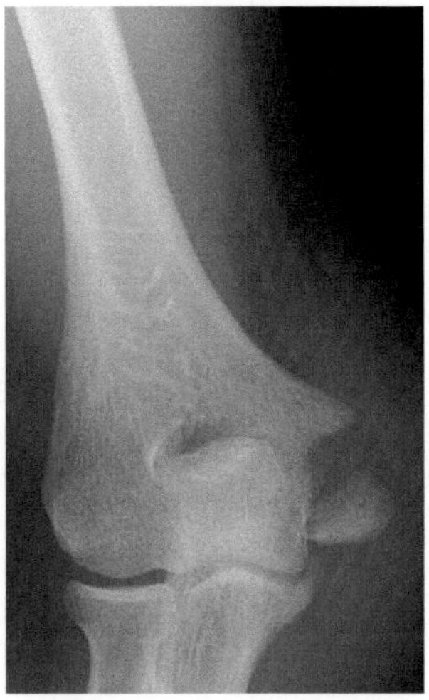

AO/OTA classification

Type A: Extra-articular fracture (13-A)

A1: Apophyseal avulsion (13-A1)

A1.2: Medial epicondyle, non-incarcerated (13-A1.2)

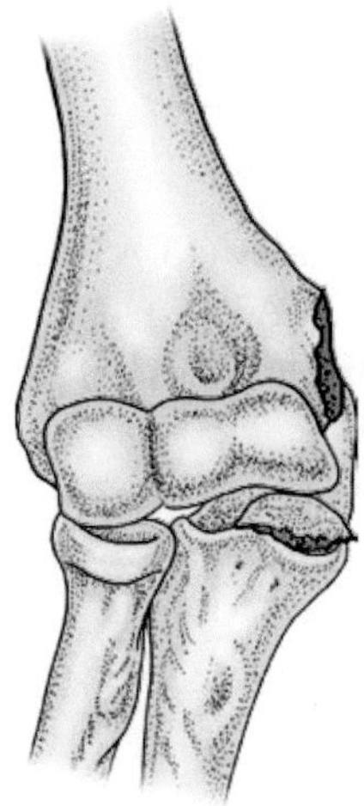

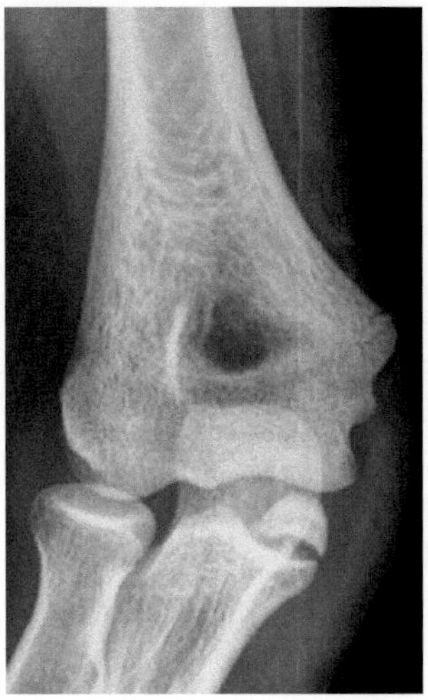

AO/OTA classification

Type A: Extra-articular fracture (13-A)

A1: Apophyseal avulsion (13-A1)

A1.3: Medial epicondyle, incarcerated (13-A1.3)

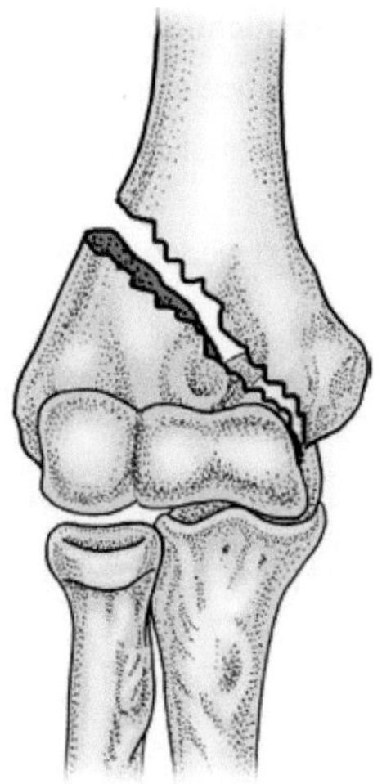

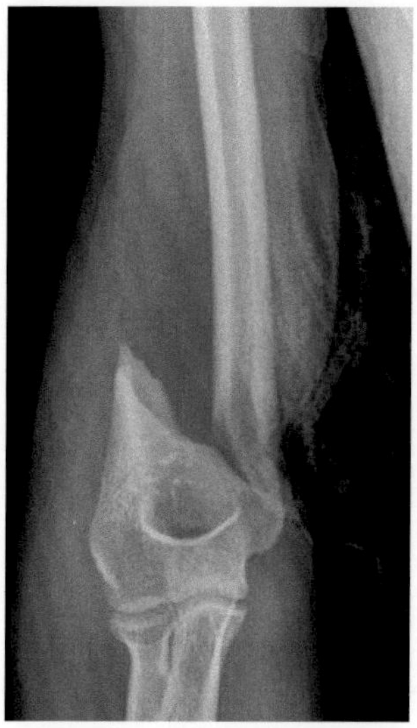

AO/OTA classification

Type A: Extra-articular fracture (13-A)

A2: Metaphyseal simple (13-A2)

A2.1: Oblique downwards and inwards (13-A2.1)

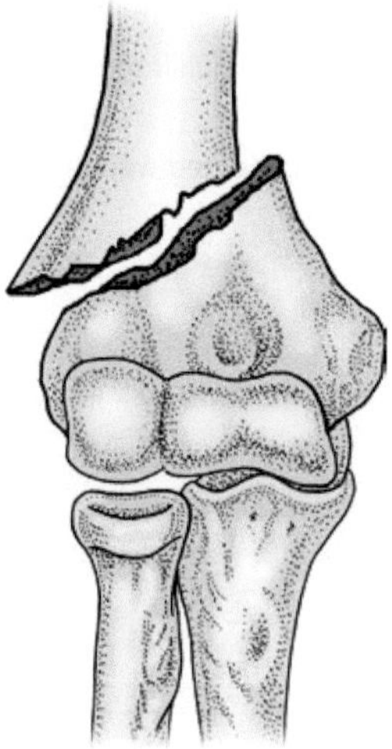

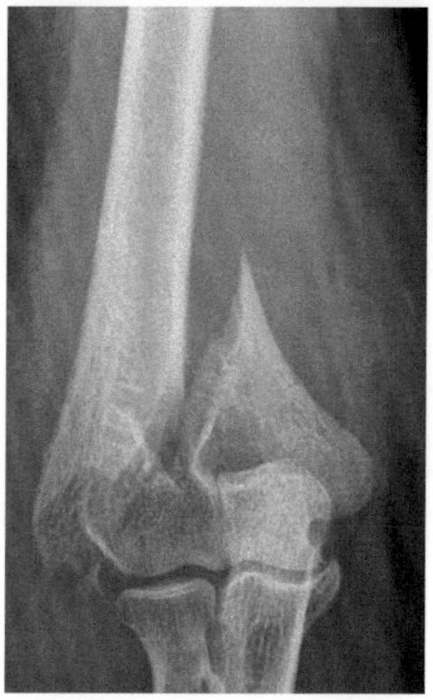

AO/OTA classification

Type A: Extra-articular fracture (13-A)

A2: Metaphyseal simple (13-A2)

A2.2: Oblique downwards and outwards (13-A2.2)

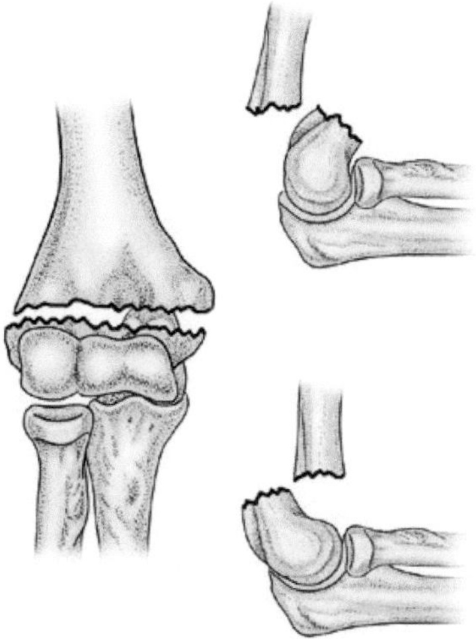

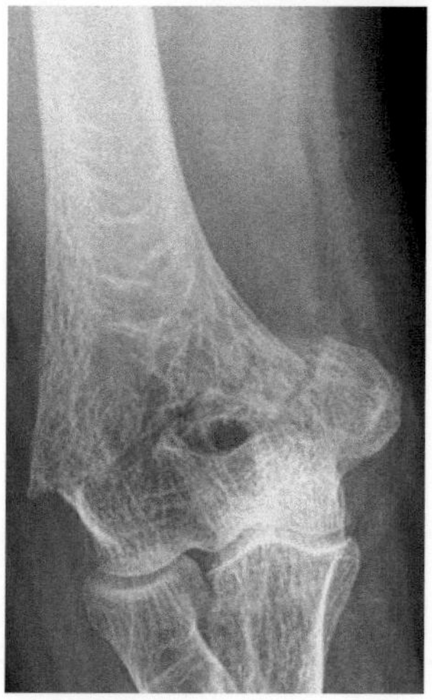

AO/OTA classification

Type A: Extra-articular fracture (13-A)

A2: Metaphyseal simple (13-A2)

A2.3: Transverse (13-A2.3)

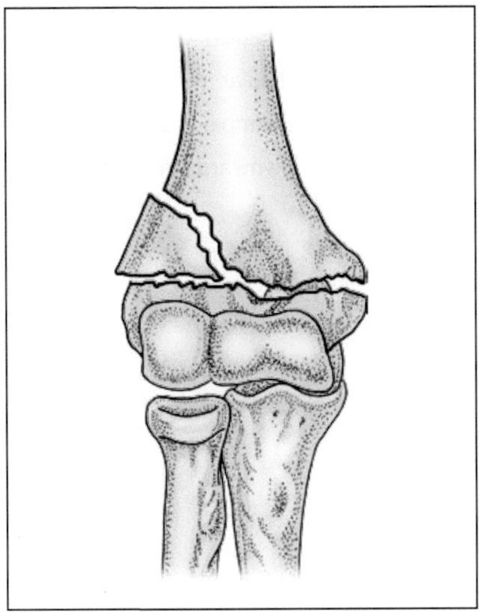

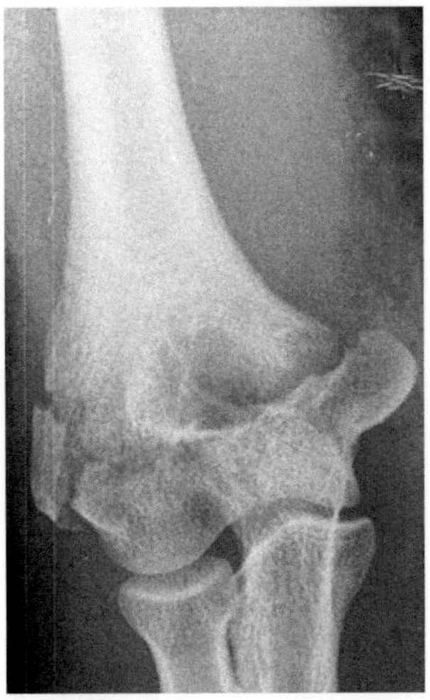

AO/OTA classification

Type A: Extra-articular fracture (13-A)

A3: Metaphyseal multifragmentary (13-A3)

A3.1: With intact wedge (13-A3.1)

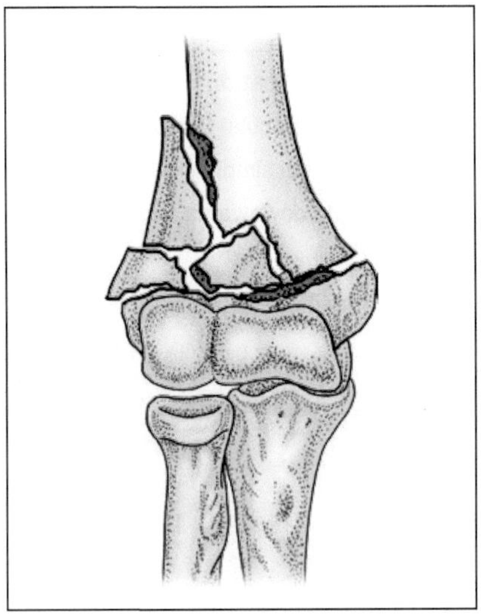

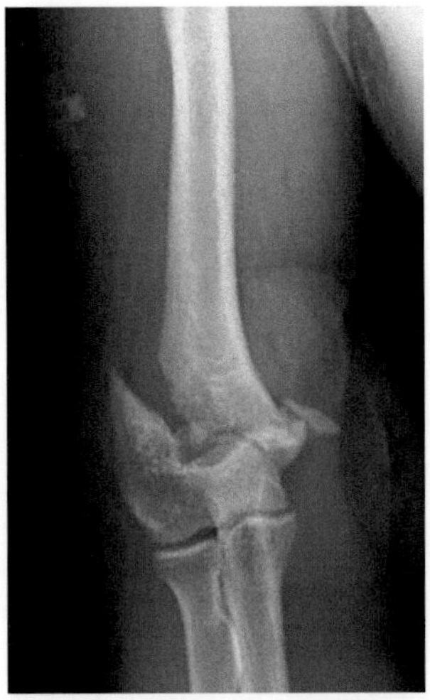

AO/OTA classification

Type A: Extra-articular fracture (13-A)

A3: Metaphyseal multifragmentary (13-A3)

A3.2: With fragmented wedge (13-A3.2)

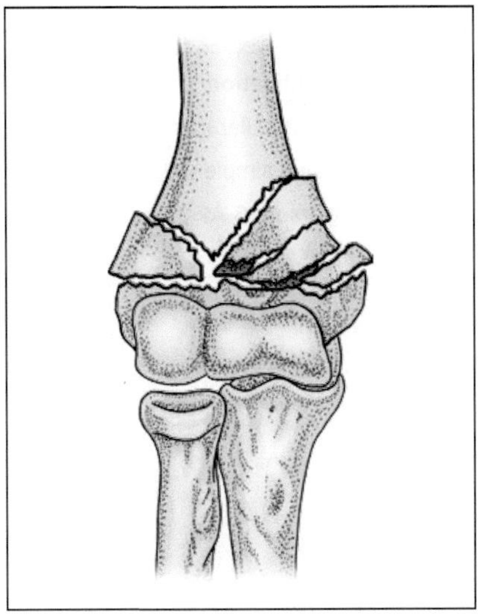

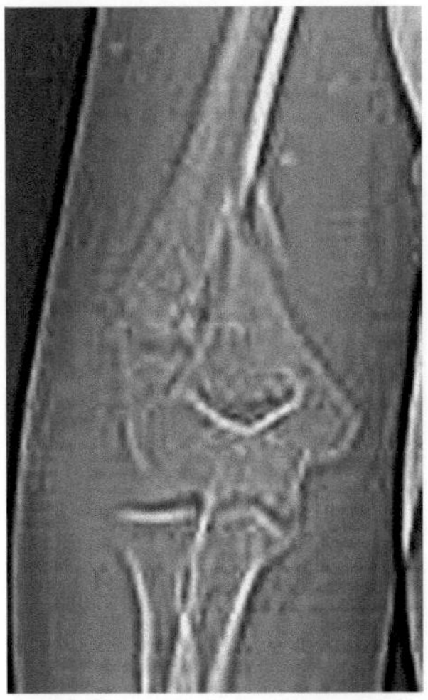

AO/OTA Classification

Type A: Extra-articular fracture (13-A).

A3: Metaphyseal multifragmentary (13-A3)

A3.3: Complex (13-A3.3)

Type B: Partial articular fracture (13-B).

B1: Lateral sagittal (13-B1):

B1.1: Capitellum (13-B1.1).

B1.2: Transtrochlear simple (13-B1.2).

B1.3: Transtrochlear multifragmentary (13-B1.3).

B2: Medial sagittal (13-B2):

B2.1: Transtrochlear simple, through medial side (Milch I) (13-B2.1).

B2.2: Transtrochlear simple, through the groove (13-B2.2).

B2.3: Transtrochlear multifragmentary (13-B2.3).

B3: Frontal (13-B3):

B3.1: Capitellum (13-B3.1).

B3.2: Trochlea (13-B3.2).

B3.3: Capitellum and trochlea (13-B3.3).

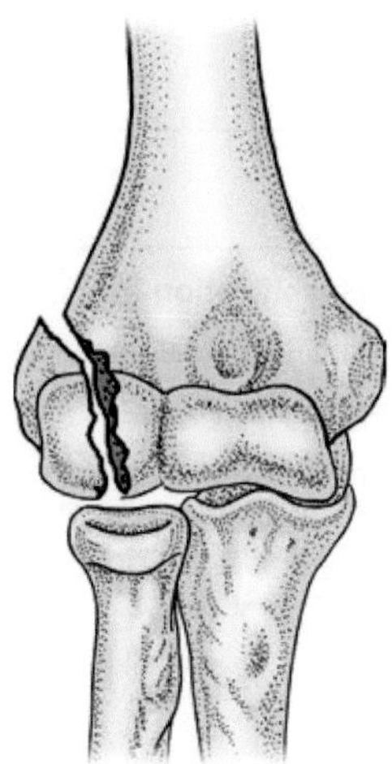

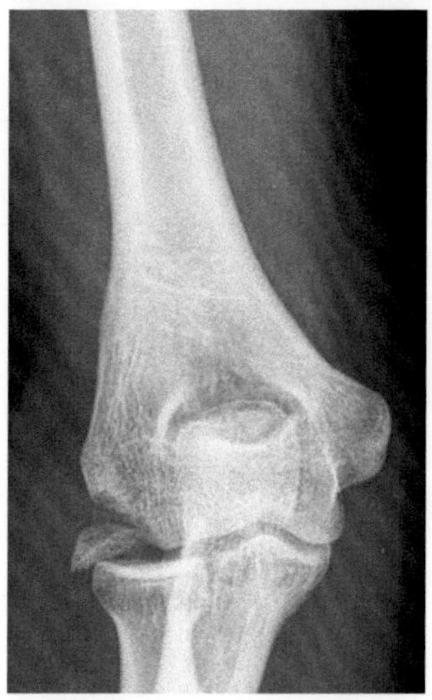

AO/OTA classification

Type B: Partial articular fracture (13-B).

B1: Lateral sagittal (13-B1).

B1.1: Capitellum (13-B1.1)

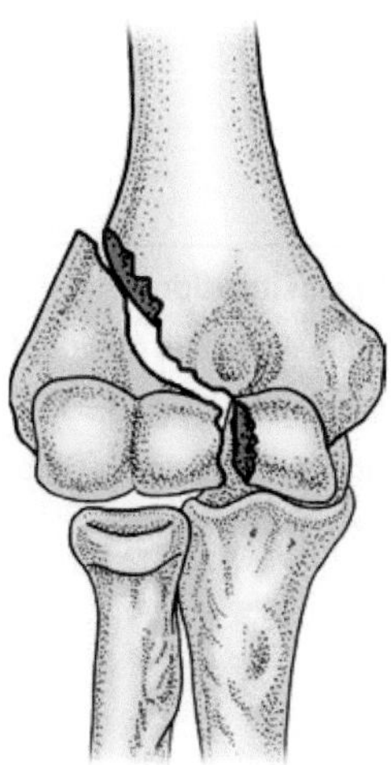

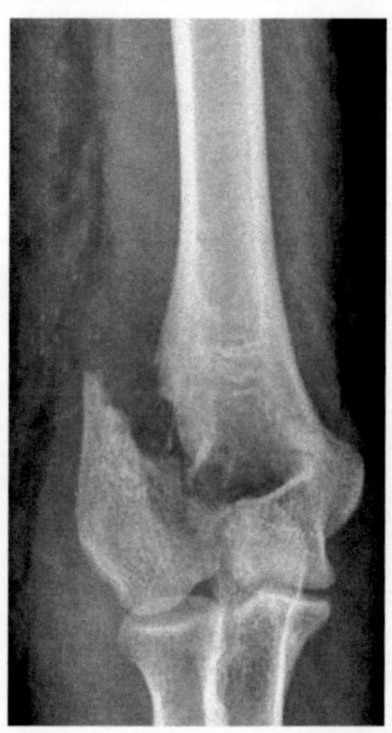

AO/OTA classification

Type B: Partial articular fracture (13-B).

B1: Lateral sagittal (13-B1).

B1.2: Transtrochlear simple (13-B1.2)

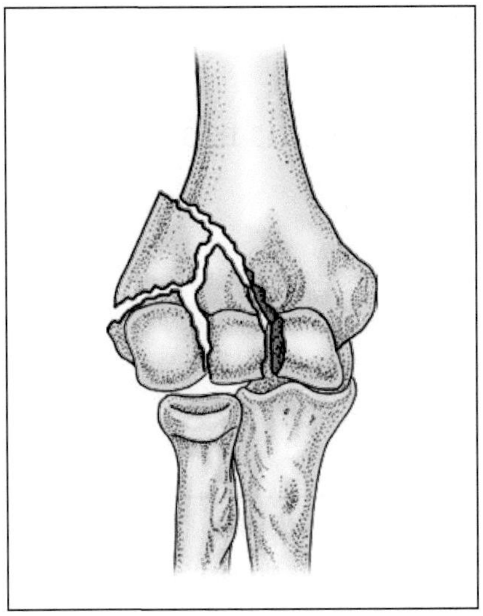

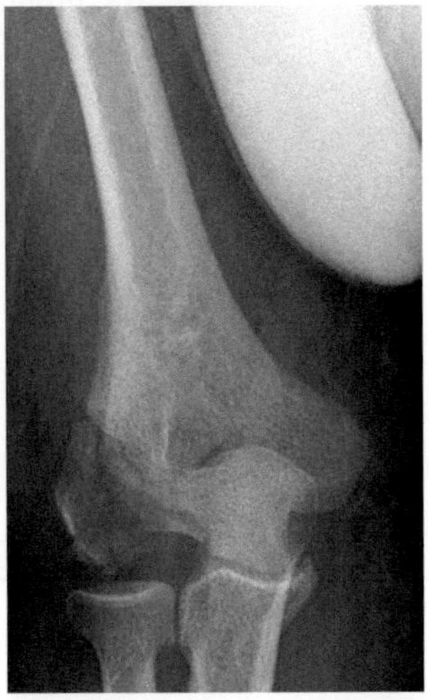

AO/OTA classification

Type B: Partial articular fracture (13-B).

B1: Lateral sagittal (13-B1).

B1.3: Transtrochlear multifragmentary (13-B1.3)

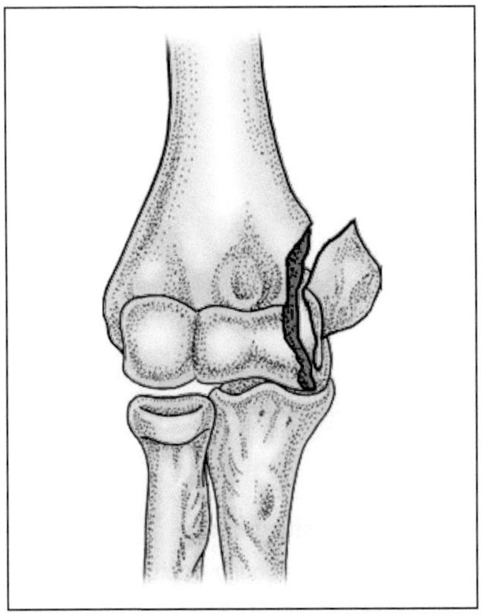

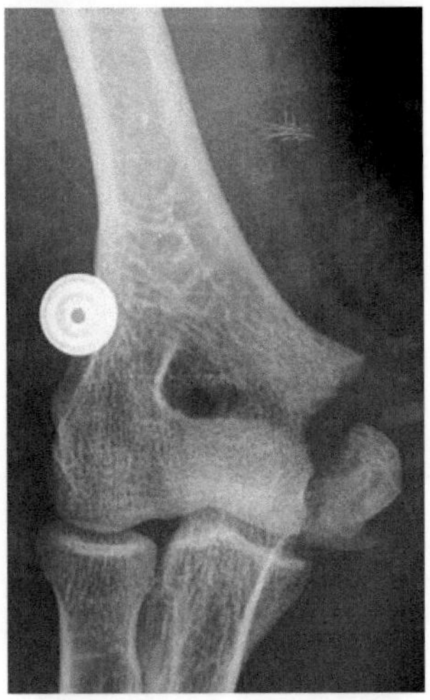

AO/OTA classification

Type B: Partial articular fracture (13-B).

B2: Medial sagittal (13-B2).

B2.1: Transtrochlear simple, through medial side (Milch I) (13-B2.1)

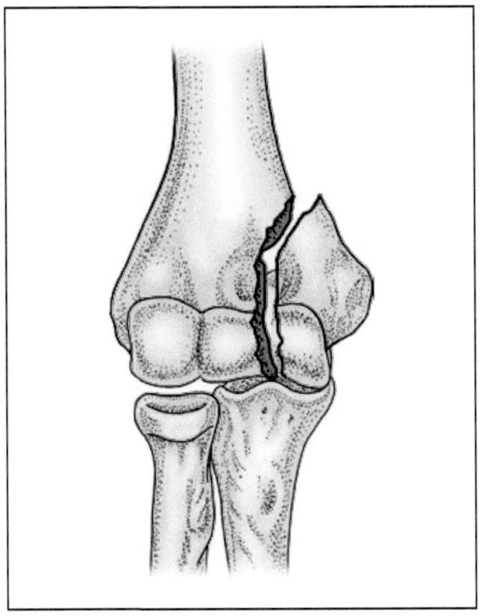

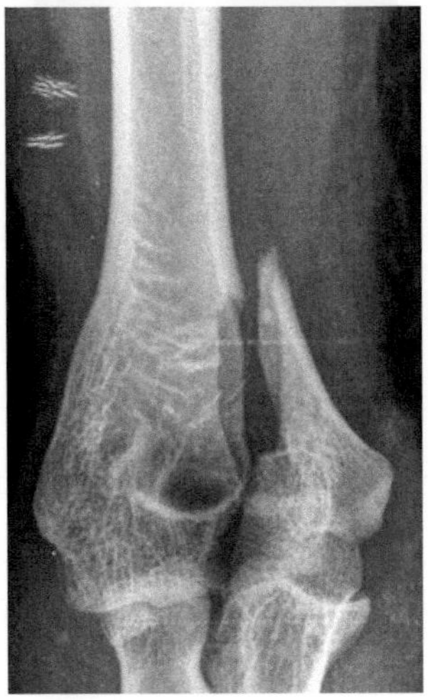

AO/OTA classification

Type B: Partial articular fracture (13-B).

B2: Medial sagittal (13-B2).

B2.2: Transtrochlear simple, through the groove (13-B2.2)

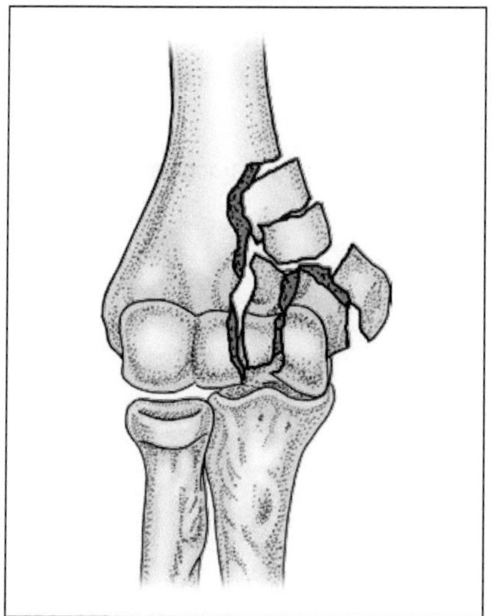

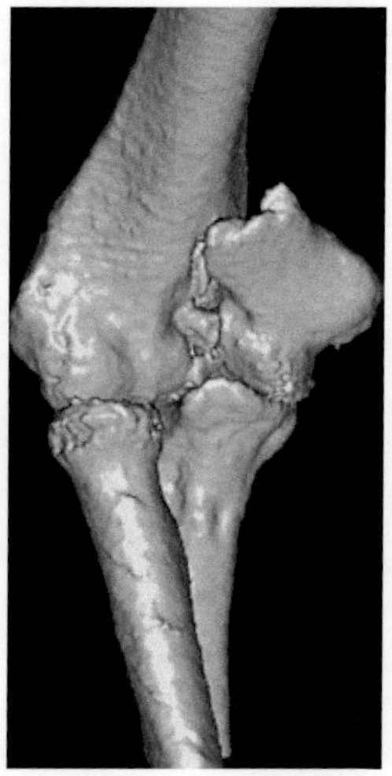

AO/OTA classification

Type B: Partial articular fracture (13-B)

B2: Medial sagittal (13-B2)

B2.3: Transtrochlear multifragmentary (13-B2.3)

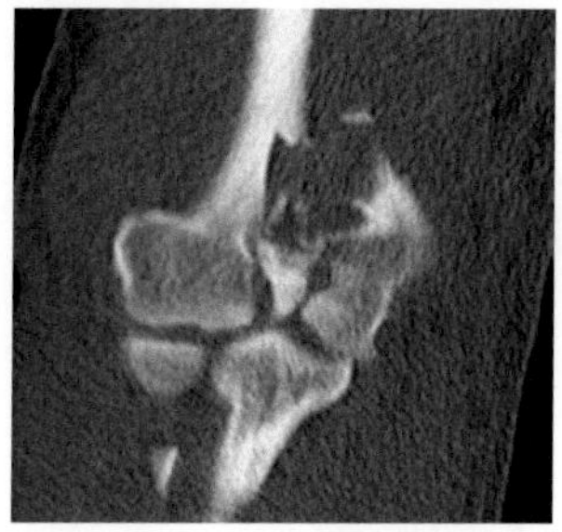

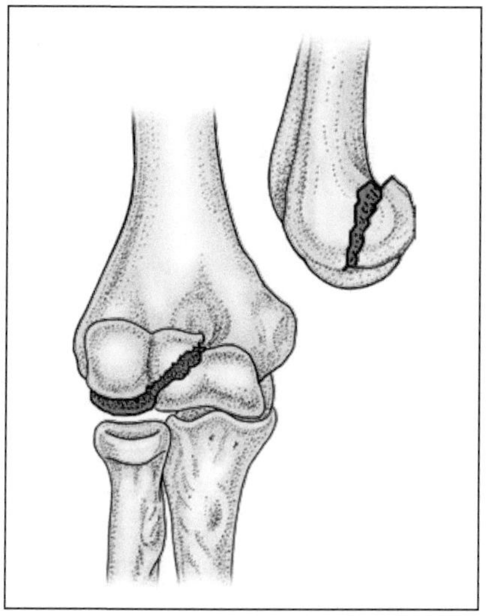

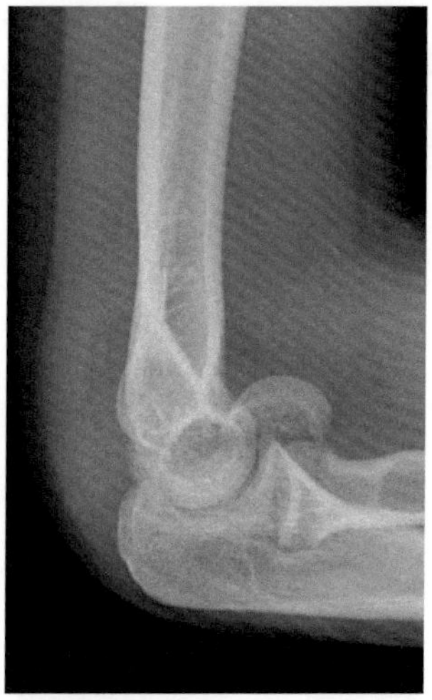

AO/OTA classification

Type B: Partial articular fracture (13-B)

B3: Frontal (13-B3).

B3.1: Capitellum (13-B3.1)

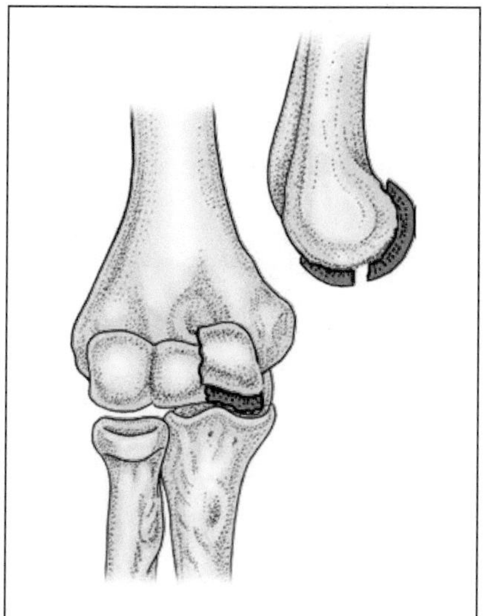

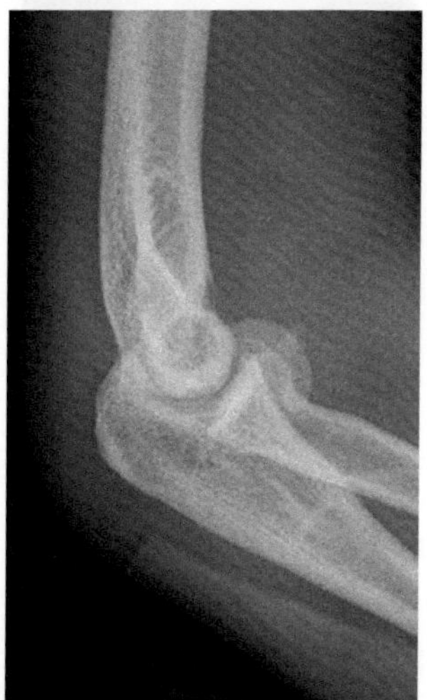

AO/OTA classification

Type B: Partial articular fracture (13-B).

B3: Frontal (13-B3)

B3.2: Trochlea (13-B3.2)

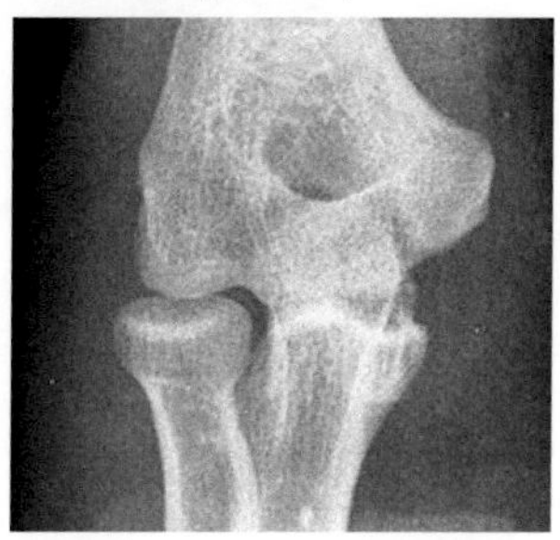

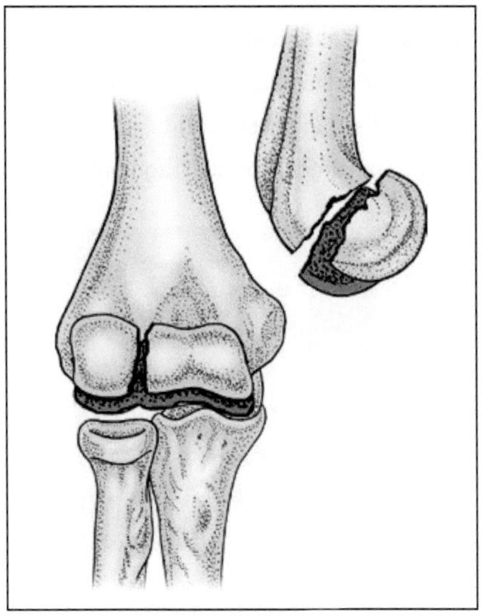

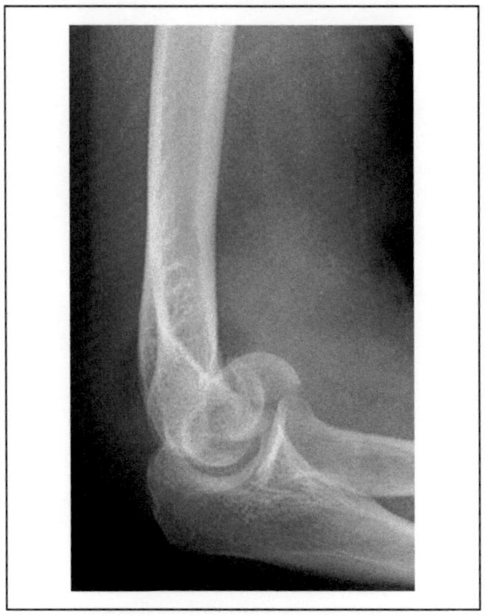

AO/OTA classification

Type B: Partial articular fracture (13-B).

B3: Frontal (13-B3).

B3.3: Capitellum and trochlea (13-B3.3)

Type C: Complete articular fracture (13-C)
- C1: Articular simple, metaphyseal simple (13-C1):
  - C1.1: With slight displacement (13-C1.1)
  - C1.2: With marked displacement (13-C1.2)
  - C1.3: T-shaped epiphyseal (13-C1.3)
- C2: Articular simple, metaphyseal multifragmentary (13-C2):
  - C2.1: With intact wedge (13-C2.1)
  - C2.2: With a fragmented wedge (13-C2.2)
  - C2.3: Complex (13-C2.3)
- C3: Articular, metaphyseal multifragmentary (13-C3):
  - C3.1: Metaphyseal simple (13-C3.1)
  - C3.2: Metaphyseal wedge (13-C3.2)
  - C3.3: Metaphyseal complex (13-C3.3)

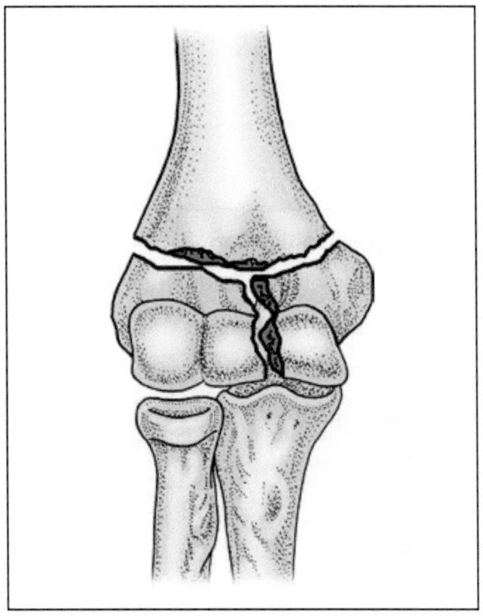

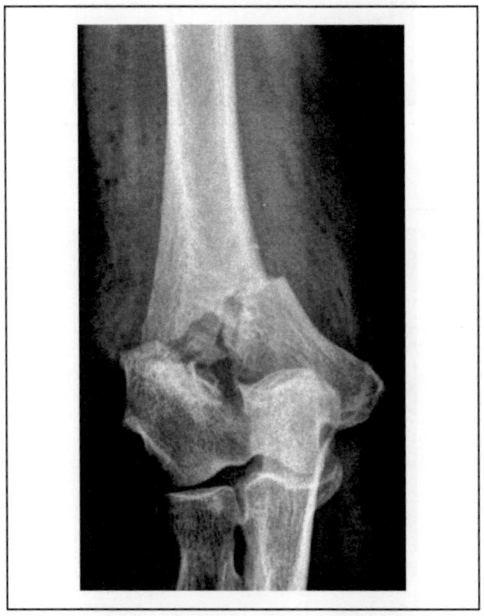

AO/OTA classification

Type C: Complete articular fracture (13-C).

C1: Articular simple, metaphyseal simple (13-C1).

C1.1: With slight displacement (13-C1.1)

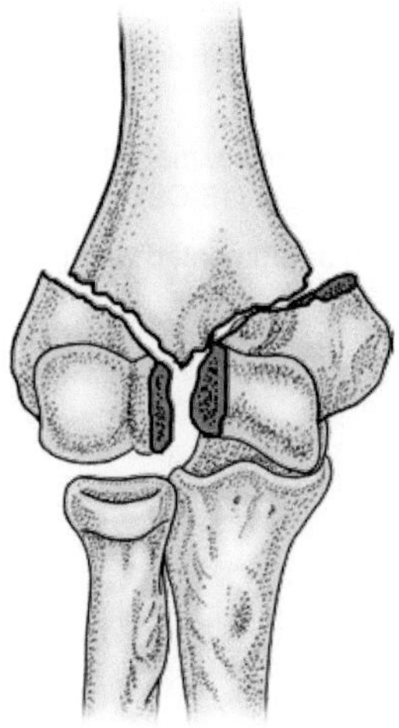

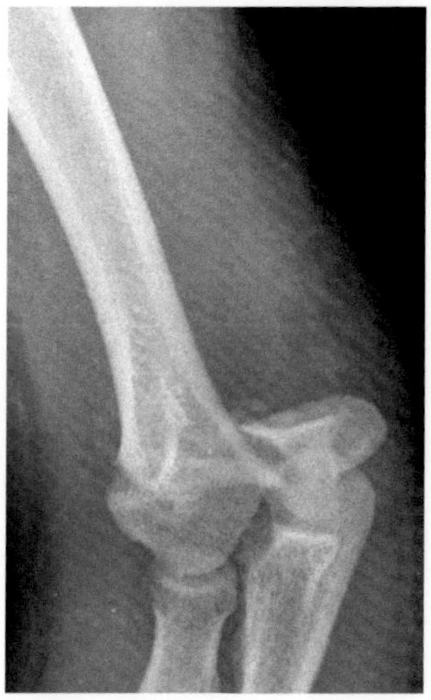

AO/OTA classification

Type C: Complete articular fracture (13-C).

C1: Articular simple, metaphyseal simple (13-C1).

C1.2: With marked displacement (13-C1.2)

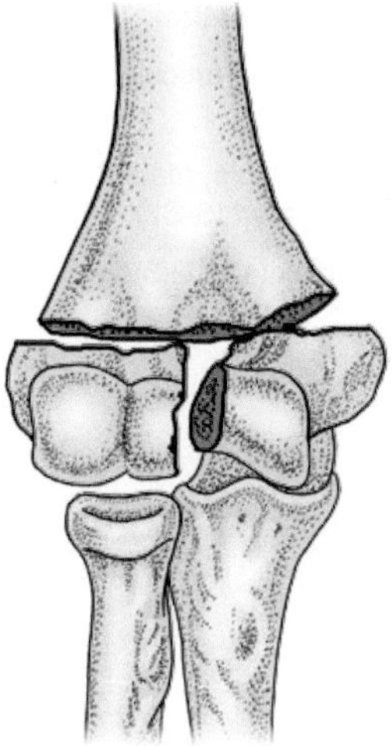

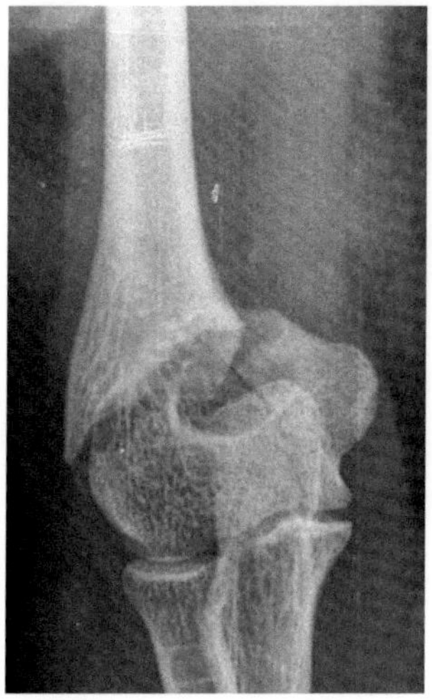

AO/OTA classification

Type C: Complete articular fracture (13-C)

C1: Articular simple, metaphyseal simple (13-C1)

C1.3: T-shaped epiphyseal (13-C1.3)

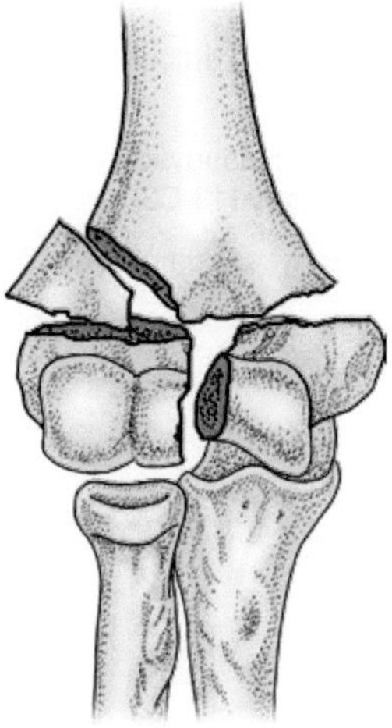

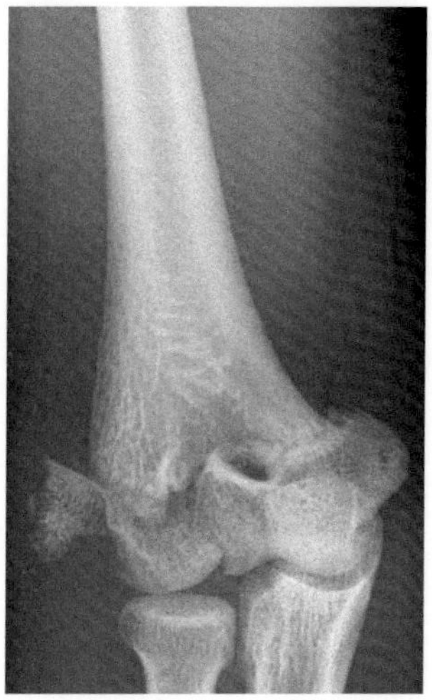

AO/OTA classification

Type C: Complete articular fracture (13-C)

C2: Articular simple, metaphyseal multifragmentary (13-C2)

C2.1: With intact wedge (13-C2.1)

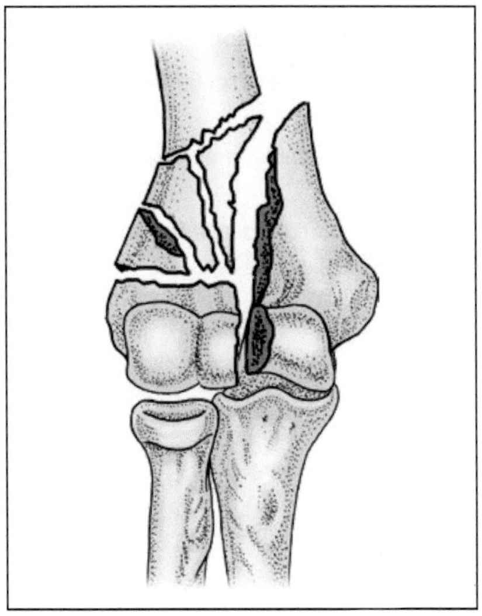

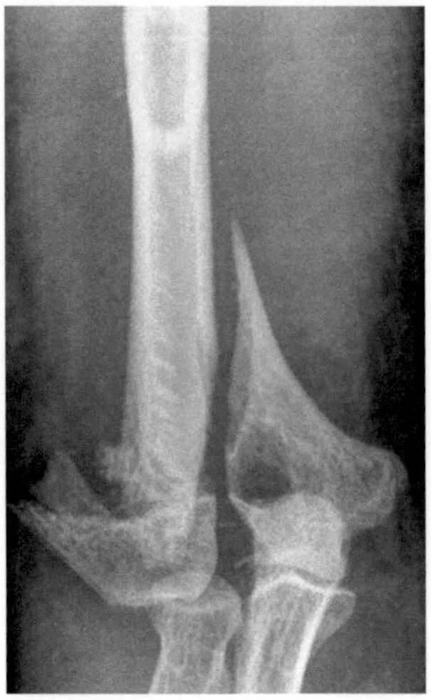

AO/OTA classification

Type C: Complete articular fracture (13-C)

C2: Articular simple, metaphyseal multifragmentary (13-C2)

C2.2: With a fragmented wedge (13-C2.2)

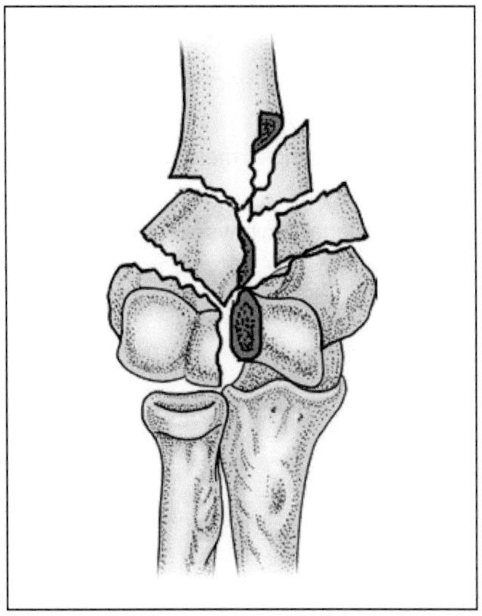

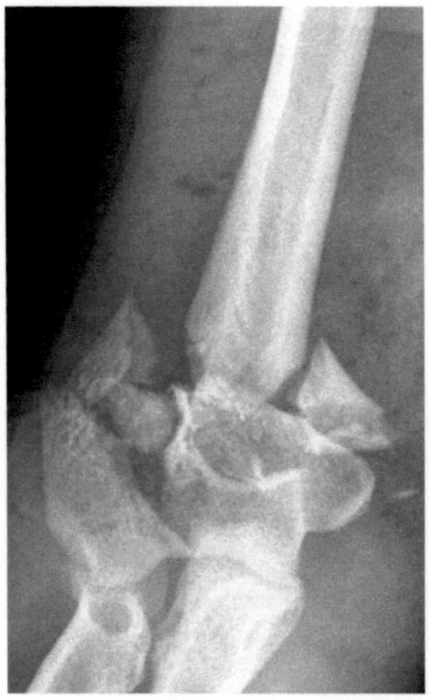

AO/OTA classification

Type C: Complete articular fracture (13-C)

C2: Articular simple, metaphyseal multifragmentary (13-C2)

C2.3: Complex (13-C2.3)

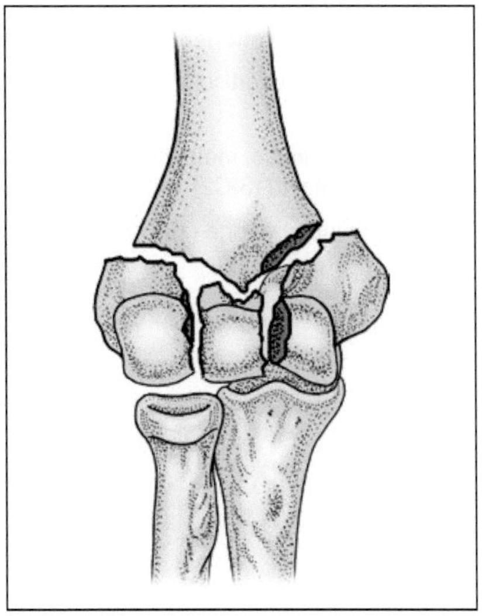

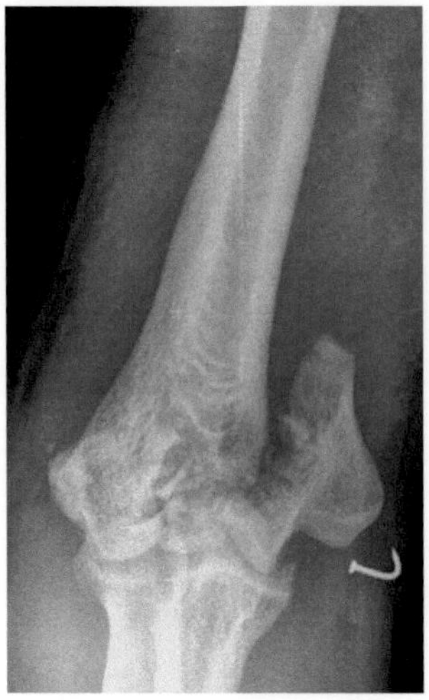

AO/OTA classification

Type C: Complete articular fracture (13-C)

C3: Articular, metaphyseal multifragmentary (13-C3)

C3.1: Metaphyseal simple (13-C3.1)

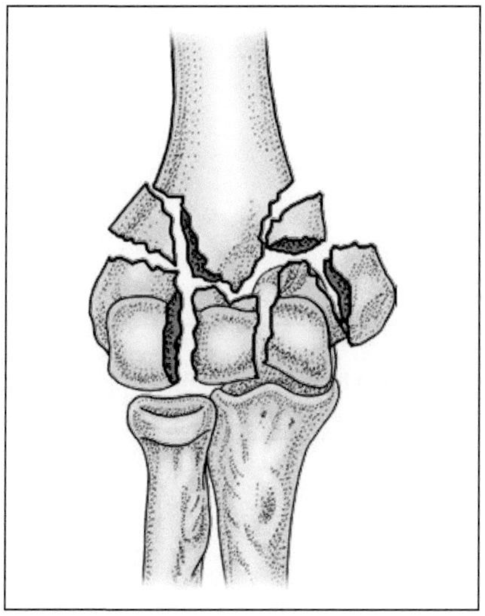

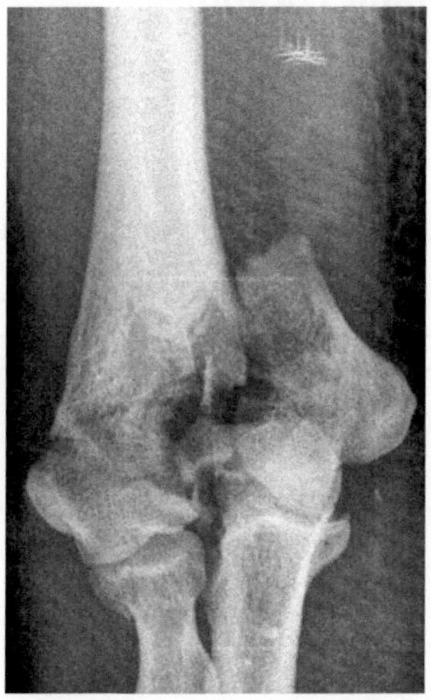

AO/OTA classification

Type C: Complete articular fracture (13-C)

C3: Articular, metaphyseal multifragmentary (13-C3)

C3.2: Metaphyseal wedge (13-C3.2)

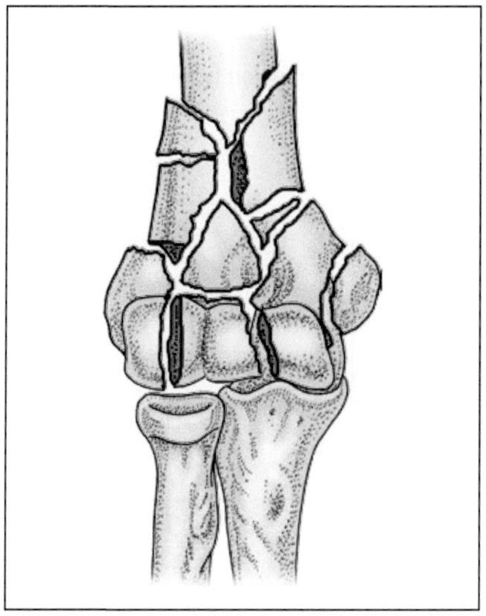

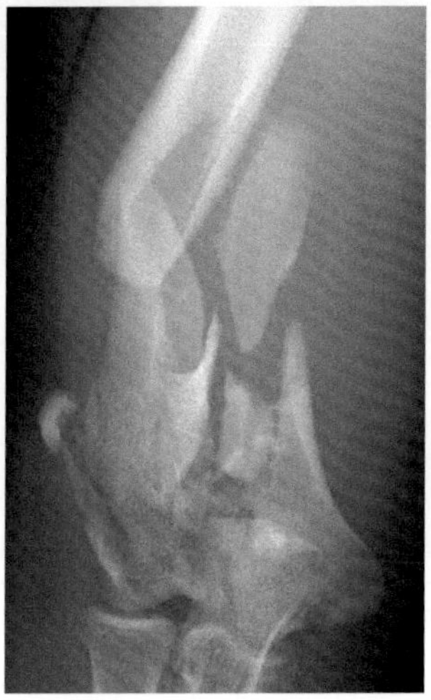

AO/OTA classification

Type C: Complete articular fracture (13-C)

C3: Articular, metaphyseal multifragmentary (13-C3)

C3.3: Metaphyseal complex (13-C3.3)

2.3.3 Classification According to Anatomic Location

2.3.3.1 Supracondylar Fractures of Humerus

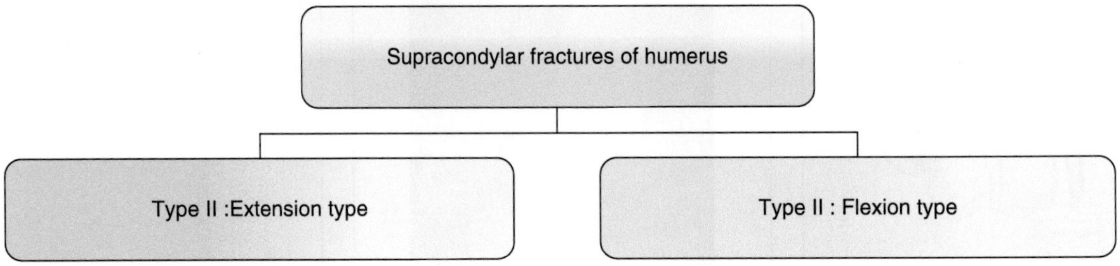

Type I: Extension type.
Type II: Flexion type.

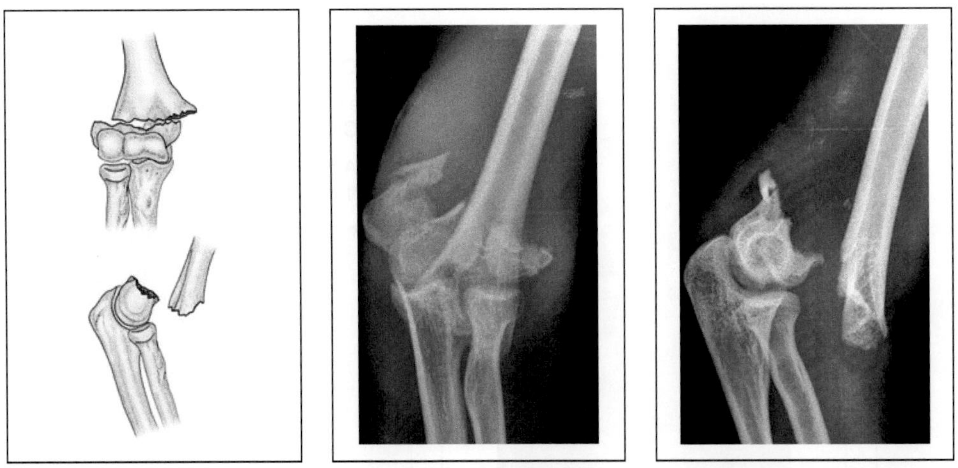

Supracondylar fractures of humerus

Extension type

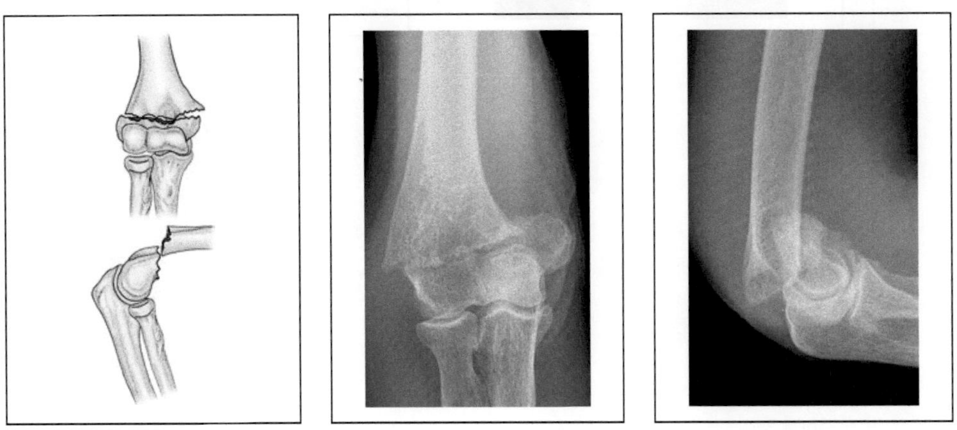

Supracondylar fractures of humerus

Flexion type

Gartland Classification System (in 1959)

Extension-type supracondylar fractures may be further classified into three types according to the Gartland classification system:

TypeI: An undisplaced fracture.
Type II: A displaced fracture with an intact posterior periosteum, posterior displacement of the distal fracture fragment.
Type III: A displaced fracture with disrupted anterior and posterior periosteum, no continuity between the proximal and distal fracture fragments.

Pirone Modified Classification (in 1988)

Pirone et al. modified Gartland classification, with type II divided into two subtypes:

Type IIa: Simple fracture with the distal fragment inclining posteriorly, and the posterior cortex bone integrated.
Type IIb: Fracture fragments laterally displaced, or with the distal fragment linking, and the broken ends of fractured bone still contact.

Mcintyre Classification (In 1994)

Mcintyre supplemented to the traditional three-type classification with every type divided into two subtypes:

Type Ia: Bone fracture fragments undisplaced, the distal fragment has a posterior inclination less than 5°.
Type Ib: Bone fracture fragments undisplaced, the posterior inclination of the distal fragment ≤15–20°, medial (lateral) separation ≤1 mm.
Type IIa: Fracture displaced 0–2 mm, the posterior inclination of the distal fragment ≤15–20°, separation at fracture site or compression distance of medial (lateral) cortex bone >1 mm.
Type IIb: Fracture displaced 2–15 mm, the broken ends of fractured bone still contact, different extent of fragment inclination.
Type IIIa: The broken ends no contact, overlap ≤20 mm or rotation >15 mm, the broken ends still contact, different extent of fragment inclination.
Type IIIb: Long distance between the broken ends or overlap >20 mm, or rotation >15 mm, with the broken ends no contact, different extent of fragment inclination.

2.3.3.2 Milch Classification of Humeral Condyle Fractures [6]

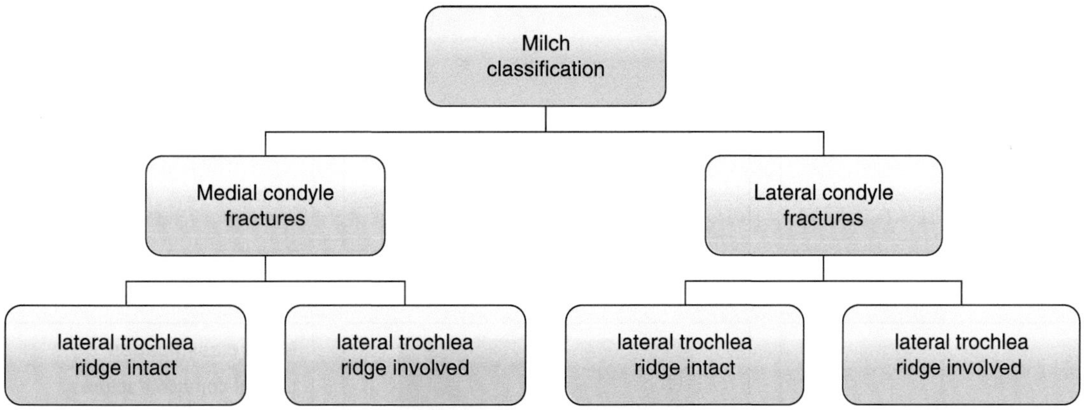

Humeral condyle fractures are divided into medial condyle fractures and lateral condyle fractures according to Milch classification, further divided into subtype depending on whether or not the lateral trochlea ridge is involved.

Medial condyle fractures:
Type I: Lateral trochlea ridge intact.
Type II: Lateral trochlea ridge involved.

Lateral condyle fractures:
Type I: Lateral trochlea ridge intact.
Type II: Lateral trochlea ridge involved.

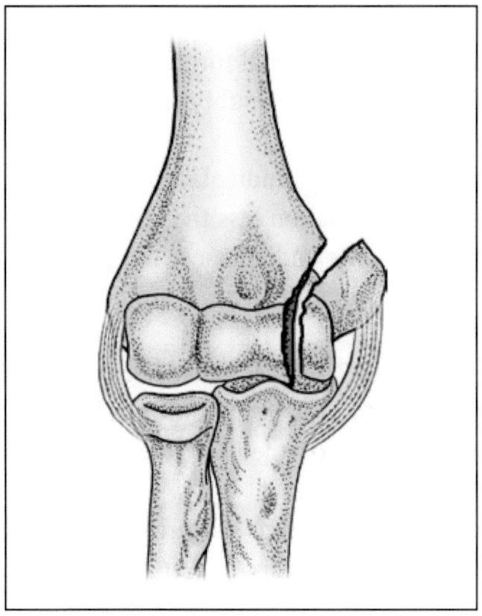

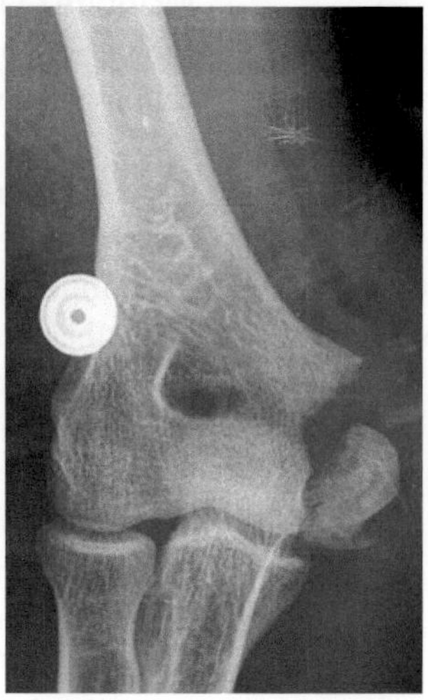

Milch classification

Medial condyle fractures

Type I: Lateral trochlea ridge intact

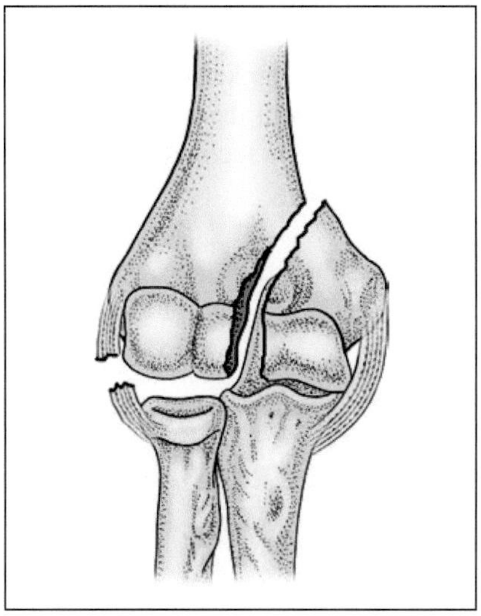

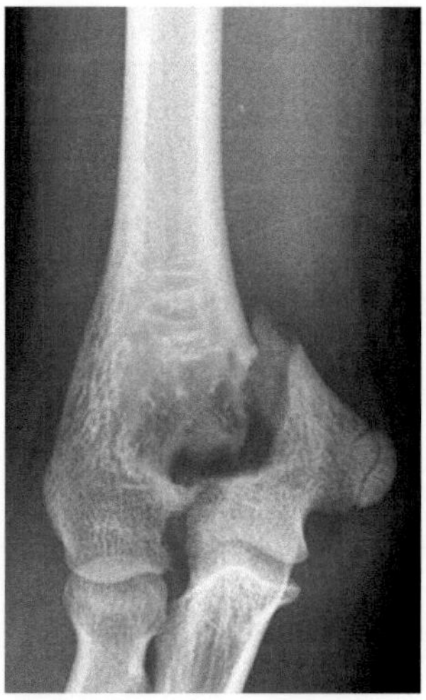

Milch classification

Medial condyle fractures

Type II: Lateral trochlea ridge involved

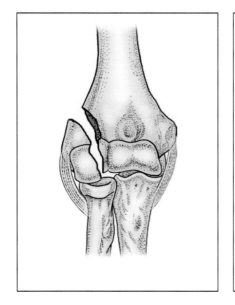

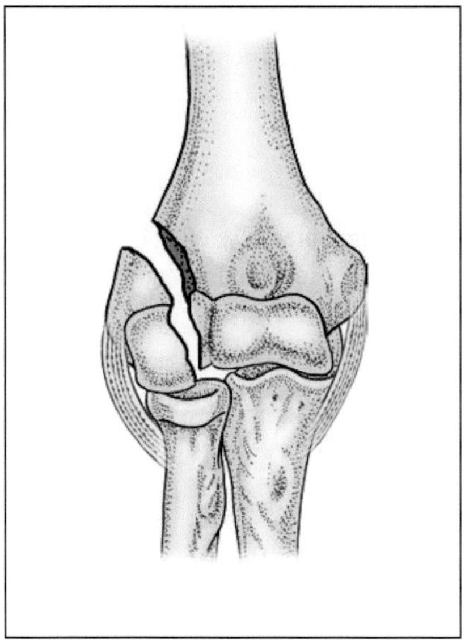

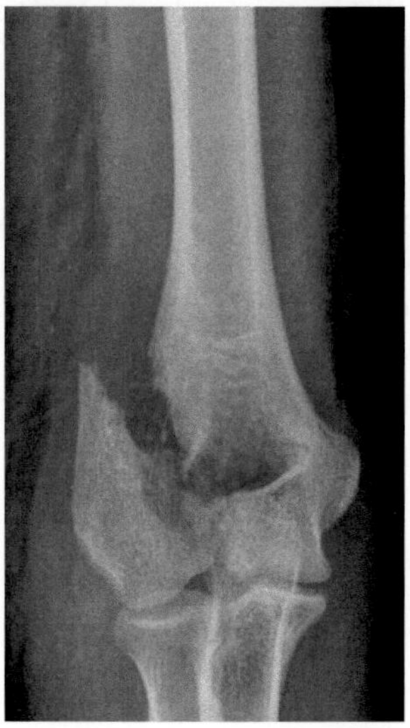

Milch classification

Lateral condyle fractures

Type I: Lateral trochlea ridge intact

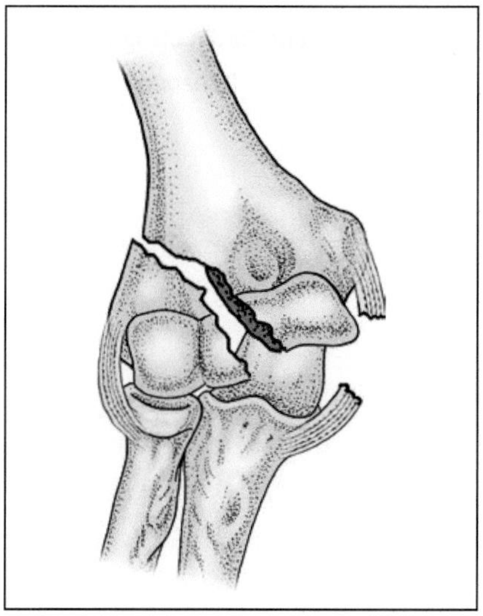

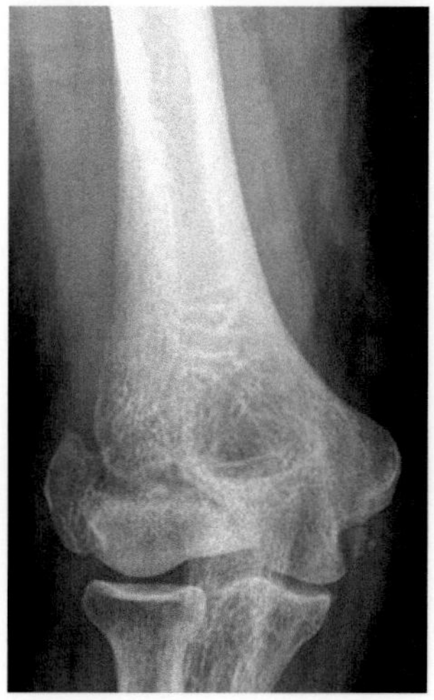

Milch classification

Lateral condyle fractures

Type II: Lateral trochlea ridge involved

2.3.3.3 Classification of Intercondylar Fractures of Humerus

Riseborough and Radin Classification [7]

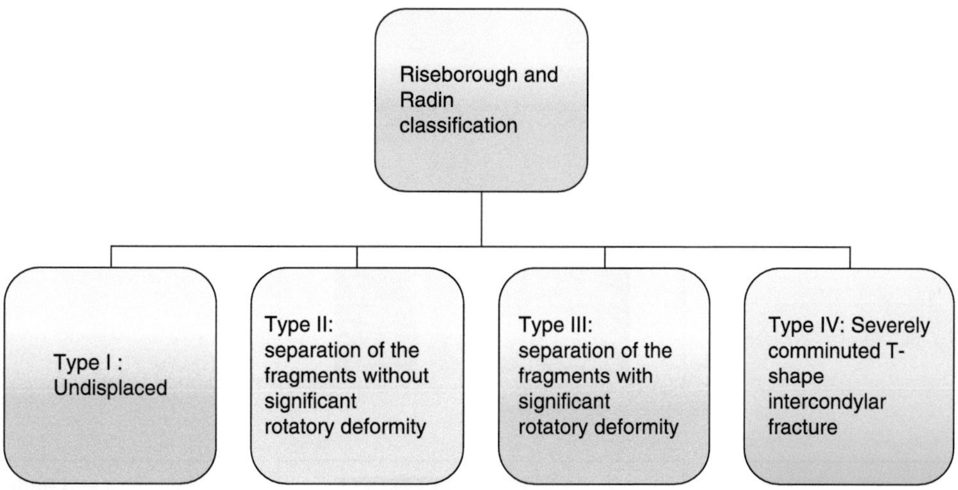

Type I: Undisplaced T-shaped intercondylar fracture.

Type II: T-shaped intercondylar fracture with separation of the fragments but without significant rotatory deformity.

Type III: T-shaped intercondylar fracture with separation of the fragments with significant rotatory deformity.

Type IV: Severely comminuted T-shape intercondylar fracture of the humerus.

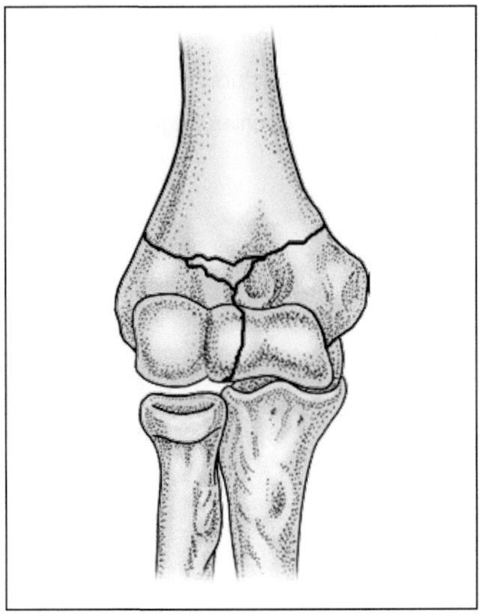

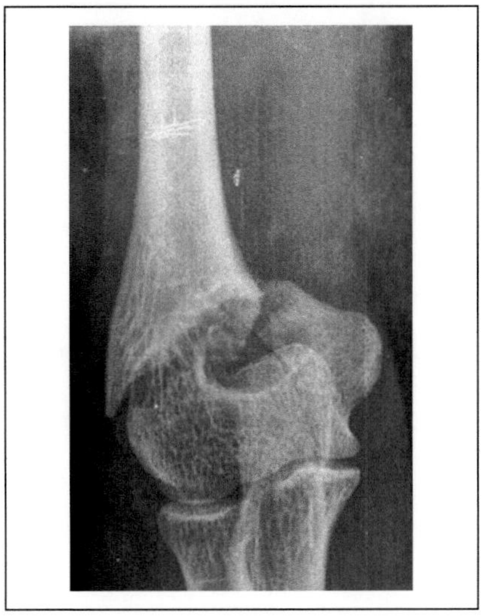

Riseborough and Radin classification

Type I: Undisplaced T-shaped intercondylar fracture

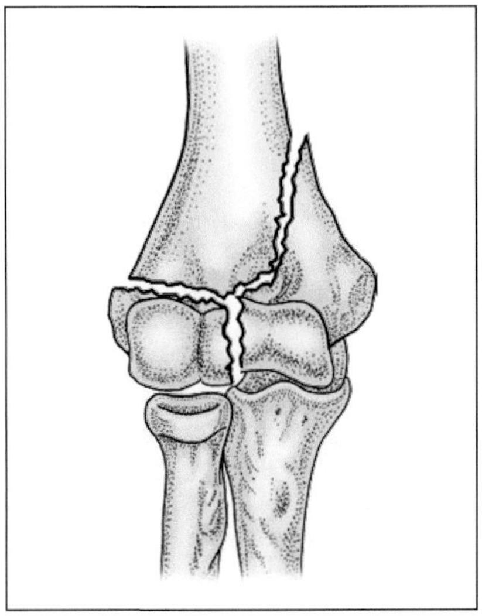

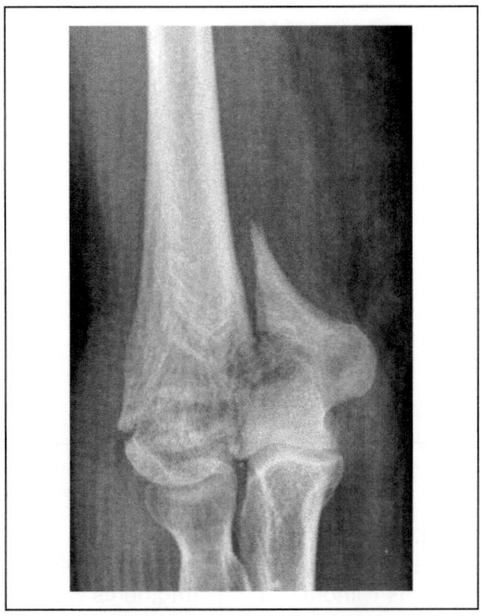

Riseborough and Radin classification

Type II: T-shaped intercondylar fracture with separation of the fragments but without significant rotatory deformity

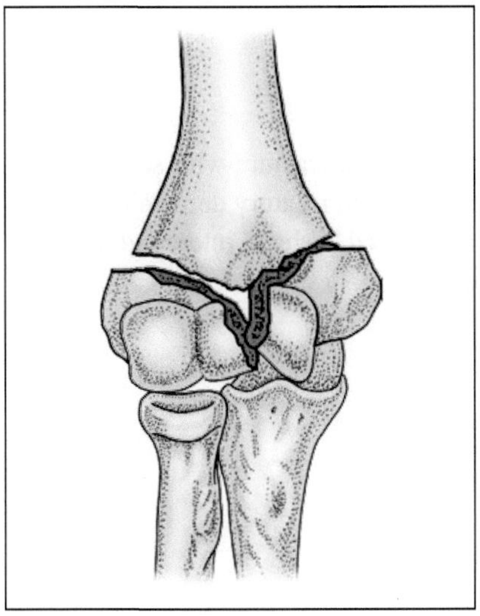

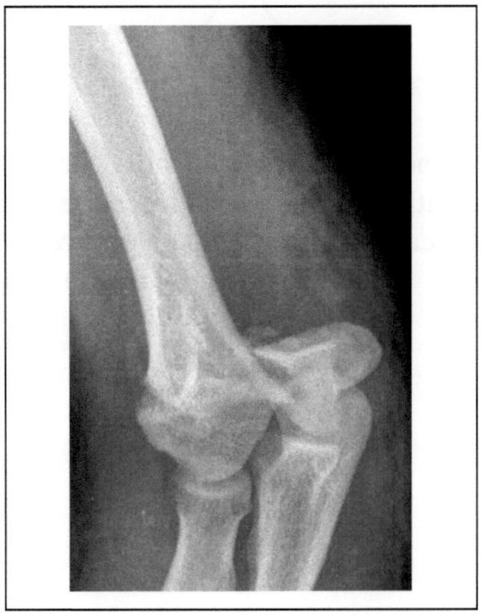

Riseborough and Radin classification

Type III: T-shaped intercondylar fracture with separation of the fragments with significant rotatory deformity

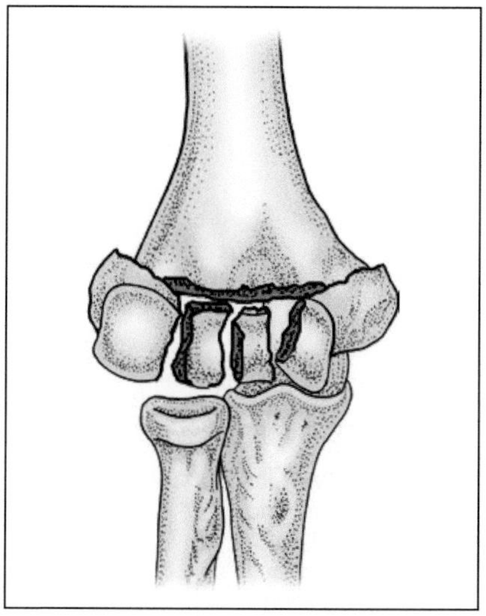

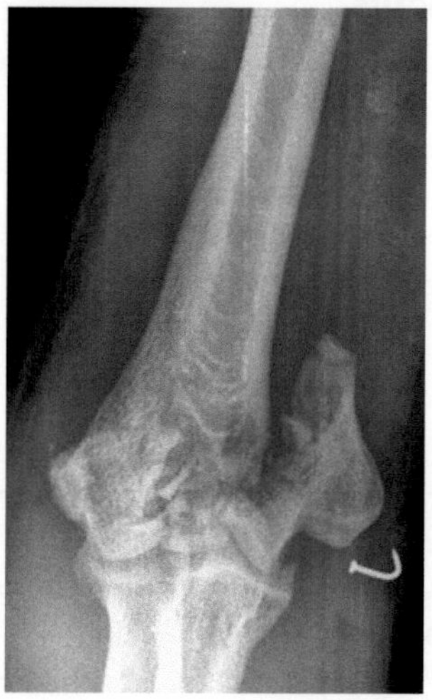

Riseborough and Radin classification

Type IV: Severely comminuted T-shape intercondylar fracture of the humerus

Men Zhenwu-Yong Yimin Classification [8]

Intercondylar fractures of the humerus are divided into two types according to the injury mechanism and direction of fracture displacement: extension introversion or flexion introversion.

Type A: Extension introversion.

The elbow is injured in an extension position, with an evident stress on elbow introversion. Fracture fragments are displaced medially and posteriorly. This type can be further divided into three degrees of injury depending on the severity of the injury.

I°: Equivalent to C1 in the AO classification; the fracture lines lie medially and extend proximally and medially, with the medial epicondyle and bone proximal to the medial epicondyle intact.

II°: More stress on elbow introversion; a wedge bone fragment exists in the medial proximal site of the fracture, which is not completely separated from the medial periosteum of the distal humerus.

III°: Most stress on elbow introversion; the medial wedge-shaped fragment is completely separated.

Type B: Flexion introversion

The elbow is injured in a flexion position, with an evident stress on elbow introversion. This type can be further divided into three degrees of injury depending on the severity of the injury.

I°: A typical T-shaped fracture with the elbow injured in a flexion position. Under the combination of flexion stress and introversion stress, a fracture similar to I° of the extension introversion type appears, except for an anterior displacement of the fragment.

II°: Under the combination of flexion stress and introversion stress, a fracture similar to II° of the extension introversion type appears, except for an anterior displacement of the fragment.

III°: The injury stress is similar to that of III° of the extension introversion type; however, the medial wedge-shaped fragment is not as typical as that in the extension type and lies in the anterior site of the elbow joint.

2.3.3.4 Lateral Condyle Fractures of Humerus

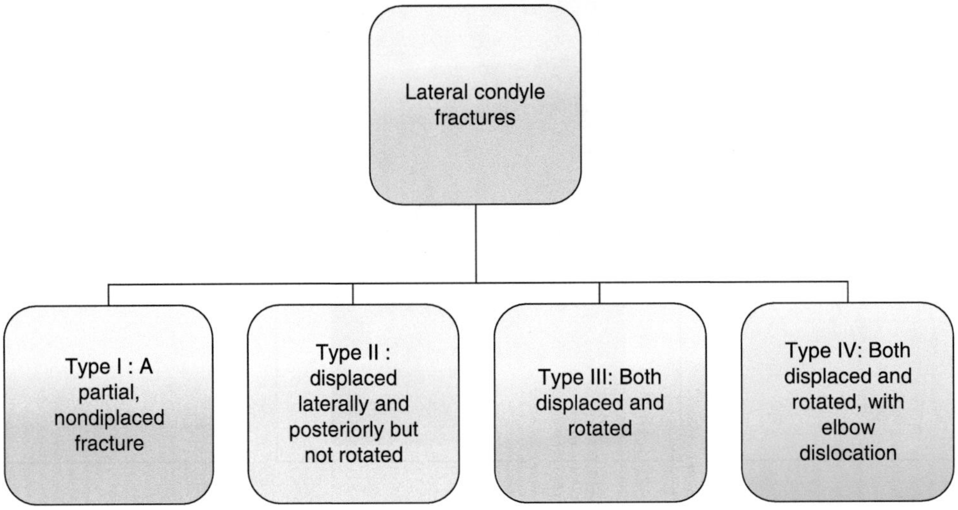

Type I: A partial, non-displaced fracture that does not traverse the entire cartilaginous epiphysis.

Type II: A complete fracture that extends through the articular surface and may be displaced laterally and posteriorly but not rotated.

Type III: Both displaced and rotated, with loss of the normal relationship of the capitellum to the proximal radius.

Type IV: Both displaced and rotated, with elbow dislocation.

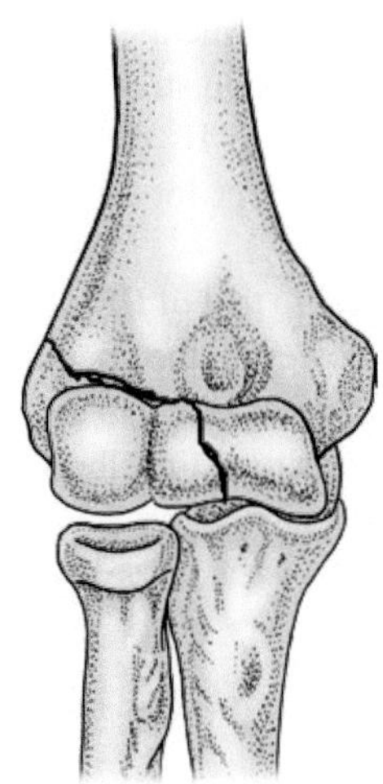

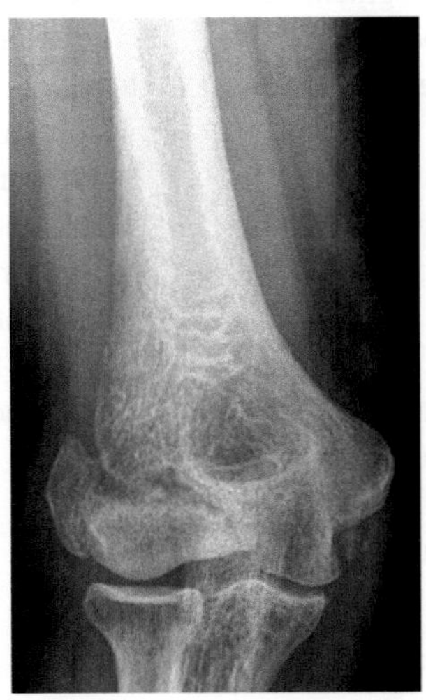

Lateral condyle fractures of humerus

Type I: A partial, non-displaced fracture

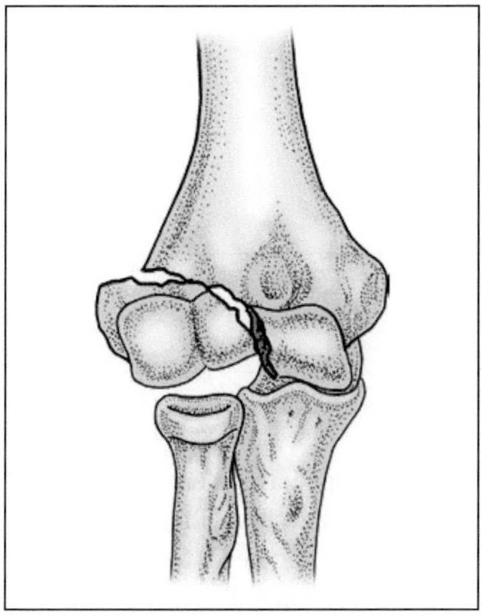

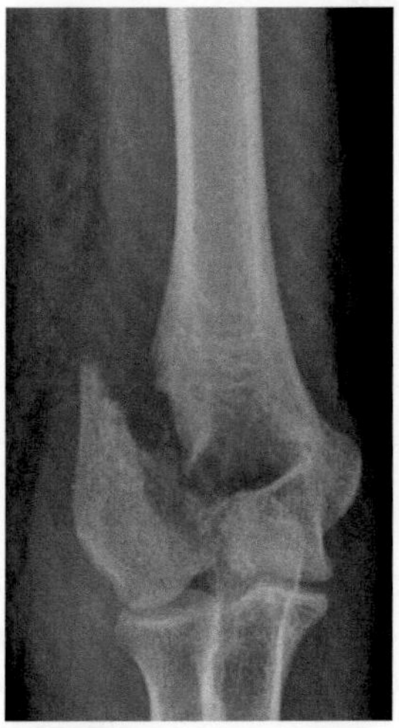

Lateral condyle fractures of humerus

Type II: Displaced laterally and posteriorly but not rotated

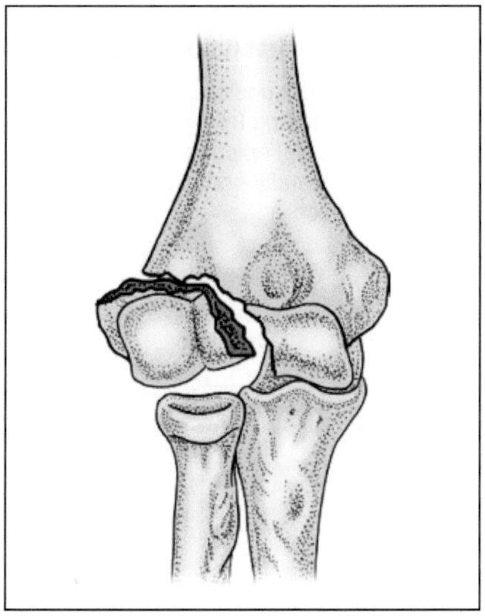

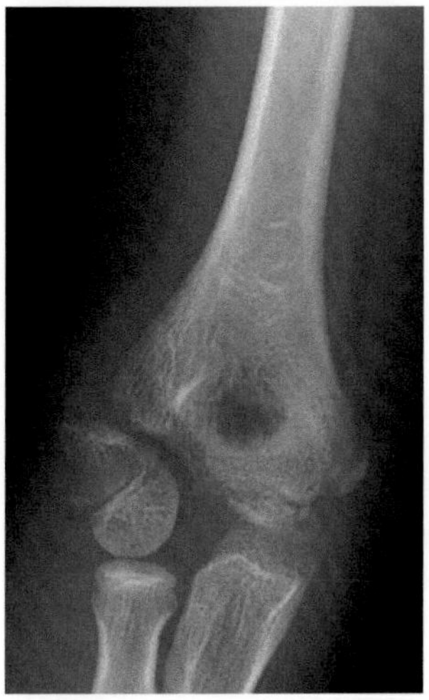

Lateral condyle fractures of humerus

Type III: Both displaced and rotated

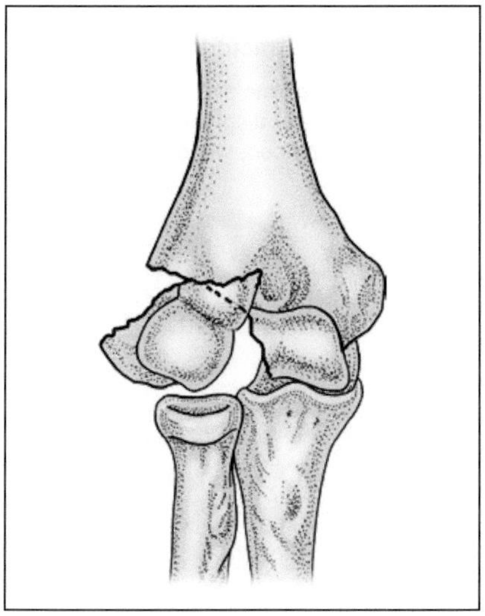

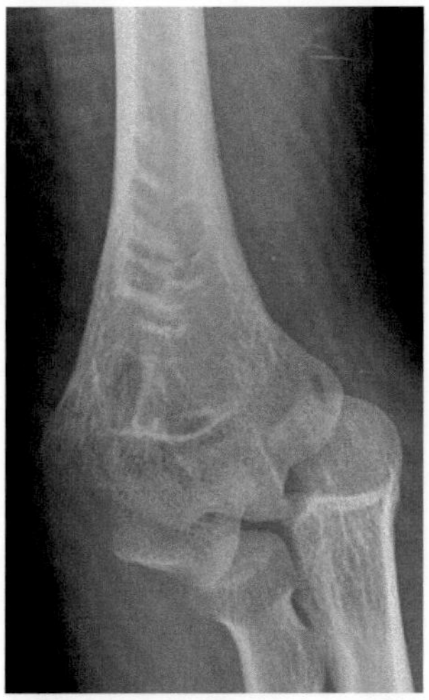

Lateral condyle fractures of humerus

Type IV: Both displaced and rotated, with elbow dislocation

2.3.3.5 Medial Condyle Fractures of Humerus

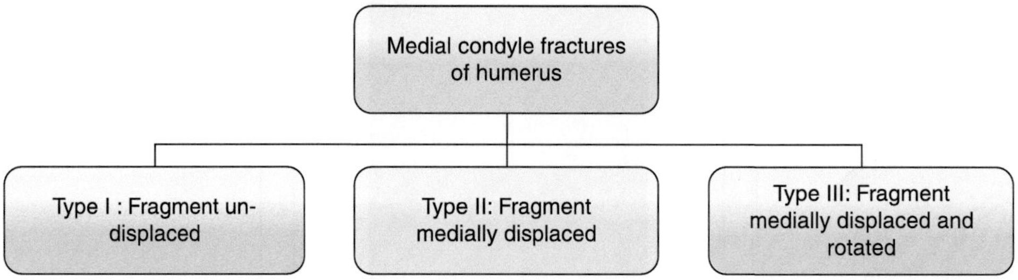

Type I: Fragment undisplaced, with the fracture line starting from proximal position of medial epicondyle towards distally and laterally ended in trochlea articular surface.

Type II: Fracture line similar to type I, fragment medially displaced or mildly proximally displaced, without rotation.

Type III: The same fracture line with type II, fragment medially or anteriorly displaced and rotated.

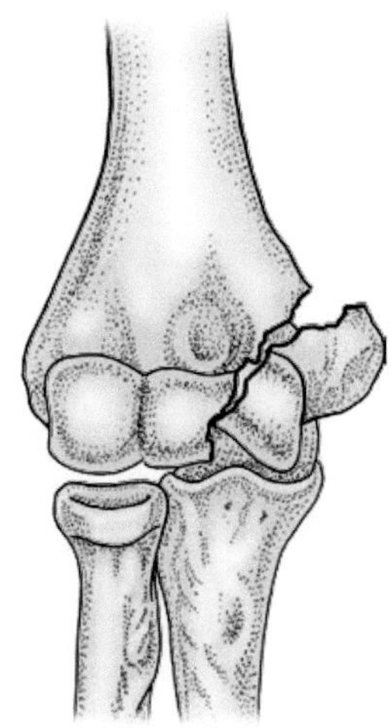

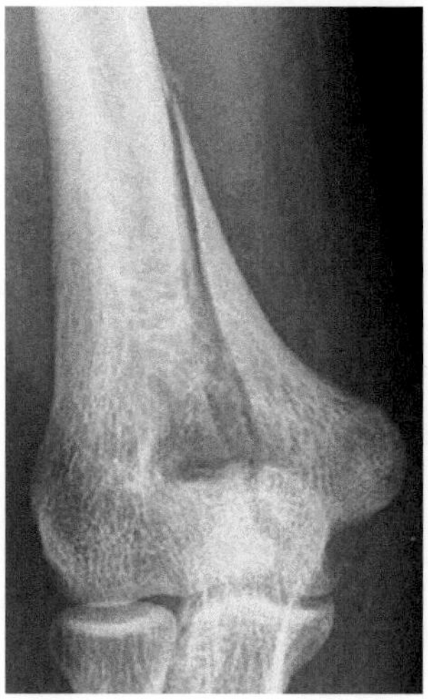

Medial condyle fractures of humerus

Type I: Fragment undisplaced, with the fracture line starting from proximal position of medial epicondyle towards distally and laterally ended in trochlea articular surface

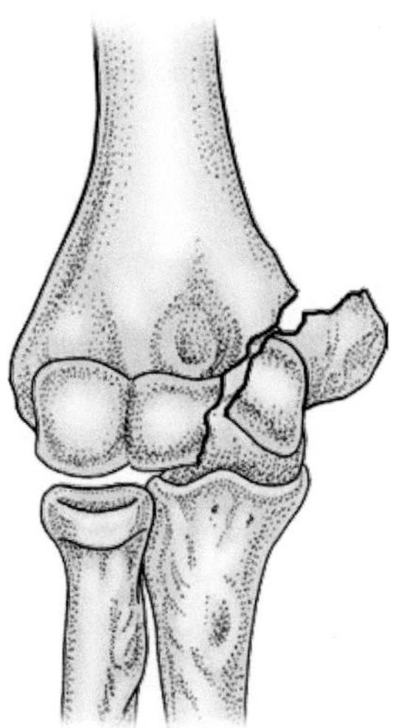

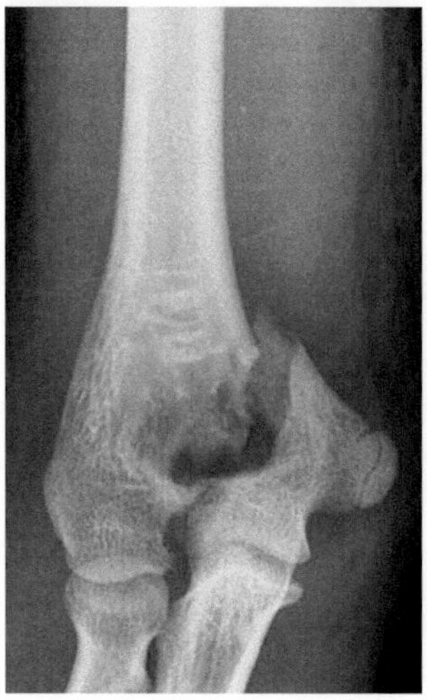

Medial condyle fractures of humerus

Type II: Fracture line similar to type I, fragment medially displaced or mildly proximally displaced, without rotation

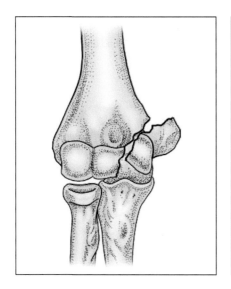

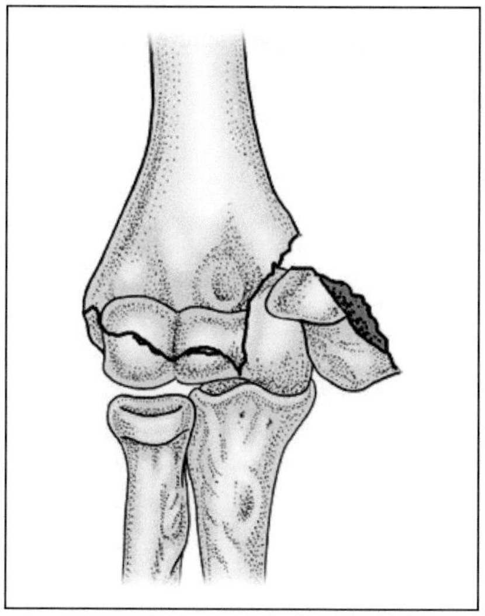

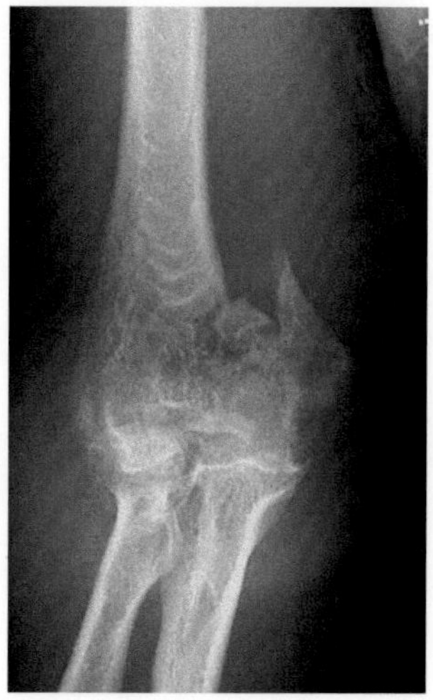

Medial condyle fractures of humerus

Type III: The same fracture line with type II, fragment medially or anteriorly displaced and rotated

2.3.3.6 Lateral Epicondyle Fractures of Humerus

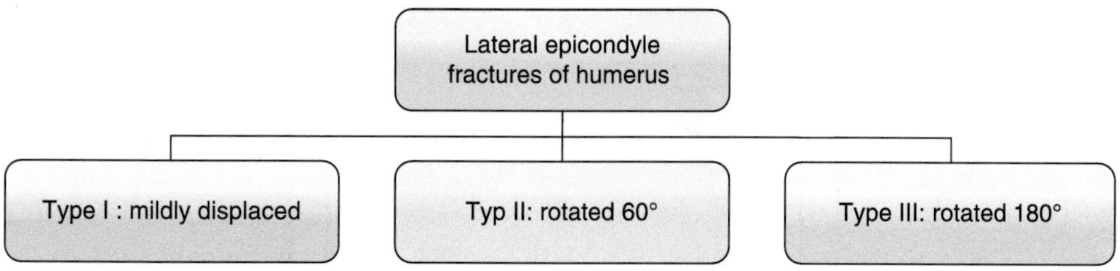

The fracture fragment could be mildly displaced, or rotated 60°–180°.

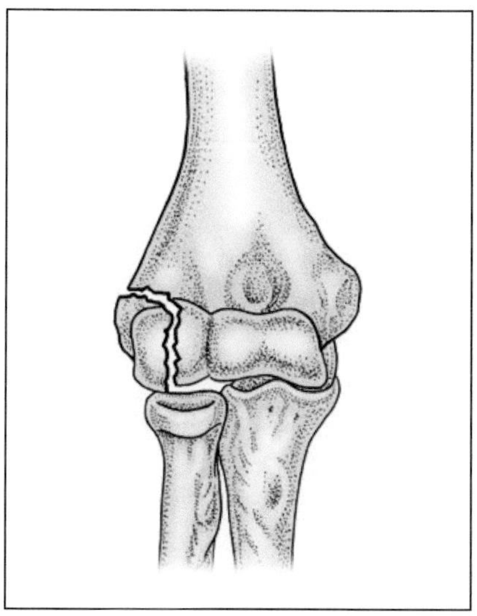

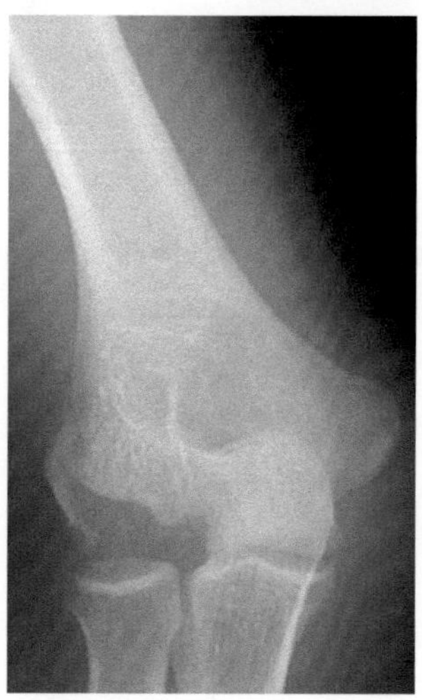

Lateral epicondyle fractures of humerus

Type I: Mildly displaced

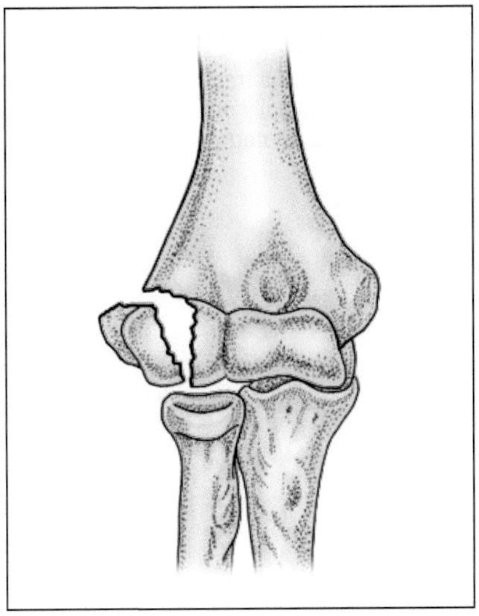

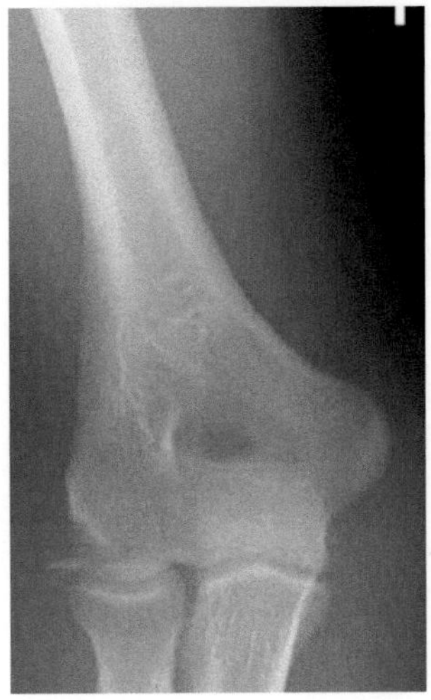

Lateral epicondyle fractures of humerus

Type II: Rotated 60°

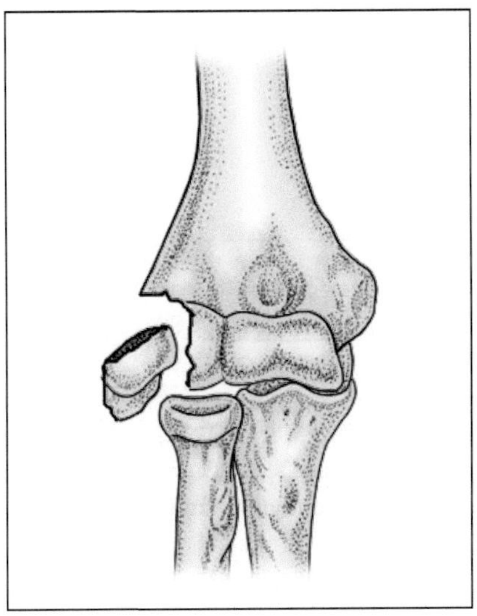

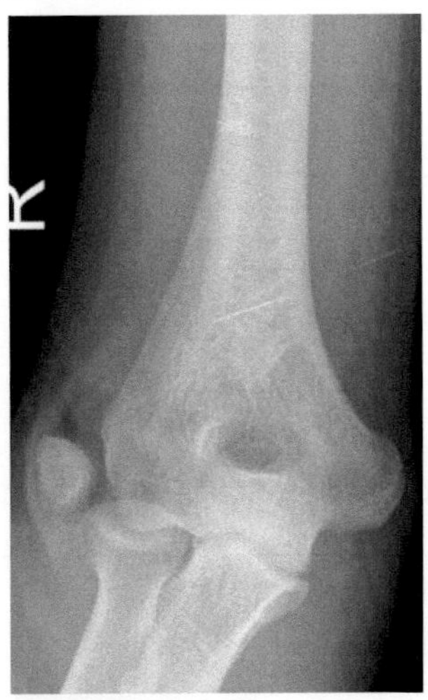

Lateral epicondyle fractures of humerus

Type III: Rotated 180°

2.3.3.7 Watson-Jones Classification of Medial Epicondyle Fractures of Humerus [9]

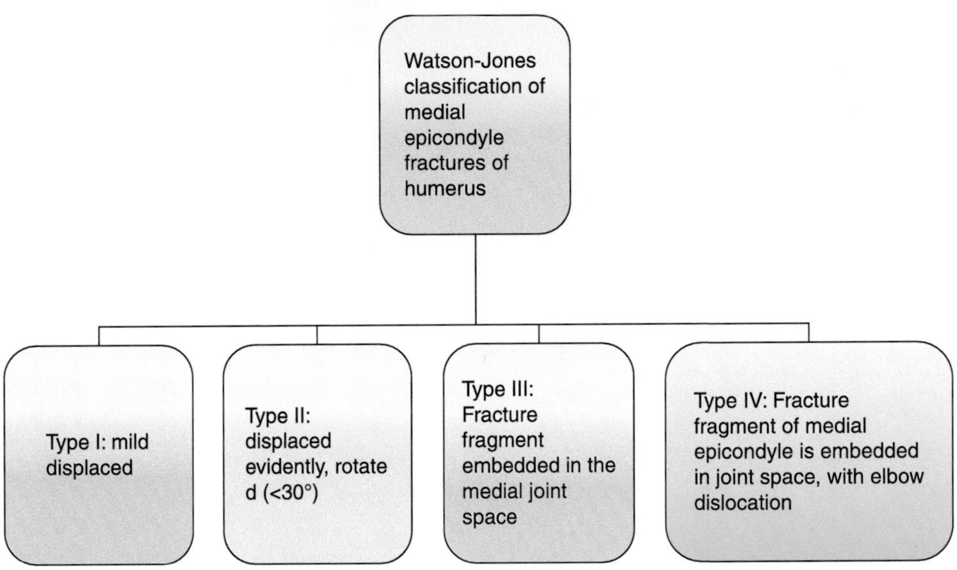

Type I: Fracture fragment of medial epicondyle mildly displaced.

Type II: Fracture fragment of medial epicondyle displaced evidently under traction, can reach the medial joint space, can be rotated (<30°).

Type III: Fracture fragment of medial epicondyle is embedded in the medial joint space, with elbow subluxation.

Type IV: Fracture fragment of medial epicondyle is embedded in joint space, with elbow dislocation.

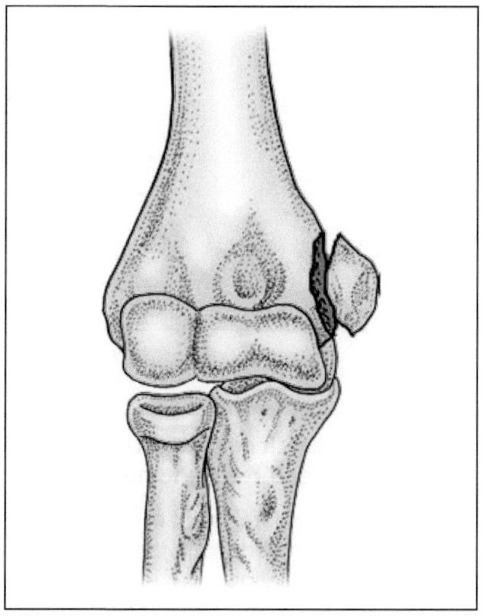

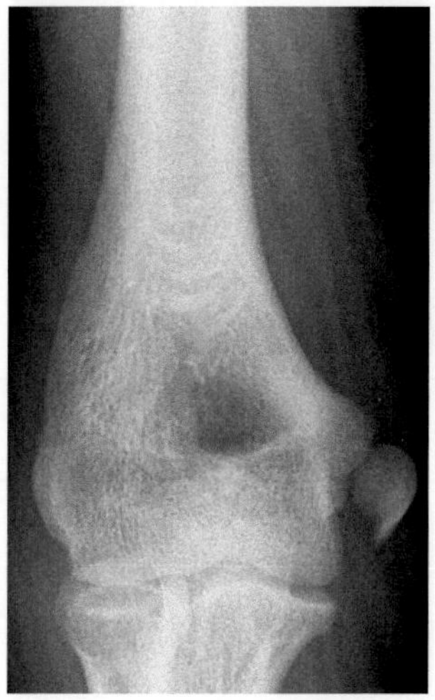

Watson-Jones classification of medial epicondyle fractures of humerus

Type I: Fracture fragment of medial epicondyle mildly displaced

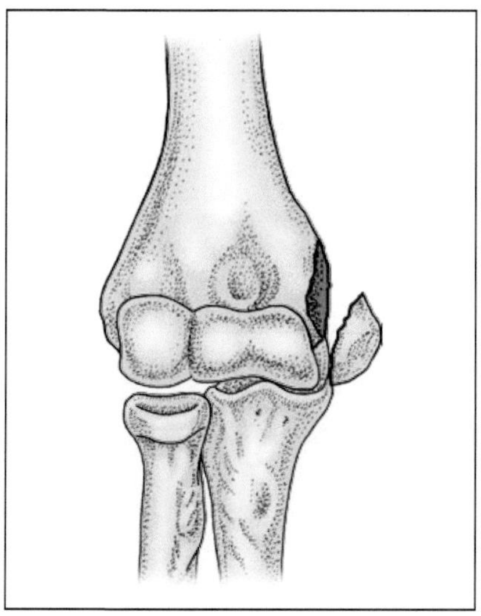

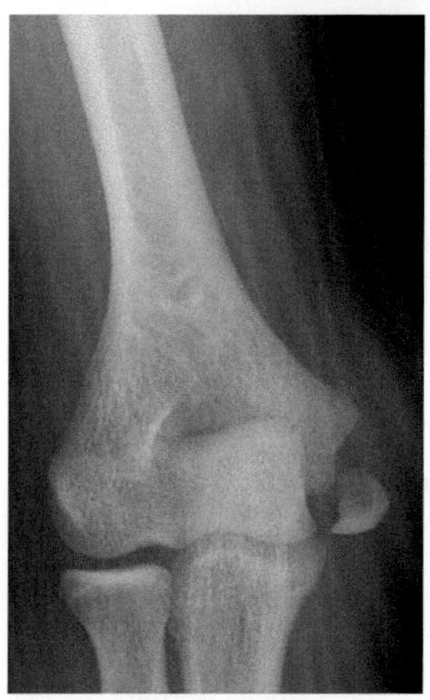

Watson-Jones classification of medial epicondyle fractures of humerus

Type II: Fracture fragment of medial epicondyle displaced evidently under traction, can reach the medial joint space, can be rotated (<30°)

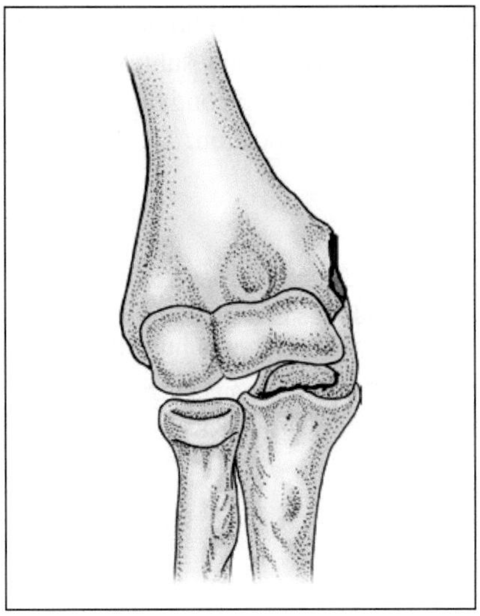

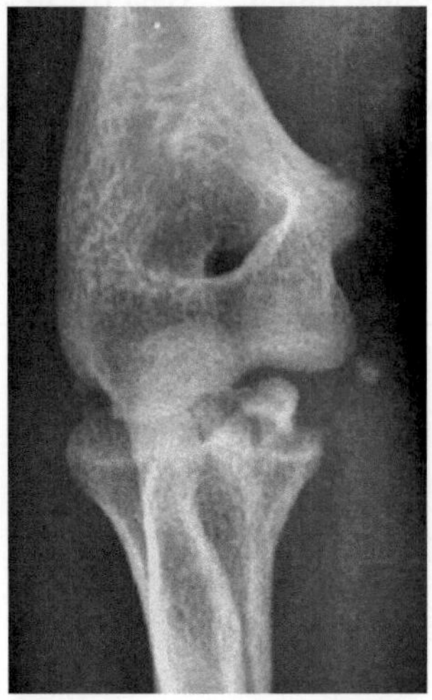

Watson-Jones classification of medial epicondyle fractures of humerus

Type III: Fracture fragment of medial epicondyle is embedded in the medial joint space, with elbow subluxation

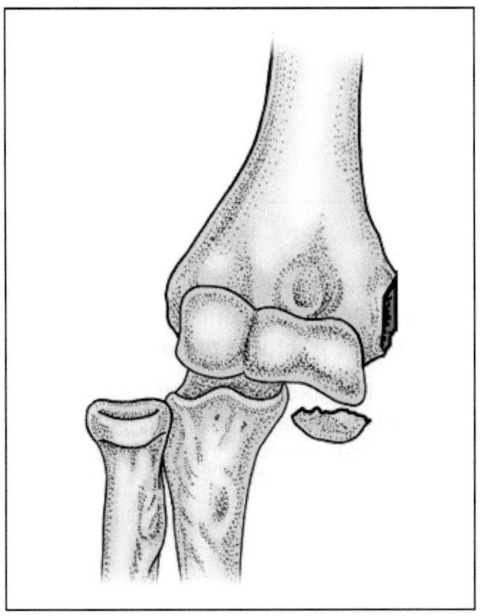

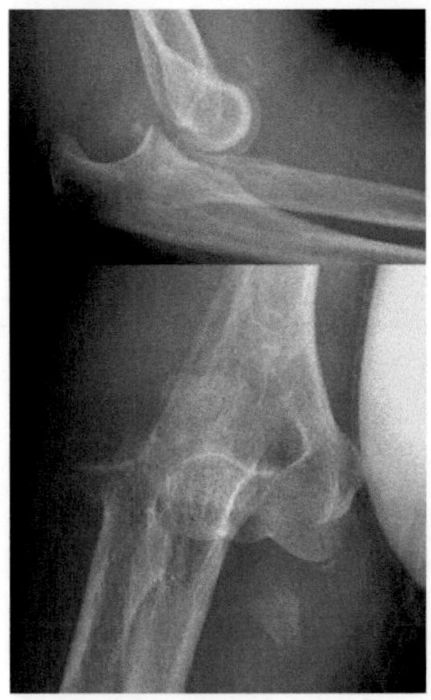

Watson-Jones classification of medial epicondyle fractures of humerus

Type IV: Fracture fragment of medial epicondyle is embedded in joint space, with elbow dislocation

2.3.3.8 Classification of Capitellar Fractures

Bryan-Morrey Classification [10]

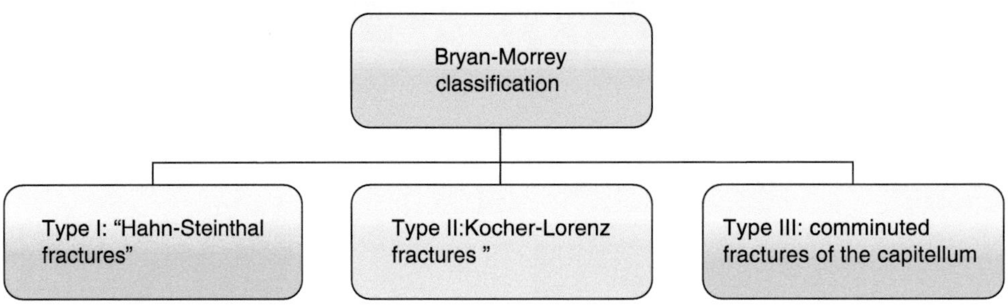

Type I: "Hahn-Steinthal fractures", involve the entire capitellum and lateral trochlear ridge.

Type II: "Kocher-Lorenz fractures", involve only the articular surface of the capitellum with subchondral bone. Sometimes a very small fragment is difficult to be detected in radiograph.

Type III: Comminuted fractures of the capitellum.

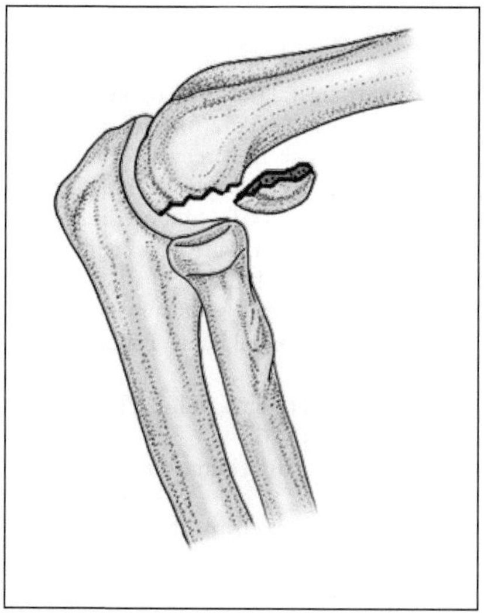

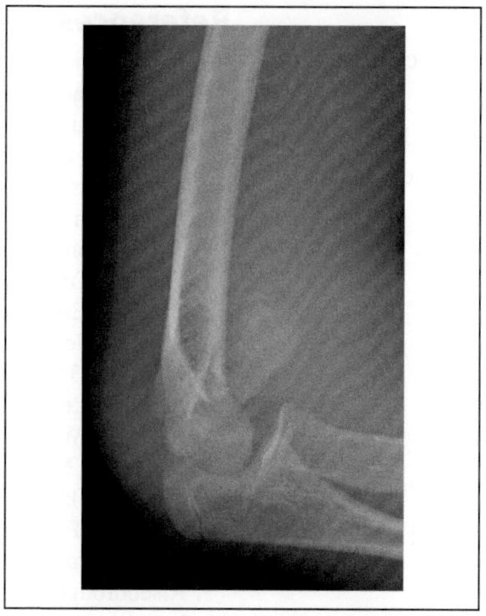

Bryan-Morrey classification

Type I: "Hahn-Steinthal fractures", involve the entire capitellum and lateral trochlear ridge

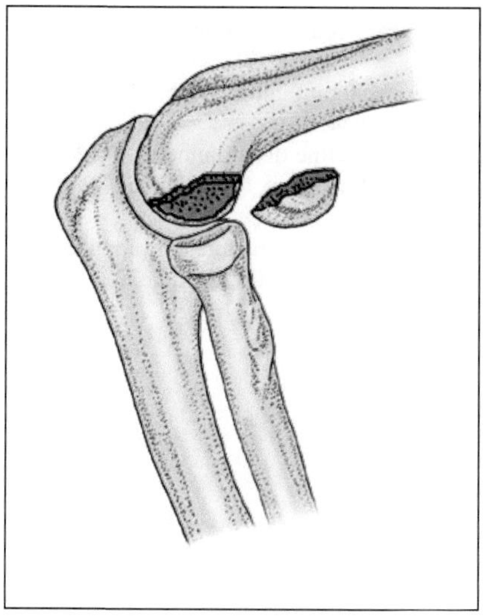

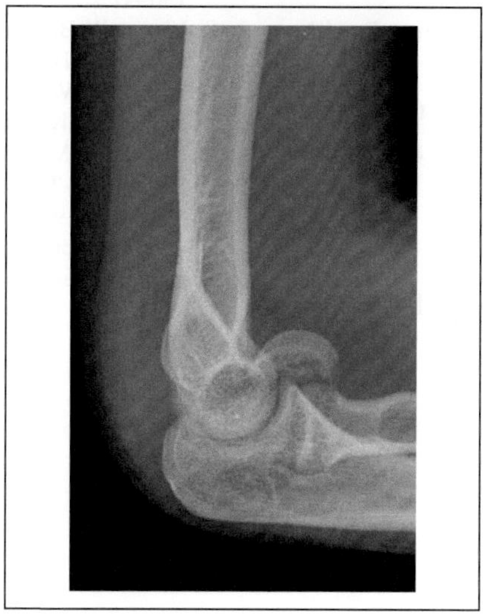

Bryan-Morrey classification

Type II: "Kocher-Lorenz fractures", involve only the articular surface of the capitellum with subchondral bone. Sometimes a very small fragment is difficult to be detected in radiograph

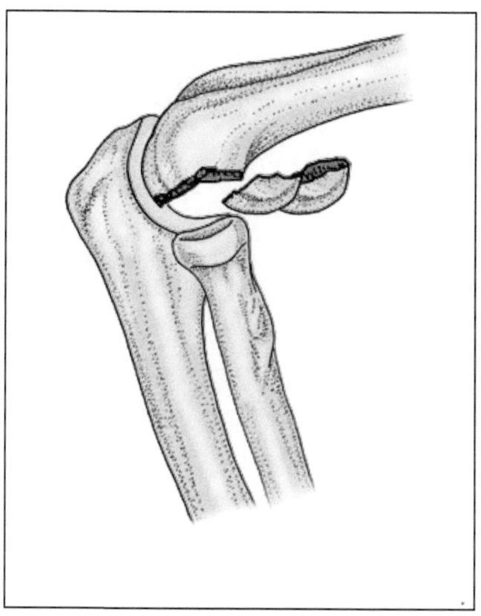

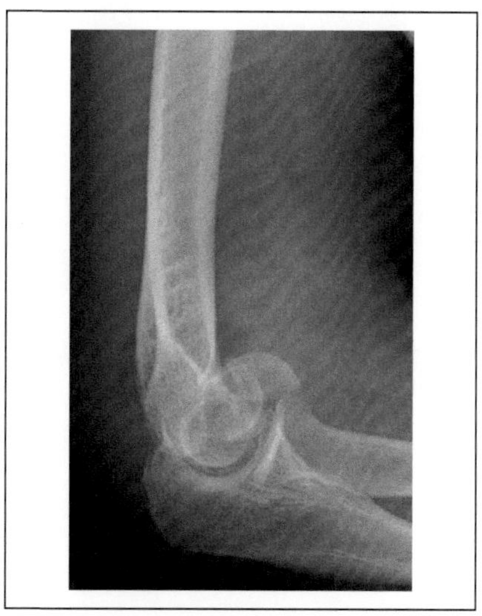

Bryan-Morrey classification

Type III: Comminuted fractures of the capitellum

Wang Chengwu Classification [8]

Type I: Complete fracture, with the fracture fragments involving the capitellum and partial trochlea.

Type II: Isolated complete fracture of the capitellum, which is sometimes difficult to detect because of the very small fracture fragments.

Type III: Cartilage shearing injury in the coronal plane of the capitellum.

2.3.4 Ring Classification [11]

Ring et al. identified five patterns of simple shearing injury of the distal humeral articular surface, on the basis of radiographs and operative findings.

Type I: A single articular fragment including the capitellum and the lateral portion of the trochlea.

Type II: A type I fracture (occasionally comminuted) with an associated fracture of the lateral epicondyle.

Type III: A type II fracture with impaction of the metaphyseal bone behind the capitellum in the distal and posterior aspect of the lateral column.

Type IV: A type III fracture with a fracture of the posterior aspect of the trochlea.

Type V: A type IV fracture with fracture of the medial epicondyle.

References

1. Neer CS 2nd. Displaced proximal humeral fractures. I. Classification and evaluation. J Bone Joint Surg Am. 1970;52(6):1077–89.
2. Marsh JL, Slongo TF, Agel J, Broderick JS, Creevey W, DeCoster TA, Prokuski L, Sirkin MS, Ziran B, Henley B, et al. Fracture and dislocation classification compendium - 2007: Orthopaedic Trauma Association classification, database and outcomes committee. J Orthop Trauma. 2007;21(10 Suppl):S1–133.
3. Codman EA. The shoulder: rupture of the supraspinatus tendon and other lesions in or about the subacromial bursa. Brooklyn, NY: Miller; 1934. p. 262–87.
4. Jupiter J, Levine A, Trafton P. Skeletal trauma, vol. 2. Philadelphia, PA/EUA: WB Saunders; 1992. p. 1146–76.
5. Jupiter JB, Mehne DK. Fractures of the distal humerus. Orthopedics. 1992;15(7):825–33.
6. Milch H. Fractures and fracture dislocations of the humeral condyles. *J Trauma*. 1964;4:592–607.
7. Riseborough EJ, Radin EL. Intercondylar T fractures of the humerus in the adult. A comparison of operative and non-operative treatment in twenty-nine cases. J Bone Joint Surg Am. 1969;51(1):130–41.
8. Yicong W. Bone and joint injuries. 3rd ed. Beijing: People's Medical Publishing House; 2001.
9. Watson J, Wilson J. Fractures and joint injuries. 5th ed. Edinburgh: Churchill Livingstone; 1976. p. 644–6.
10. Bryan RS, Morrey BF. Fractures ofthe distal humerus. In: Morrey BF, editor. The elbow and its disorders. Philadelphia, PA: WB Saunders; 1985. p. 302–39.
11. Ring D, Jupiter JB, Gulotta L. Articular fractures of the distal part of the humerus. J Bone Joint Surg Am. 2003;85-A(2):232–8.

Classifications of Radius and Ulna Fractures

3

Yingze Zhang and Juan Wang

3.1 Section 1 Classifications of Proximal Radius and Ulna Fractures

In 1924, Speed first classified radial head fractures [1]. Currently, over ten classifications have been reported in relation to proximal radius and ulna fractures [2]. According to the reports published in resent 5 years, AO classification is the most commonly used system in scientific research [3]. In clinical practice, Morrey classification is the most commonly used system for olecranon fractures, and Mason and modified Mason classifications for radial head fractures [4–6].

3.1.1 Classification of Olecranon Fractures

3.1.1.1 Morrey and Mayo Classification [7, 8]

Type I: Olecranon fractures: Stable and nondisplaced fractures
  Type IA: Noncomminuted fracture.
  Type IB: Comminuted fracture.
Type II: Olecranon fractures: Stable fractures with a displacement >3 mm
  Type IIA: Noncomminuted fracture, transversal fracture, or oblique fracture.
  Type IIB: Comminuted fracture.
Type III: Olecranon fractures: Unstable and displaced fractures.
  Type IIIA: Noncomminuted fracture.
  Type IIIB: Comminuted fracture.

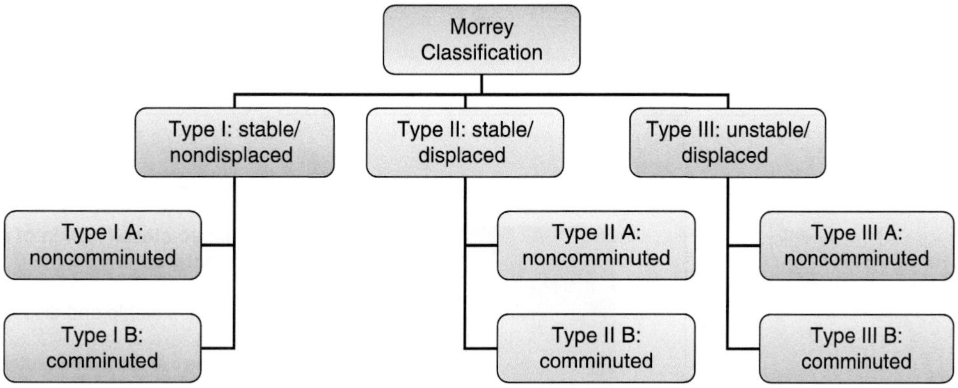

Y. Zhang (✉) • J. Wang
Department of Orthopedics,
The Third Hospital of Hebei Medical University,
Shijiazhuang, China
e-mail: yzzhangdr@126.com, yzling_liu@163.com

Y. Zhang (ed.), *Clinical Classification in Orthopaedics Trauma*, https://doi.org/10.1007/978-981-10-6044-1_3

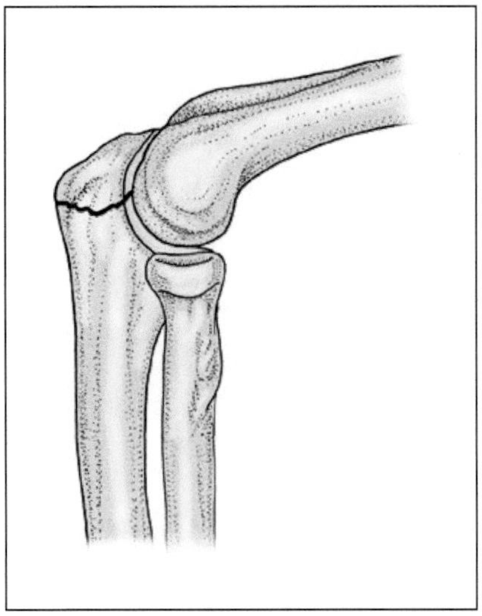

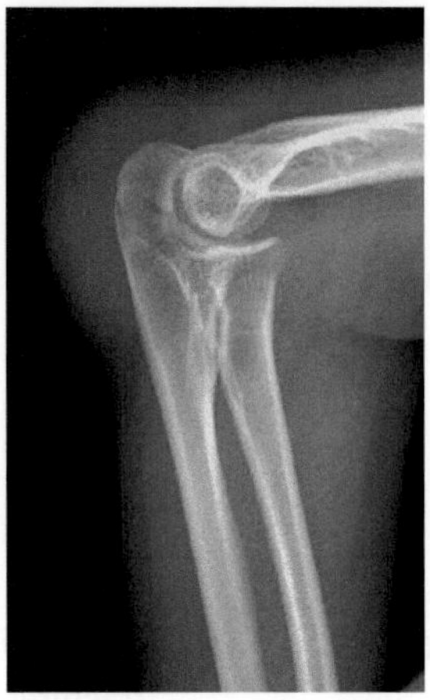

Mayo classification of olecranon fractures

Type I: stable and nondisplaced.

Type I A: noncomminuted

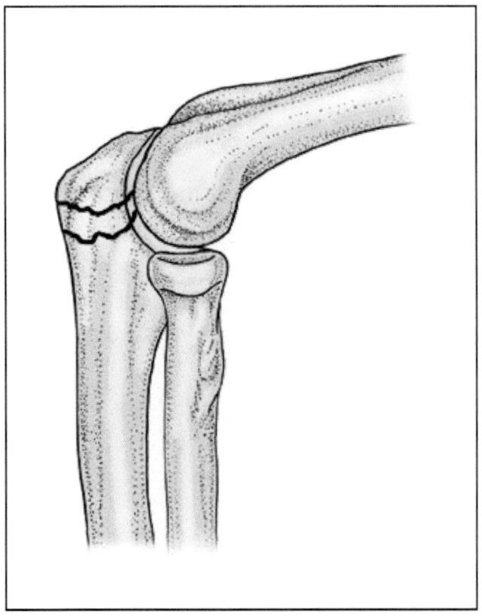

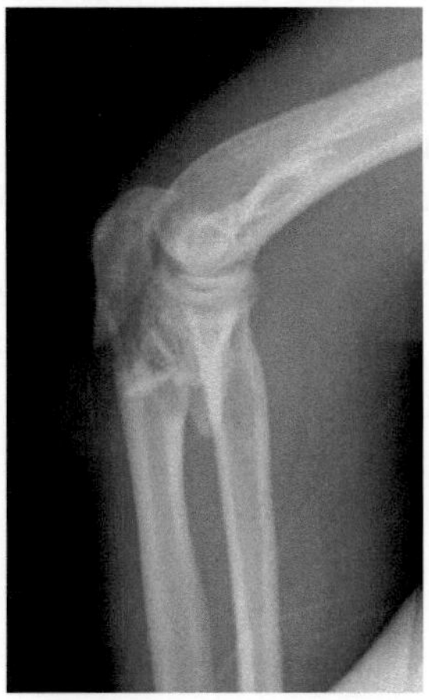

Mayo classification of olecranon fractures

Type I: stable and nondisplaced.

Type I B: comminuted

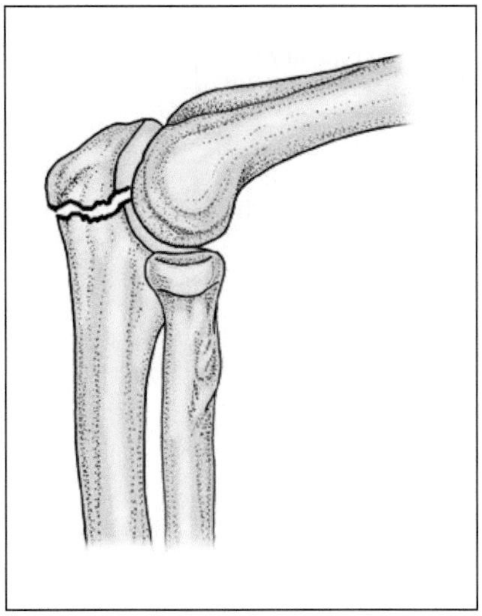

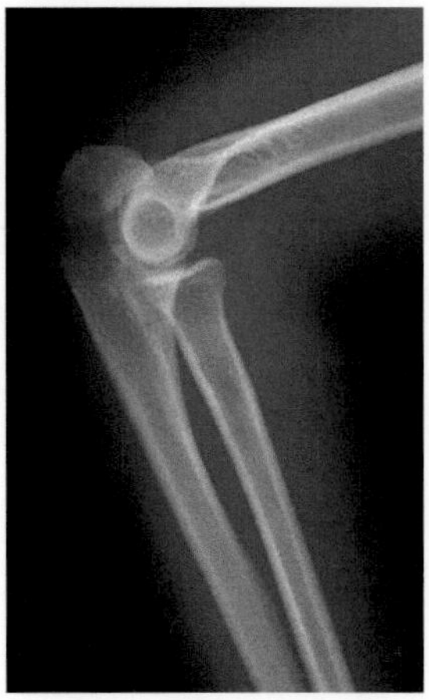

Mayo classification of olecranon fractures

Type I: stable and displaced.

Type I A: noncomminuted

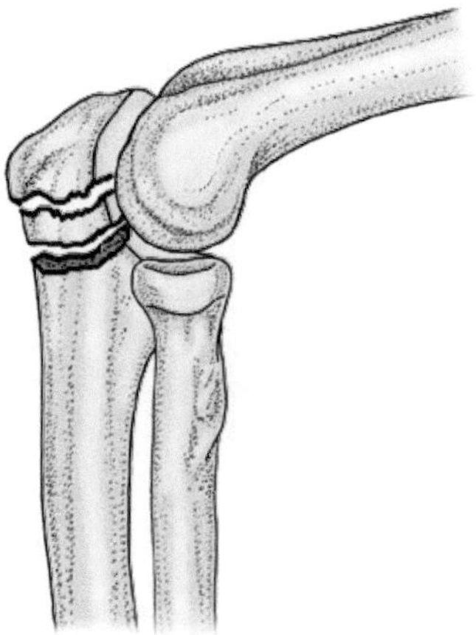

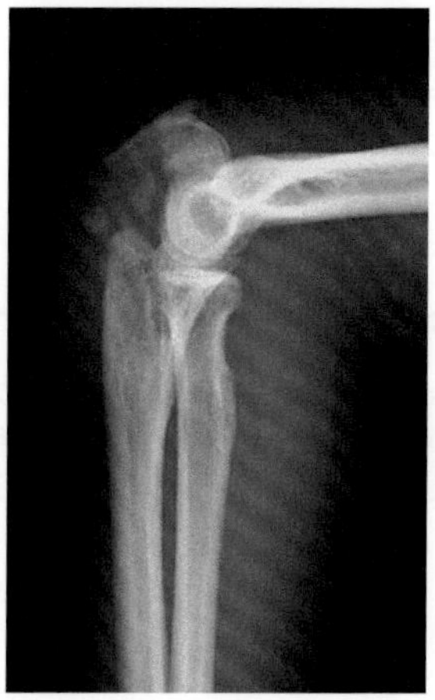

Mayo classification of olecranon fractures

Type II: stable and displaced.

Type II B: comminuted

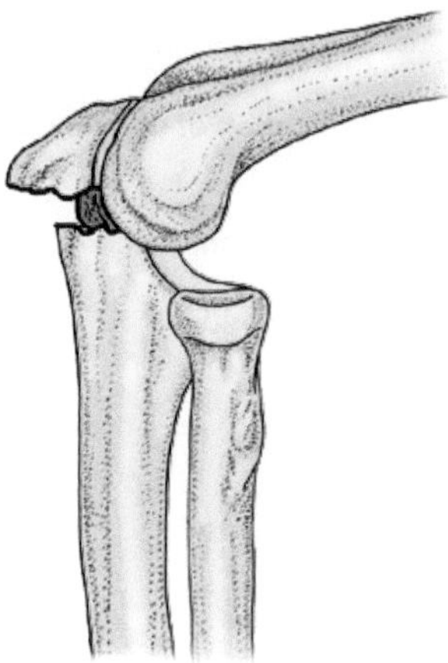

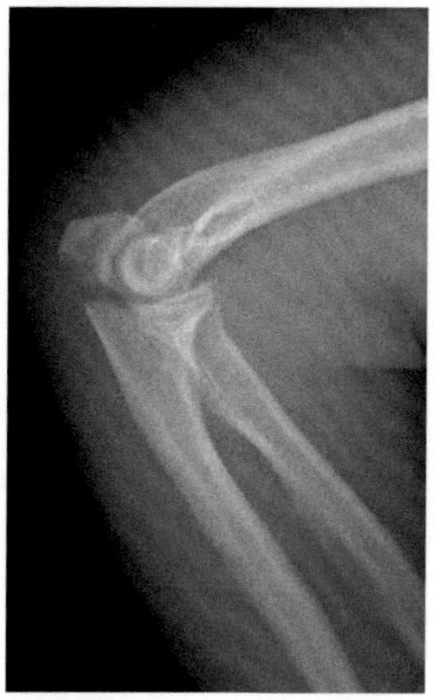

Mayo classification of olecranon fractures

Type III: unstable and displaced.

Type IIIA: noncomminuted

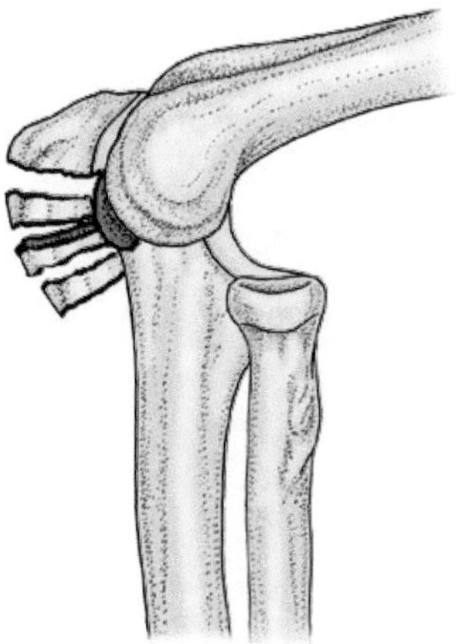

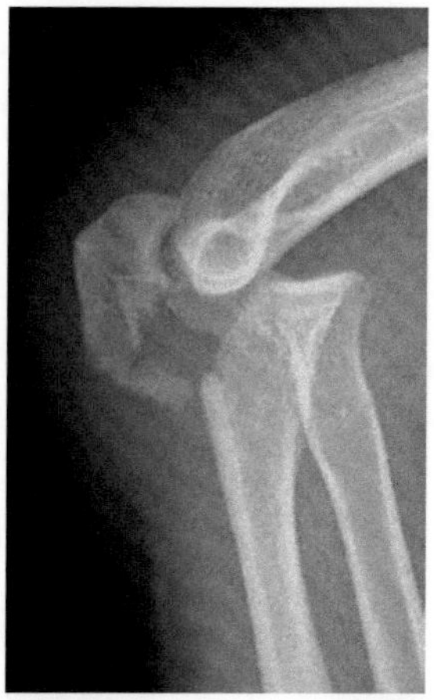

Mayo classification of olecranon fractures

Type III: unstable and displaced.

Type IIIB: comminuted

3.1.1.2 Colton Classification [9]

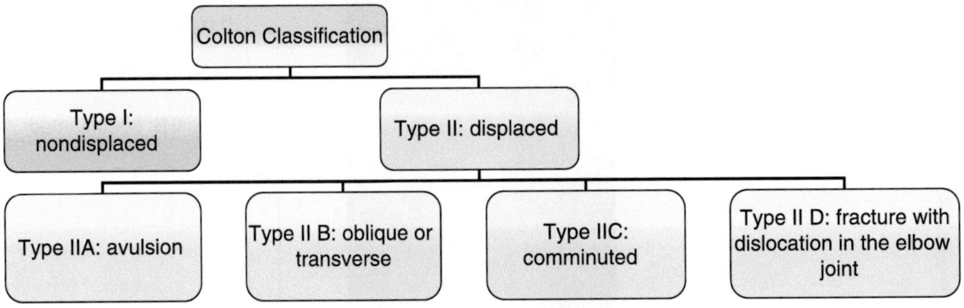

Type I: Undisplaced and stable; or displacement <2 mm, displacement does not increase with elbow flexion.

Type II: Displaced

- Type IIA: Avulsion fracture.
- Type IIB: Oblique or transverse fracture.
- Type IIC: Comminuted fracture.
- Type IID: Fracture with dislocation in the elbow joint

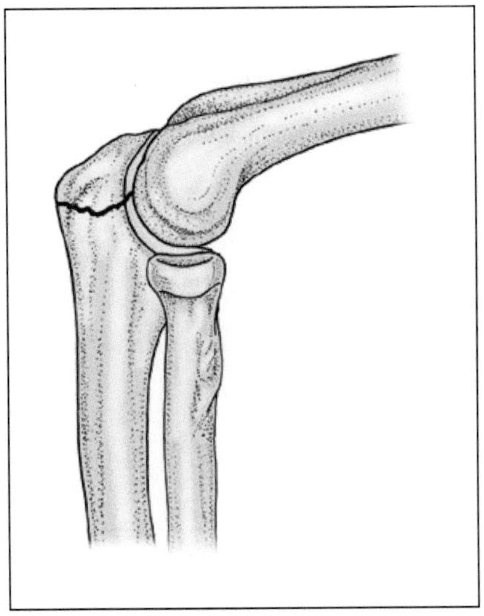

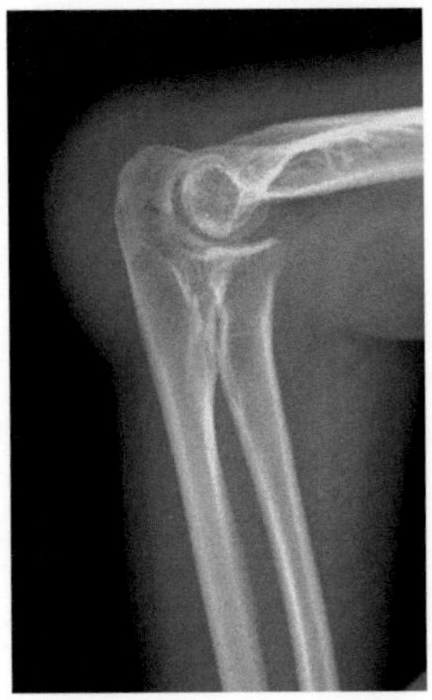

Colton classification of olecranon fractures

Type I : undisplaced and stable

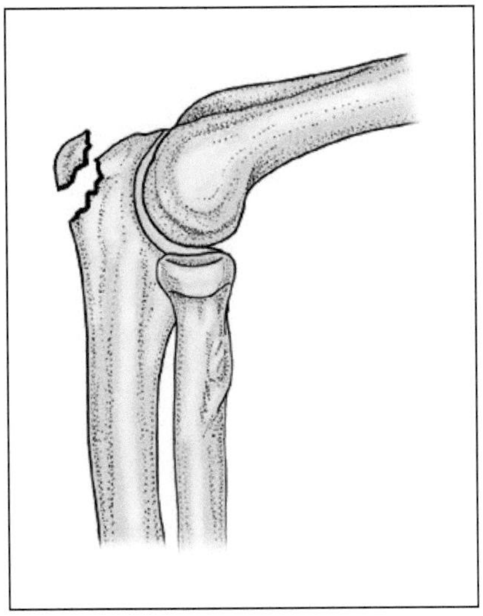

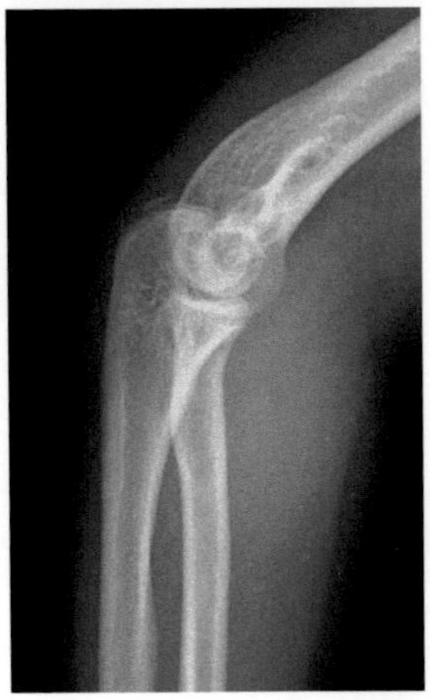

Colton classification of olecranon fractures

Type II : displaced.

Type II A: avulsion

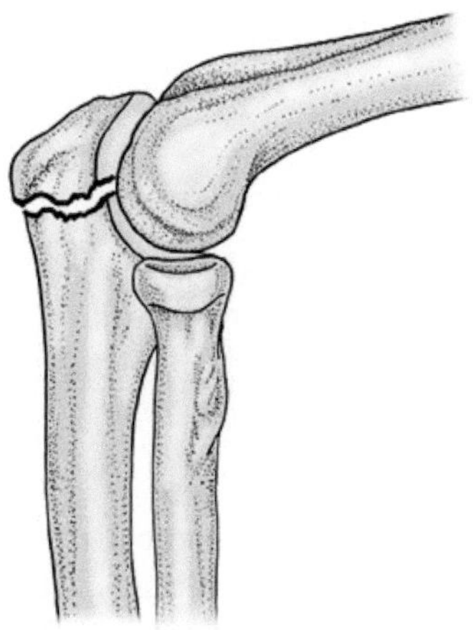

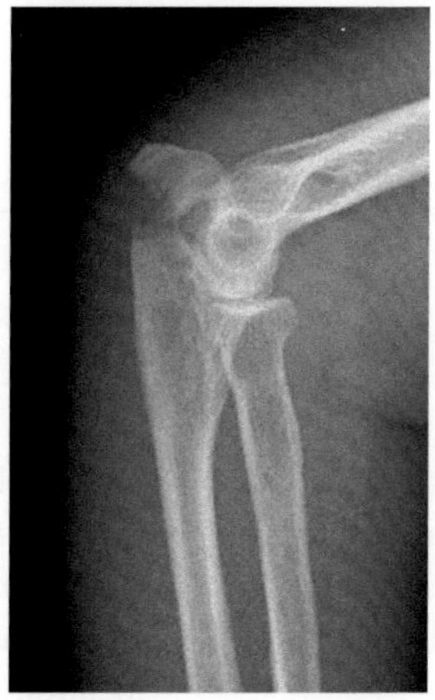

Colton classification of olecranon fractures

Type II : displaced.

Type II B: oblique or transverse

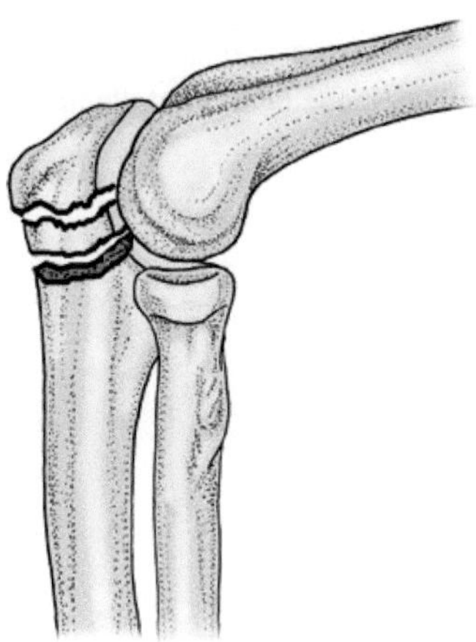

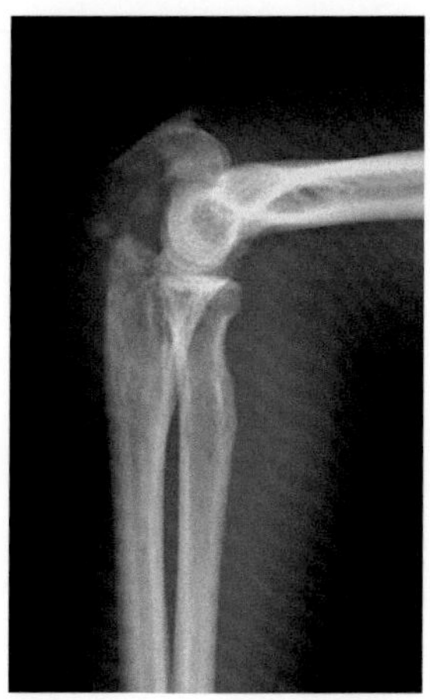

Colton classification of olecranon fractures

Type II : displaced.

Type II C: comminuted

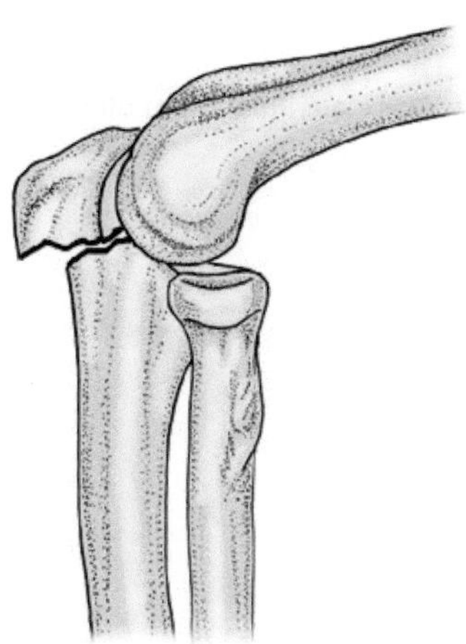

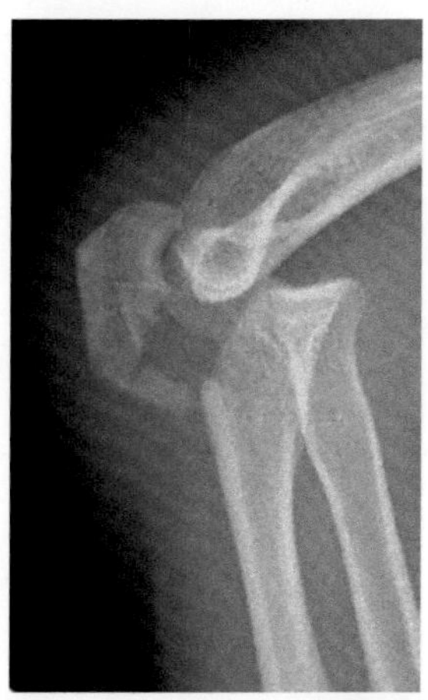

Colton classification of olecranon fractures

Type II : displaced.

Type II D: fracture with dislocation in the elbow joint

3.1.1.3 Schatzker Classification [10]

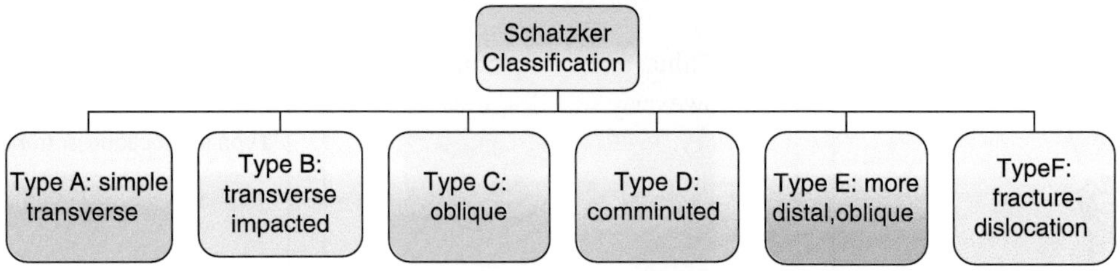

Schatzker classification is the modification of Colton classification. Owing to consideration of biomechanical characteristics of olecranon fractures, Schatzker classification benefits preoperative selection of implant selection and placement planning. Six types are included.

Type A: Simple transverse fracture.
Type B: Transverse impacted fracture.
Type C: Oblique fracture.
Type D: Comminuted fracture.
Type E: More distal oblique fracture, extra-articular.
Type F: Fracture–dislocation. Olecranon fractures with dislocation of elbow joint are often combined with Mason type III radial head fractures.

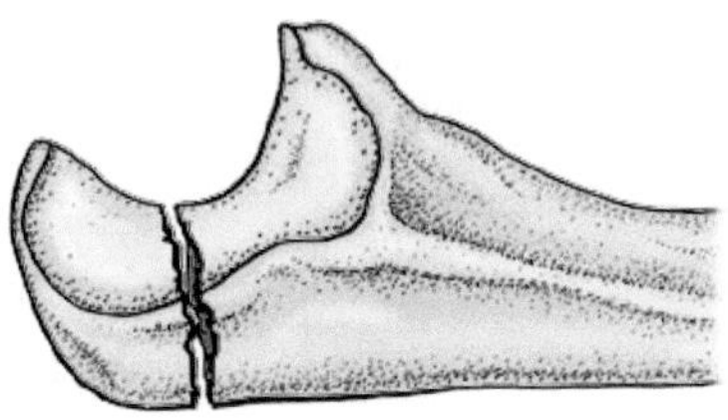

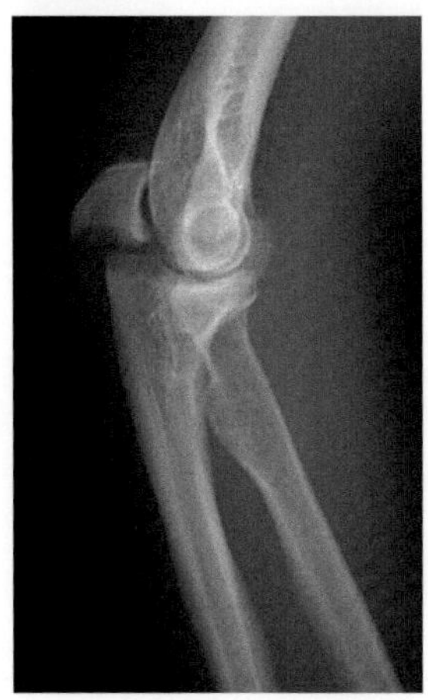

Schatzker classification of olecranonf ractures

Type A: simple transverse

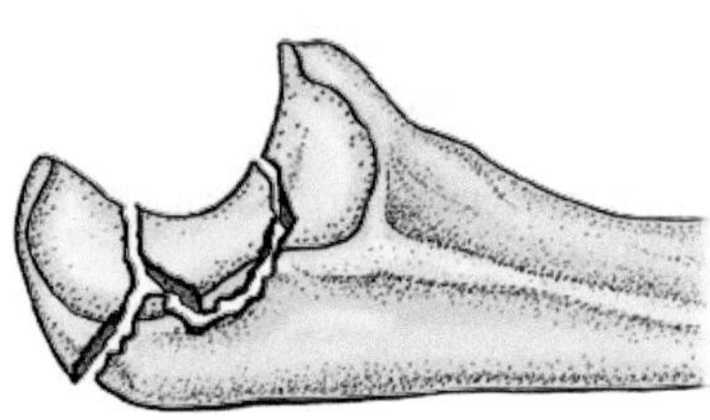

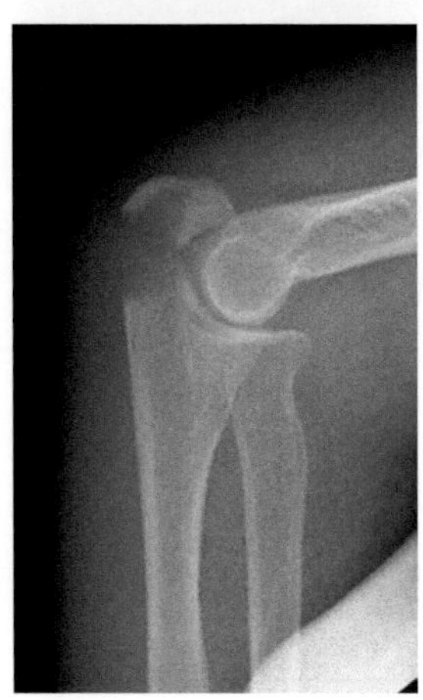

Schatzker classification of olecranon fractures

Type B: transverse impacted

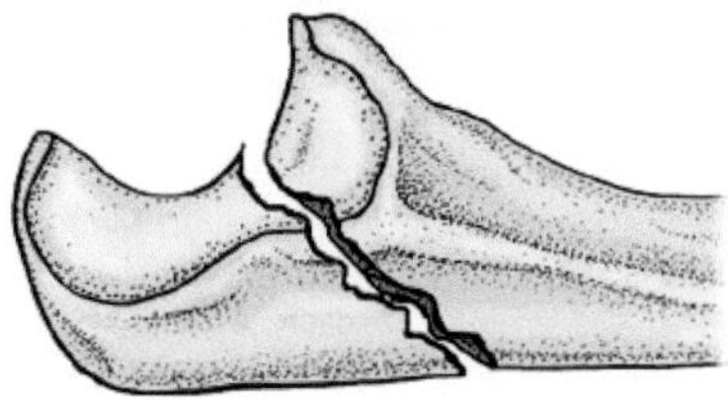

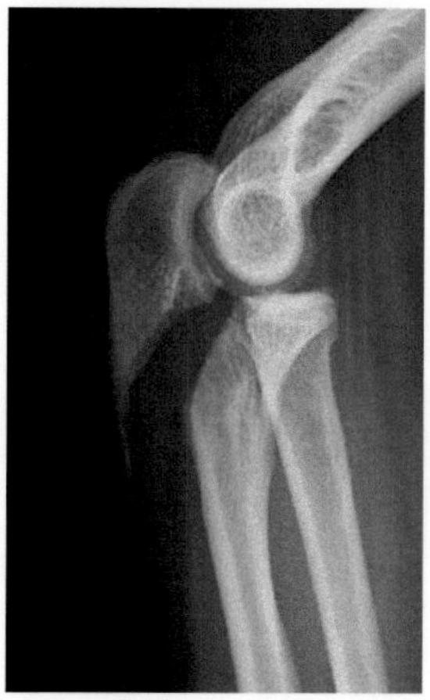

Schatzker classification of olecranon fractures

Type C: oblique fracture line across the center of trochlear notch

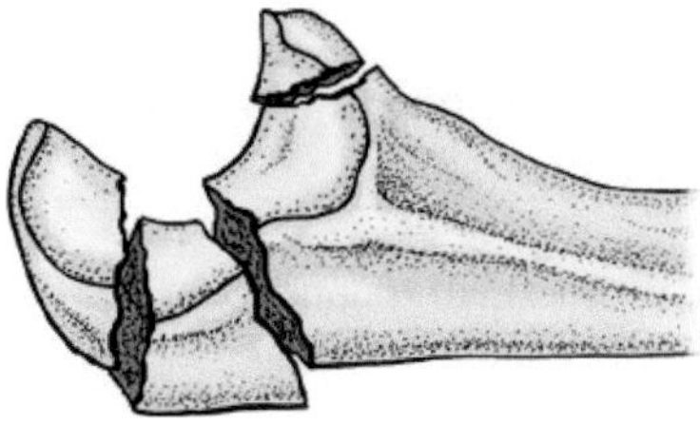

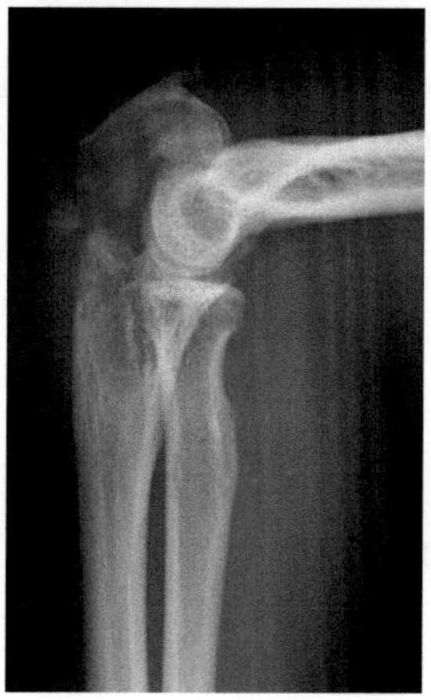

Schatzker classification of olecranon fractures

Type D: comminuted

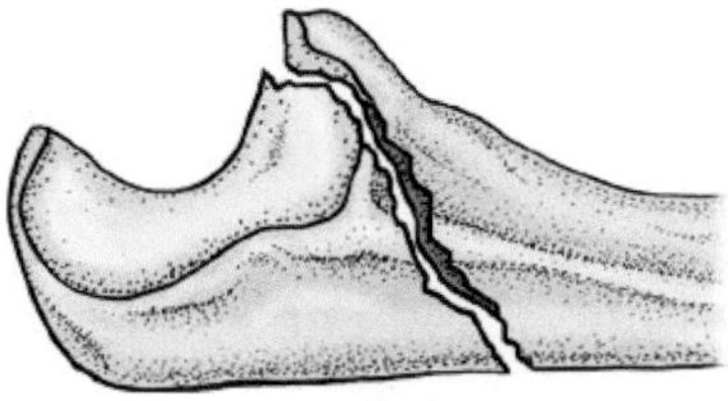

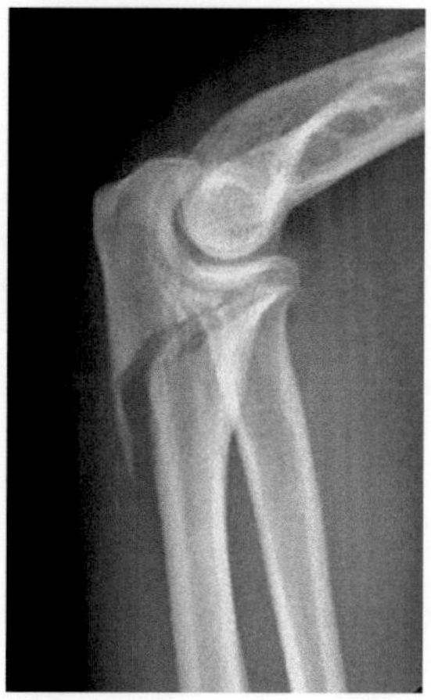

Schatzker classification of olecranon fractures

Type E: more distal, oblique

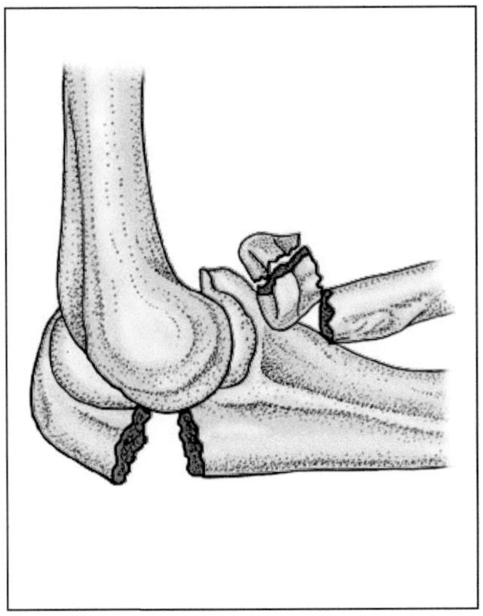

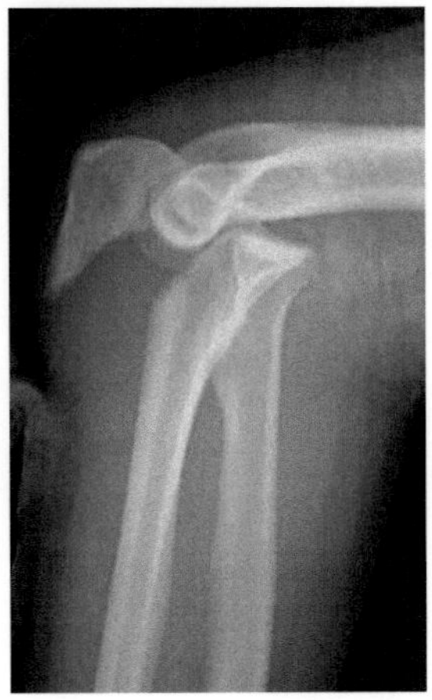

Schatzker classification of olecranon fractures

Type F: olecranon fracture with dislocation of elbow joint or even Mason Type III radial head fractures

3.1.1.4 Horne-Tanzer Classification [11]

The system includes three types:

Type I: Transverse intra-articular, proximal 1/3 of olecranon articular surface or short oblique extra-articular, involving the tip of the olecranon.

Type II: Oblique or transverse, involving middle 1/3 of greater sigmoid notch:

- Type IIA: Simple fracture.
- Type IIB: Complex fracture.

Type III: Involving distal 1/3 of the greater sigmoid notch with or without coronoid fracture.

3.1.1.5 Wadsworth Classification [12]

The system includes three types:

Type I: Avulsed fracture with a small fragment.
Type II: Simple fracture with a large fragment.
Type III: Comminuted fracture.

3.1.2 Classification of Coronoid Fractures

3.1.2.1 Regan and Morrey Classification [13]

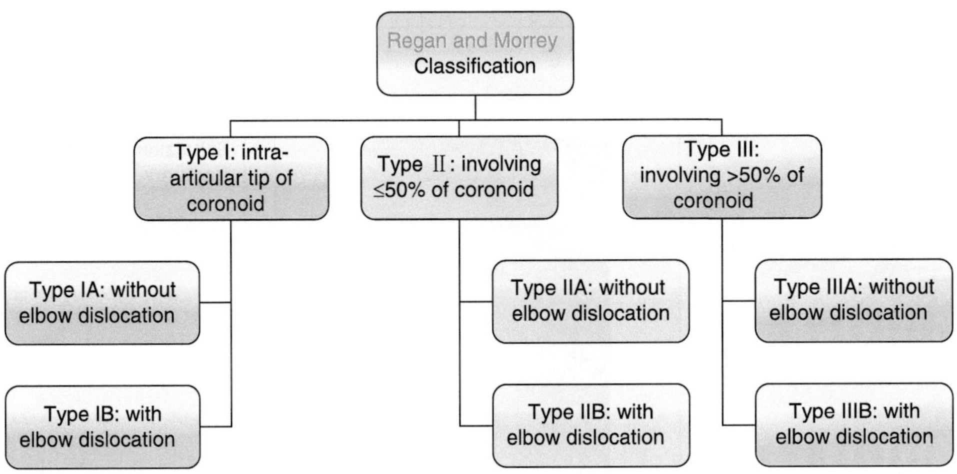

Type I: Fracture of the intra-articular tip of the coronoid

- Type IA: Without dislocation of elbow joint.
- Type IB: With dislocation of elbow joint.

Type II: Fracture involving half or less of the coronoid.

- Type IIA: Without dislocation of elbow joint.
- Type IIB: With dislocation of elbow joint.

Type III: Fracture involving more than 50% of the coronoid process.

- Type IIIA: Without dislocation of elbow joint.
- Type IIIB: With dislocation of elbow joint.

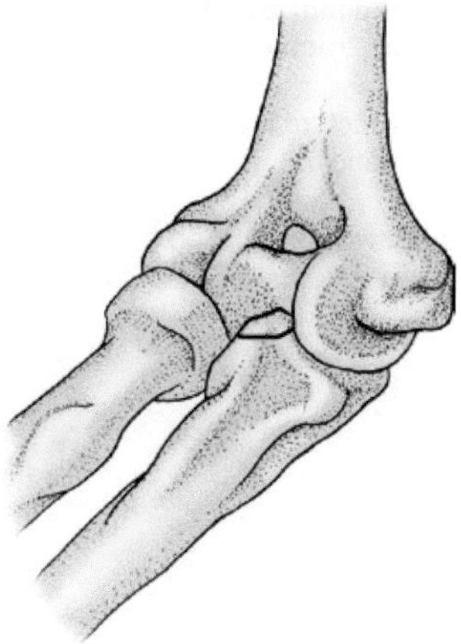

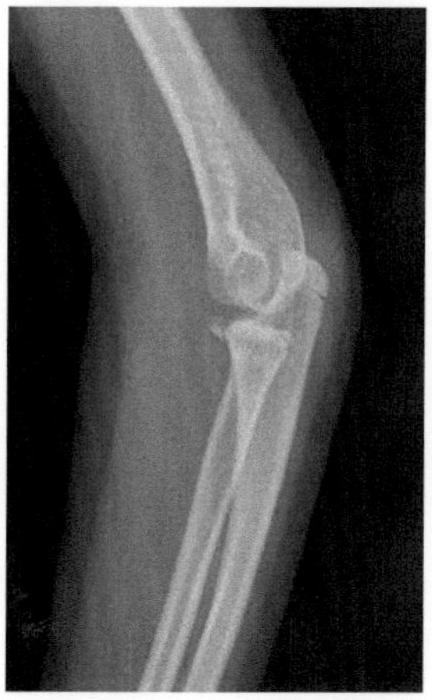

Regan and Morrey Classification of Coronoid Fractures

Type I : Fracture of the intra-articular tip of the coronoid.

Type I A: without dislocation of elbow joint

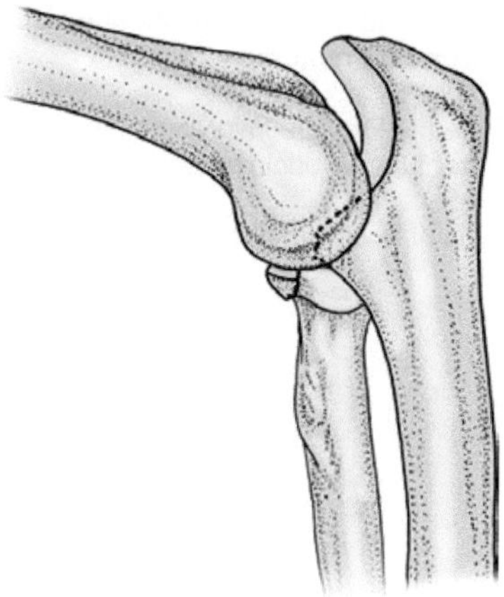

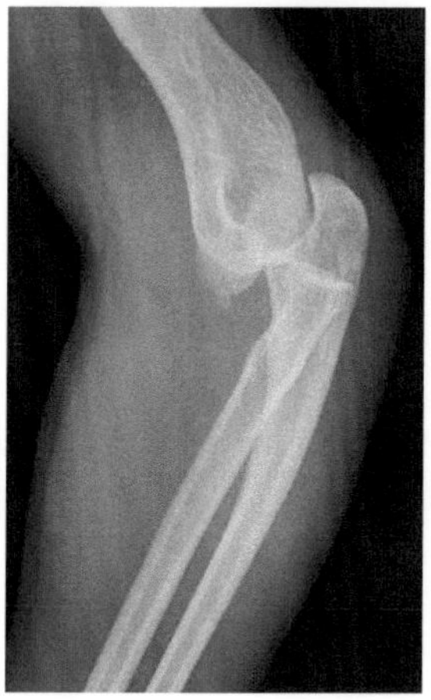

Regan and Morrey Classification of Coronoid Fractures

Type I: Fracture of the intra-articular tip of the coronoid.

Type I B: with dislocation of elbow joint

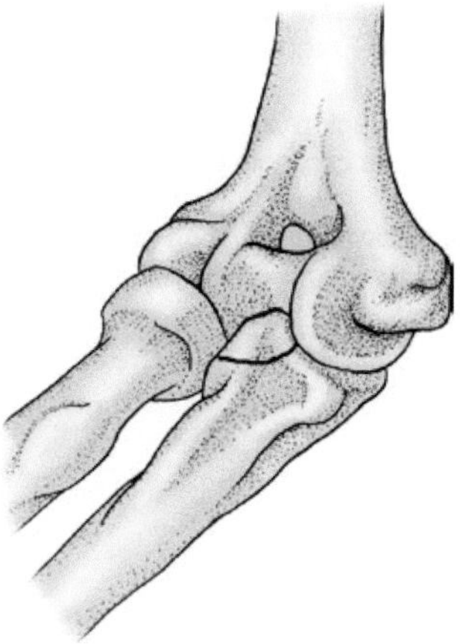

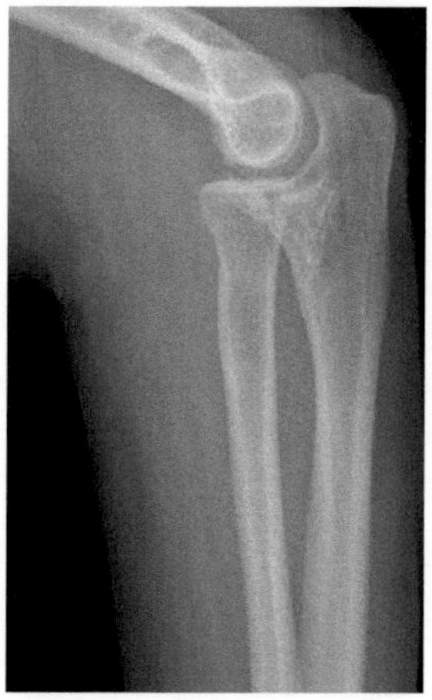

Regan and Morrey Classification of Coronoid Fractures

Type II : Fracture involving half or less of the coronoid.

Type II A: without dislocation of elbow joint

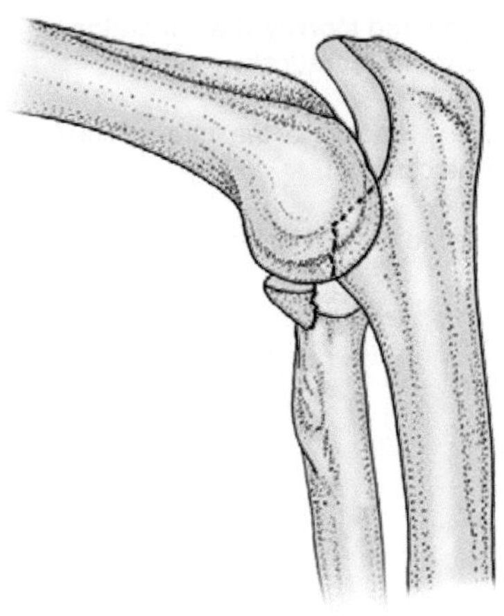

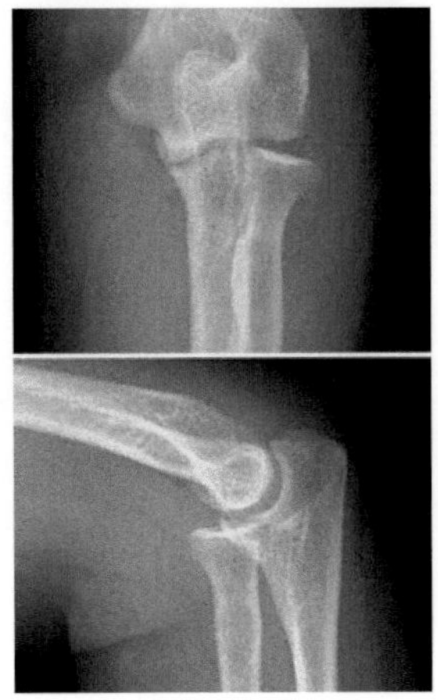

Regan and Morrey Classification of Coronoid Fractures

Type II : Fracture involving half or less of the coronoid.

Type II B: with dislocation of elbow joint

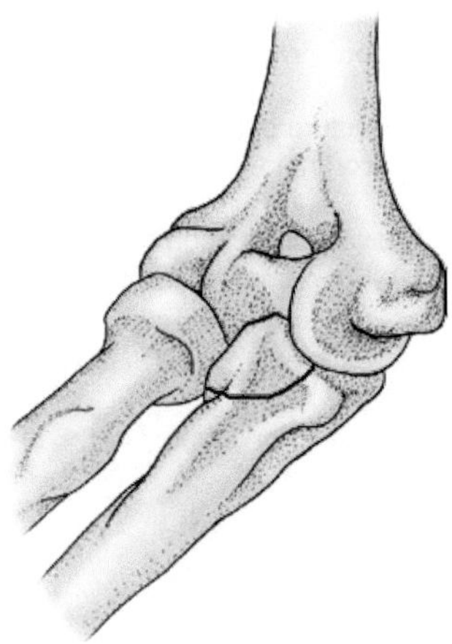

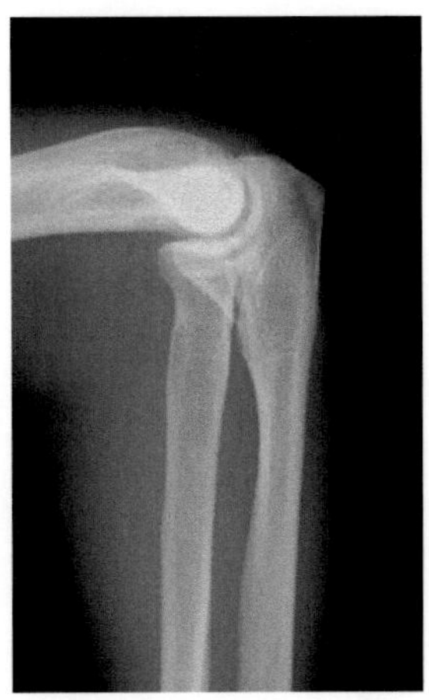

Regan and Morrey Classification of Coronoid Fractures

Type III : Fracture involving more than 50% of the coronoid process.

Type IIIA: without dislocation of elbow joint

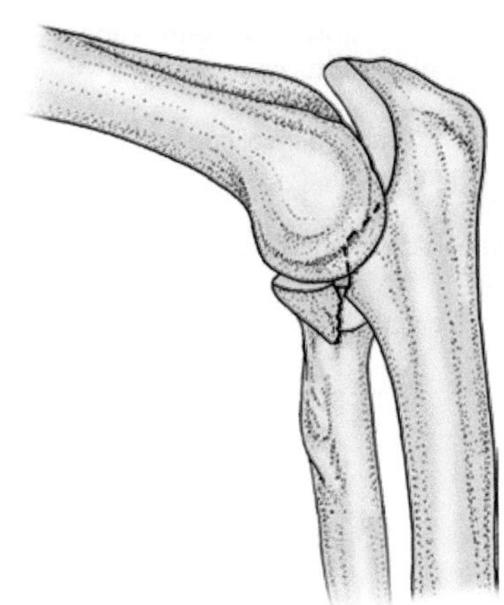

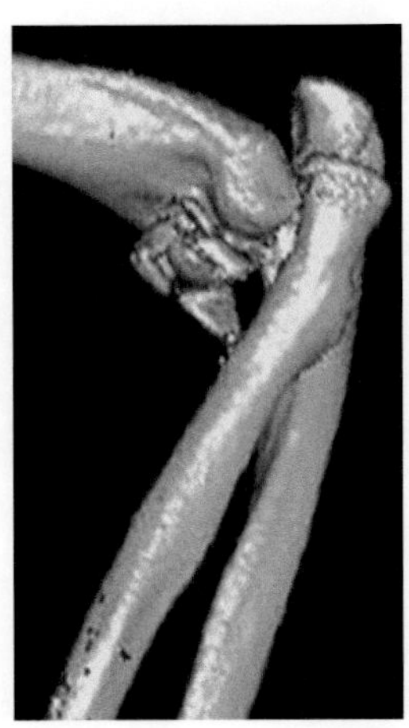

Regan and Morrey Classification of Coronoid Fractures

Type III: Fracture involving more than 50% of the coronoid process.

Type IIIB: with dislocation of elbow joint

3.1.2.2 Wang Classification [14]

Wang et al. [13] divided coronoid fractures into four types based on fracture site, involvement of ulnar collateral ligament, and stability of the elbow joint.

Type I: Fracture <50% of coronoid.

Type II: Unstable fracture at 50% of coronoid; often involvement of ulnar collateral ligament.

Type III: Basal fracture often associated with dislocation or subluxation of the elbow joint, occasionally with injury of the anterior band of ulnar collateral ligament.

Type IV: Severe comminuted fracture with instability of the elbow joint.

3.1.3 Classification of Radial Head Fractures

3.1.3.1 Mason-Johnston Classification [15]

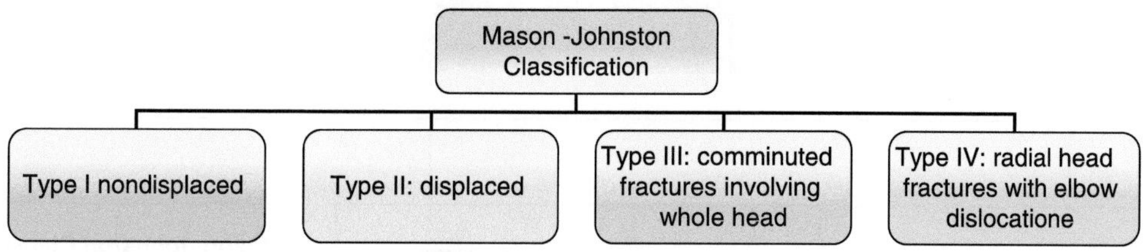

Radial head fractures are divided into three types, and Johnston added a fourth type:

Type I: Partial head fractures without displacement.
Type II: Partial head fractures involving 30–50% of radial head with displacement.
Type III: Comminuted fractures involving the whole head.
Type IV: Radial head fracture associated with an elbow dislocation (added by Johnston).

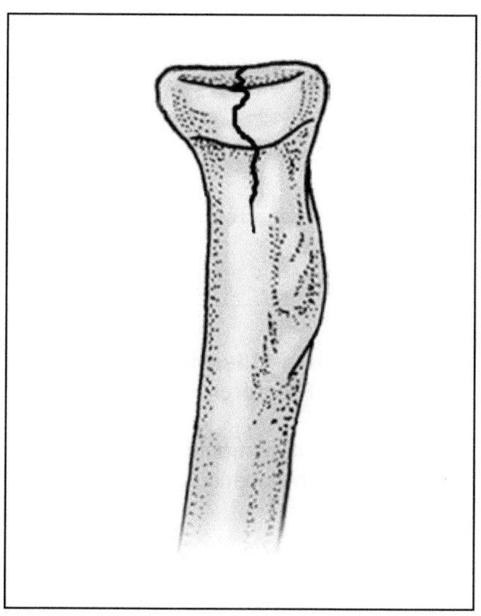

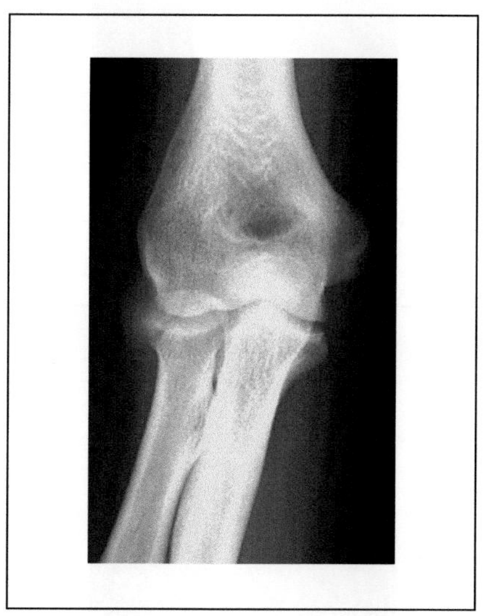

Mason-Johnston Classification of Radial Head Fractures

Type I : partial head fractures without displacement

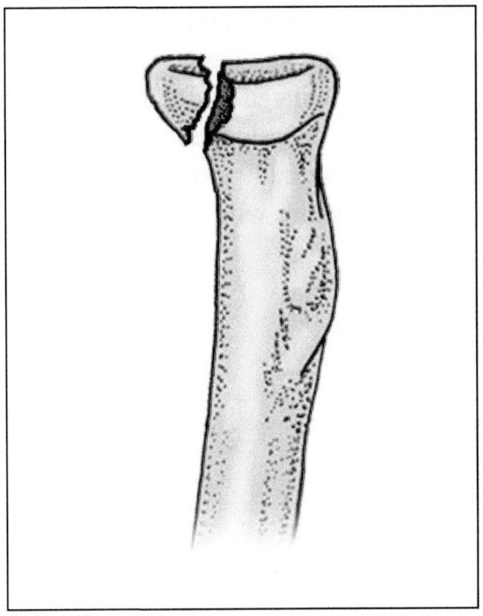

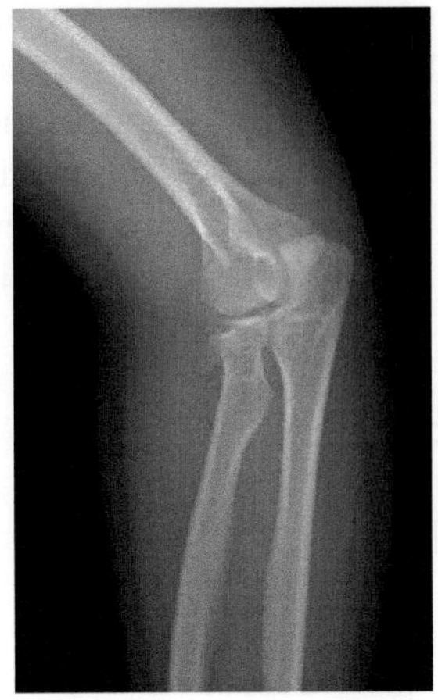

Mason-Johnston Classification of Radial Head Fractures

Type II : partial head fractures involving 30-50% of radial head with displacement

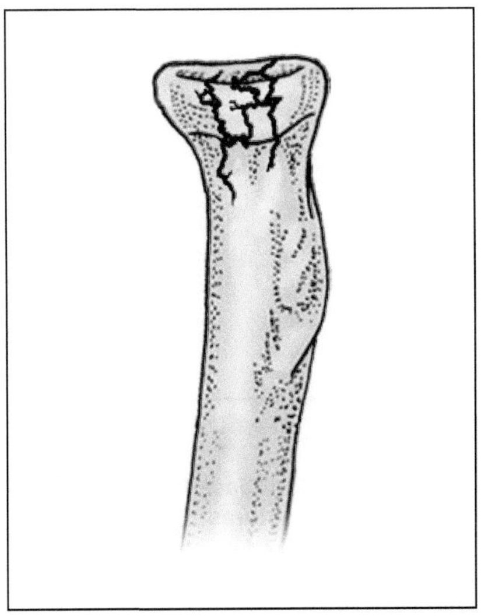

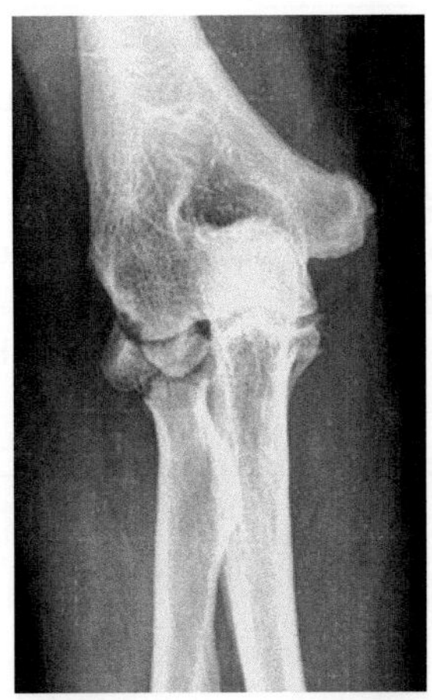

Mason-Johnston Classification of Radial Head Fractures

Type III : comminuted fractures involving the whole head

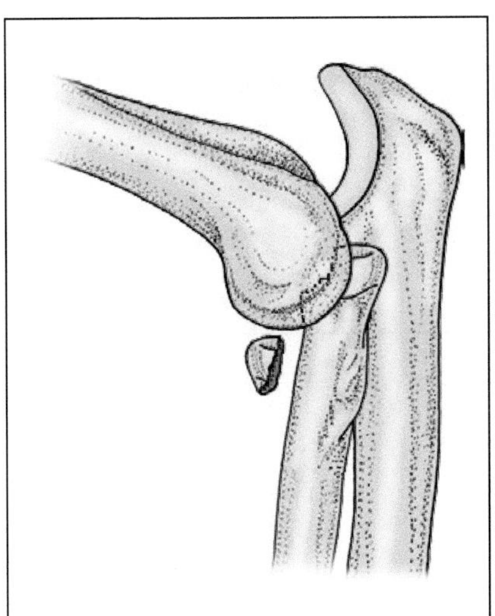

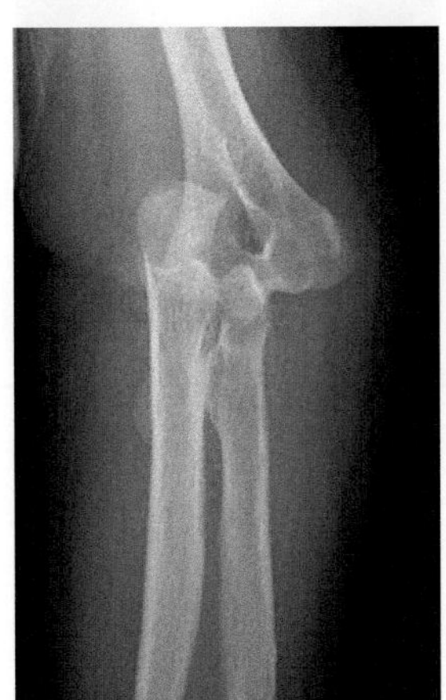

Mason-Johnston Classification of Radial Head Fractures

Type IV: radial head fracture associated with an elbow dislocation (added by Johnston)

3.1.3.2 Hotchkiss Modification of Mason Classification [16]

Hotchkiss modified Mason classification.

Type I: Minimal fracture displacement, no mechanical block to forearm rotation, and intra-articular displacement less than 2 mm are treated by nonoperative treatment.
Type II: Fracture displaced more than 2 mm or angulated and possible mechanical block to forearm rotation are treated by open reduction and internal fixation.
Type III: Severely comminuted fracture, with mechanical block to motion, is treated by radial head arthroplasty.

3.1.3.3 Mason Classification [17]

Radial head fractures are divided into three types based on displacement and complex of the fractures:

Type I: Partial head fractures without displacement.
Type II: Partial head fractures involving 30–50% of radial head with displacement.
Type III: Comminuted fractures involving the whole head.

3.1.3.4 Bakalim Classification [18]

Type I: Undisplaced marginal head fracture.
Type II: Displaced marginal head fracture.
Type III: Comminuted head fracture.
Type IV: Undisplaced neck fracture.
Type V: Displaced neck fracture.

3.1.3.5 Schatzker-Tile Classification [19]

Type I: Displaced or undisplaced marginal head fractures.
Type II: Impaction fractures: In this pattern part of the head and neck remains intact. The portion involved in the fracture is tilted and impacted.
Type III: Severely comminuted fractures involving radial neck and articular surface.

3.1.3.6 Mayo Extended Classification (Modified Mason Classification by van Riet and Morrey) [20]

Type I: Non-displaced.
Type II: Displaced more than 2 mm.
Type III: Comminuted, non-reconstructible radial head.

The Mayo extended classification then adds a suffix to the fracture type to show any associated injuries.

Suffix:

"c" associated coronoid fracture. "C"—if operative treatment was done.

"o" associated olecranon fractures. "O"—if operative treatment was done.

"m" for medial collateral ligament (MCL) injury. "M"—if operative repair was done.

"l" for the lateral collateral ligament (LCL) injury. "L"—if operative repair was done.

"d" for longitudinal distal radioulnar joint (DRUJ) dissociation. "D"—if operative treatment done.

"X" added for radial head excision.

"F" if radial head was fixed and "A" if arthroplasty was done.

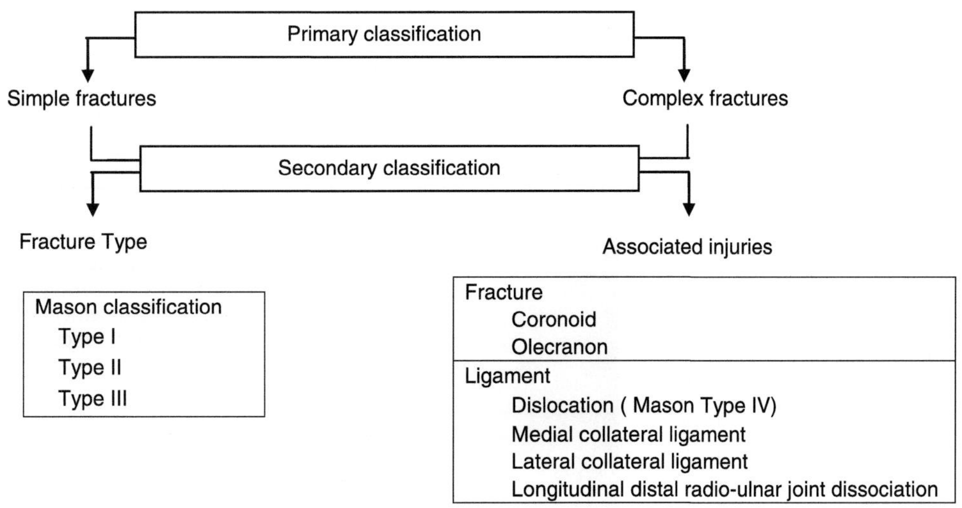

3.1.3.7 **Speed Classification** [1]

The first classification of radial head fractures. The system includes complete and incomplete fractures of the head and neck.

3.1.4 **Judet Classification of Radial Neck Fractures** [21]

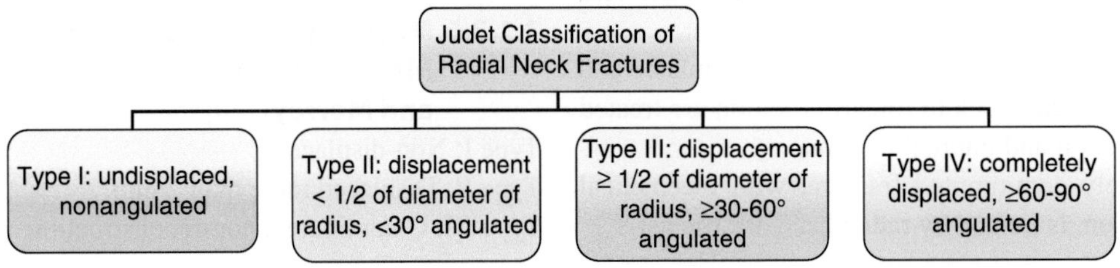

Type I: Undisplaced, nonangulated.
Type II: Displacement <1/2 of diameter of radius, <30° angulated.
Type III: Displacement ≥1/2 of diameter of radius, ≥30–60° angulated.
Type IV: Completely displaced, ≥60–90° angulated.

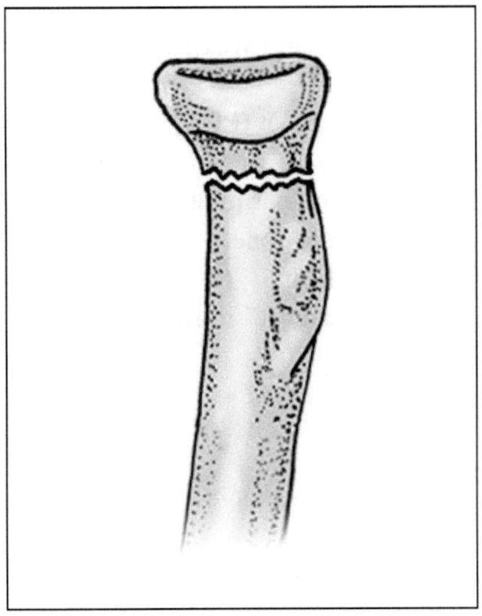

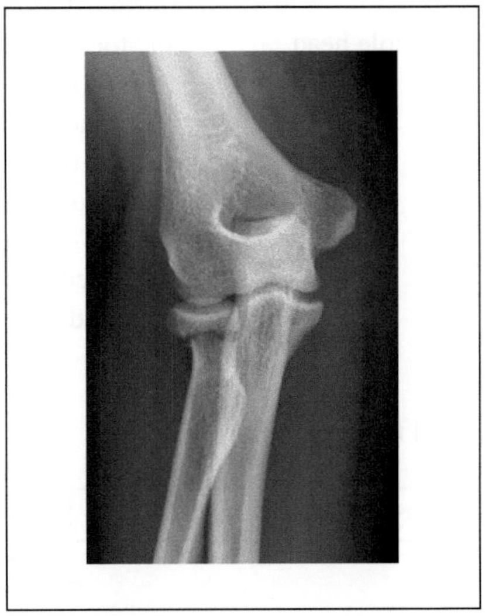

Judet Classification of Radial Neck Fractures

Type I : undisplaced, nonangulated

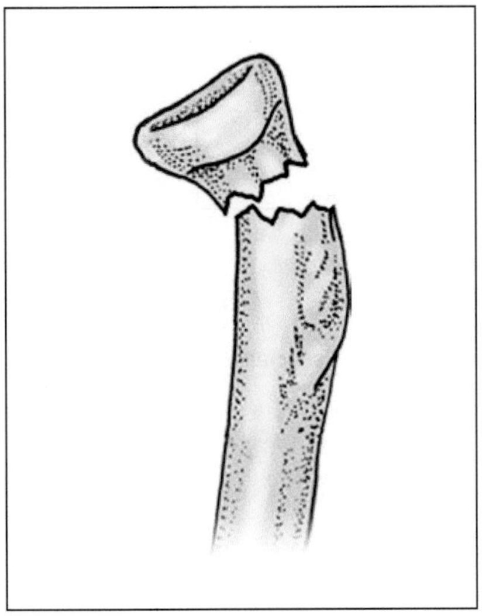

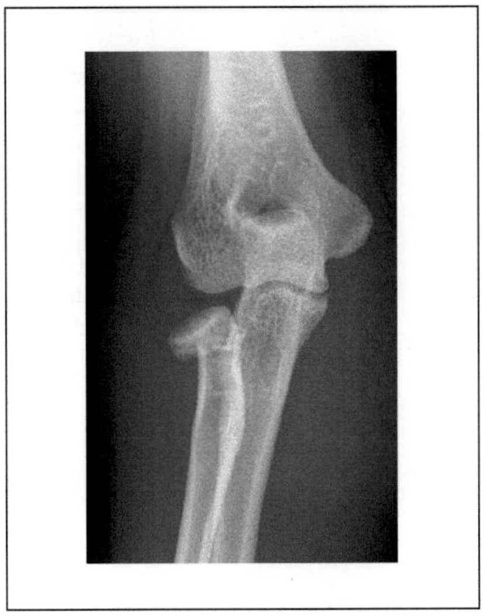

Judet Classification of Radial Neck Fractures

Type II: displacement < 1/2 of diameter of radius, <30° angulated

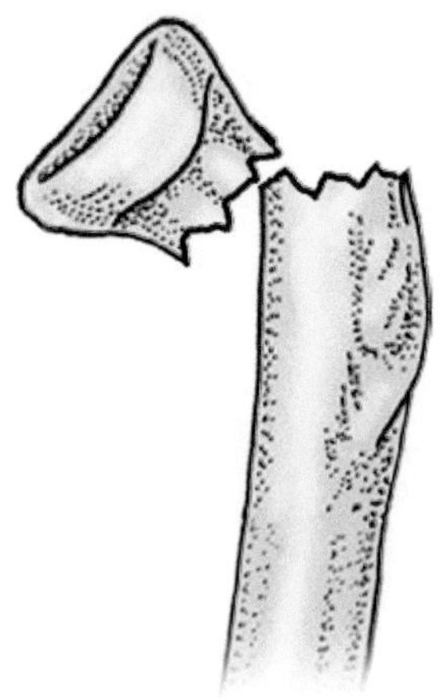

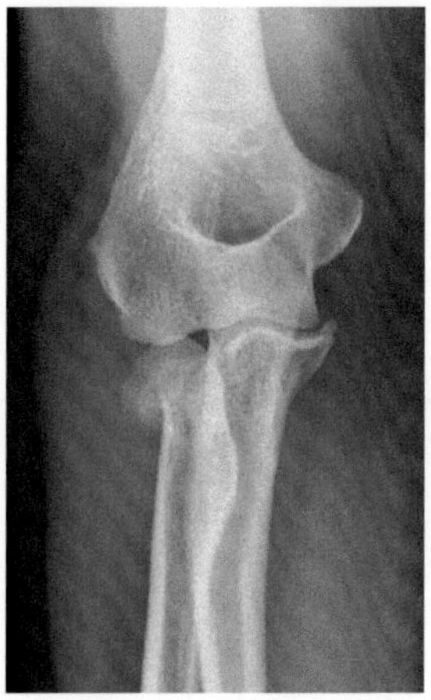

Judet Classification of Radial Neck Fractures

Type III: displacement ≥ 1/2 of diameter of radius, ≥30-60° angulated

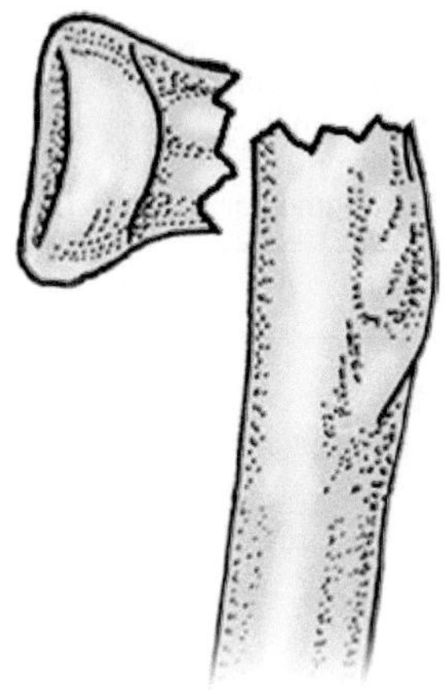

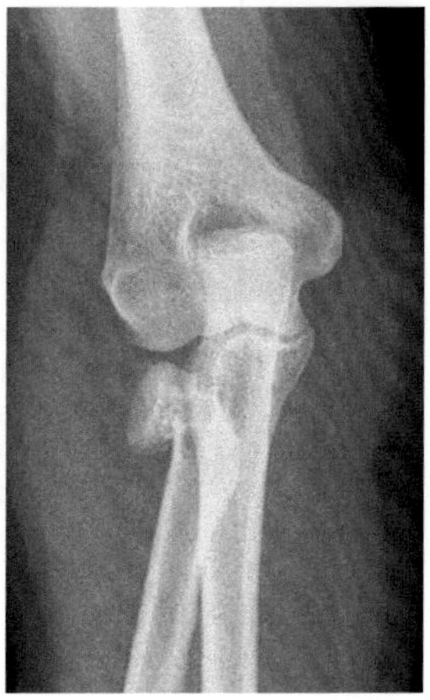

Judet Classification of Radial Neck Fractures

Type IV: completely displaced, ≥60-90° angulated

3.1.5 AO/OTA Classification of Proximal Radius and Ulna fractures [22, 23]

In 1987, Muller and the AO foundation published the widely accepted AO/OTA universal classifications, and modified it in 2007. Every major bone and each bone segment are numbered.

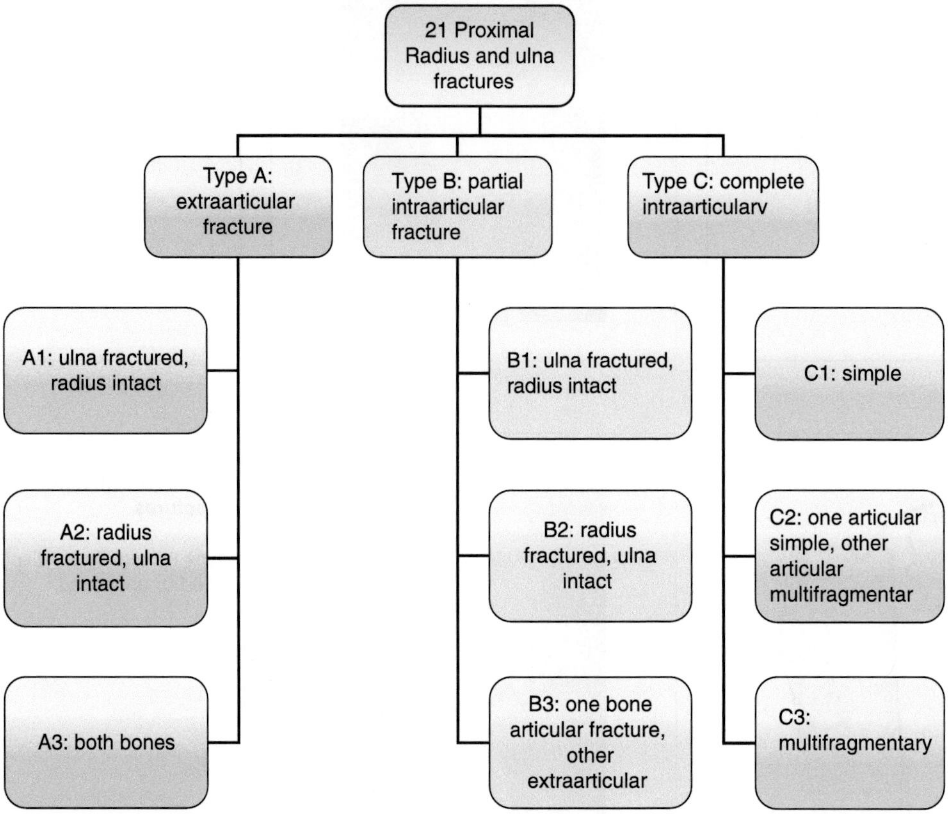

21-A: Extra-articular fracture:

- A1: Ulna fractured, radius intact:
  - A1.1: Avulsion fracture at triceps tendon insertion into the olecranon.
  - A1.2: Simple proximal metaphyseal fracture of ulna.
  - A1.3: Comminuted proximal metaphyseal fracture of ulna.
- A2: Radius fractured, ulna intact:
  - A2.1: Avulsion fracture of biceps tendon from radial tuberosity.
  - A2.2: Simple radial neck fracture.
  - A2.3: Comminuted radial neck fracture.
- A3: Fractures of both bones:
  - A3.1: Simple fractures of both bones.
  - A3.2: Comminuted fracture of one bone and simple fracture of another bone.
  - A3.3: Comminuted fractures of both bones.

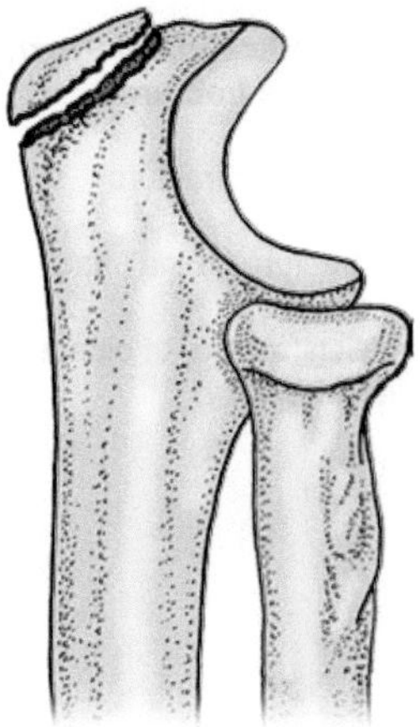

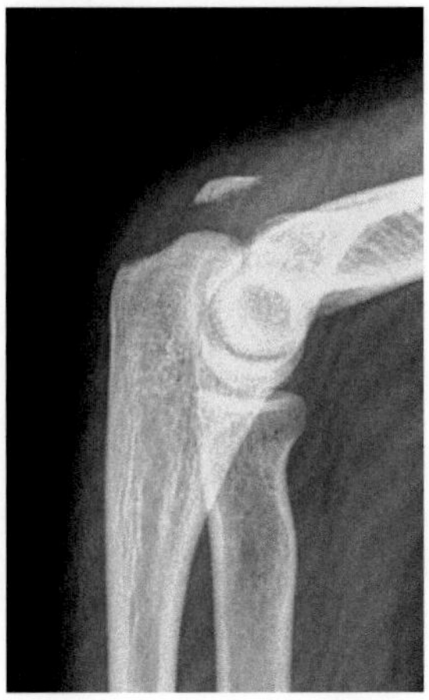

AO/OTA Classification of Proximal Radius and ulna fractures

21-A: extraarticular fracture

A1: ulna fractured, radius intact

A1.1: avulsion fracture at triceps tendon insertion into the olecranon

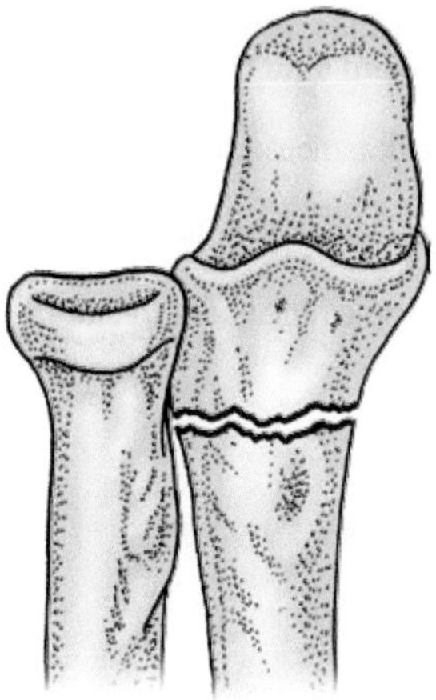

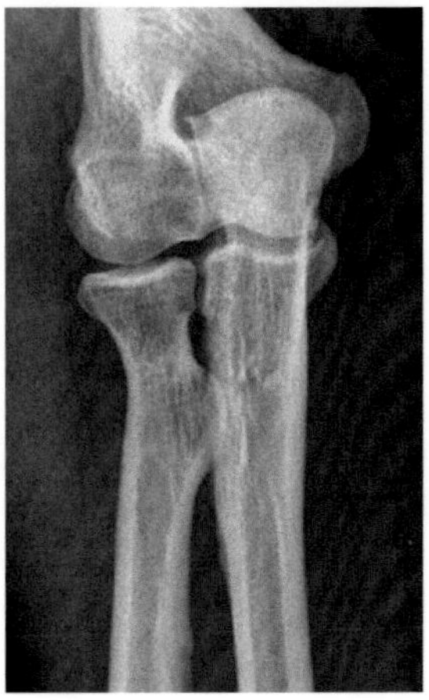

AO/OTA Classification of Proximal Radius and ulna fractures

21-A: extraarticular fracture

A1: ulna fractured, radius intact

A1.2: simple proximal metaphyseal fracture of ulna

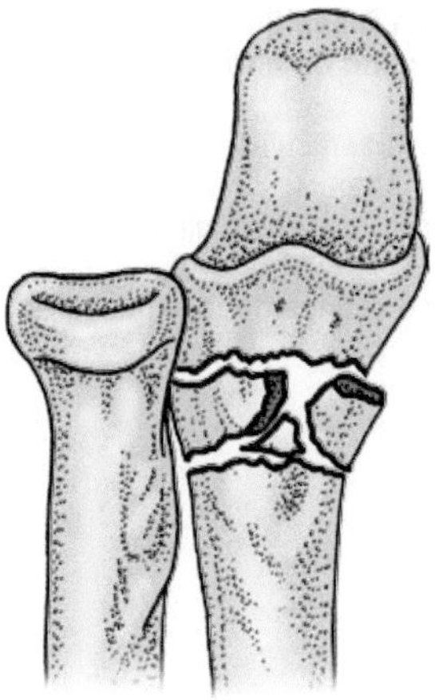

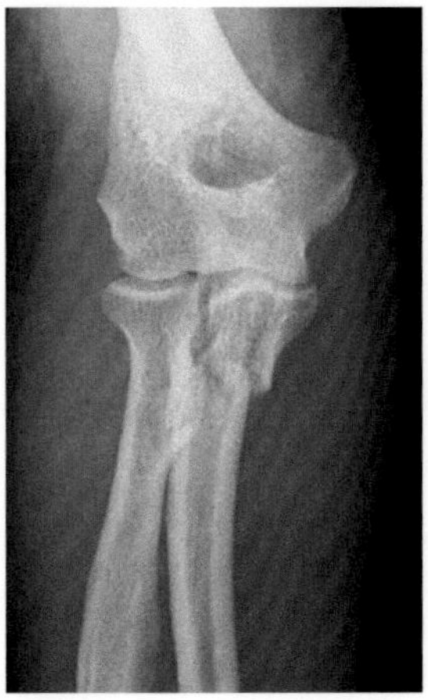

AO/OTA Classification of Proximal Radius and ulna fractures

21-A: extraarticular fracture

A1: ulna fractured, radius intact

A1.3: comminuted proximal metaphyseal fracture of ulna

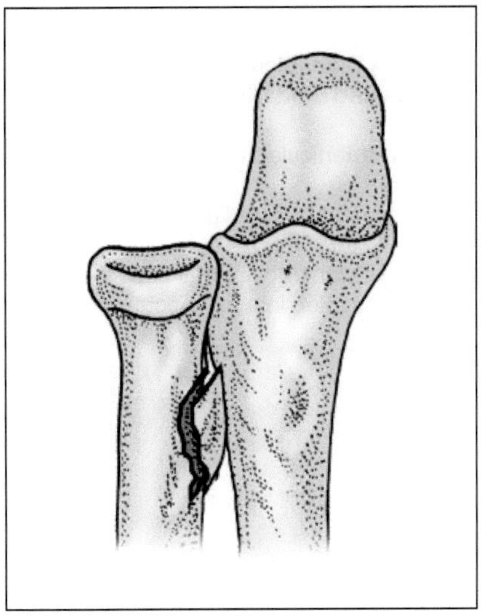

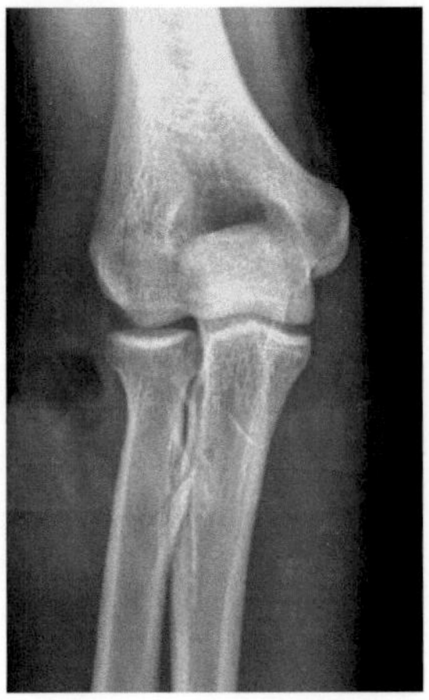

AO/OTA Classification of Proximal Radius and ulna fractures

21-A: extraarticular fracture

A2: radius fractured, ulna intact

A2.1: avulsion fracture of biceps tendon from radial tuberosity

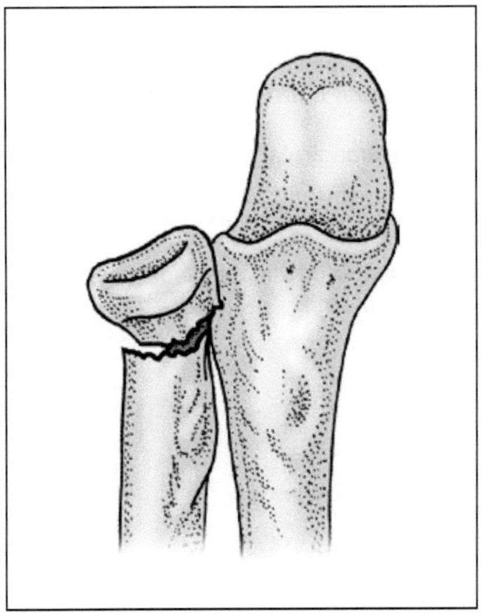

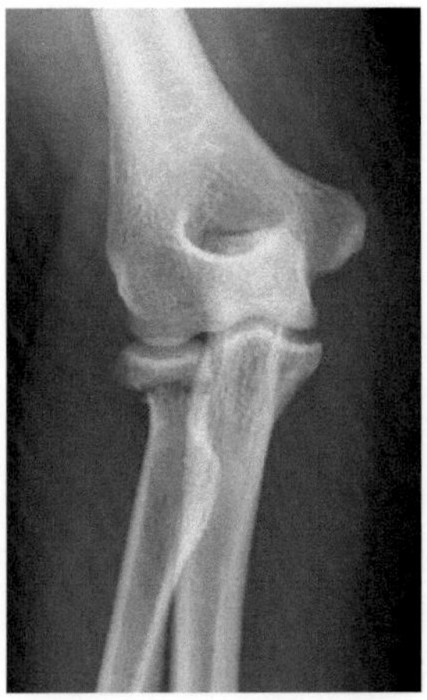

AO/OTA Classification of Proximal Radius and ulna fractures

21-A: extraarticular fracture

A2: radius fractured, ulna intact

A2.2: simple radial neck fracture

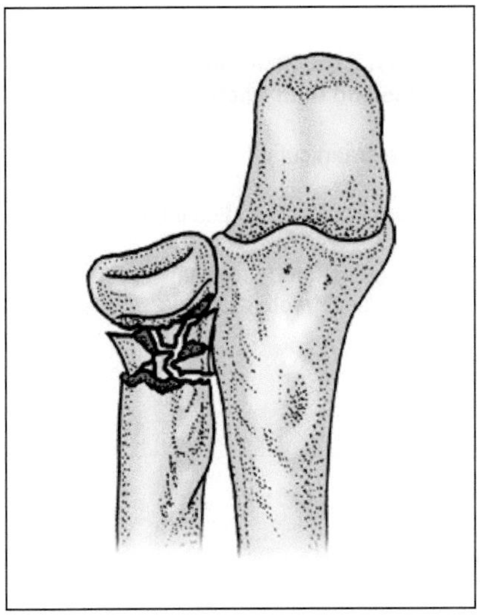

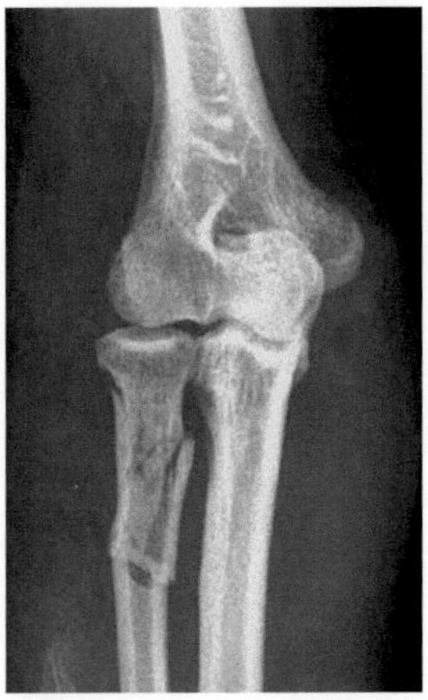

AO/OTA Classification of Proximal Radius and ulna fractures

21-A: extraarticular fracture

A2: radius fractured, ulna intact

A2.3: comminuted radial neck fracture

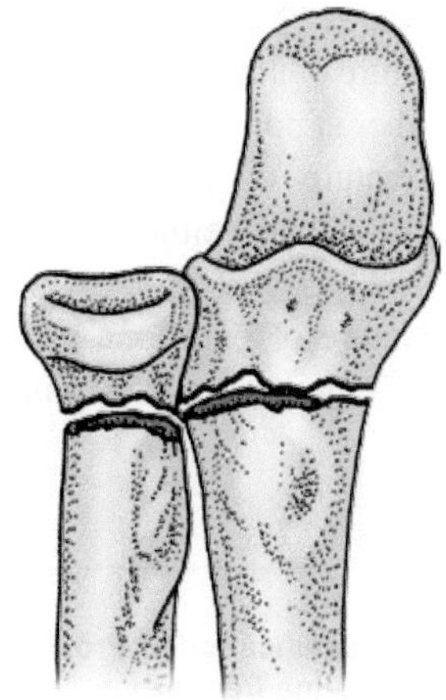

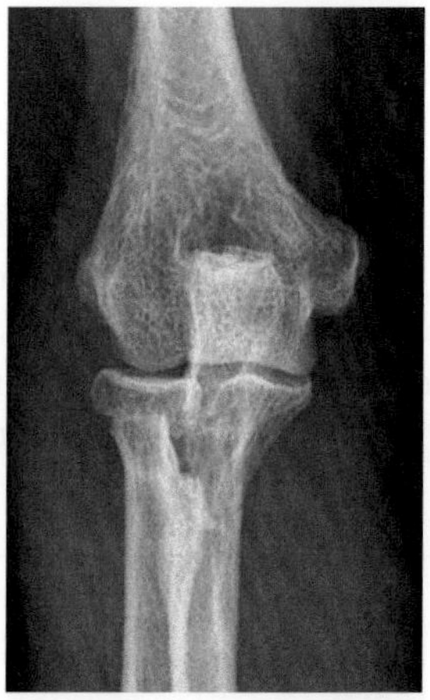

AO/OTA Classification of Proximal Radius and ulna fractures

21-A: extraarticular fracture

A3: fractures of both bones

A3.1: simple fractures of both bones

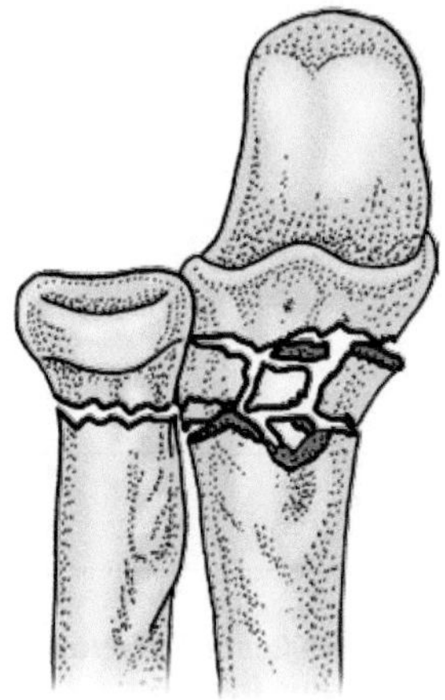

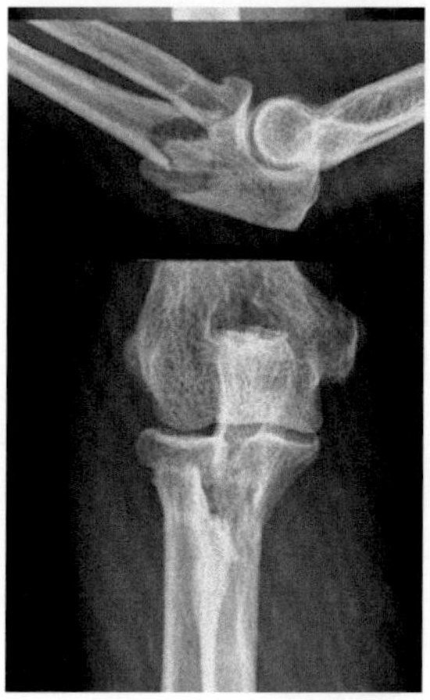

AO/OTA Classification of Proximal Radius and ulna fractures

21-A: extraarticular fracture

A3: fractures of both bones

A3.2: comminuted fracture of one bone and simple fracture of another bone

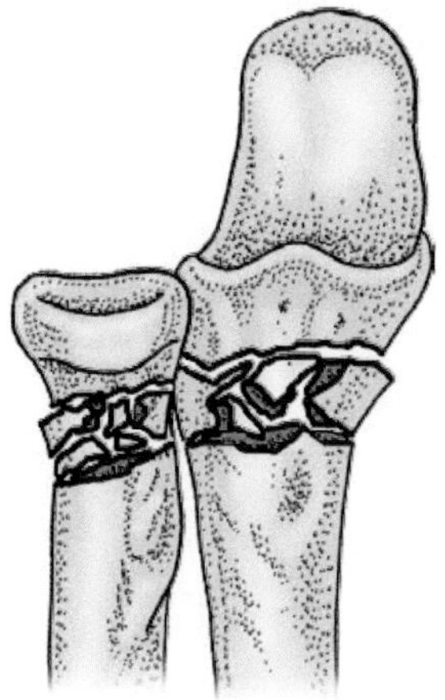

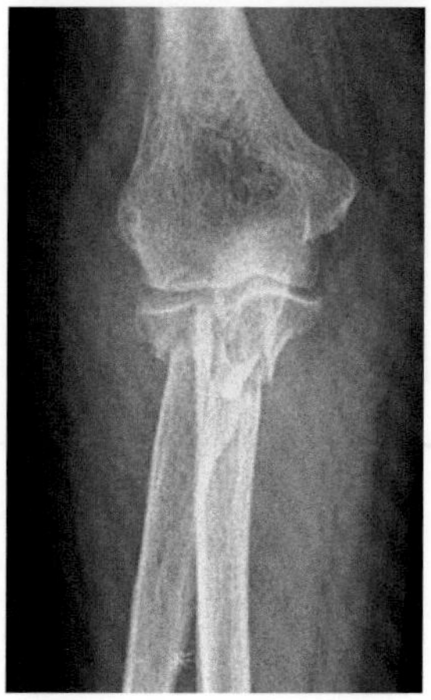

AO/OTA Classification of Proximal Radius and ulna fractures

21-A: extraarticular fracture

A3: fractures of both bones

A3.3: comminuted fractures of both bones

21-B: Articular fracture.

- B1: Ulna fractured, radius intact.
  - B1.1: One simple fracture.
  - B1.2: Two simple fractures.
  - B1.3: Comminuted fractures.
- B2: Radius fractured, ulna intact.
  - B2.1: Intra-articular fracture of radius.
  - B2.2: Comminuted fractures without compression.
  - B2.3: Comminuted fracture of radius with compression.
- B3: One bone articular fracture, another extra-articular fracture.
  - B3.1: Intra-articular fracture of ulna and extra-articular fracture of radius, either simple or comminuted.
  - B3.2: Intra-articular fracture of radius and extra-articular fracture of ulna, either simple or comminuted.
  - B3.3: Intra-articular fracture of one bone and extra-articular fracture of another, either simple or comminuted.

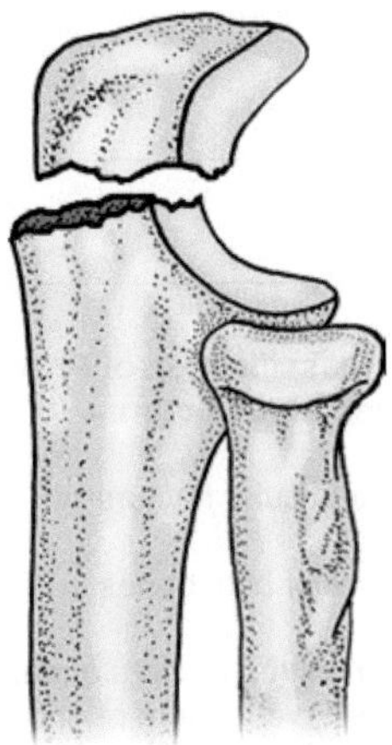

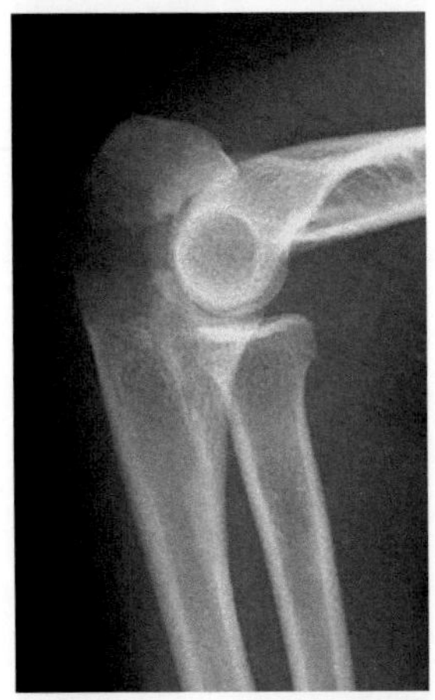

AO/OTA Classification of Proximal Radius and ulna fractures

21-B: articular fracture

B1: ulna fractured, radius intact

B1.1: one simple fracture

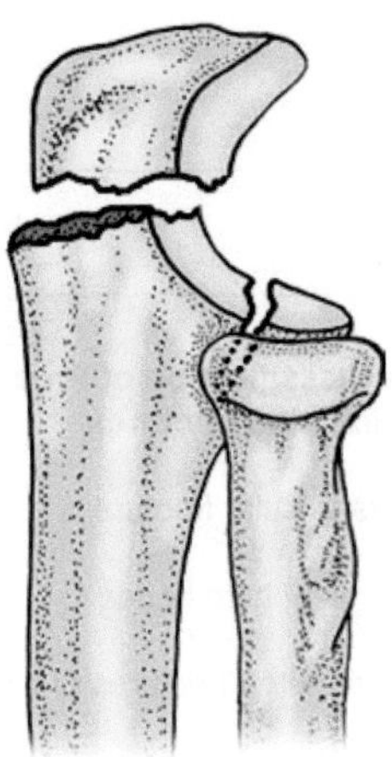

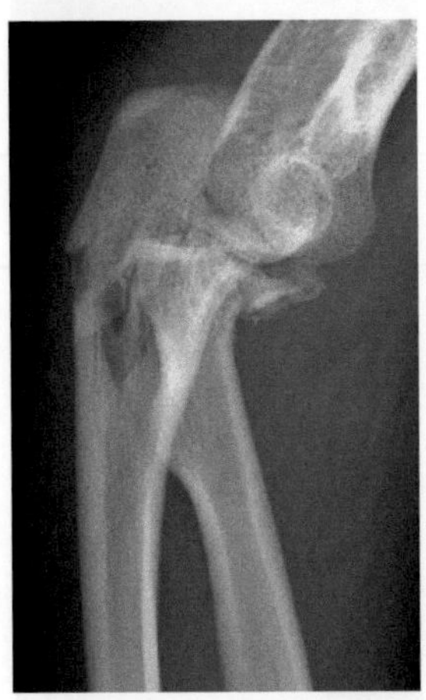

AO/OTA Classification of Proximal Radius and ulna fractures

21-B: articular fracture

B1: ulna fractured, radius intact

B1.2: two simple fractures

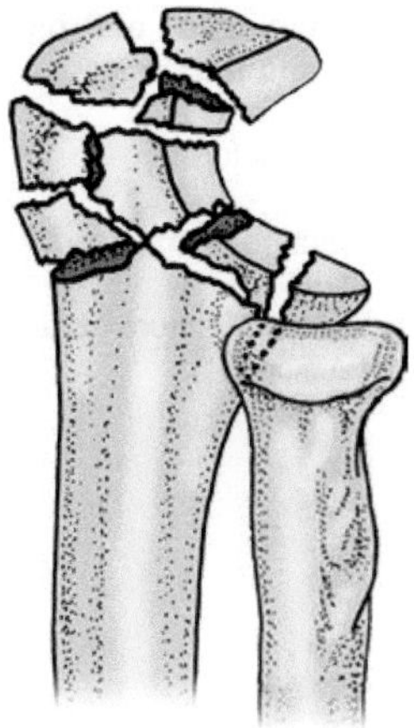

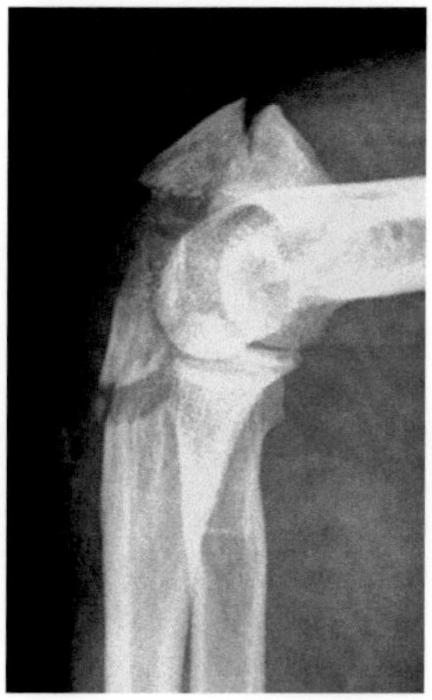

AO/OTA Classification of Proximal Radius and ulna fractures

21-B: articular fracture

B1: ulna fractured, radius intact

B1.3: comminuted fractures

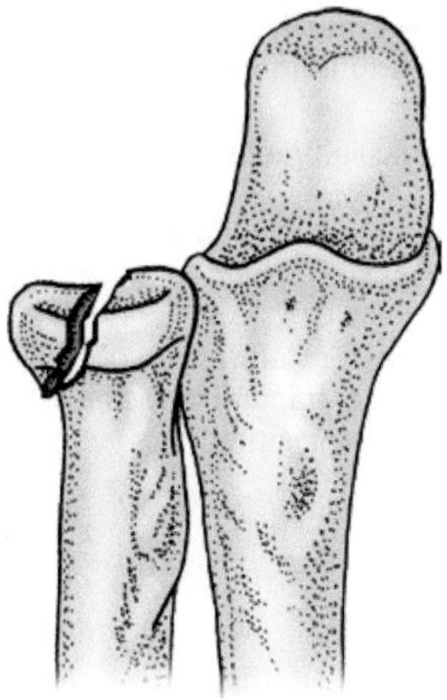

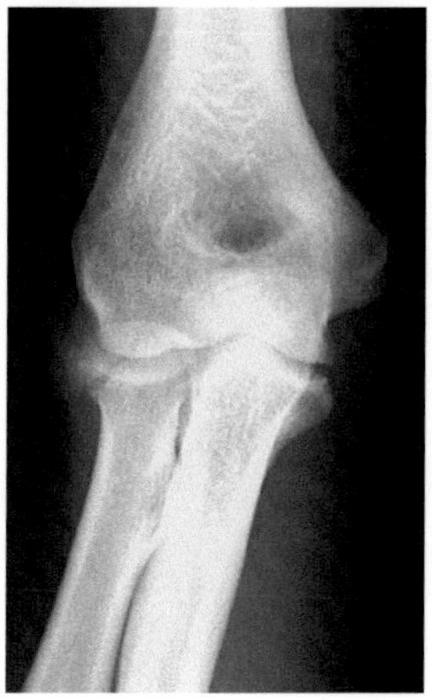

AO/OTA Classification of Proximal Radius and ulna fractures

21-B: articular fracture

B2: radius fractured, ulna intact

B2.1: intraarticular fracture of radius

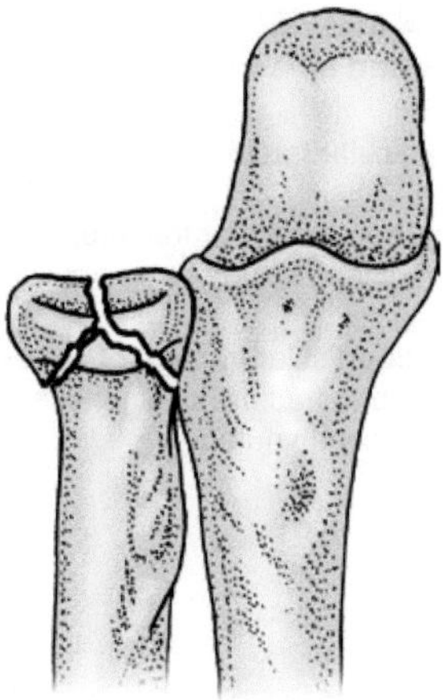

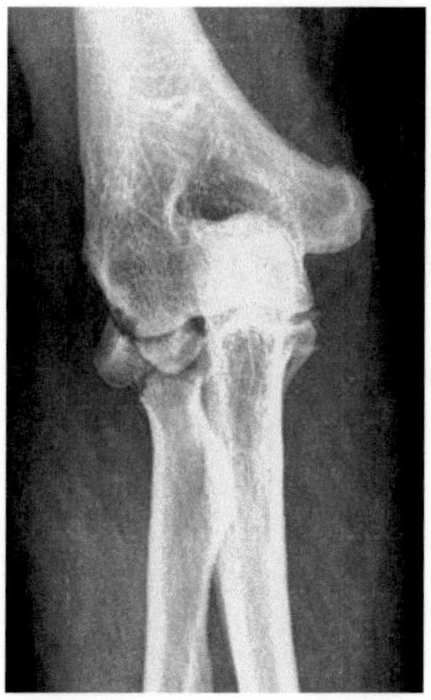

AO/OTA Classification of Proximal Radius and ulna fractures

21-B: articular fracture

B2: radius fractured, ulna intact

B2.2: comminuted fractures without compression

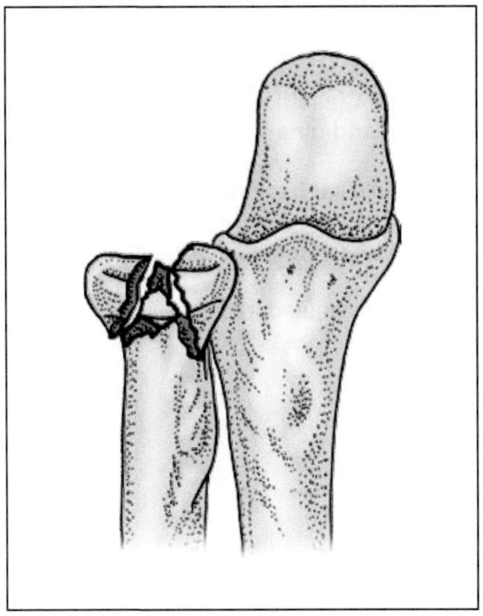

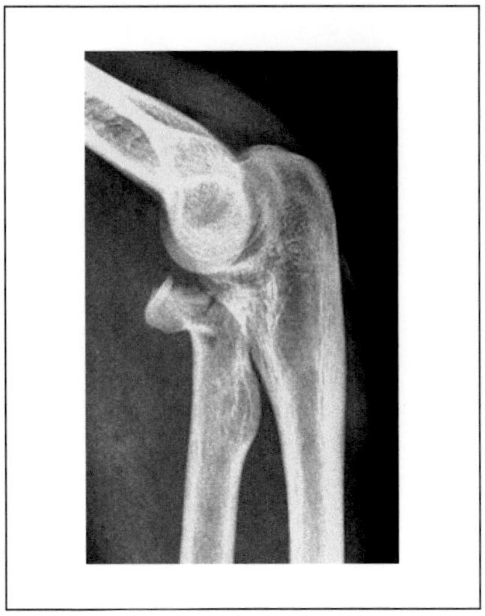

AO/OTA Classification of Proximal Radius and ulna fractures

21-B: articular fracture

B2: radius fractured, ulna intact

B2.3: comminuted fracture of radius with compression

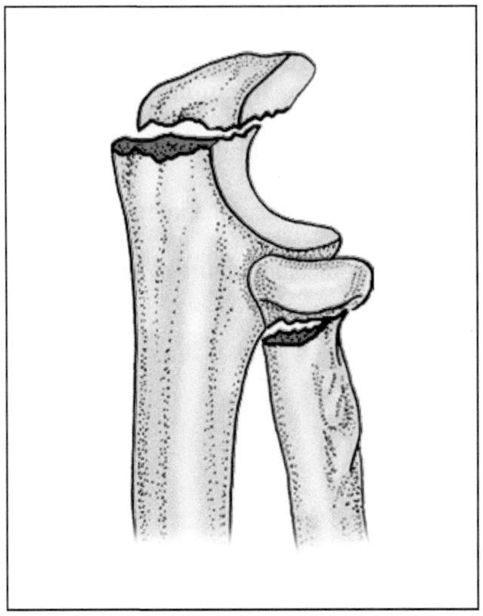

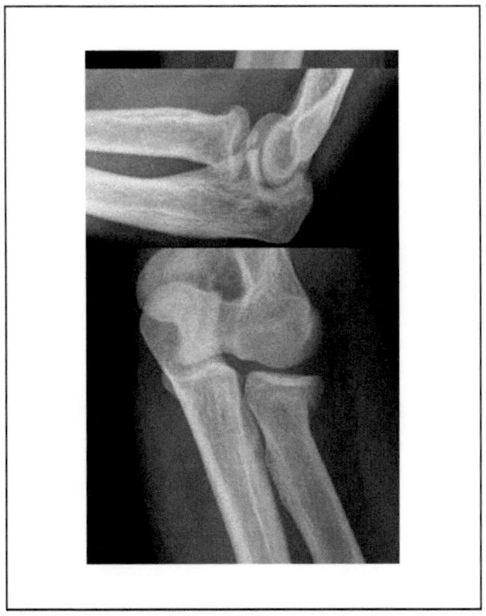

AO/OTA Classification of Proximal Radius and ulna fractures

21-B: articular fracture

B3: one bone articular fracture, another extraarticular fracture

B3.1: intraarticular fracture of ulna and extraarticular fracture of radius, either simple or comminuted

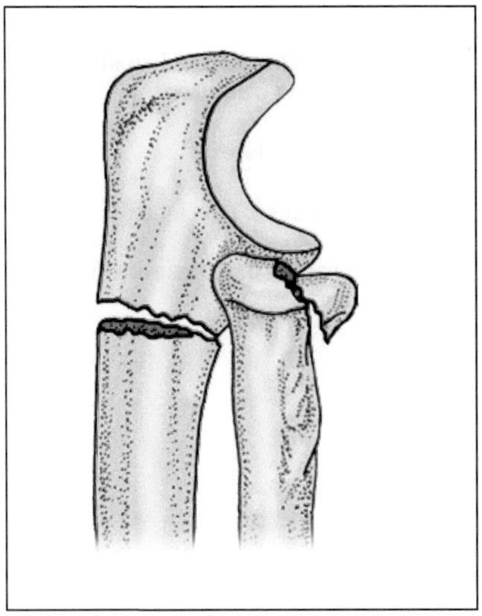

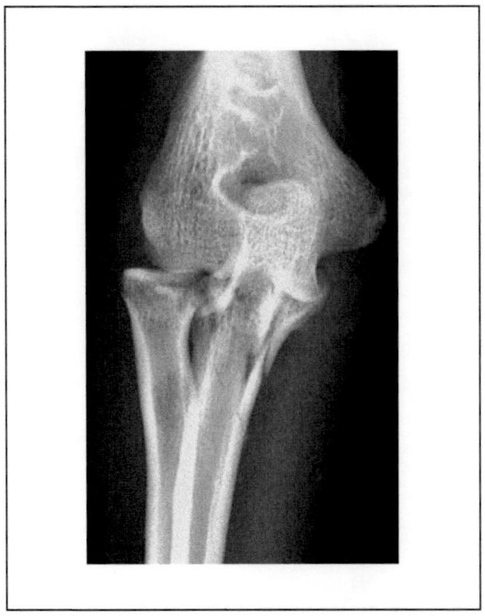

AO/OTA Classification of Proximal Radius and ulna fractures

21-B: articular fracture

B3: one bone articular fracture, another extraarticular fracture

B3.2: intraarticular fracture of radius and extraarticular fracture of ulna, either simple or comminuted

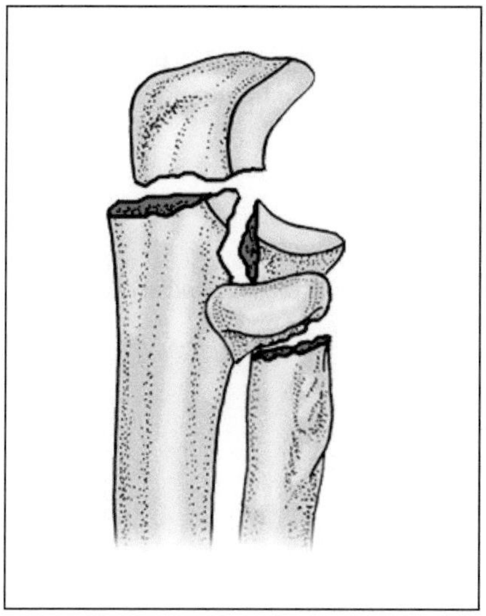

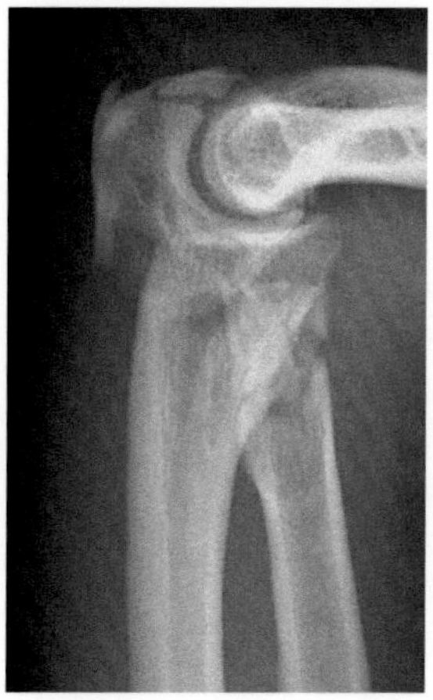

AO/OTA Classification of Proximal Radius and ulna fractures

21-B: articular fracture

B3: one bone articular fracture, another extraarticular fracture

B3.3: intraarticular fracture of one bone and extraarticular fracture of another, either simple or comminuted

21-C: Articular fracture of both bones:
- C1: Simple:
  - C1.1: Olecranon, radial head.
  - C1.2: Coronoid process, radial head.
- C2: One articular simple, another articular multifragmentary:
  - C2.1: Comminuted olecranon, simple radial head.
  - C2.2: Simple olecranon, comminuted radial head.
  - C2.3: Simple coronoid process, comminuted radial head.
- C3: Multifragmentary:
  - C3.1: Three fragments of each bone.
  - C3.2: Four or more fragments of ulna, three or more fragments of radius.
  - C3.3: Four or more fragments of radius, three or more fragments of ulna.

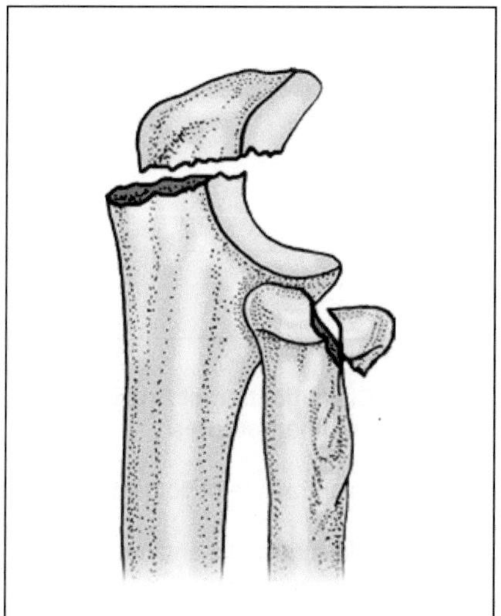

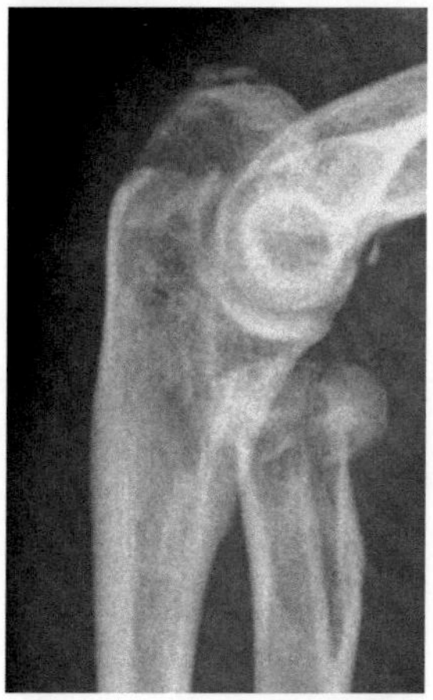

AO/OTA Classification of Proximal Radius and ulna fractures

21-C: articular fracture of both bones

C1: simple

C1.1: olecranon, radial head

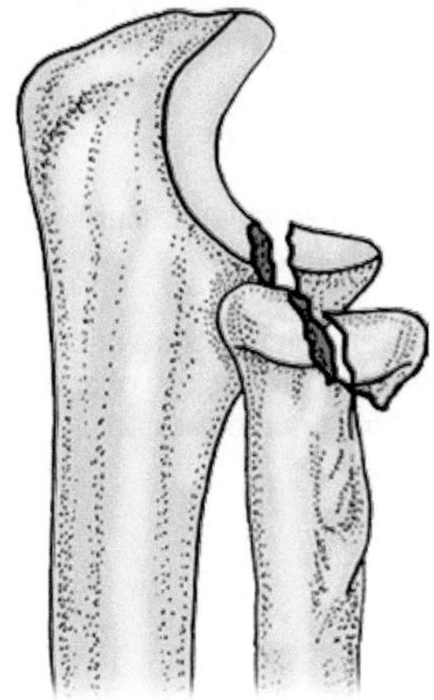

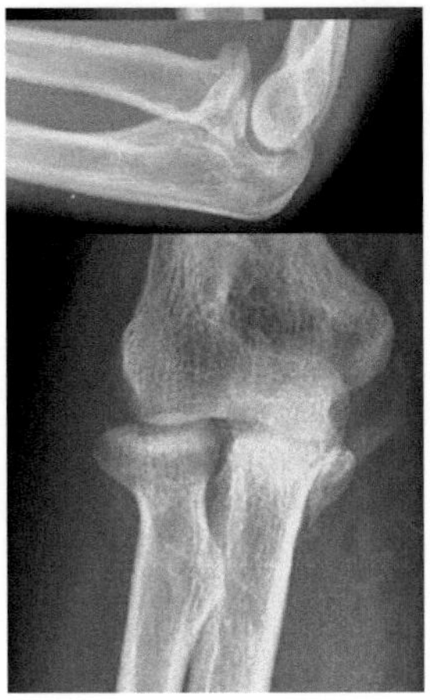

AO/OTA Classification of Proximal Radius and ulna fractures

21-C: articular fracture of both bones

C1: simple

C1.2: coronoid process, radial head

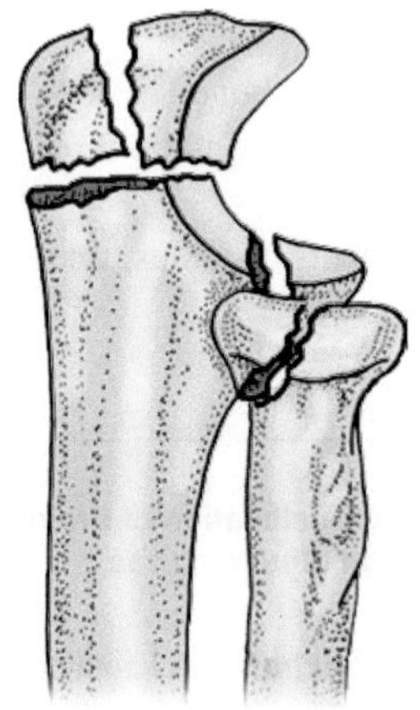

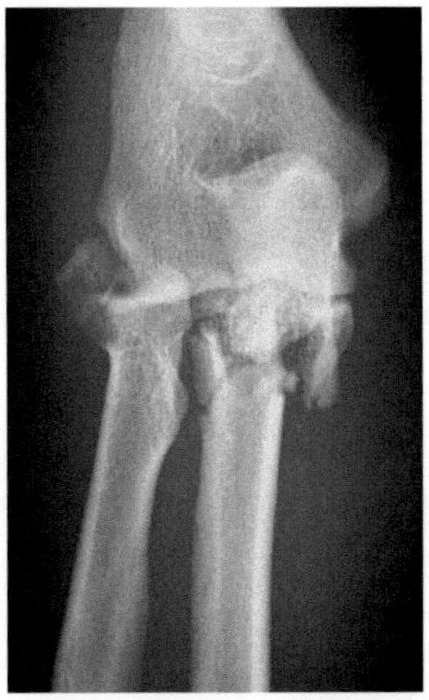

AO/OTA Classification of Proximal Radius and ulna fractures

21-C: articular fracture of both bones

C2: one articular simple, another articular multifragmentary

C2.1: comminuted olecranon, simple radial head

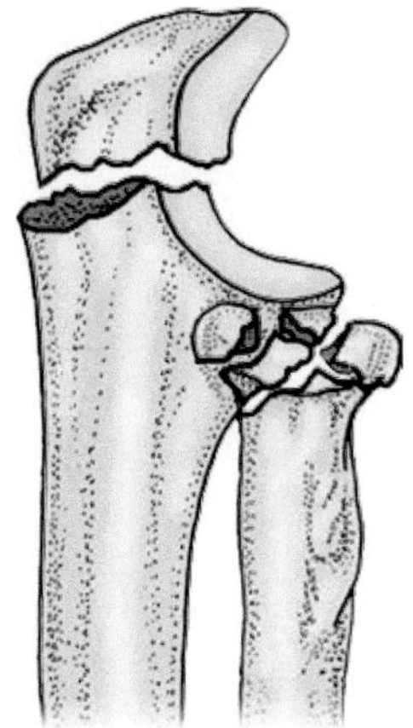

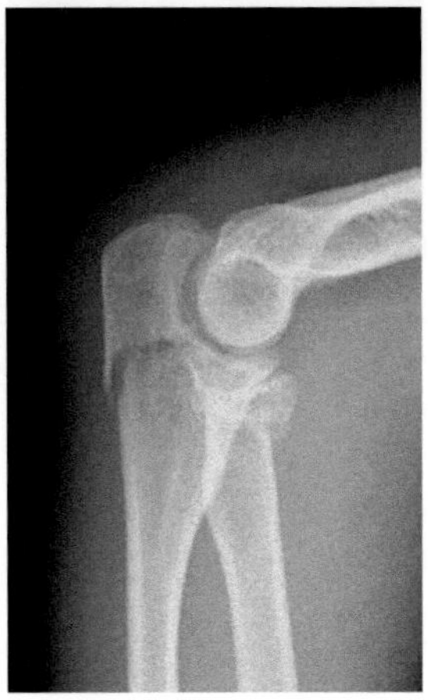

AO/OTA Classification of Proximal Radius and ulna fractures

21-C: articular fracture of both bones

C2: one articular simple, another articular multifragmentary

C2.2: simple olecranon, comminuted radial head

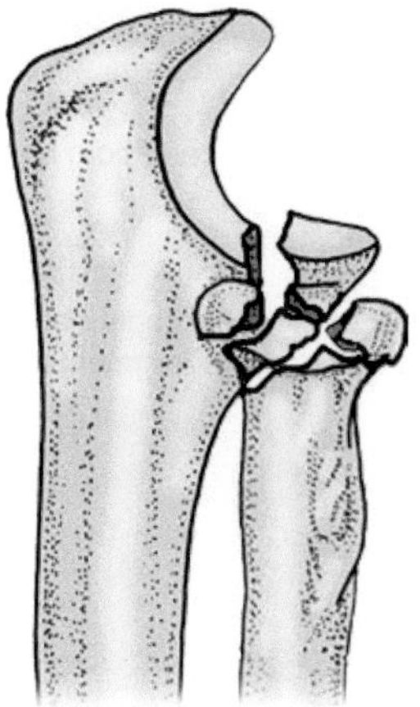

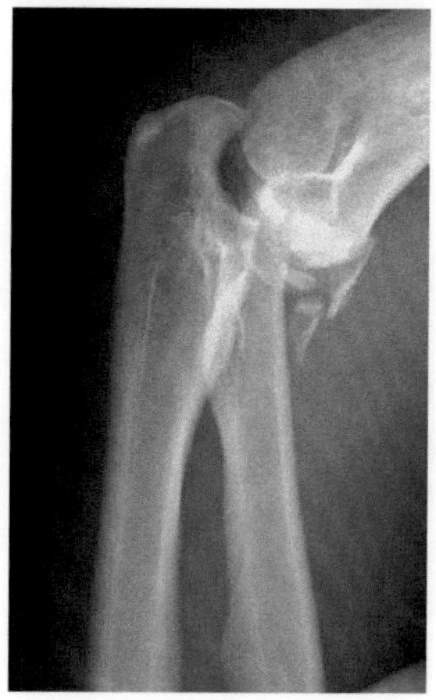

AO/OTA Classification of Proximal Radius and ulna fractures

21-C: articular fracture of both bones

C2: one articular simple, another articular multifragmentary

C2.3: simple olecranon, comminuted radial head

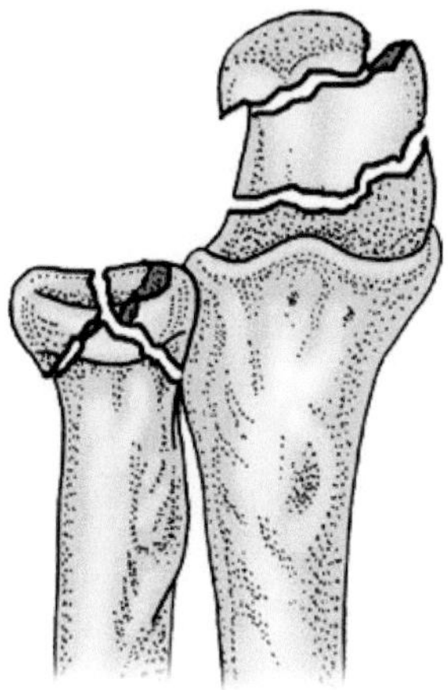

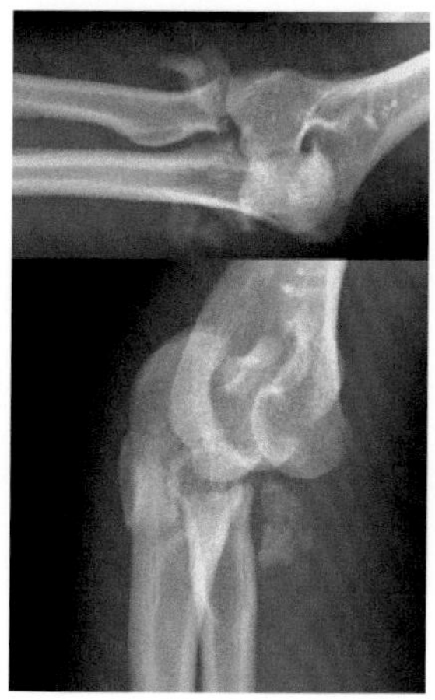

AO/OTA Classification of Proximal Radius and ulna fractures

221-C: articular fracture of both bones

C3: multifragmentary

C3.1: three fragments of each bone

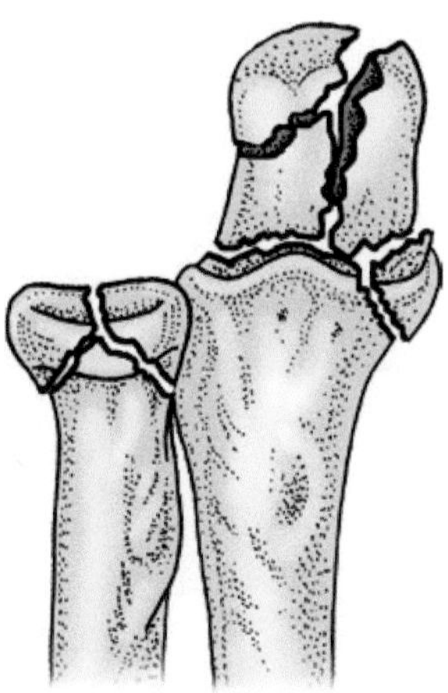

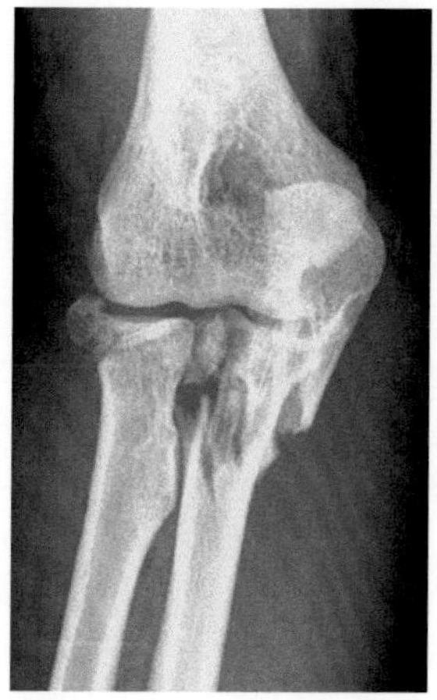

AO/OTA Classification of Proximal Radius and ulna fractures

21-C: articular fracture of both bones

C3: multifragmentary

C3.2: four or more fragments of ulna, three or more fragments of radius

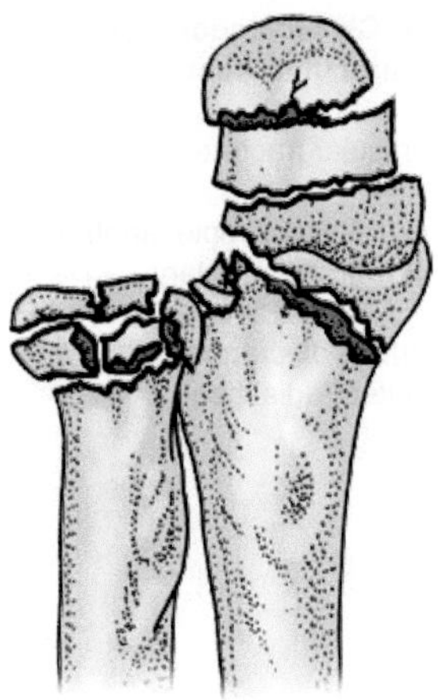

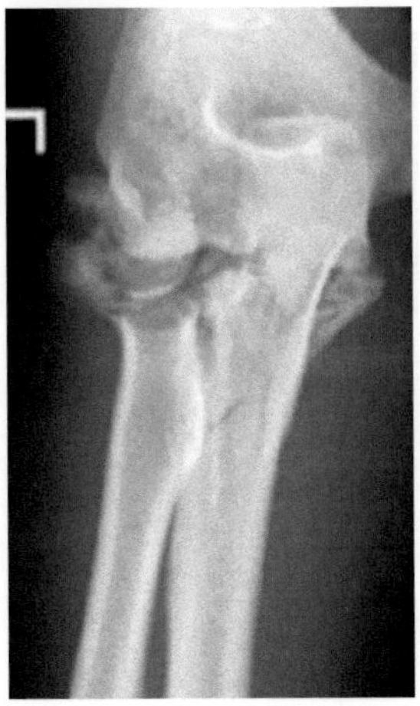

AO/OTA Classification of Proximal Radius and ulna fractures

21-C: articular fracture of both bones

C3: multifragmentary

C3.3: four or more fragments of radius, three or more fragments of ulna

3.2 Section 2 Classifications of Diaphyseal Radius and Ulna Fractures

3.2.1 Diaphyseal Radius and Ulna Fractures

Several classifications have been reported, including AO/OTA, Mason, and Gustilo-Anderson classifications. The fractures are also classified according to fracture site involved, fracture patterns, and absence or presence of wounds that communicate with fracture. AO/OTA classification is the most commonly used system in recent 5 years.

3.2.1.1 AO/OTA Classification [24]

Muller classification of long bone fractures was first reported in 1987 [25], and modified in 2007 [26]. AO trauma developed AO/OTA classification system based on Muller classification.

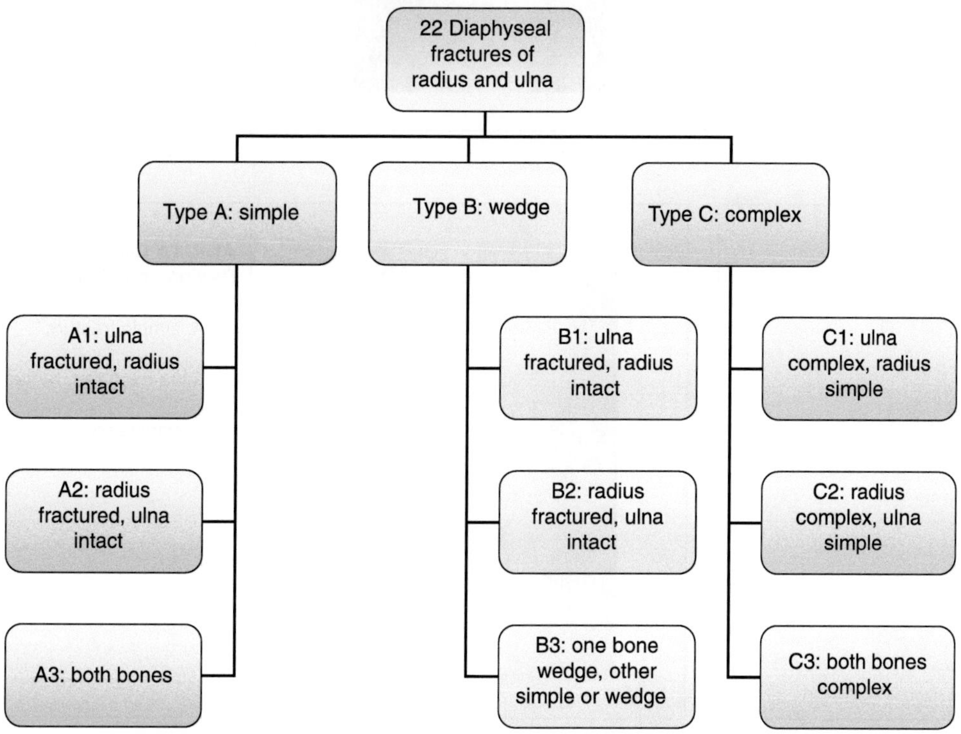

22-A: Simple fracture:
- A1: Ulna fractured, radius intact:
  - A1.1: Oblique.
  - A1.2: Transverse.
  - A1.3: With dislocation of radial head (Monteggia fracture–dislocation).
- A2: Radius fractured, ulna intact:
  - A2.1: Oblique.
  - A2.2: Transverse.
  - A2.3: With dislocation of the distal radioulnar joint (Galeazzi fracture–dislocation).
- A3: Both bones:
  - A3.1: Radius, proximal zone.
  - A3.2: Radius, middle zone.
  - A3.3: Radius, distal zone.

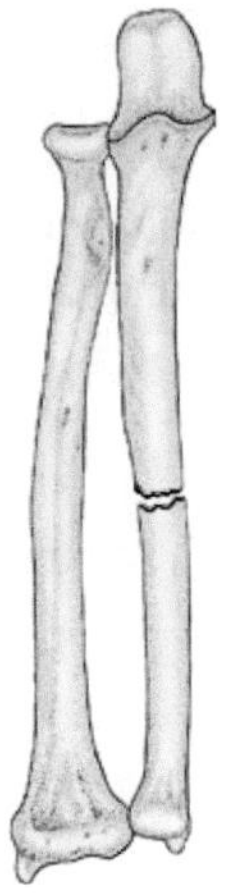

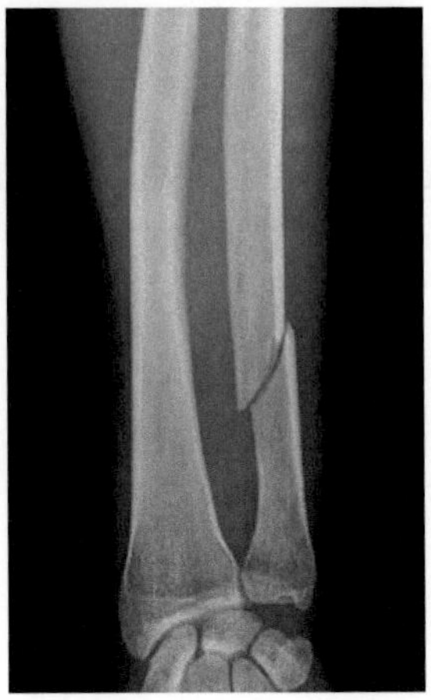

AO/OTA Classification of Diaphyseal Radius and ulna fractures

22-A: simple fracture

A1: ulna fractured, radius intact

A1.1: oblique

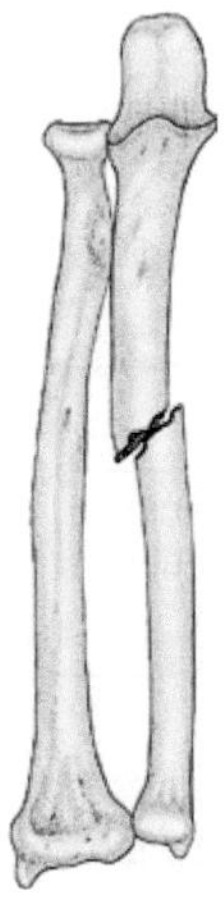

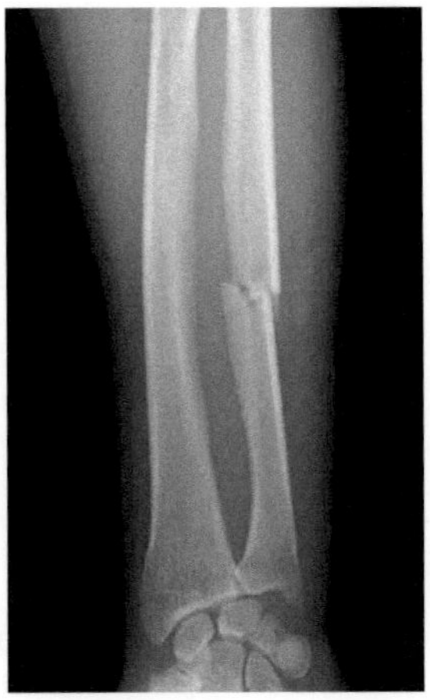

AO/OTA Classification of Diaphyseal Radius and ulna fractures

22-A: simple fracture

A1: ulna fractured, radius intact

A1.2: transverse

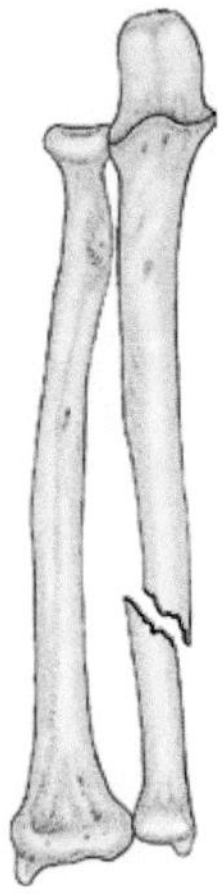

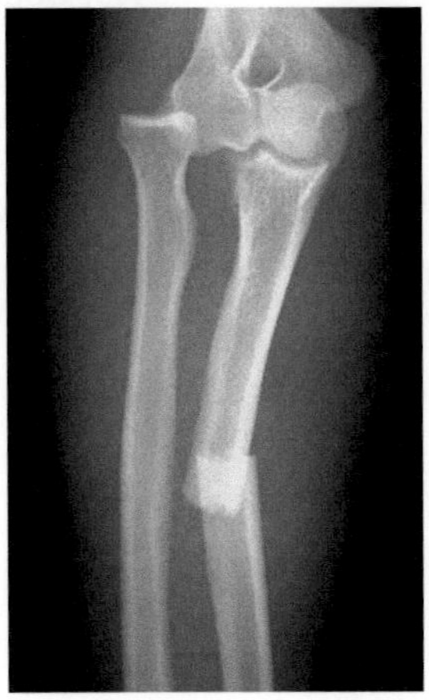

AO/OTA Classification of Diaphyseal Radius and ulna fractures

22-A: simple fracture

A1: ulna fractured, radius intact

A1.3: with dislocation of radial head (Monteggia)

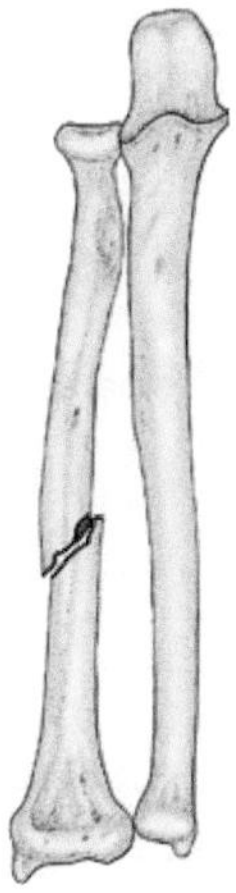

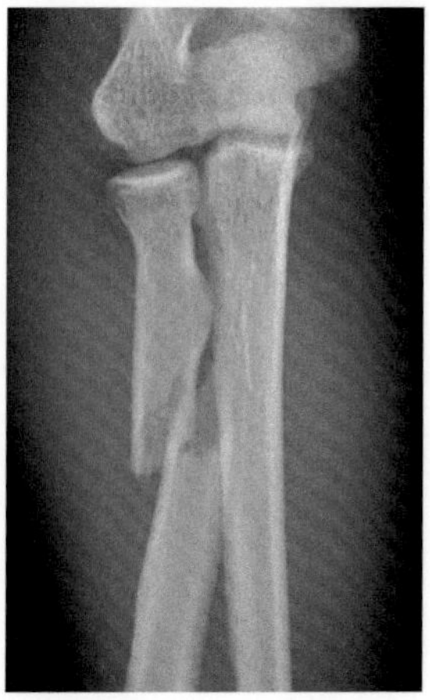

AO/OTA Classification of Diaphyseal Radius and ulna fractures

22-A: simple fracture

A2: radius fractured, ulna intact

A2.1: oblique

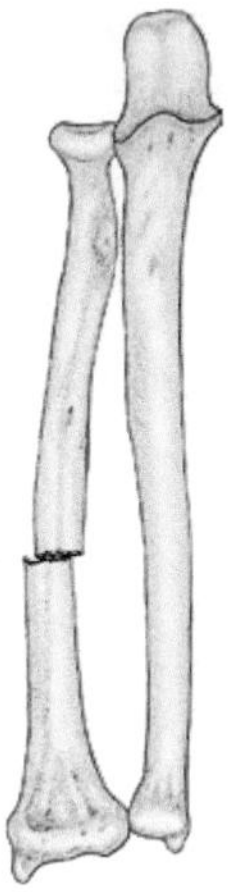

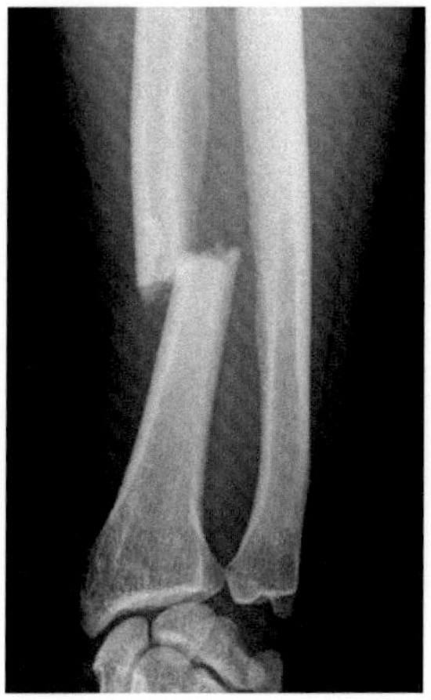

AO/OTA Classification of Diaphyseal Radius and ulna fractures

22-A: simple fracture

A2: radius fractured, ulna intact

A2.2: transverse

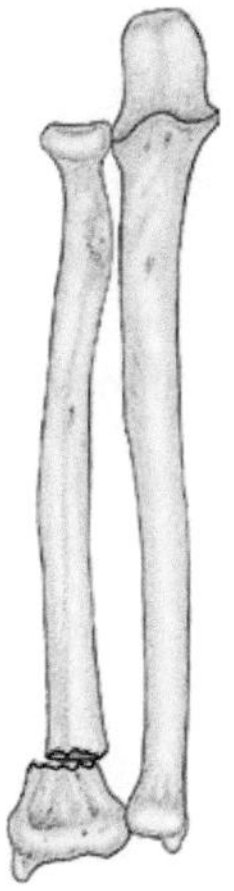

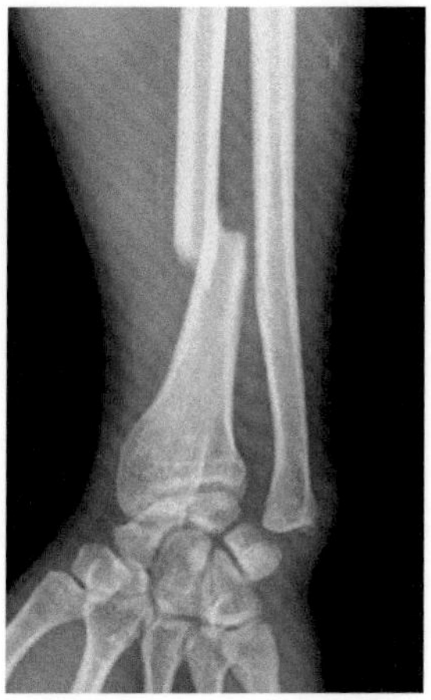

AO/OTA Classification of Diaphyseal Radius and ulna fractures

22-A: simple fracture

A2: radius fractured, ulna intact

A2.3: with dislocation of the distal radioulnar joint (Galeazzi)

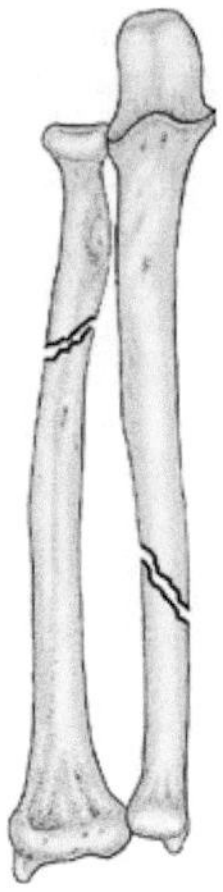

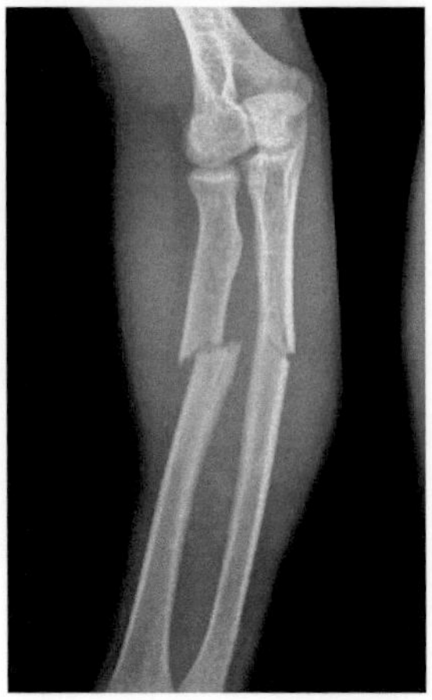

AO/OTA Classification of Diaphyseal Radius and ulna fractures

22-A: simple fracture

A3: both bones

A3. 1: radius, proximal zone

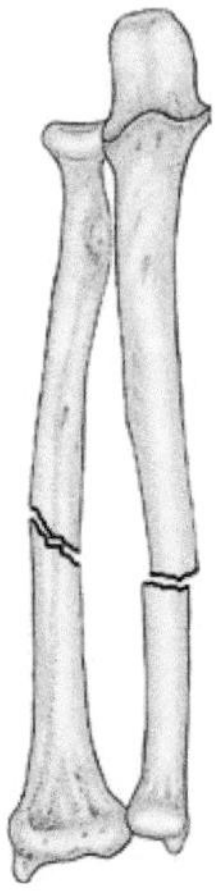

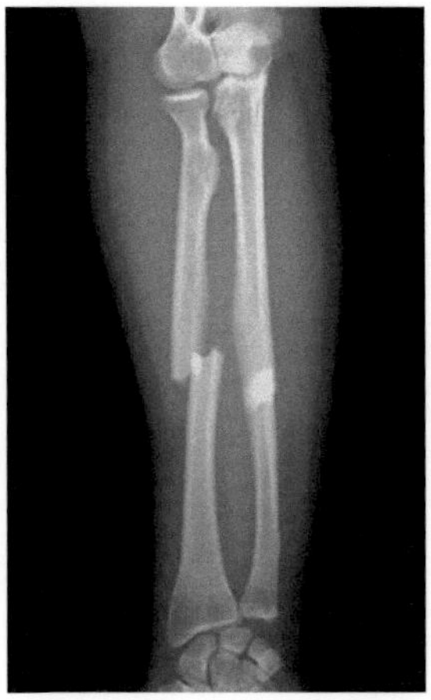

AO/OTA Classification of Diaphyseal Radius and ulna fractures

22-A: simple fracture

A3: both bones

A3.2: radius, middle zone

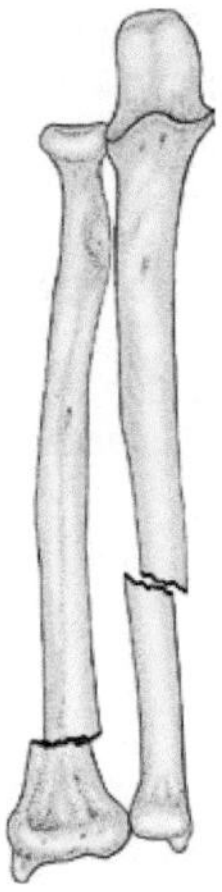

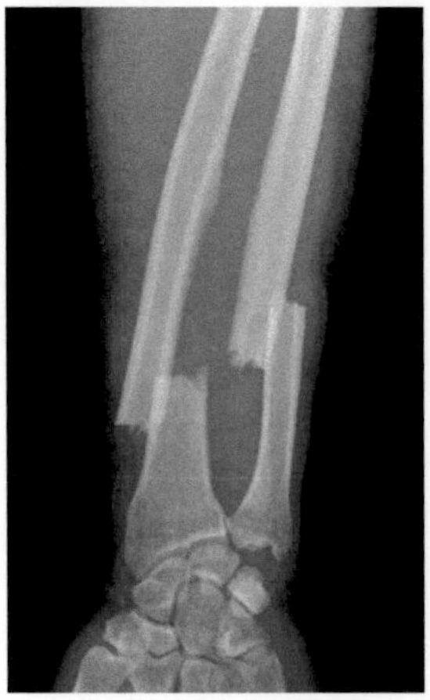

AO/OTA Classification of Diaphyseal Radius and ulna fractures

22-A: simple fracture

A3: both bones

A3.3: radius, distal zone

22-B: Wedge fracture:
- B1: Ulna fractured, radius intact:
  - B1.1: Intact wedge.
  - B1.2: Fragmented wedge.
  - B1.3: With dislocation of radial head (Monteggia fracture–dislocation).
- B2: Radius fractured, ulna intact:
  - B2.1: Intact wedge.
  - B2.2: Fragmented wedge.
  - B2.3: Associated with dislocation of the distal radioulnar joint (Galeazzi fracture-dislocation).
- B3: One bone wedge, other simple or wedge:
  - B3.1: Ulnar wedge, radial simple.
  - B3.2: Radial wedge, ulnar simple.
  - B3.3: Radial and ulnar wedge.

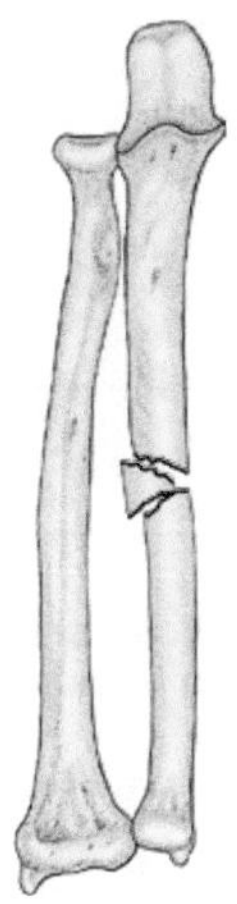

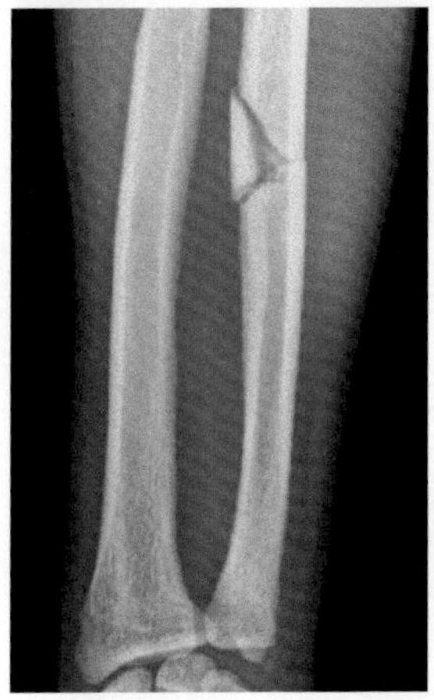

AO/OTA Classification of Diaphyseal Radius and ulna fractures

22-B: wedge fracture

B1: ulna fractured, radius intact

B1.1: intact wedge

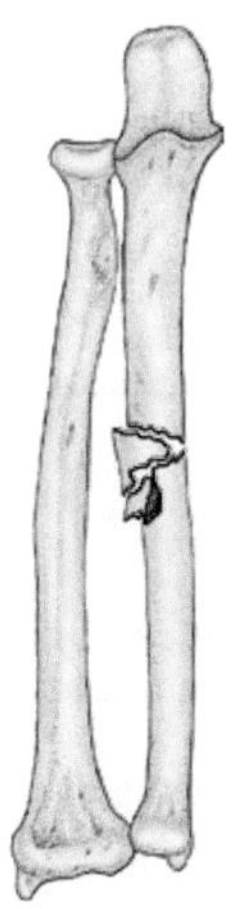

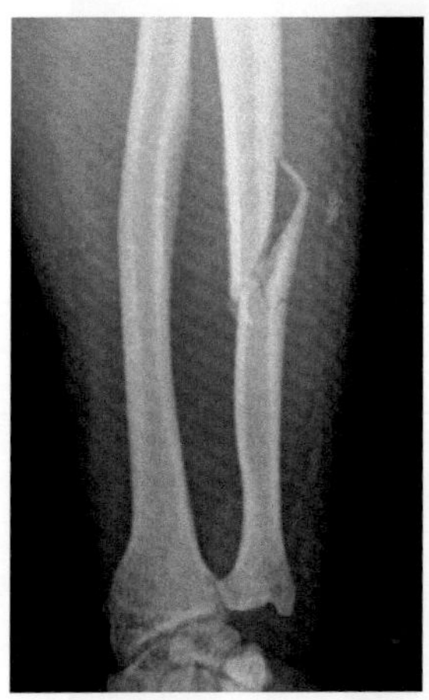

Diaphyseal Radius and ulna fractures

22-B: wedge fracture

B1: ulna fractured, radius intact

B1.2: fragmented wedge

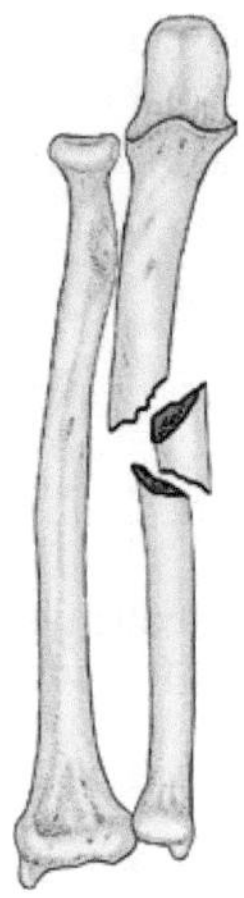

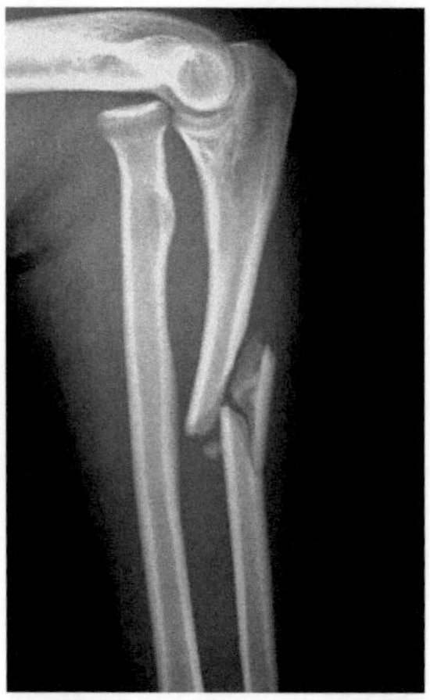

Diaphyseal Radius and ulna fractures

22-B: wedge fracture

B1: ulna fractured, radius intact

B1.3: with dislocation of radial head (Monteggia)

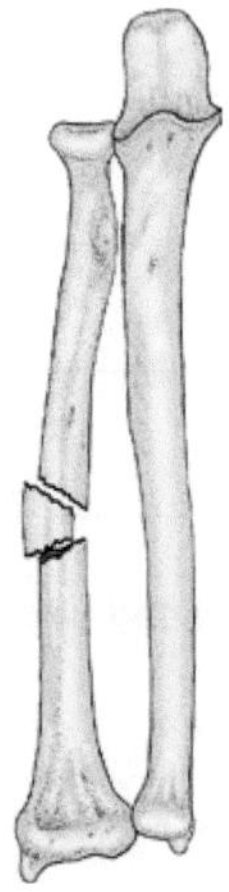

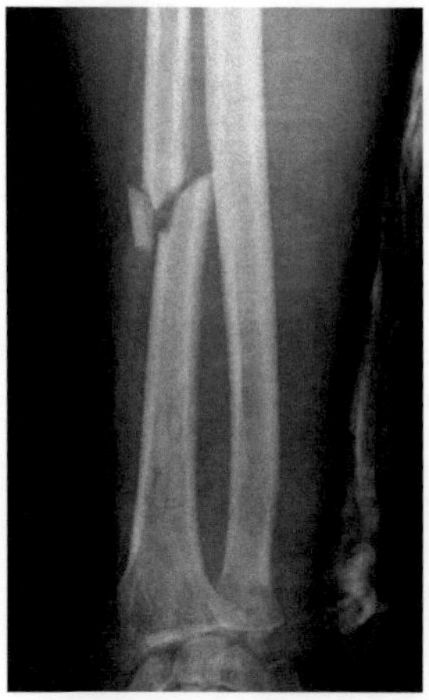

AO/OTA Classification of Diaphyseal Radius and ulna fractures

22-B: wedge fracture

B2: radius fractured, ulna intact

B2. 1: intact wedge

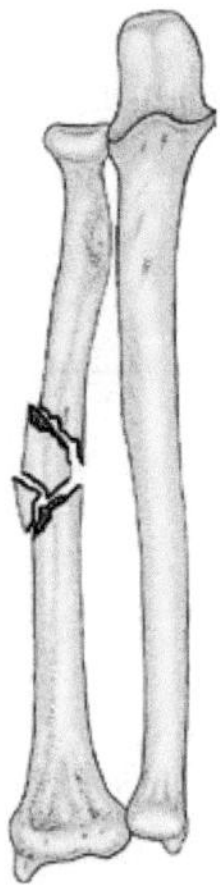

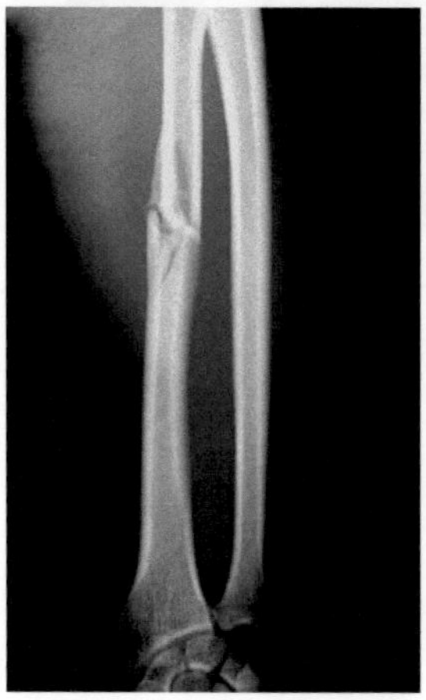

AO/OTA Classification of Diaphyseal Radius and ulna fractures

22-B: wedge fracture

B1: ulna fractured, radius intact

B1.2: fragmented wedge

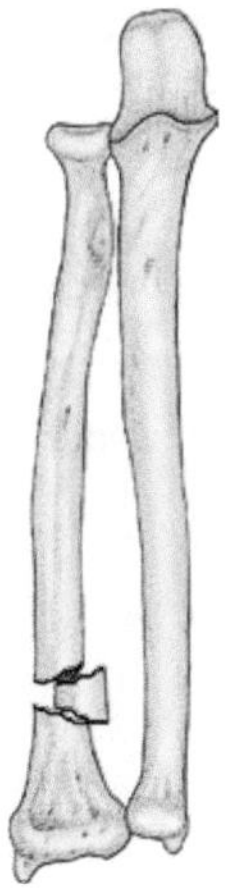

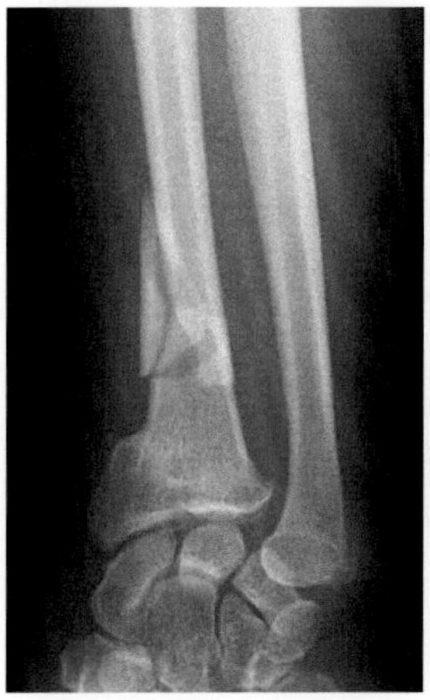

AO/OTA Classification of Diaphyseal Radius and ulna fractures

22-B: wedge fracture

B2: radius fractured, ulna intact

B2.3: associated with dislocation of the distal radioulnar joint (Galeazzi)

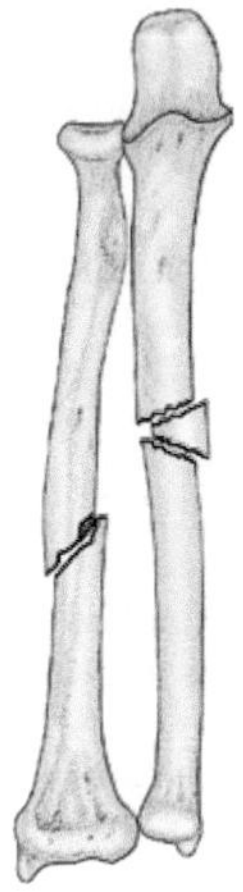

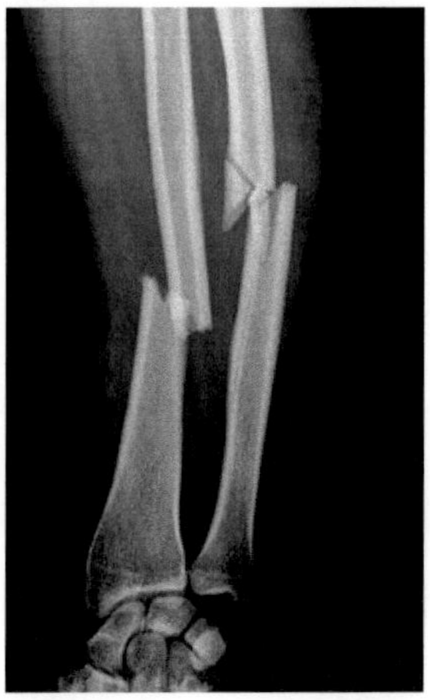

AO/OTA Classification of Diaphyseal Radius and ulna fractures

22-B: wedge fracture

B3: one bone wedge, other simple or wedge

B3.1: ulnar wedge, radial simple

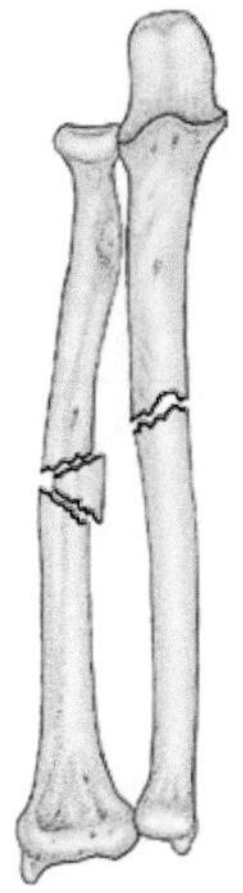

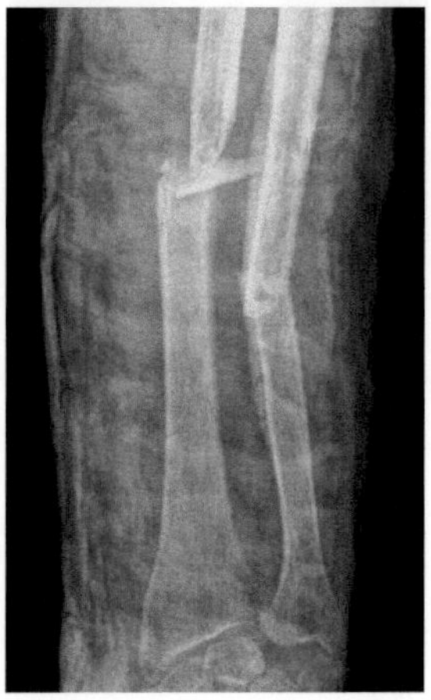

AO/OTA Classification of Diaphyseal Radius and ulna fractures

22-B: wedge fracture

B3: one bone wedge, other simple or wedge

B3.2: radial wedge, ulnar simple

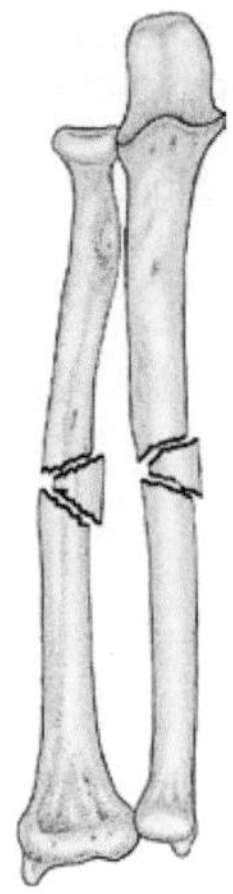

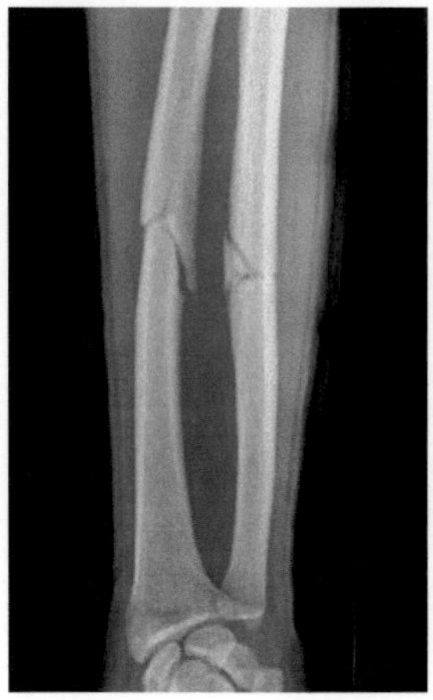

AO/OTA Classification of Diaphyseal Radius and ulna fractures

22-B: wedge fracture

B3: one bone wedge, other simple or wedge

B3.3: radial and ulnar wedge

22-C: Complex fracture:
- C1: Ulna complex, radius simple:
  - C1.1: Bifocal, radius intact.
  - C1.2: Bifocal with radius fracture.
  - C1.3: Irregular of ulna.
- C2: Radius complex, ulna simple:
  - C2.1: Bifocal, ulna intact.
    - C2.1.1: Without dislocation.
    - C2.1.2: With dislocation of distal radioulnar joint.
  - C2.2: Bifocal, ulna fracture.
  - C2.3: Irregular.
- C3: Both bones complex:
  - C3.1: Bifocal.
  - C3.2: Bifocal of one, irregular of other.
  - C3.3: Irregular.

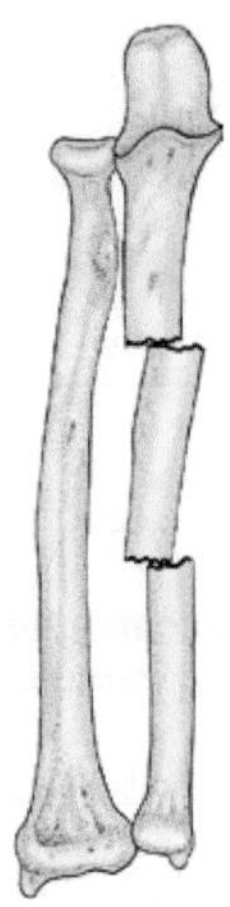

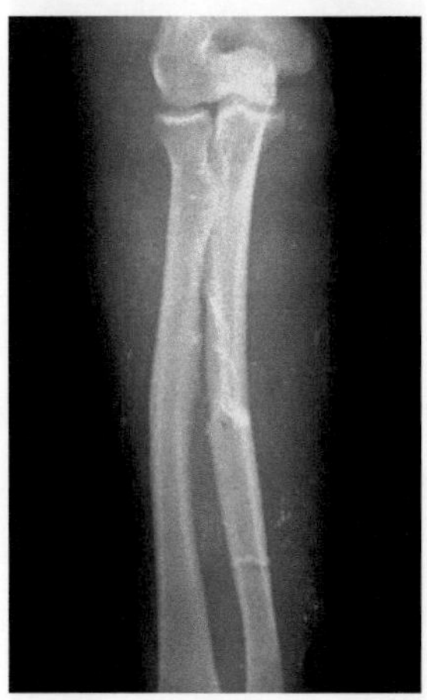

AO/OTA Classification of Diaphyseal Radius and ulna fractures

22-C: complex fracture

C1: ulna complex, radius simple

C1.1: bifocal, radius intact

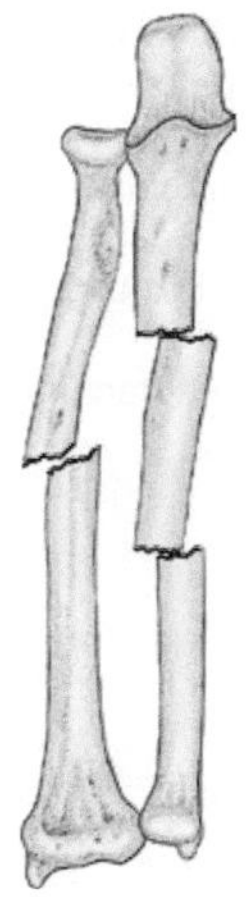

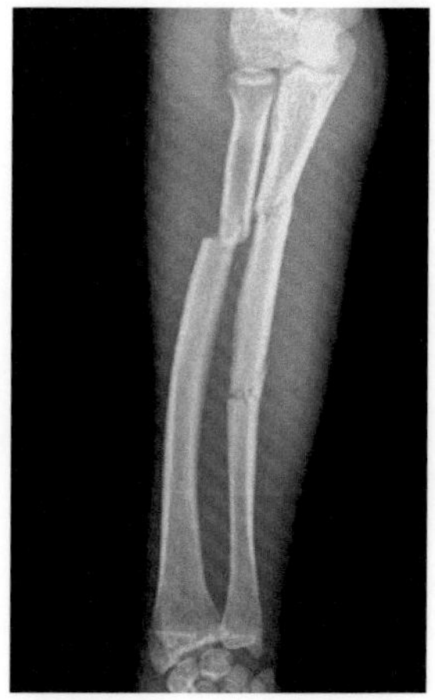

AO/OTA Classification of Diaphyseal Radius and ulna fractures

22-C: complex fracture

C1: ulna complex, radius simple

C1.2: bifocal with radius fracture

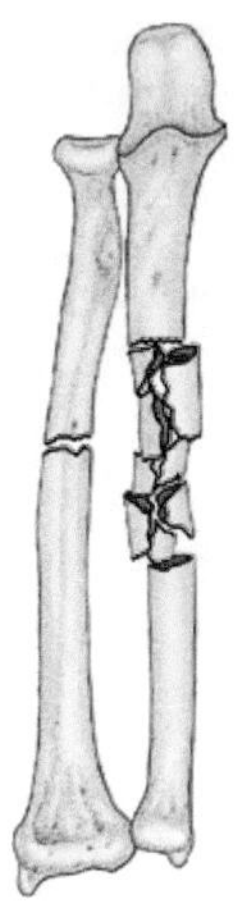

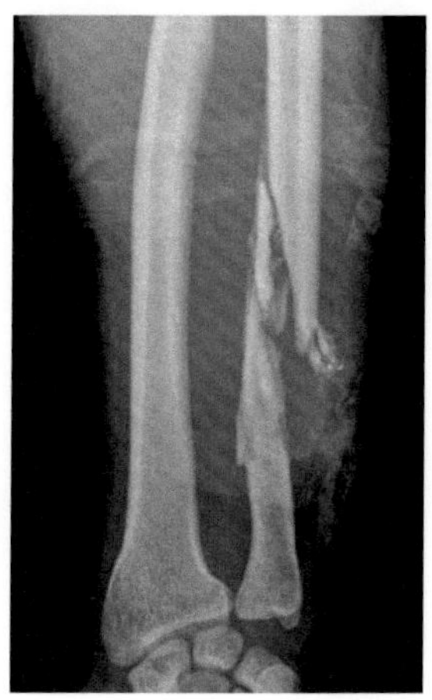

AO/OTA Classification of Diaphyseal Radius and ulna fractures

22-C: complex fracture

C1: ulna complex, radius simple

C1.3: irregular of ulnavv

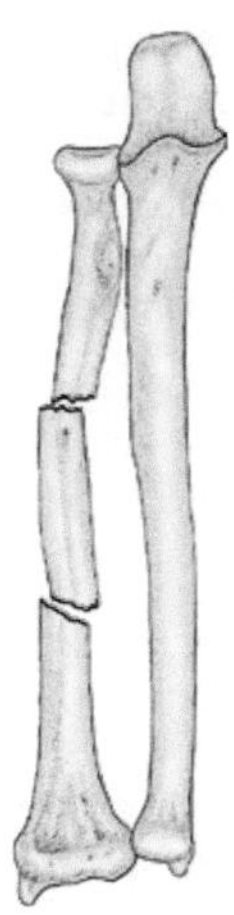

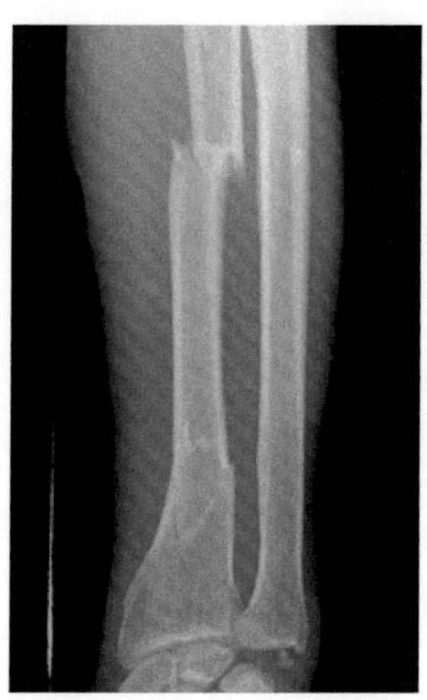

AO/OTA Classification of Diaphyseal Radius and ulna fractures

22-C: complex fracture

C2: radius complex, ulna simple

C2.1: bifocal, ulna intact

C2.1.1: without dislocation

C2.1.2: with dislocation of distal radioulnar joint (Galeazzi)

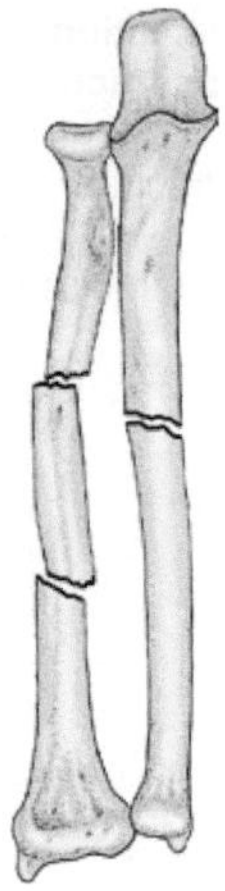

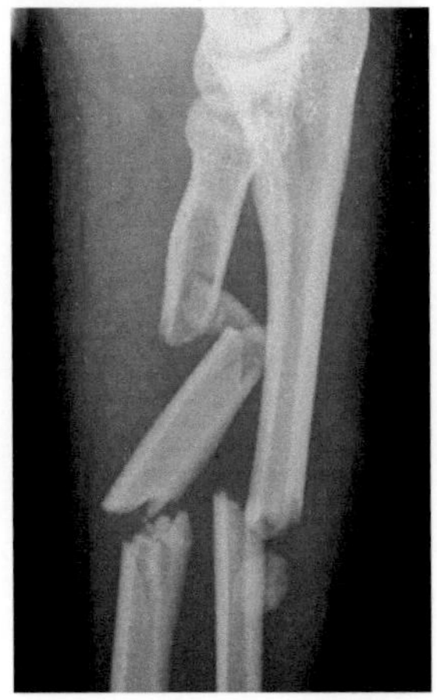

AO/OTA Classification of Diaphyseal Radius and ulna fractures

22-C: complex fracture

C2: radius complex, ulna simple

C2.2: bifocal, ulna fracture

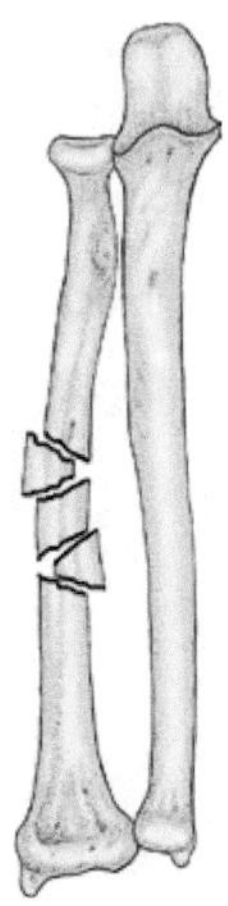

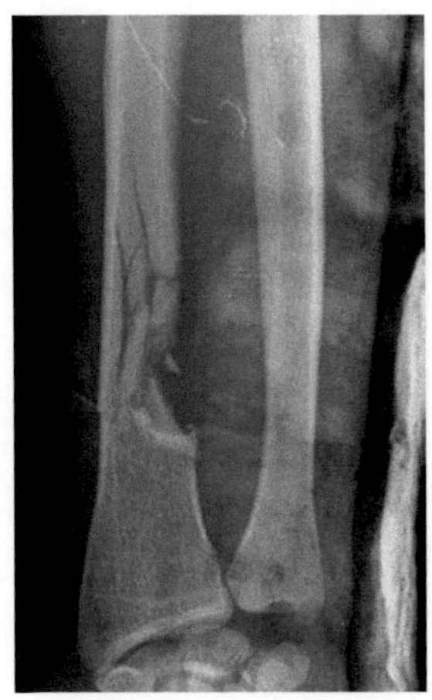

AO/OTA Classification of Diaphyseal Radius and ulna fractures

22-C: complex fracture

C2: radius complex, ulna simple

C2.3: irregular

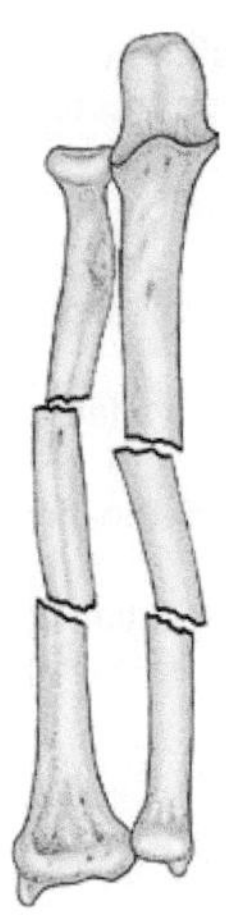

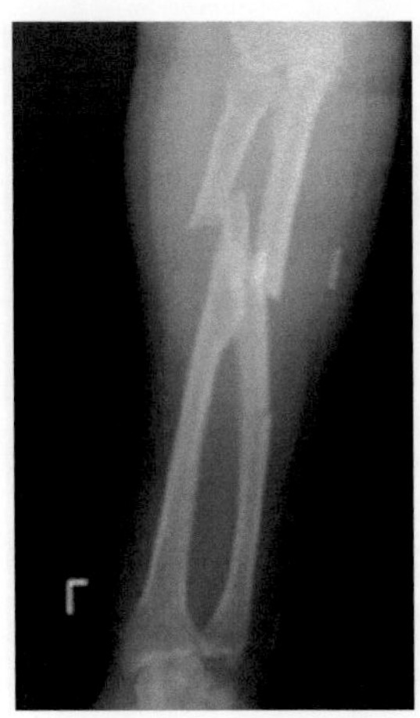

AO/OTA Classification of Diaphyseal Radius and ulna fractures

222-C: complex fracture

C3: both bones complex

C3.1: bifocal

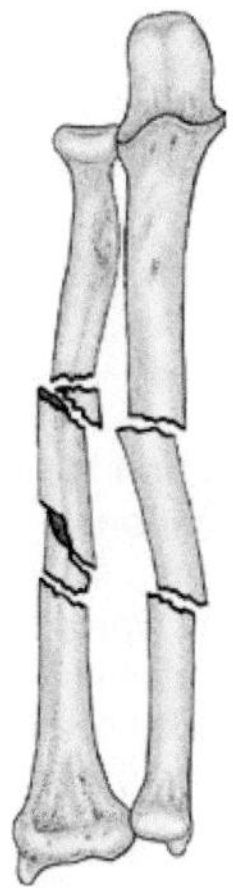

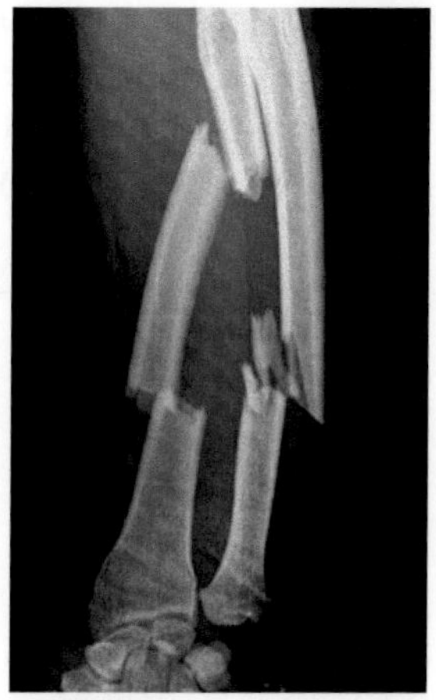

AO/OTA Classification of Diaphyseal Radius and ulna fractures

22-C: complex fracture

C3: both bones complex

C3.2: bifocal of one, irregular of other

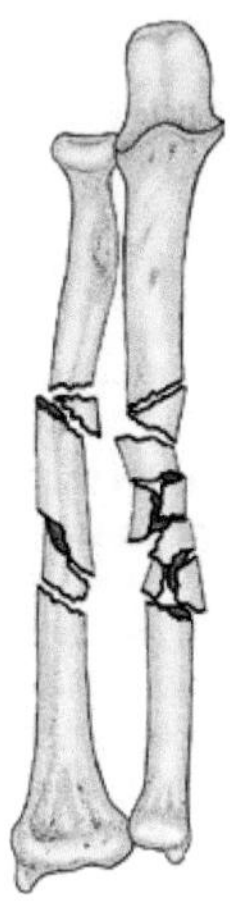

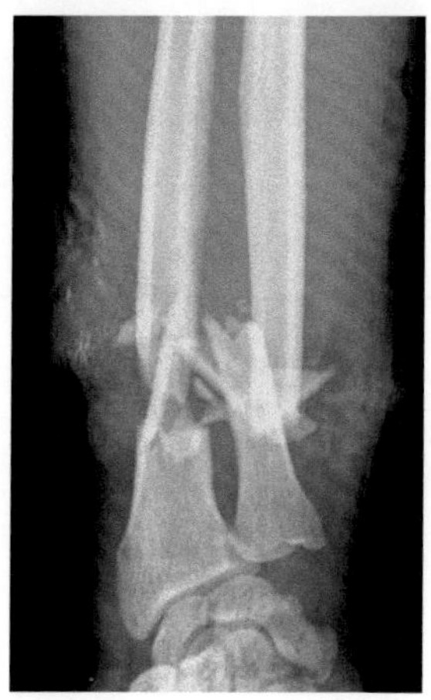

AO/OTA Classification of Diaphyseal Radius and ulna fractures

22-C: complex fracture

C3: radius complex, ulna simple

C3.3: irregular

3.2.1.2 Bado Classification for Monteggia Fracture–Dislocations [27]

Bado classification includes four types based on displacement of the radial head.

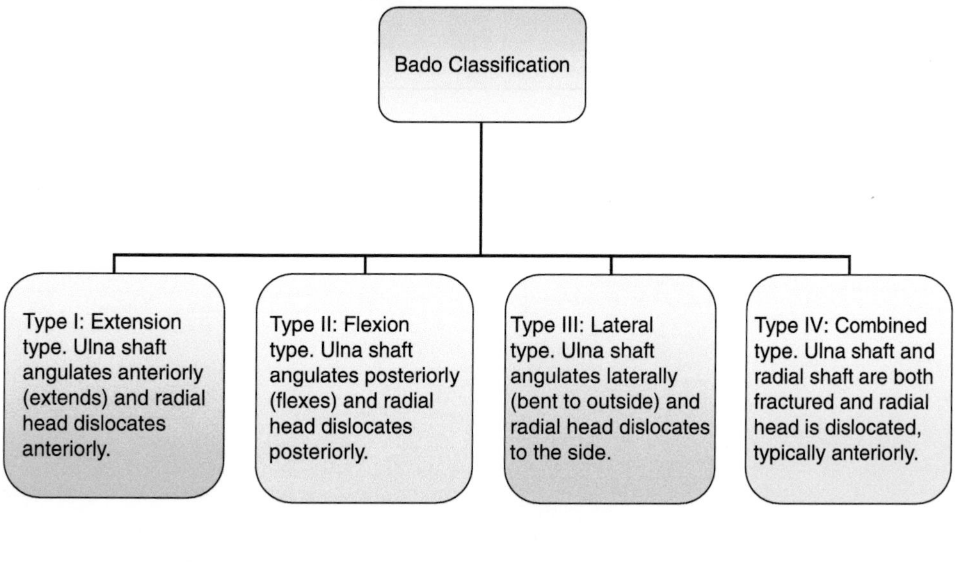
Bado Classification
Type I: Extension type. Ulna shaft angulates anteriorly (extends) and radial head dislocates anteriorly.
Type II: Flexion type. Ulna shaft angulates posteriorly (flexes) and radial head dislocates posteriorly.
Type III: Lateral type. Ulna shaft angulates laterally (bent to outside) and radial head dislocates to the side.
Type IV: Combined type. Ulna shaft and radial shaft are both fractured and radial head is dislocated, typically anteriorly.

Type I: Extension type: Ulna shaft angulates anteriorly (extends) and radial head dislocates anteriorly.

Type II: Flexion type: Ulna shaft angulates posteriorly (flexes) and radial head dislocates posteriorly.

Type III: Lateral type: Ulna shaft angulates laterally (bent to outside) and radial head dislocates to the side.

Type IV: Combined type: Ulna shaft and radial shaft are both fractured and radial head is dislocated, typically anteriorly.

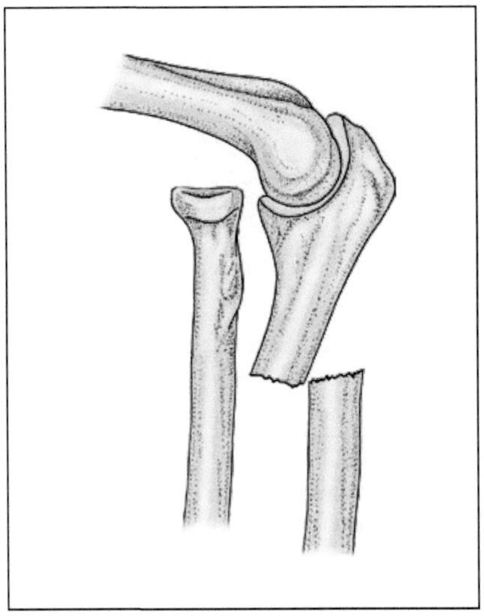

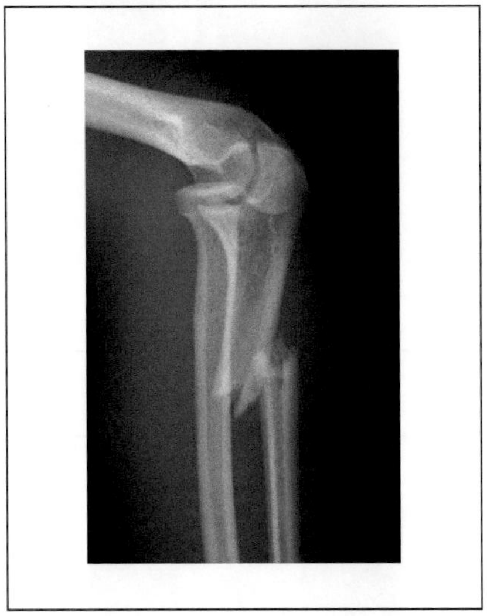

Bado Classification for Monteggia Fracture-Dislocations

Type I: Extension type.
Ulna shaft angulates anteriorly (extends) and radial head dislocates anteriorly.

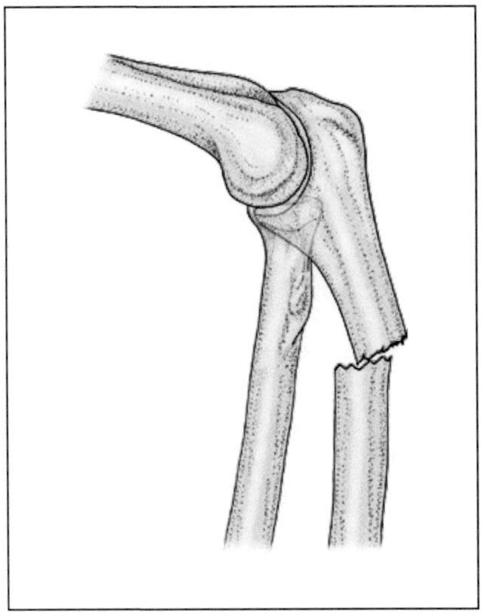

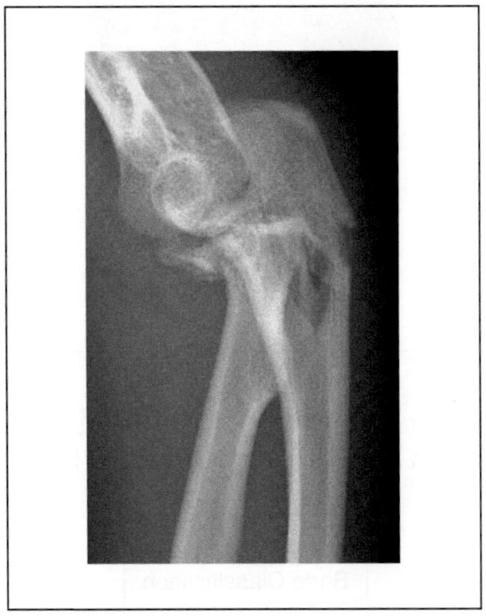

Bado Classification for Monteggia Fracture-Dislocations

Type II: Flexion type. Ulna shaft angulates posteriorly (flexes) and radial head dislocates posteriorly

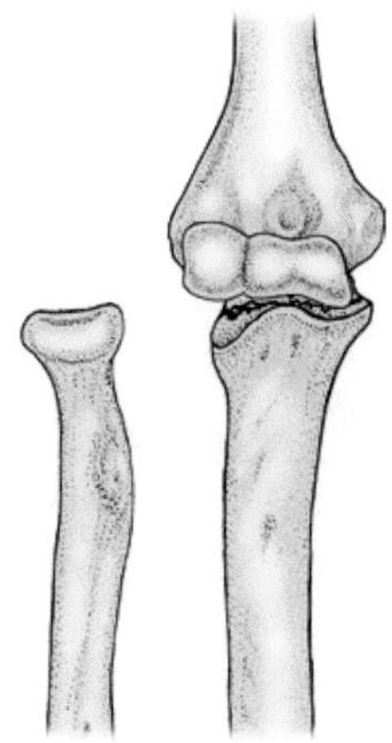

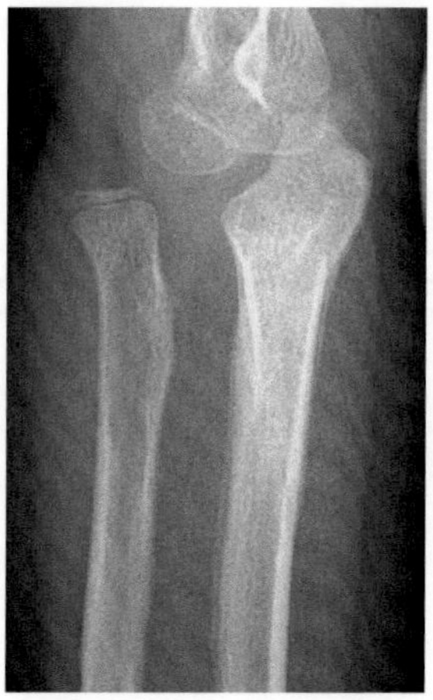

Bado Classification for Monteggia Fracture-Dislocations

Type III: Lateral type. Ulna shaft angulates laterally (bent to outside) and radial head dislocates to the side.

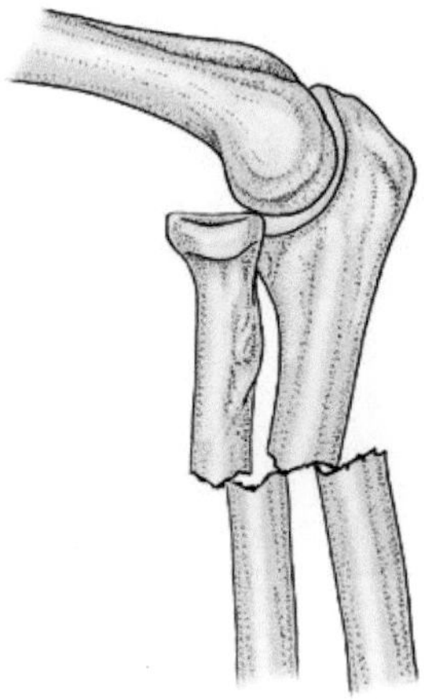

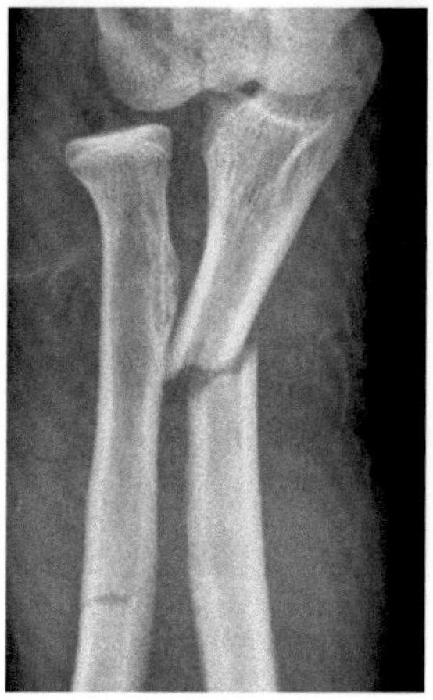

Bado Classification for Monteggia Fracture-Dislocations

Type IV: Combined type.
Ulna shaft and radial shaft are both fractured and radial head is dislocated, typically anteriorly.

3.2.1.3 Classification of Galeazzi Fracture–Dislocation [28]

Galeazzi fracture was first described by Sir Astley Cooper in 1822, but was named after the Italian surgeon Riccardo Galeazzi, who presented 18 cases of this fracture in 1934. It classically involves an isolated fracture of the junction of the distal third and middle third of the radius with associated subluxation or dislocation of the distal radioulnar joint [29].

Classification of Galeazzi fractures according to Macule et al. [30]

Type I: Fracture of radius occurs between 0 and 10 cm from the styloid process.
Type II: Fracture of radius occurs between 10 and 15 cm from the styloid process.
Type III: Fracture of radius occurs more than 15 cm from the styloid process.

3.2.1.4 Galeazzi Classification [31]

In 1934, Galeazzi classified the distal 1/3 radius fractures into three types based on displacement and stability after reduction.

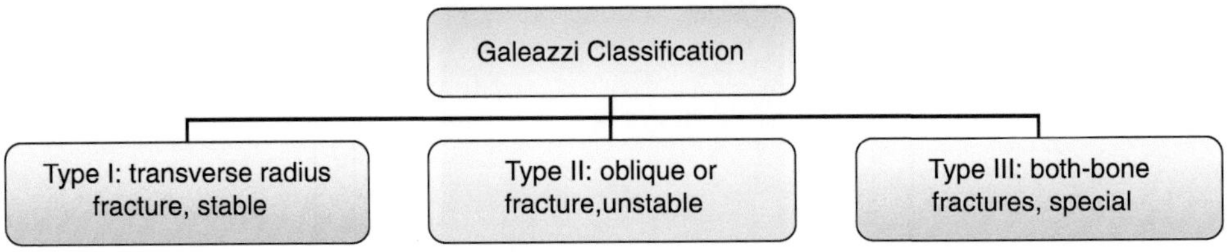

Type I: Transverse radius fracture, stable.
Type II: Oblique or comminuted radius fracture, unstable.
Type III: Both bone fractures, special.

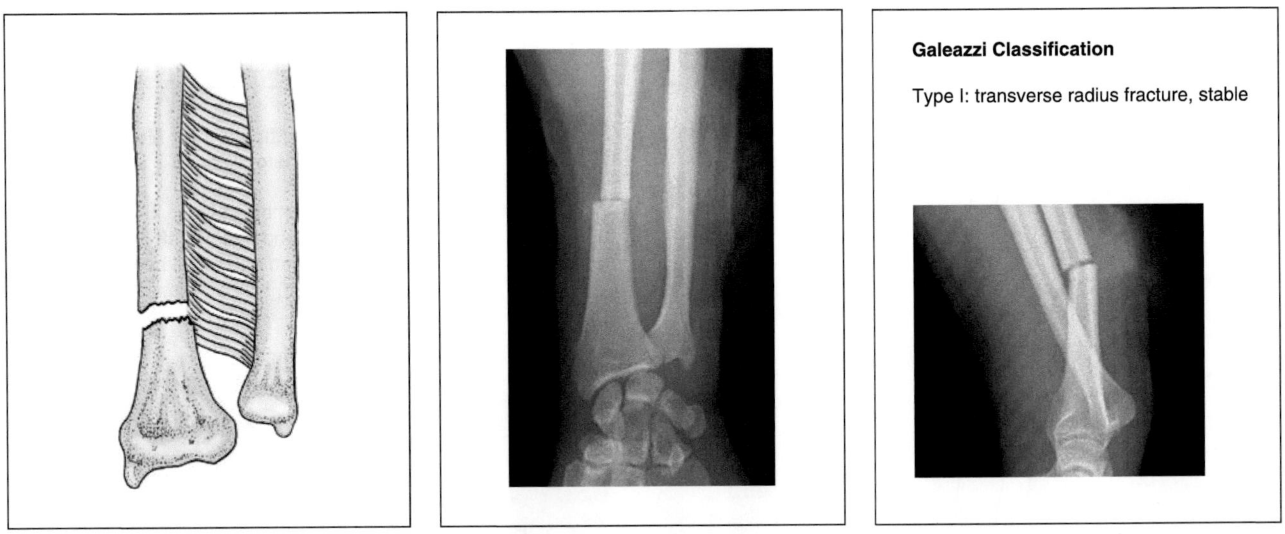

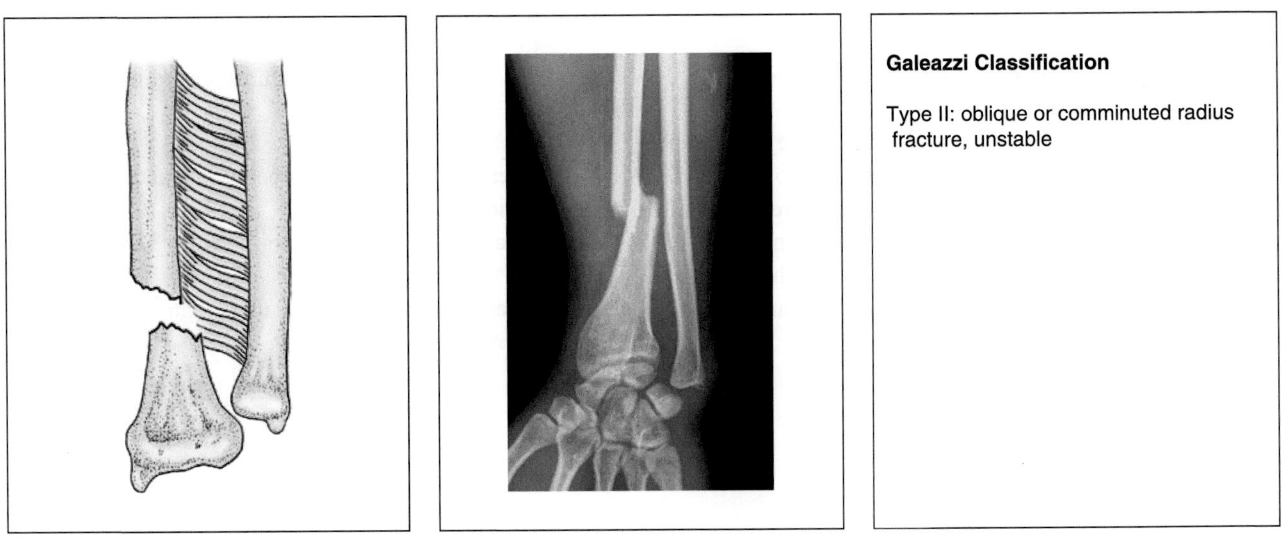

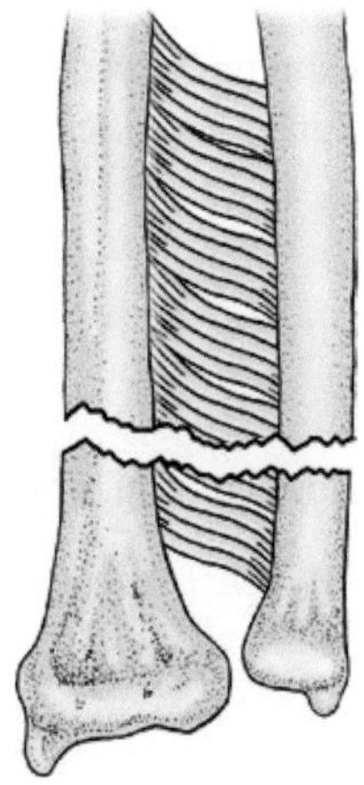

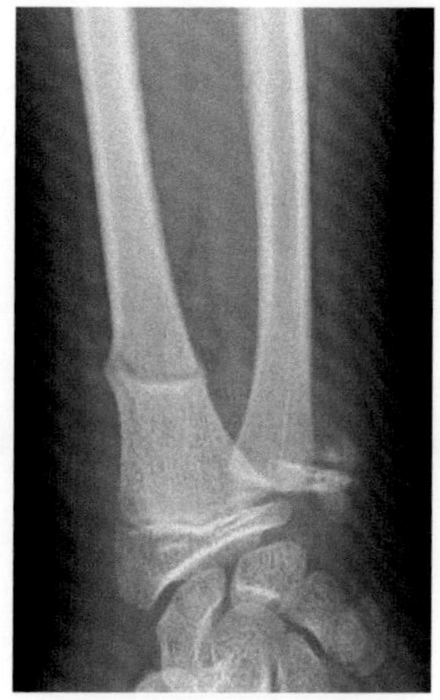

Galeazzi Classification

Type III: both-bone fractures, special

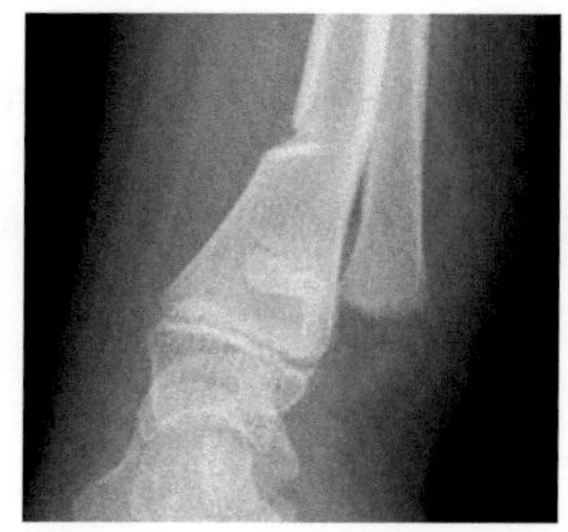

3.2.1.5 Classification of Galeazzi Fracture–Dislocation by Rettig and Raskin [32]

Type I: Distance between the midarticular surface of the distal radius and the fracture is within 7.5 cm. DRUJ joint more unstable, when tested intraoperatively.

Type II: Distance between the midarticular surface of the distal radius and the fracture is more than 7.5 cm. Only 6% of patients required ORIF of the DRUJ.

3.2.1.6 Classification Based on Fracture Site

Fractures are classified into proximal 1/3, middle 1/3, and distal 1/3 fractures.

3.2.1.7 Classification Based on Fracture Patterns

Fractures are classified into transverse, oblique, spiral, and comminuted fractures.

3.2.1.8 Classification Based on Wound

Fractures are classified into open and closed fractures according to absence or presence of wounds that communicate with fracture, respectively.

3.3 Section 3 Classifications of Distal Radius and Ulna Fractures

Common descriptive names of distal radius fractures include Colles, Smith, Barton, and Hutchinson fractures. Over 20 classification systems are available for distal radius and ulna fractures. Cooney, AO/OTA, and Frykman classifications are the most commonly used systems in recent 5 years.

3.3.1 Cooney Classification [33]

Fractures are classified according to extra-articular or intra-articular (radiocarpal joint, distal radioulnar joint, or both) types.

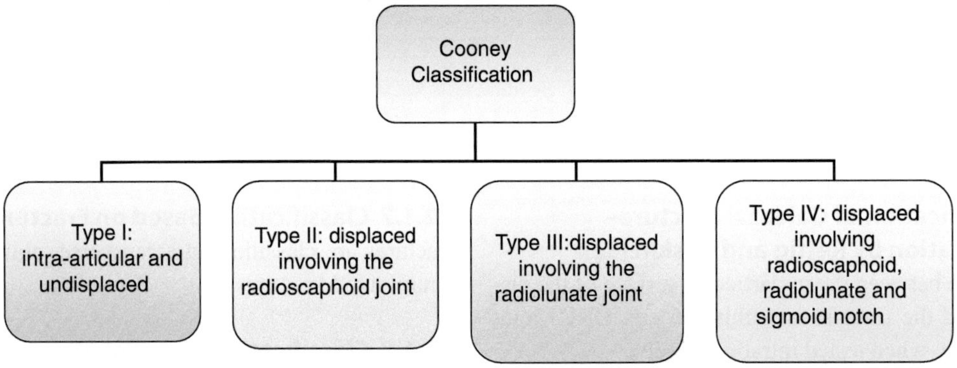

Type I: Intra-articular and undisplaced.
Type II: Displaced involving the radioscaphoid joint.
Type III: Displaced involving the radiolunate joint.
Type IV: Displaced involving radioscaphoid, radiolunate, and sigmoid notch.

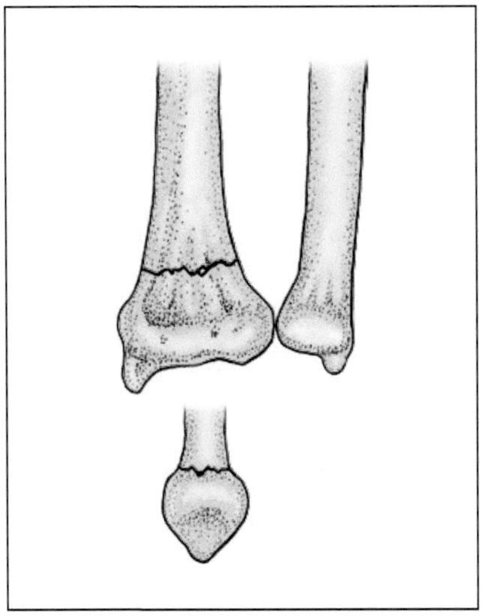

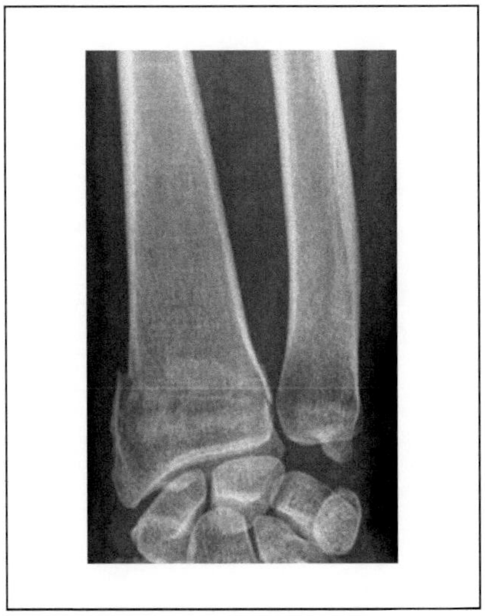

Cooney Classification of Distal Radius and ulna fractures

Type I: intra-articular and undisplaced

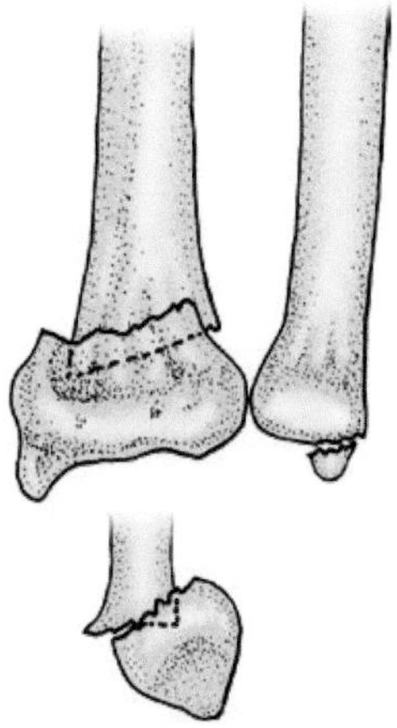

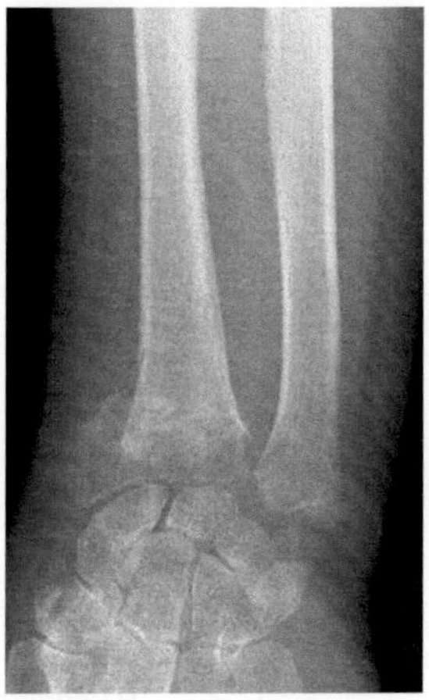

Cooney Classification of Distal Radius and ulna fractures

Type II: displaced involving the radioscaphoid joint

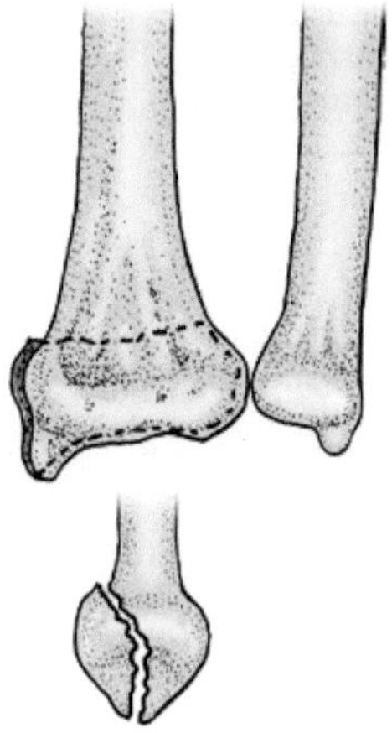

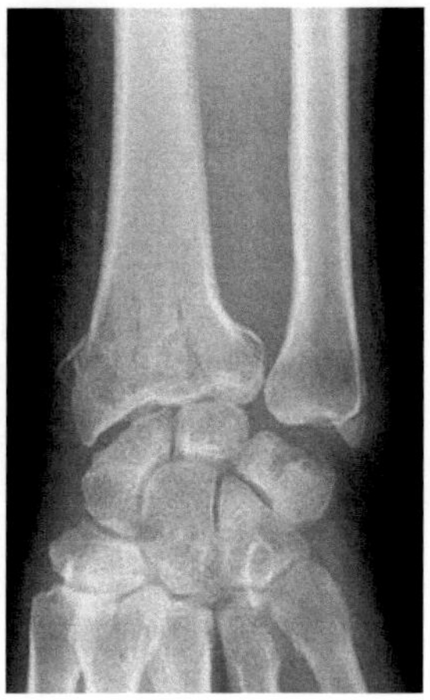

Cooney Classification of Distal Radius and ulna fractures

Type III: displaced involving the radiolunate joint

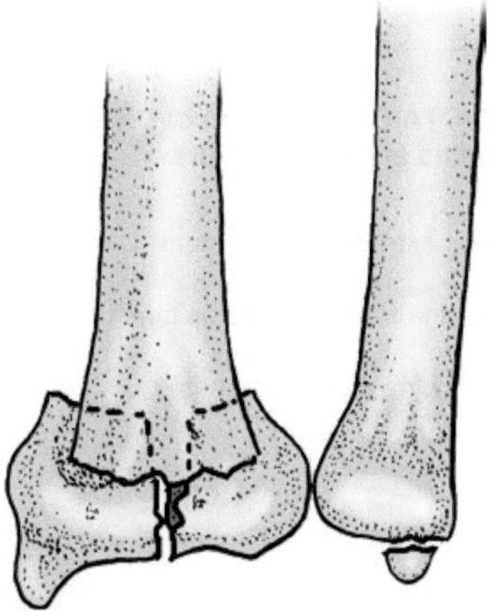

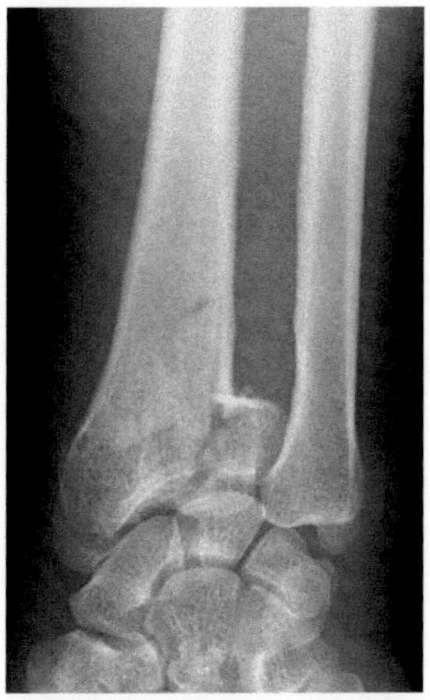

Cooney Classification of Distal Radius and ulna fractures

Type IV: displaced involving radioscaphoid, radiolunate and sigmoid notch

3.3.2 AO/OTA Classification [24]

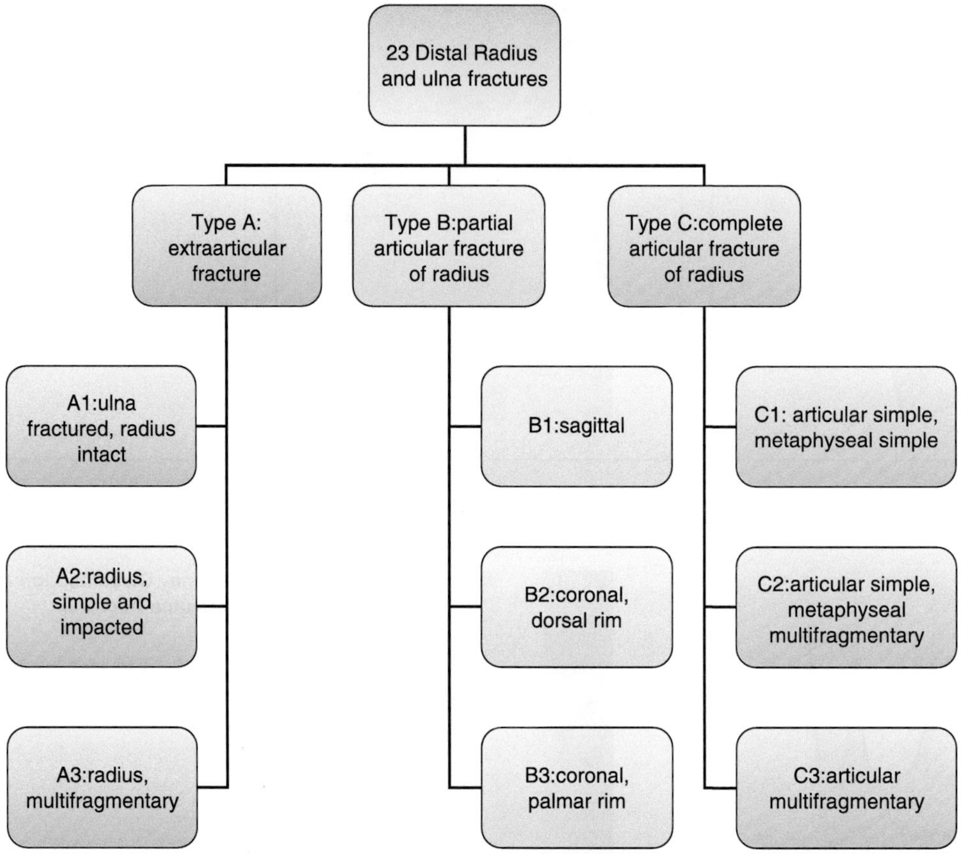

23-A: Extra-articular fracture:
- A1: Ulna fractured, radius intact:
  - A1.1: Ulna styloid process.
  - A1.2: Metaphyseal simple.
  - A1.3: Metaphyseal multifragmentary.
- A2: Radius, simple, and impacted:
  - A2.1: Transverse, no tilt, but may be axially shortened.
  - A2.2: With dorsal tilt, oblique fracture upward and back (Pouteau-Colles).
  - A2.3: Volar tilt, oblique upwards and forward (Goyrand-Smith).
- A3: Radius, multifragmentary:
  - A3.1: Impacted with axial shortening.
  - A3.2: With a wedge.
  - A3.3: Complex.

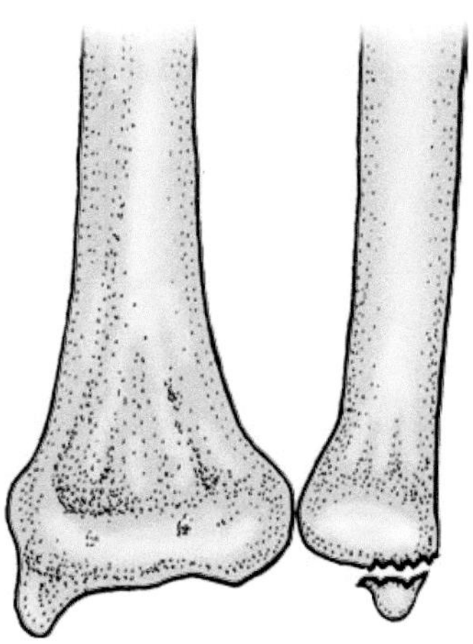

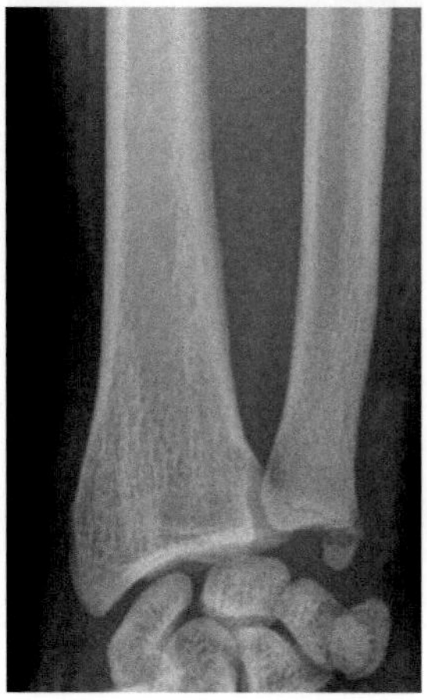

AO/OTA Classification of Distal Radius and ulna fractures

23-A: extraarticular fracture

A1: ulna fractured, radius intact

A1.1: ulna styloid process

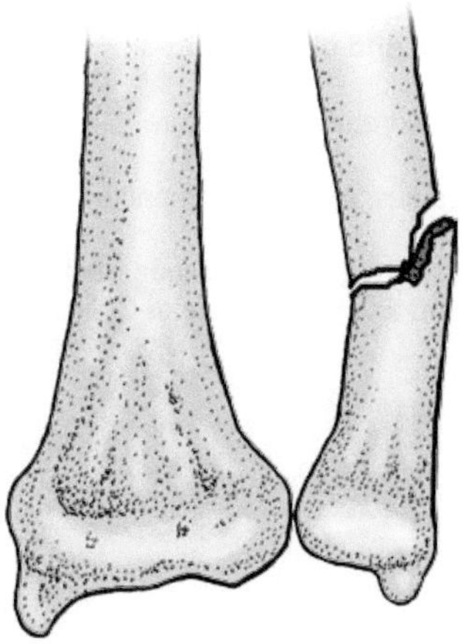

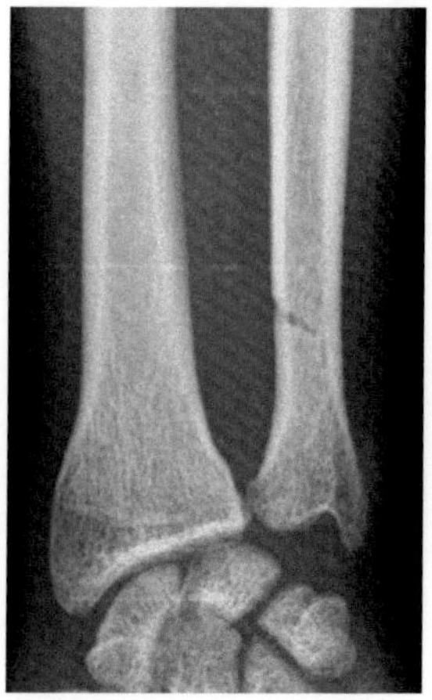

AO/OTA Classification of Distal Radius and ulna fractures

23-A: extraarticular fracture

A1: ulna fractured, radius intact

A1.2: metaphyseal simple

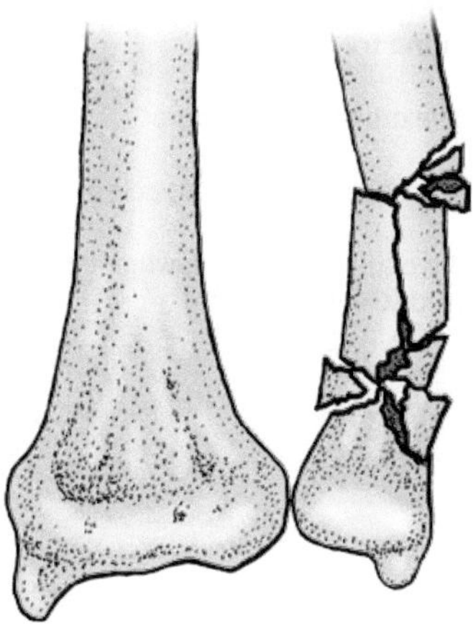

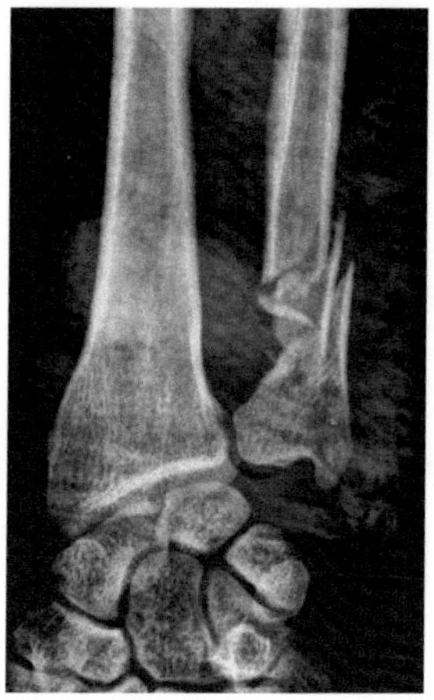

AO/OTA Classification of Distal Radius and ulna fractures

23-A: extraarticular fracture

A1: ulna fractured, radius intact

A1.3: metaphyseal multifragmentary

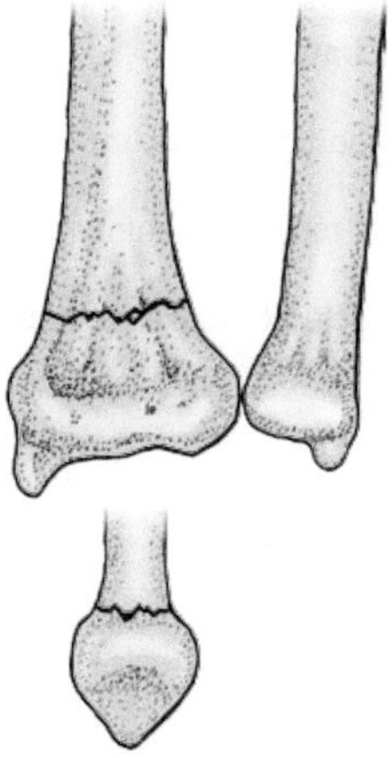

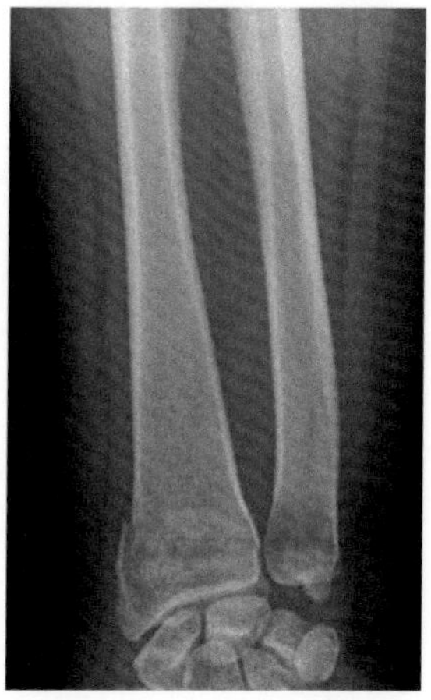

AO/OTA Classification of Distal Radius and ulna fractures

23-A: extraarticular fracture

A2: radius, simple and impacted

A2.1: transverse, no tilt, but may be axially shortened

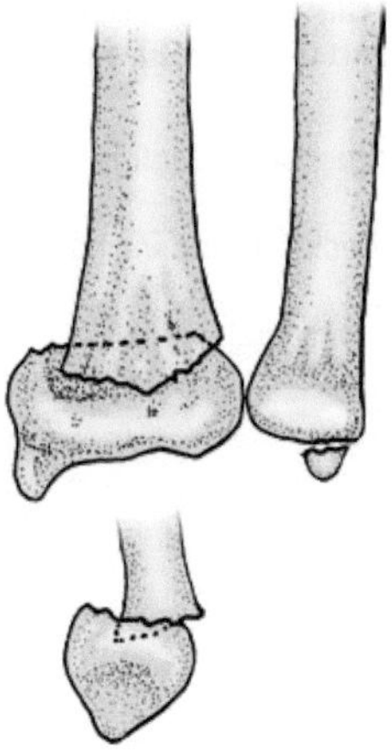

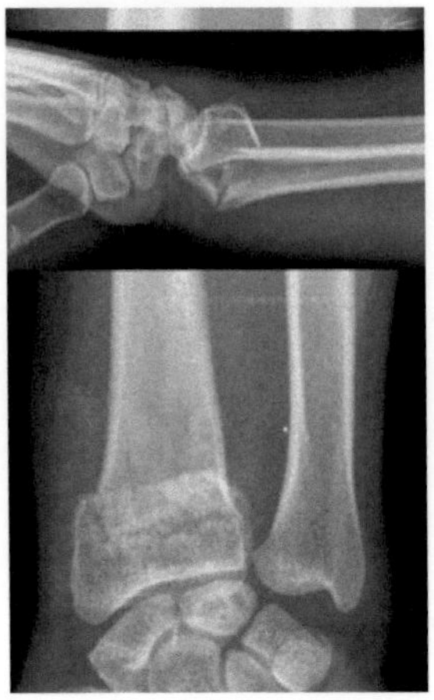

AO/OTA Classification of Distal Radius and ulna fractures

23-A: extraarticular fracture

A2: radius, simple and impacted

A2.2: with dorsal tilt, oblique fracture upward and back (Pouteau-Colles)

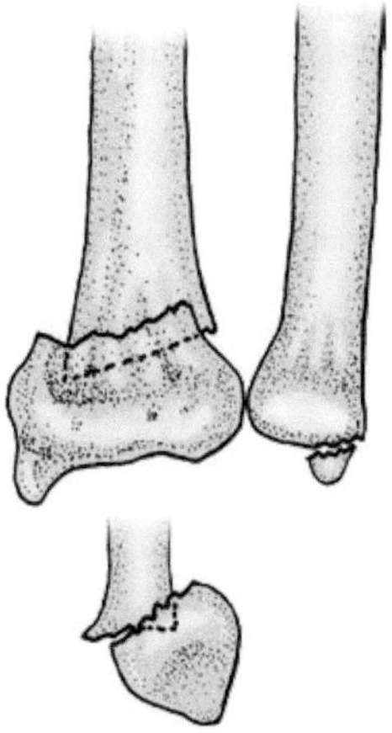

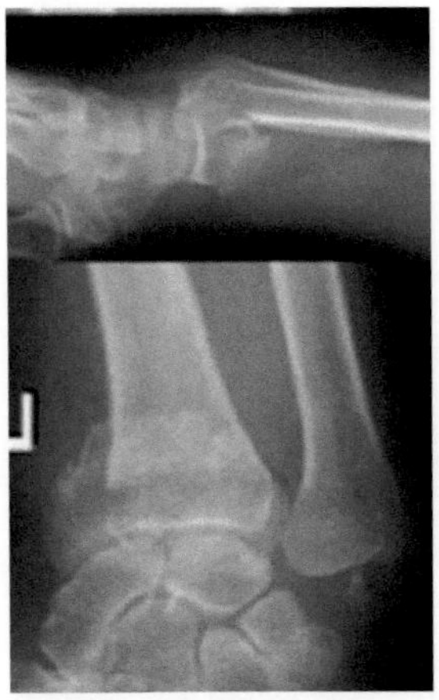

AO/OTA Classification of Distal Radius and ulna fractures

23-A: extraarticular fracture

A2: radius, simple and impacted

A2.3: volar tilt, oblique upwards and forward (Goyrand-Smith)

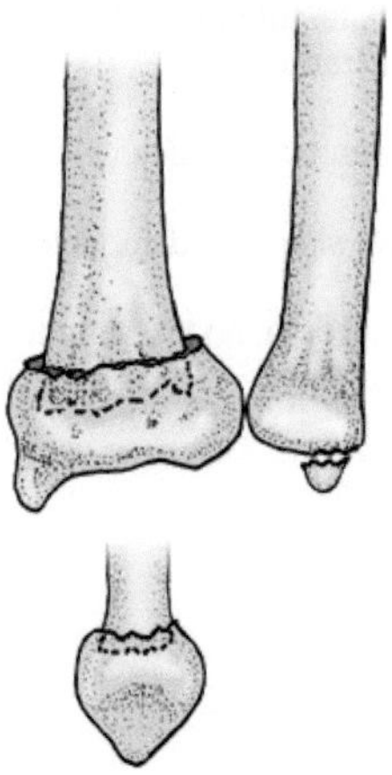

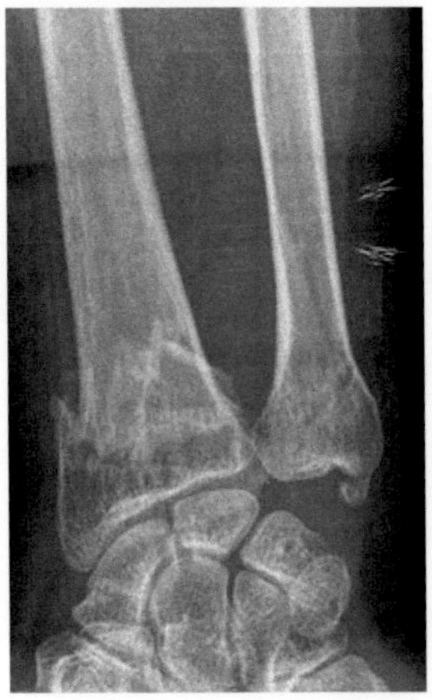

AO/OTA Classification of Distal Radius and ulna fractures

23-A: extraarticular fracture

A3: radius, multifragmentary

A3.1: impacted with axial shortening

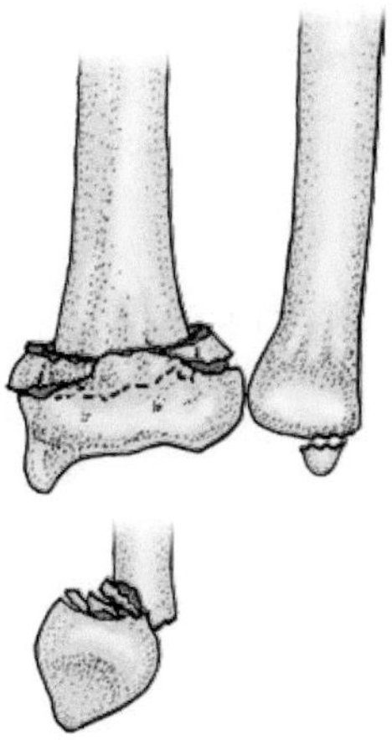

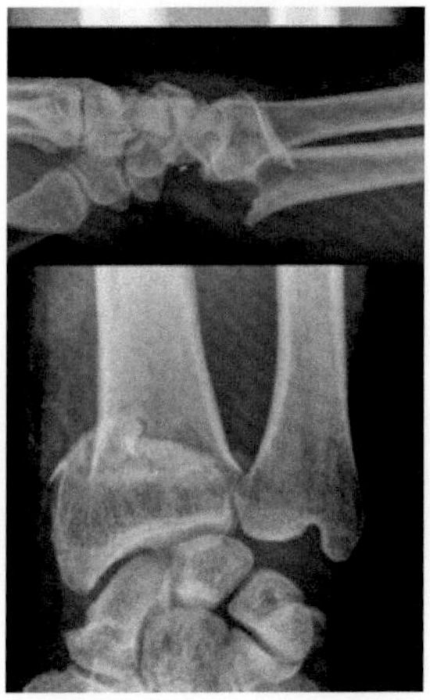

AO/OTA Classification of Distal Radius and ulna fractures

23-A: extraarticular fracture

A3: radius, multifragmentary

A3.2: with a wedge

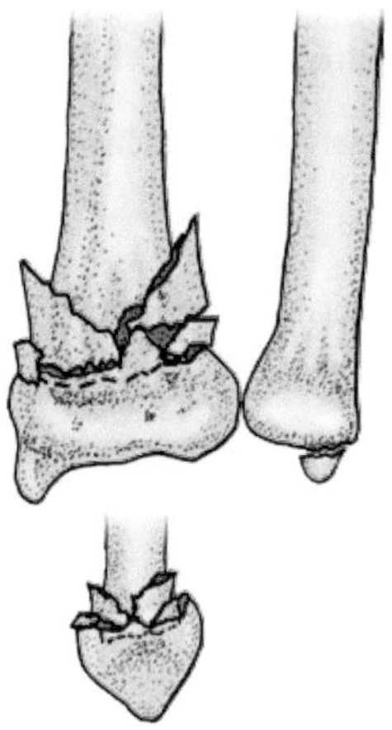

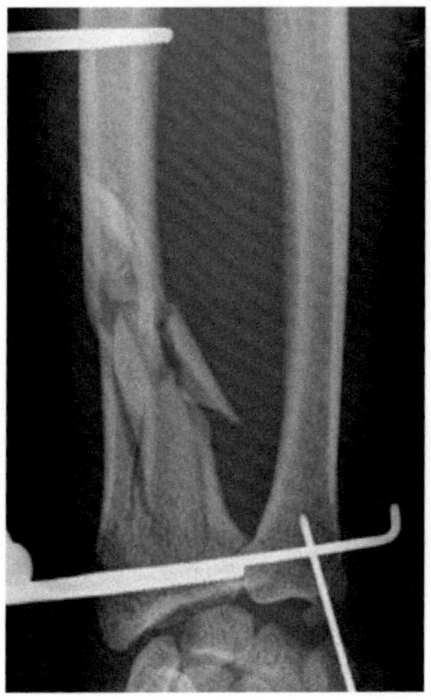

AO/OTA Classification of Distal Radius and ulna fractures

23-A: extraarticular fracture

A3: radius, multifragmentary

A3.3: complex

23-B: Partial articular fracture of radius:
- B1: Sagittal:
  - B1.1: Lateral simple.
  - B1.2: Lateral multifragmentary.
  - B1.3: Medial.
- B2: Coronal, dorsal rim:
  - B2.1: Simple with small fragment.
  - B2.2: Simple with larger fragment.
  - B2.3: Multifragmentary.
- B3: Coronal, palmar rim:
  - B3.1: Simple with small fragment.
  - B3.2: Simple with larger fragment.
  - B3.3: Multifragmentary.

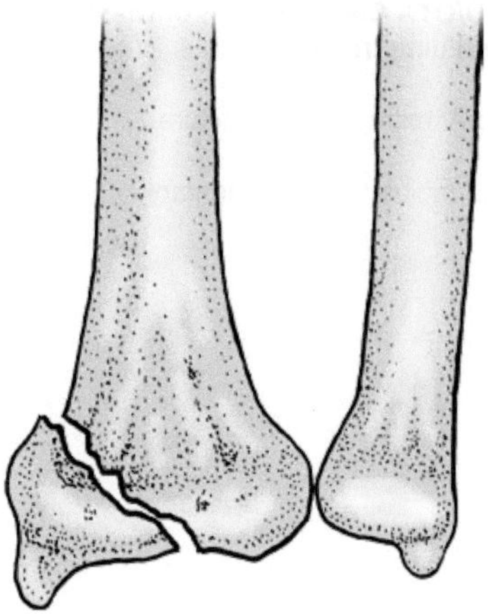

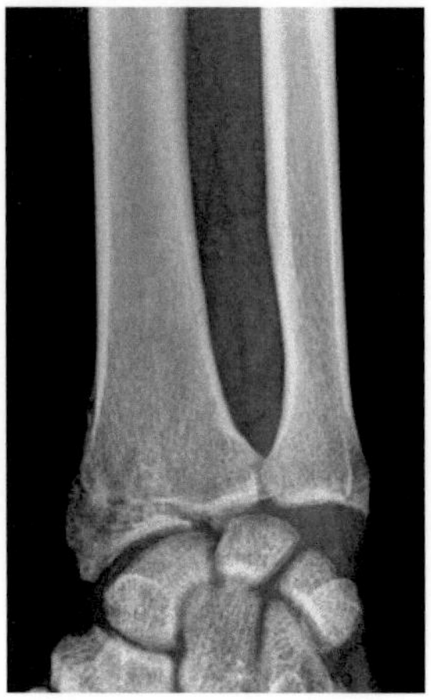

AO/OTA Classification of Distal Radius and ulna fractures

23-B: partial articular fracture of radius

B1: sagittal

B1.1: lateral simple

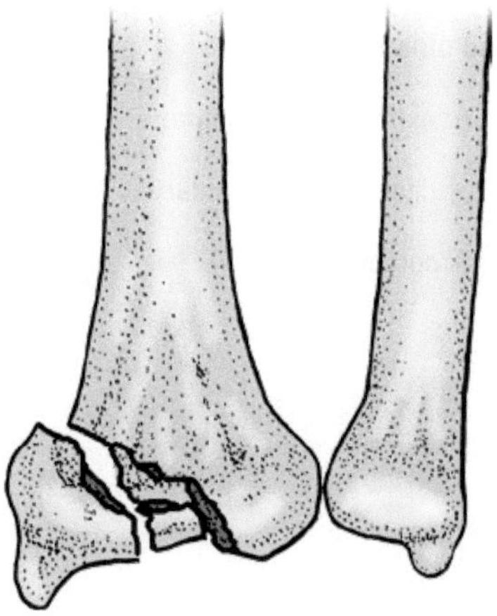

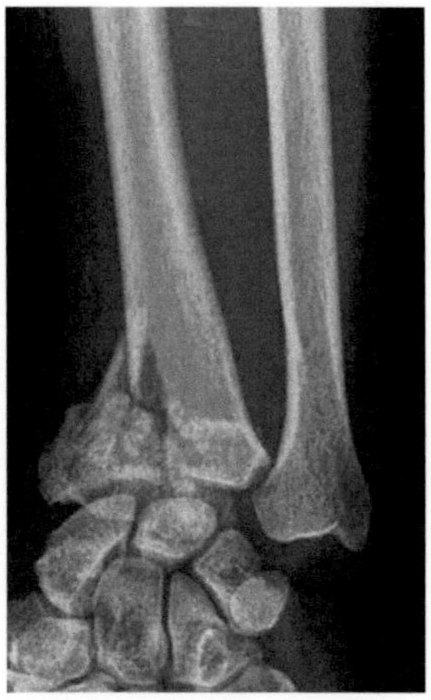

AO/OTA Classification of Distal Radius and ulna fractures

23-B: partial articular fracture of radius

B1: sagittal

B1.2: lateral multifragmentary

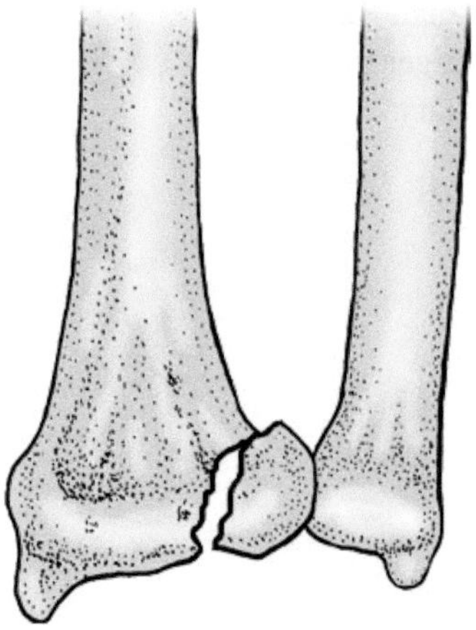

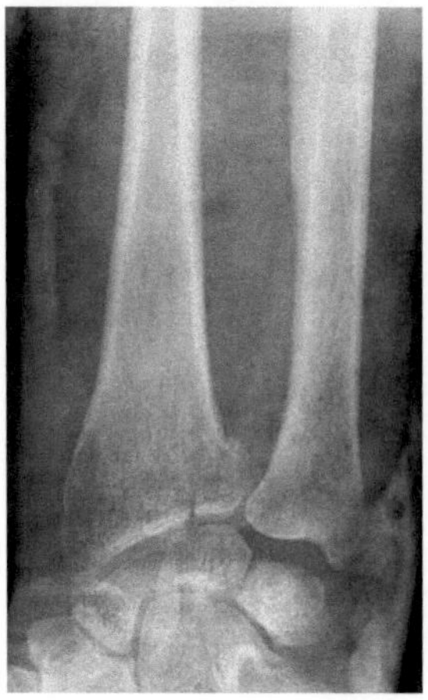

AO/OTA Classification of Distal Radius and ulna fractures

23-B: partial articular fracture of radius

B1: sagittal

B1.3: medial

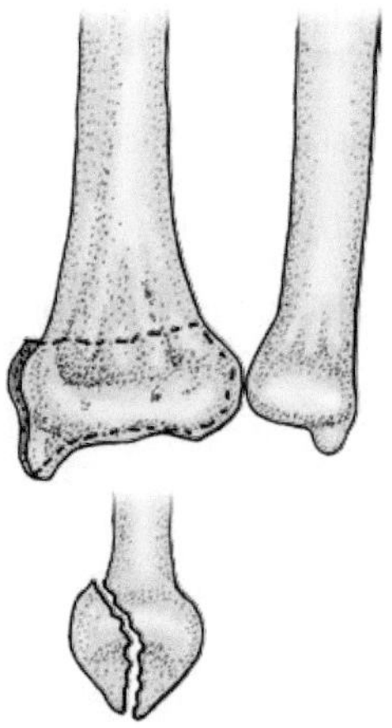

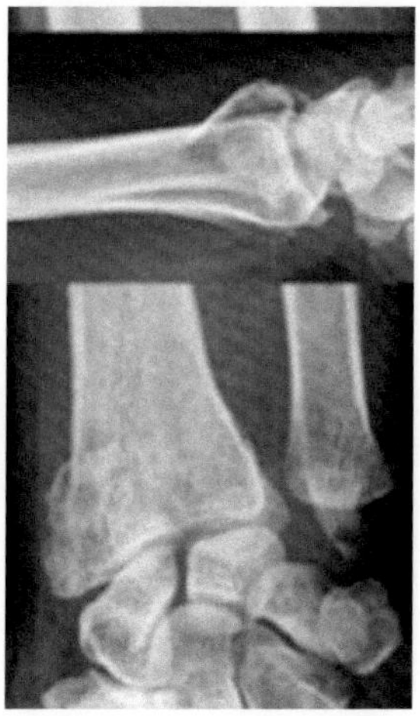

AO/OTA Classification of Distal Radius and ulna fractures

23-B: partial articular fracture of radius

B2: coronal, dorsal rim

B2.1: simple with small fragment

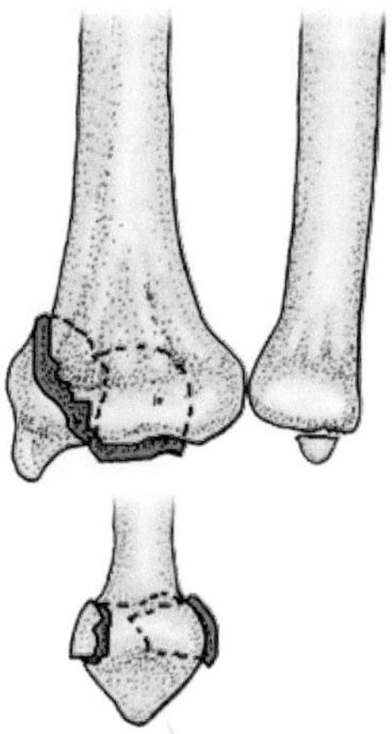

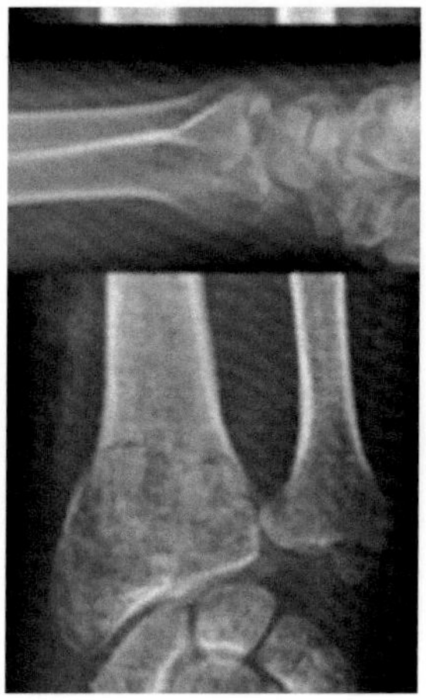

AO/OTA Classification of Distal Radius and ulna fractures

23-B: partial articular fracture of radius

B2: coronal, dorsal rim

B2.2: simple with larger fragment

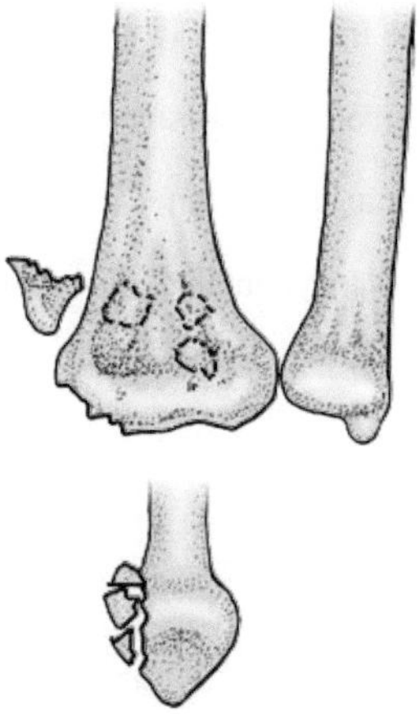

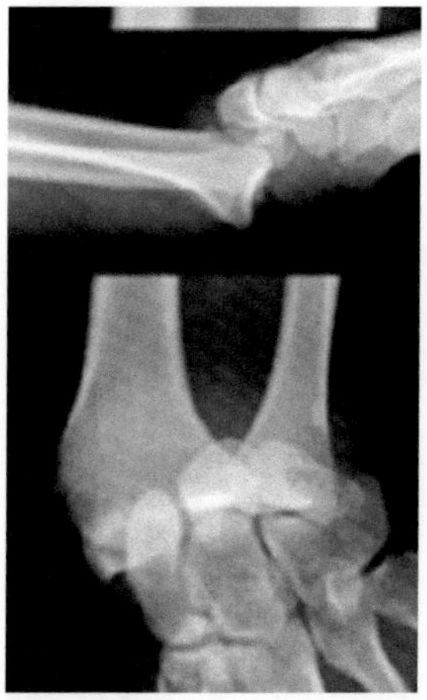

AO/OTA Classification of Distal Radius and ulna fractures

23-B: partial articular fracture of radius

B2: coronal, dorsal rim

B2.3: multifragmentary

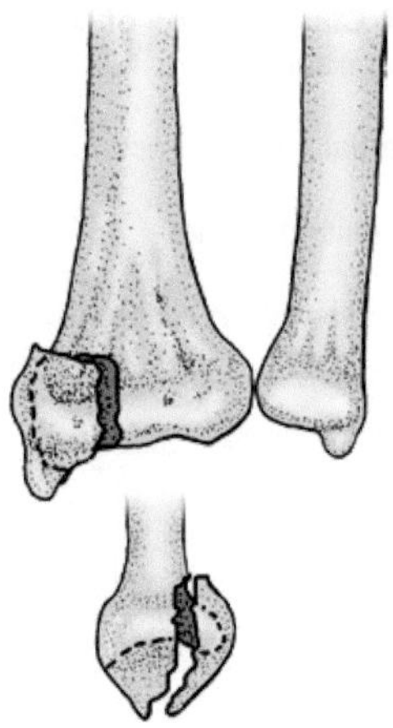

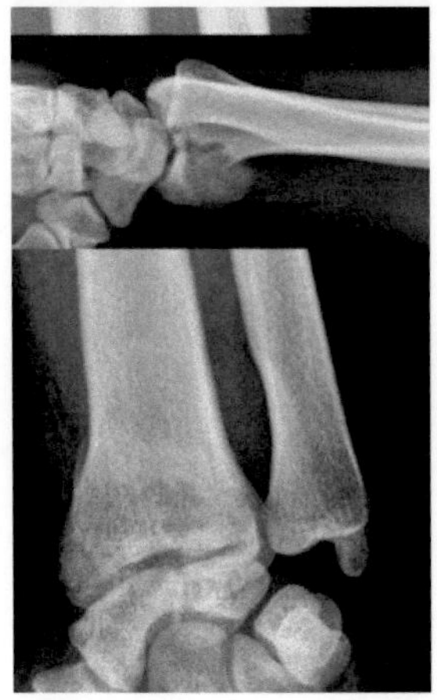

AO/OTA Classification of Distal Radius and ulna fractures

23-B: partial articular fracture of radius

B3: coronal, palmar rim

B3.1: simple with small fragment

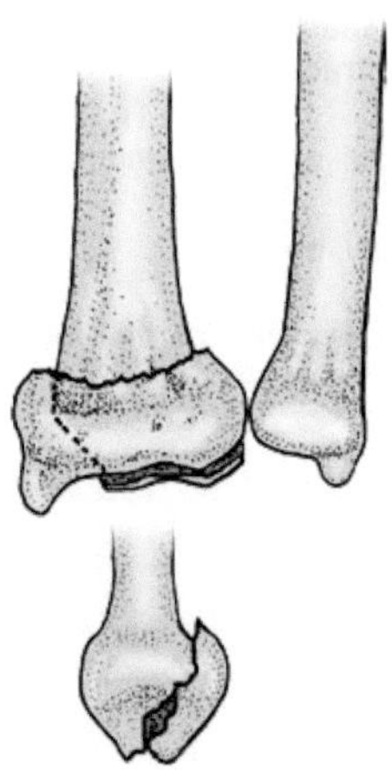

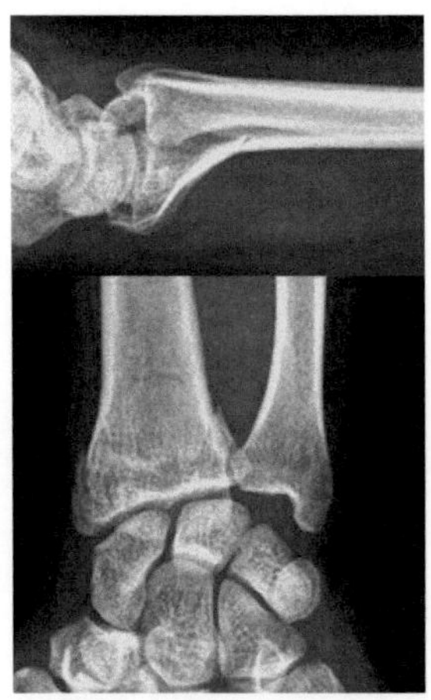

AO/OTA Classification of Distal Radius and ulna fractures

23-B: partial articular fracture of radius

B3: coronal, palmar rim

B3.2: simple with larger fragment

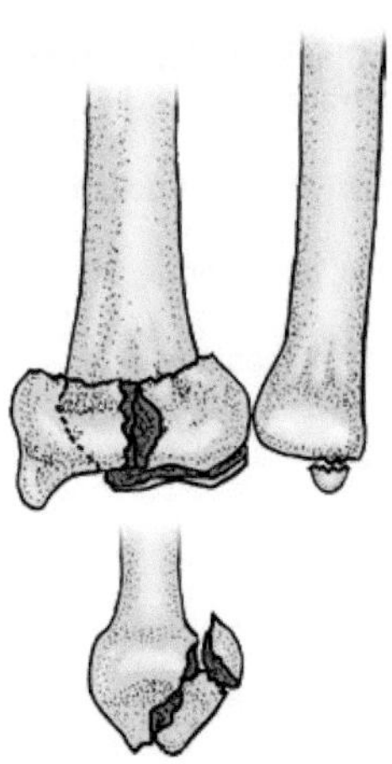

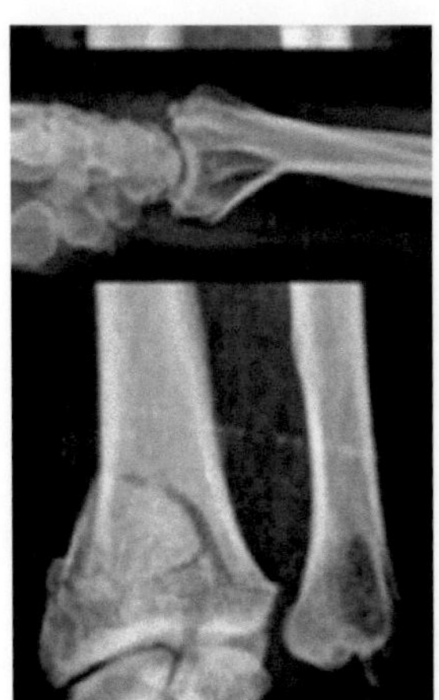

AO/OTA Classification of Distal Radius and ulna fractures

23-B: partial articular fracture of radius

B3: coronal, palmar rim

B3.3: multifragmentary

23-C: Complete articular fracture of radius:
- C1: Articular simple, metaphyseal simple:
  - C1.1: Posteromedial articular fragment.
  - C1.2: Sagittal articular fracture line.
  - C1.3: Frontal articular fracture line.
- C2: Articular simple, metaphyseal multifragmentary:
  - C2.1: Sagittal articular fracture line.
  - C2.2: Frontal articular fracture line.
  - C2.3: Extending into diaphysis.
- C3: Articular multifragmentary:
  - C3.1: Metaphyseal simple.
  - C3.2: Metaphyseal multifragmentary.
  - C3.3: Extending into diaphysis.

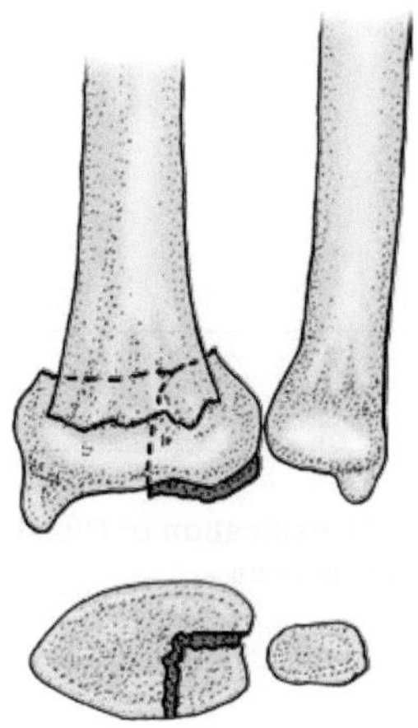

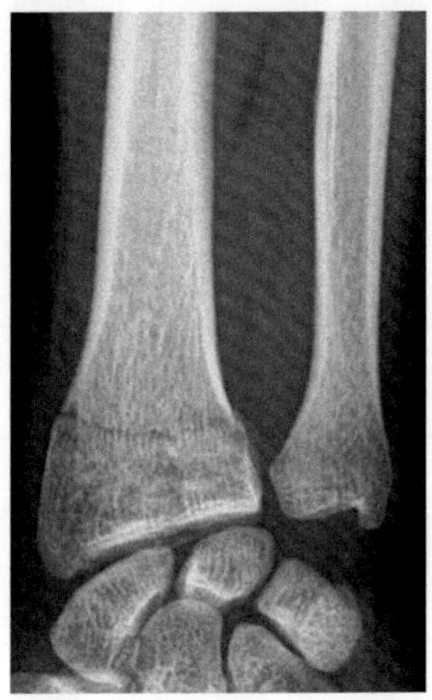

AO/OTA Classification of Distal Radius and ulna fractures

C: complete articular fracture of radius

C1: articular simple, metaphyseal simple

C1.1: posteromedial articular fragment

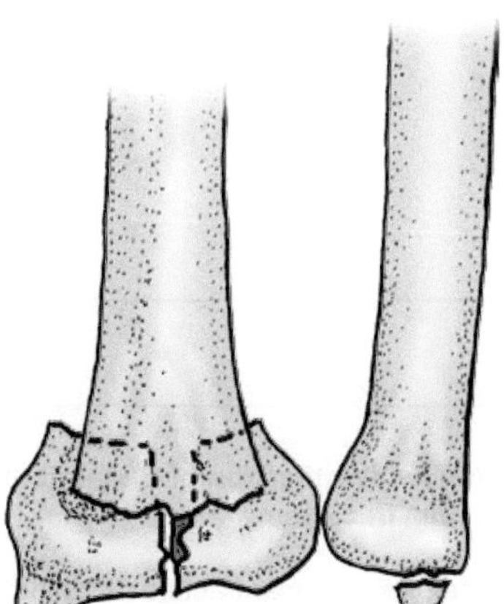

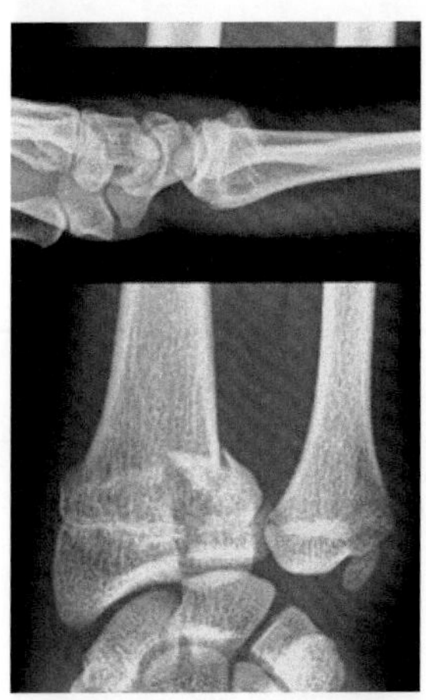

AO/OTA Classification of Distal Radius and ulna fractures

C: complete articular fracture of radius

C1: articular simple, metaphyseal simple

C1.2: sagittal articular fracture line

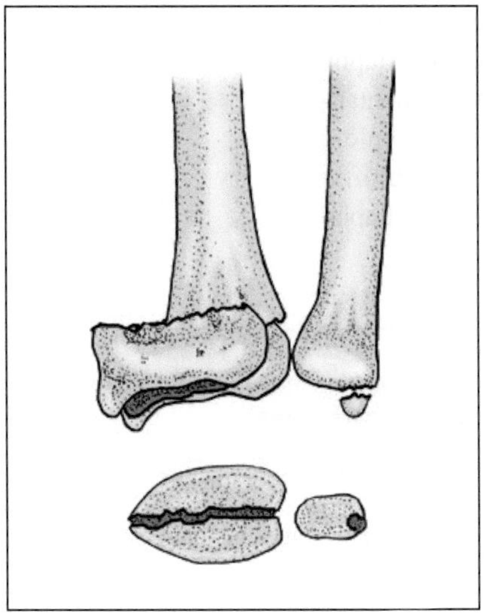

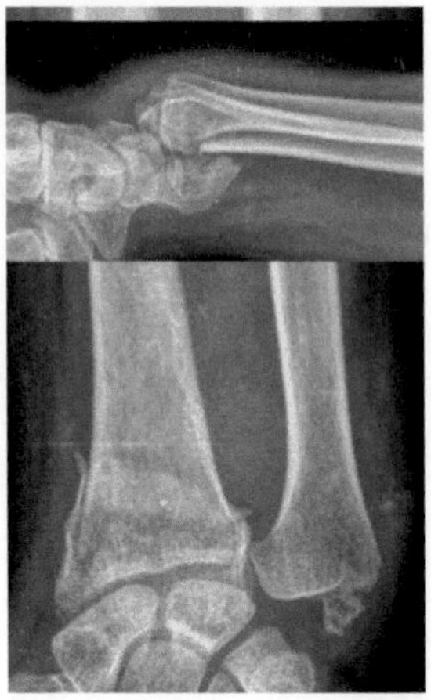

AO/OTA Classification of Distal Radius and ulna fractures

C: complete articular fracture of radius

C1: articular simple, metaphyseal simple

C1.3: frontal articular fracture line

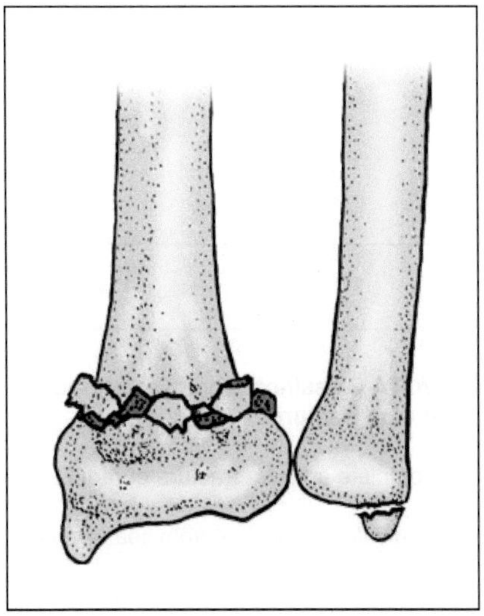

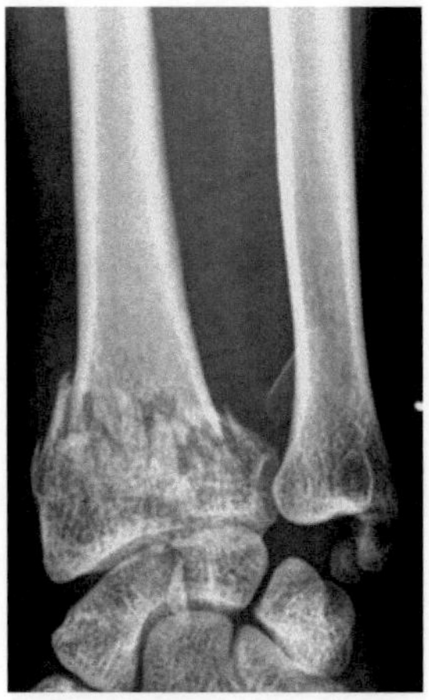

AO/OTA Classification of Distal Radius and ulna fractures

C: complete articular fracture of radius

C2: articular simple, metaphyseal multifragmentary

C2.1: sagittal articular fracture line

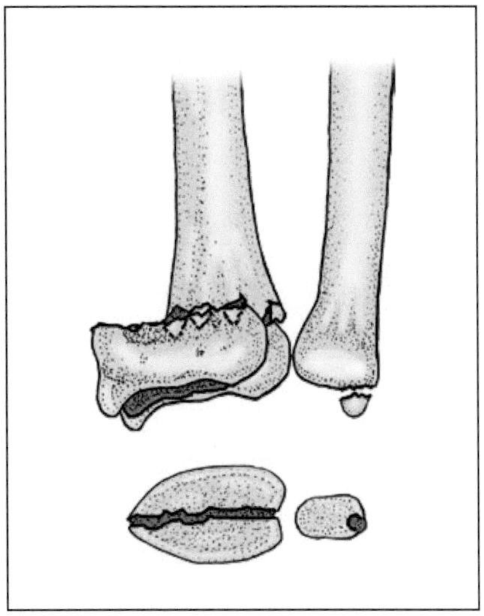

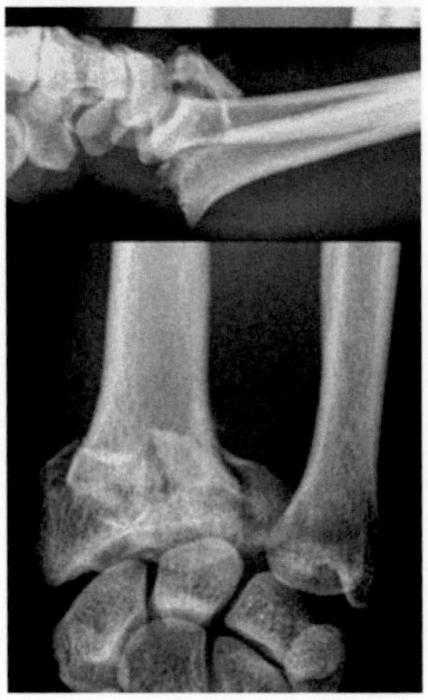

AO/OTA Classification of Distal Radius and ulna fractures

C: complete articular fracture of radius

C2: articular simple, metaphyseal multifragmentary

C2.2: frontal articular fracture line

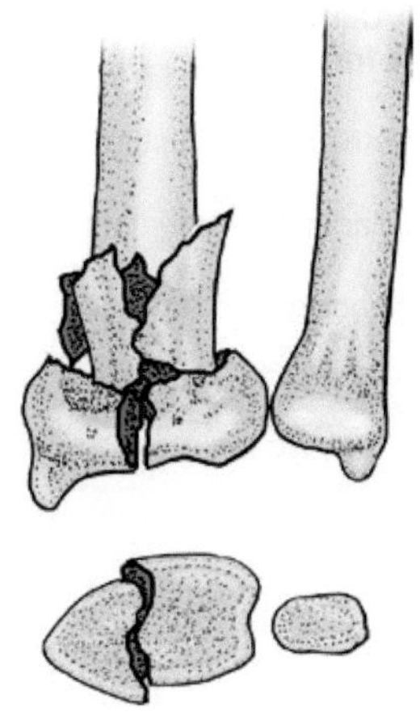

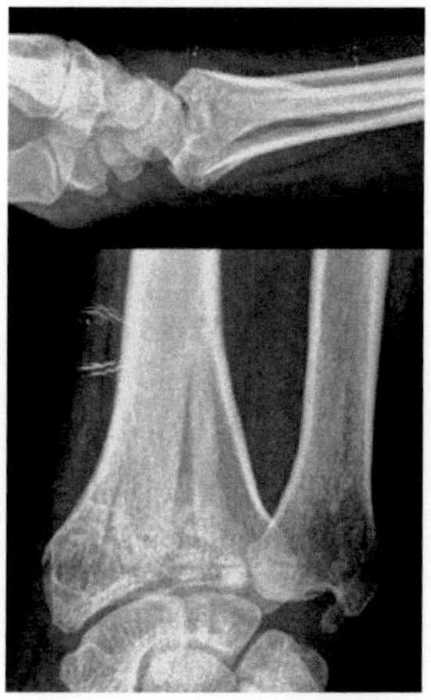

AO/OTA Classification of Distal Radius and ulna fractures

C: complete articular fracture of radius

C2: articular simple, metaphyseal multifragmentary

C2.3: extending into diaphysis

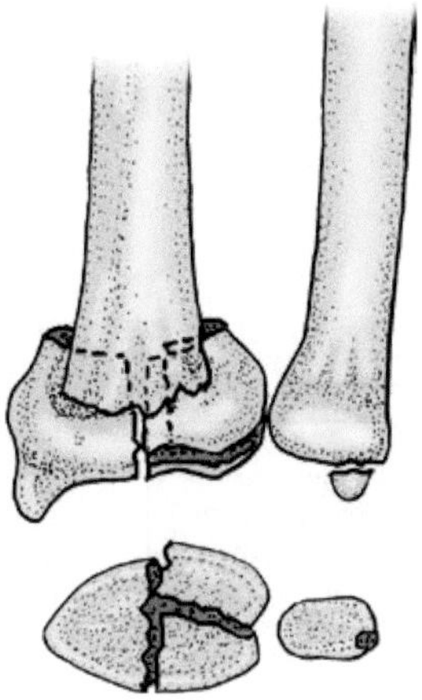

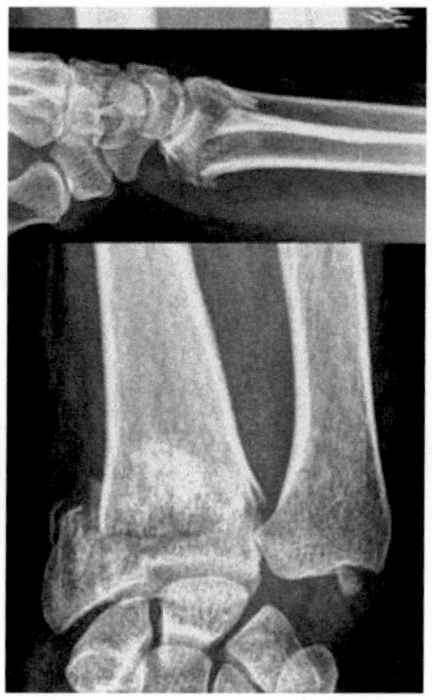

AO/OTA Classification of Distal Radius and ulna fractures

C: complete articular fracture of radius

C3: articular multifragmentary

C3.1: metaphyseal simple

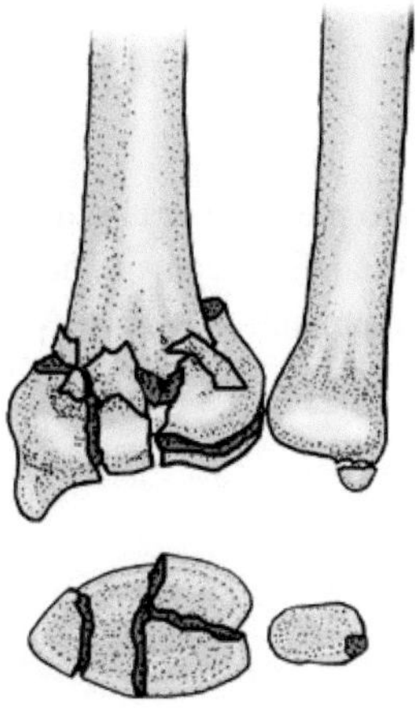

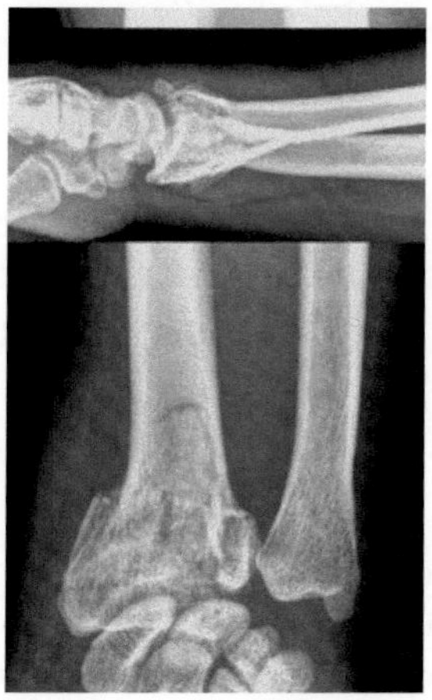

AO/OTA Classification of Distal Radius and ulna fractures

C: complete articular fracture of radius

C3: articular multifragmentary

C3.2: metaphyseal multifragmentary

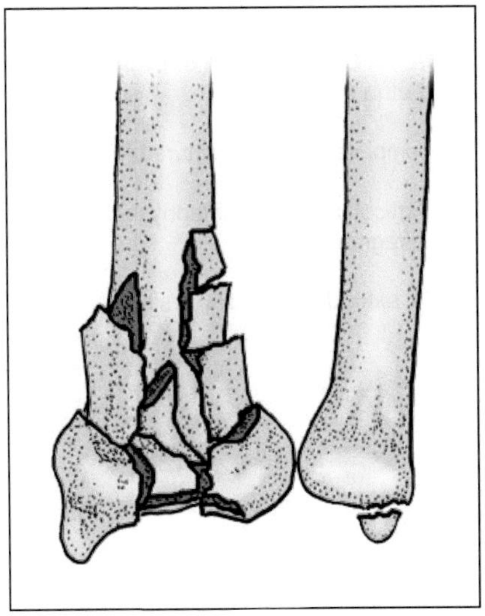

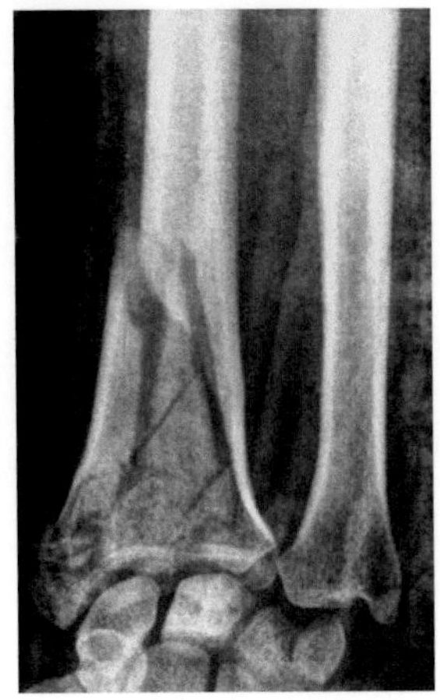

AO/OTA Classification of Distal Radius and ulna fractures

C: complete articular fracture of radius

C3: articular multifragmentary

C3.3: extending into diaphysis

3.3.3 Frykman Classification [34]

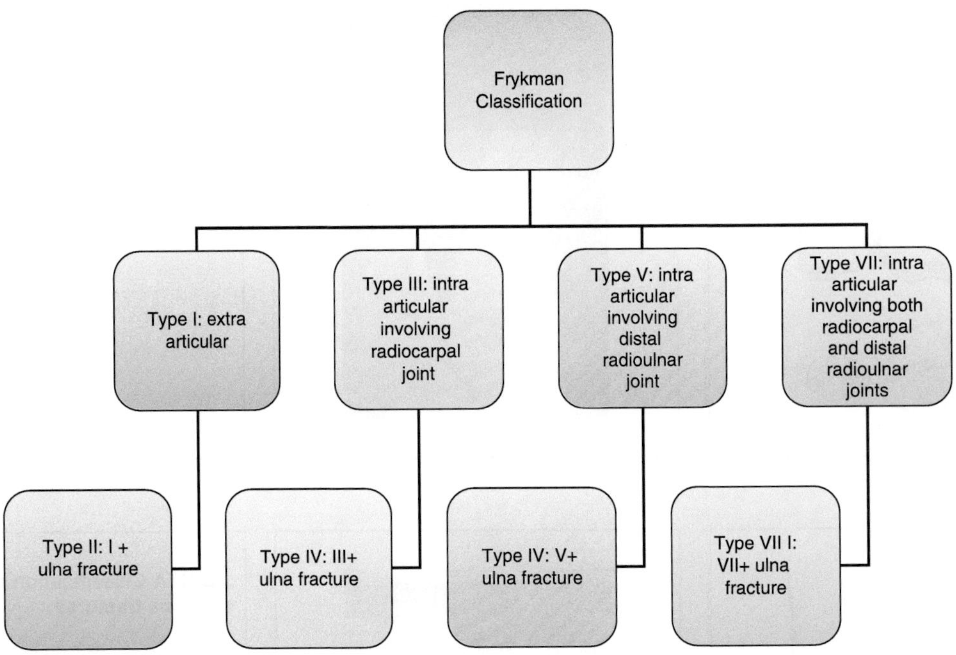

Frykman classification considers involvement of radiocarpal and radioulnar joint, in addition to presence or absence of fracture of ulnar styloid process. Since the classification does not include extent or direction of initial displacement, dorsal comminution, or shortening of the distal fragment, it is less useful in evaluating the outcome of treatment.

	Ulna fracture	
Radius fracture	Absent	Present
Extra-articular	I	II
Intra-articular involving radiocarpal joint	III	IV
Intra-articular involving distal radio-ular joint	V	VI
Intra-articular involving both radiocarpal and distal radioulnar joints	VII	VIII

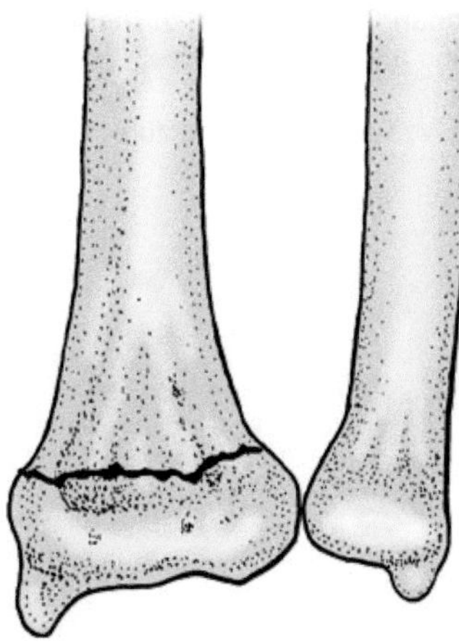

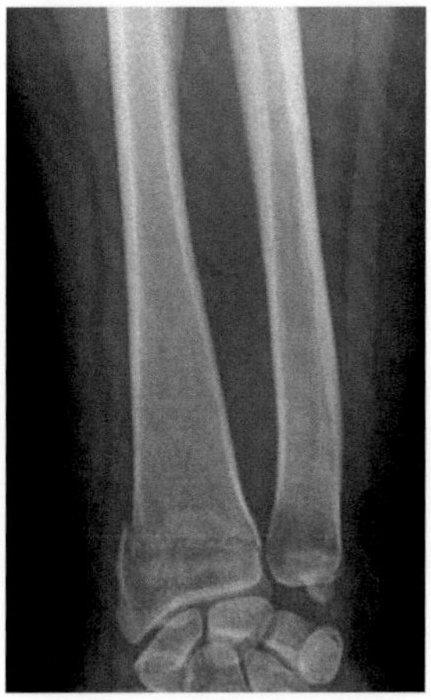

Frykman Classification of Distal Radius and ulna fractures

Type I: extra articular

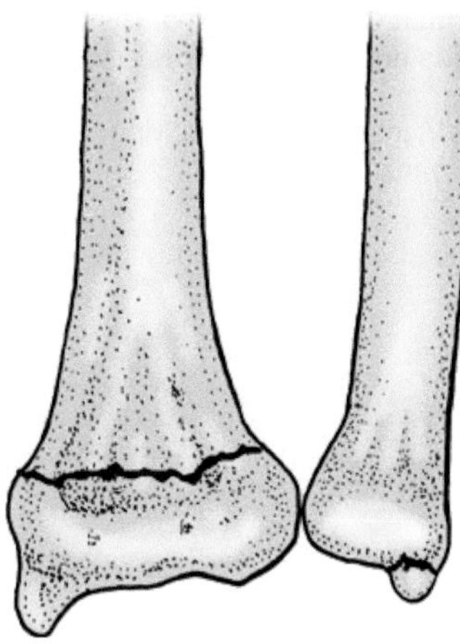

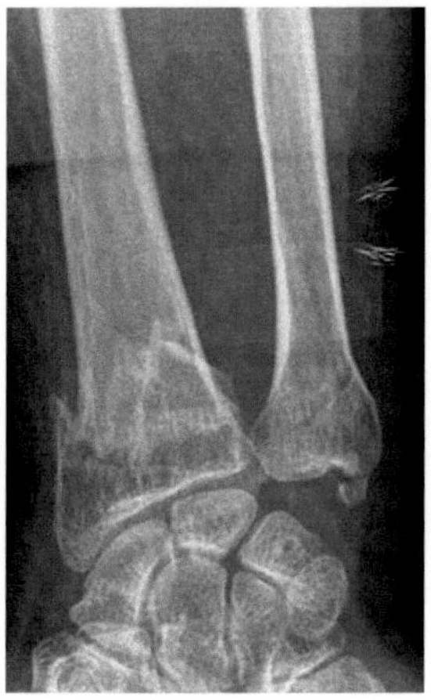

Frykman Classification of Distal Radius and ulna fractures

Type II: Type I + ulna fracture

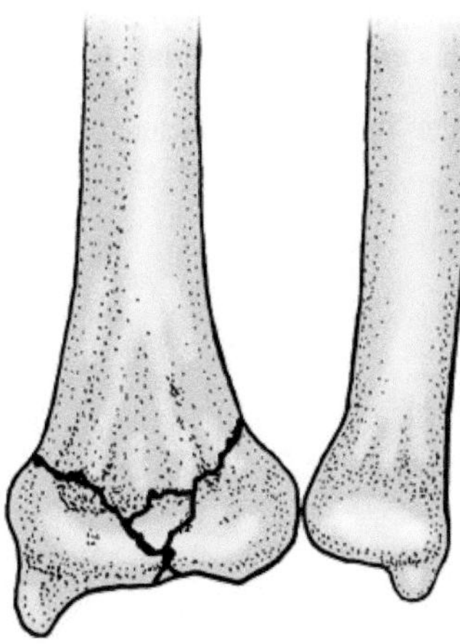

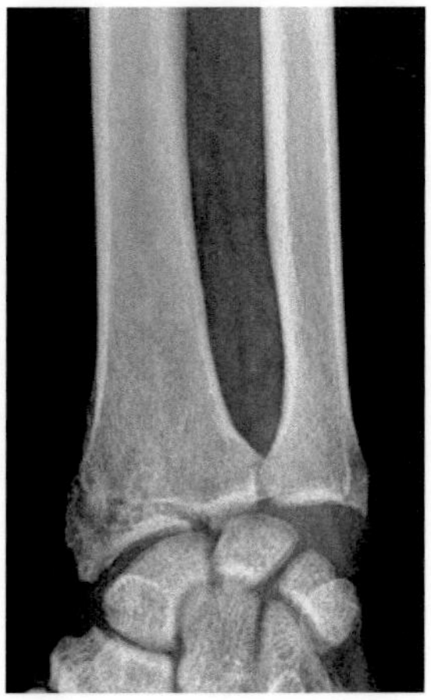

Frykman Classification of Distal Radius and ulna fractures

Type III: intra-articular involving radiocarpal joint

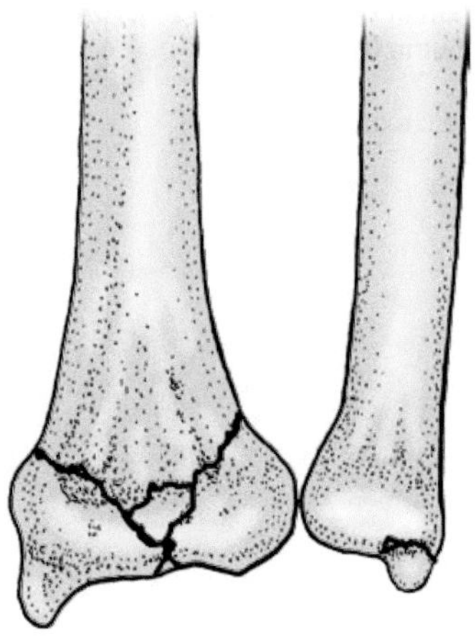

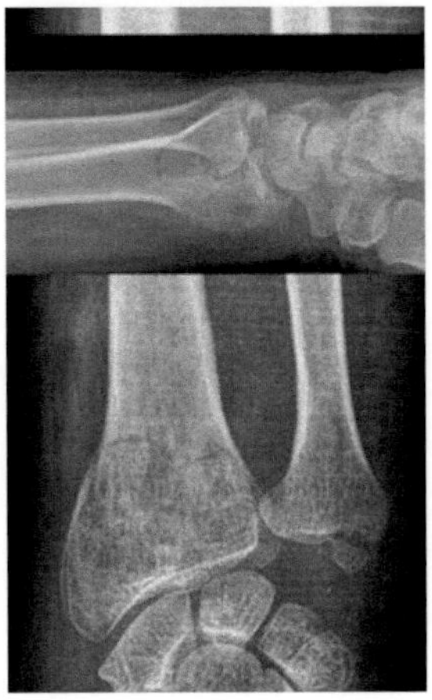

Frykman Classification of Distal Radius and ulna fractures

Type IV: Type III+ ulna fracture

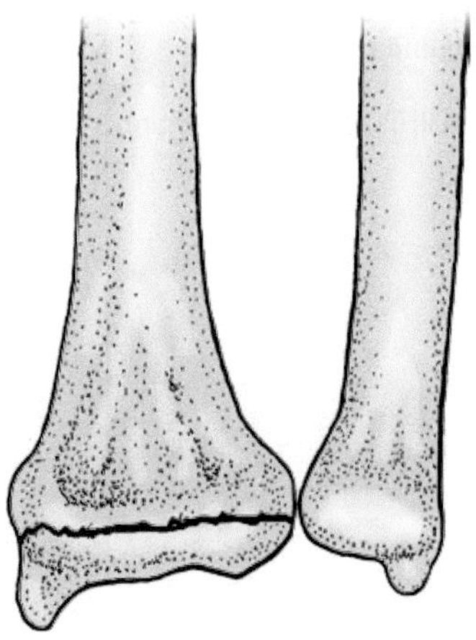

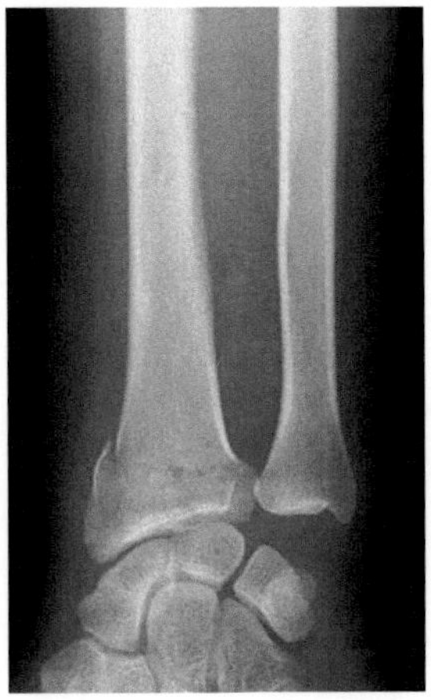

Frykman Classification of Distal Radius and ulna fractures

Type V: intra articular involving distal radioulnar joint.

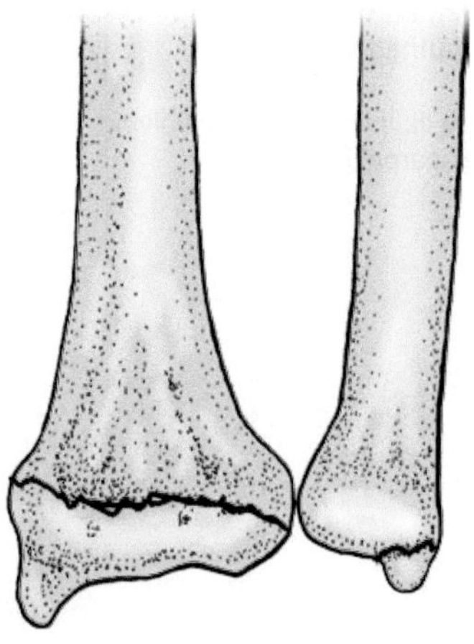

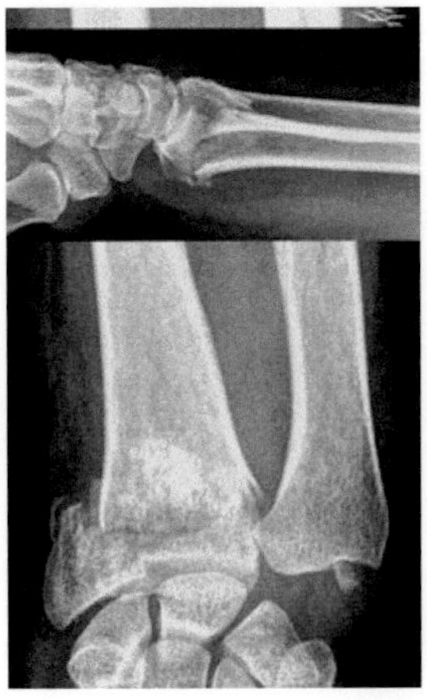

Frykman Classification of Distal Radius and ulna fractures

Type VI: Type V+ ulna fracture

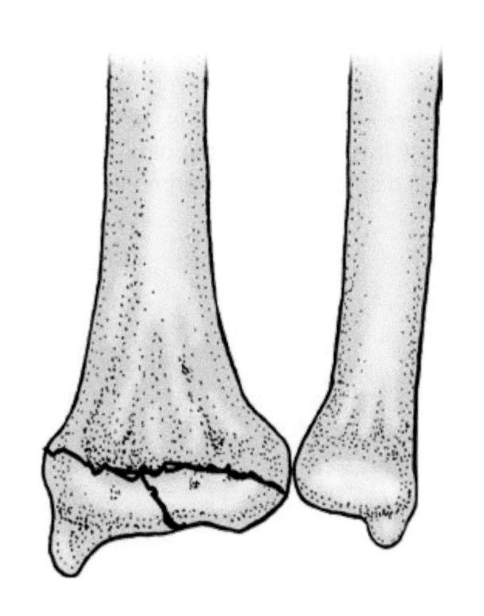

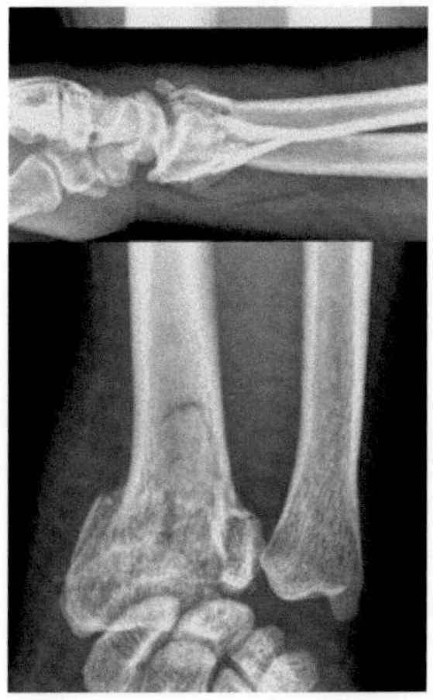

Frykman Classification of Distal Radius and ulna fractures

Type VII: intra articular involving both radiocarpal & distal radioulnar joints

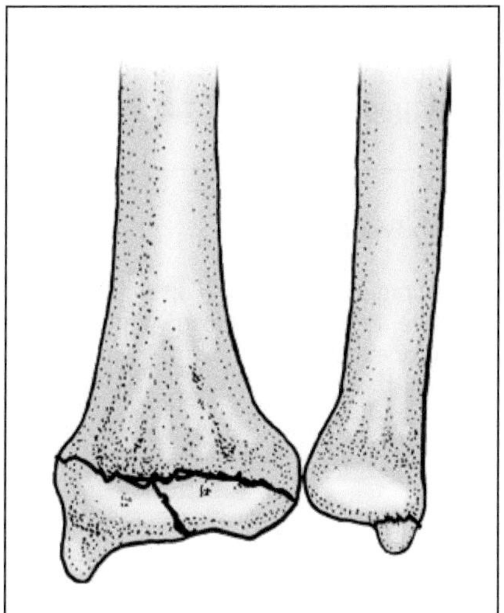

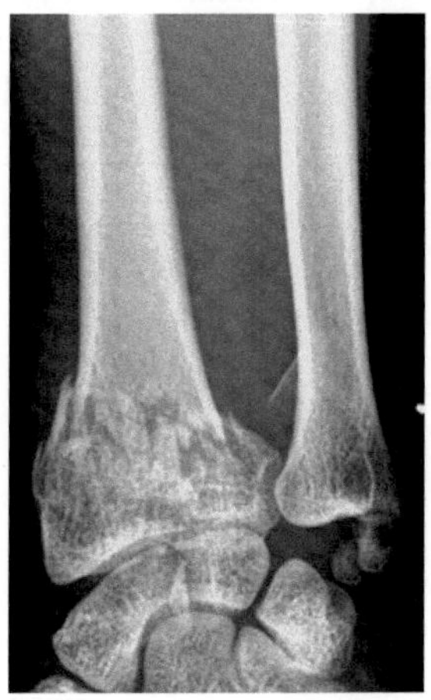

Frykman Classification of Distal Radius and ulna fractures

Type VIII: Type VII+ ulna fracture

3.3.4 Eponymic Distal Radius and Ulna Fractures

There are five commonly used classifications named after the people who first described their existence. The most commonly used fracture eponyms are Colles [35], Smith [36], and Barton [37] that correspond to extension, flexion, and intra-articular fractures, respectively. Chauffeur fracture [38] (also known as Hutchinson fractures or backfire fractures) is an intra-articular fracture of the radial styloid process. The radial styloid is within the fracture fragment, although the fragment can vary markedly in size. Rutherford or Cotton [39, 40] fractures refer to compression fractures involving central part of radius, especially the lunate facet of the distal radius articular surface.

Eponymic classifications of distal radius and ulna fractures can typically plan treatment strategies. However, the classifications do not include all fracture patterns, which may mislead diagnosis, treatments, and assessments.

3.3.4.1 Colles Fracture

A Colles fracture (also called Pouteau fracture or Pouteau-Colles fracture in French literature) is a fracture at the distal end (usually 2–3 cm) of the radius with dorsal and radial displacement [41]. It is named after Abraham Colles (1773–1843), an Irish surgeon who first described it in 1814 by simply looking at the classical deformity before the advent of X-rays.

Colles described it as a fracture that "takes place at about an inch and a half (38mm) above the carpal extremity of the radius" and "the carpus and the base of metacarpus appears to be thrown backward". Currently, the term tends to be used loosely to describe any fracture of the distal radius, with or without involvement of the ulna, with dorsal displacement of fragments [42].

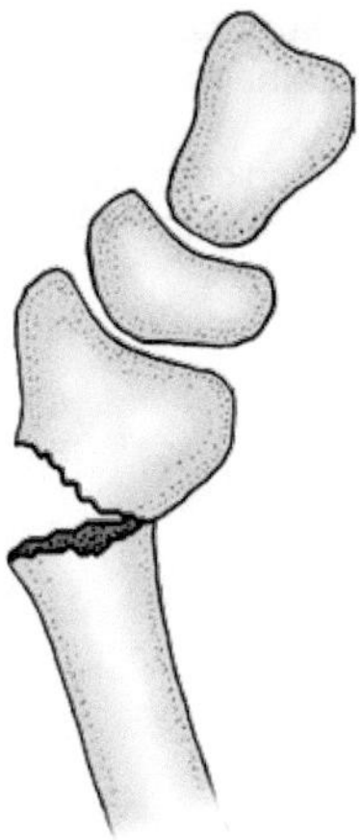

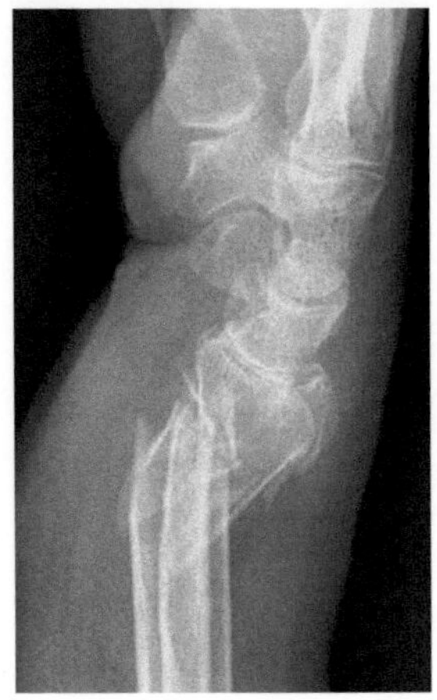

Colles Fracture

Fracture of the distal radius, with or without involvement of the ulna, with dorsal displacement of fragments.

3.3.4.2 Smith Fracture

A Smith fracture, also called reverse Colles fracture, is a fracture of the distal radius with distal fracture fragment displaced volarly. It is caused by a direct blow to the dorsal forearm or falling onto flexed wrists, as opposed to a Colles fracture which occurs as a result of falling onto wrists in extension. This fracture is named after Robert William Smith (1807–1873) [43].

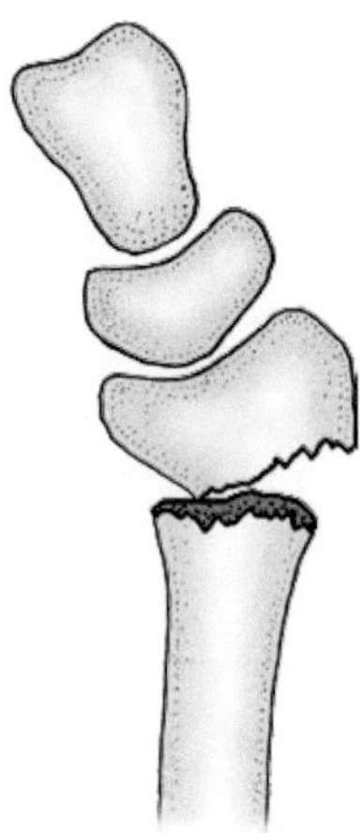

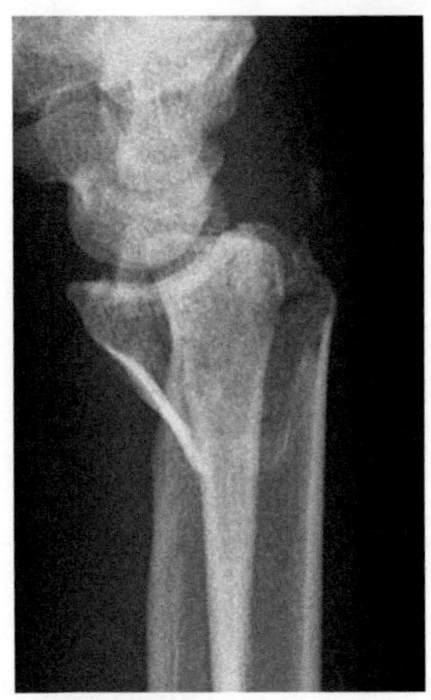

Smith Fracture

Distal radius fracture with distal fracture fragment displaced volarly, intra- or extraarticular

3.3.4.3 Barton Fracture

A Barton fracture is an intra-articular fracture of the distal radius with dislocation of the radiocarpal joint. The term is named after John Rhea Barton (1794–1871), an American surgeon who first described this in 1838 [44].

Typically, Barton fractures are classified into two types according to involvement of palmar or dorsal rim of the radius.

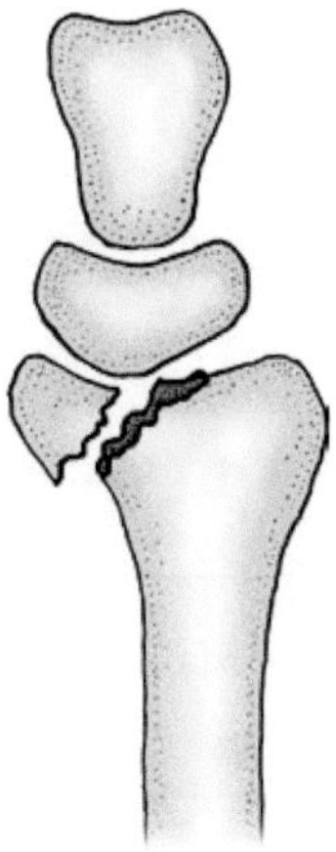

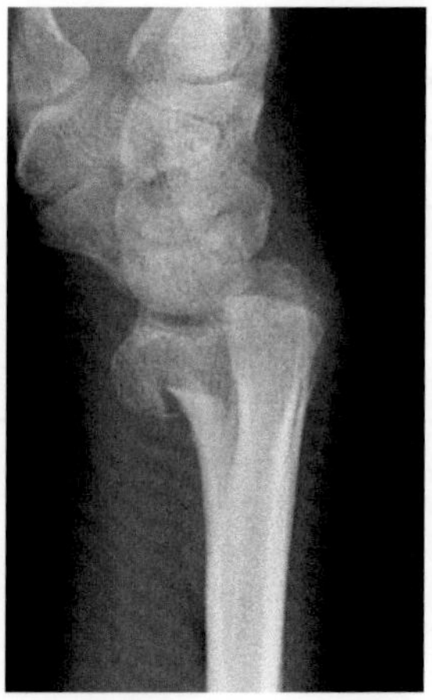

Barton Fracture

involvement of palmar rim

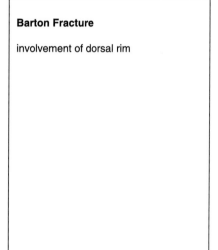

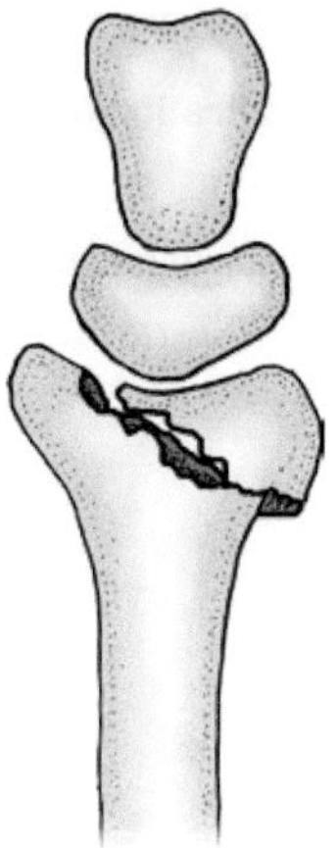

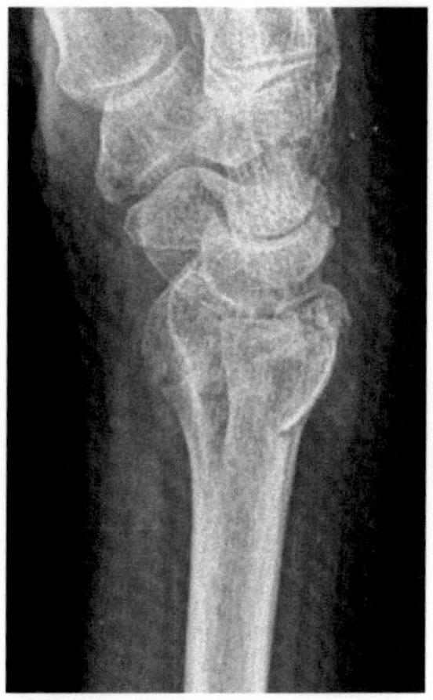

Barton Fracture

involvement of dorsal rim

3.3.4.4 Chauffeur Fracture

In 1910, Chauffeur first described radial styloid fracture with ulnar displacement of the wrist. Owing to involvement of dislocation of the carpal bones and rupture of the ligaments, prognosis is usually poor.

3.3.4.5 Rutherford Fracture or Cotton Fracture

Rutherford or Cotton [39, 40] fractures are compression fractures involving central part of radius, especially the lunate facet of the distal radius articular surface. Owing to lack of soft-tissue attachment, closed reduction of the fractures often fails.

3.3.5 Other Classifications

3.3.5.1 Thomas Classification for Smith Fractures [45]

Smith fractures are classified as Thomas classification into three types as follows:

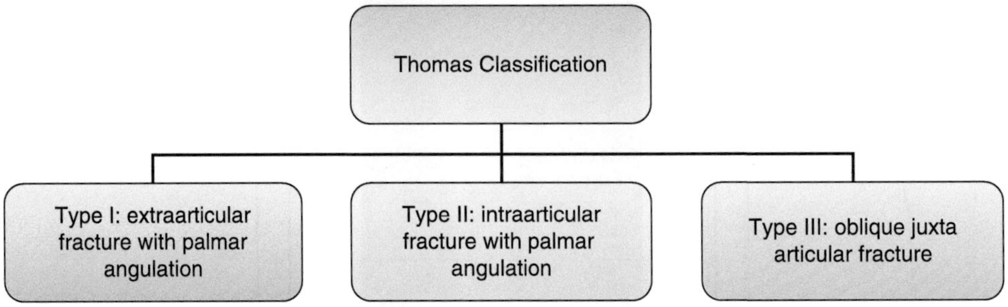

Type I: Extra-articular fracture with palmar angulation.
Type II: Intra-articular fracture with palmar angulation.
Type III: Oblique juxta-articular fracture.

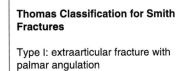

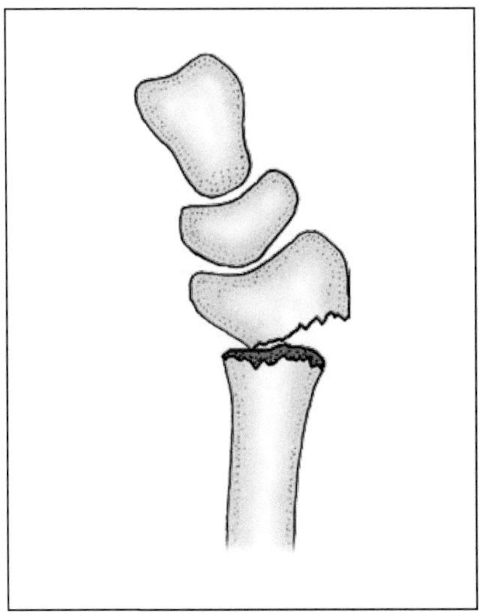

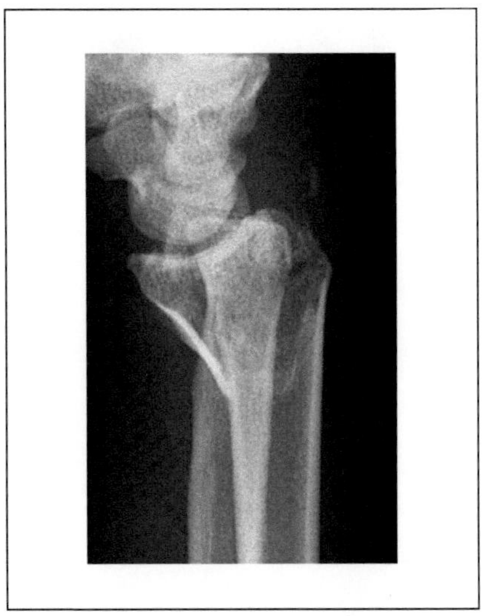

Thomas Classification for Smith Fractures

Type I: extraarticular fracture with palmar angulation

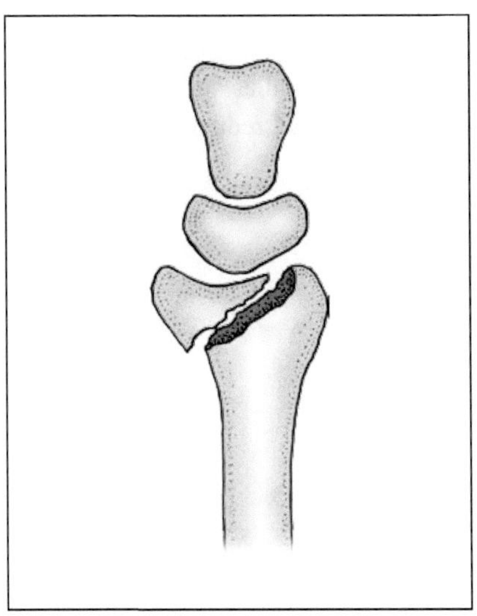

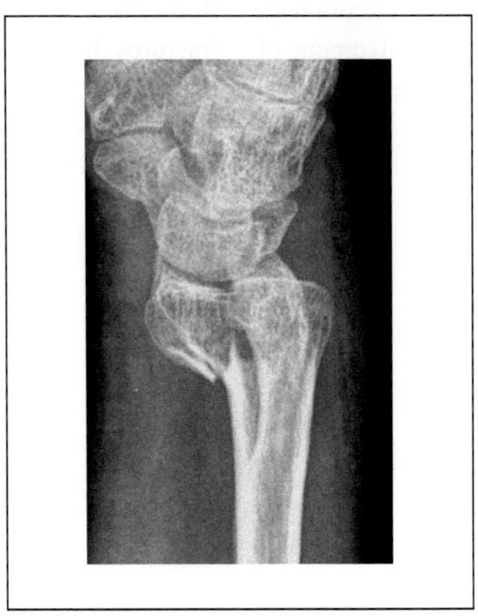

Thomas Classification for Smith Fractures

Type II: intraarticular fracture with palmar angulation

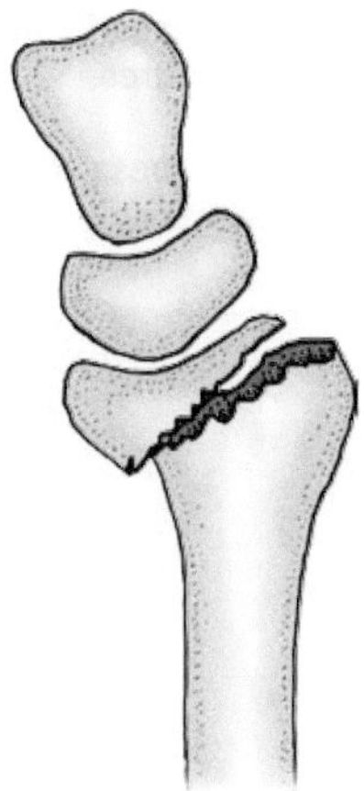

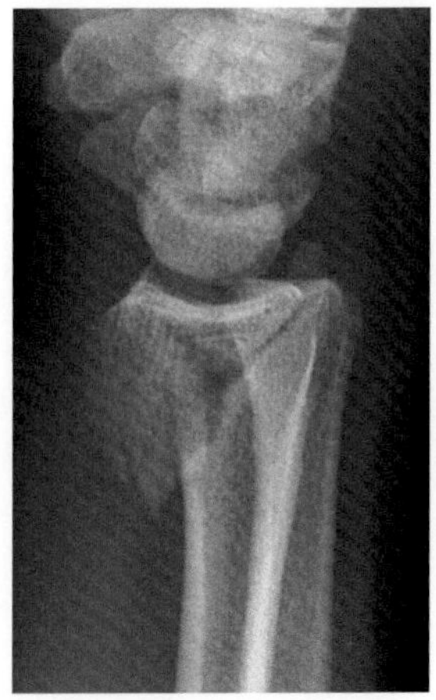

Thomas Classification for Smith Fractures

Type III: oblique juxta articular fracture

3.3.5.2 Lozano-Calderon Classification for Dorsal Barton Fractures [46]

Type I: Palmar compression: Involvement of both dorsal and palmar lips with palmar fragments compressed dorsally.

Type II: Palmar displacement and rotation: Involvement of both dorsal and palmar lip.

Type III: Central compression without involvement of palmar lip.

Type VI: Radiocarpal dislocation with involvement of dorsal lip.

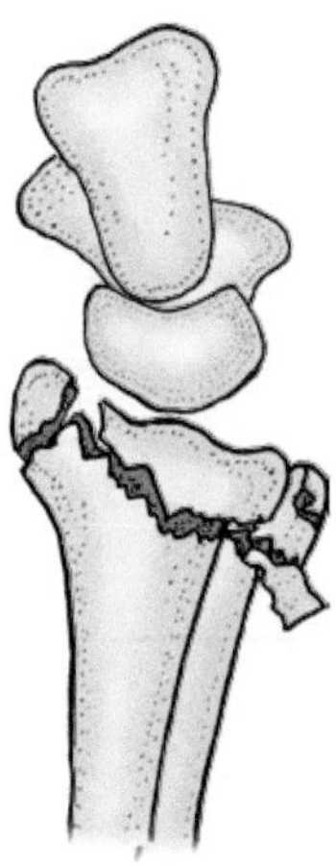

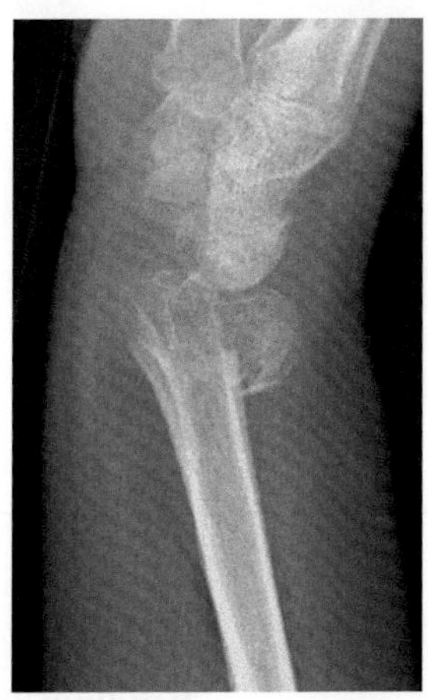

Lozano-Calderon Classification for Dorsal Barton Fractures

Type I: Palmar compression. Involvement of both dorsal and palmar lips with palmar fragments compressed dorsally

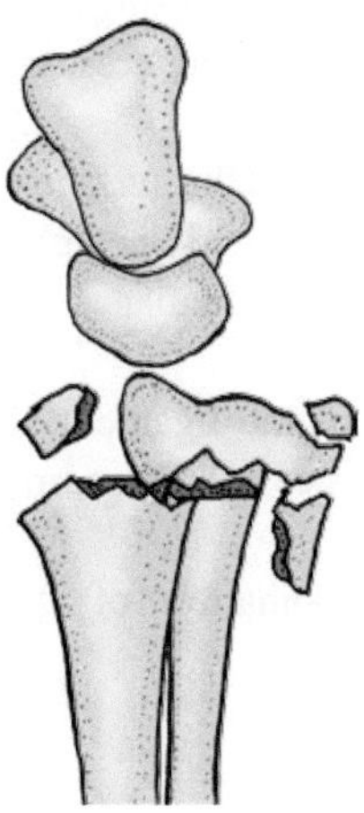

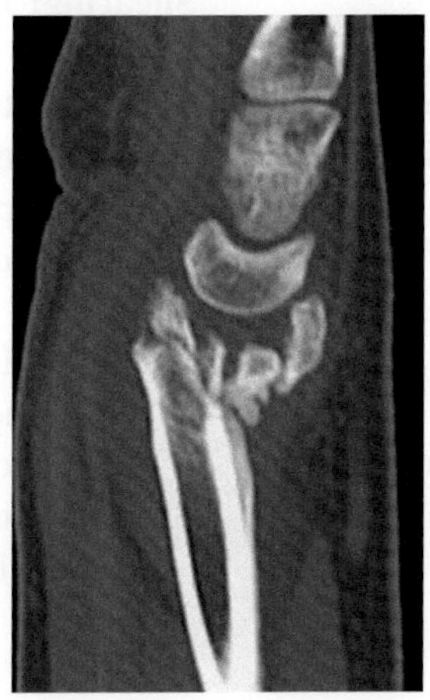

Lozano-Calderon Classification for Dorsal Barton Fractures

Type II: Palmar displaced and rotation. Involvement of both dorsal and palmar lip

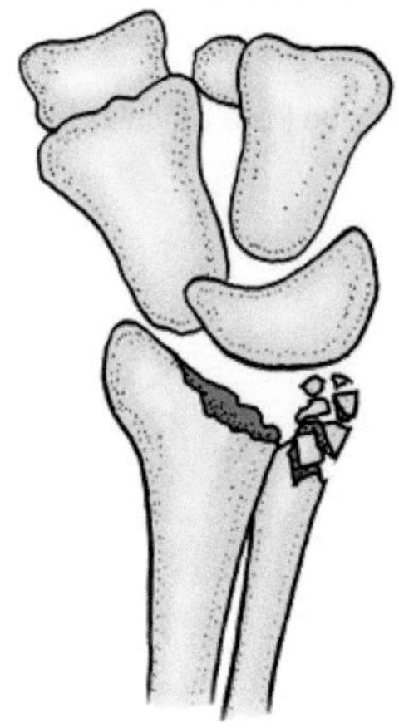

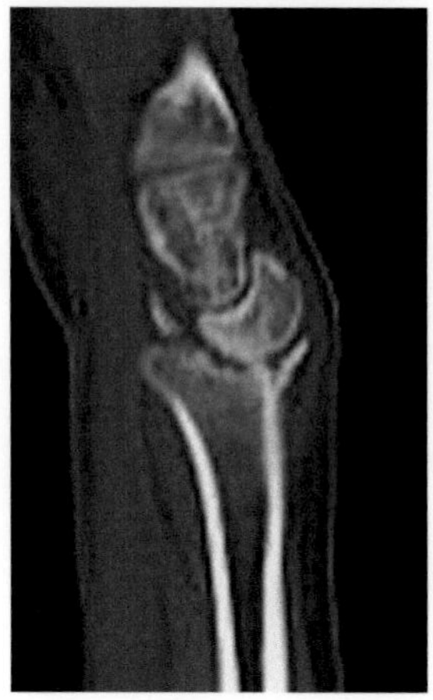

Lozano-Calderon Classification for Dorsal Barton Fractures

Type III: Central compression without involvement of palmar lip

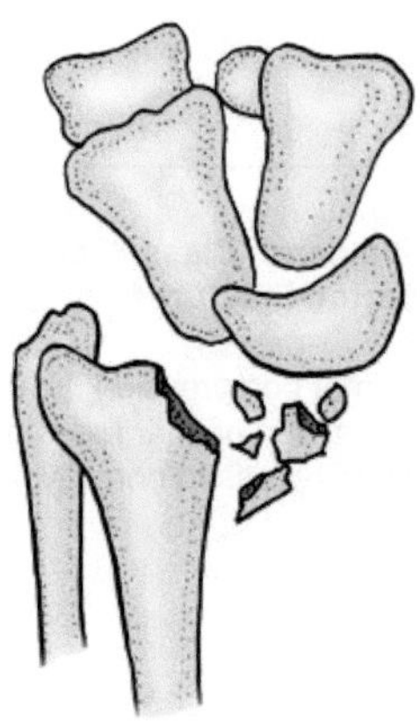

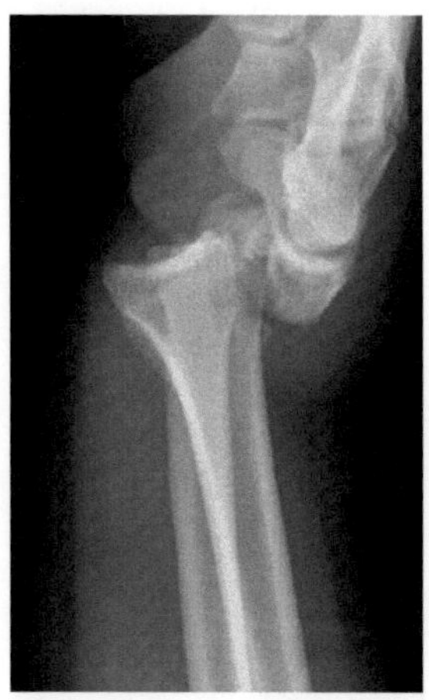

Lozano-Calderon Classification for. Dorsal Barton Fractures

Type VI: Radiocarpal dislocation with involvement of dorsal lip

3.3.5.3 Mayo Classification [47]/Missakian Classification [33]

Intra-articular fractures:

Type I: Extra-articular radiocarpal, intra-articular radioulnar.

Type II: Intra-articular scaphoid fossa of distal radius.

Type III: Intra-articular lunate fossa of distal radius +/− sigmoid fossa.

Type IV: Intra-articular, scaphoid fossa, lunate fossa, and a sigmoid fossa of the distal radius.

3.3.5.4 Fernandez Classification [48]

In 1993, Fernandez classified distal radial fractures into five types based on mechanism of injury.

Bending: Type I—One cortex of the metaphysis fails due to tensile stress (Colles and Smith fractures), and the opposite undergoes a certain degree of comminution.

Shearing: Type II—Fracture of the joint surface—Barton's, reversed Barton's, styloid process fractures, simple articular fracture.

Compression: Type III—Fracture of the surface of the joint with impaction of subchondral and metaphyseal bone (die-punch fracture), intra-articular comminuted fracture.

Avulsion: Type IV—Fracture of the ligament attachments ulnar and radial styloid process, radiocarpal fracture dislocation.

Combinations: Type V—Combination of types, high-velocity injuries.

3.3.5.5 Fernandez-Jupiter Classification [49]

Type I: Bending: Colles, Smith.

Type II: Shearing: Barton, reversed Barton's, simple articular fracture.

Type III: Compression: Intra-articular comminuted fractures, die-punch fractures.

Type IV: Avulsion: Radiocarpal fracture dislocation.

Type V: Combinations: High-energy injuries.

3.3.5.6 Gartland and Werley Classification [50]

In 1951, Gartland and Werley published a detailed evaluation and classification system based on metaphysical comminution, intra-articular extension, and displacement.

Type I: Simple Colles fracture with no involvement of the radial articular surface.

Type II: Comminuted Colles fracture with involvement of the radial articular surface.

Type III: Comminuted Colles fracture with involvement of the radial articular surface with displacement of the fragments.

Type IV: Extra-articular, non-displaced (added by Solgaard in 1985).

3.3.5.7 Older Classification [51]

Type I: Non-displaced—up to 5° dorsal angulation, radial articular surface at least 2 mm distal ulnar head,

Type II: Displaced with minimal comminution—dorsal angulation or displacement, radial articular surface no lower than 3 m proximal to the ulnar head, minimal comminution of dorsal radius.

Type III: Displaced with comminution of dorsal radius—comminution of dorsal radius; radial articular surface proximal to ulnar head; minimal comminution of distal fragment.

Type VI: Displaced with severe comminution of radial head—marked comminution of dorsal and distal radius; radial articular surface 2–8 mm proximal to ulnar head.

3.3.5.8 Jenkins Classification [52]

Type I: No radiographically visible comminution.

Type II: Comminution of the dorsal radial cortex without comminution of the fracture fragment.

Type III: Comminution of the fracture fragment without significant involvement of the dorsal cortex.

Type IV: Comminution of both the distal fragment and the dorsal cortex.

3.3.5.9 Lidstrom Classification [53]

Type I: Undisplaced.

Type IIa: Dorsal angulation, extra-articular.

Type IIb: Dorsal angulation, intra-articular but without gross separation of fragments.

Type IIc: Dorsal angulation plus dorsal displacement, extra-articular.

Type IId: Dorsal angulation plus dorsal displacement, intra-articular but without gross separation of fragments.

Type IIe: Dorsal angulation plus dorsal displacement, intra-articular with separation of fragments.

3.3.5.10 Melone Classification [54]

This classification includes the following components: shaft, radial styloid, and dorsal medial and palmar medial parts.

Type I:

- Colles frx equiv.: Undisplaced and minimally comminuted.

Type II:

- Die-punch fracture: Unstable with moderate-to-severe displacement.
- Similar to Mayo class II: Displaced fracture involving radioscaphoid joint.
- Radioscaphoid joint fracture: Involves more than radial styloid (Chauffeur fracture) fracture) and has significant dorsal angulation and radial shortening.
- Requires stabilization provided by external fixators, along with percutaneous pins, to maintain an accurate reduction.

Type IIb (irreducible):

- This is a double die-punch fracture which is an irreducible injury.
- Dorsal medial component fragmentation.
- Persistent radiocarpal incongruity greater than 2 mm.
- Radial shortening >3–5 mm.
- Dorsal tilting and displacement > of 10°.
- Radiocarpal step off >5 mm (on a lateral view).
- Requires open treatment for restoration of articular congruity.
- Requires ORIF of radiocarpal articular surface, supplementary external fixation, and iliac bone grafting.

Type III:

- Is die-punch or lunate load fracture, and is often irreducible by traction alone.
- Involves additional fracture from shaft of radius that projects into flexor compartment.
- Mayo equivalent: Are displaced involving the radiolunate joint.
- This may require fixation w/ small screws or wires in conjunction with closed or limited open articular surgery.

Type IV:

- Transverse split of articular surfaces w/ rotational displacement.
- Mayo equivalent is a displaced fracture involving both radioscaphoid and lunate joints, and the sigmoid fossa of the distal radius.
- Is often a more comminuted fracture involving all of major joint articular surfaces, and almost always includes fracture component into distal radioulnar joint.

3.3.5.11 Nissen-Lie Classification [55]

Type I: A fracture at the junction of the shaft and distal extremity of the radius, i.e., somewhat more proximal than the most common fractures. Frequently it is associated with a fracture of the ulna. This type occurs only in children aged 1–15 years and is often of the green-stick type.

Type II: Slipping of the epiphysis with dorsal displacement, often with a dorsally avulsed triangular fragment of the radius. Occurs in the age range 10–20 years.

Type III: Fracture through the distal end of the radius with negligible displacement. The fracture line runs transversely through the radius, about 1 cm proximal to the articular surface and is often visible only as an irregularity on the dorsal aspect. Occurs in adults of all ages.

Type IV: The typical radial fracture with dorsal and radial displacement. Frequently this fracture is comminuted with small fragments dorsally.

Type V: The typical radial fracture with splintering of the distal fragment. This fracture is always intra-articular, T- or Y-shaped. Common in elderly and aged persons.

Type VI: Isolated fracture through the styloid process of the radius. Very rarely displaced. Seen most commonly in men aged 20–50.

Type VII: All fractures with volar displacement, i.e., Smith's fracture, as well as epiphysiolysis with volar displacement.

3.3.5.12 McMurtry Classification [56]

Nissen-Lie classified the displacement of the fractures by measuring the angle made by the distal articular surface of the radius in relation to the longitudinal axis, partly in the lateral view.

Type I: Two parts: The opposite portion of the radiocarpal joint remains intact dorsal Barton, palmar Barton, Chauffeur, die punch.

Type II: Three parts: The lunate and scaphoid facets separate from each other and the proximal portion of the radius.

Type III: Four parts: The same plus lunate facet fractured in dorsal and volar fragment.

Type IV: Five parts or more.

3.3.5.13 Castaing Classification [57]

Type I: Compression—extension (posterior displacement) (Pouteau, Colles with posteromedial fragment complex, (a) sagittal T, (b) with medial component, (c) with lateral component, (d) posterolateral rim isolated or complex, (e) frontal T, (f) cross lines in two planes, (g) comminuted, (h) undisplaced).

Type II: Compression—flexion (Goyrand-Smith, anterior rim isolated or anterolateral, complex anterior rim).

Type III: Associated osteoarticular injuries (ulnar styloid, ulnar head, ulnar neck, radioulnar dislocation, radioulnar diastasis, carpal injuries, other injuries of the upper limb, open fracture, and bilateral).

Type IV: Non-classified.

3.3.5.14 Jakim Classification [58]

Type	Distal segment	Articular components
1	Undisplaced	Undisplaced
2	Displaced	Undisplaced
3	Displaced	≤2 mm displacement
4	Displaced	>2 mm displacement and/or rotation
5	Gross comminution, extending into the metaphysis, with severe soft-tissue damage	

3.3.5.15 Doi Classification [59]

On the basis of 3D CT scanning, Doi classified intra-articular distal radius fractures into 2, 3, and 4 part types, according to the number of main fracture fragments involved in the joint surface. This classification benefits for arthroscopic surgery:

Two-part fractures: (a) vertical line; (b) horizontal line; (c) dorsal line.

Three-part fractures.

Four-part fractures.

3.3.5.16 Saito Classification [60] (1989)

Type I: Chauffeur fracture.

Type II: Medial wedge.

Type III: Dorsal Barton.

Type IV: Palmar Barton.

Type V: Comminuted Colles.

Type VI: Comminuted Smith.

Type VII: Dorsal Barton and Chauffeur fracture.

Type VII: Palmar Barton and Chauffeur fracture.

Type I–IV: Simple intra-articular fractures.

Type V–VII: Comminuted intra-articular fractures.

3.3.5.17 Mathoulin-Lestrsne-Saffar Classification [60]

Type I: One articular line in the coronal plane—Barton, reverse Barton's.

Type II: One articular line in the sagittal plane involving (a) scaphoid facet, (b) lunate facet, (c) radioulnar joint.

Type III: Two lines associated: (a) one extra-articular horizontal, (b) one intra-articular = type 2a, b ± other fragments or dorsal comminution (T-fractures, die punch).

Type IV: Three lines associated: (a) one extra-articular horizontal, (b) two articular, one coronal, one sagittal (posteromedial fragments, T-frontal, and sagittal).

References

1. Speed K. Traumatic lesions of the head of the radius: relation to elbow joint dysfunction. Surg Clin North Am. 1924;4:651–6.
2. Giannicola G, Scacchi M, Sacchetti FM, Cinotti G. Clinical usefulness of proximal ulnar and radius fracture-dislocation comprehensive classification system (PURCCS): prospective study of 39 cases. J Shoulder Elbow Surg. 2013;22:1729–36.
3. Newey ML, Ricketts D, Roberts L. The AO classification of long bone fractures: an early study of its use in clinical practice. Injury. 1993;24:309–12.
4. van Riet RP, Morrey BF, O'Driscoll SW, van Glabbeek F. Associated injuries complicating radial head fractures: a demographic study. Clin Orthop Relat Res. 2005;441:351–5.
5. Morgan SJ, Itamura JM, Shankwiller J, Brien WW, Kuschner SH. Reliability evaluation of classifying radial head fractures by the system of Mason. Bull Hosp Jt Dis. 1997;56(2):95–8.
6. Sheps DM, Kiefer KR, Boorman RS, Donaghy J, Lalani A, Walker R, Hildebrand KA. The interobserver reliability of classification systems for radial head fractures: the Hotchkiss modification of the Mason classification and the AO classification systems. Can J Surg. 2009;52:277–82.
7. Morrey BF. Instructional course lecture. Current concepts in the treatment of fractures of the radial head, the olecranon and the coronoid. J Bone Joint Surg Am. 1995;77:316–27.
8. Veillette CJ, Steinmann SP. Olecranon fractures. Orthop Clin North Am. 2008;39:229–36.
9. Colton CL. Fractures of the olecranon in adults: classification and management. Injury. 1973;5:121–9.
10. Schatzker J. Olecranon fractures. In: Schatzker J, Tile M, editors. The rational basis of operative fracture care. New York: Springer; 1987. p. 31–48.
11. Horne JG, Tanzer TL. Olecranon fractures: a review of 100 cases. J Trauma. 1981;21:469–72.
12. Wadsworth TG. Screw fixation of the olecranon after fracture or osteotomy. Clin Orthop Relat Res. 1976;119:197–201.
13. Regan W, Morrey B. Fractures of the coronoid process of the ulna. J Bone Joint Surg Am. 1989;71:1348–54.
14. Wang Y, Liu P, Zhou Z. Classification and treatments of coronoid fractures. Chinese. J Orthop. 2006;26:361–5.
15. Johnston GW. A follow-up of one hundred cases of fracture of the head of the radius with a review of the literature. Ulster Med J. 1962;31:51–6.
16. Hotchkiss RN. Displaced fractures of the radial head: internal fixation or excision? J Am Acad Orthop Surg. 1997;5:1–10.
17. Mason ML. Some observations on fractures of the head of the radius with a review of one hundred cases. Br J Surg. 1954;42:123–32.
18. Bakalim G. Fractures of the radial head and their treatment. Acta Orthop Scand. 1970;41:320–31.
19. Hotchkiss RN. Fractures and dislocations of the elbow. In: Rockwood Jr CA, Green DP, Bucholz RW, Heckman JD, editors. Rockwood and Green's fractures in adults, vol. 1. 4th ed. Philadelphia, PA: Lippincott-Raven; 1996. p. 929–1024.
20. van Riet RP, Morrey BF. Documentation of associated injuries occurring with radial head fracture. Clin Orthop Relat Res. 2008;466:130–4.
21. van Vugt AB. Surgical treatment of fractures of the proximal end of the radius in childhood. Arch Orthop Trauma Surg. 1985;104:37–41.
22. Müller ME, Nazarian S, Koch P. Classification AO des fractures. Tome I. Les os longs. 1st ed. Berlin: Springer; 1987.
23. Müller ME, Nazarian S, Koch P, et al. The comprehensive classification of fractures of long bones. 1st ed. Berlin/Heidelberg/New York: Springer; 1990.
24. Journal of Orthopaedic Trauma. 2007; 21 supplement. http://ota.org/media/23048/97042.1TOC-i-iv.pdf.
25. Müller ME, Nazarian S, Koch P. Classification AO des fractures. Tome I. Les os longs. Springer: Berlin; 1987.
26. JL M, Slongo TF, Agel J, Broderick JS, Creevey W, DeCoster TA, Prokuski L, Sirkin MS, Ziran B, Henley B, Audigé L. Fracture and dislocation classification compendium - 2007: orthopaedic trauma association classification, database and outcomes committee. J Orthop Trauma. 2007;21(10 Suppl):S1–133.
27. Bado JL. The Monteggia lesion. Clin Orthop Relat Res. 1967;50:71–86.
28. Galeazzi R. Über ein besonderes Syndrom bei Verletzungen im Bereich der Unterarmknochen. Arch Orthop Unfallchir. 1934;35:557–62.
29. Mikic ZD. Galeazzi fracture-dislocations. J Bone Joint Surg Am. 1975;57:1071–80.
30. Maculé Beneyto F, Arandes Renú JM, Ferreres Claramunt A, Ramón Soler R. Treatment of Galeazzi fracture dislocations. J Trauma. 1994;36:352–5.
31. Galeazzi R. Concerning a particular syndrome of injury of the forearm. Bones Arch orthop Unfall; 1934.
32. Rettig ME, Raskin KB. Galeazzi fracture-dislocation: a new treatment oriented classification. J Hand Surg Am. 2001;26:228–35.
33. Cooney WP. Fractures of the distal radius. A modern treatment-based classification. Orthop Clin North Am. 1993;24:211–6.
34. Frykman GK. Fracture of the distal radius including sequelae: shoulder hand finger syndrome; disturbance in the distal radioulnar joint and impairment of nerve function: a clinical and experimental study. Acta Orthop Scand Suppl. 1967;108:1–155.
35. Macdonald JA. On Colles' fracture of the radius, and its treatment. Br Med J. 1873;1:223–4.
36. Peltier LF. Eponymic fractures: Robert William Smith and Smith's fracture. Surgery. 1959;45:1035–42.
37. Peltier LF. Eponymic fractures: John Rhea Barton and Barton's fractures. Surgery. 1953;34:960–70.
38. Lund FB. Fractures of the radius in starting automobiles. Boston Med Surg J. 1904;151:481–3.
39. Cotton FJ. VIII. The pathology of fracture of the lower extremity of the radius. Ann Surg. 1900;32:388–415.
40. Cotton FJ. III. The pathology of fracture of the lower extremity of the radius. Ann Surg. 1900;32:194–218.
41. Louis S, David W, Selvadurai N. Apley's system of orthopaedics and fractures. 9th ed. London: Hodder Education; 2010. p. 772.
42. Colles A. On the fracture of the carpal extremity of the radius. Edinb Med Surg J. 1814;10:181. Clin Orthop Relat Res. 2006;445:5–7.
43. Stead LG, Stead SM, Kaufman MS. First aid: emergency medicine. 2nd ed. New York, NY: McGraw-Hill; 2006. p. 395–6.
44. Barton JR. Views and treatment of an important injury of the wrist. Med Exam. 1838;1:365–8.
45. Thomas FB. Reduction of Smith's fracture. J Bone Joint Surg Br. 1957;39:463–70.
46. Lozano-Calderón SA, Doornberg J, Ring D. Fractures of the dorsal articular margin of the distal part of the radius with dorsal radiocarpal subluxation. J Bone Joint Surg Am. 2006;88:1486–93.
47. Missakian ML, Cooney WP, Amadio PC, Glidewell HL. Open reduction and internal fixation for distal radius fractures. J Hand Surg Am. 1992;17:745–55.
48. Fernández DL. Fractures of the distal radius: operative treatment. Instr Course Lect. 1993;42:73–88.

49. Jupiter JB, Fernandez DL. Comparative classification for fractures of the distal end of the radius. J Hand Surg Am. 1997;22:563–71.
50. Gartland JJ, Werley CW. Evaluation of healed Colles' fractures. J Bone Joint Surg Am. 1951;33:895–907.
51. Older TM, Stabler EV, Cassebaum WH. Colles fracture: evaluation and selection of therapy. J Trauma. 1965;5:469–76.
52. Jenkins NH. The unstable Colles' fracture. J Hand Surg Br. 1989;14:149–54.
53. Lidstrom A. Fractures of the distal end of the radius. A clinical and statistical study of end results. Acta Orthop Scand Suppl. 1959;41:1–118.
54. Melone CP Jr. Articular fractures of the distal radius. Orthop Clin North Am. 1984;15:217–36.
55. Nissen-Lie HS. Fracturea Radii "Typica". Nord Med. 1939;1:293–303.
56. McMurtry RY, Jupiter JB. Fractures of the distal radius. In: Browner BD, Jupiter JB, Levine AM, Trafton PG, editors. Skeletal trauma. Philadelphia, PA: W.B. Saunders; 1992. p. 1063–94.
57. Castaing J. Recent fractures of the lower extremity of the radius in adults. Rev Chir Orthop Reparatrice Appar Mot. 1964;50:581–696.
58. Jakim I, Pieterse HS, Sweet MB. External fixation for intra-articular fractures of the distal radius. J Bone Joint Surg Br. 1991;73:302–6.
59. Doi K, Hattori Y, Otsuka K, Abe Y, Yamamoto H. Intra-articular fractures of the distal aspect of the radius: arthroscopically assisted reduction compared with open reduction and internal fixation. J Bone Joint Surg Am. 1999;81:1093–110.
60. Saito H, Shibata M. Classification of fracture at the distal end of the radius with reference to treatment of comminuted fractures. In: Boswick JA, editor. Current concepts in hand surgery. Philadelphia, PA: Lea & Febiger; 1983. p. 129–45.

Classifications of Hand and Wrist Fractures

4

Yingze Zhang and Xin Xing

4.1 Section 1 Classifications of Hand Bone Fractures

Over ten classifications have been reported, and majority of fractures are classified according to location of the fractures.

4.1.1 Classification of Fractures of Hand Bones

4.1.1.1 Classification Based on Fracture Configuration

Usually descriptive types.

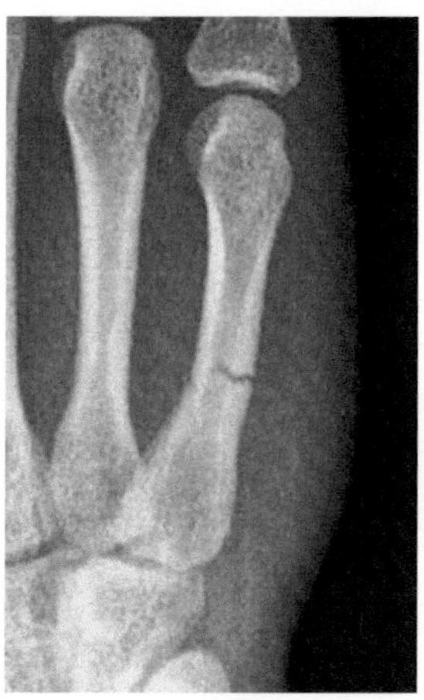

Transverse

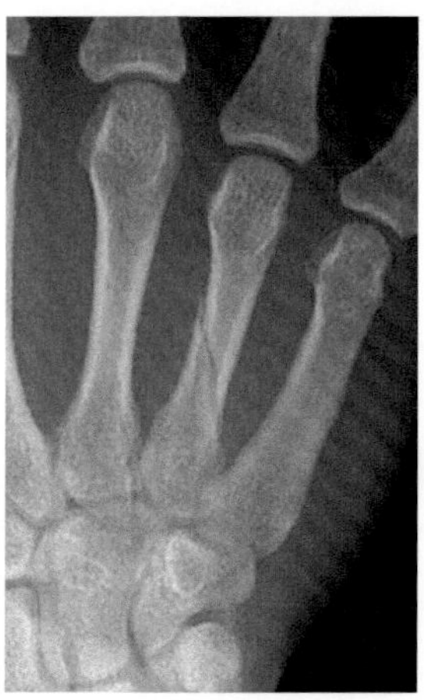

Oblique

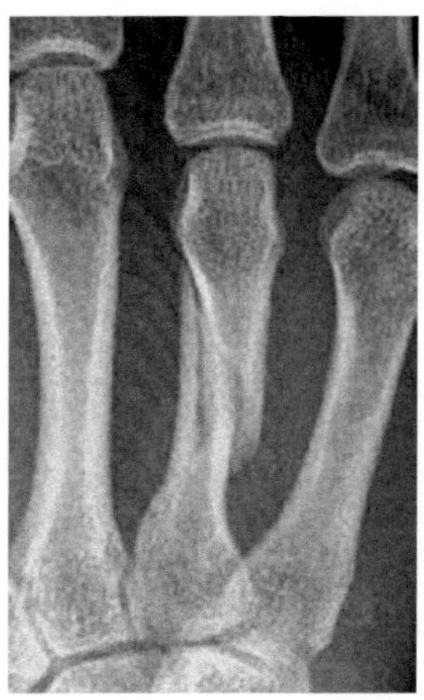

Spiral

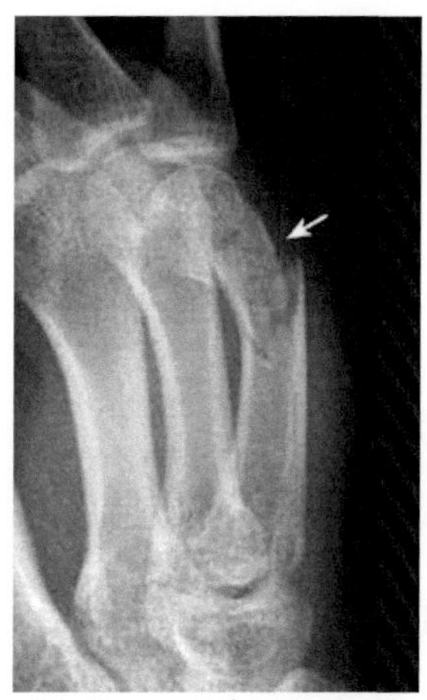

Displacement/angulation/ shortening

Y. Zhang (✉) • X. Xing
Department of Orthopedics,
The Third Hospital of Hebei Medical University,
Shijiazhuang, China
e-mail: yzzhangdr@126.com, yzling_liu@163.com

Y. Zhang (ed.), *Clinical Classification in Orthopaedics Trauma*, https://doi.org/10.1007/978-981-10-6044-1_4

4.1.1.2 Classification Based on Location of Fracture

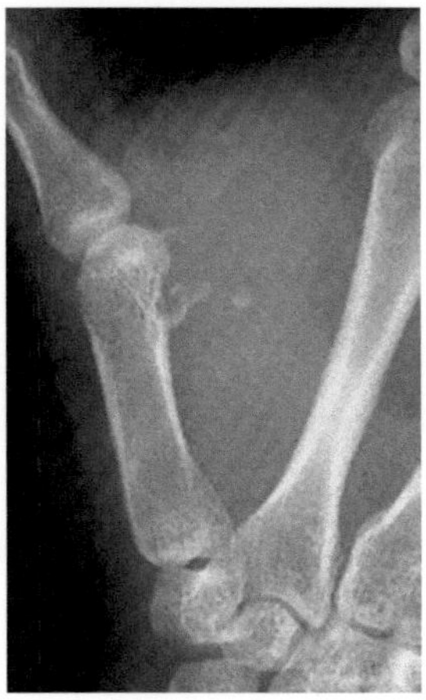

Head fracture

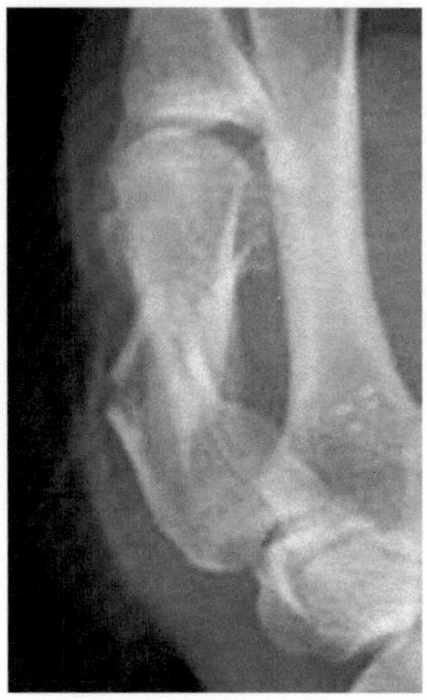

Shaft fracture

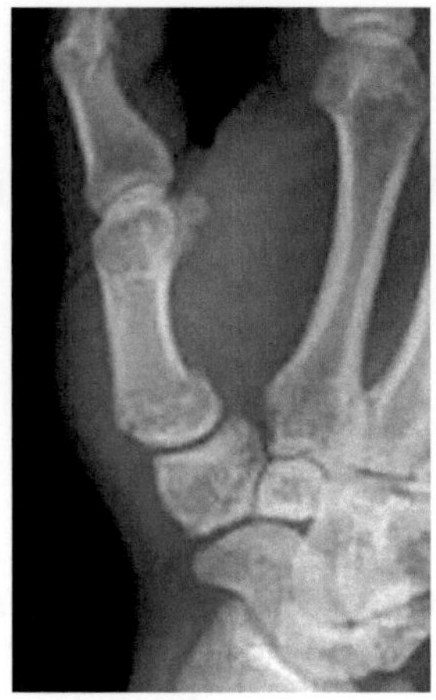

Basal fracture

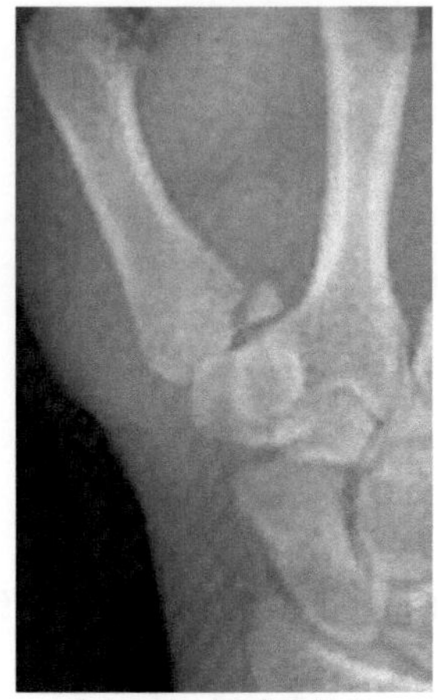

Intaarticular fracture (Bennett)

4.1.1.3 Green Classification of Thumb Metacarpal [1]

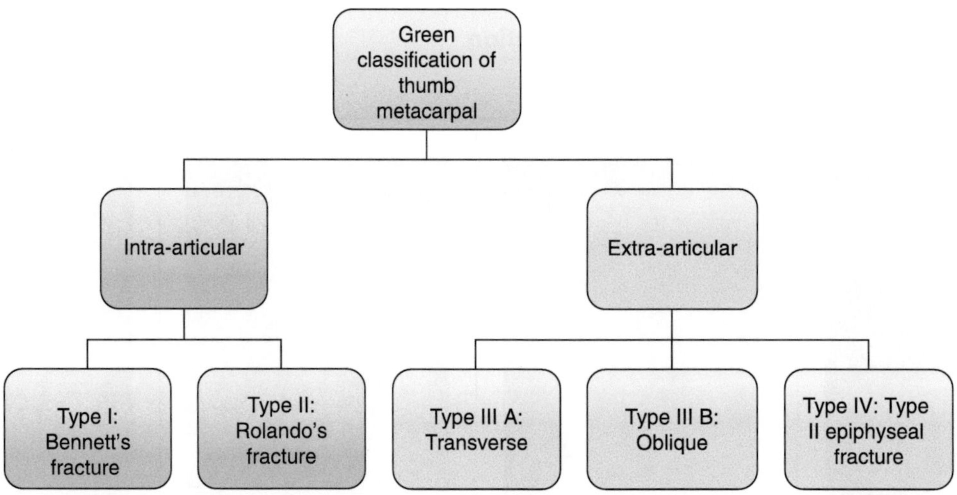

Also named Green and O'Brien classification.

Type I: Bennett's fracture.
Type II: Rolando's fracture.
Type IIIA: Transverse extra-articular.
Type IIIB: Oblique extra-articular.
Type IV: Type II epiphyseal fracture (paediatric).

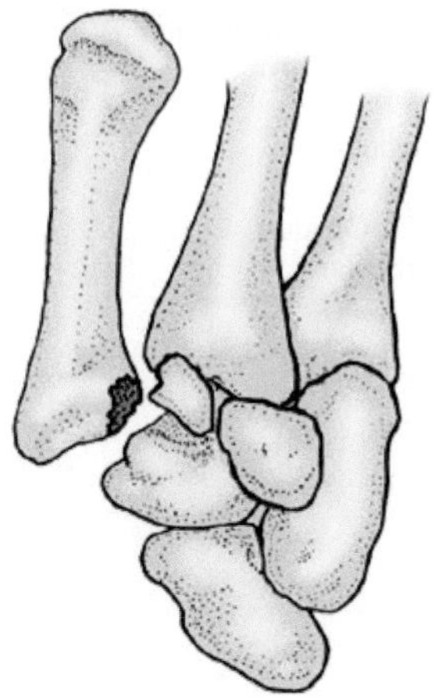

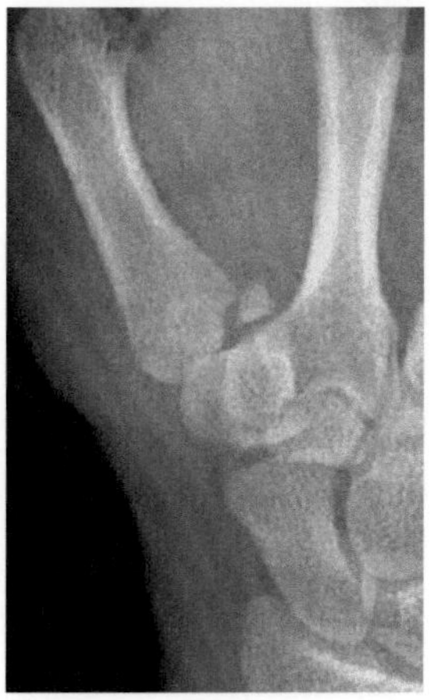

Green Classification of Thumb Metacarpal

Intraarticular.

Type I: Bennett's fracture

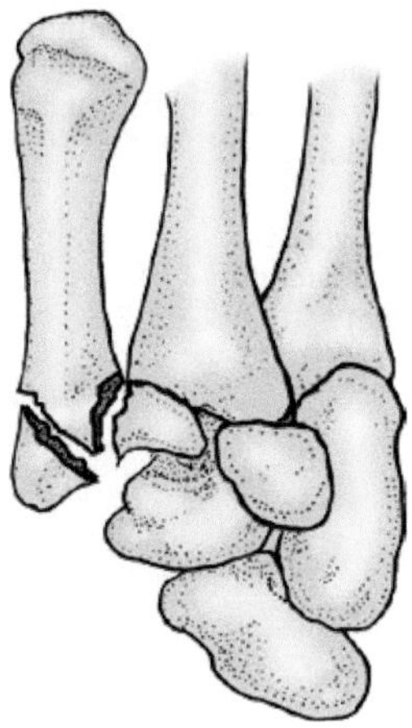

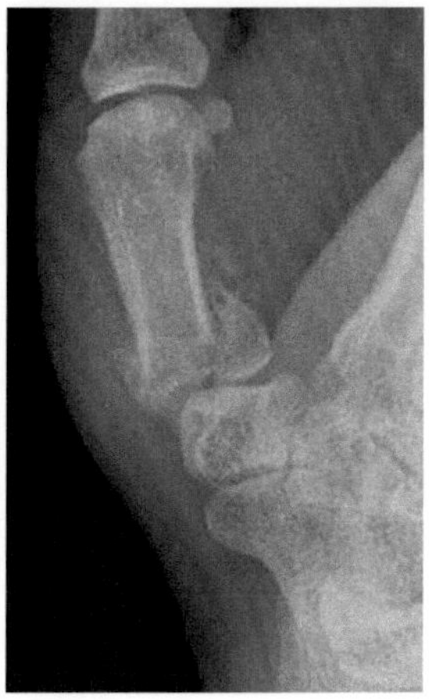

Green Classification of Thumb Metacarpal

Intraarticular.

Type II: Rolando's fracture

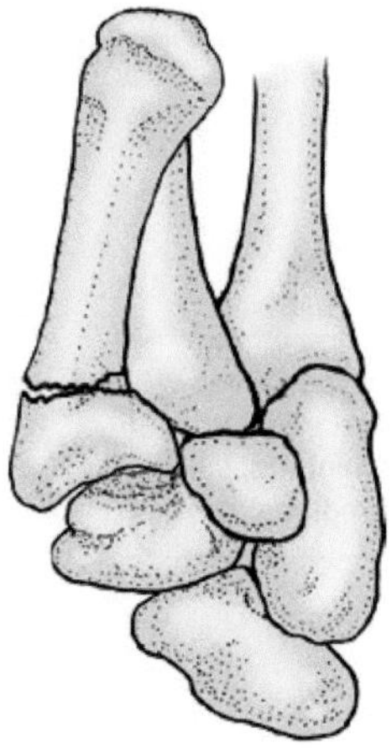

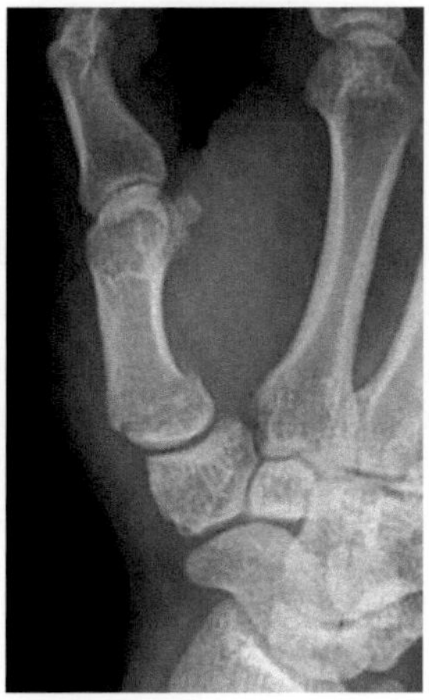

Green Classification of Thumb Metacarpal

Extraarticular.

Type IIIA: Transverse extra-articular

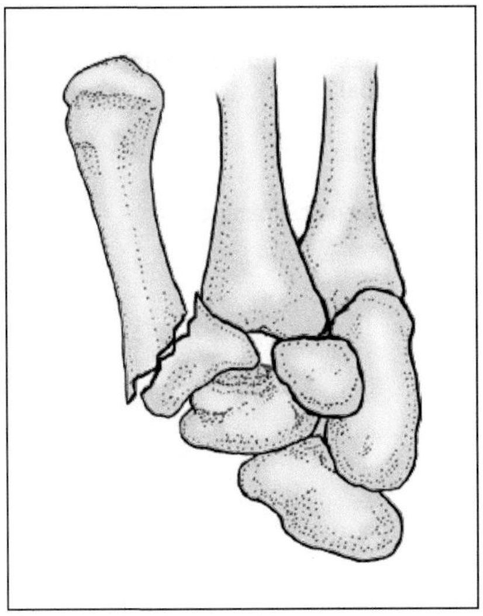

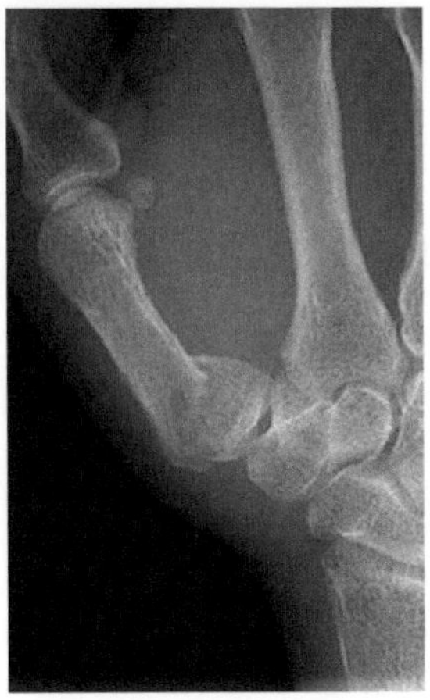

Green Classification of Thumb Metacarpal

Extraarticular.

Type IIIB: Oblique extra-articular

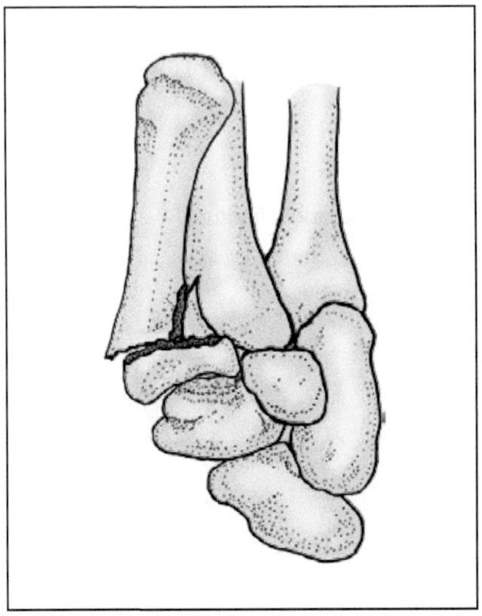

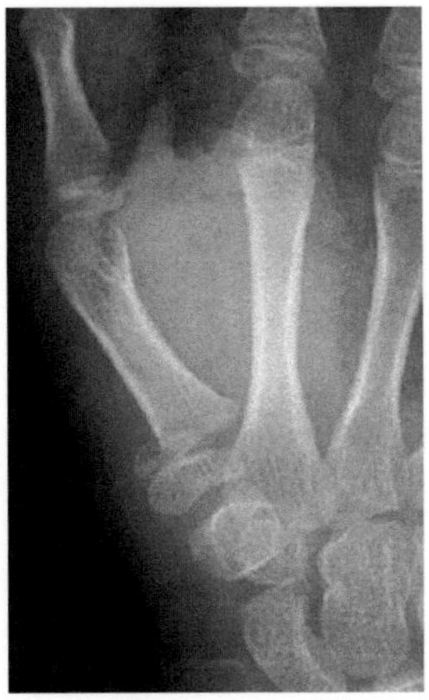

Green Classification of Thumb Metacarpal

Extraarticular.

Type IV : Type II epiphyseal fracture (paediatric)

4.1.1.4 Classification of the Fifth Metacarpal Base Fracture [2]

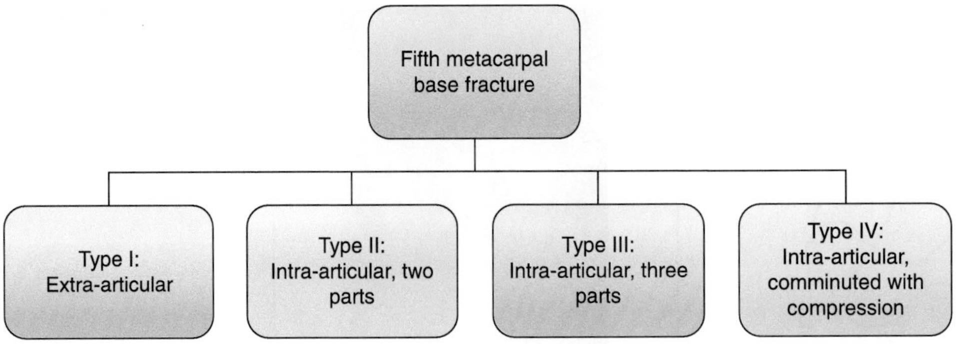

Type I: Extra-articular.
Type II: Intra-articular, two parts.
Type III: Intra-articular, three parts.
Type IV: Intra-articular, comminuted with compression.

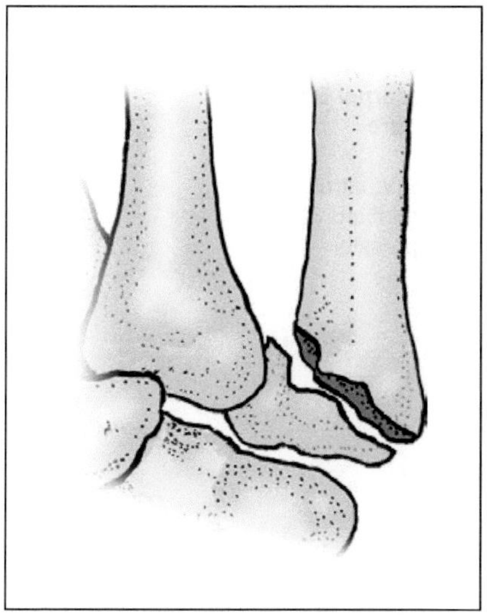

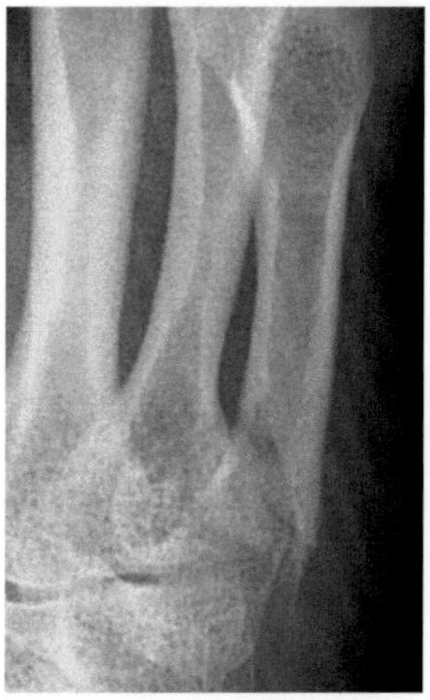

Classification of Fifth Metacarpal Base Fracture

Type I: extraarticular

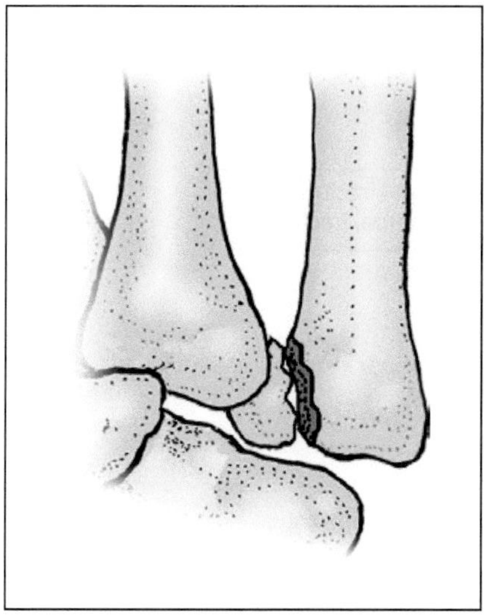

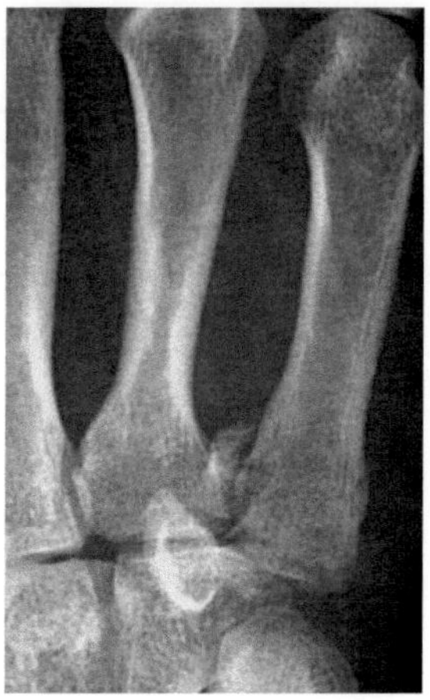

Classification of Fifth Metacarpal Base Fracture

Type II: intraarticular, two parts

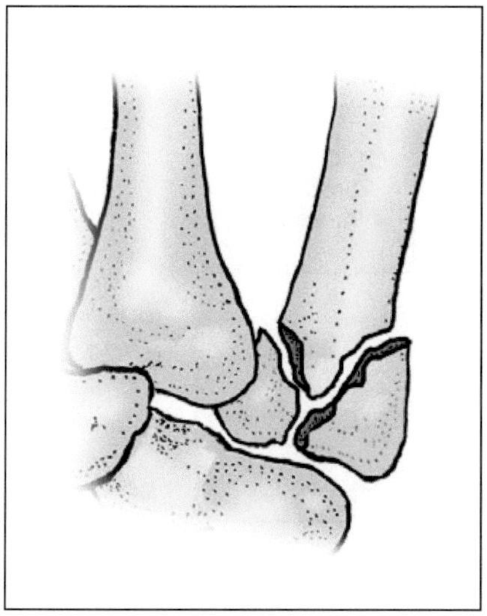

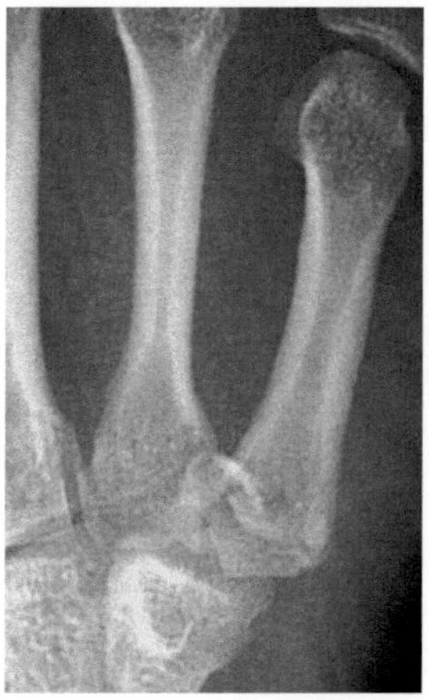

Classification of Fifth Metacarpal Base Fracture

Type III: intraarticular, three parts

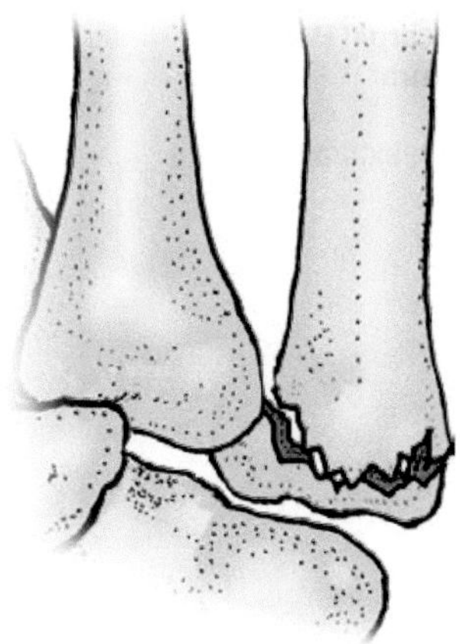

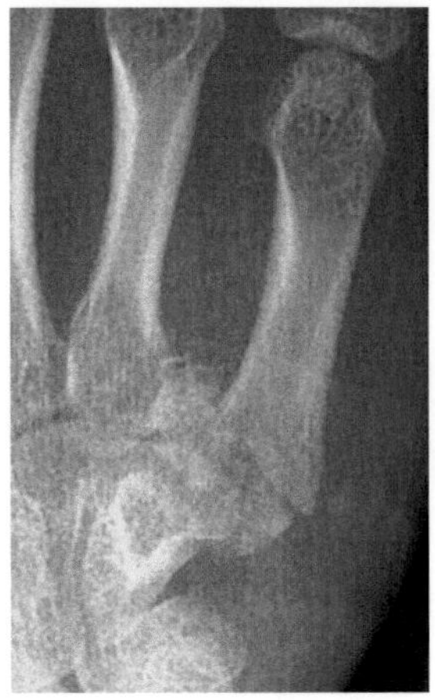

Classification of Fifth Metacarpal Base Fracture

Type IV: intraarticular, comminuted with compression

4.1.1.5 AO/OTA Classification of Metacarpal Fractures

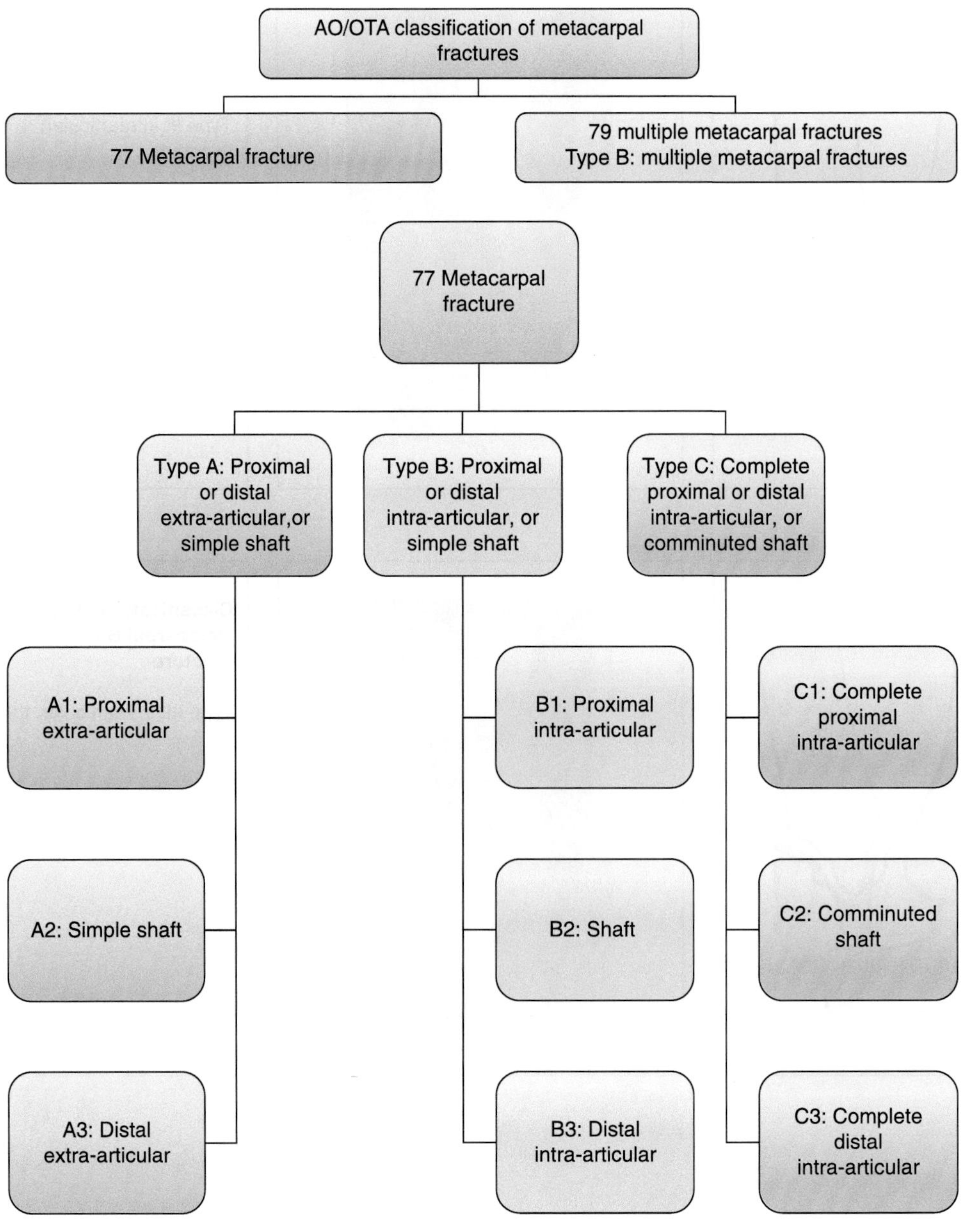

77 Metacarpal fracture:
- Type A: Proximal or distal extra-articular, or simple shaft:
  - A1: Proximal extra-articular:
    - A1.1: Simple extra-articular.
    - A1.2: Extra-articular wedge or comminuted.
  - A2: Simple shaft:
    - A2.1: Spiral.
    - A2.2: Oblique.
    - A2.3: Transverse.
  - A3: Distal extra-articular:
    - A3.1: Simple extra-articular.
    - A3.2: Extra-articular comminuted.

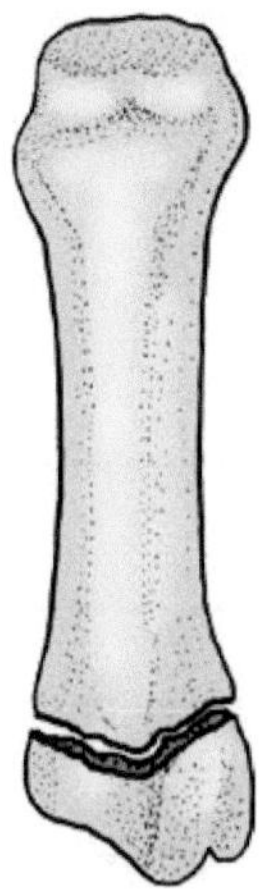

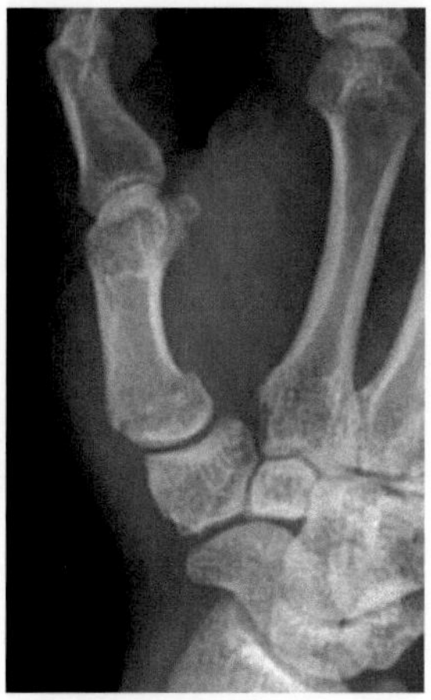

AO/OTA Classification of Hand Bone Fractures

77 Metacarpal fracture.

Type A: proximal or distal extraarticular, or simple shaft.

A1: proximal extraarticular.

A1.1: simple extraarticular

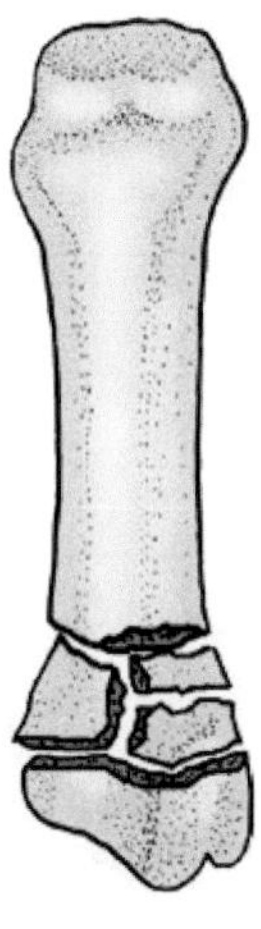

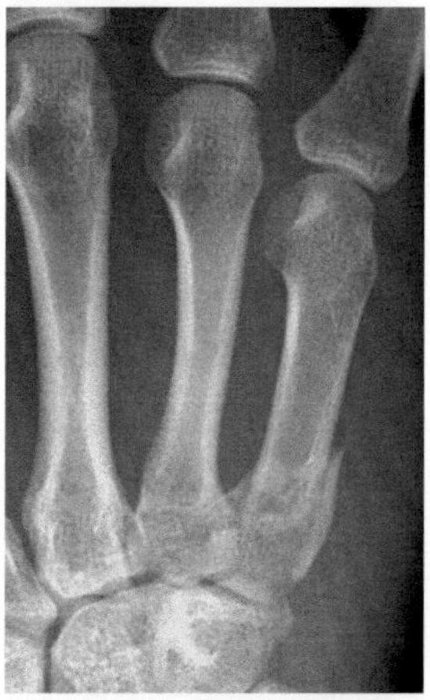

AO/OTA Classification of Hand Bone Fractures

77 Metacarpal fracture.

Type A: proximal or distal extraarticular, or simple shaft.

A1: proximal extraarticular.

A1.2: extraarticular wedge or comminuted

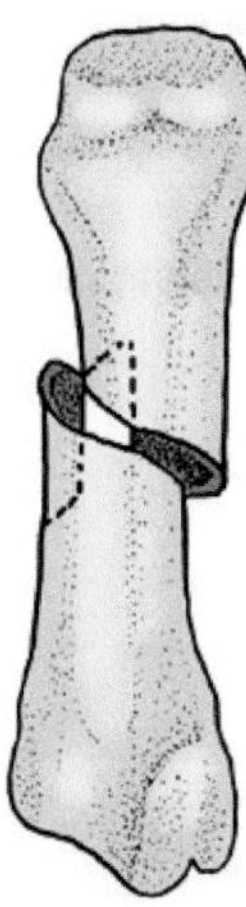

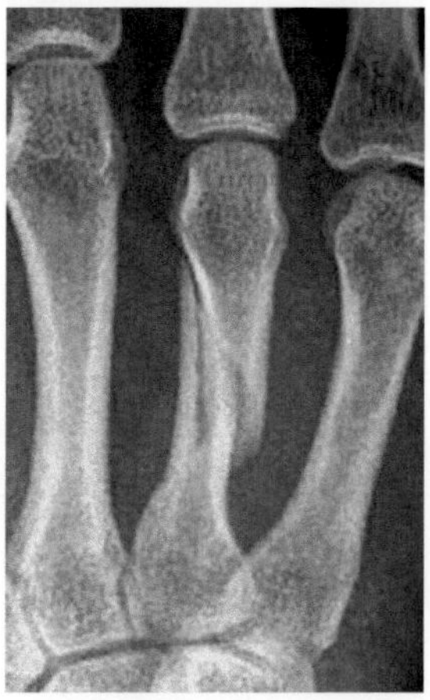

AO/OTA Classification of Hand Bone Fractures

77 Metacarpal fracture.

Type A: proximal or distal extraarticular, or simple shaft.

A2: simple shaft.

A2.1: spiral

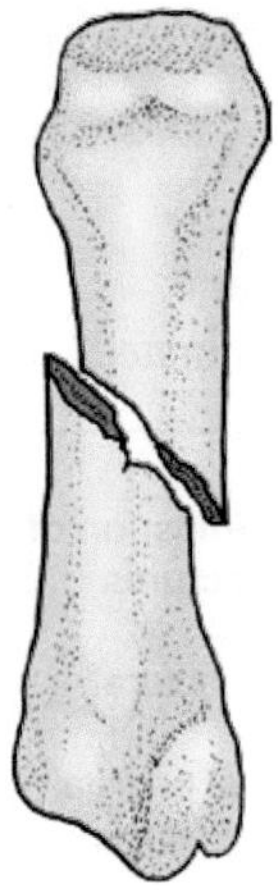

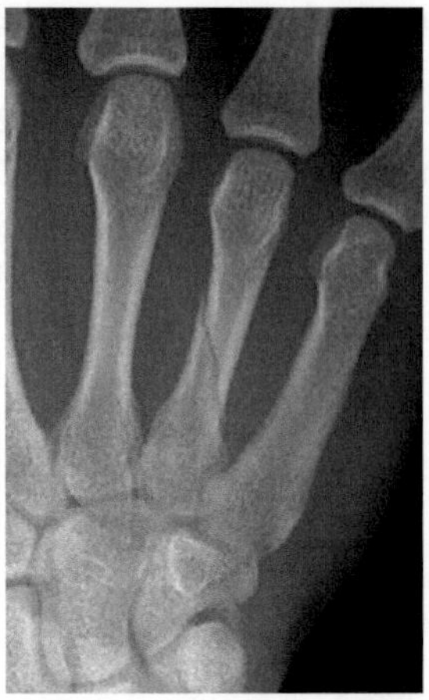

AO/OTA Classification of Hand Bone Fractures

77 Metacarpal fracture.

Type A: proximal or distal extraarticular, or simple shaft.

A2: simple shaft.

A2.:2 oblique

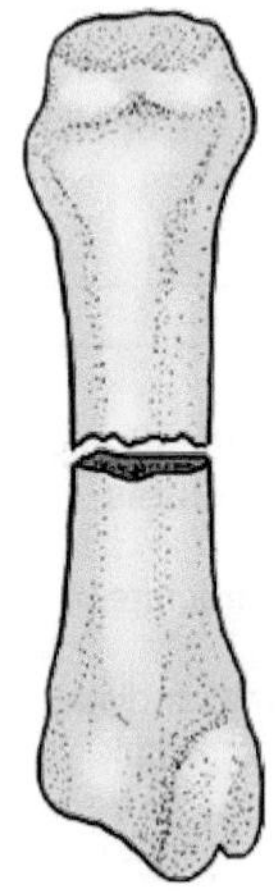

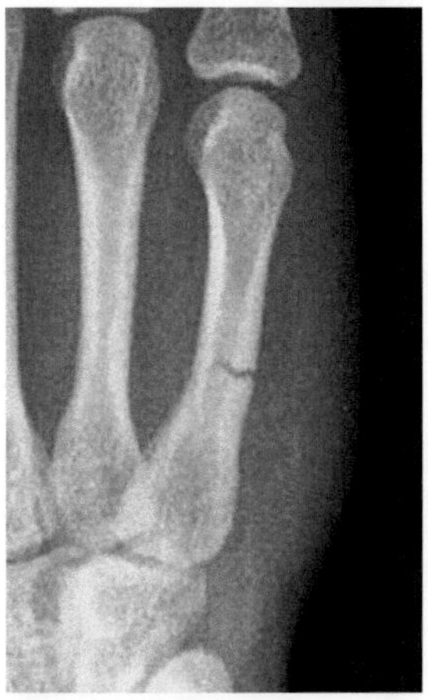

AO/OTA Classification of Hand Bone Fractures

77 Metacarpal fracture.

Type A: proximal or distal extraarticular, or simple shaft.

A2: simple shaft.

A2.3: transverse

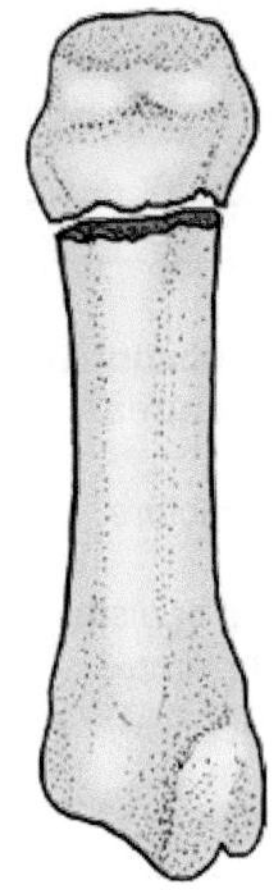

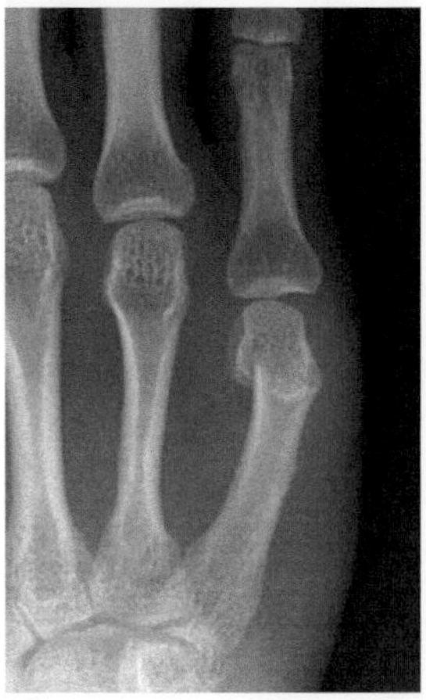

AO/OTA Classification of Hand Bone Fractures

77 Metacarpal fracture.

Type A: proximal or distal extraarticular, or simple shaft.

A3: distal extraarticular.

A3.1: simple extraarticular

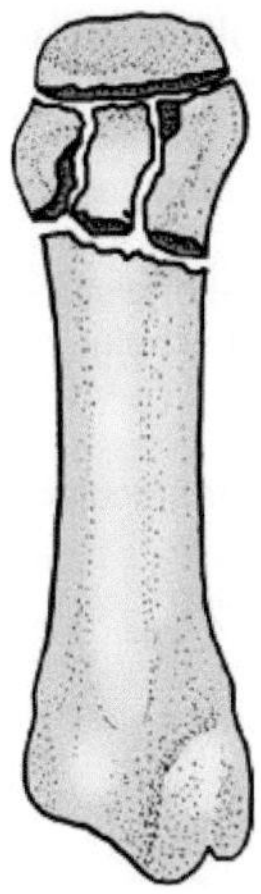

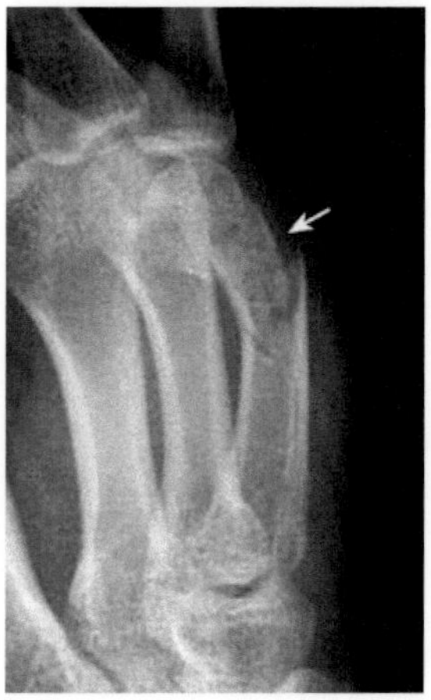

AO/OTA Classification of Hand Bone Fractures

77 Metacarpal fracture.

Type A: proximal or distal extraarticular, or simple shaft.

A3: distal extraarticular.

A3.2: extraarticular comminuted

Type B: Proximal or distal intra-articular, or simple shaft:
- B1: Proximal intra-articular:
  - B1.1: Avulsion or spilt.
  - B1.2: Compression.
  - B1.3: Spilt with compression.
- B2: Shaft:
  - B2.1: Spiral wedge.
  - B2.2: Long oblique wedge.
  - B2.3: Fragmented.
- B3: Distal intra-articular:
  - B3.1: Avulsion or spilt.
  - B3.2: Compression.
  - B3.3: Spilt with compression.

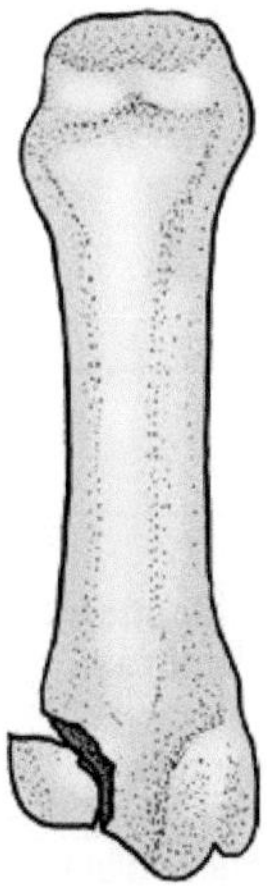

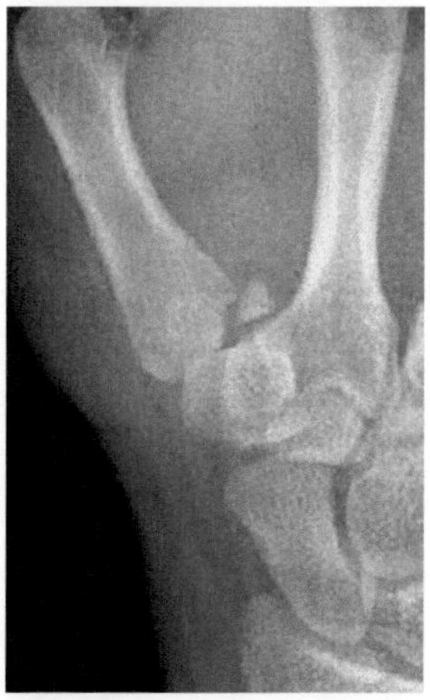

AO/OTA Classification of Hand Bone Fractures

77 Metacarpal fracture.

Type B: proximal or distal intraarticular, or simple shaft.

B1: proximal intraarticular.

B1.1: avulsion or spilt

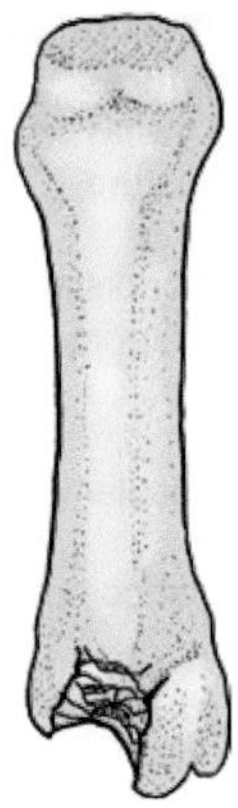

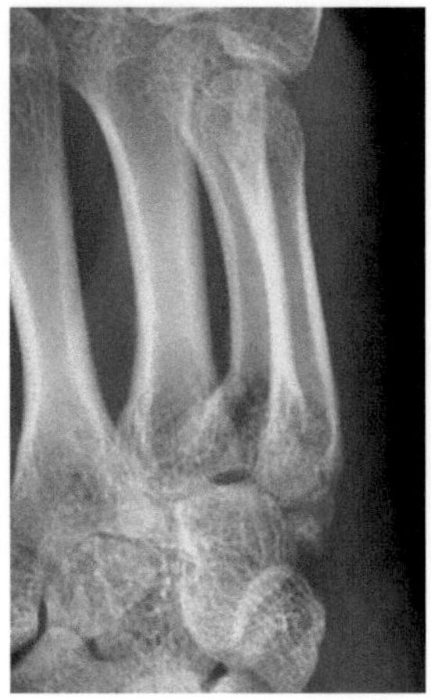

AO/OTA Classification of Hand Bone Fractures

77 Metacarpal fracture.

Type B: proximal or distal intraarticular, or simple shaft.

B1: proximal intraarticular.

B1.2: compression

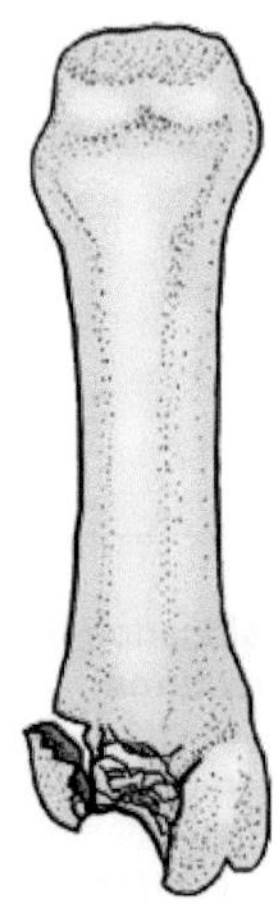

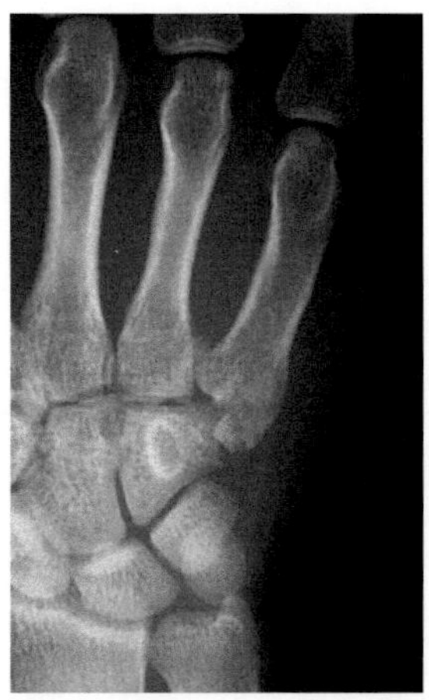

AO/OTA Classification of Hand Bone Fractures

77 Metacarpal fracture.

Type B: proximal or distal intraarticular, or simple shaft.

B1: proximal intraarticular.

B1.3: spilt with compression.

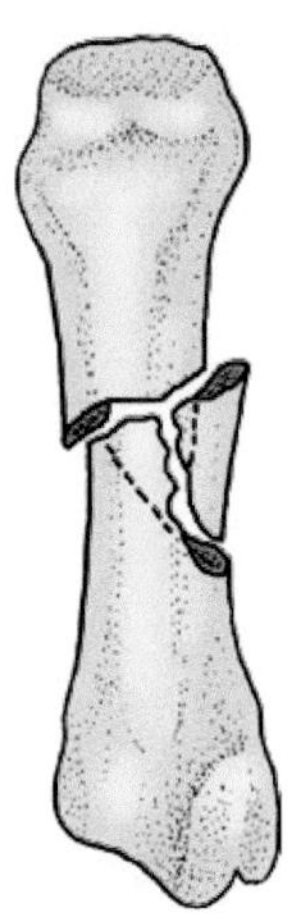

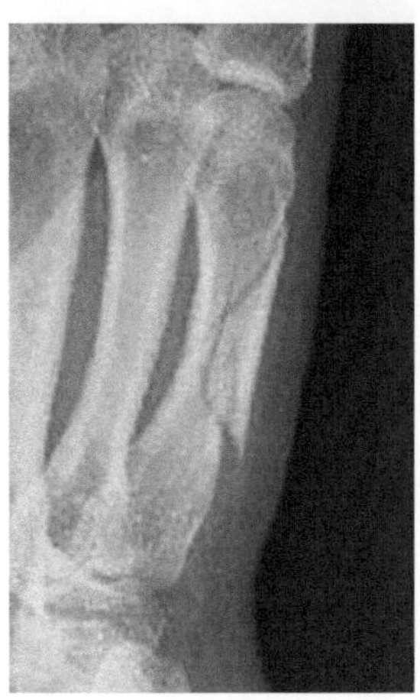

AO/OTA Classification of Hand Bone Fractures

77 Metacarpal fracture.

Type B: proximal or distal intraarticular, or simple shaft.

B2: shaft.

B2.1: spiral wedge

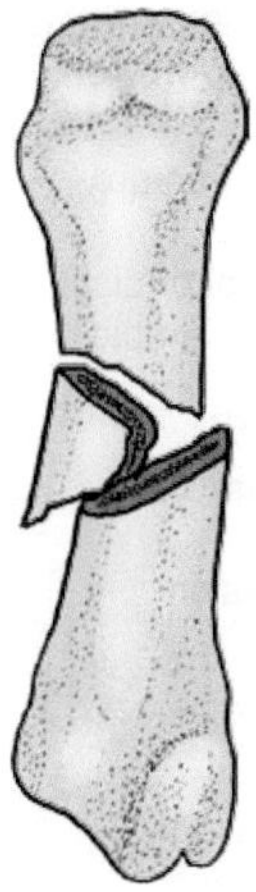

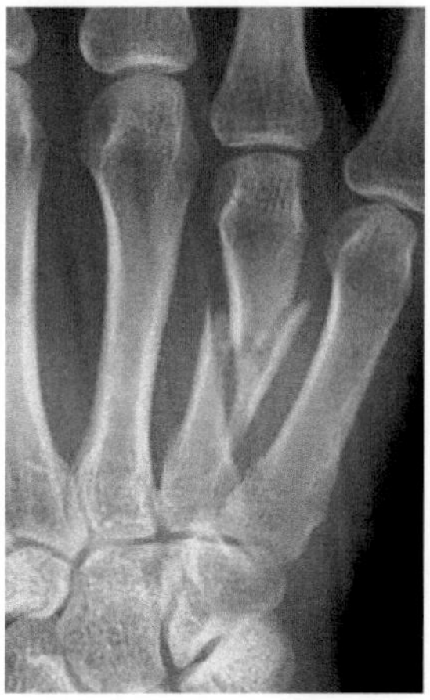

AO/OTA Classification of Hand Bone Fractures

77 Metacarpal fracture.

Type B: proximal or distal intraarticular, or simple shaft.

B2: shaft.

B2.2: long oblique wedge.

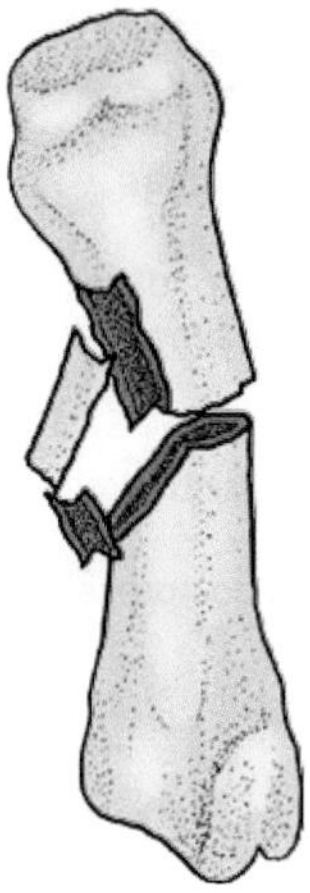

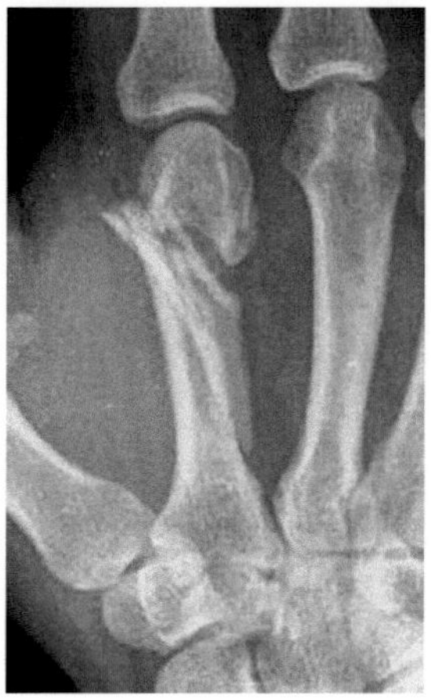

AO/OTA Classification of Hand Bone Fractures

77 Metacarpal fracture.

Type B: proximal or distal intraarticular, or simple shaft.

B2: shaft.

B2.3: fragmented

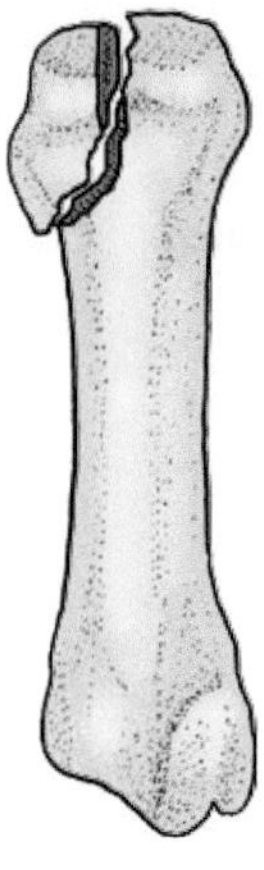

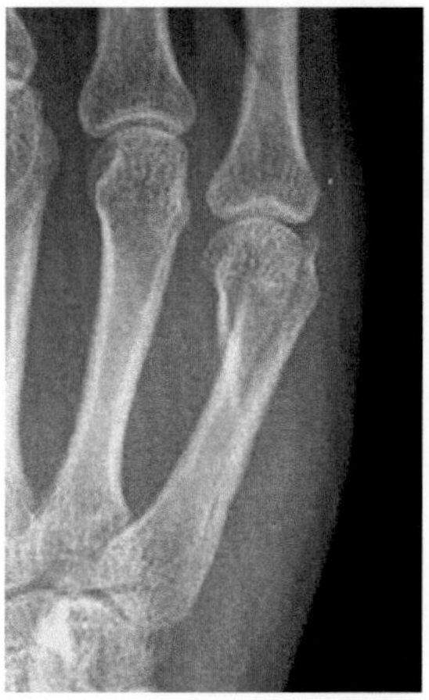

AO/OTA Classification of Hand Bone Fractures

77 Metacarpal fracture.

Type B: proximal or distal intraarticular, or simple shaft.

B3: distal intraarticular.

B3.1: avulsion or spilt

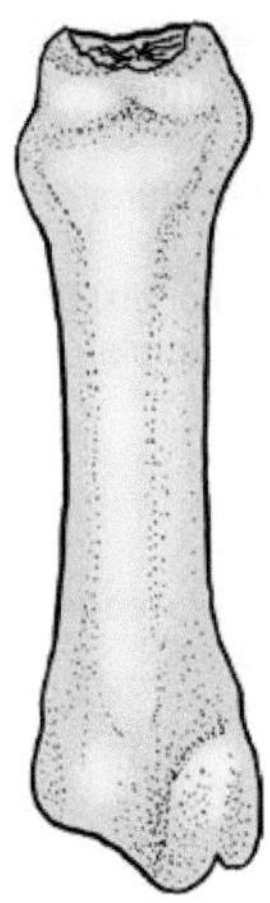

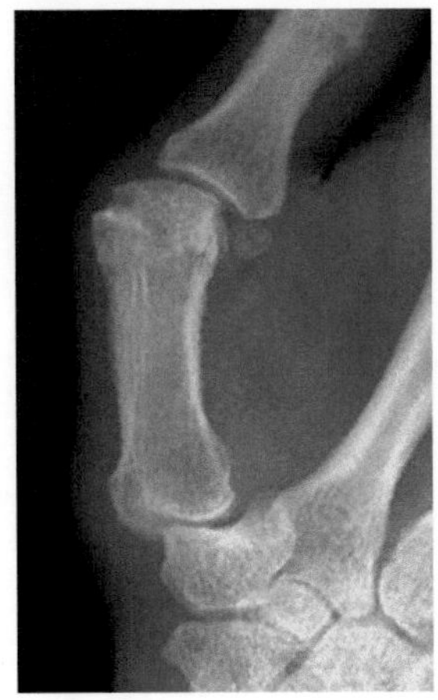

AO/OTA Classification of Hand Bone Fractures

77 Metacarpal fracture.

Type B: proximal or distal intraarticular, or simple shaft.

B3: distal intraarticular.

B3.2: compression

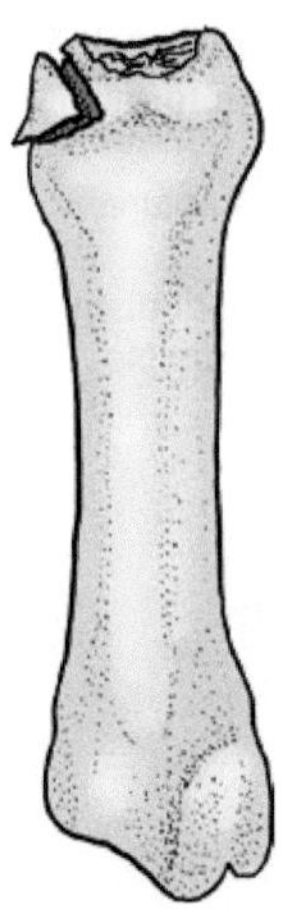

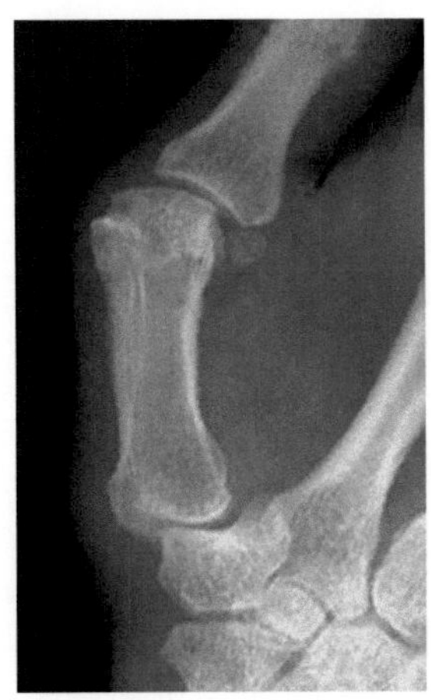

AO/OTA Classification of Hand Bone Fractures

77 Metacarpal fracture.

Type B: proximal or distal intraarticular, or simple shaft.

B3: distal intraarticular.

B3.3: spilt with compression

Type C: Complete proximal or distal intra-articular, or comminuted shaft:
- C1: Complete proximal intra-articular:
  - C1.1: Simple intra-articular, simple metaphyseal.
  - C1.2: Intra-articular comminuted, metaphyseal comminuted.
  - C1.3: Intra-articular comminuted.
- C2: Comminuted shaft:
  - C2.1: Segmental.
  - C2.2: Complex.
- C3: Complete distal intra-articular:
  - C3.1: Simple intra-articular, simple metaphyseal.
  - C3.2: Simple intra-articular, metaphyseal comminuted.
  - C3.3: Intra-articular comminuted.

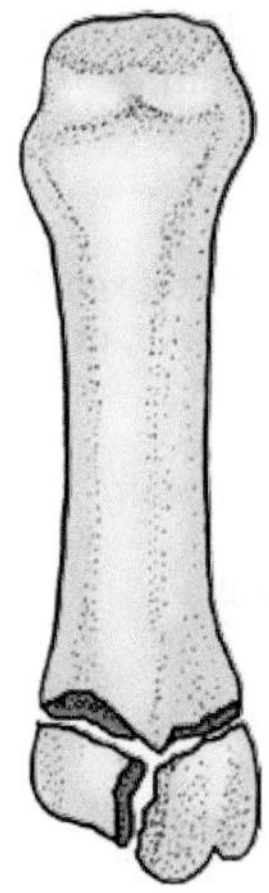

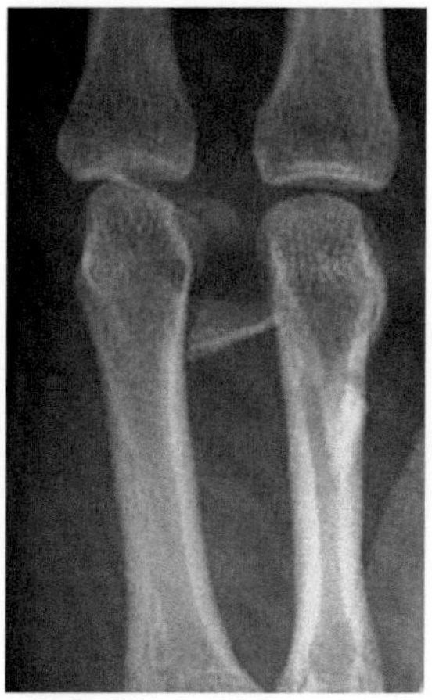

AO/OTA Classification of Hand Bone Fractures

77 Metacarpal fracture.

Type C: complete proximal or distal intraarticular, or comminuted shaft.

C1: complete proximal intraarticular.

C1.1: simple intraarticular, simple metaphyseal

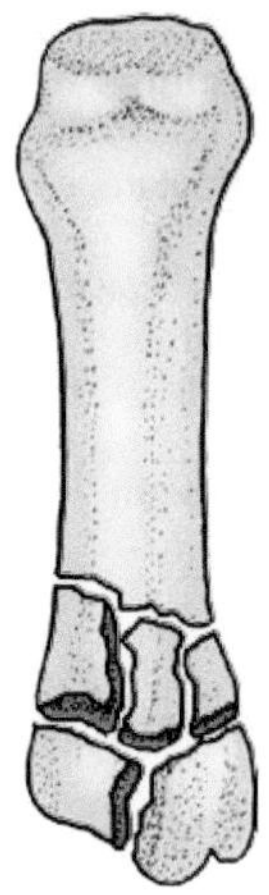

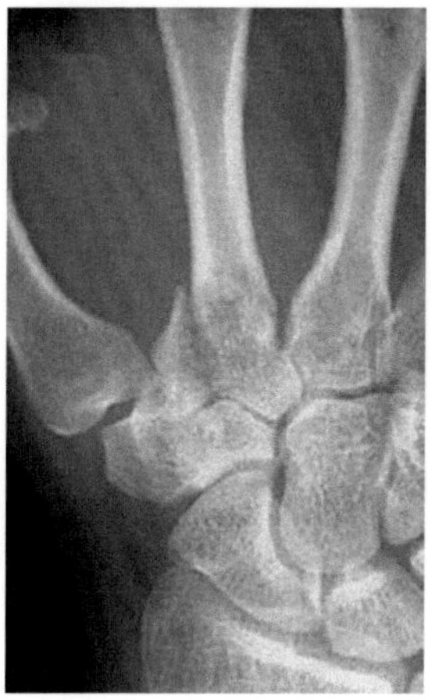

AO/OTA Classification of Hand Bone Fractures

77 Metacarpal fracture.

Type C: complete proximal or distal intraarticular, or comminuted shaft.

C1: complete proximal intraarticular.

C1.2: intraarticular comminuted, metaphyseal comminuted

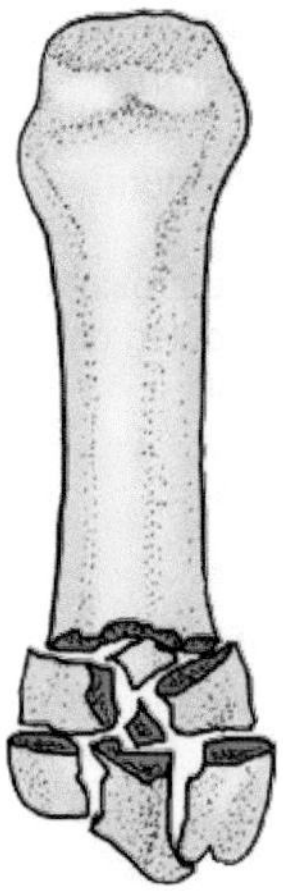

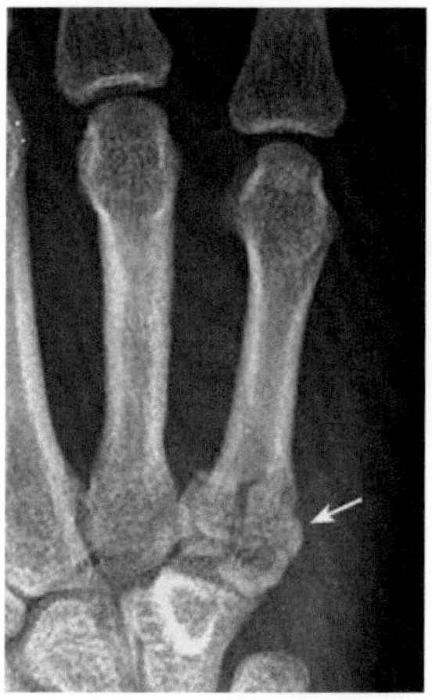

AO/OTA Classification of Hand Bone Fractures

77 Metacarpal fracture.

Type C: complete proximal or distal intraarticular, or comminuted shaft.

C1: complete proximal intraarticular.

C1.3: intraarticular comminuted

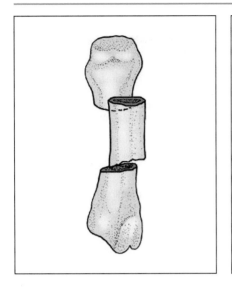

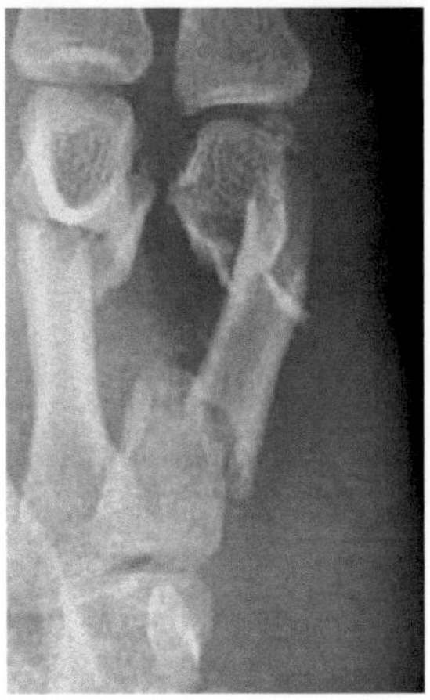

AO/OTA Classification of Hand Bone Fractures

77 Metacarpal fracture.

Type C: complete proximal or distal intraarticular, or comminuted shaft.

C2: comminuted shaft.

C2.1: segmental

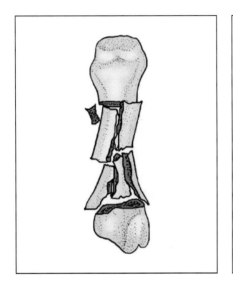

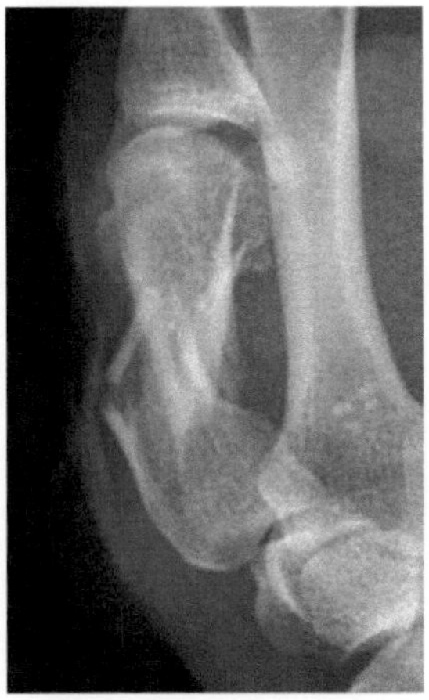

AO/OTA Classification of Hand Bone Fractures

77 Metacarpal fracture.

Type C: complete proximal or distal intraarticular, or comminuted shaft.

C2: comminuted shaft.

C2.2: complex

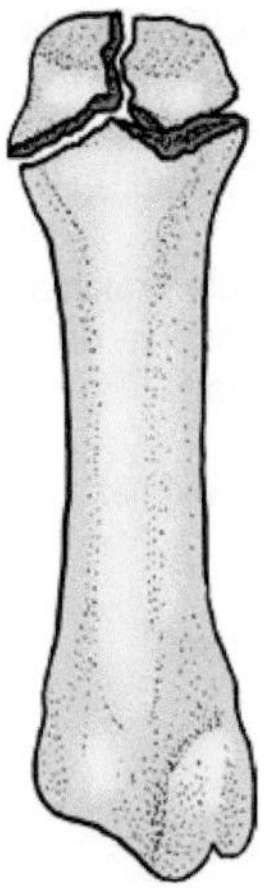

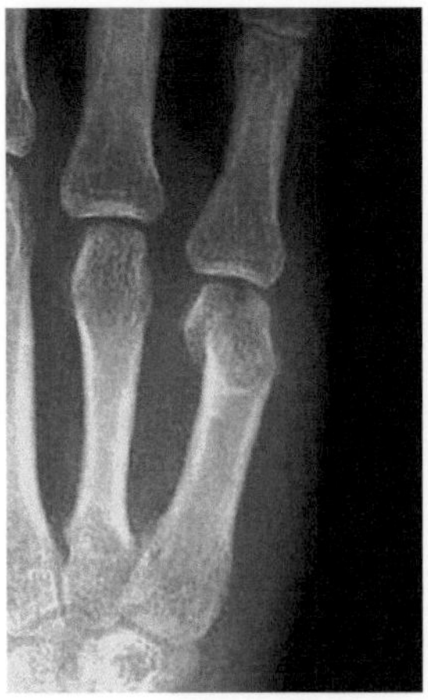

AO/OTA Classification of Hand Bone Fractures

77 Metacarpal fracture.

Type C: complete proximal or distal intraarticular, or comminuted shaft.

C3: complete distal intraarticular.

C3.1: simple intraarticular, simple metaphyseal

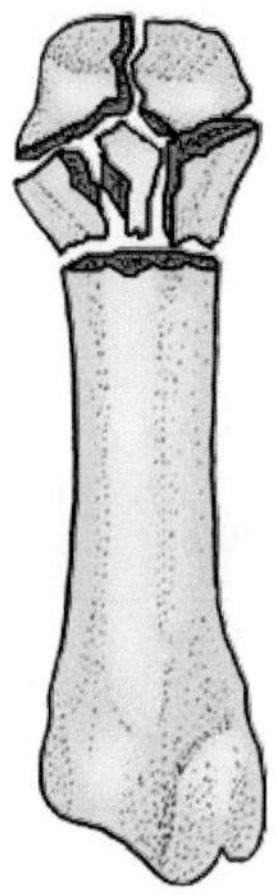

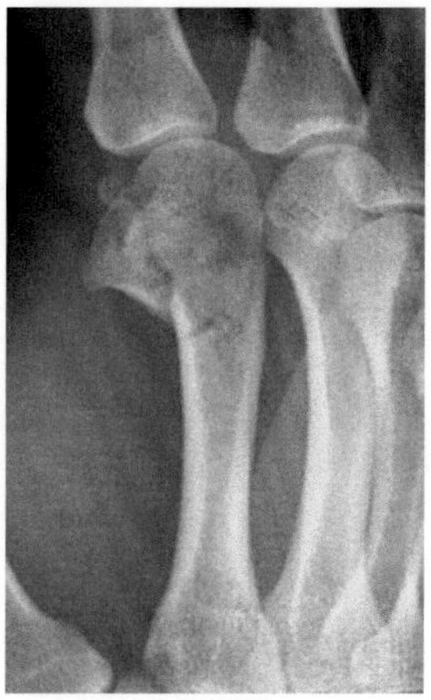

AO/OTA Classification of Hand Bone Fractures

77 Metacarpal fracture.

Type C: complete proximal or distal intraarticular, or comminuted shaft.

C3: complete distal intraarticular.

C3.2: simple intraarticular, metaphyseal comminuted

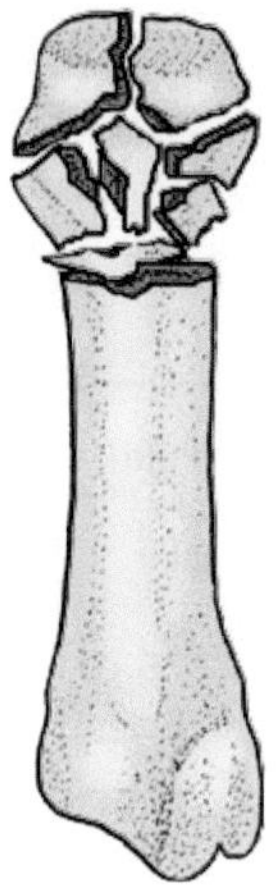

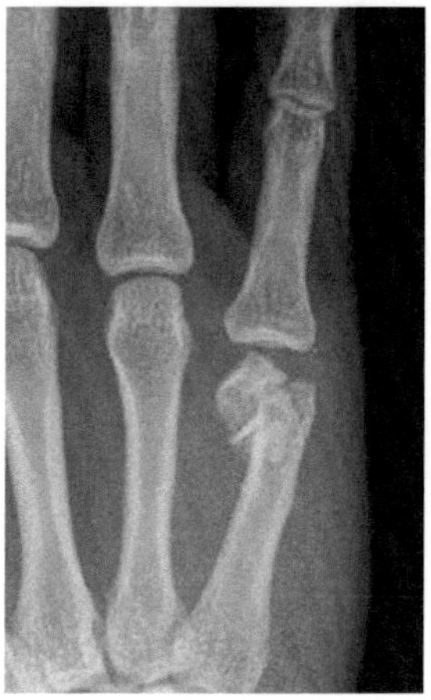

AO/OTA Classification of Hand Bone Fractures

77 Metacarpal fracture.

Type C: complete proximal or distal intraarticular, or comminuted shaft.

C3: complete distal intraarticular.

C3.3: intraarticular comminuted

79 Multiple fractures.

Type B: Multiple fractures of metacarpal.

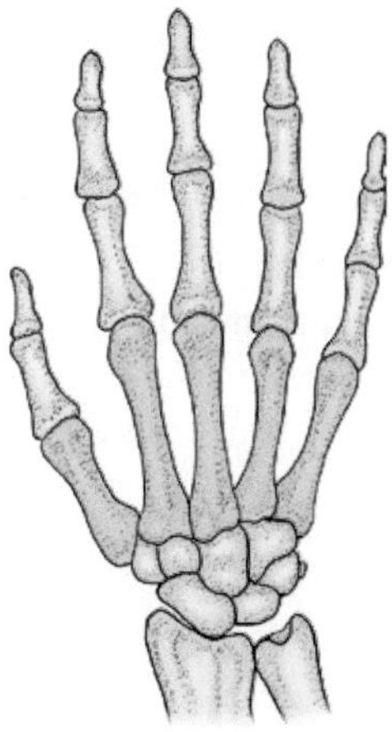

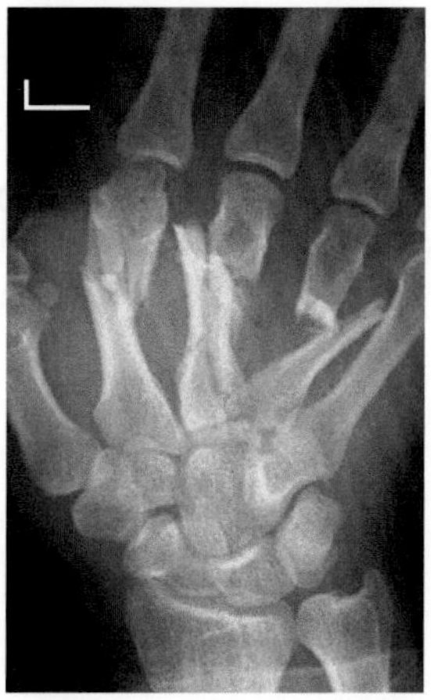

AO/OTA Classification of Hand Bone Fractures

79 Multiply Fractures.

Type B: Multiply fractures of metacarpal

4.1.2 Classification of Fractures of Phalanx

4.1.2.1 AO/OTA Classification of Phalangeal Fractures

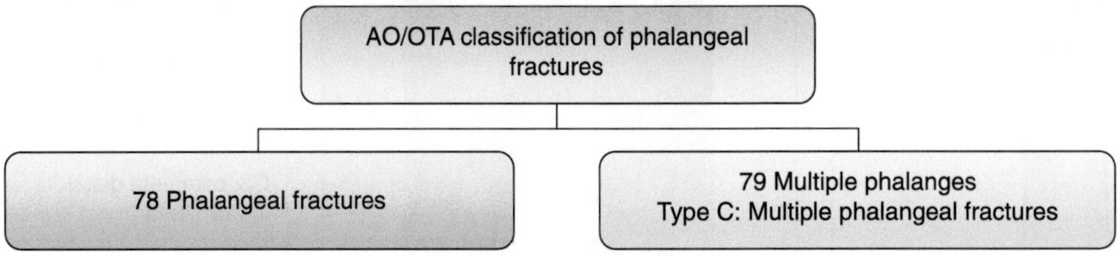

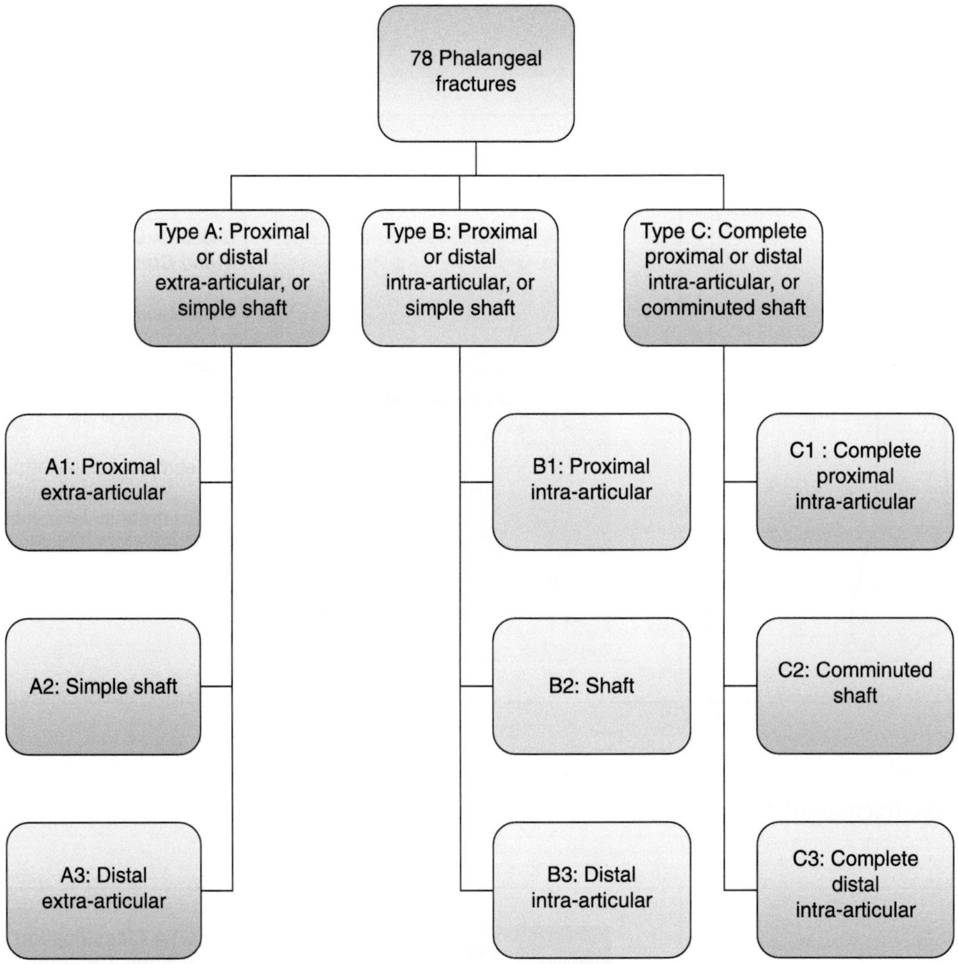

78 Phalangeal fractures.
- Type A: Proximal or distal extra-articular, or simple shaft:
  - A1: Proximal extra-articular:
    - A1.1: Simple extra-articular.
    - A1.2: Extra-articular comminuted.
  - A2: Simple shaft:
    - A2.1: Spiral.
    - A2.2: Oblique.
    - A2.3: Transverse.
  - A3: Distal extra-articular:
    - A3.1: Simple extra-articular.
    - A3.2: Extra-articular comminuted.

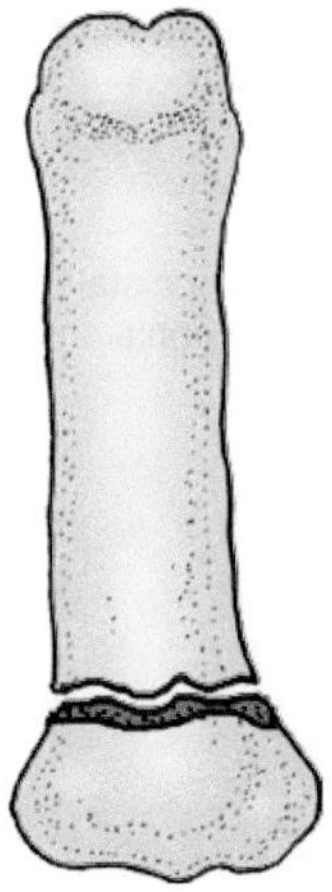

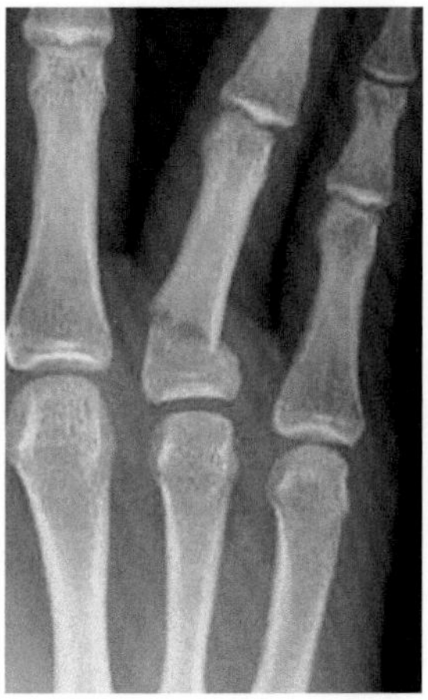

AO/OTA Classification of Hand Bone Fractures

78 Phalangeal fracture.

Type A: proximal or distal extraarticular, or simple shaft.

A1: proximal extraarticular.

A1.1: simple extraarticular

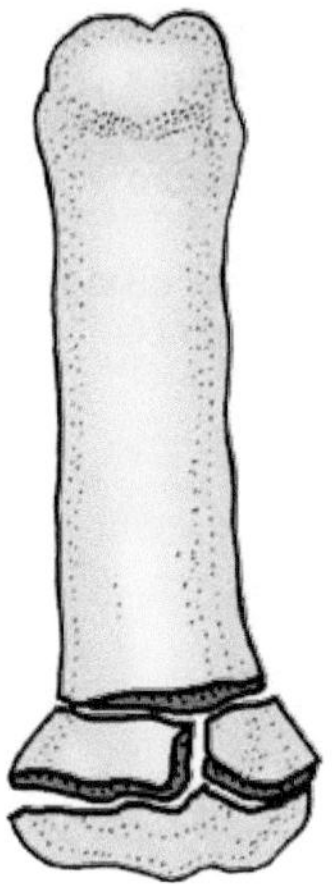

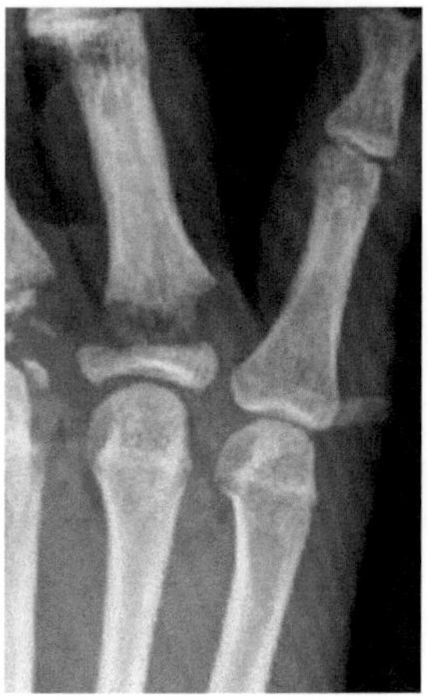

AO/OTA Classification of Hand Bone Fractures

78 Phalangeal fracture.

Type A: proximal or distal extraarticular, or simple shaft.

A1: proximal extraarticular.

A1.2 – extraarticular comminuted

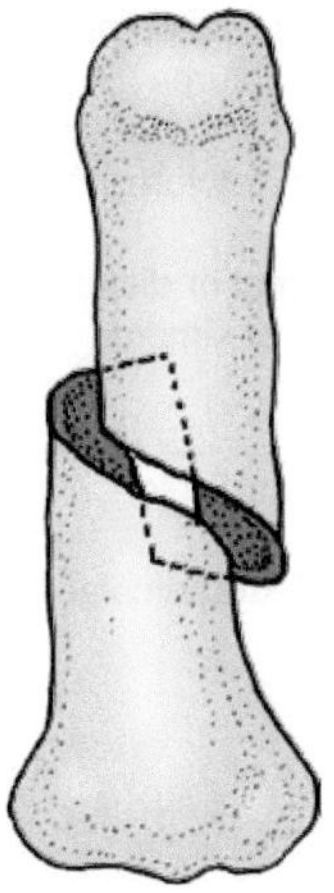

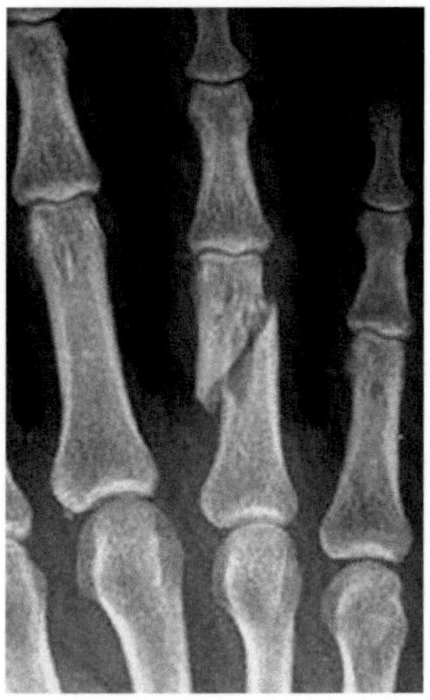

AO/OTA Classification of Hand Bone Fractures

78 Phalangeal fracture.

Type A: proximal or distal extraarticular, or simple shaft.

A2: simple shaft.

A2.1: spiral

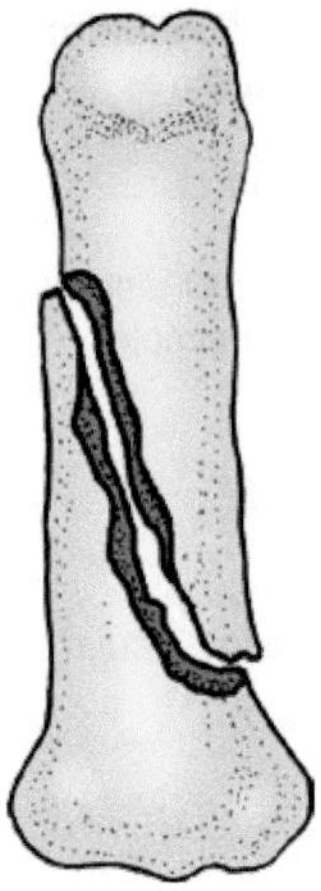

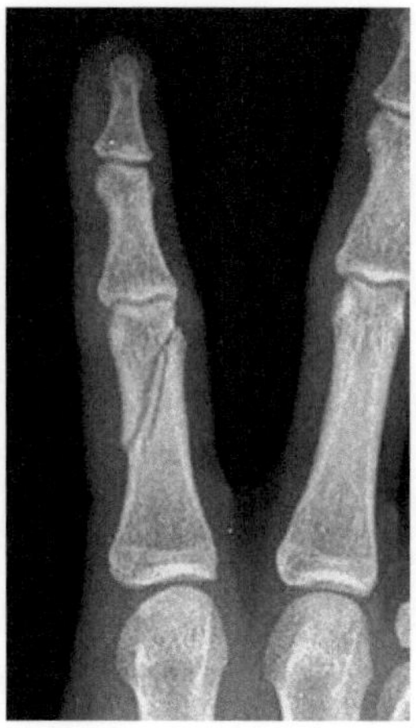

AO/OTA Classification of Hand Bone Fractures

78 Phalangeal fracture.

Type A: proximal or distal extraarticular, or simple shaft.

A2: simple shaft.

A2.2: oblique

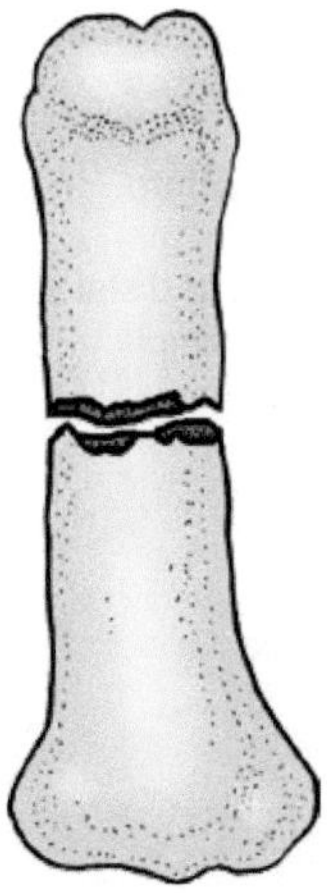

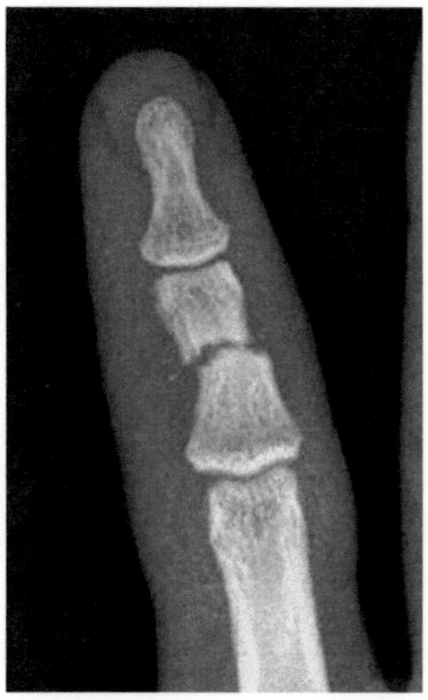

AO/OTA Classification of Hand Bone Fractures

78 Phalangeal fracture.

Type A: proximal or distal extraarticular, or simple shaft.

A2: simple shaft.

A2.3: transverse

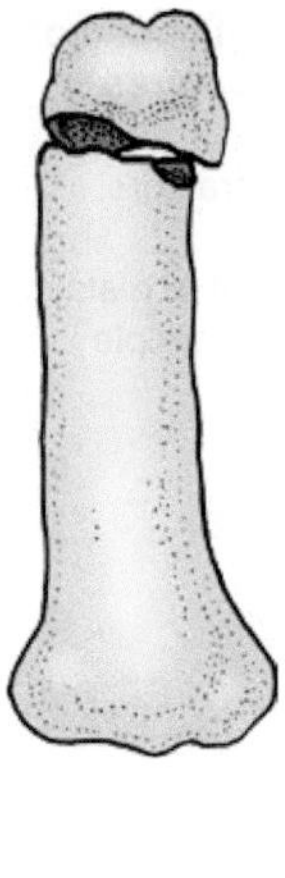

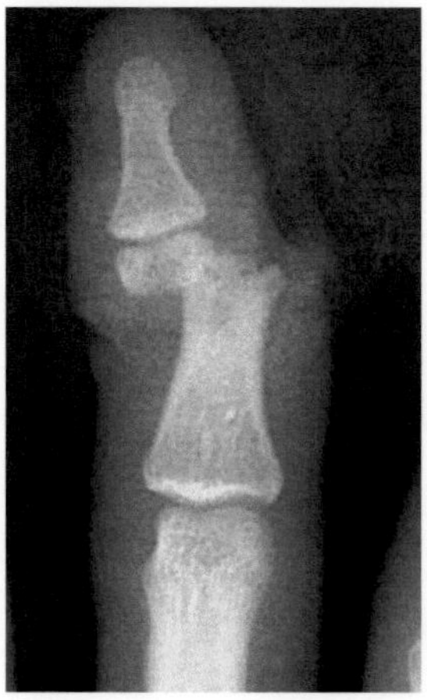

AO/OTA Classification of Hand Bone Fractures

78 Phalangeal fracture.

Type A: proximal or distal extraarticular, or simple shaft.

A3: distal extraarticular.

A3.1: simple extraarticular

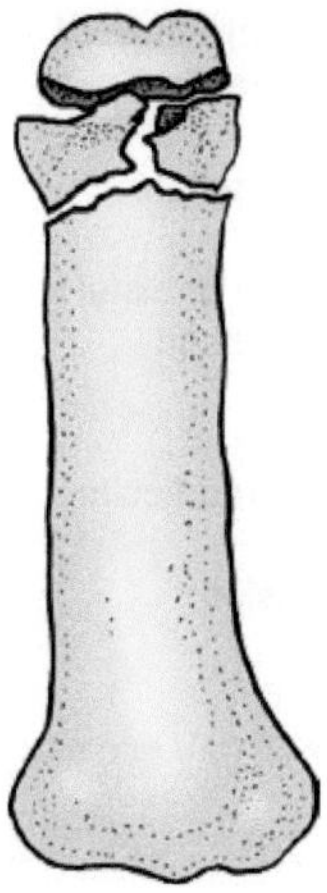

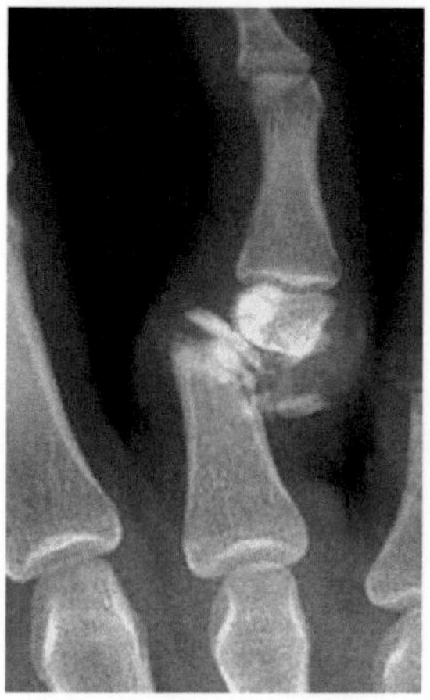

AO/OTA Classification of Hand Bone Fractures

78 Phalangeal fracture.

Type A: proximal or distal extraarticular, or simple shaft.

A3: distal extraarticular.

A3.2: extraarticular comminuted

Type B: Proximal or distal intra-articular, or shaft wedge:
- B1: Proximal intra-articular:
  - B1.1: Avulsion or spilt.
  - B1.2: Compression.
  - B1.3: Spilt with compression.
- B2: Shaft:
  - B2.1: Spiral wedge.
  - B2.2: Long oblique wedge.
  - B2.3: Fragmented.
- B3: Distal intra-articular:
  - B3.1: Avulsion or spilt.
  - B3.2: Compression.
  - B3.3: Spilt with compression.

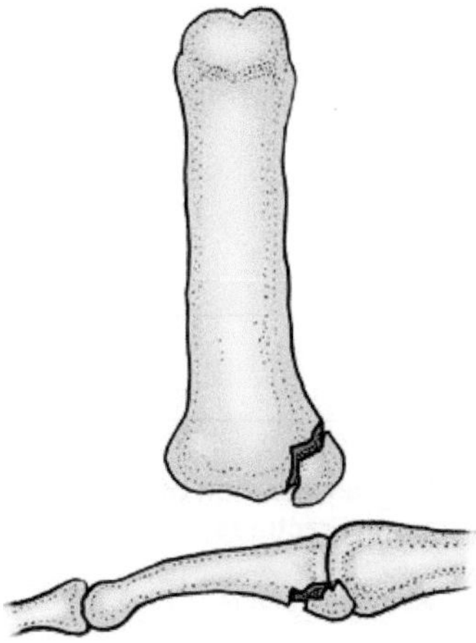

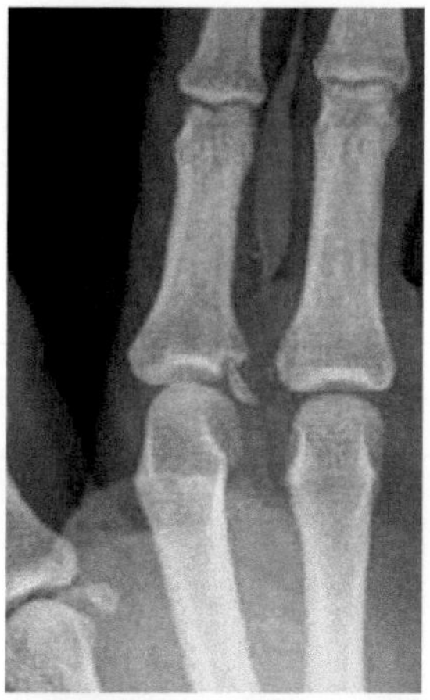

AO/OTA Classification of Hand Bone Fractures

78 Phalangeal fracture.

Type B: proximal or distal intraarticular, or shaft wedge.

B1: proximal intraarticular.

B1.1: avulsion or spilt

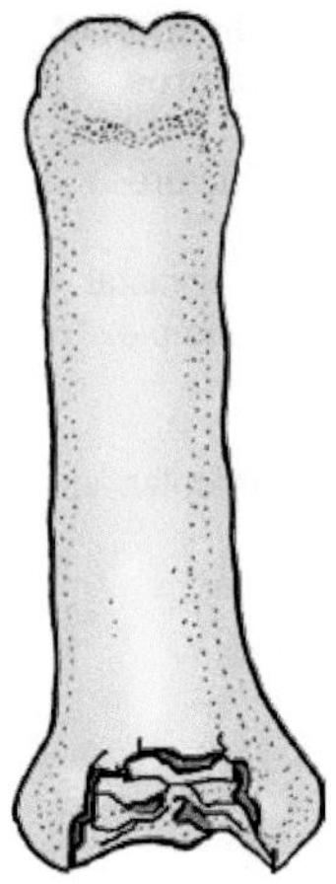

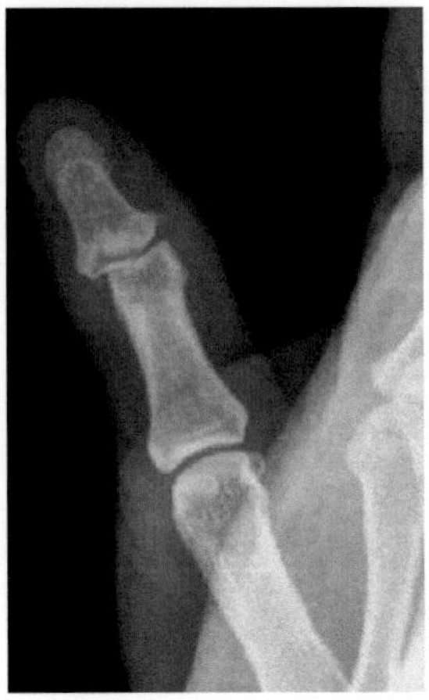

AO/OTA Classification of Hand Bone Fractures

78 Phalangeal fracture.

Type B: proximal or distal intraarticular, or shaft wedge.

B1: proximal intraarticular.

B1.2: compression.

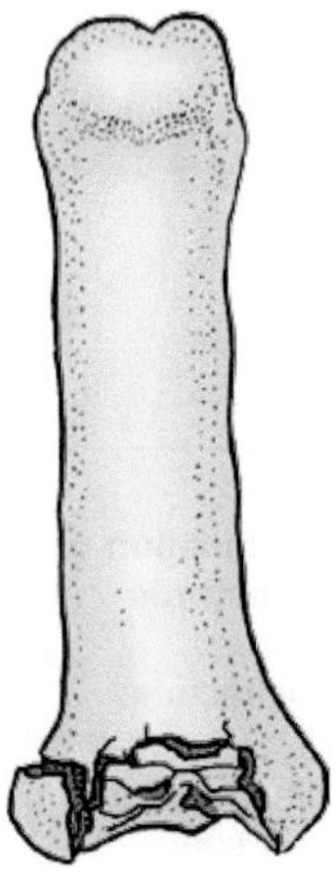

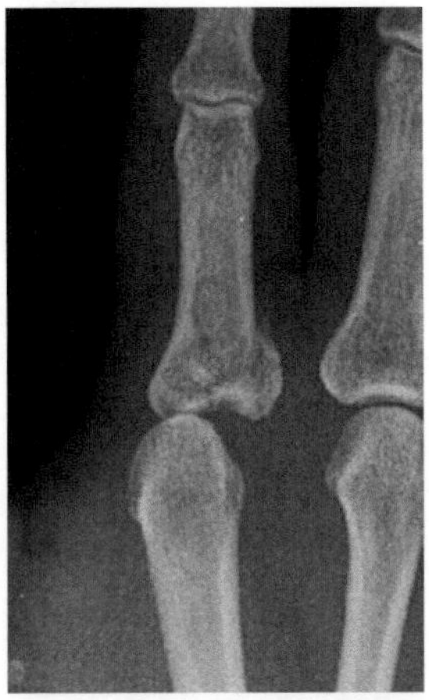

AO/OTA Classification of Hand Bone Fractures

78 Phalangeal fracture.

Type B: proximal or distal intraarticular, or shaft wedge.

B1: proximal intraarticular.

B1.3: spilt with compression.

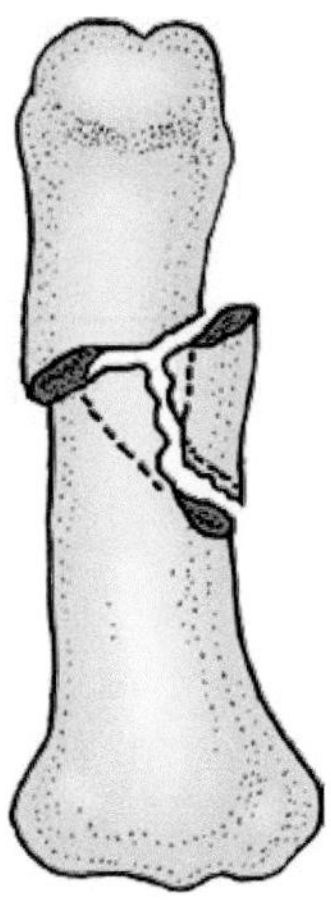

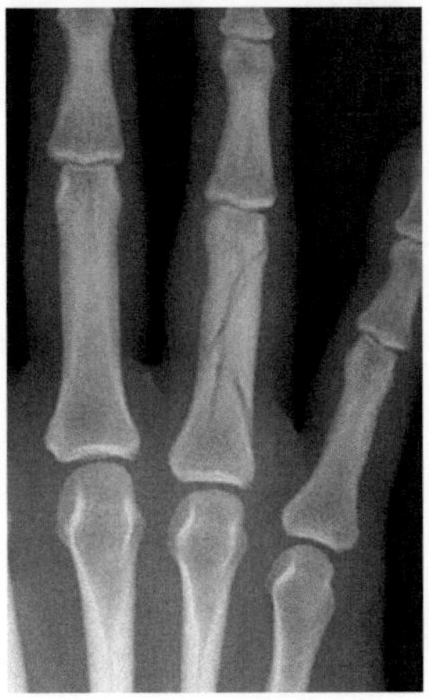

AO/OTA Classification of Hand Bone Fractures

78 Phalangeal fracture.

Type B: proximal or distal intraarticular, or shaft wedge.

B2: shaft wedge

B2.1: spiral wedge

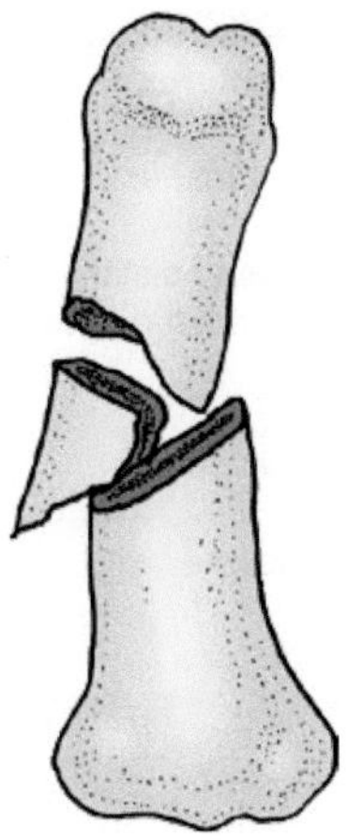

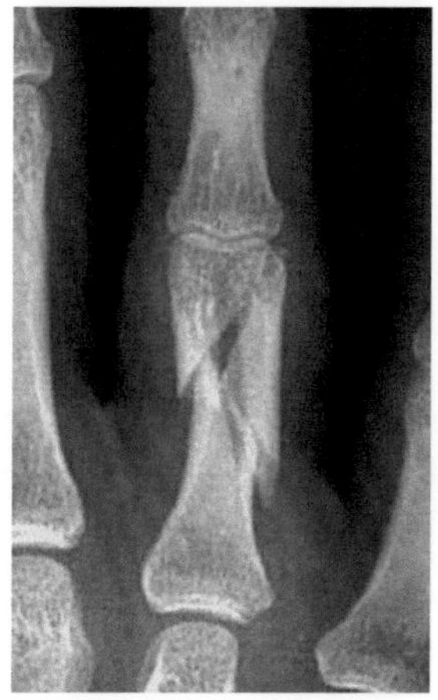

AO/OTA Classification of Hand Bone Fractures

78 Phalangeal fracture.

Type B: proximal or distal intraarticular, or shaft wedge.

B2: shaft wedge

B2.2: long oblique wedge

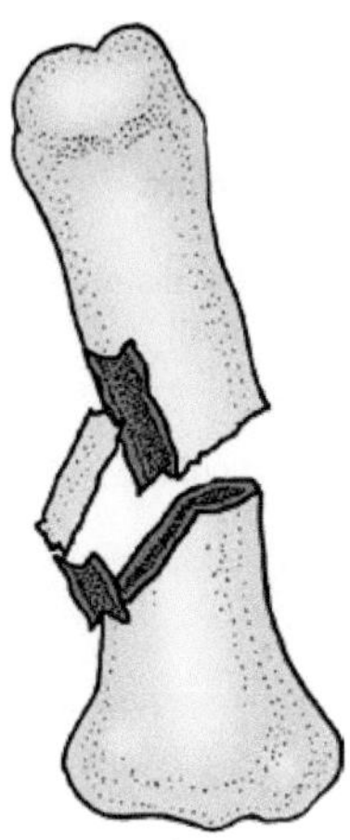

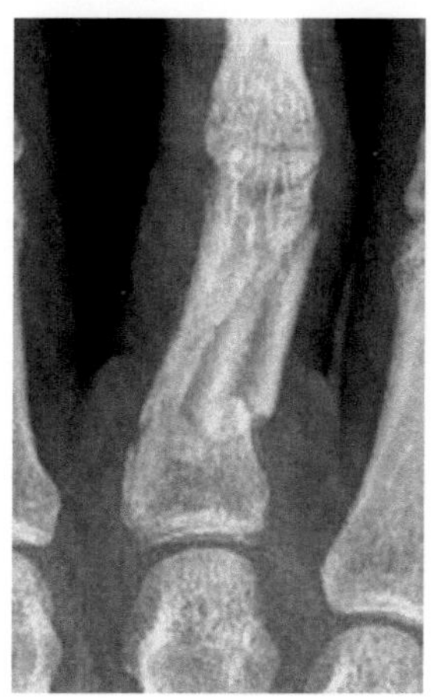

AO/OTA Classification of Hand Bone Fractures

78 Phalangeal fracture.

Type B: proximal or distal intraarticular, or shaft wedge.

B2: shaft wedge

B2.3: shaft wedge fragmented

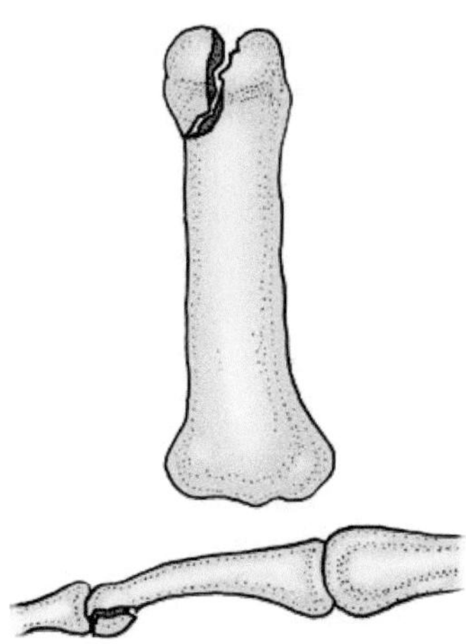

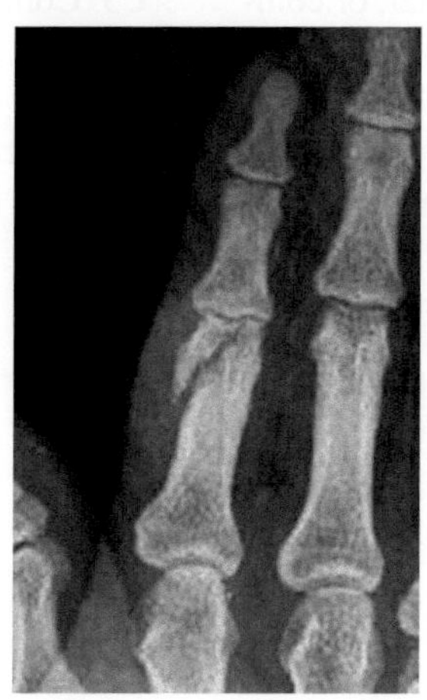

AO/OTA Classification of Hand Bone Fractures

78 Phalangeal fracture.

Type B: proximal or distal intraarticular, or shaft wedge.

B3: distal intraarticular.

B3.1: avulsion or spilt

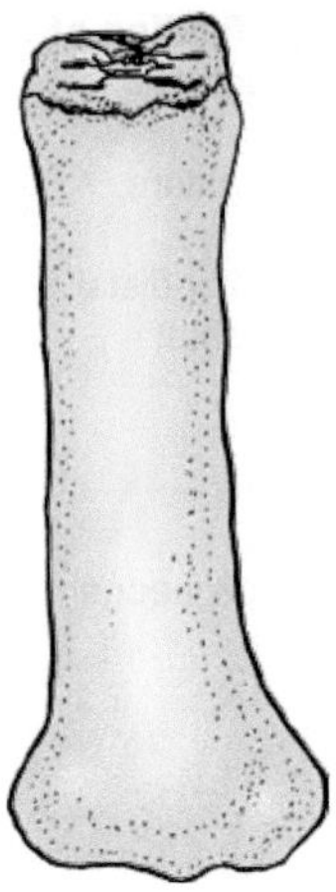

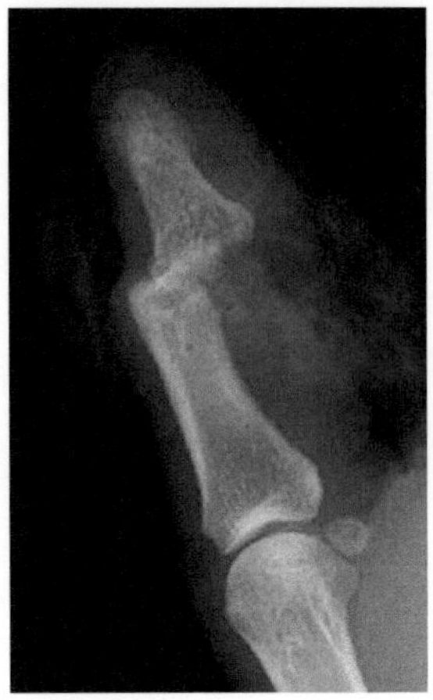

AO/OTA Classification of Hand Bone Fractures

78 Phalangeal fracture.

Type B: proximal or distal intraarticular, or shaft wedge.

B3: distal intraarticular.

B3.2: compression

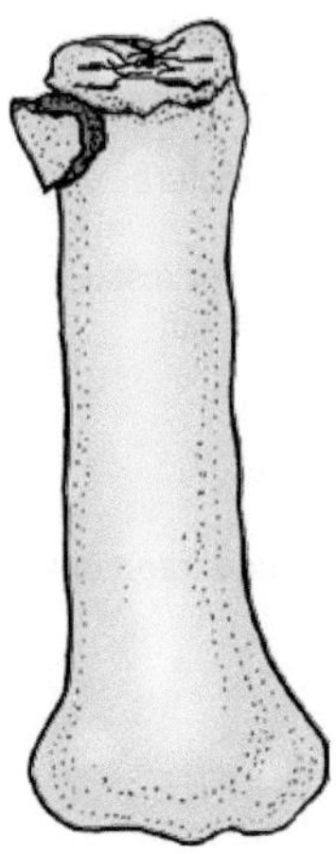

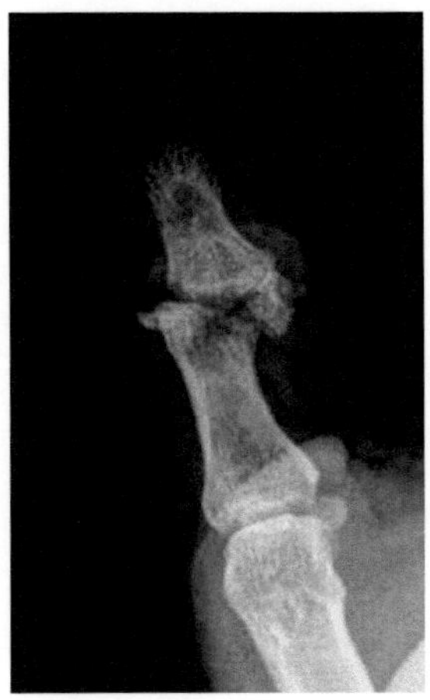

AO/OTA Classification of Hand Bone Fractures

78 Phalangeal fracture.

Type B: proximal or distal intraarticular, or shaft wedge.

B3: distal intraarticular.

B3.3: spilt with compression

Type C: Complete proximal or distal intra-articular, or comminuted shaft:
- C1: Complete proximal intra-articular:
  - C1.1: Simple intra-articular, simple metaphyseal.
  - C1.2: Intra-articular in-/un-comminuted, metaphyseal comminuted.
  - C1.3: Intra-articular comminuted.
- C2: Comminuted shaft:
  - C2.1: Segmental.
  - C2.2: Complex.
- C3: Complete distal intra-articular:
  - C3.1: Simple intra-articular, simple metaphyseal.
  - C3.2: Simple intra-articular, metaphyseal comminuted.
  - C3.3: Intra-articular comminuted.

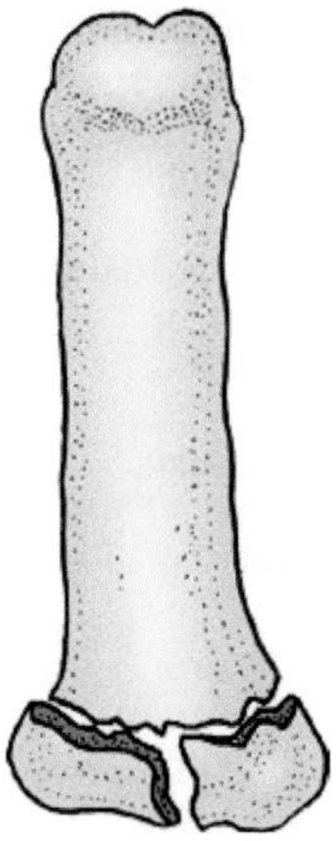

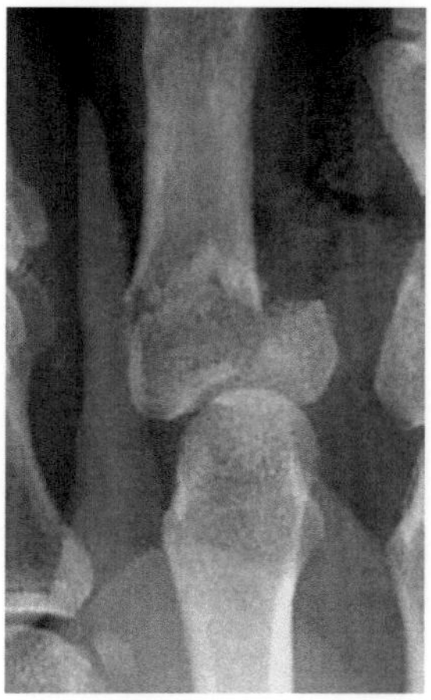

AO/OTA Classification of Hand Bone Fractures

78 Phalangeal fracture.

Type C: complete proximal or distal intraarticular, or comminuted shaft.

C1: complete proximal intraarticular.

C1.1: simple intraarticular, simple metaphyseal

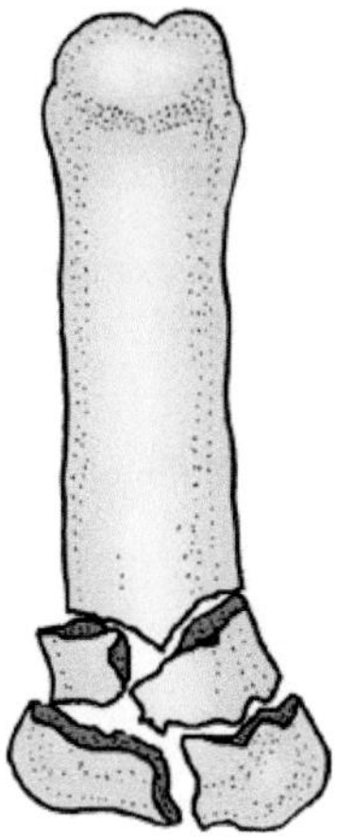

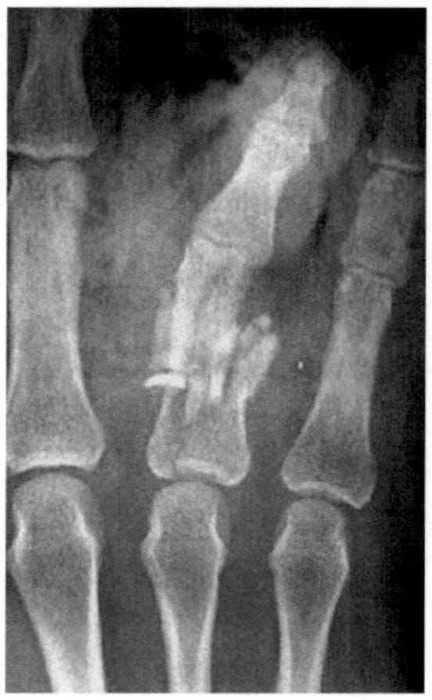

AO/OTA Classification of Hand Bone Fractures

78 Phalangeal fracture.

Type C: complete proximal or distal intraarticular, or comminuted shaft.

C1: complete proximal intraarticular.

C1.2: intraarticular in-/un-comminuted, metaphyseal comminuted

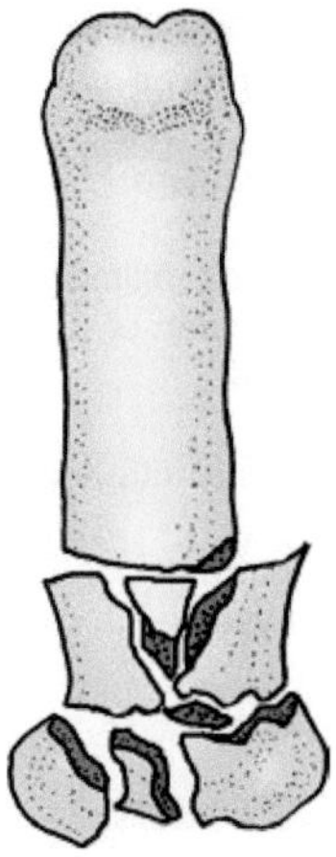

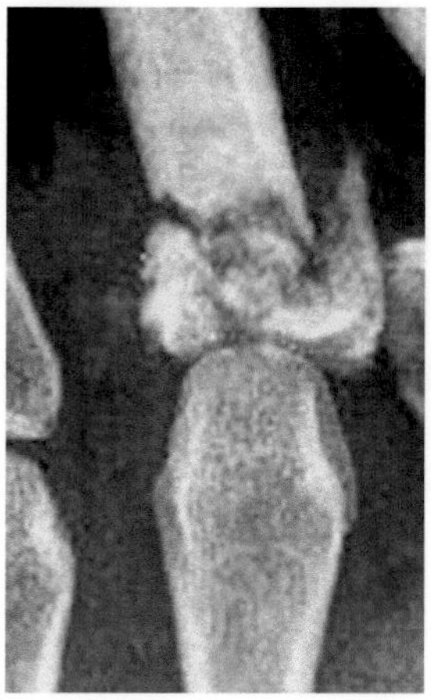

AO/OTA Classification of Hand Bone Fractures

78 Phalangeal fracture.

Type C: complete proximal or distal intraarticular, or comminuted shaft.

C1: complete proximal intraarticular.

C1.3: intraarticular comminuted

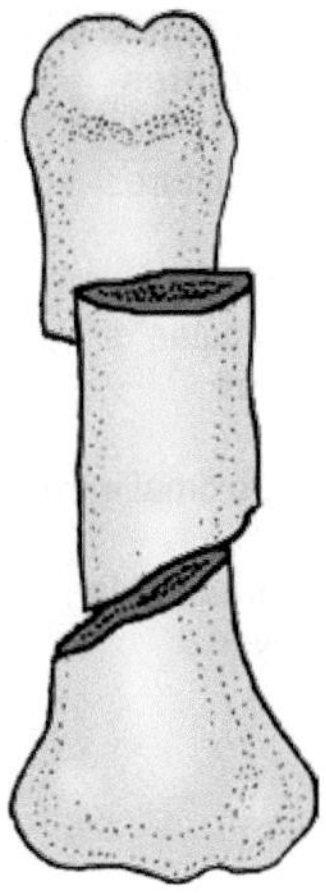

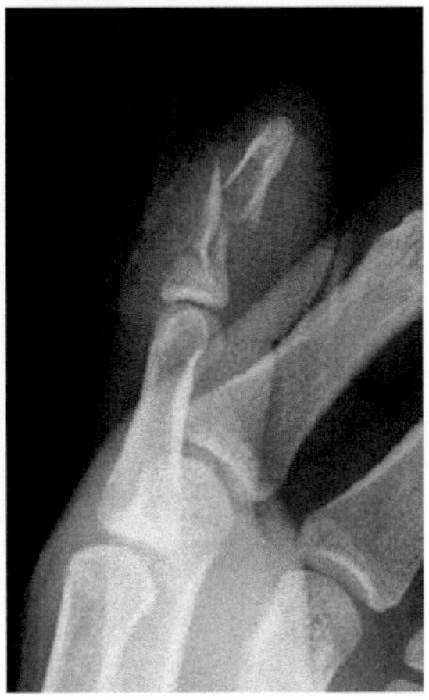

AO/OTA Classification of Hand Bone Fractures

78 Phalangeal fracture.

Type C: complete proximal or distal intraarticular, or comminuted shaft.

C2: comminuted shaft.

C2.1: segmental

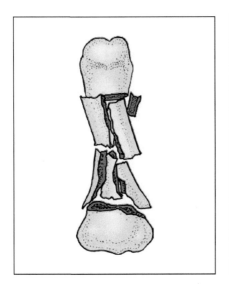

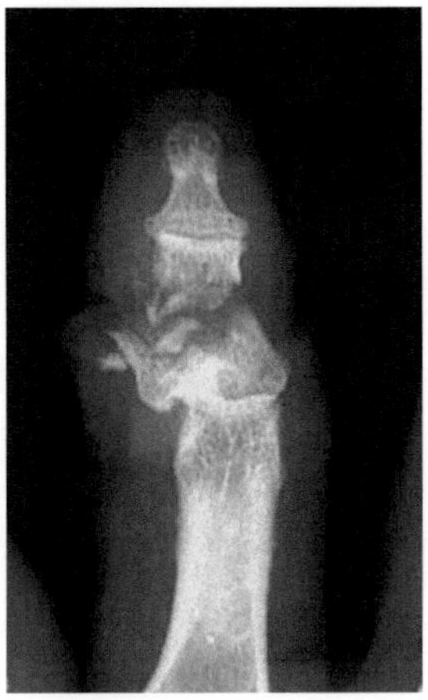

AO/OTA Classification of Hand Bone Fractures

78 Phalangeal fracture.

Type C: complete proximal or distal intraarticular, or comminuted shaft.

C2: comminuted shaft.

C2.2: complex

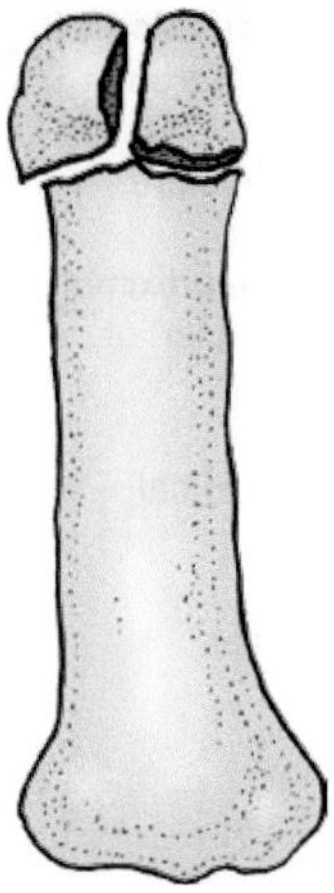

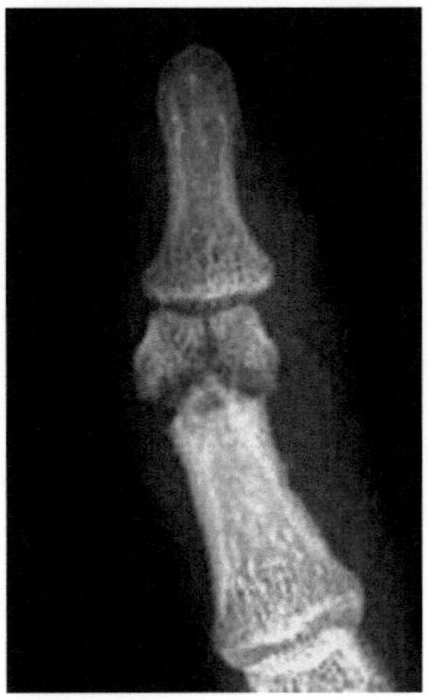

AO/OTA Classification of Hand Bone Fractures

78 Phalangeal fracture.

Type C: complete proximal or distal intraarticular, or comminuted shaft.

C3: complete distal intraarticular.

C3.1: simple intraarticular, simple metaphyseal

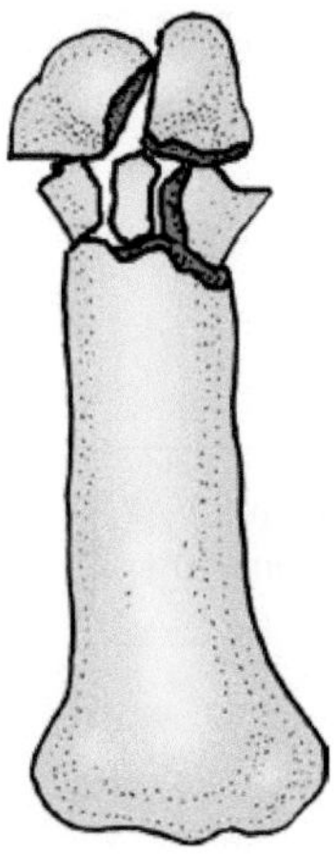

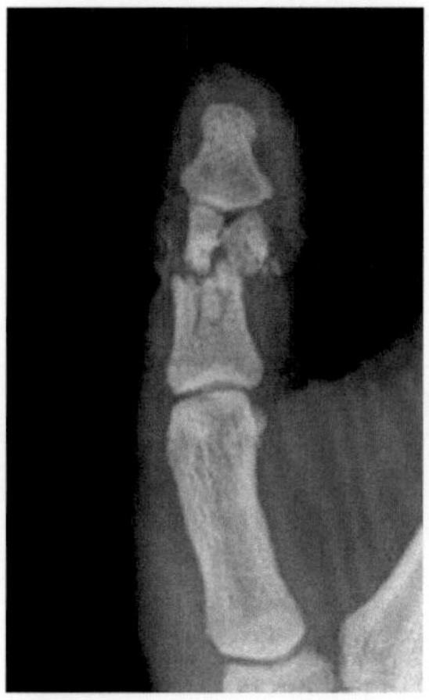

AO/OTA Classification of Hand Bone Fractures

78 Phalangeal fracture.

Type C: complete proximal or distal intraarticular, or comminuted shaft.

C3: complete distal intraarticular.

C3.2: simple intraarticular, metaphyseal comminuted

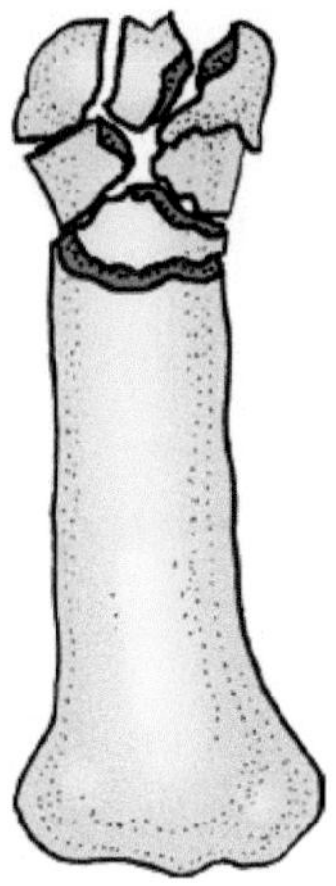

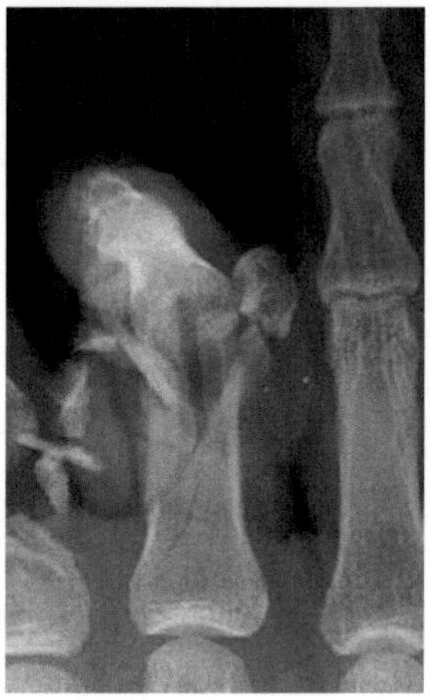

AO/OTA Classification of Hand Bone Fractures

78 Phalangeal fracture.

Type C: complete proximal or distal intraarticular, or comminuted shaft.

C3: complete distal intraarticular.

C3.3: intraarticular comminuted

79 Multiple phalanges
Type C: Multiple phalangeal fractures

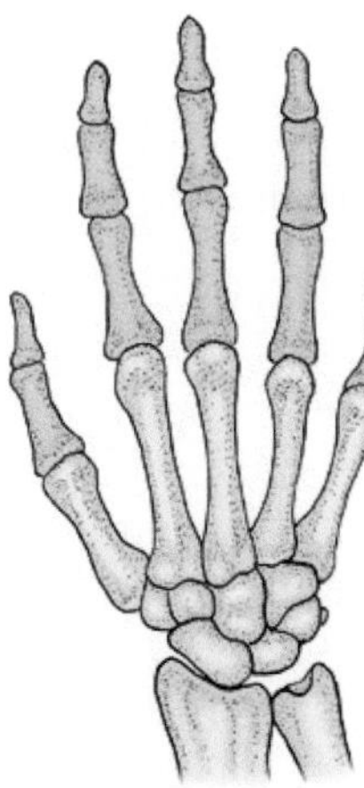

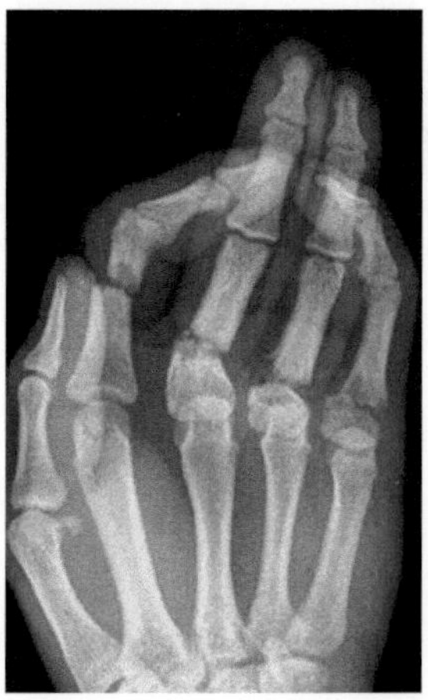

AO/OTA Classification of Hand Bone Fractures

79 Multiple Phalanges.

Type C: Multiple phalangeal fractures

4.1.2.2 Schenck Classification of Fractures of Interphalangeal Joint [3]

The classification expresses as a percentage of articular involvement.

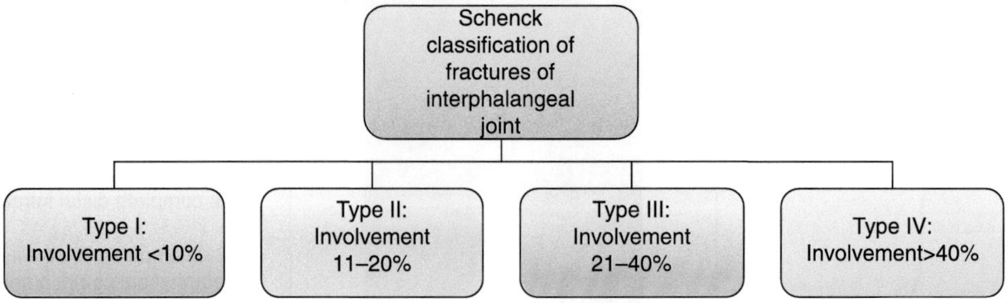

Type I: Involvement <10%.
Type II: Involvement 11–20%.
Type III: Involvement 21–40%.
Type IV: Involvement >40%.

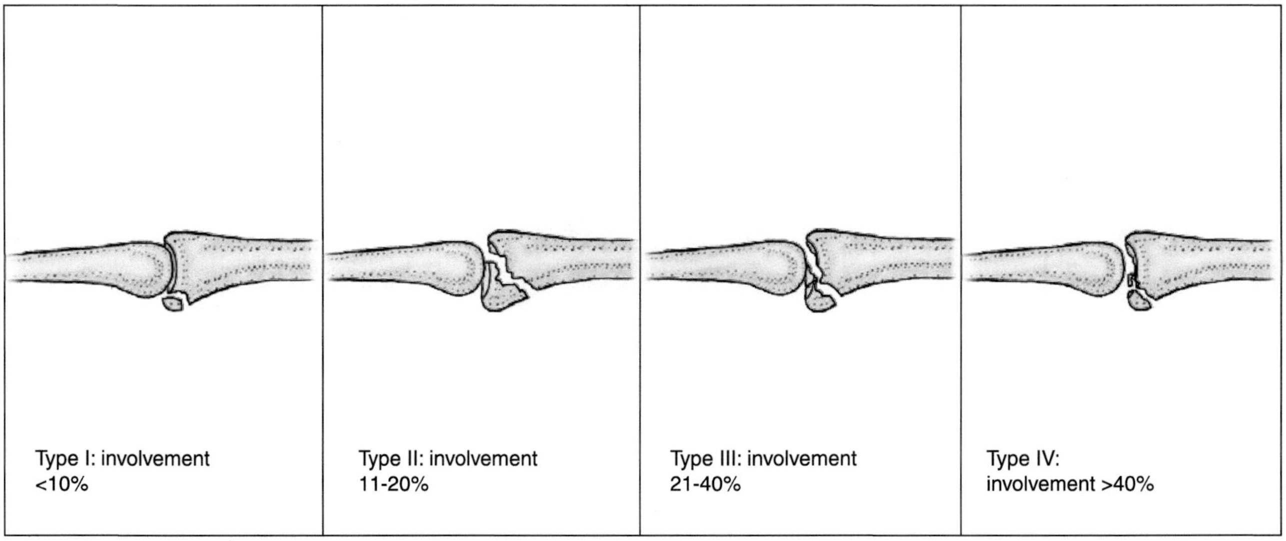

4.1.2.3 London Classification of Condyle Fracture [4]

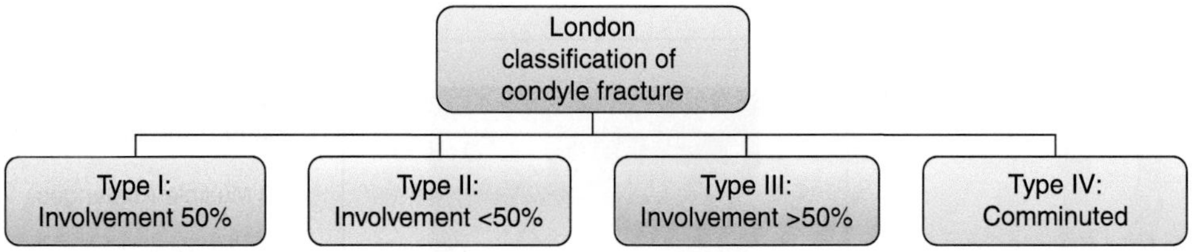

Type I: Involvement 50%.
Type II: Involvement <50%.
Type III: Involvement >50%.
Type IV: Comminuted.

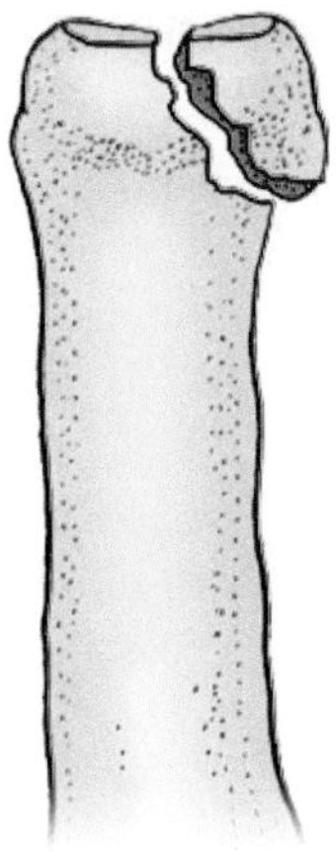

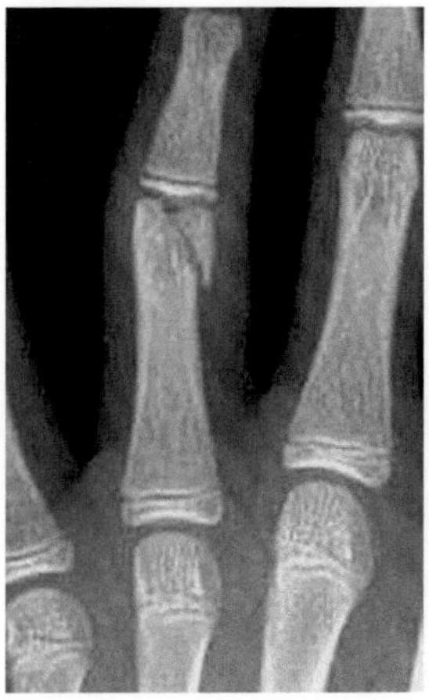

London Classification of Condyle Fracture

Type I: involvement 50%

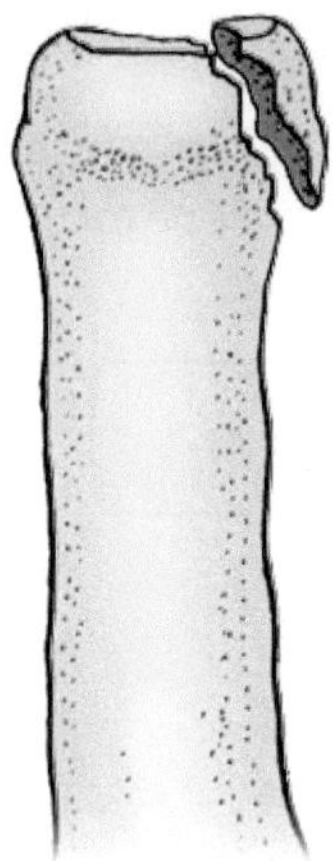

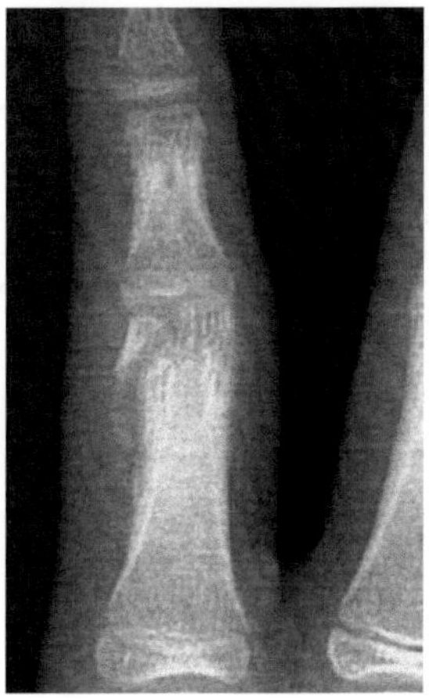

London Classification of Condyle Fracture

Type II: involvement <50%

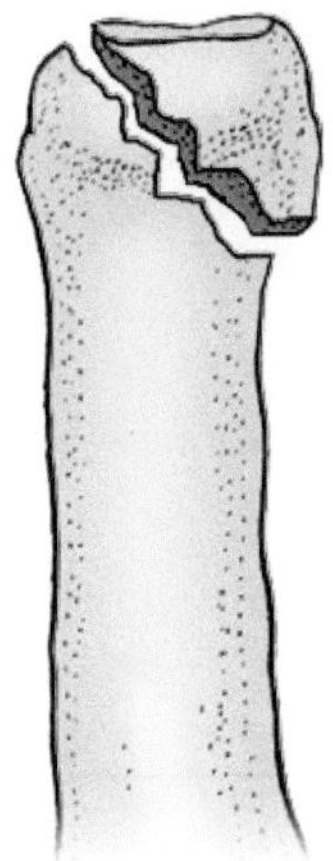

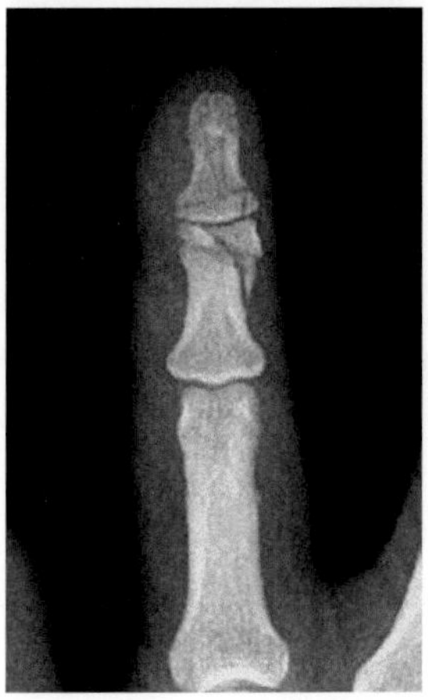

London Classification of Condyle Fracture

Type III: involvement >50%

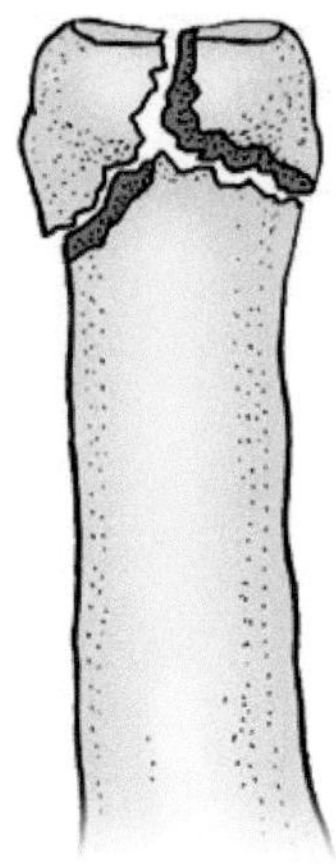

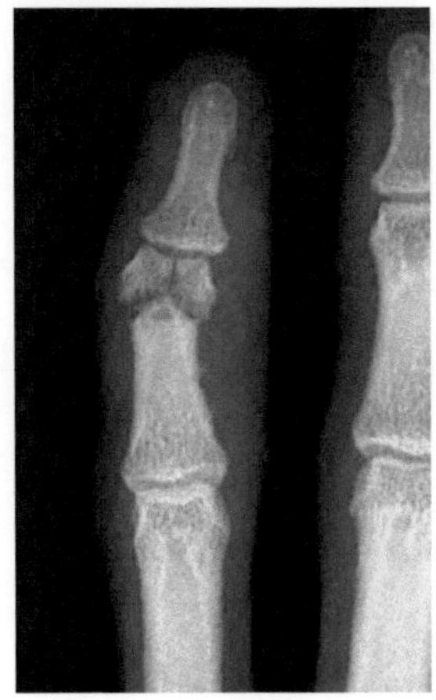

London Classification of Condyle Fracture

Type IV: comminuted

4.1.2.4 Classification of Distal Phalangeal Fracture

Kaplan Classification of Distal Phalangeal Fracture [5]

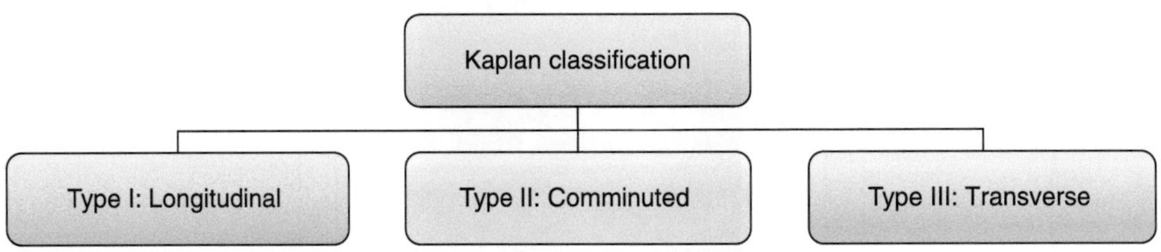

Type I: Longitudinal.
Type II: Comminuted.
Type III: Transverse.

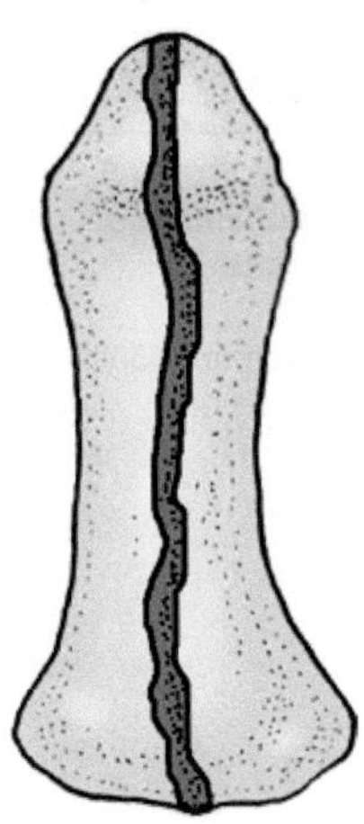

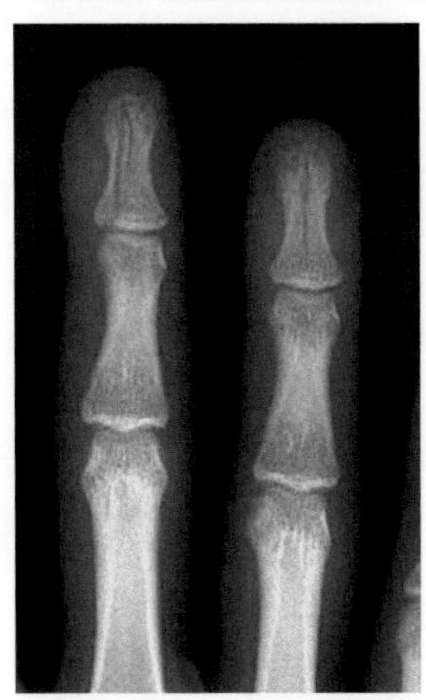

Kaplan Classification of Distal Phalangeal Fracture

Type I: longitudinal

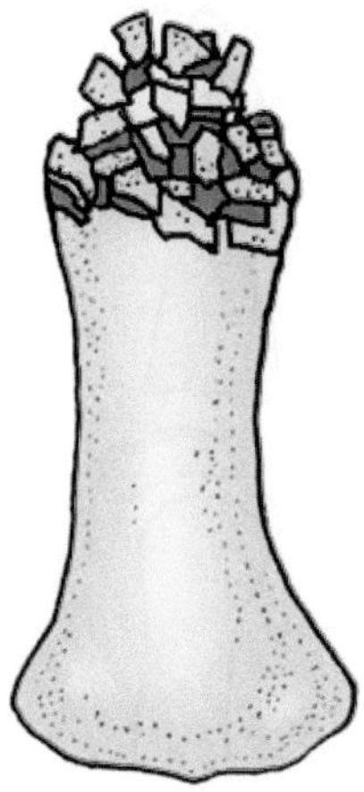

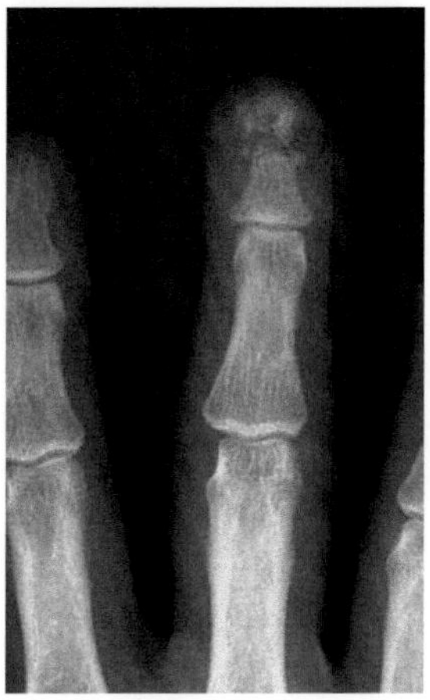

Kaplan Classification of Distal Phalangeal Fracture

Type II: comminuted

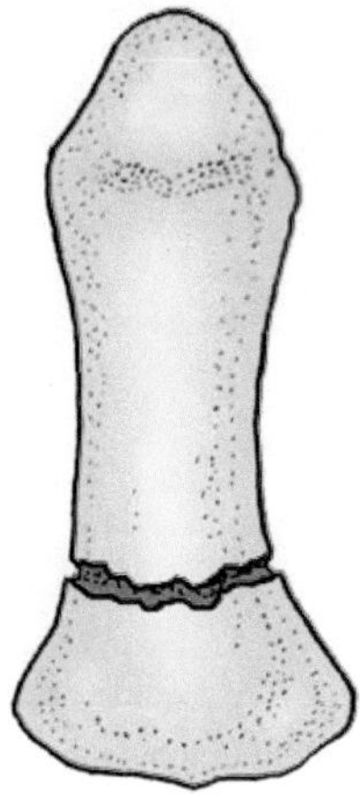

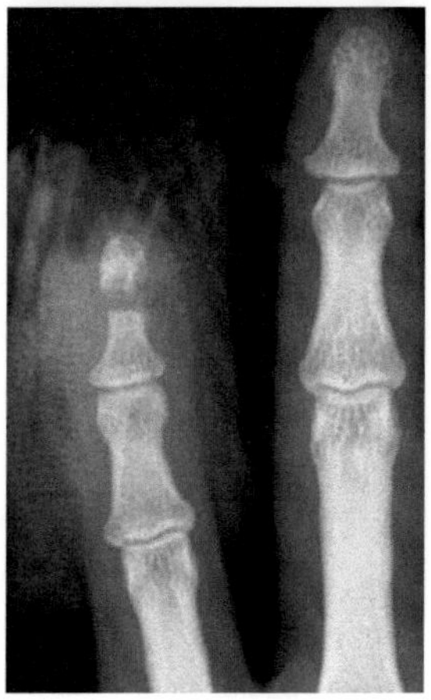

Kaplan Classification of Distal Phalangeal Fracture

Type III: transverse

Dobyns Classification of Distal Phalangeal Fracture [6]

Location	Closed	Open
Tip	Stable	Probably unstable with nailbed injuries
Shaft	Non-displaced	Probably unstable with nailbed injuries
Base	Probably unstable	Probably with rotation or angulation and with nailbed injuries

Wehbe-Schneider Classification of Bony Mallet Fractures [7]

Type	Description
I ABC	No DIP joint subluxation
II ABC	DIP joint subluxation
III ABC	Epiphyseal and physeal injuries
Subtype	Articular involvement
A	1/3
B	1/3–2/3
C	>2/3

DIP distal interphalangeal

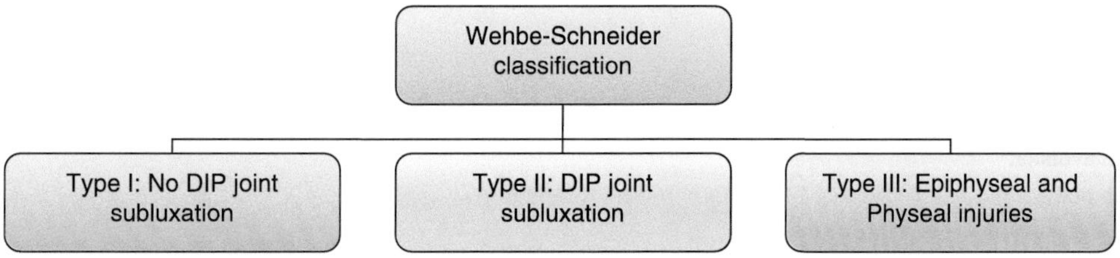

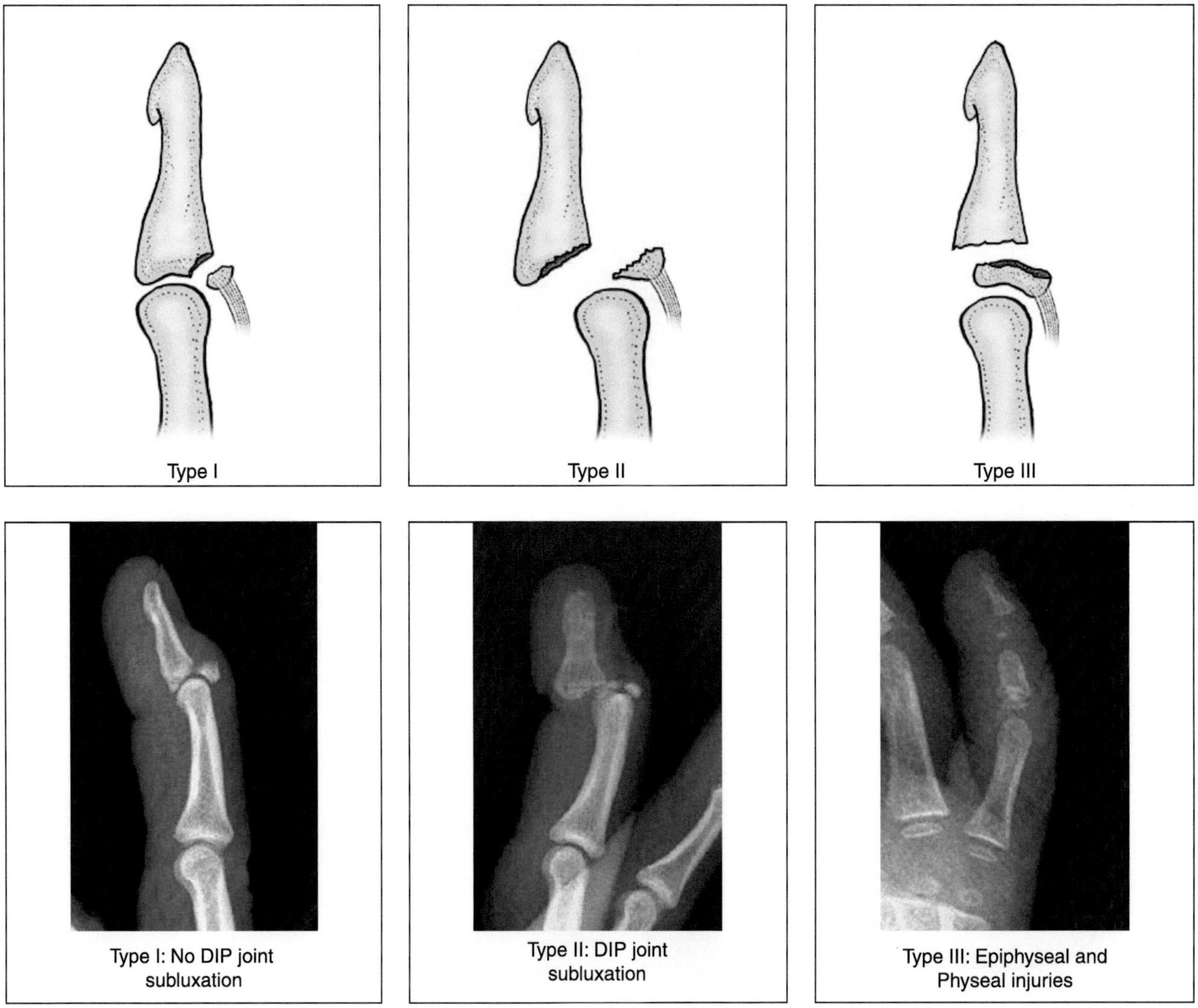

Classification of Mallet Injuries

Mallet injury classification			
I	Closed—tendon rupture		
II	Laceration		
III	Abrasion with tissue loss		
IV	With fracture	**IVa**	Without joint subluxation
		IVb	With joint subluxation
Also note:		Extension lag active___passive___	
		Swan neck? Y___N___	
		X-ray abnormalities:	

Distal Interphalangeal Base Fracture

DIP Base Fractures

Profundus tendon avulsion
Mallet injuries
Collateral ligament avulsion
Comminuted/combined
Epiphyseal

Distal Interphalangeal Joint Injury

DIP Joint Fractures

Middle phalangeal head fractures
Distal phalangeal base fractures
DIP biarticular fractures

Distal Phalanx Fracture Staging

Distal phalanx fractures		
Beneath sterile matrix	Simple	Non-displaced
		Displaced

4.1.3 Classification of Injuries of Hand

4.1.3.1 Duncan Open Phalangeal Fracture Wound Classification

Type I	Tidy laceration less than 1 cm in length, no soiling, no soft-tissue loss or crush. Basically a puncture wound from within or without
Type II	Tidy laceration less than 2 cm in length, from outside in, no soiling, no soft-tissue crush or loss. Partial muscle laceration
Type IIIA	Laceration greater than 2 cm. Penetrating or puncturing projectile wound. Any frankly soiled wound
Type III B	Same as IIIA + any periosteal elevation or stripping
Type IIIC	Same as IIIB + neurovascular injury

4.1.3.2 Blast Injuries of the Hand [8]

Type I	Distal phalanx or soft tissue only
Type II	Flexor tendon zone II fracture or web space laceration
Type III	Zone II Amp/degloved/devascularized or tendon injury
Type IV	Carpal or metacarpal fracture/dislocation/amputation

4.1.3.3 Tic Tac Toe Classification

Mutilating hand injuries may be classified by this scheme of orientation, wound type, and zone of injury:

Orientation		Wound subtype	
Type I	Dorsal	Type A	Soft-tissue loss
Type II	Palmar	Type B	Bony loss
Type III	Ulnar	Type C	Combined tissue loss
Type IV	Radial	1	Vascularized
Type V	Transverse	2	Devascularized
Type VI	Degloving		
Type VII	Combined		

Zone of injury

Zone	Radial	Central	Ulnar
Distal	I	II	III
	Thumb P1, P2	Index, MIDDLE P1, P2, P3	Ring, small P1, P2, P3
Central	IV	V	VI
	Thumb metacarpal	Index, middle metacarpal	Ring, small metacarpal
Proximal	VII	VII	IX
	Scaphoid, trapezium, trapezoid	Capitate, lunate	Hamate, triquetrum, pisiform

4.1.3.4 Wound Classification

Tidy	Incised	
	Sliced	With flaps
		With tissue loss
Untidy	Contusion	
	Burn	Thermal
		Chemical
		Mechanical/abrasion
	Contortion	Crush
		Avulsion
		Torsion
		Traction
	Toothed blade	
	Injection	
	Multiple level	
	Indeterminate viabil	

4.1.3.5 Gustilo Classification of Open Fracture

Type I	Low energy, wound less than 1 cm	
Type II	Wound greater than 1 cm with moderate soft-tissue damage	
Type III	High-energy wound greater than 1 cm with extensive soft-tissue damage	
	IIIA	Adequate soft-tissue cover
	IIIB	Inadequate soft-tissue cover
	IIIC	Associated with arterial injury

4.2 Section 2 Classifications of Carpal Bone Fractures

Over ten classifications of carpal bone fractures have been reported. AO/OTA classification is the most commonly used in clinical practice.

4.2.1 AO/OTA Classification of Carpal Bone Fractures

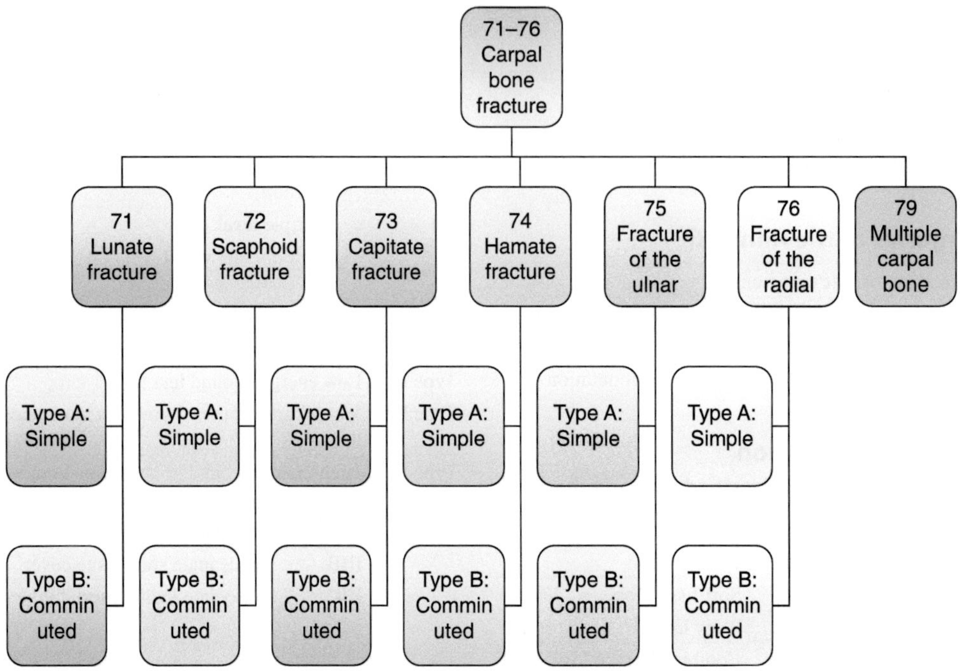

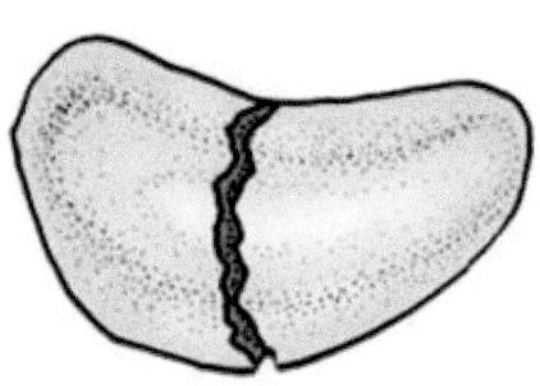

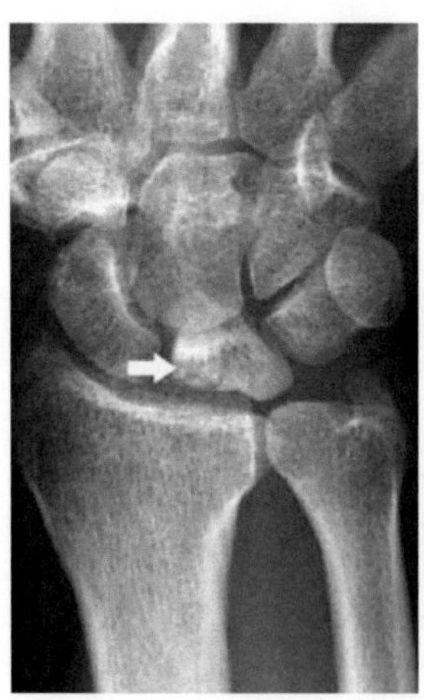

AO/OTA Classification of Carpal Bone Fractures

71 Lunate fracture.

Type A: Simple

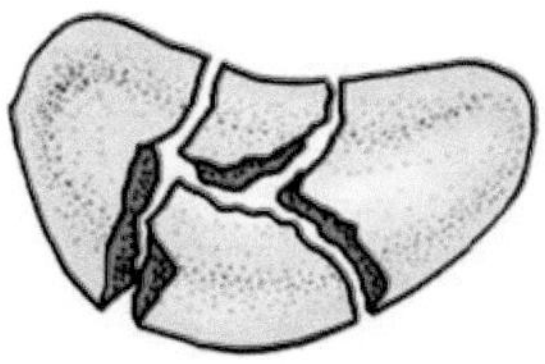

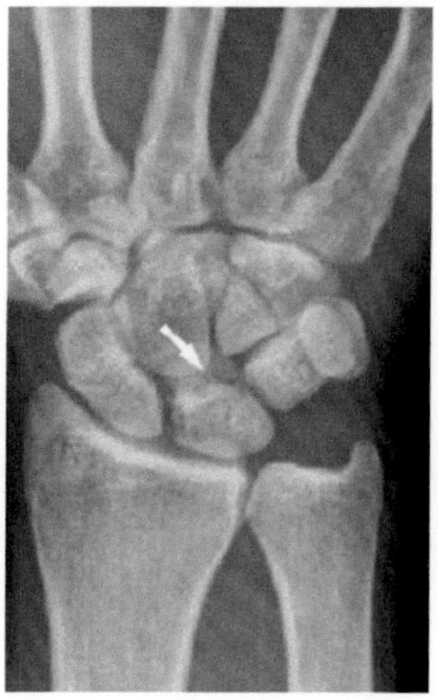

AO/OTA Classification of Carpal Bone Fractures

71 Lunate fracture.

Type B: Comminuted

72 Scaphoid fracture:
- Type A: Simple:
  - A1: Proximal pole.
  - A2: Waist.
  - A3: Distal pole.
- Type B: Comminuted:
  - B1: Proximal pole.
  - B2: Waist.
  - B3: Distal pole.

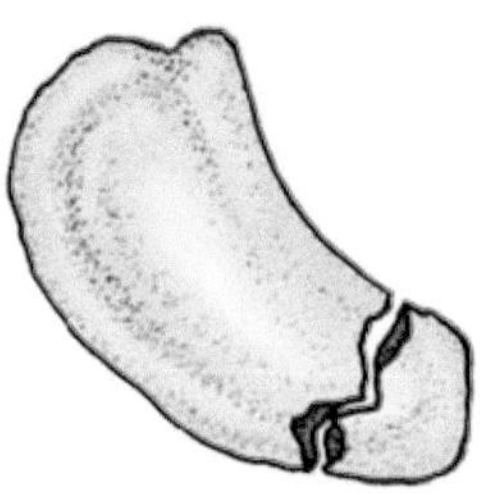

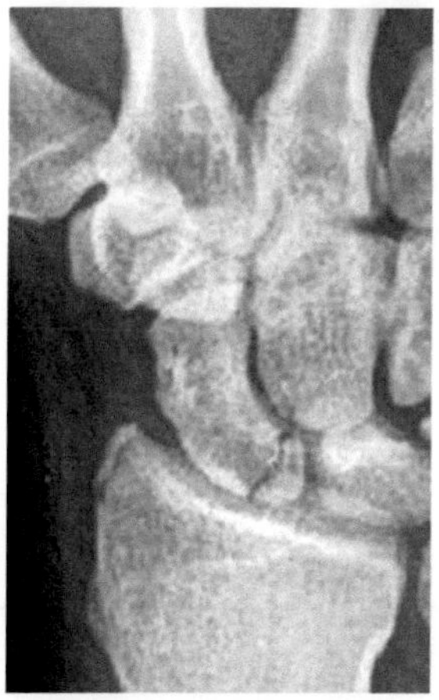

AO/OTA Classification of Carpal Bone Fractures

72 Scaphoid fracture.

Type A: Simple.

A1: proximal pole

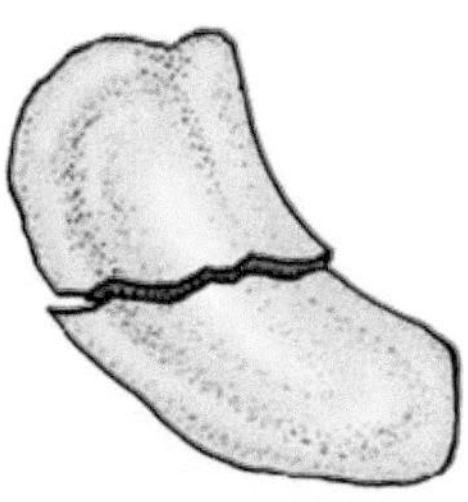

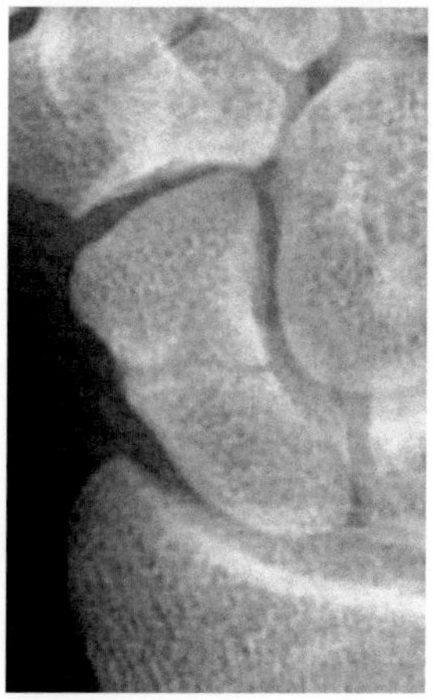

AO/OTA Classification of Carpal Bone Fractures

72 Scaphoid fracture.

Type A: Simple.

A2: waist

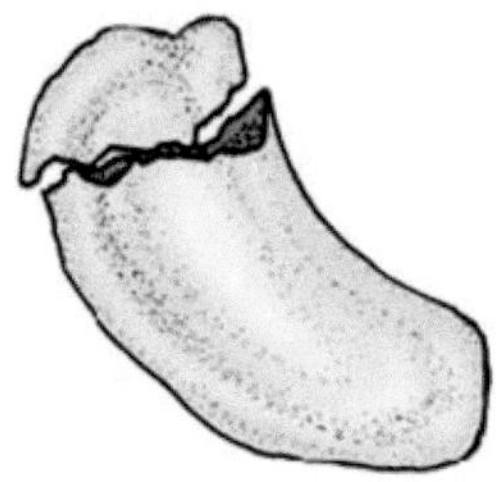

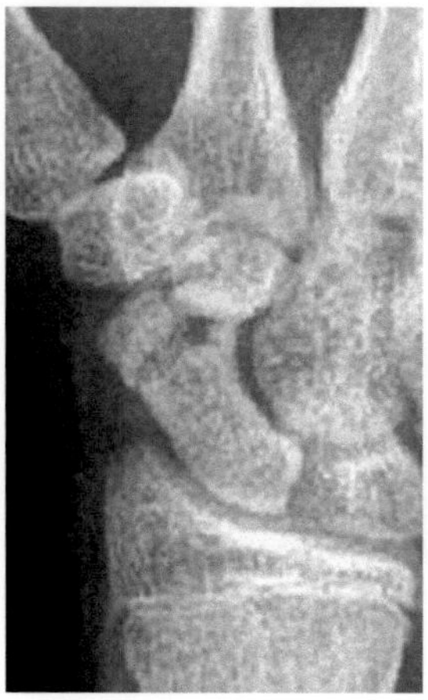

AO/OTA Classification of Carpal Bone Fractures

72 Scaphoid fracture.

Type A: Simple.

A3: distal pole

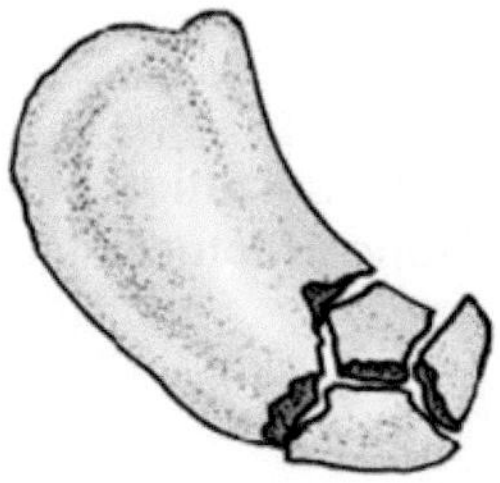

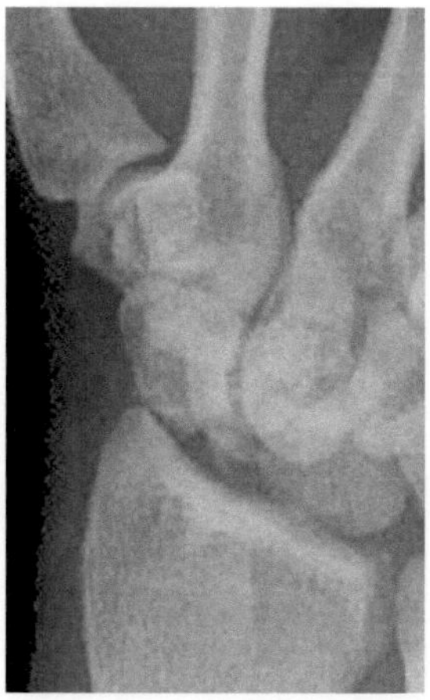

AO/OTA Classification of Carpal Bone Fractures

72 Scaphoid fracture.

Type B: Comminuted.

B1: proximal pole

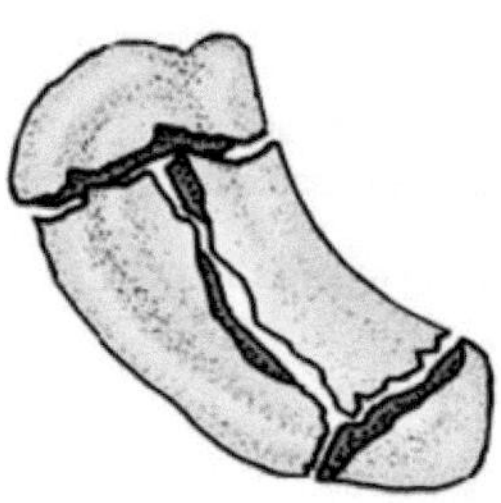

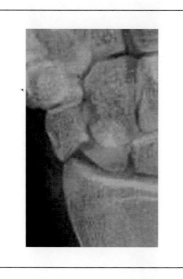

AO/OTA Classification of Carpal Bone Fractures

72 Scaphoid fracture.

Type B: Comminuted.

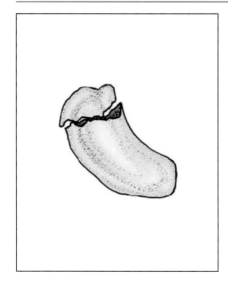

B2: waist

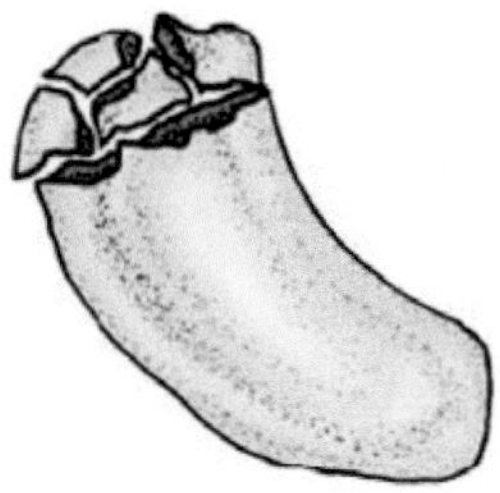

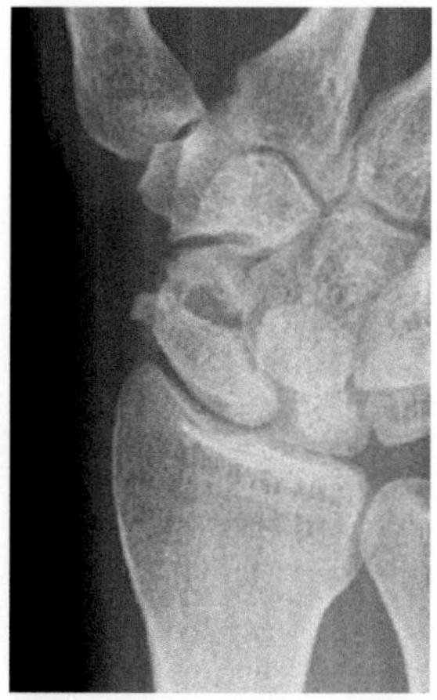

AO/OTA Classification of Carpal Bone Fractures

72 Scaphoid fracture.

Type B: Comminuted.

B3: distal pole

73 Capitate fracture:
Type A: Simple.
Type B: Comminuted.

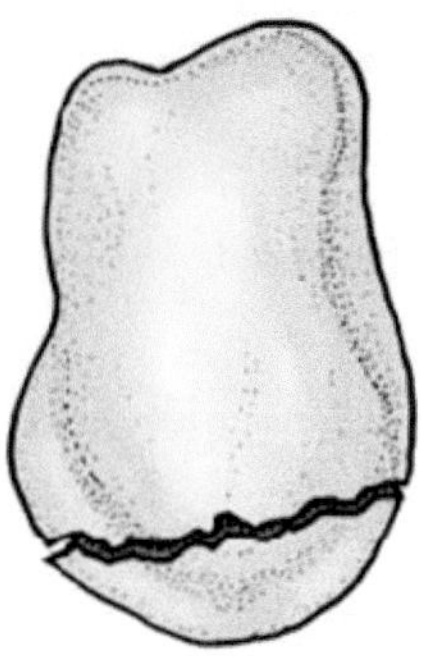

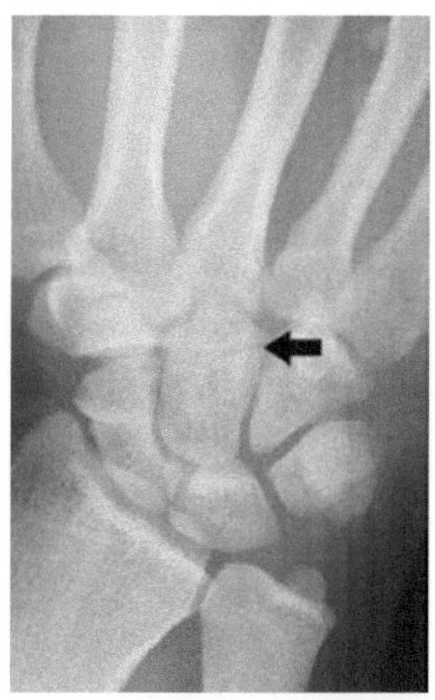

AO/OTA Classification of Carpal Bone Fractures

73 Capitate fracture.

Type A: Simple

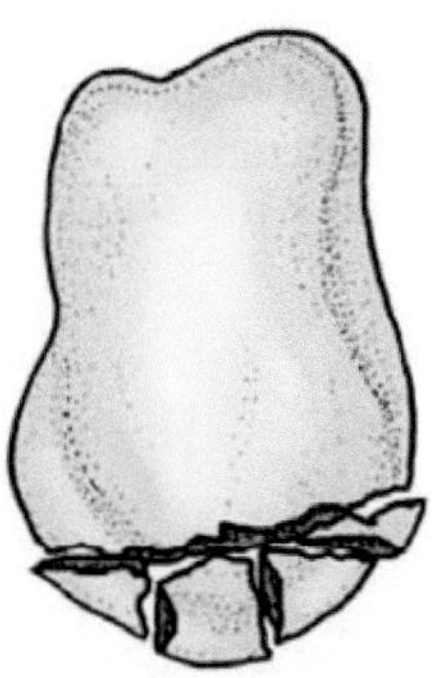

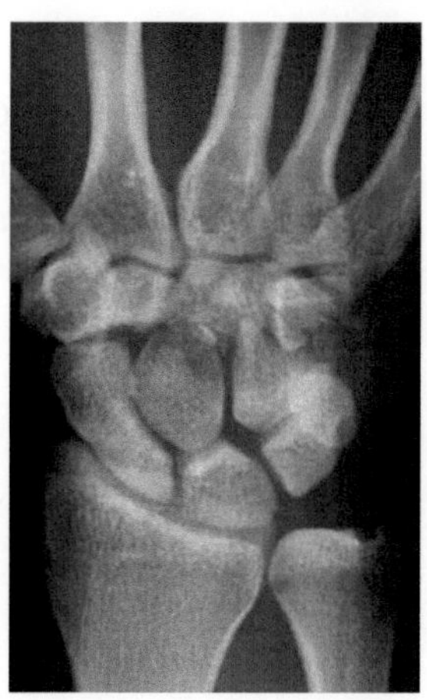

AO/OTA Classification of Carpal Bone Fractures

73 Capitate fracture.

Type B: Comminuted

74 Hamate fracture:
Type A: Simple.
Type B: Comminuted.

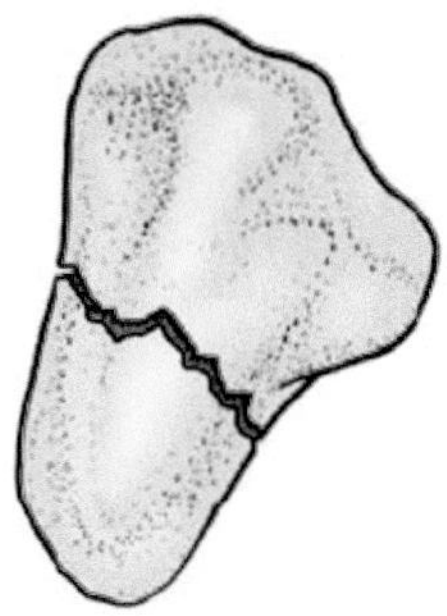

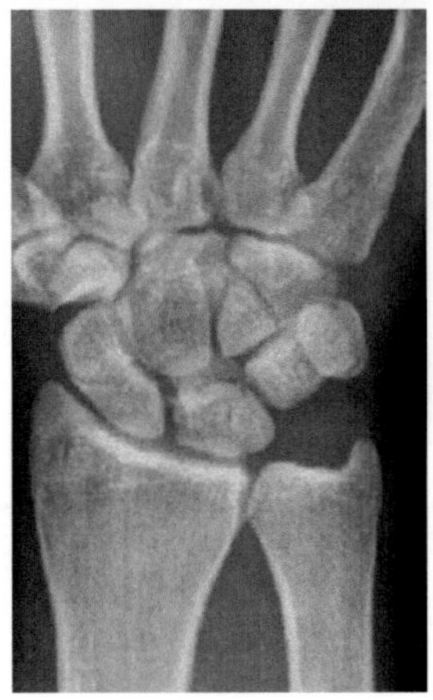

AO/OTA Classification of Carpal Bone Fractures

74 Hamate fracture.

Type A: Simple

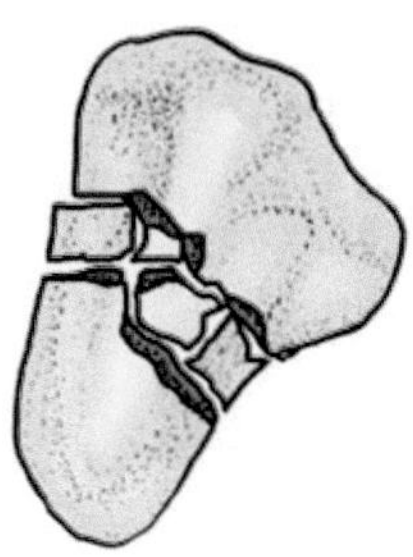

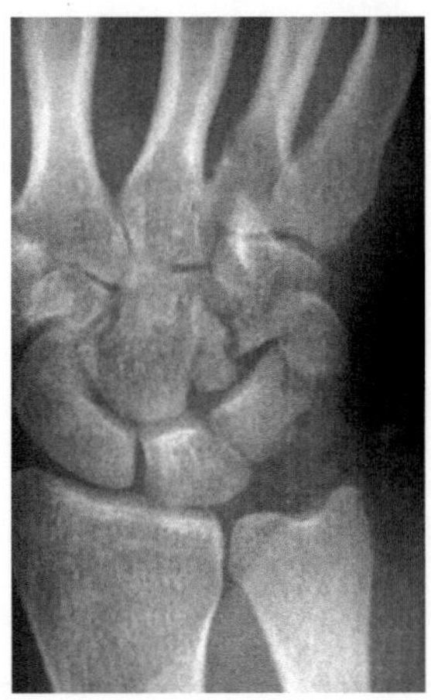

AO/OTA Classification of Carpal Bone Fractures

74 Hamate fracture.

Type B: Comminuted

75 Fracture of the ulnar carpal bone:
Type A: Simple:
A1: Pisiform fracture.
A2: Triquetral fracture.
Type B: Comminuted:
B1: Pisiform comminuted fracture.
B2: Triquetral comminuted fracture.

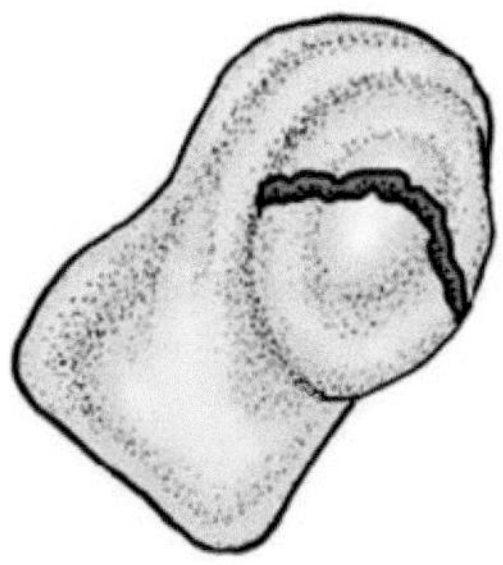

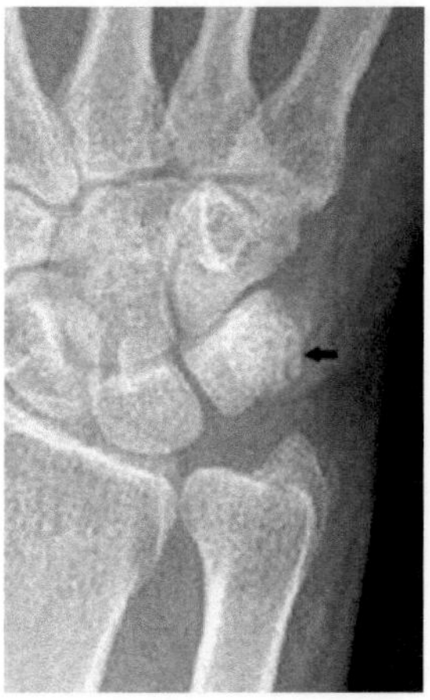

AO/OTA Classification of Carpal Bone Fractures

75 Fracture of the ulnar carpal bone.

Type A: Simple.

A1: pisiform fracture

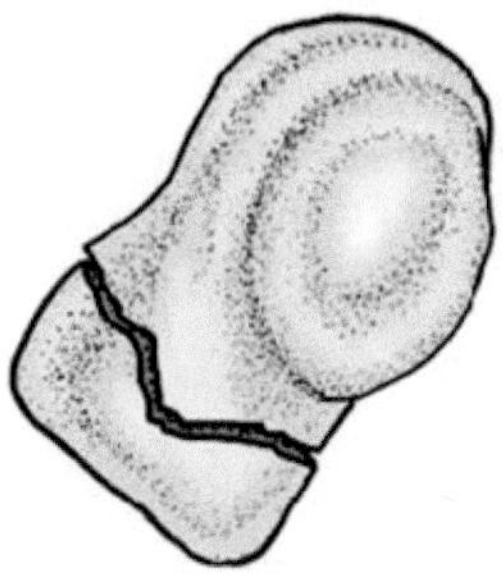

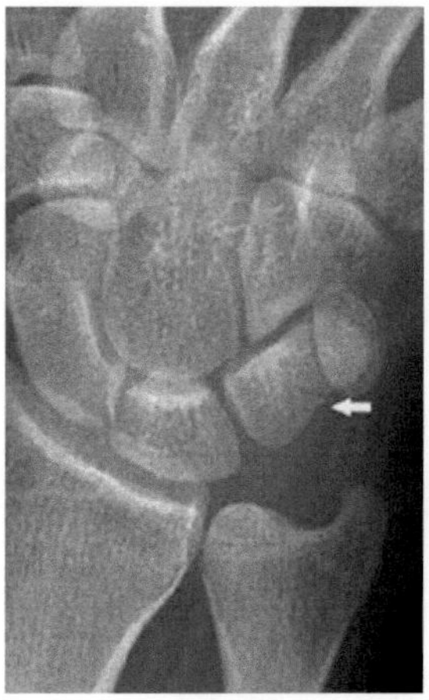

AO/OTA Classification of Carpal Bone Fractures

75 Fracture of the ulnar carpal bone.

Type A: Simple.

A2: triquetral fracture

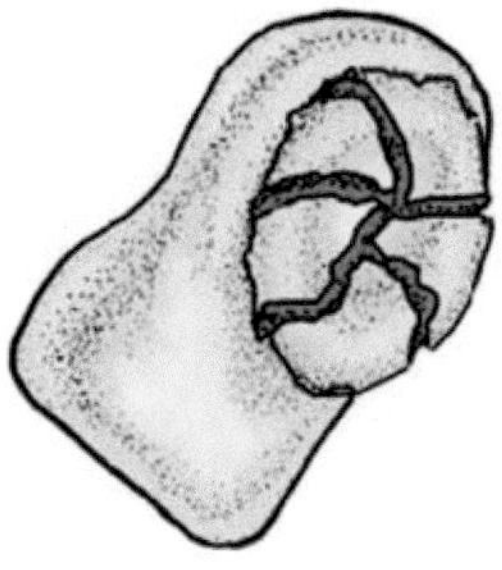

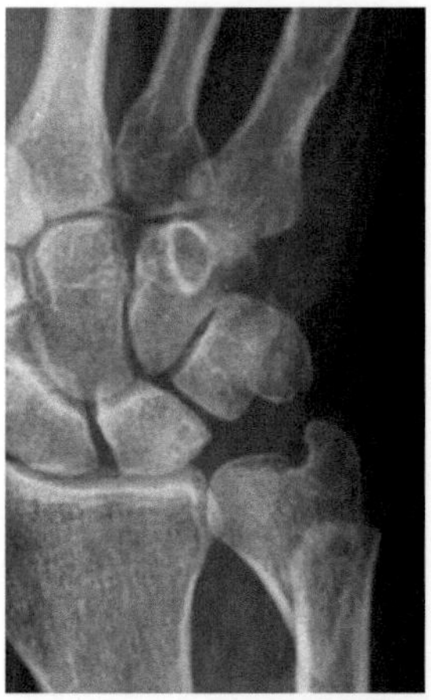

AO/OTA Classification of Carpal Bone Fractures

75 Fracture of the ulnar carpal bone.

Type B: Comminuted.

B1: pisiform comminuted fracture

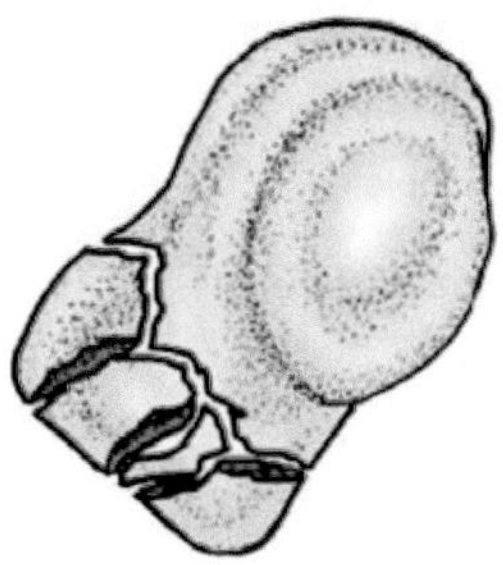

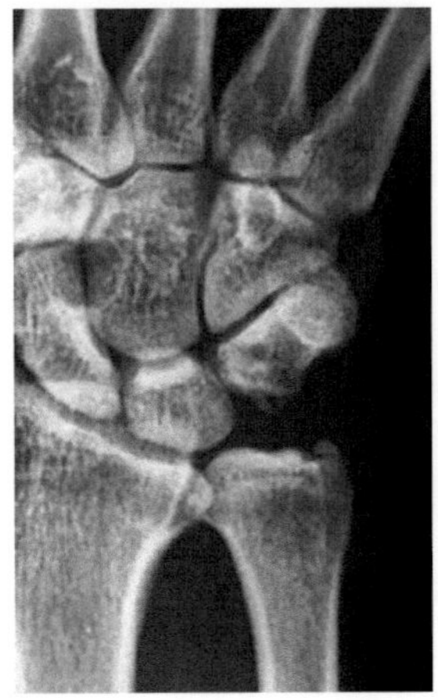

AO/OTA Classification of Carpal Bone Fractures

75 Fracture of the ulnar carpal bone.

Type B: Comminuted.

B2: triquetral comminuted fracture

76 Fracture of the radial carpal bone:
- Type A: Simple:
  - A1: Trapezium fracture.
  - A2: Trapezoid fracture.
- Type B: Comminuted:
  - B1: Trapezium fracture.
  - B2: Trapezoid fracture.

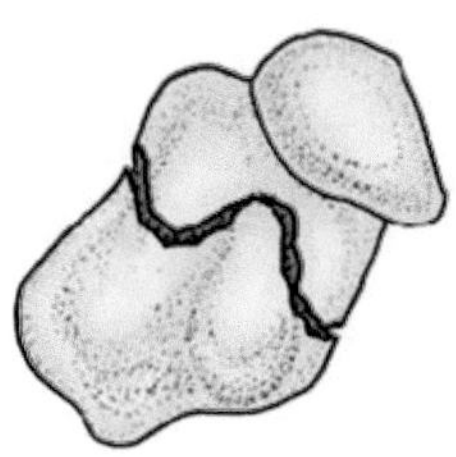

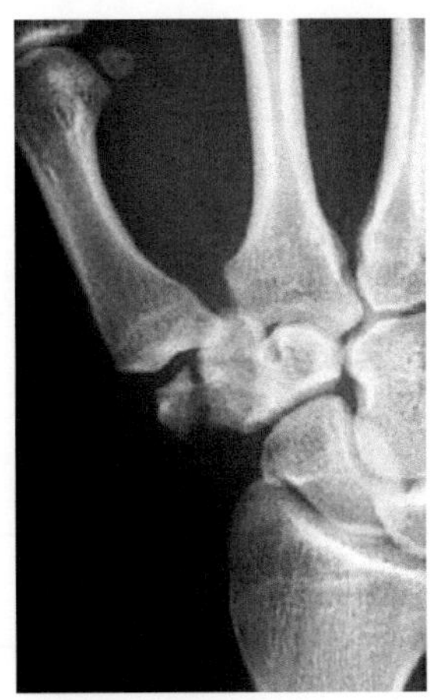

AO/OTA Classification of Carpal Bone Fractures

76 Fracture of the radial carpal bone.

Type A: Simple.

A1: trapezium fracture

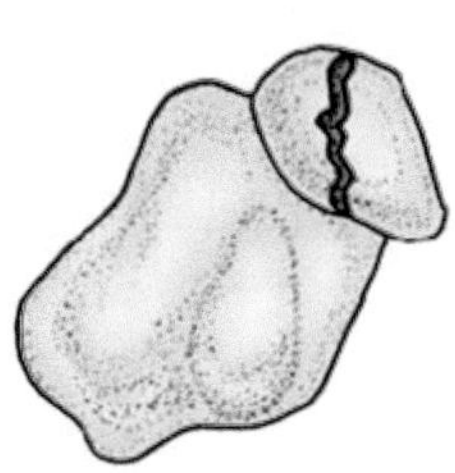

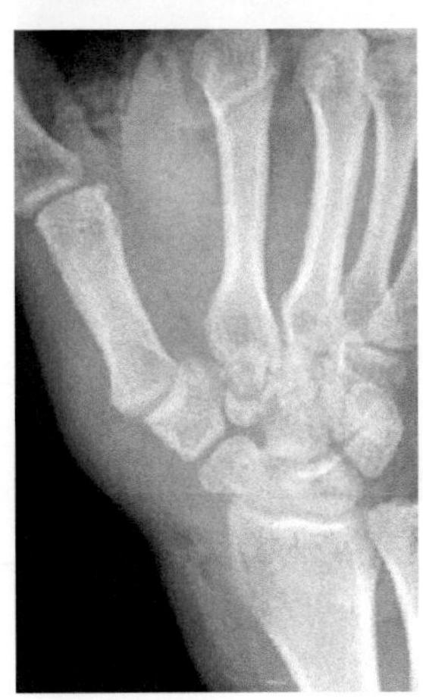

AO/OTA Classification of Carpal Bone Fractures

76 Fracture of the radial carpal bone.

Type A: Simple.

A2: trapezoid fracture

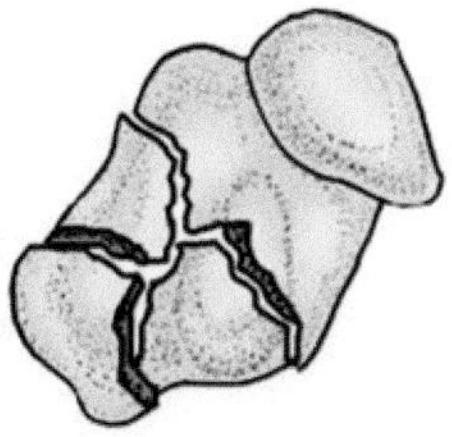

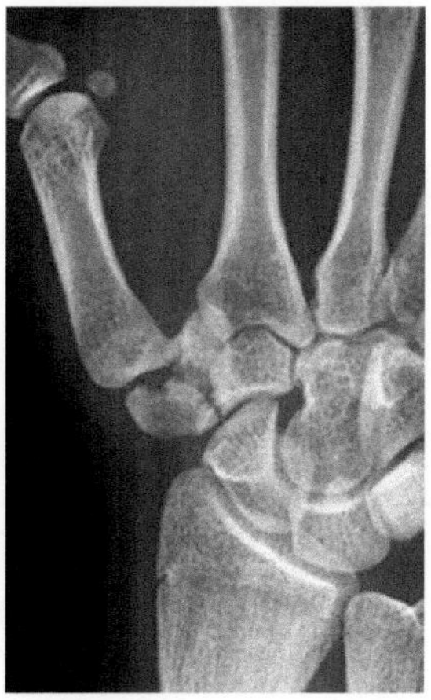

AO/OTA Classification of Carpal Bone Fractures

76 Fracture of the radial carpal bone.

Type B: Comminuted.

B1: trapezium comminuted fracture

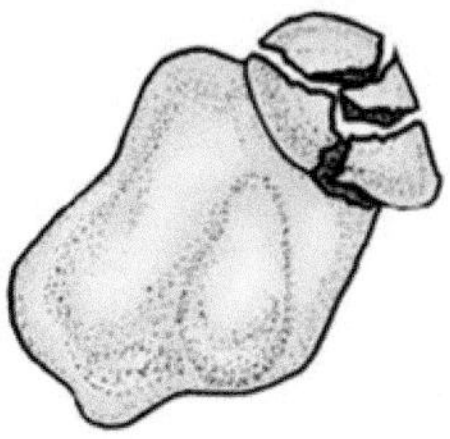

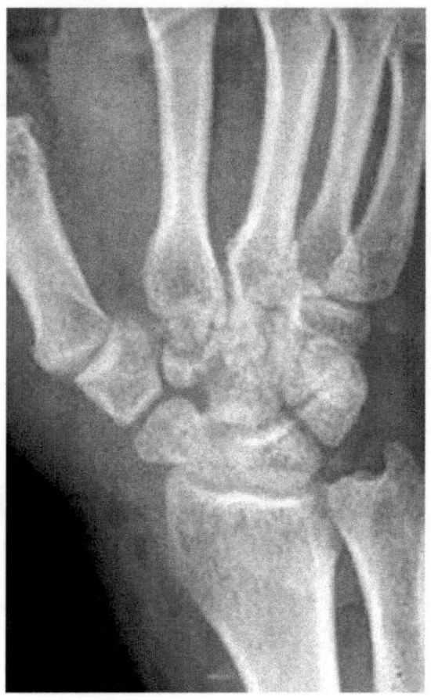

AO/OTA Classification of Carpal Bone Fractures

76 Fracture of the radial carpal bone.

Type B: Comminuted.

B2: trapezoid comminuted fracture

79 Multiple carpal bone fractures (type A)
Type A Multiple fractures

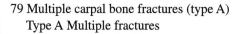

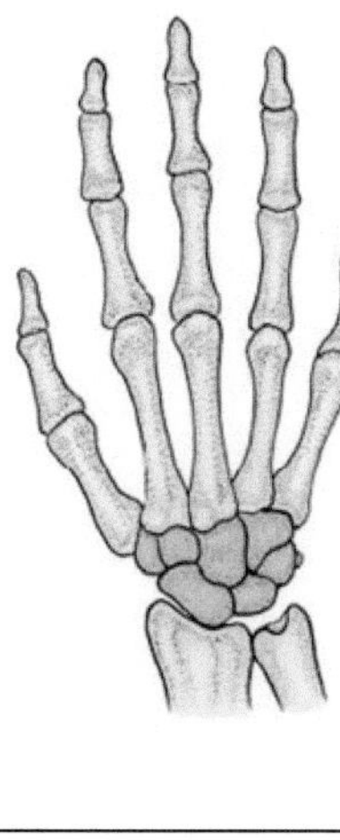

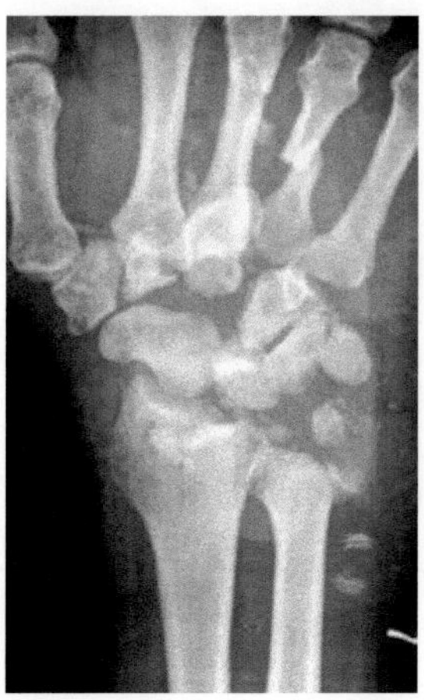

AO/OTA Classification of Carpal Bone Fractures

79 Multiple carpal bone fractures.

Type A: Multiple fractures

4.2.2 Classification of Carpal Bone Fracture

4.2.2.1 Scaphoid Fracture

Herbert Classification of Scaphoid Fracture [9]

Scaphoid fractures are classified based on stability of fracture. Unstable fractures are characterized by a displacement over 1 mm or an angulation over 5 degrees.

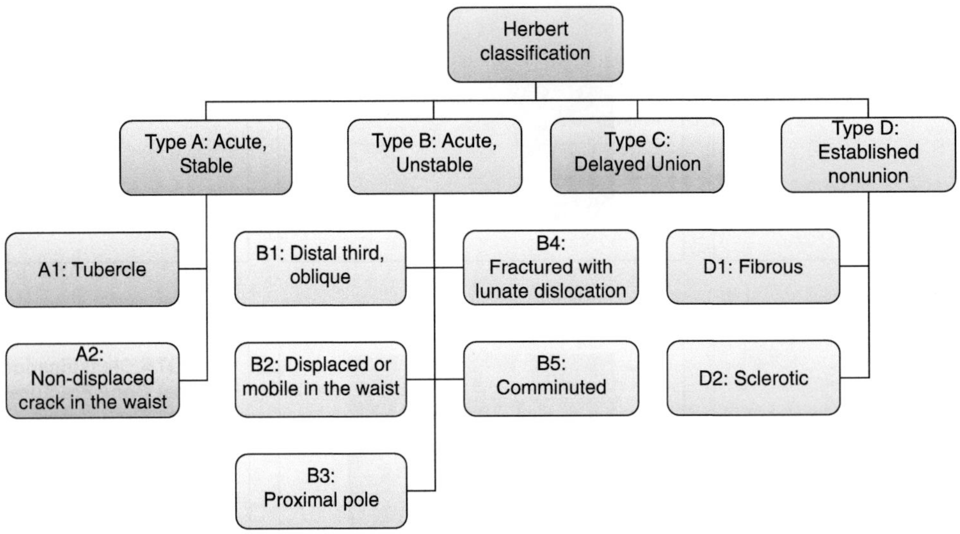

Type A: Acute, stable:
- A1: Tubercle.
- A2: Non-displaced crack in the waist.

Type B: Acute, unstable:
- B1: Oblique, distal third.
- B2: Displaced or mobile, waist.
- B3: Proximal pole.
- B4: Fracture–dislocation.
- B5: Comminuted.

Type C: Delayed union.

Type D: Established nonunion:
- D1: Fibrous.
- D2: Sclerotic.

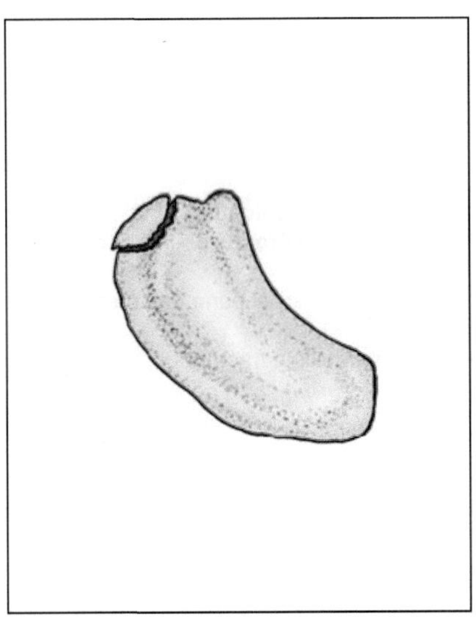

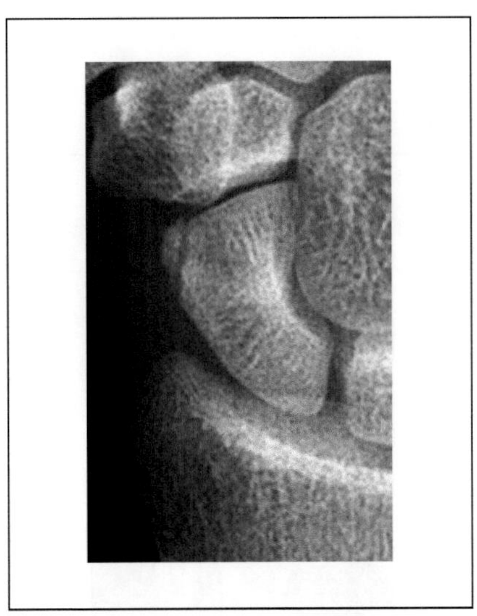

Herbert Classification of Scaphoid Fracture

Type A: Acute, Stable.

A1: Tubercle

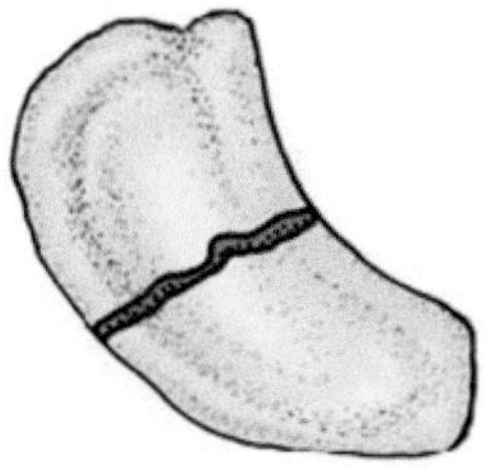

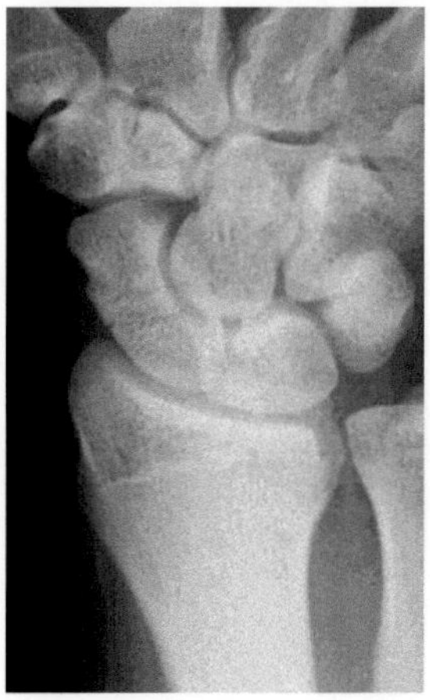

Herbert Classification of Scaphoid Fracture

Type A: Acute, Stable.

A2: Nondisplaced crack in the waist

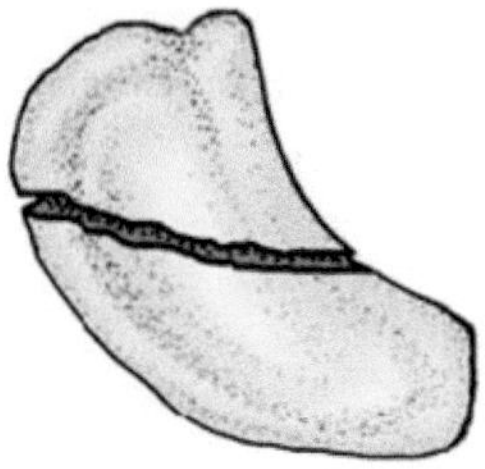

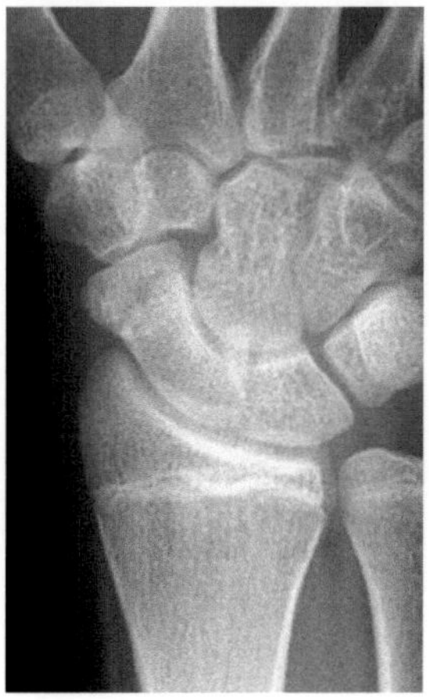

Herbert Classification of Scaphoid Fracture

Type B: Acute, Unstable.

B1: Distal third, oblique

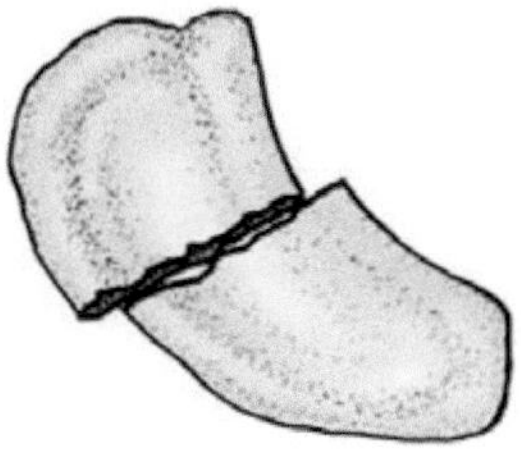

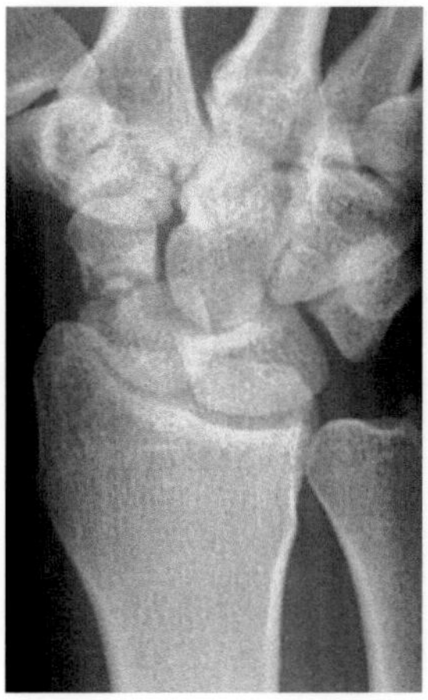

Herbert Classification of Scaphoid Fracture

Type B: Acute, Unstable.

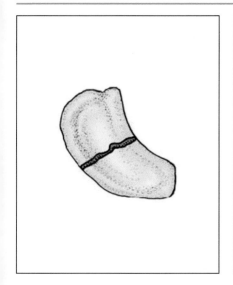

B2: Displaced or mobile, waist

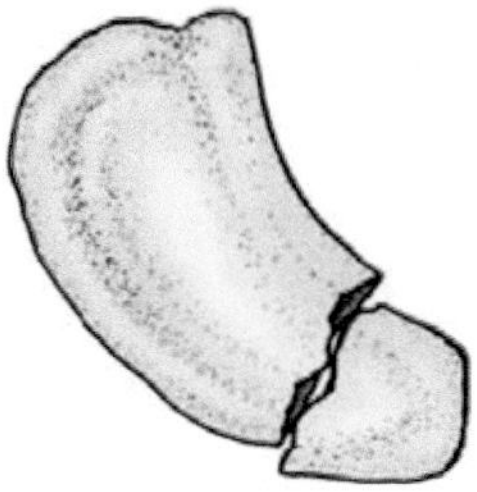

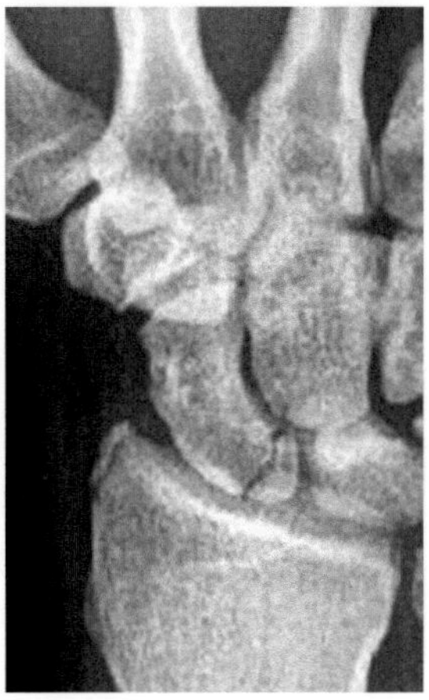

Herbert Classification of Scaphoid Fracture

Type B: Acute, Unstable.

B3: Proximal pole

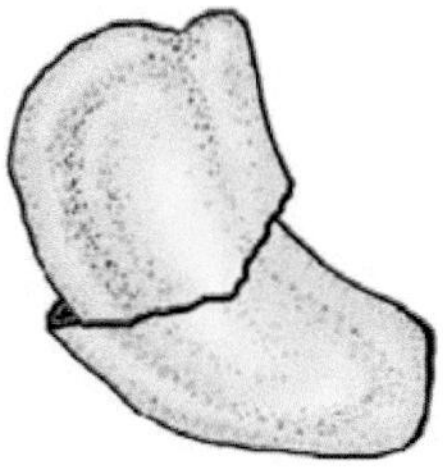

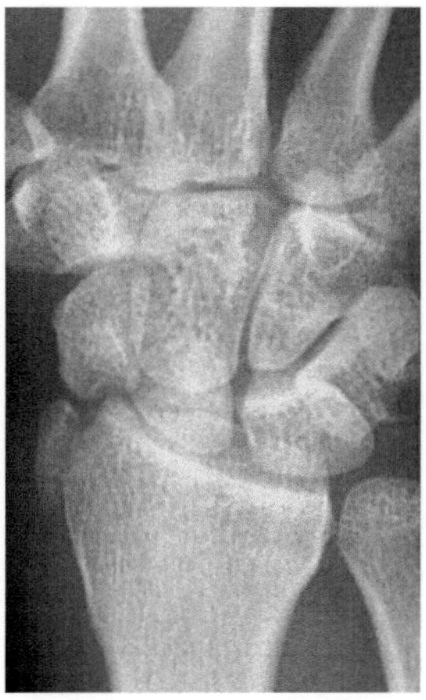

Herbert Classification of Scaphoid Fracture

Type B: Acute, Unstable.

B4: Fracture with lunate Dislocation

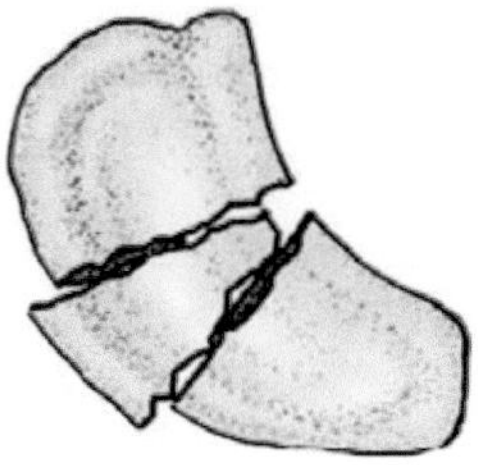

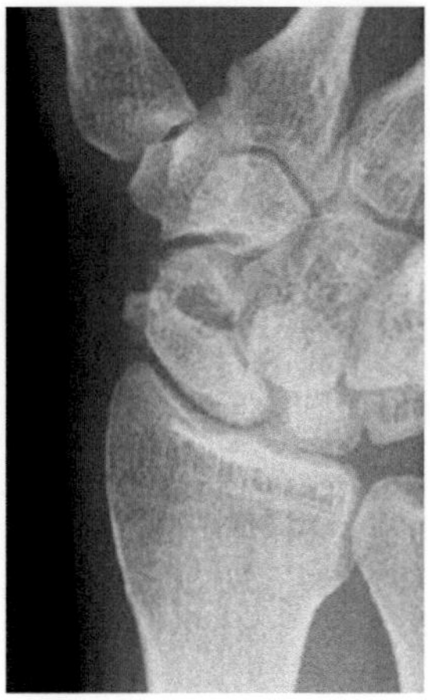

Herbert Classification of Scaphoid Fracture

Type B: Acute, Unstable.

B5: Comminuted

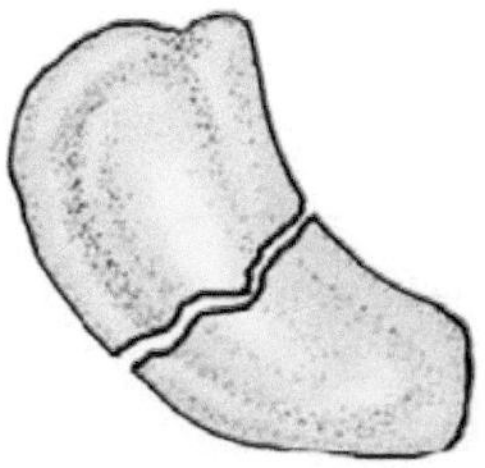

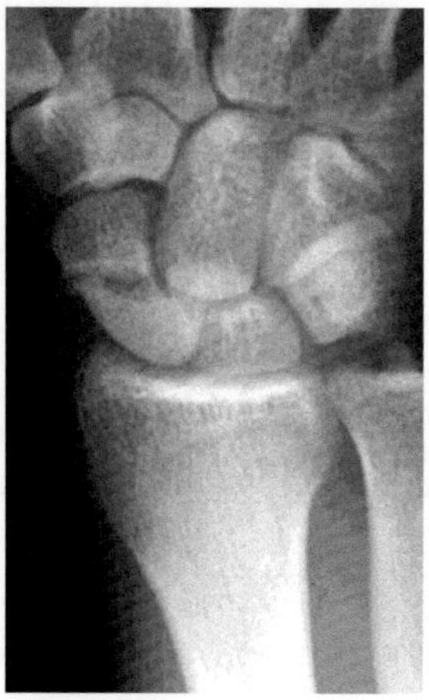

Herbert Classification of Scaphoid Fracture

Type C: Delayed Union

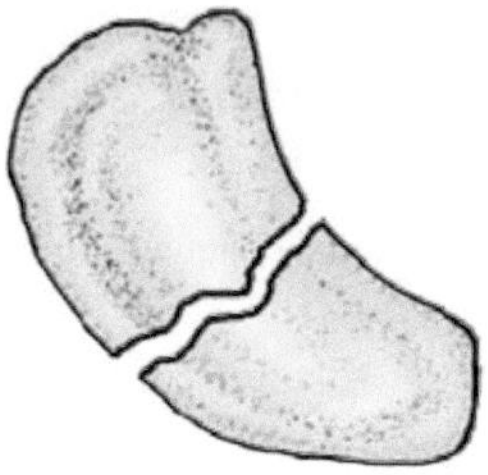

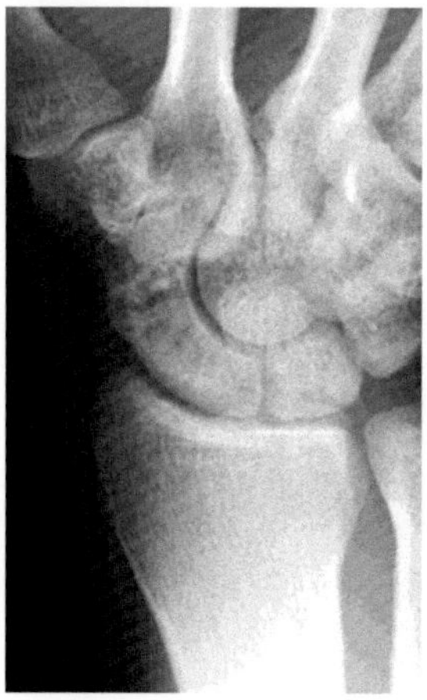

Herbert Classification of Scaphoid Fracture

Type D: Established nonunion.

D1: Fibrous

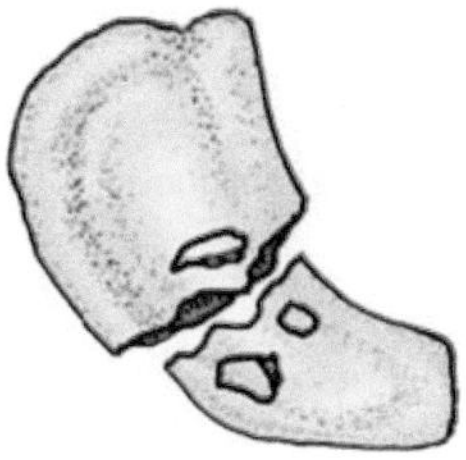

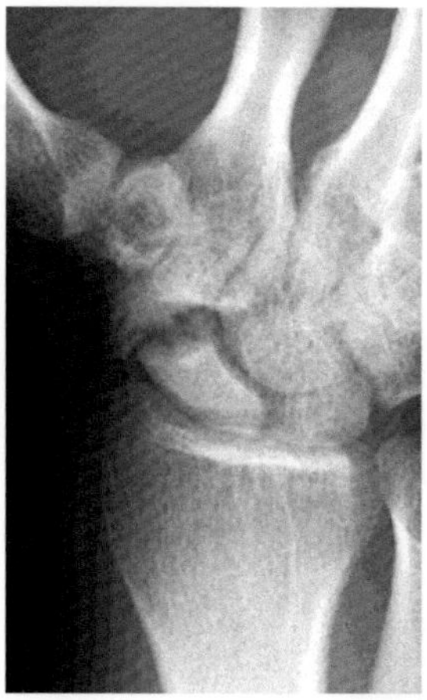

Herbert Classification of Scaphoid Fracture

Type D: Established nonunion.

D2: Sclerotic

Russe Classification of Scaphoid Fracture [10]

Russe classification uses the inclination of the fracture line to guide the risk of fracture instability.

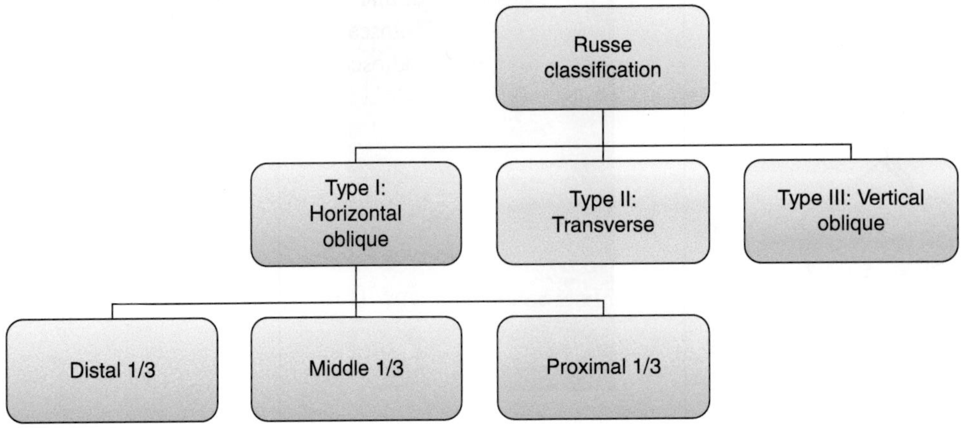

Type I: Horizontal oblique.
- Distal 1/3.
- Middle 1/3.
- Proximal 1/3.

Type II: Transverse.

Type III: Vertical oblique.

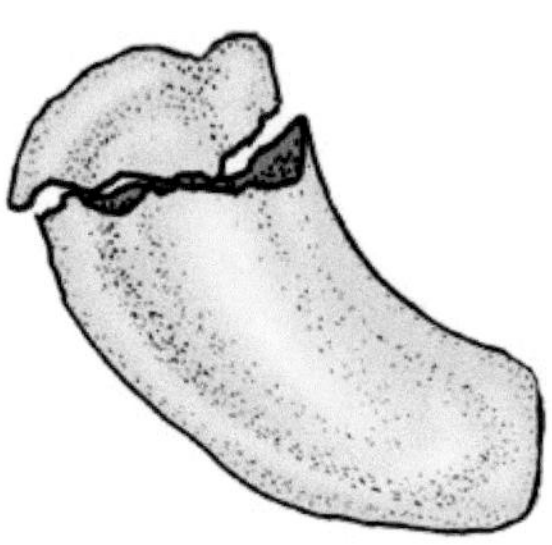

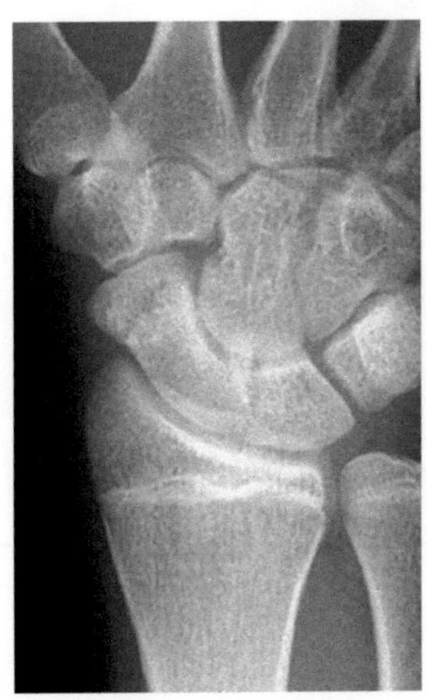

Russe Classification of Scaphoid Fracture

Type I: Horizontal oblique.

Distal 1/3

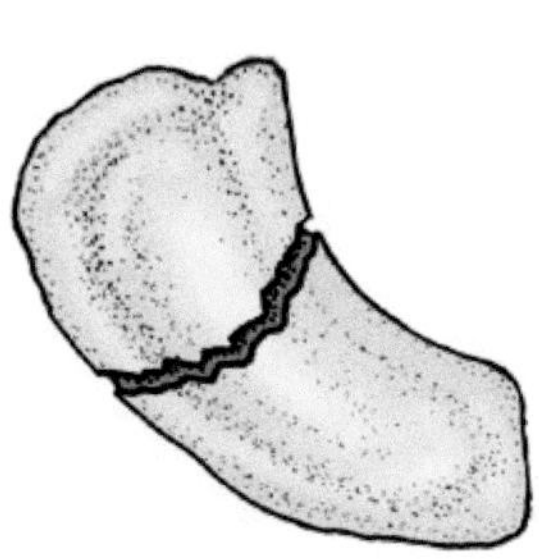

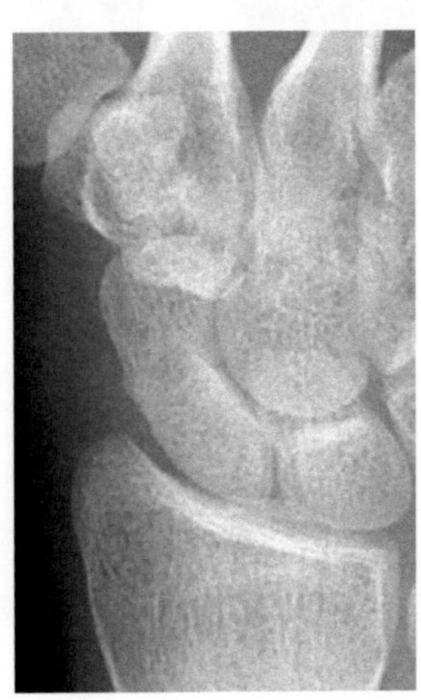

Russe Classification of Scaphoid Fracture

Type I: Horizontal oblique.

Middle 1/3

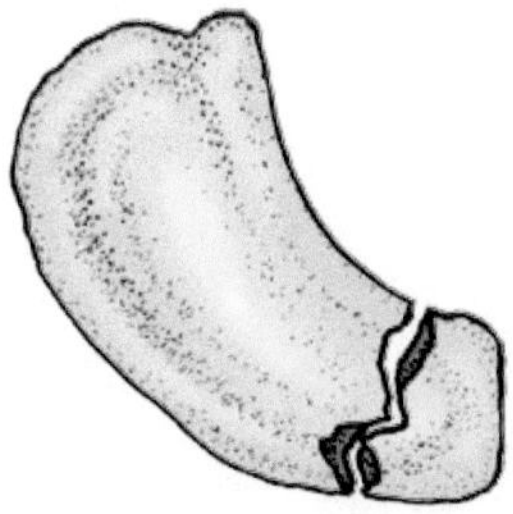

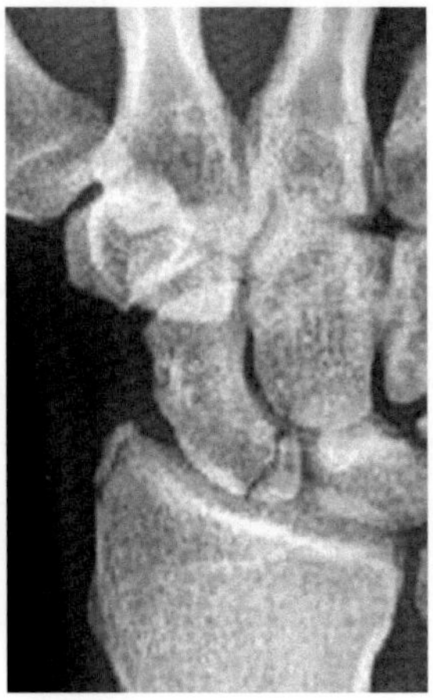

Russe Classification of Scaphoid Fracture

Type I: Horizontal oblique.

Proximal 1/3

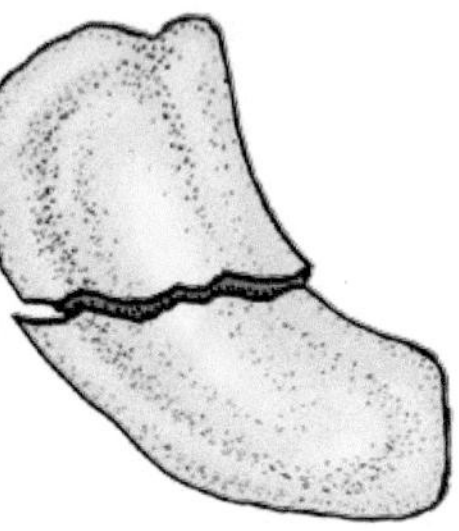

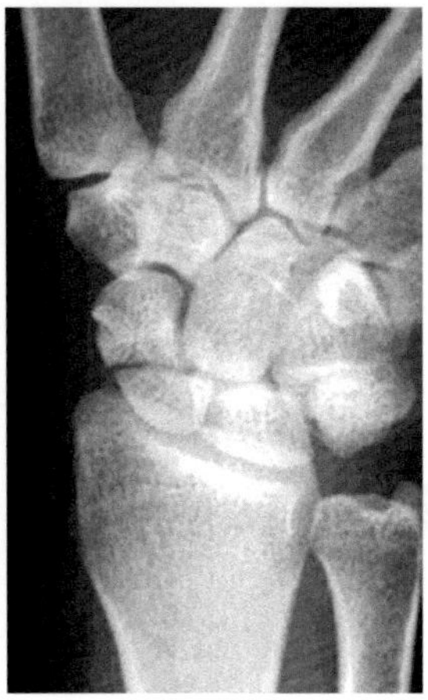

Russe Classification of Scaphoid Fracture

Type II: Transverse

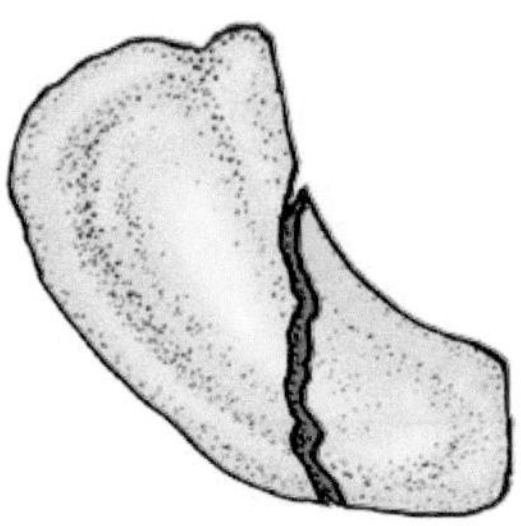

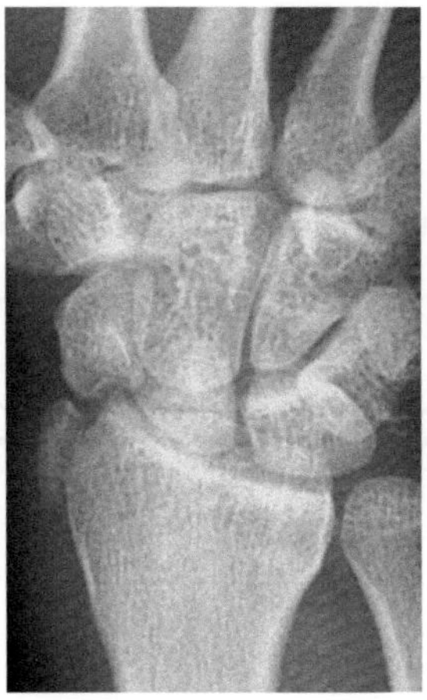

Russe Classification of Scaphoid Fracture

Type III: Vertical oblique

Mayo Classification of Scaphoid Fracture [11]

Mayo classification sets out criteria aimed at predicting instability and guiding management and includes fracture malalignment.

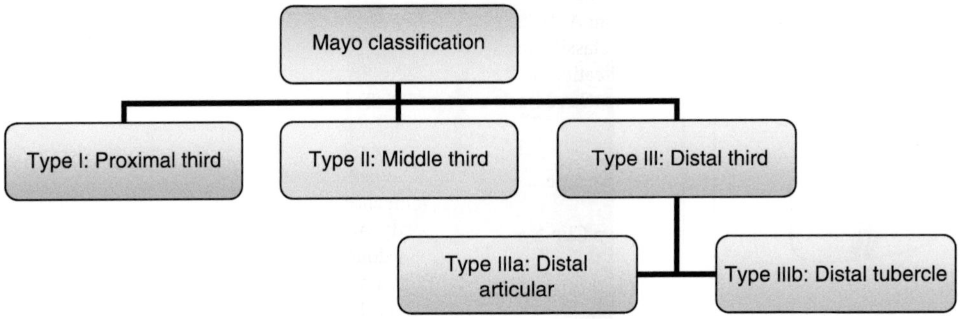

Type	Description
Proximal third	Fracture of the proximal third of the scaphoid bone
Middle third	Fracture of the middle third of the scaphoid bone
Distal third	Fracture of the distal third of the scaphoid bone:
	a: Fracture of the distal articular
	b: Fracture of the distal tubercle

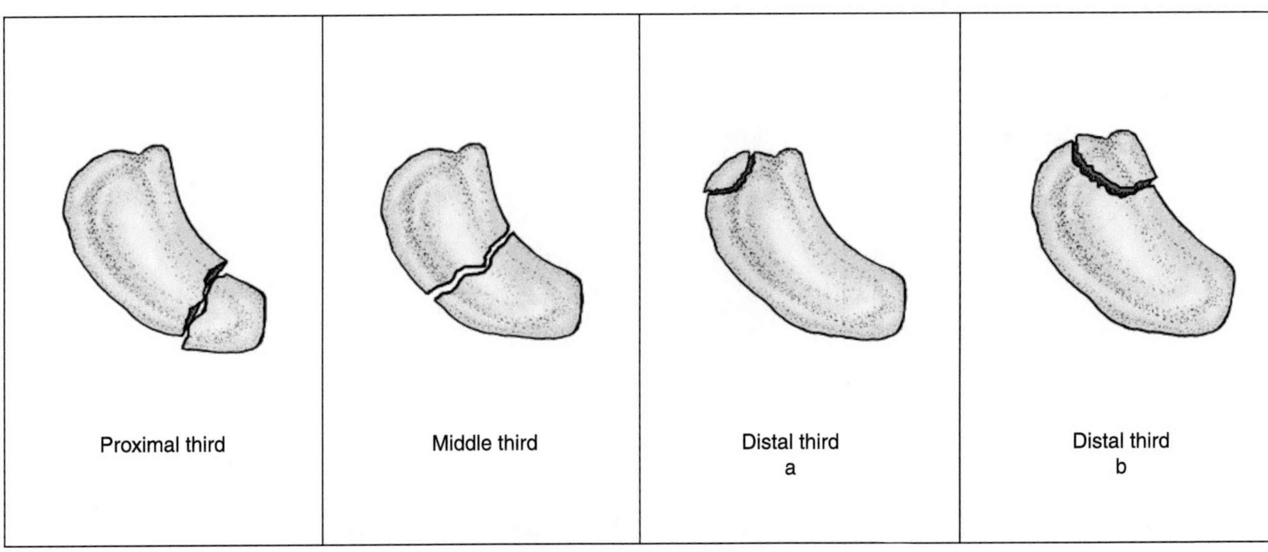

AO/OTA Classification of Scaphoid Fracture [12]

AO/OTA classification divides fractures into location (distal pole, waist, proximal pole) and comminution.

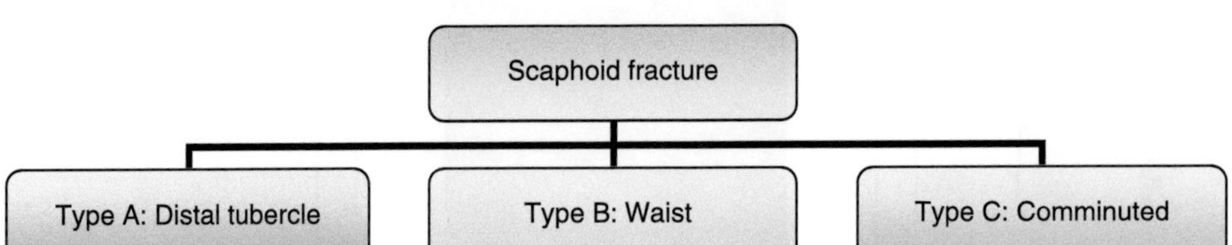

Type A: Distal tubercle.

Type B: Waist.

Type C: Comminuted.

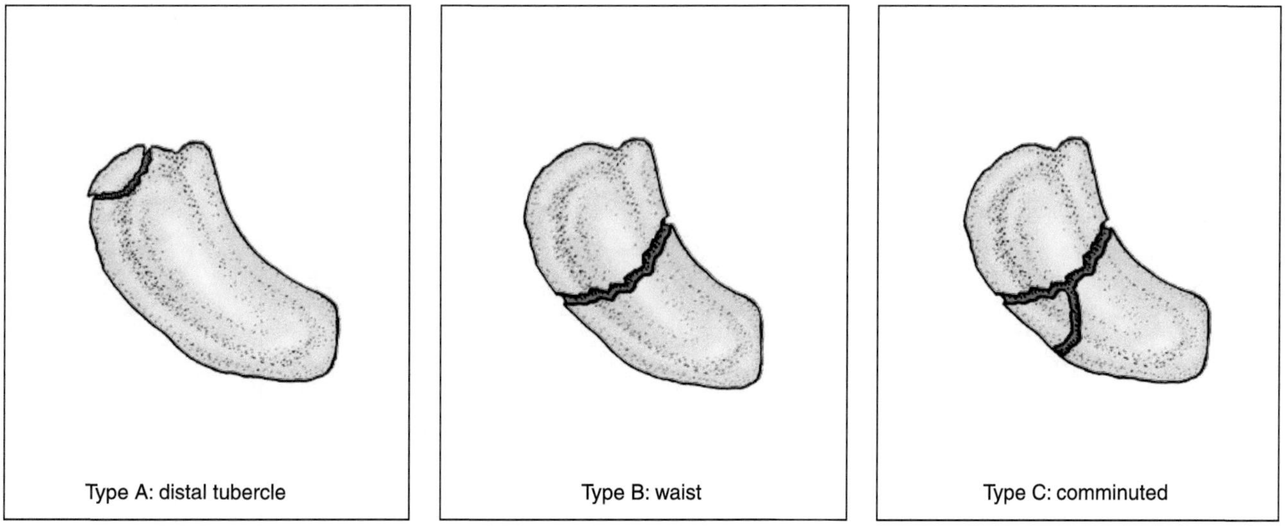

Rockwood-Green Classification of Scaphoid Fracture [13]

65%: Waist.

15%: Proximal pole.

10%: Distal body.

8%: Tuberosity.

2%: Distal articular surface.

4.2.2.2 Teisen and Hjarkbeak Classification of Lunate Fracture [14]

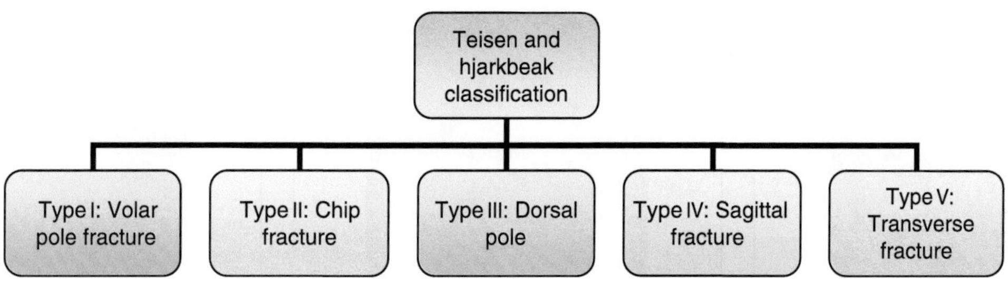

Type	Description
I	Volar pole fracture
II	Chip fracture not affecting blood supply
III	Fracture of dorsal pole
IV	Sagittal fracture through body
V	Transverse fracture through body

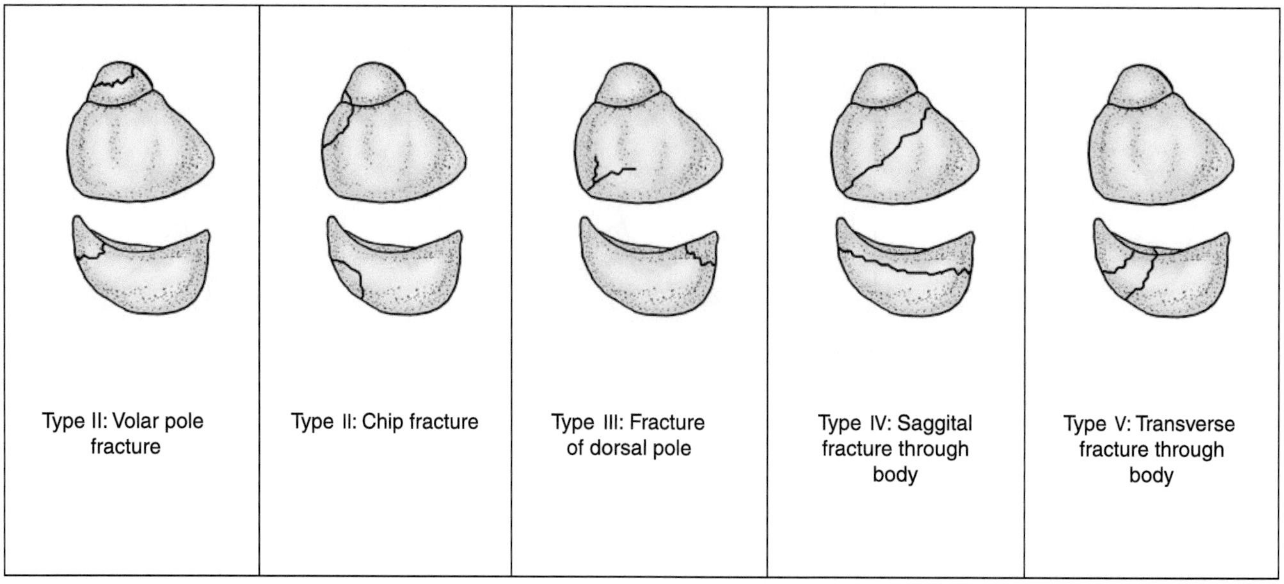

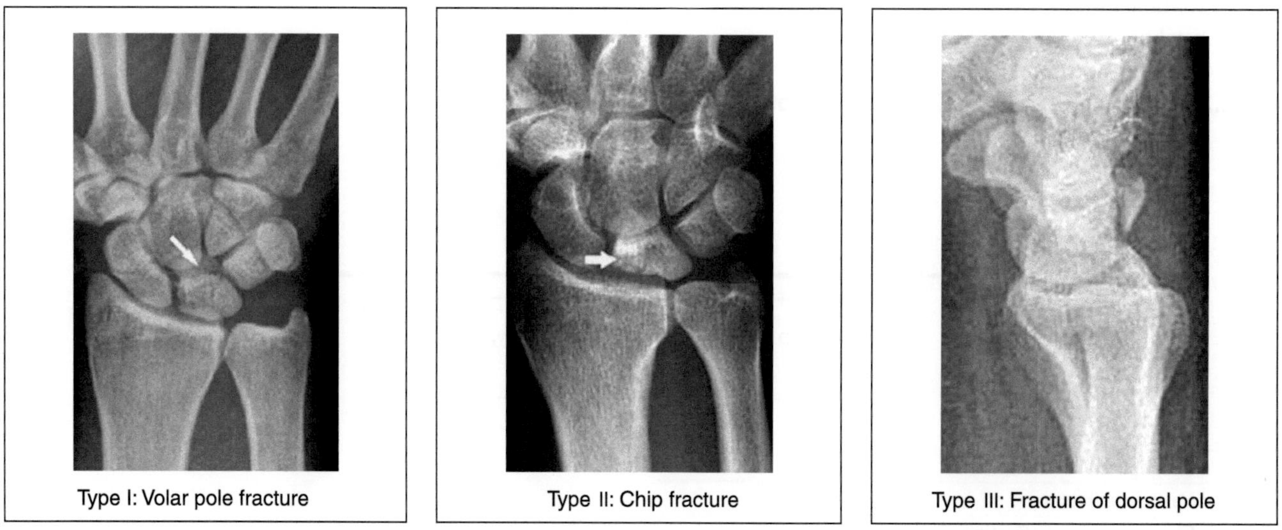

References

1. Green DP, O'Brien ET. Fractures of the thumb metacarpal. South Med J. 1972;65:807–14.
2. Calif E, Stahl S. The surgical treatment of fractures of the base of the fifth metacarpal bone. Harefuah. 2001;140:813–5. 896.
3. Schenck RR. Classification of fractures and dislocations of the proximal interphalangeal joint. Hand Clin. 1994;10: 179–85.
4. London PS. Sprains and fractures involving the interphalangeal joints. Hand. 1971;3:155–8.
5. Kaplan L. Treatment of fractures and dislocations of the hand and fingers. Surg Clin North Am. 1940;20:1695–720.
6. Cannon B, May LW. Skin contractures of the hand. In: Flynn JE, editor. Hand surgery. 3rd ed. Baltimore, MD: Williams and Wilkins; 1982. p. 111–80.
7. Wehbé MA, Schneider LH. Mallet fractures. J Bone Joint Surg Am. 1984;66:658–69.
8. Kleinert H E, Williams D J. Blast injuries of the hand.[J]. Journal of Trauma, 1962, 2(1):10.
9. Herbert TJ, Fisher WE. Management of the fractured scaphoid using a new bone screw. J Bone Joint Surg Br. 1984;66:114–23.
10. Russe O. Fracture of the carpal navicular. Diagnosis, non-operative treatment, and operative treatment. J Bone Joint Surg Am. 1960;42:759–68.
11. Cooney WP 3rd. Scaphoid fractures: current treatments and techniques. Instr Course Lect. 2003;52:197–208.
12. Neuhaus V, Jupiter JB. Current concepts review: carpal injuries - fractures, ligaments, dislocations. Acta Chir Orthop Traumatol Cechoslov. 2011;78:395–403.
13. Charles AR, David PG. Rockwood and green's fractures in adults. Philadelphia, PA: Lippincott-Raven; 1996.
14. Teisen H, Hjarbaek J. Classification of fresh fractures of the lunate. J Hand Surg Br. 1988;13:458–62.

Classification of Dislocation of Shoulder and Upper Limb

5

Yingze Zhang and Wenjuan Wu

5.1 Section 1: Classification of Dislocation of Shoulder

5.1.1 Classification of Acromioclavicular Joint Dislocation

5.1.1.1 The Rockwood Classification (1996, Fractures in Adult. 4nd Ed. Philadelphia Lippincott-Raven Publishers, 1341–1414)

Allman and Tossy initially proposed a three-grade classification that Rockwood expanded to six types of injury. Grades I and II are the same in both classification schemes, with grade III in the Tossy classification subdivided into grades III, IV, V, and VI in the Rockwood classification.

The Rockwood classification is as follows:

Type I: Minor sprain of AC ligament, the joint capsule, coracoclavicular ligament, triangular ligament, trapezoid ligament intact.

Type II: Acromioclavicular ligament and joint capsule rupture, the acromioclavicular joint space widen, the coracoclavicular ligament injury but the coracoclavicular joint space was normal, triangular ligament, trapezoid ligament mild tear.

Type III: Acromioclavicular ligament, joint capsule, ligament rupture, complete separation of acromioclavicular joint, triangular ligament, and trapezoid ligament tear.

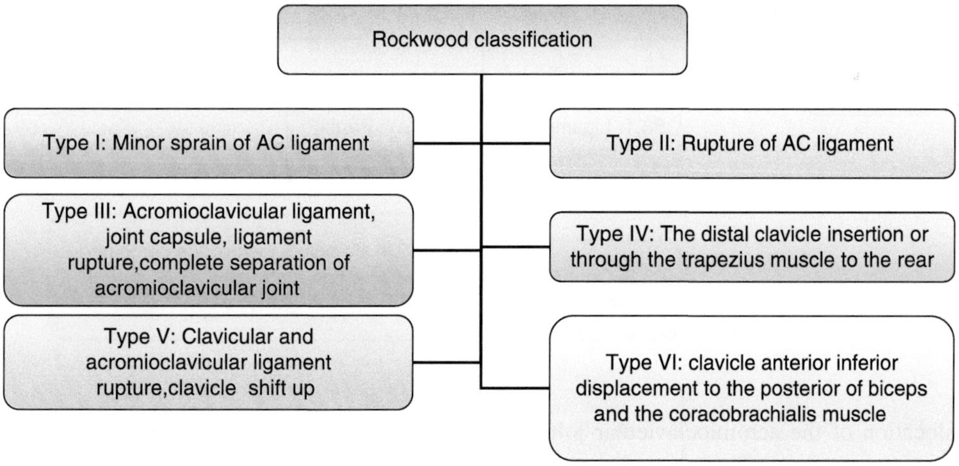

Y. Zhang (✉) • W. Wu
Department of Orthopedics,
The Third Hospital of Hebei Medical University,
Shijiazhuang, China
e-mail: yzzhangdr@126.com, yzling_liu@163.com

Y. Zhang (ed.), *Clinical Classification in Orthopaedics Trauma*, https://doi.org/10.1007/978-981-10-6044-1_5

Type IV: Acromioclavicular ligament, joint capsule, ligament rupture, clavicle moves backward to the trapezius muscle.

Type V: Acromioclavicular ligament, joint capsule, ligament rupture, clavicle moves backward, triangular ligament, trapezoid ligament tear.

Type VI: Acromioclavicular ligament, joint capsule, ligament rupture, clavicle moves down and forward to the biceps and the coracobrachialis muscle.

5.1.1.2 Tossy Classification (1963, CORR, 28: 111–119)

Type I: Contusion of acromioclavicular ligament, radiographically normal.

Type II: Local pain and swelling. Subluxation of acromioclavicular joint, clavicle shifts up half of the space. The coracoclavicular space widened, coracoclavicular ligament partial tear.

Type III: Dislocation of the acromioclavicular joint, clavicle shifts up more than half of the joint space. And coracoclavicular space severely widens, coracoclavicular ligament completely ruptured.

5.1.1.3 Allman Classification (1967, J Bone Joint Surg (Am), 49:774–784)

Type I: Acromioclavicular joint ligament and capsule contusion, no laxity, X-ray normal.

Type II: Acromioclavicular joint ligament and capsule rupture, no rupture of coracoclavicular, laxity is present in the joint, roentgenography reveals the distal clavicle upward displacement;

Type III: The ligament rupture on both the acromioclavicular and coracoclavicular, the joint complete dislocation.

5.1.1.4 AO/CTA Classification (2007 revise, Journal of Orthopaedic Trauma. 21 Supplement)

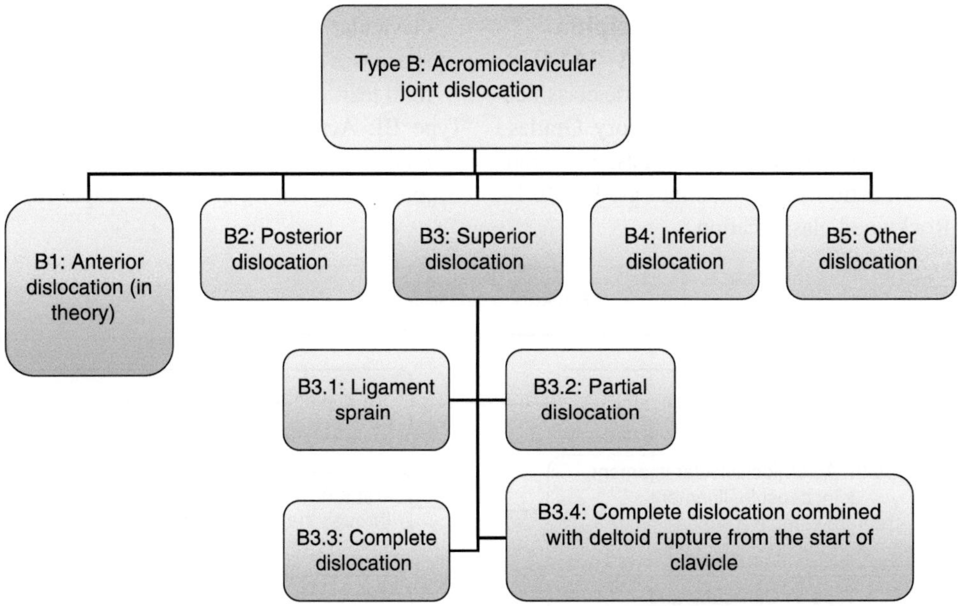

B1: Anterior dislocation of the acromioclavicular joint (in theory).

B2: Posterior dislocation of acromioclavicular joint.

B3: Superior dislocation of acromioclavicular joint, including

B3.1: Ligament sprain.

B3.2: Partial dislocation.

B3.3: Complete dislocation.

B3.4: Complete dislocation combined with deltoid rupture from the start of clavicle.

B4: Inferior dislocation of the acromioclavicular joint.

B5: Other dislocation.

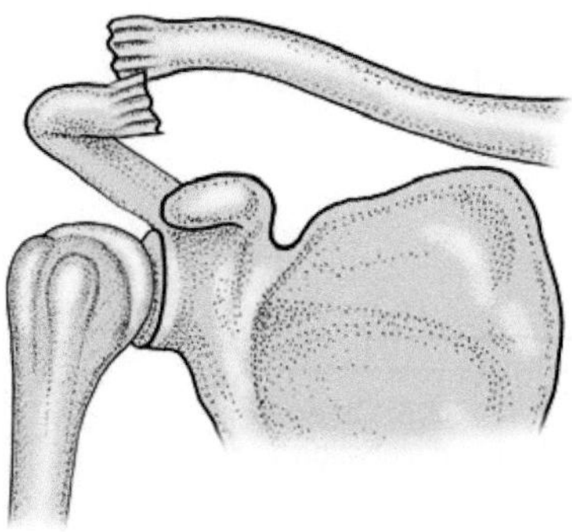

10-B2

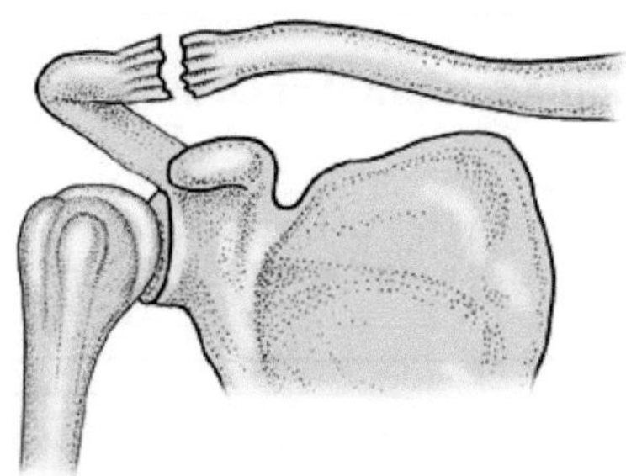

10-B3.1

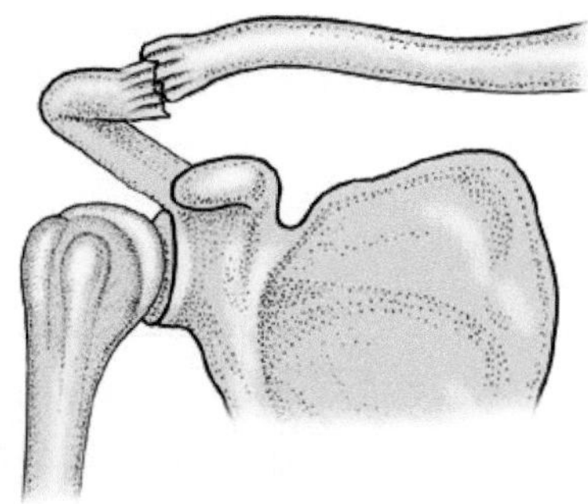

10-B3.2

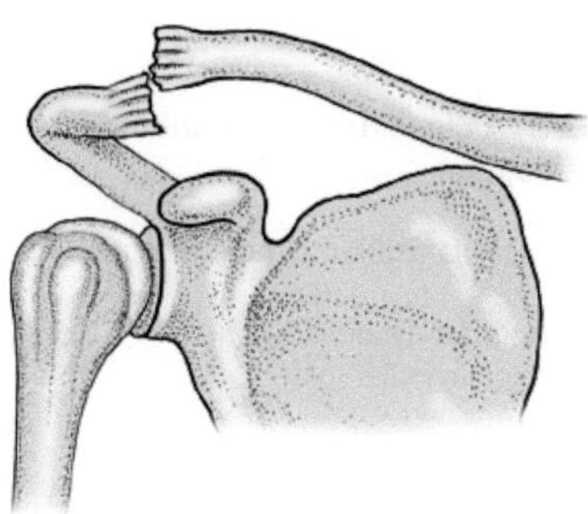

10-B3.3

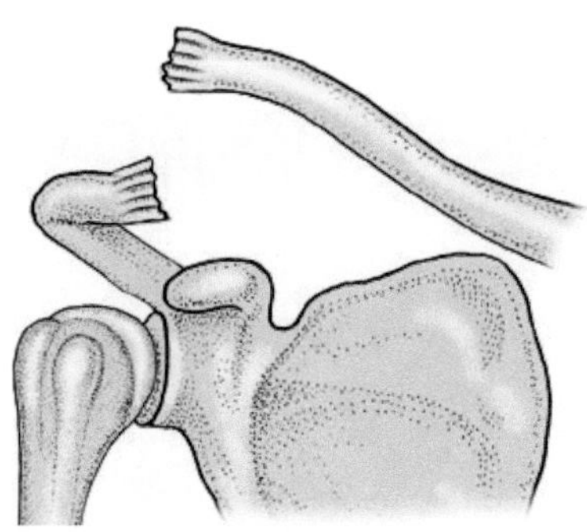

10-B3.4

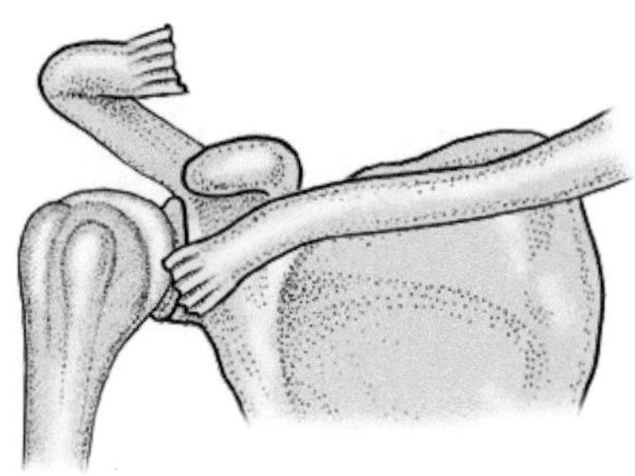

10-B4

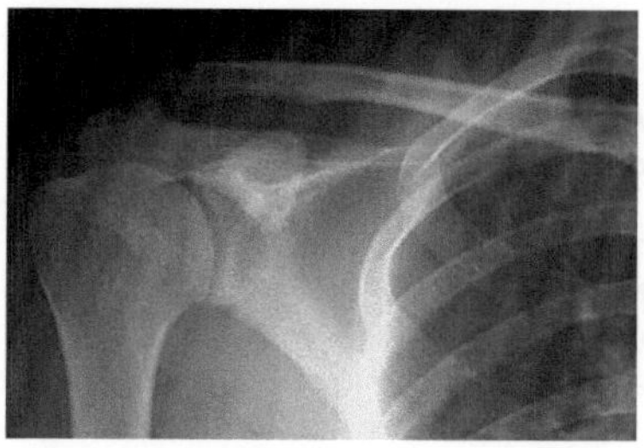

10-B3.2

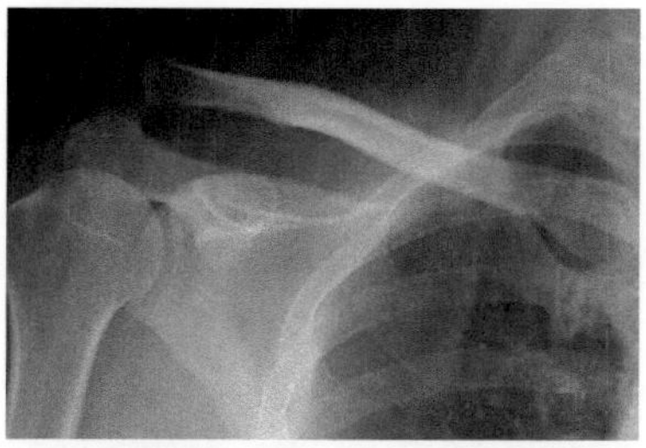

10-B3.3

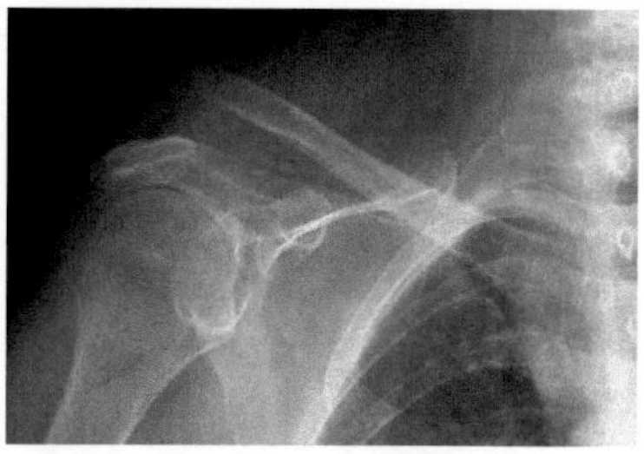

10-B3.4

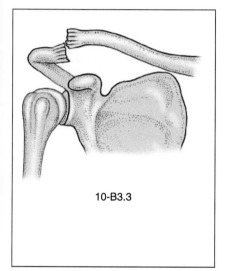

5.1.2 Classification of Sternoclavicular Joint Dislocation

5.1.2.1 AO/OTA Classification (2007 modified, Journal of Orthopaedic Trauma. 21 Supplement)

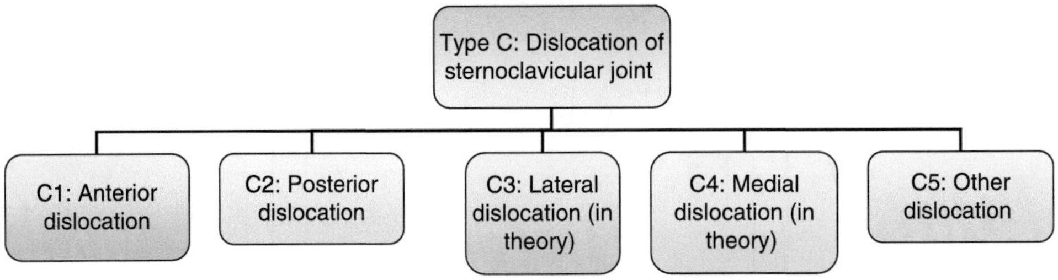

C1: Anterior dislocation of sternoclavicular joint.
C2: Posterior dislocation of sternoclavicular joint.
C3: Lateral dislocation of sternoclavicular joint (in theory).
C4: Medial dislocation of sternoclavicular joint (in theory).
C5: Other dislocation.

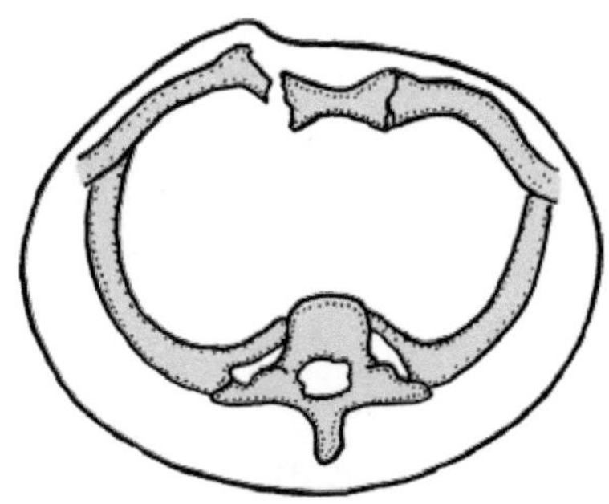

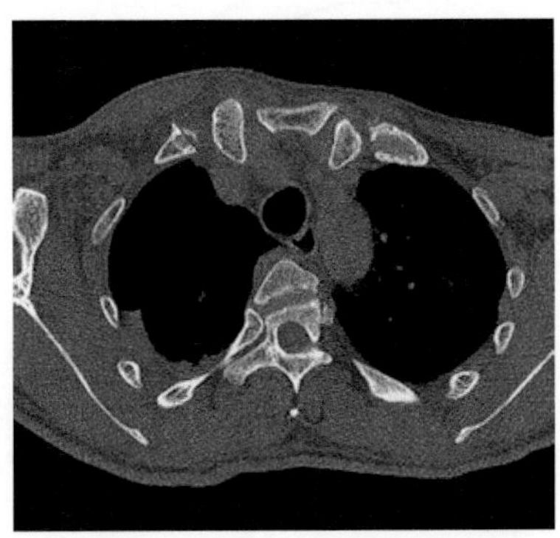

AO/OTA classification of shoulder dislocation

Type C: Dislocation of acromioclavicular joint.
C1: Anterior dislocation of acromioclavicular joint

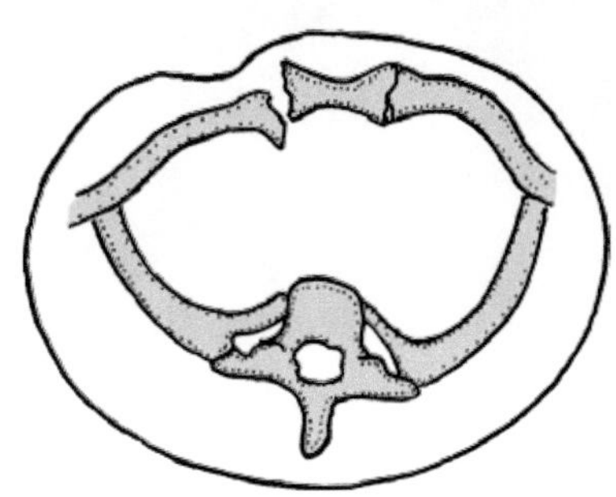

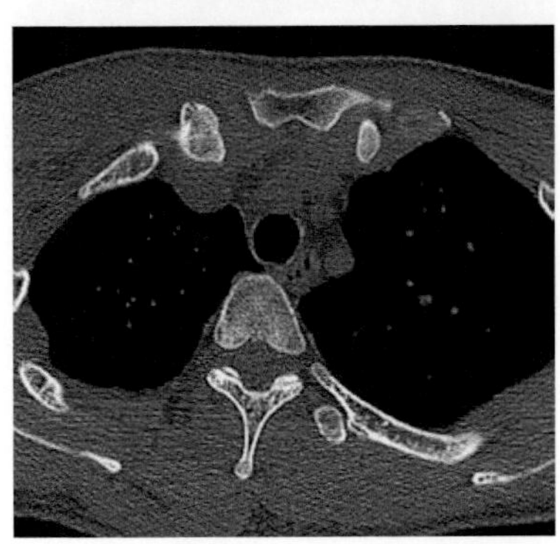

AO/OTA classification of shoulder dislocation

Type C: Dislocation of acromioclavicular joint.
C2: Posterior dislocation of the acromioclavicular joint

5.1.2.2 Rockwood Classification (1996, Fractures in Adult. 4th Ed. Philadelphia Lippincott Raven Publishers)

Anatomic Classification

Type I: Anterior dislocation. The most common one, the proximal part of the clavicle located at the front or the anterosuperior of manubrium sterni leading edge.

Type II: Posterior dislocation. The rare ones, the proximal end of the clavicle located in the posterior or posterosuperior part of the posterior border of the manubrium sterni.

Pathogeny Classification

Type A: Traumatic dislocation, further divided into:

A1: Sprain or subluxation.
A2: Acute dislocation.
A3: Recurrent dislocation.
A4: Irreducible dislocation.

Type B: Nontraumatic dislocation, further divided into:

B1: Spontaneous subluxation or dislocation.
B2: Congenital or developmental dislocation.

Type C: Arthritic dislocation.

Type D: Infective dislocation.

5.1.3 Classification of Glenohumeral Dislocation

5.1.3.1 According to the Joint Classification Orientation

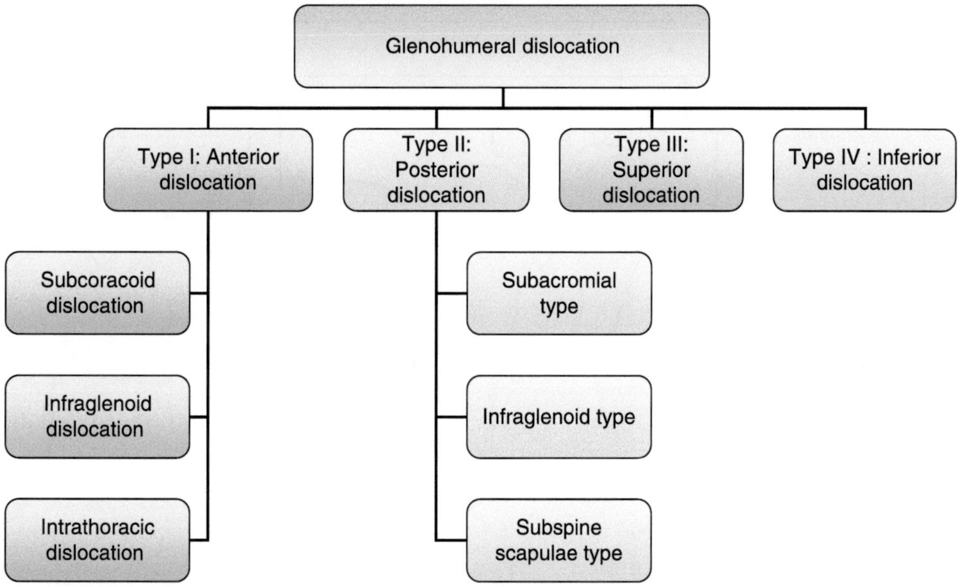

Glenohumeral Joint Anterior Dislocation

Further divided into:

Ia: Subcoracoid dislocation.
Ib: Infraglenoid dislocation.
Ic: Intrathoracic dislocation.

Glenohumeral Joint Posterior Dislocation

Further divided into:

Subacromial type (98%): Articular surface moves backward, lesser humeral tubercle usually occupies the glenoid fossa, often with the anterior humeral head impacted fracture.

Infraglenoid type (rare): The humeral head in the lower back of glenoid fossa.

Subspinous type (extremely rare): The humeral head located in the medial side of acromion, below the spine scapula.

Glenohumeral Joint Superior Dislocation

Glenohumeral Joint Inferior Dislocation

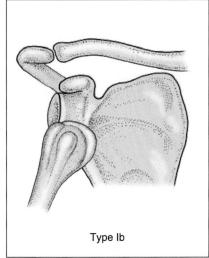

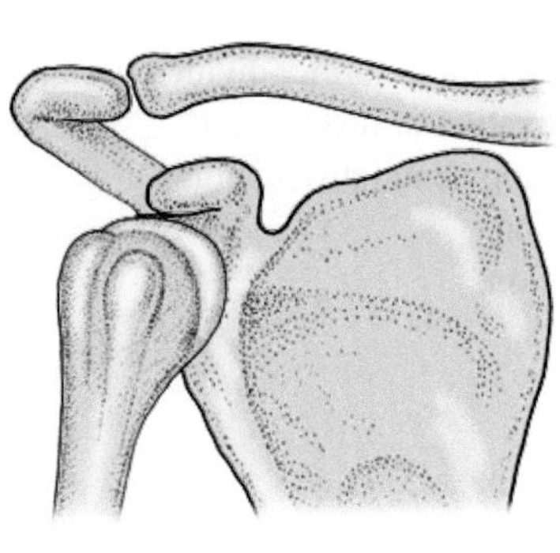

Type Ia

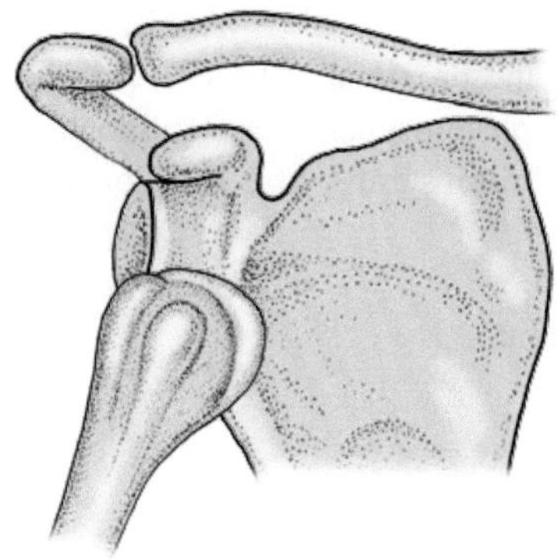

Type Ib

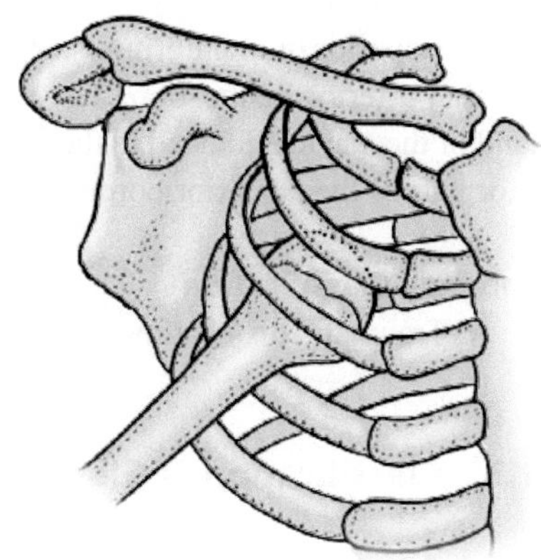

Type Ic

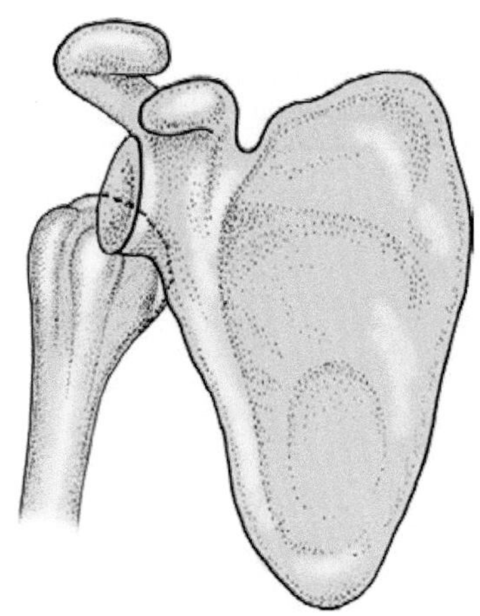

Type II

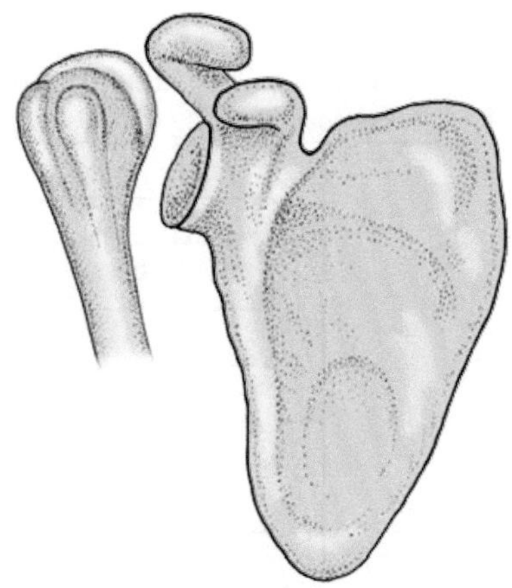

Type III

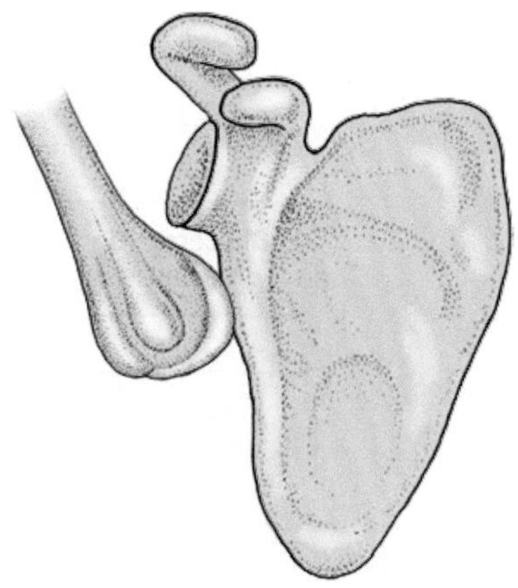

Type IV

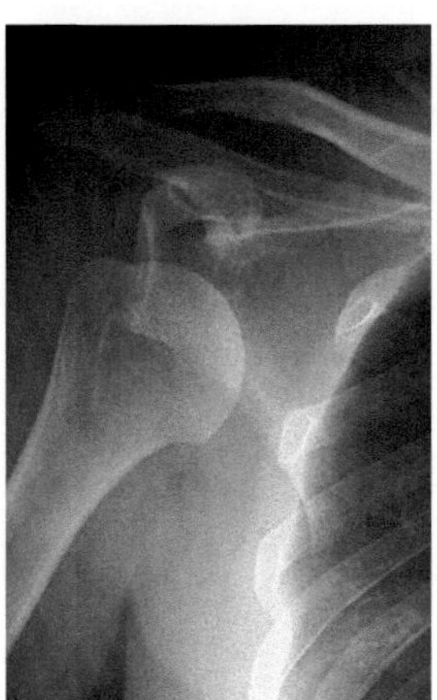

Type Ia : Subcoracoid dislocation

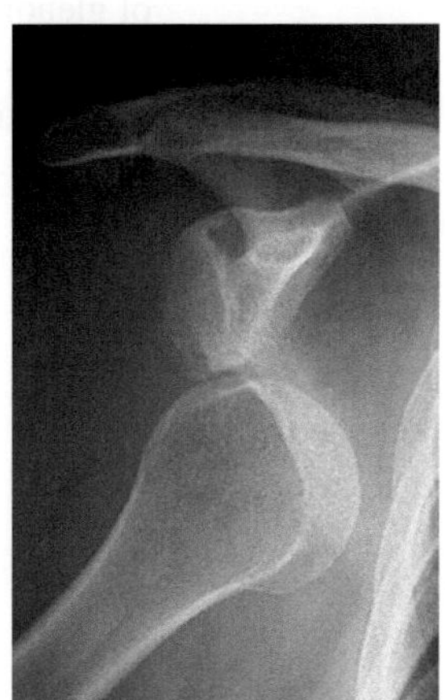

Type Ib: Infraglenoid dislocation

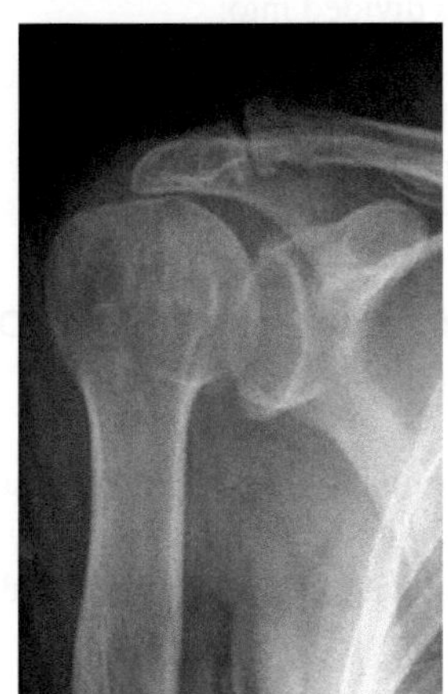

Type II: Posterior dislocation

5.1.3.2 AO/OTA Classification (2007 modified, Journal of Orthopaedic Trauma. 21 Supplement)

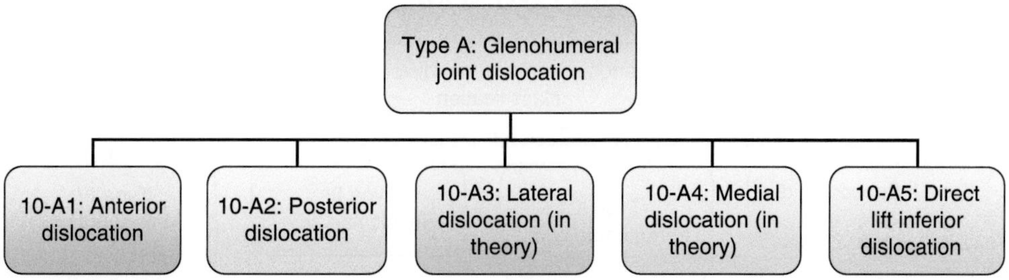

A1: Shoulder joint anterior dislocation.
A2: Shoulder joint posterior dislocation.
A3: Lateral dislocation (in theory).
A4: Medial dislocation (in theory).
A5: Direct lift inferior dislocation.

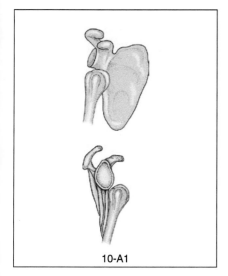

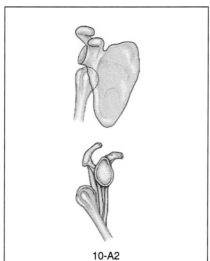

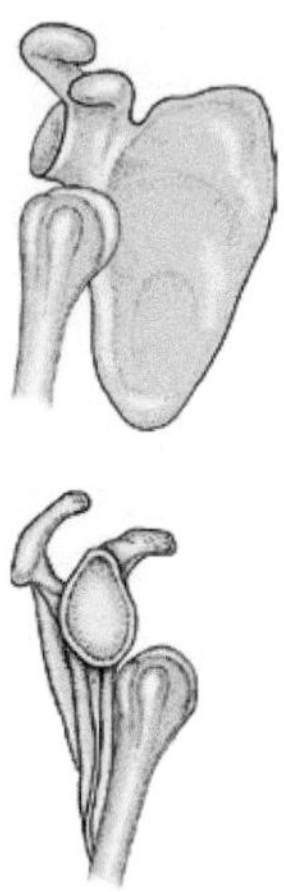
10-A1

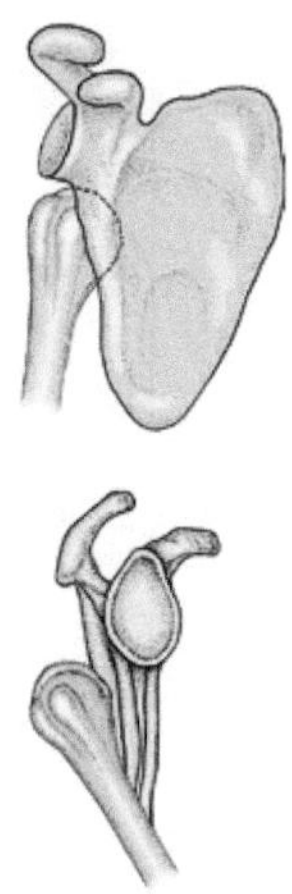
10-A2

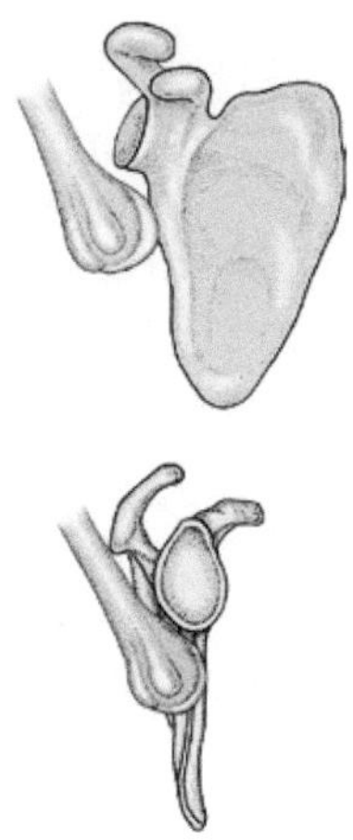
10-A5

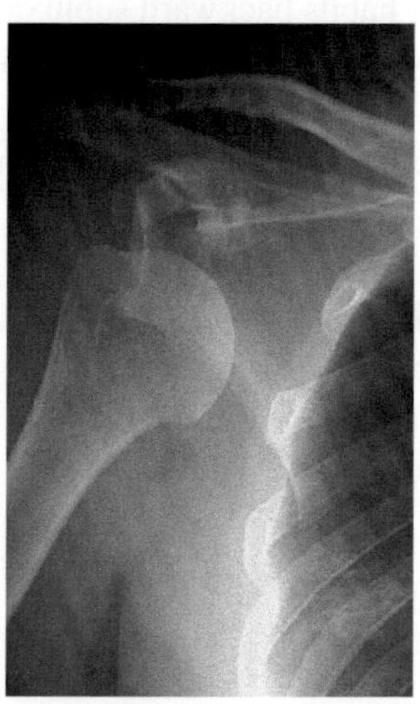
10-A1

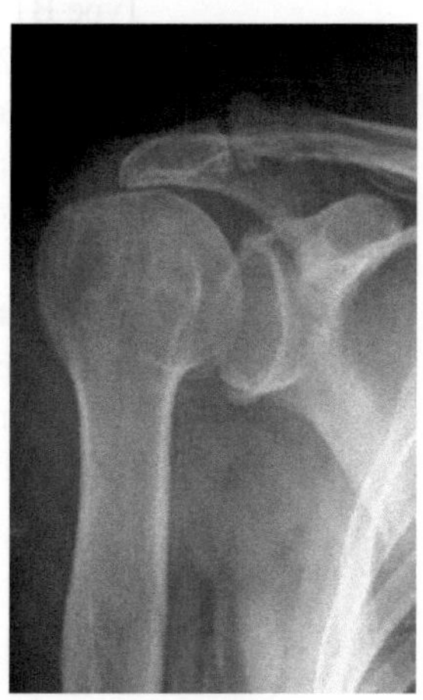
10-A2

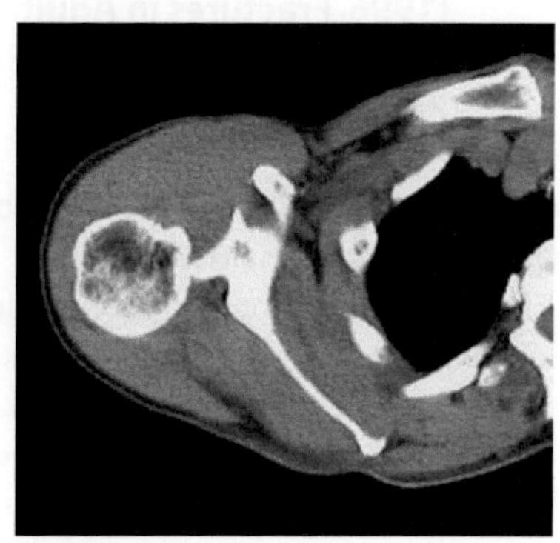
10-A2

5.1.3.3 Glenohumeral Anterior Dislocation Classification (2001, Wang Yicong editor, Bone and Joint Injury. Third edition, Beijing: People's Medical Publish House, 2001, 514–514)

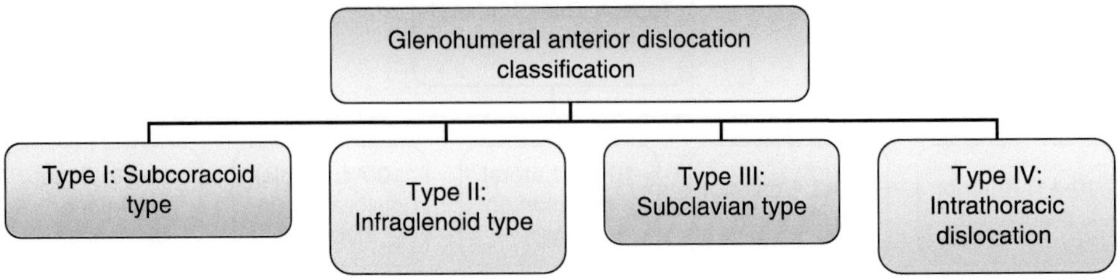

Type I: Subcoracoid type. Humeral head dislocates below to the coracoid process.

Type II: Infraglenoid type. Humeral head anterior dislocation to the inferior margin of the glenoid fossa.

Type III: Subclavian type. Humeral head shifts medially after dislocation to the medial side of coracoid process and the inferior side of clavicle.

Type IV: Intrathoracic dislocation. The humeral head dislocates into the chest through muscle. This type rare, common combined pulmonary and vascular nerve injury.

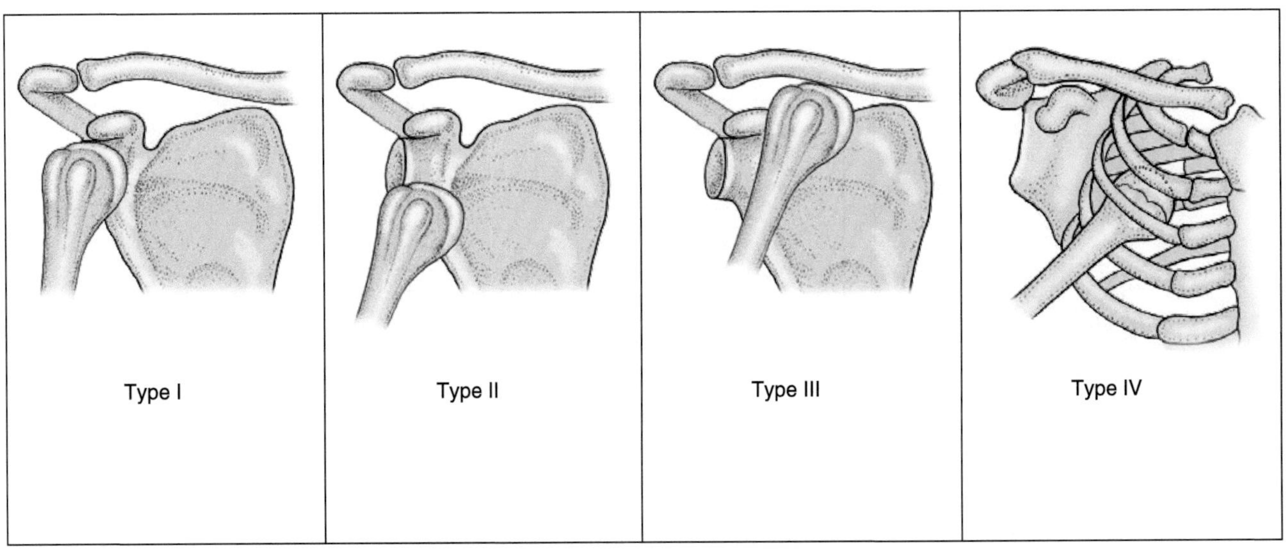

5.1.3.4 Glenohumeral Joint Posterior Dislocation (1996, Fractures in Adult. 4th Ed. Philadelphia Lippincott Raven Publishers)

According to Pathology Classification

Type A: Traumatic injuries.
- Type A1: Contusion of posterior shoulder.
- Type A2: Acute shoulder joint back subluxation.
- Type A3: Acute shoulder joint back luxation.
- Type A4: Recurrent back subluxation or luxation.
- Type A5: Irreducible posterior luxation.

Type B: Nontraumatic injuries.
- Type B1: Spontaneous or habits backward subluxation.
- Type B2: Non-spontaneous backward subluxation or luxation.
- Type B3: Hereditary or developmental backward subluxation or luxation.

According to the Anatomical Classification

Type A: Subacromial dislocation.
Type B: Infraglenoid dislocation.
Type C: Subspinous dislocation.

5.1.4 AO/OTA Classification of Scapular Dislocation (2007 modified, Journal of Orthopaedic Trauma. 21 Supplement)

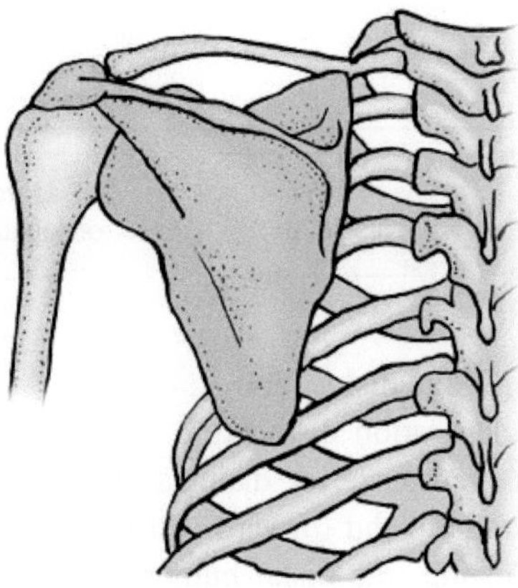

AO/OTA classification of scapular dislocation 10-D scapular dislocation

5.2 Section 2. The Classification of Elbow Joint Dislocation

5.2.1 Browner Classification (1998, Skeletal Trauma. 2nd Harcourt Publishers Limited)

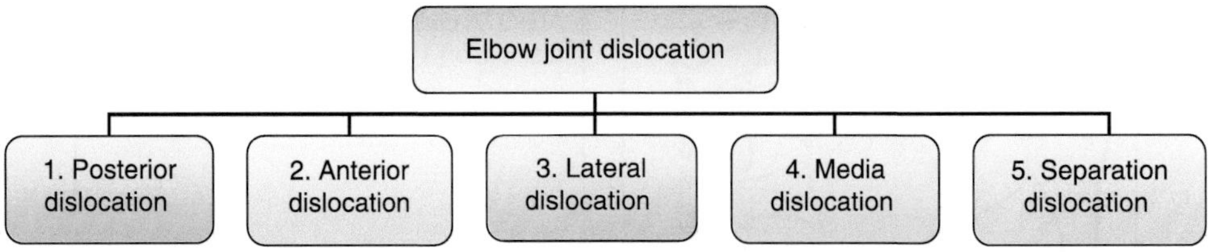

1. Posterior dislocation: More than 80% were posterolateral dislocation, and some cases were posteromedial dislocation.
2. Anterior dislocation: Anterior dislocation of ulna and radius
3. Lateral dislocation
4. Medial dislocation
5. Separation dislocation (very rare): Further divided into anteroposterior dislocation (ulan backward dislocation, radial head forward dislocation) and mediolateral dislocation (the distal humerus is inserted between the ulna and radius)

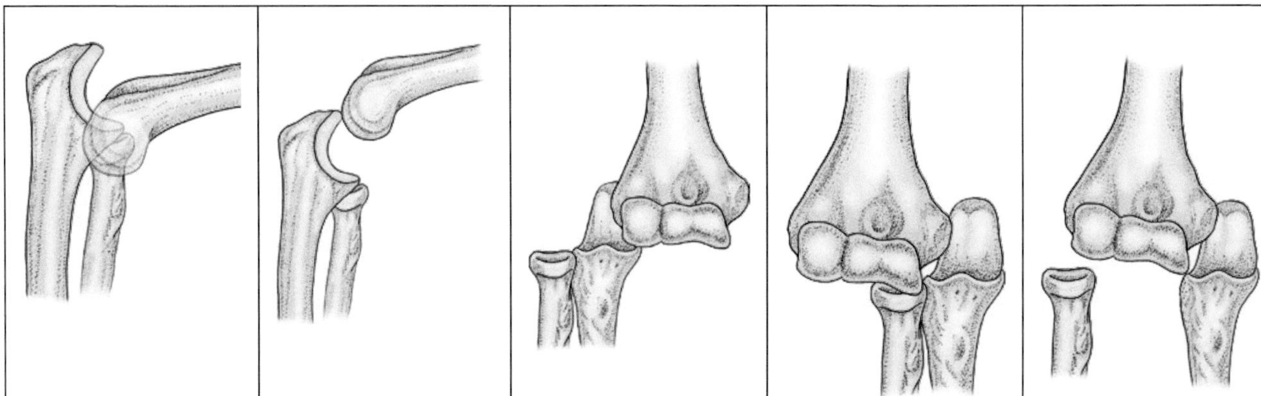

1.elbow joint posterior dislocation	2.elbow joint anterior dislocation	3.elbow joint lateral. dislocation	4.elbow joint medial dislocation	5.elbow joint separation dislocation

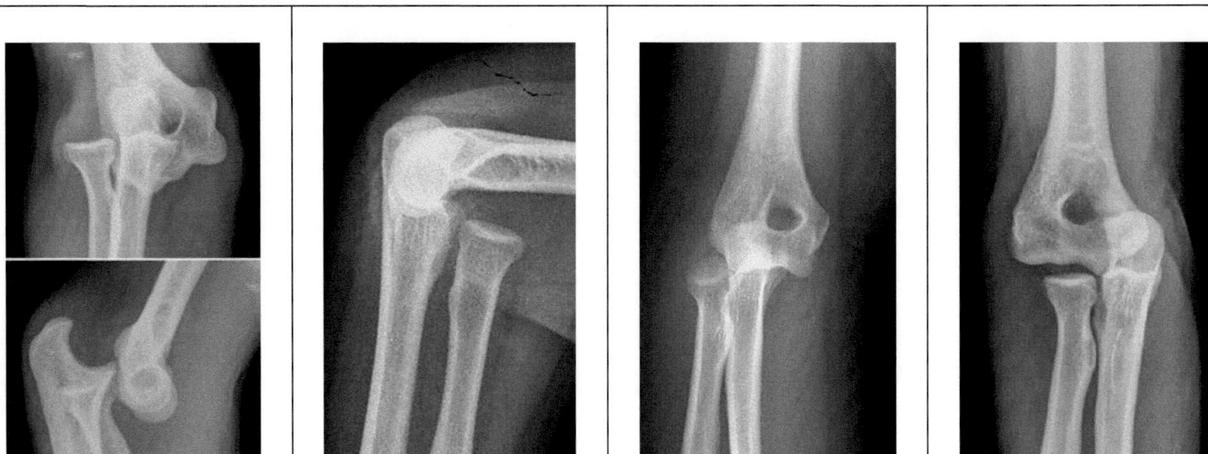

1.elbow joint posterior dislocation	2.elbow joint anterior dislocation	3.elbow joint lateral dislocation	4.elbow joint medial dislocation

5.2.2 O'Driscoll-Morrey Classification (1992, Clin Orthop Relat Res. 280:186–197)

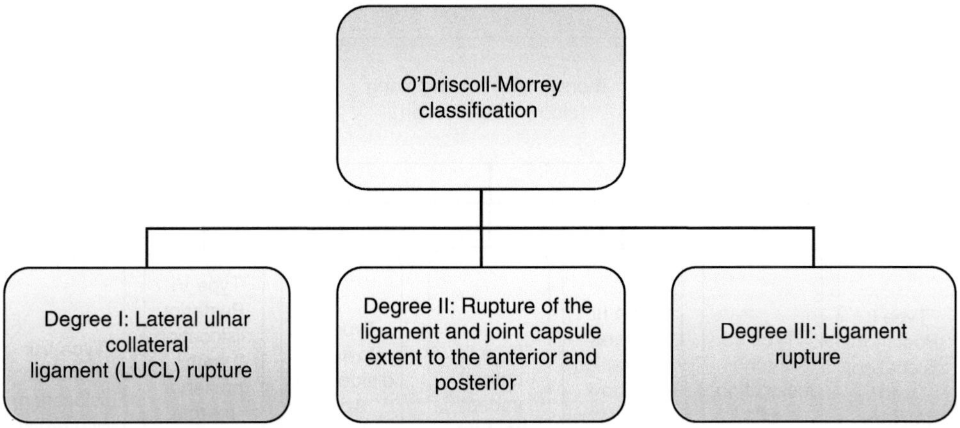

Degree I: Lateral ulnar collateral ligament (LUCL) rupture, the other part of the ligament can be intact, or break, caused elbow joint posterolateral rotatory subluxation, but the subluxation can be automatic reduction.

Degree II: Rupture of the ligament and joint capsule extent to the anterior and posterior, the elbow joint is in the condition of incomplete posterolateral dislocation, trochlear is ride on the coronoid process.

Degree III:

IIIa: Almost all soft tissue and ligaments around the elbow were torn, including posterior bundle of ulnar collateral ligament, only the anterior bundle of the ulnar collateral ligament not injured, leading to posterior dislocation of the elbow, the ulnar collateral ligament becomes the point of elbow rotation.

IIIb: Medial collateral ligament totally tears.

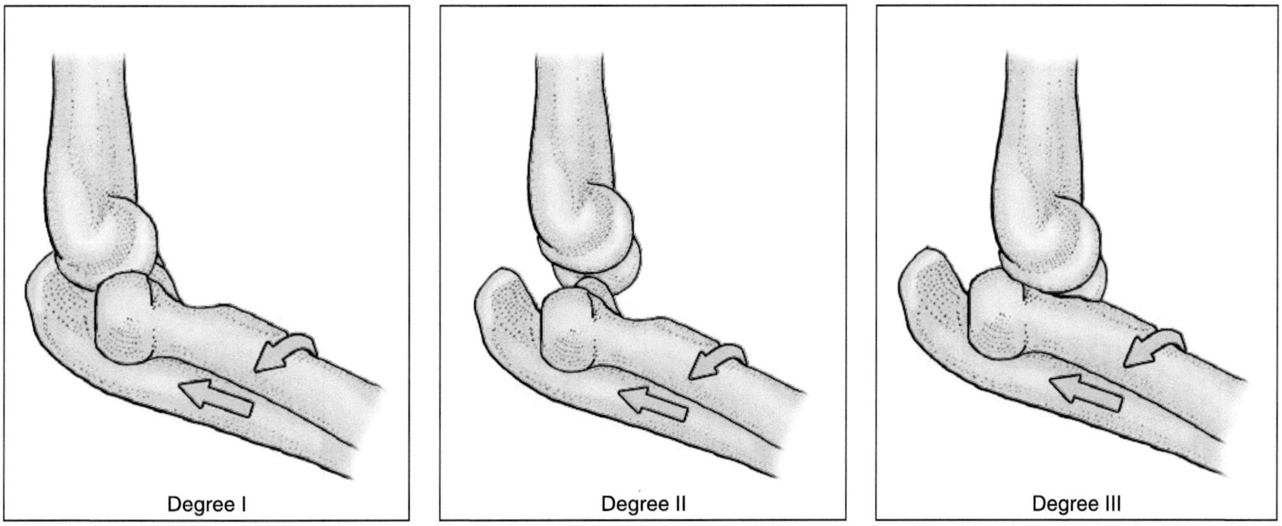

5.2.3 Elbow Zhenwu Men-Yiming Yong Classification (Yicong Wang, Bone and joint injury, The Third Edition. Beijing: People's Medical Publishing House, 2001, 623–625)

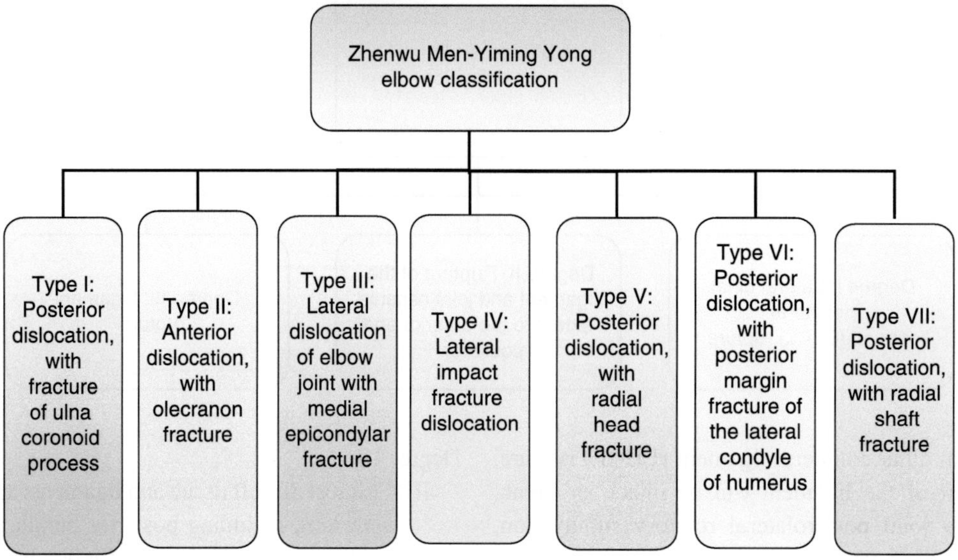

Type I: Posterior dislocation, with fracture of ulna coronoid process.
Type II: Anterior dislocation, with olecranon fracture.
Type III: Lateral dislocation, with medial epicondylar fracture.
Type IV: Lateral impact fracture dislocation.
Type V: Posterior dislocation, with radial head fracture
Type VI: Posterior dislocation, with posterior margin fracture of the lateral condyle of humerus.
Type VII: Posterior dislocation, with radial shaft fracture.

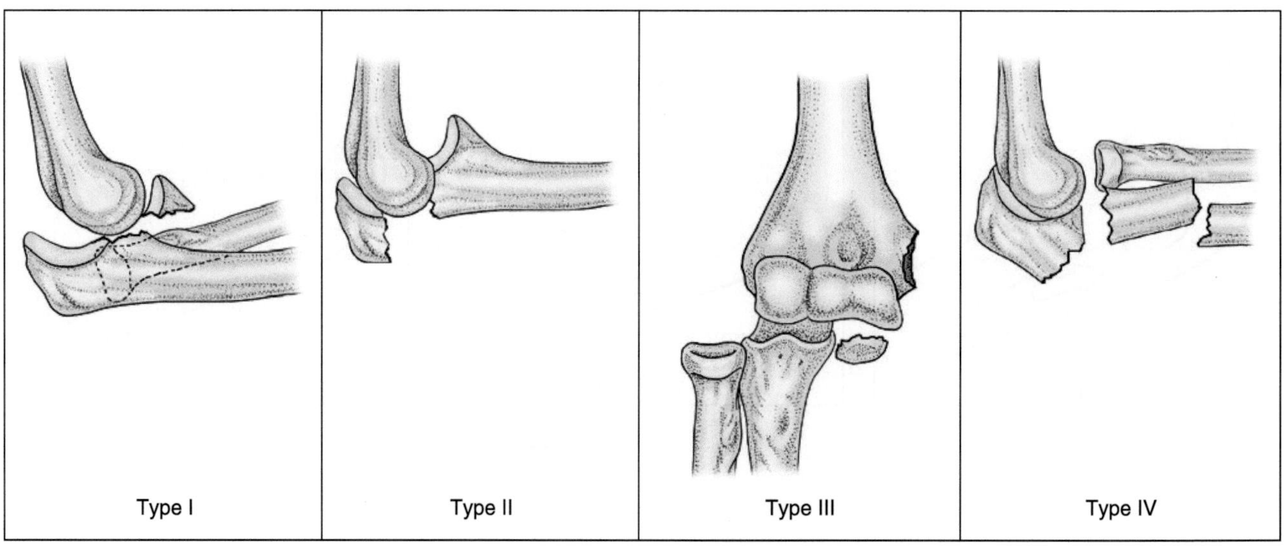

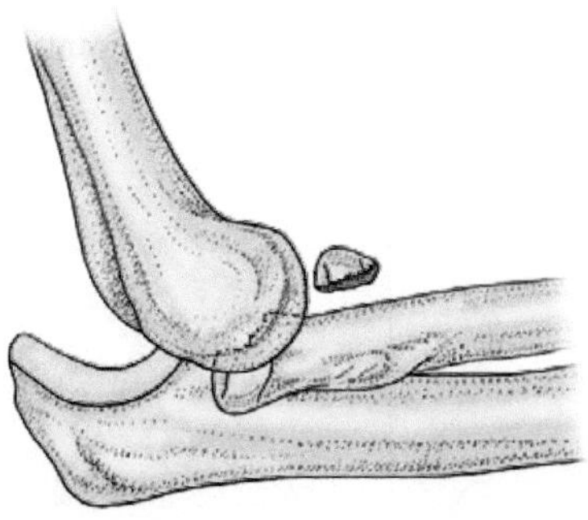
Type V

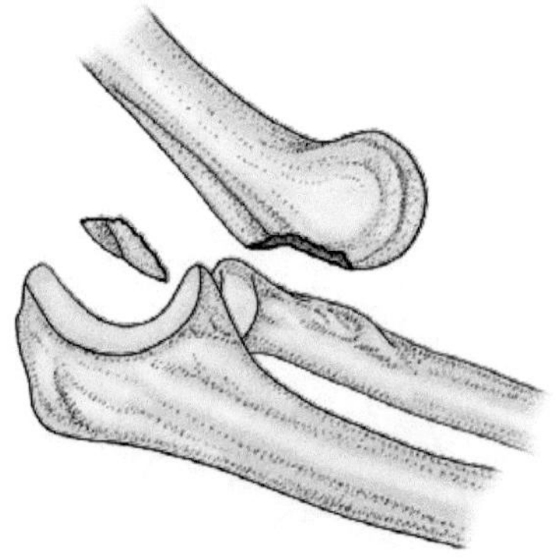
Type VI

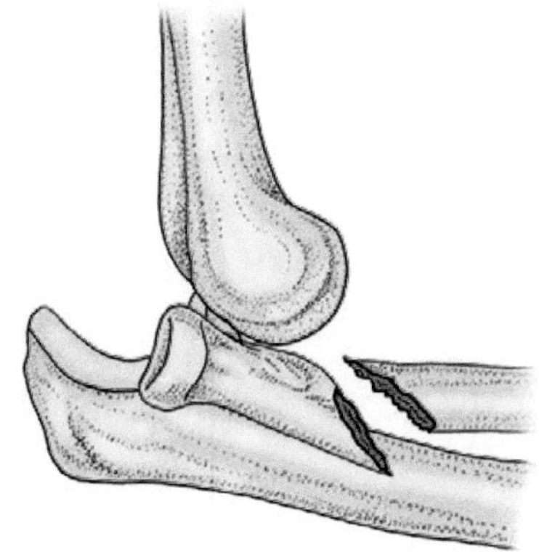
Type VII

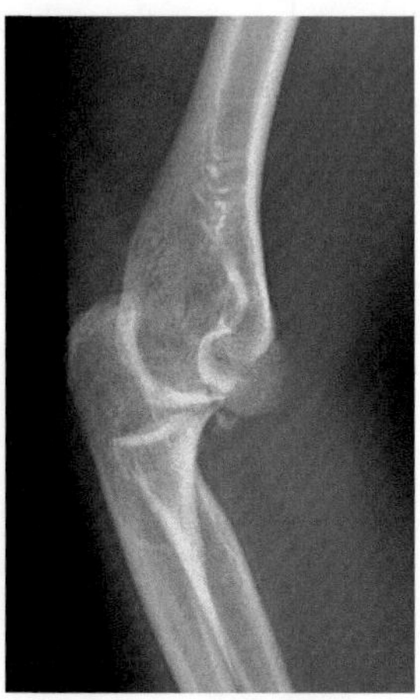
Type I

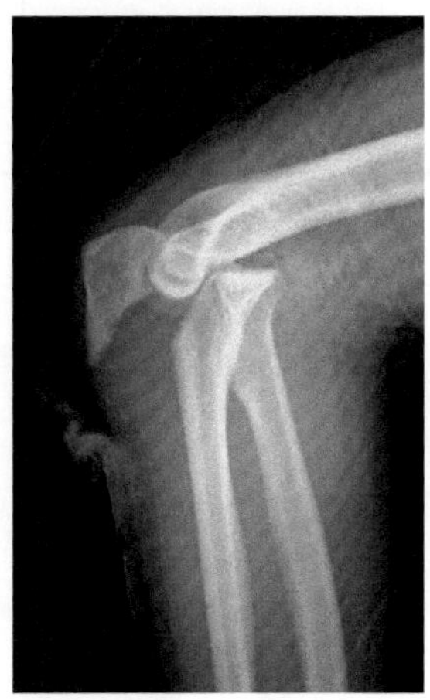
Type II

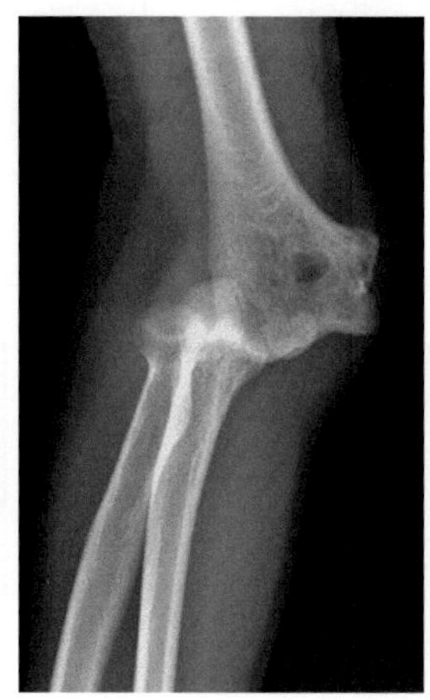
Type III

5.2.4 AO/OTA Classification (2007 modified, Journal of Orthopaedic Trauma. 21 Supplement)

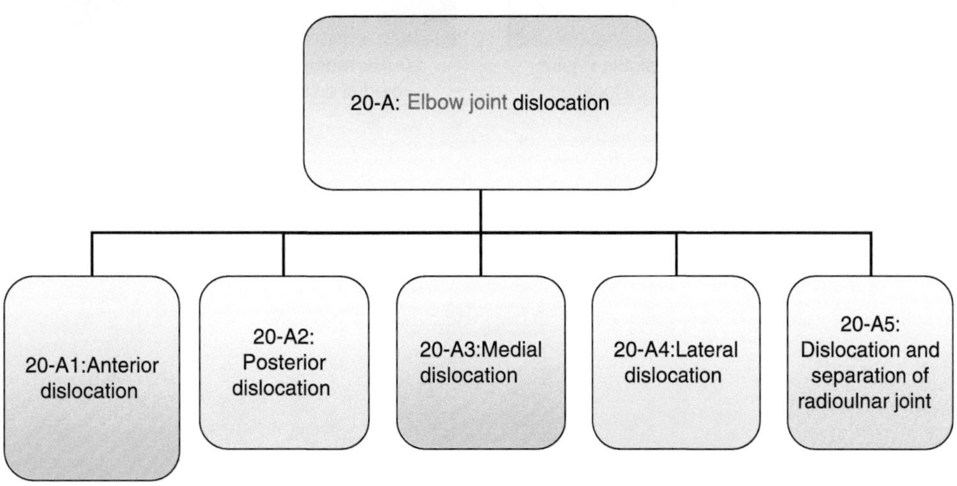

20-A: Dislocation of radioulnar joint.

20-A1: Anterior dislocation of radioulnar joint.

20-A2: Posterior dislocation of radioulnar joint.

20-A3: Medial dislocation of radioulnar joint.

20-A4: Lateral dislocation of radioulnar joint.

20-A5: Dislocation and separation of radioulnar joint.

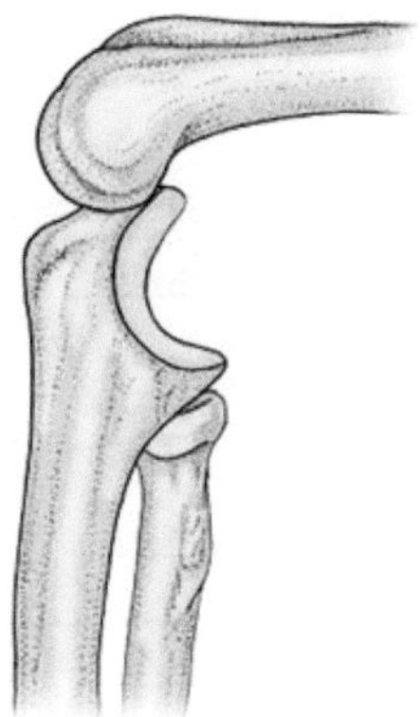

20-A1: radioulnar joint anterior dislocation

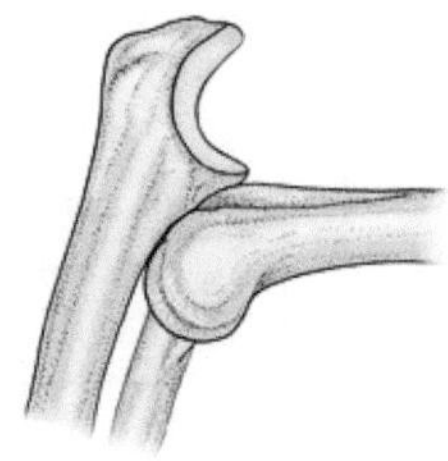

20-A2: radioulnar joint posterior dislocation

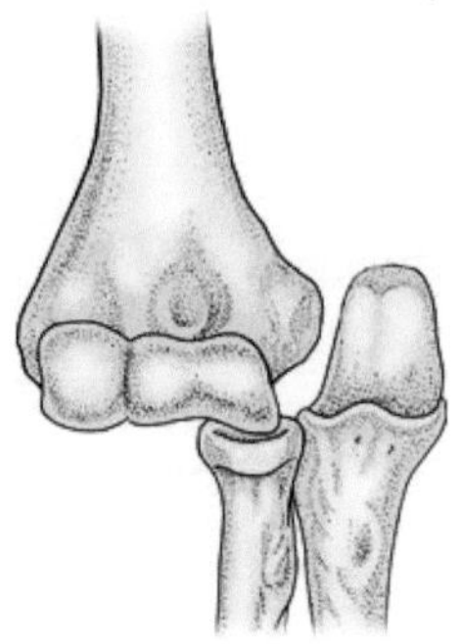

20-A3: radioulnar joint medial dislocation

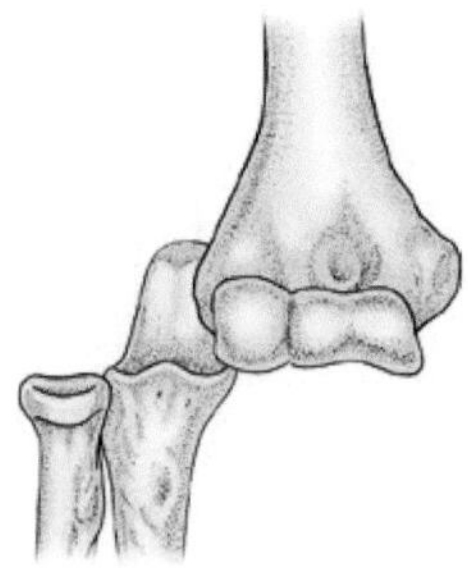

20-A4: radioulnar joint lateral dislocation

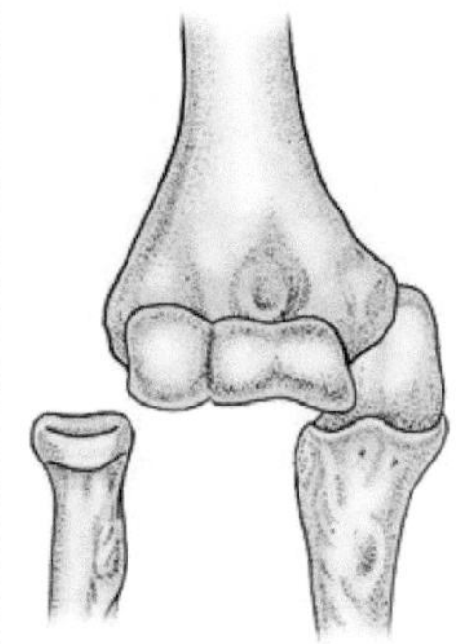

20-A5: radioulnar joint separation dislocation

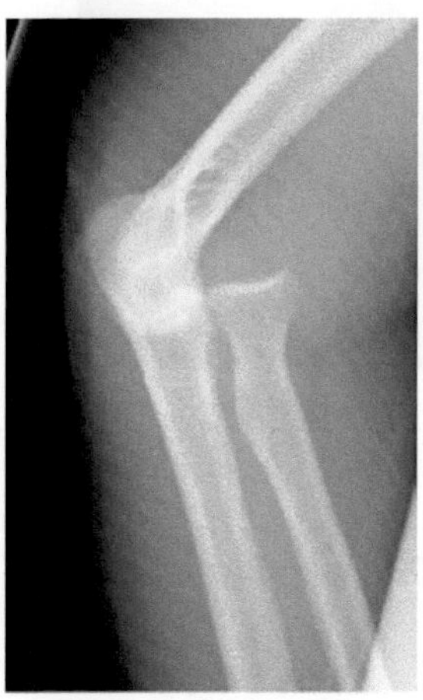

20-A1: radioulnar joint anterior dislocation

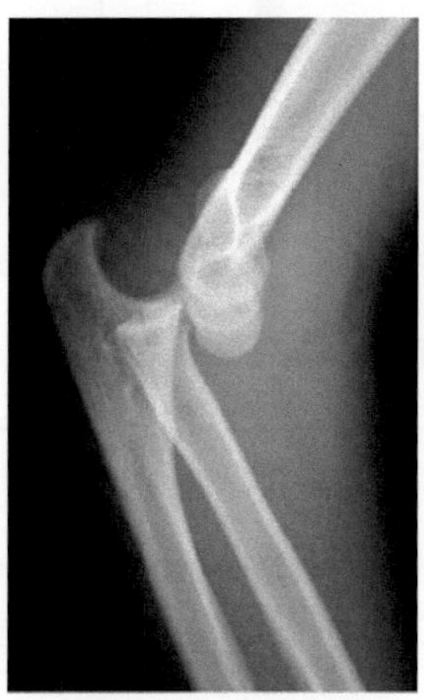

20-A2: radioulnar joint posterior dislocation

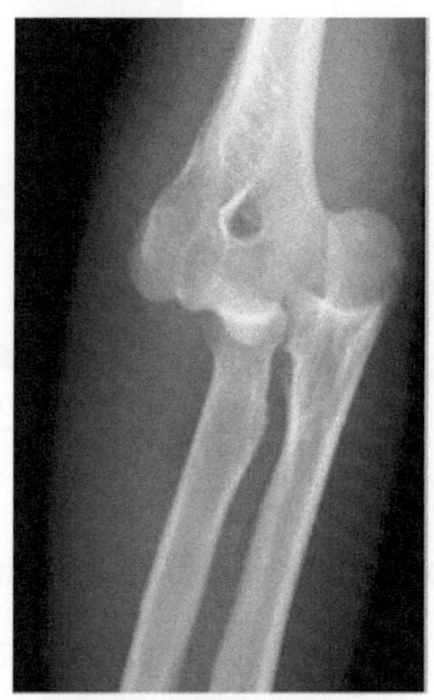

20-A3: radioulnar joint medial dislocation

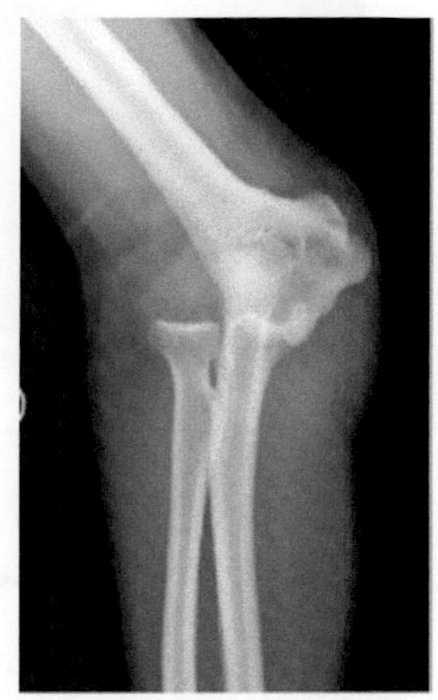

20-A4: radioulnar joint separation dislocation

5.2.5 AO/OTA Classification of the Dislocation of the Single Radial Joint (2007 modified, Journal of Orthopaedic Trauma. 21 Supplement)

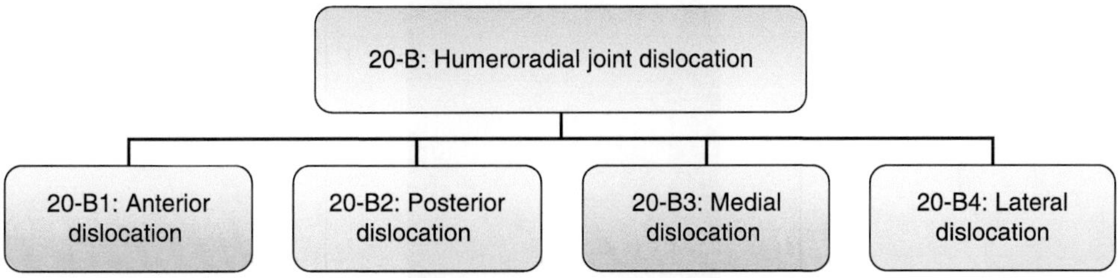

20-B1: Anterior dislocation.
20-B2: Posterior dislocation.
20-B3: Medial dislocation.
20-B4: Lateral dislocation.

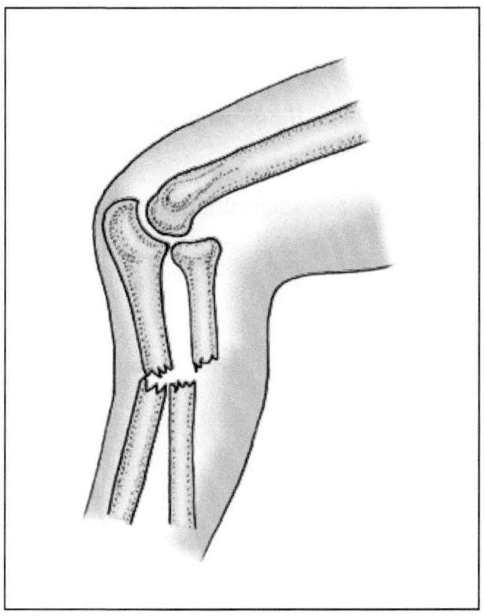

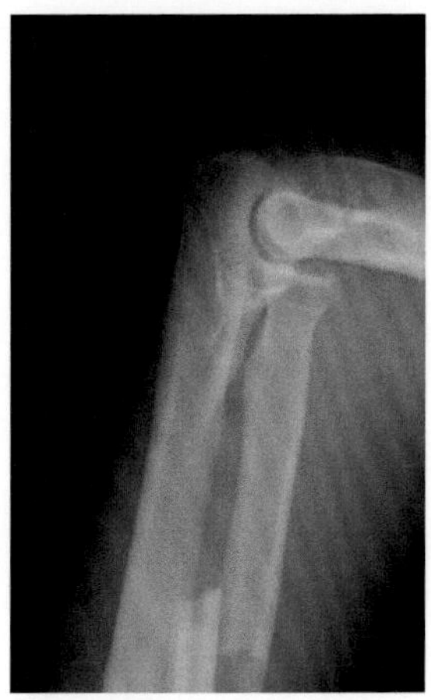

AO/OTA classification of elbow dislocation

20-B: Humeroradial joint dislocation.

20-B1: anterior dislocation

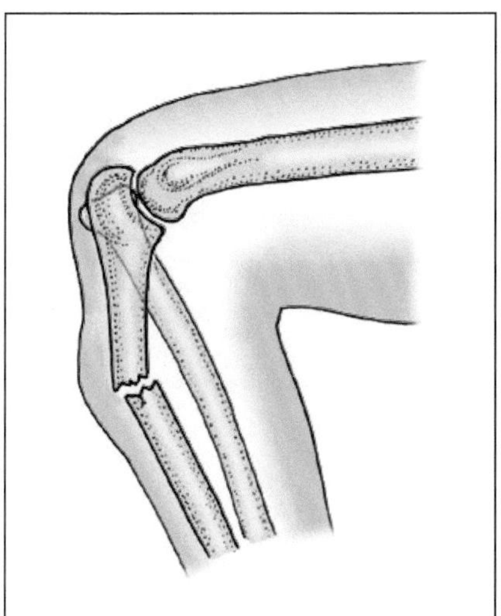

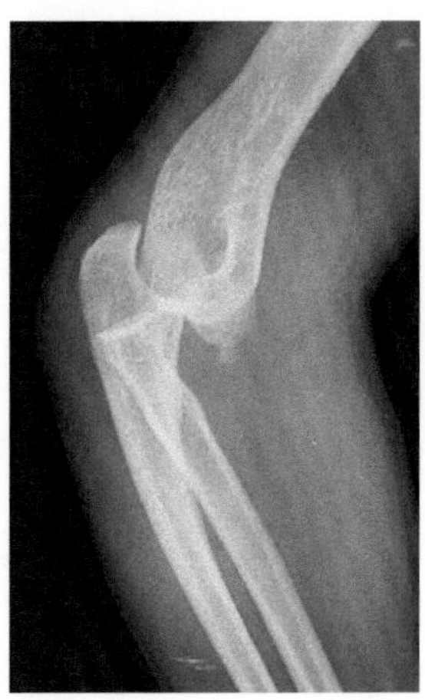

AO/OTA classification of elbow dislocation

20-B: Humeroradial joint dislocation.

20-B2: posterior dislocation

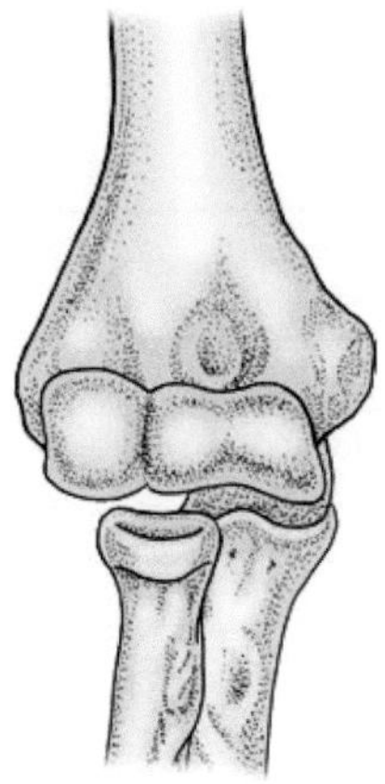

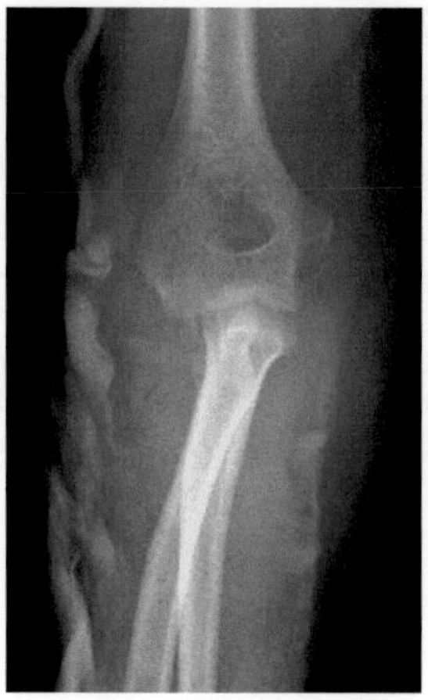

AO/OTA classification of elbow dislocation

20-B: Humeroradial joint dislocation.

20-B3: medial dislocation

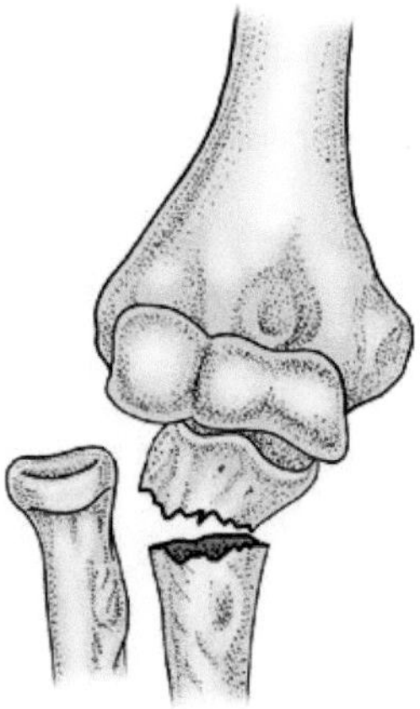

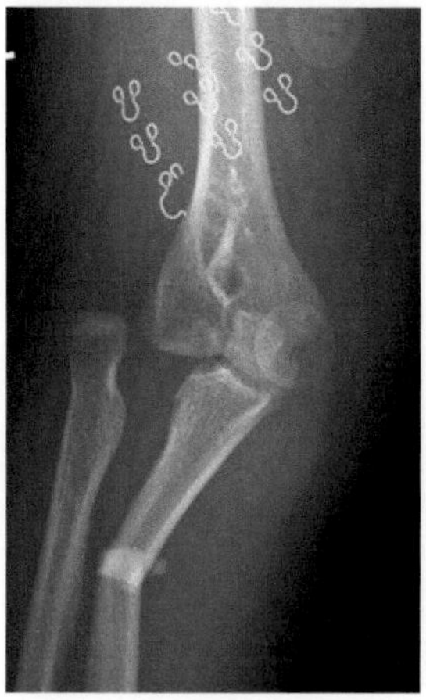

AO/OTA classification of elbow dislocation

20-B: Humeroradial joint dislocation.

20-B4: lateral dislocation

5.3 Section 3. Wrist Dislocation Classification

5.3.1 AO/OTA Classification of Dislocation of Inferior Radioulnar Joint (2007 modified, Journal of Orthopaedic Trauma. 21 Supplement)

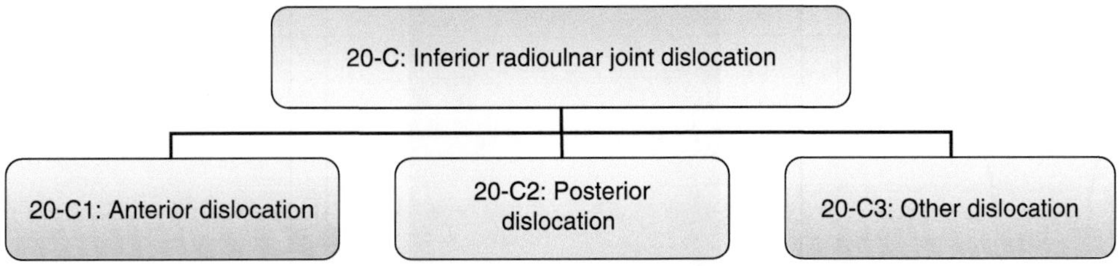

20-C1: Inferior radioulnar joint anterior dislocation.
20-C2: Inferior radioulnar joint posterior dislocation.
20-C3: Other dislocation of inferior radioulnar.

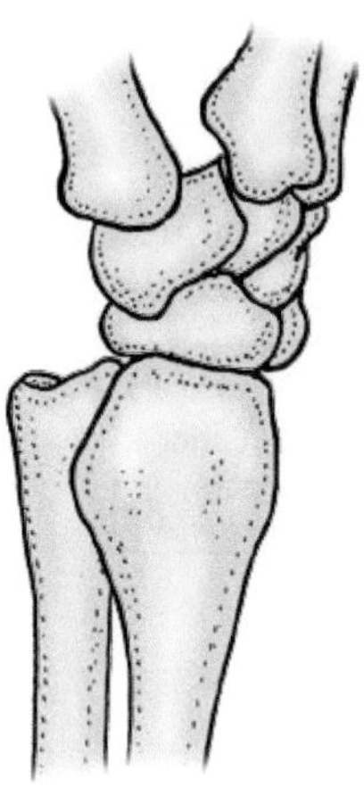

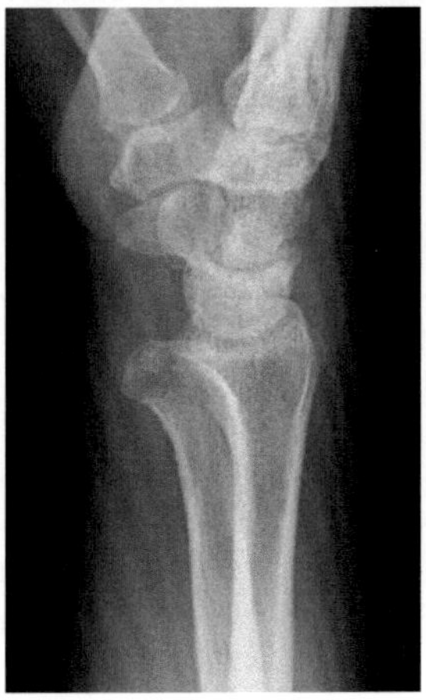

20-C: AO/OTA classification of dislocation of inferior radioulnar joint.
20-C1: anterior dislocation

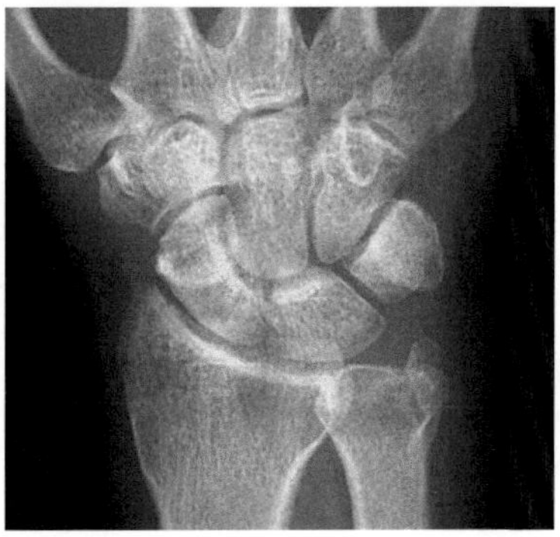

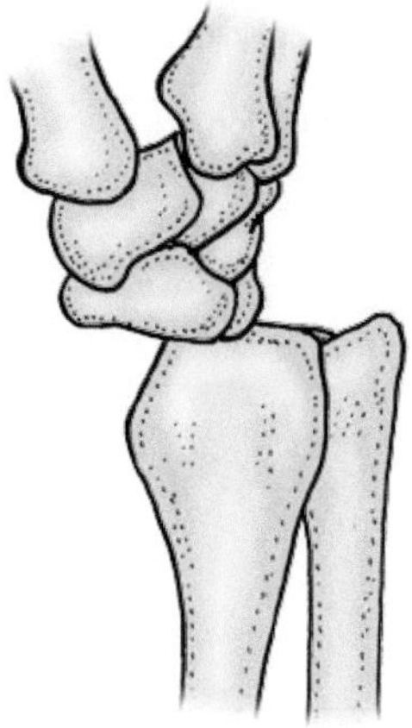

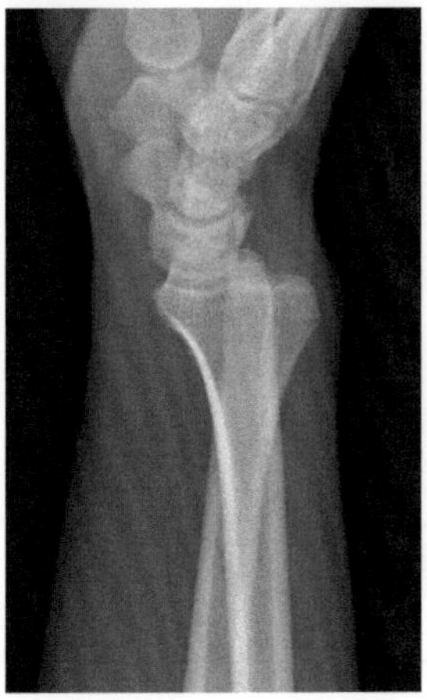

20-C: AO/OTA classification of dislocation of inferior radioulnar joint.

20-C2: posterior dislocation

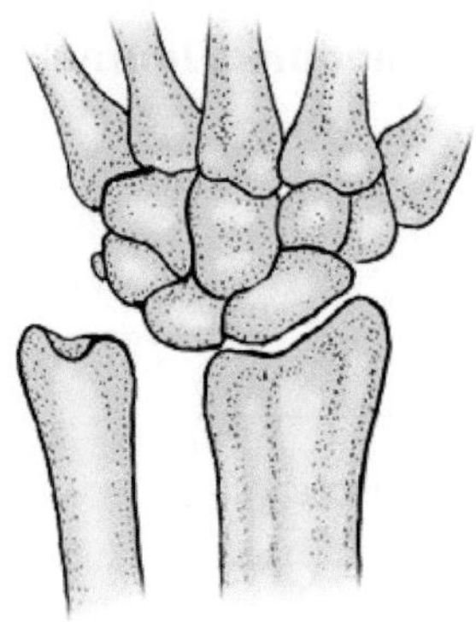

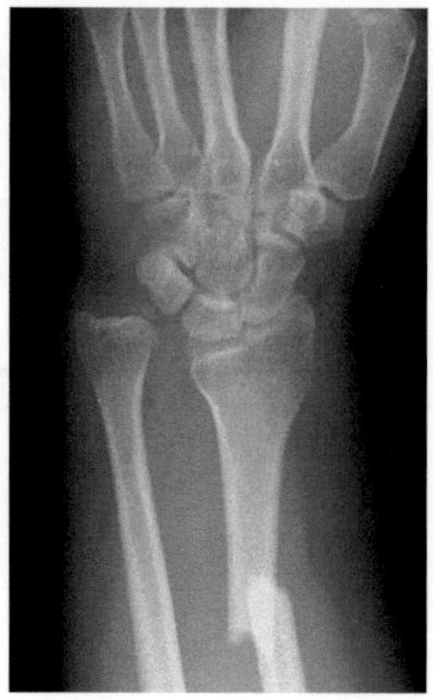

20-C: AO/OTA classification of dislocation of inferior radioulnar joint.

20-C3: Other dislocation

5.3.2 OA/OTA Classification of Radiocarpal Joint Dislocation (2007 modified, Journal of Orthopaedic Trauma. 21 Supplement)

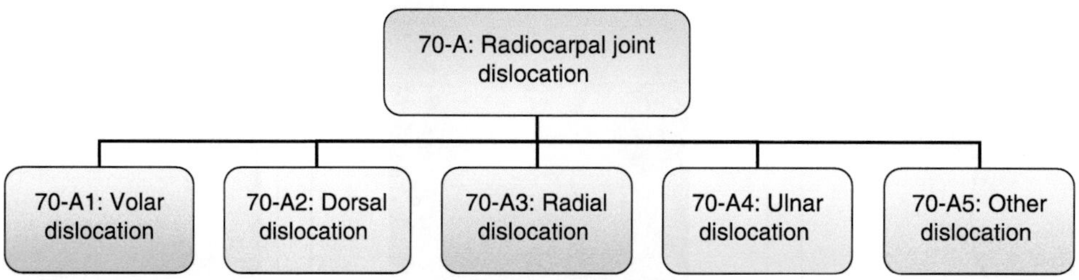

70-A1: Volar dislocation.
70-A2: Dorsal dislocation.
70-A3: Radial dislocation.
70-A4: Ulnar dislocation.
70-A5: Other dislocation.

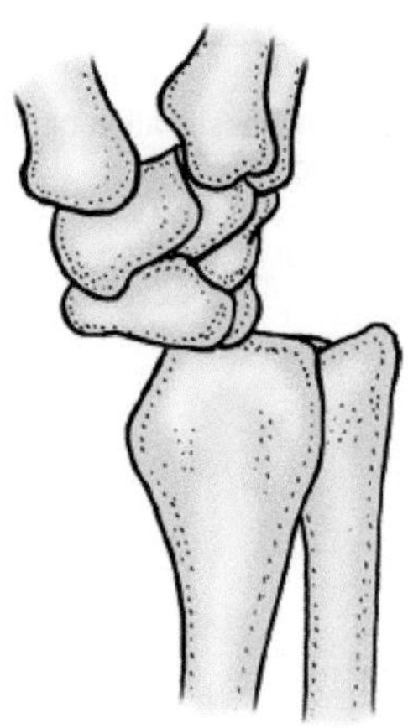

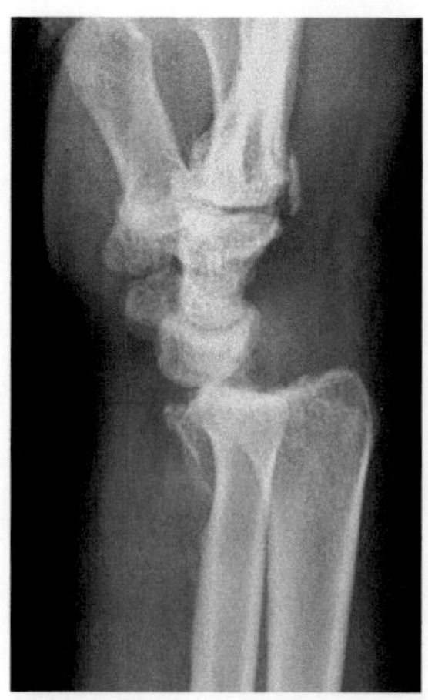

AO/OTA clssification of hand-wrist dislocation

70-A: radiocarpal joint dislocation.

A1: Volar dislocation

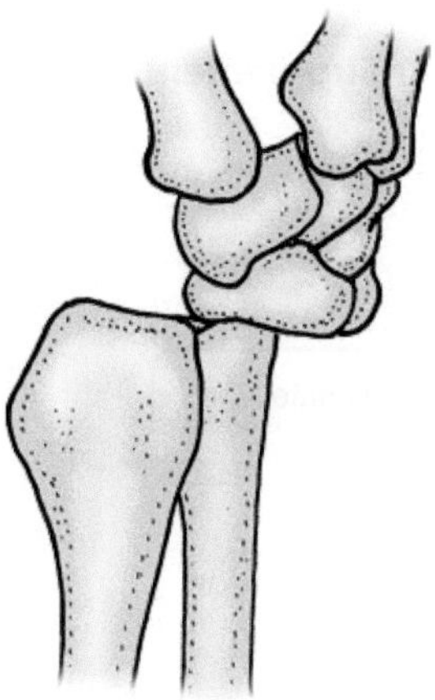

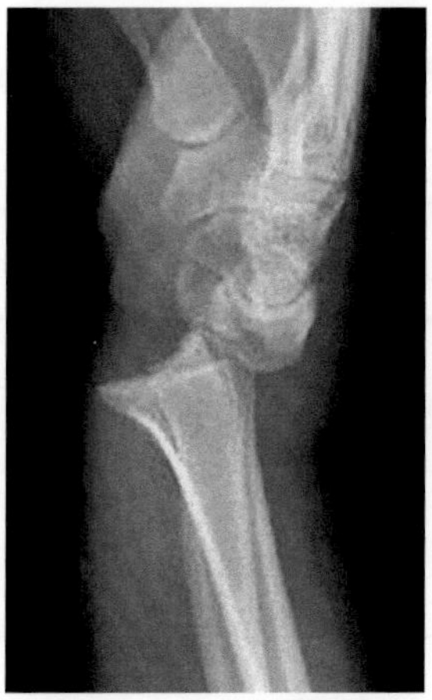

AO/OTA clssification of hand-wrist dislocation

70-A: radiocarpal joint dislocation.

A2: Dorsal dislocation

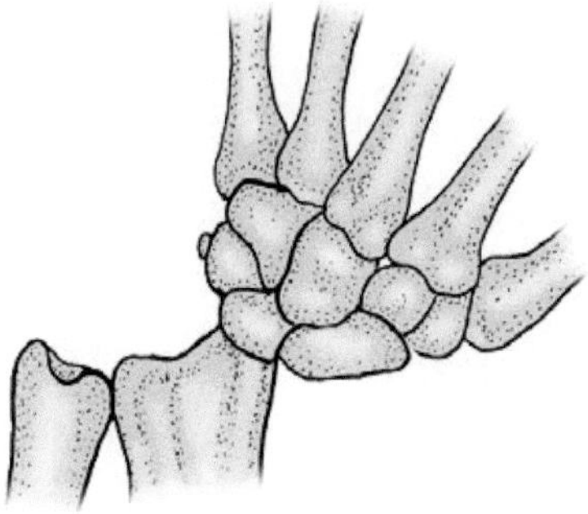

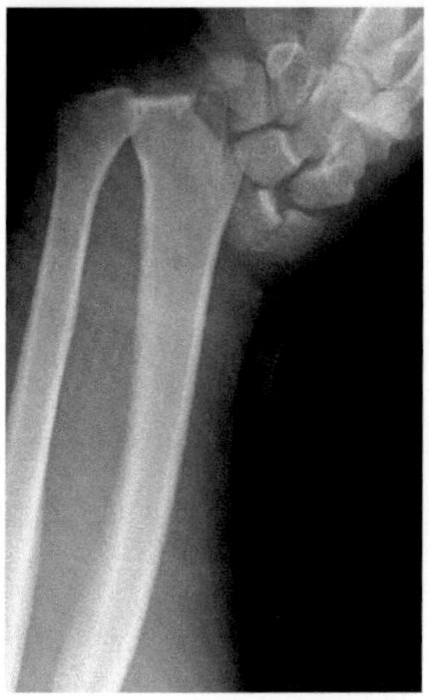

AO/OTA clssification of hand-wrist dislocation

70-A: radiocarpal joint dislocation.

A3: Radial dislocation

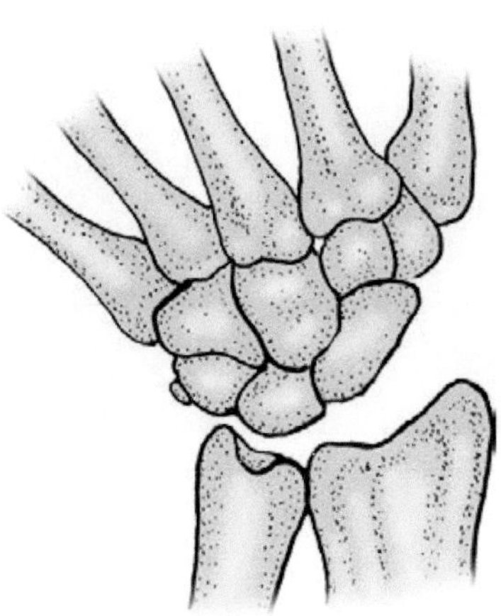

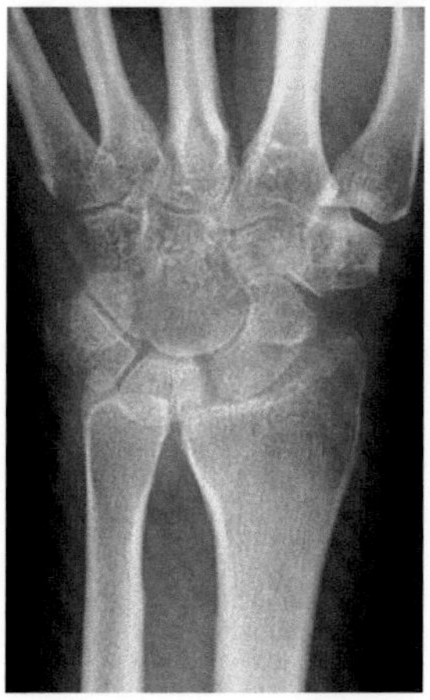

AO/OTA clssification of hand-wrist dislocation

70-A: radiocarpal joint dislocation.

A4: Ulnar dislocation

5.3.3 Midcarpal Joint Dislocation

5.3.3.1 AO/OTA Classification (2007 modified, Journal of Orthopaedic Trauma. 21 Supplement)

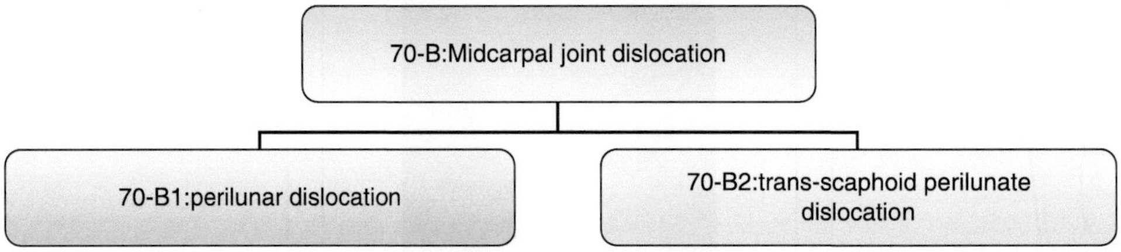

70-B: Midcarpal joint dislocation, including perilunar dislocation or trans-scaphoid perilunate dislocation.

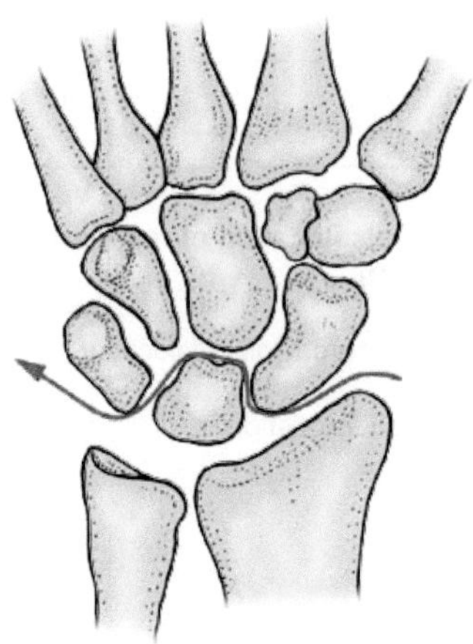

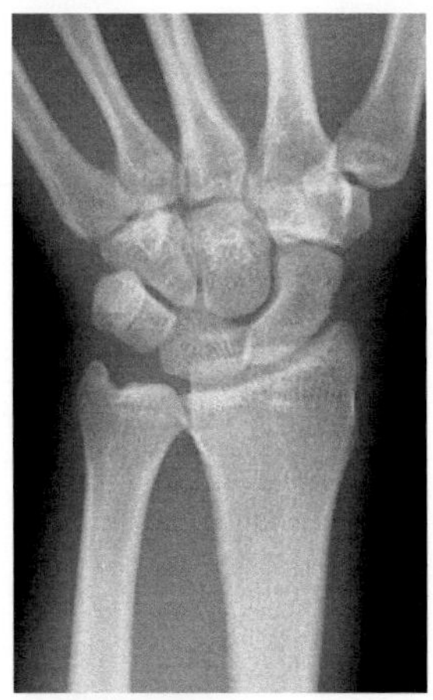

AO/OTA clssification of hand-wrist dislocation

70-B1: Midcarpal joint dislocation. perilunar dislocation

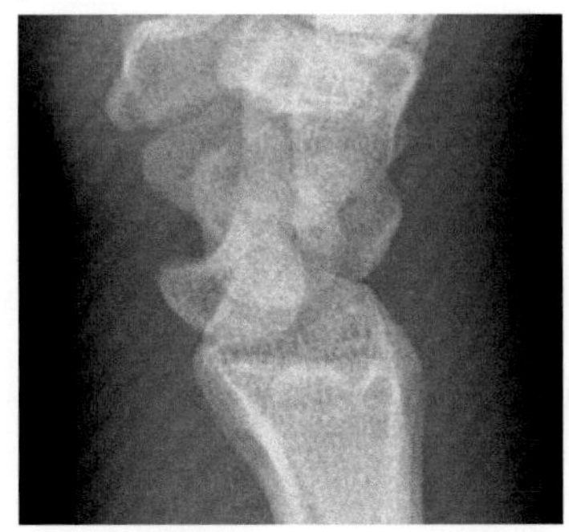

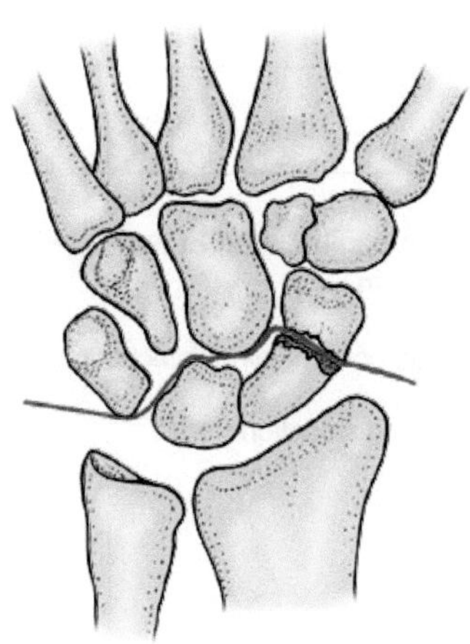

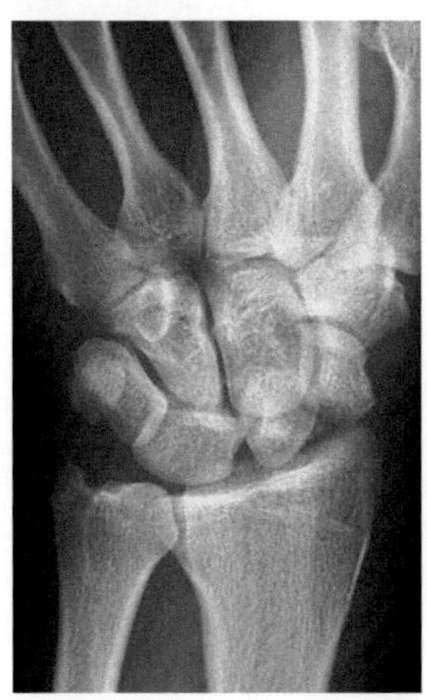

AO/OTA clssification of hand-wrist dislocation

70-B2: Midcarpal joint dislocation. trans-scaphoid perilunate dislocation

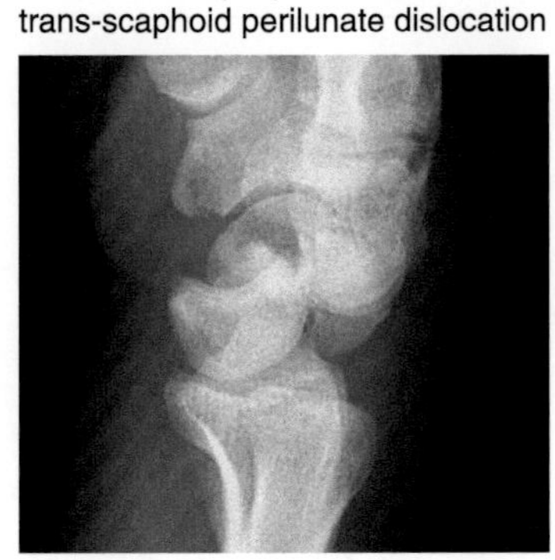

5.3.3.2 Other Type of Perilunar Dislocation

Tang Jinpo Classification (Gu Yudong, Wang Shuhuan, Shi de. Hand Surgery. Shang Hai: Shanghai Science and Technology Press 2002)

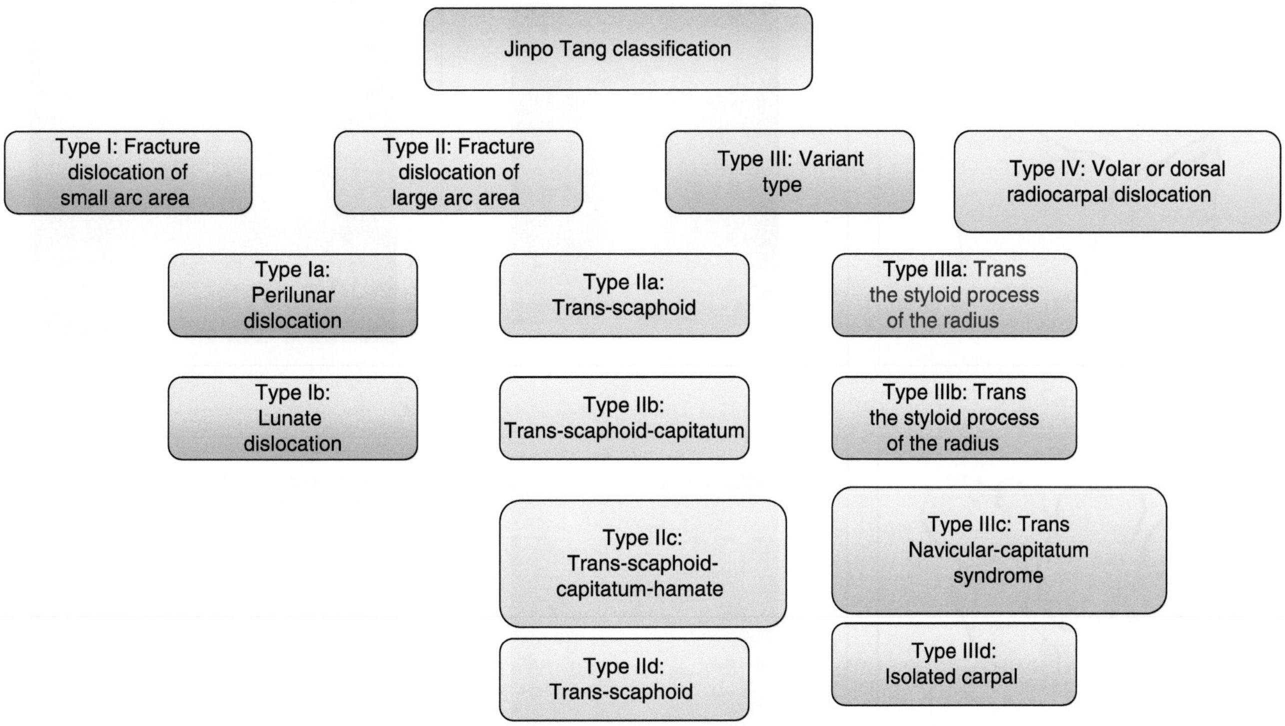

Type I: Fracture dislocation of small arc area, divided into:
- Ia: Perilunar dislocation.
- Ib: Lunate dislocation.

Type II: Fracture dislocation of large arc area, divided into:
- IIa: Trans-scaphoid perilunate fracture dislocations.
- IIb: Trans-scaphoid-capitatum perilunate fracture dislocations.
- IIc: Trans-scaphoid-capitatum-hamate-triquetrum perilunate dislocations.
- IId: Trans-scaphoid lunate volar fracture dislocations.

Type III: Variant type, divided into:
- IIIa: Trans the styloid process of the radius perilunate fracture dislocations.
- IIIb: Trans the styloid process of the radius-scaphoid perilunate fracture dislocations.
- IIIc: Navicular-capitatum syndrome.
- IIId: Isolated carpal dislocation.

Type IV: Volar or dorsal radiocarpal dislocation.

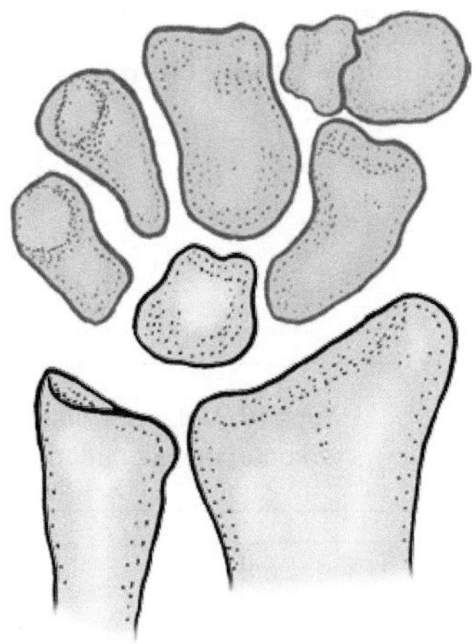

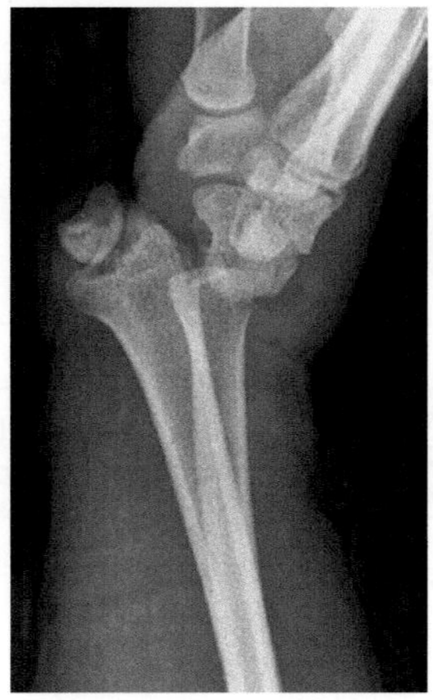

Jinpo Tang classification of perilunar dislocation
Type I: Fracture dislocation of small arc area.
Type Ia: Perilunar dislocation

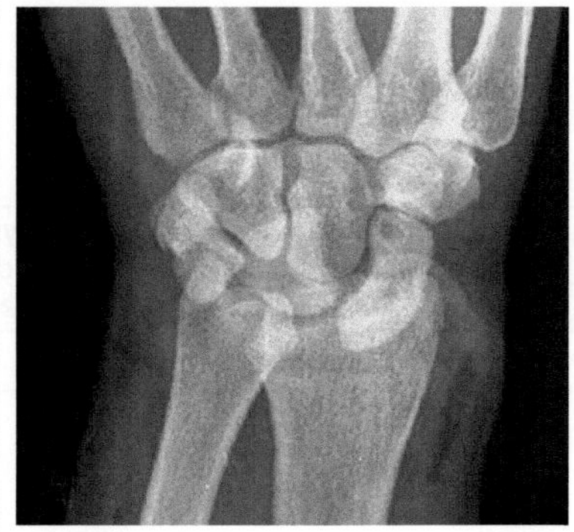

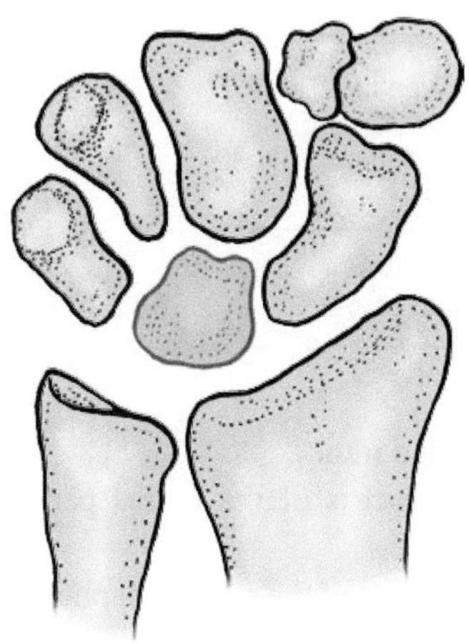

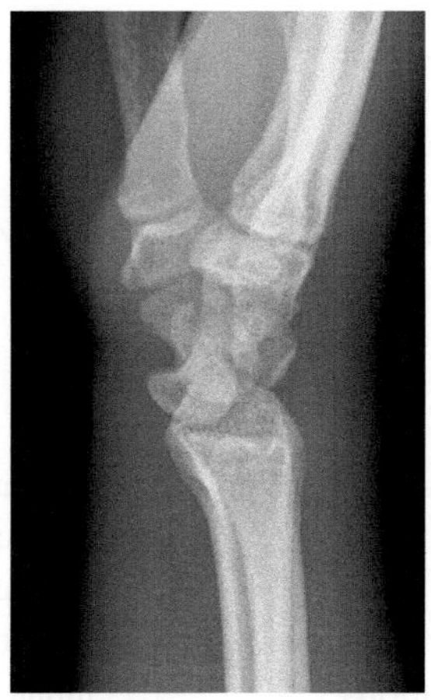

Jinpo Tang classification of perilunar dislocation
Type I: Fracture dislocation of small arc area.
Type Ib: Lunate dislocation

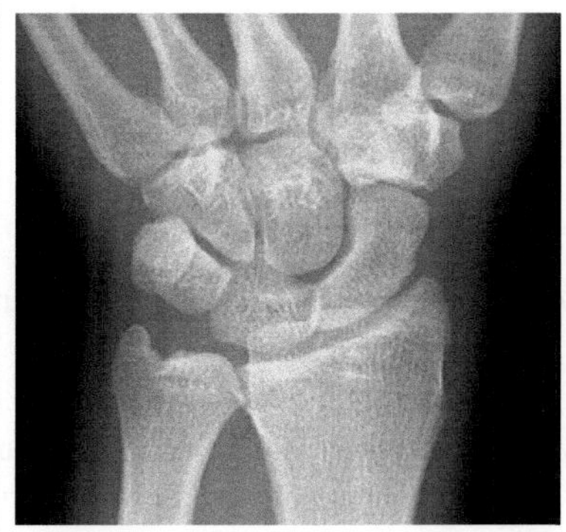

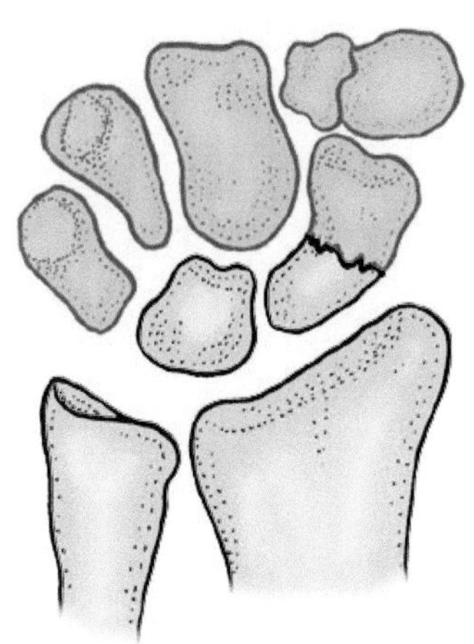

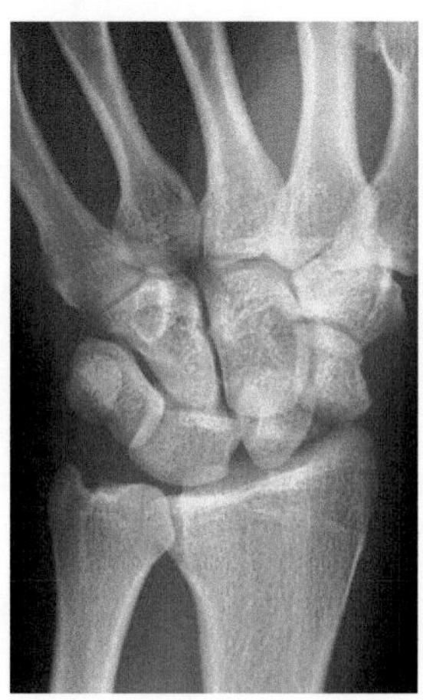

Jinpo Tang classification of perilunar dislocation
Type II: Fracture dislocation of large arc area.
Type IIa: Trans-scaphoid perilunate fracture dislocations

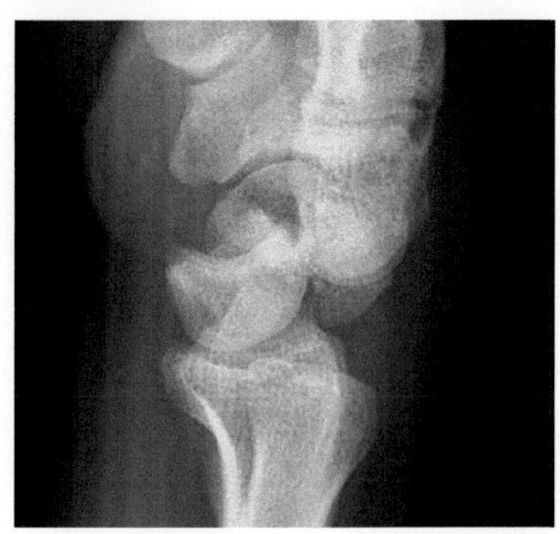

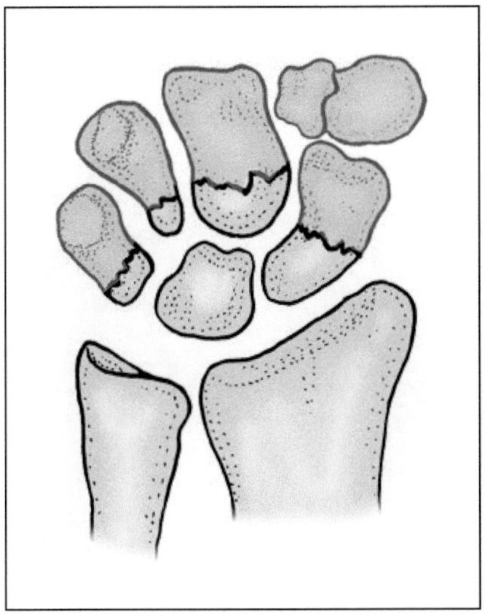

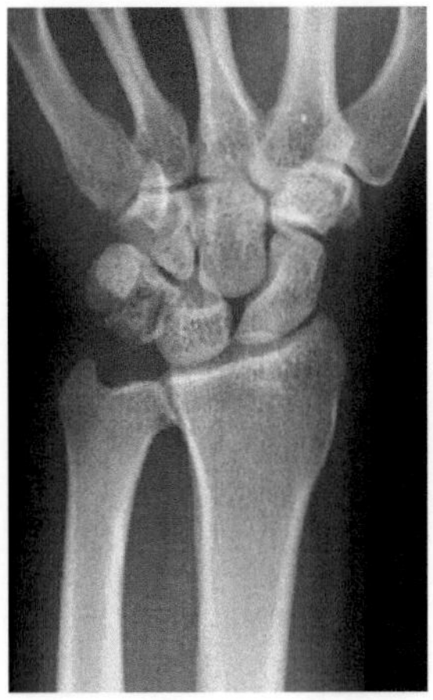

Jinpo Tang classification of perilunar dislocation
Type II: Fracture dislocation of large arc area.
Type IIc: Trans-scaphoid-capitatum perilunate dislocations

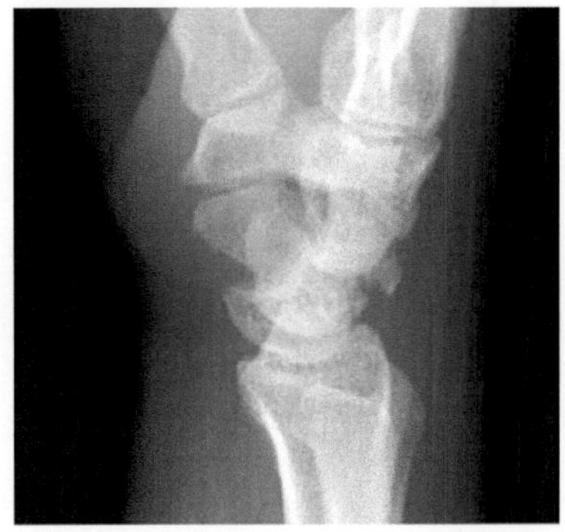

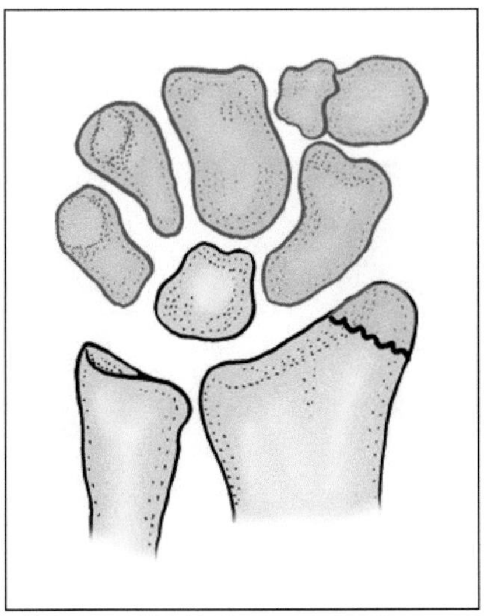

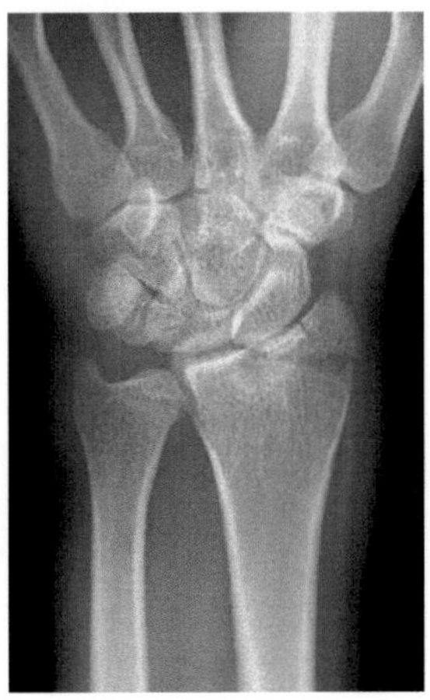

Jinpo Tang classification of perilunar dislocation
Type III: Variant type.
Type IIIa: Trans the styloid process of the radius perilunate fracture dislocations

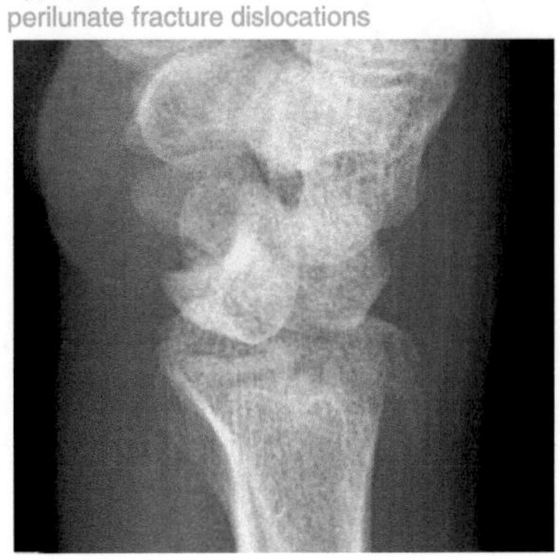

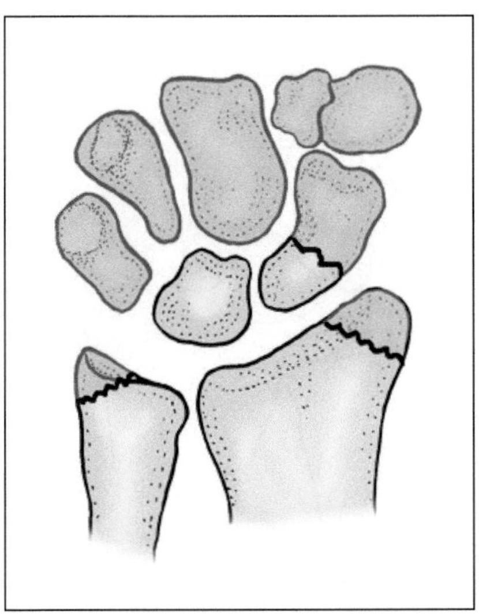

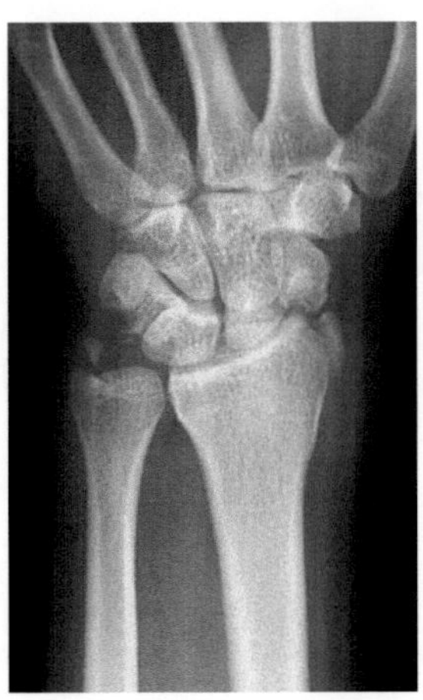

Jinpo Tang classification of perilunar dislocation
Type III: Variant type.
Type IIIb: Trans the styloid process of the radius -scaphoid perilunate fracture dislocations

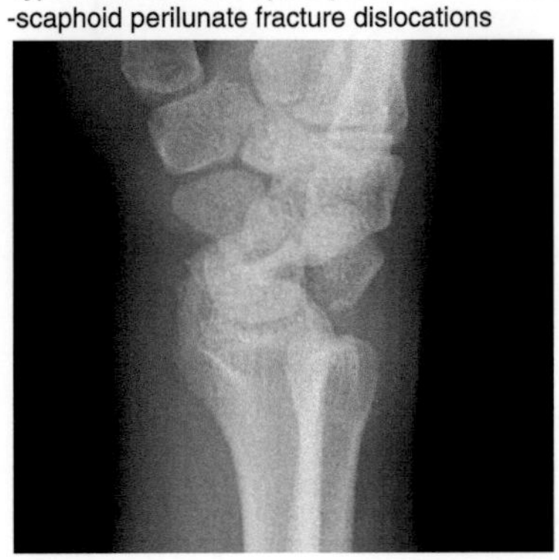

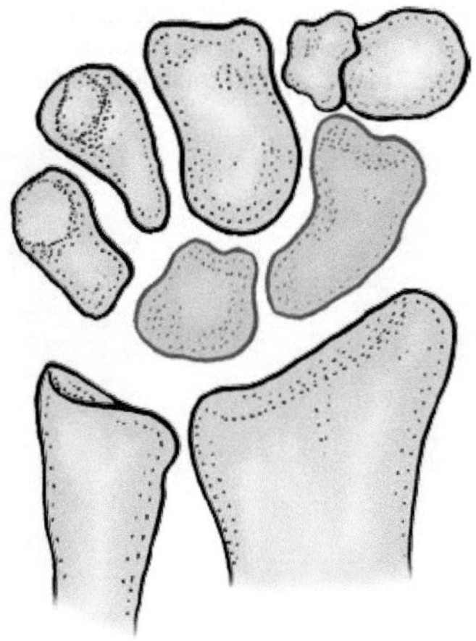

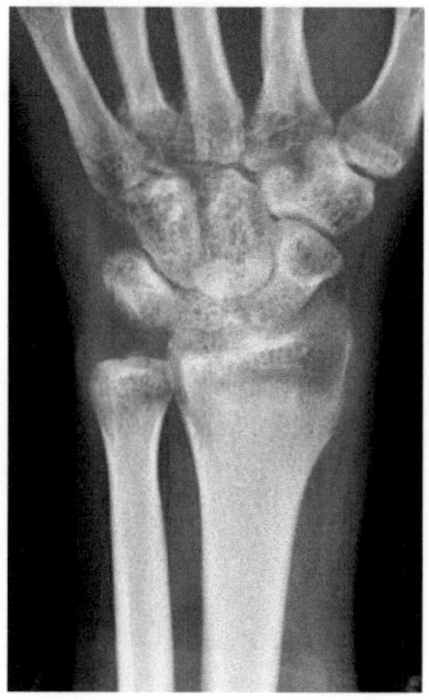

Jinpo Tang classification of perilunar dislocation
Type III: Variant type.
Type IIId: Isolated carpal dislocation

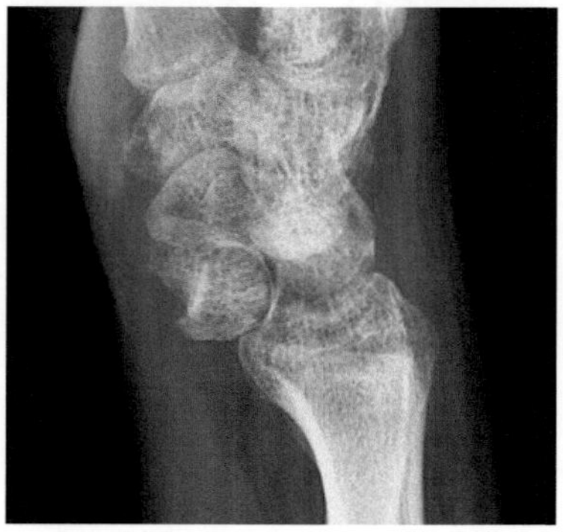

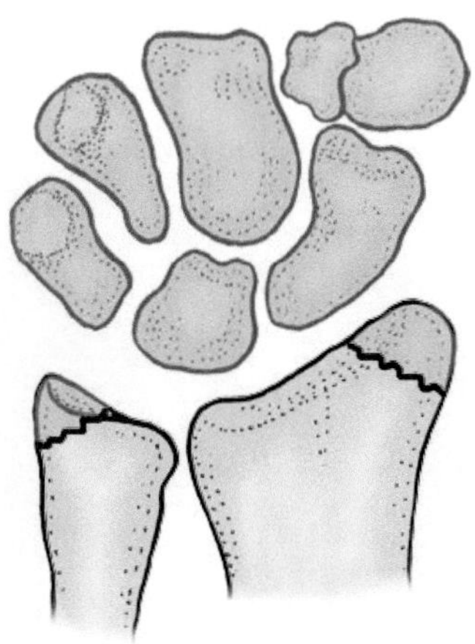

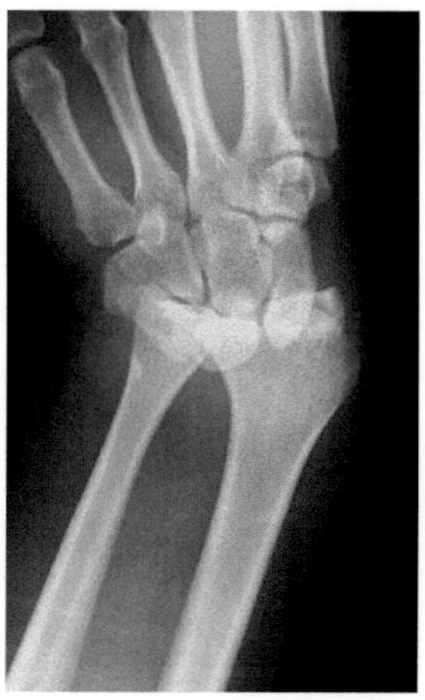

Jinpo Tang classification of perilunar dislocation
Type IV: dorsal radiocarpal joint dislocation

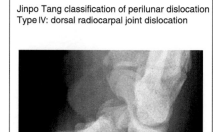

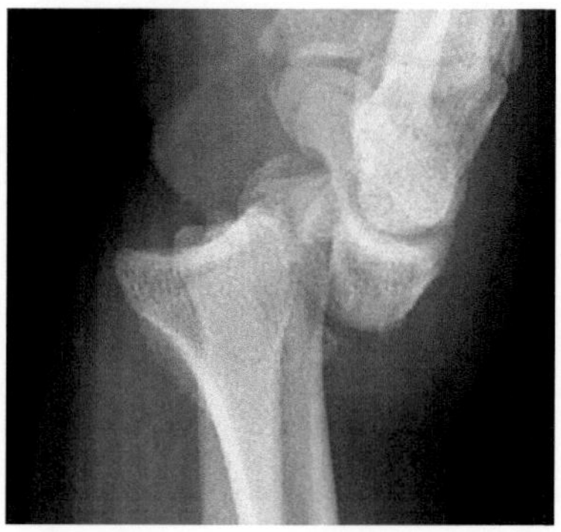

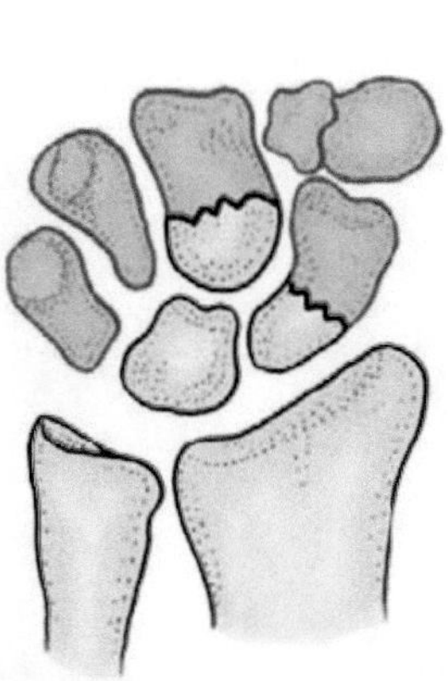

Jinpo Tang classification of perilunar dislocation
Type II: Fracture dislocation of large arc area.
Type IIb: Trans-scaphoid-capitatum perilunate fracture dislocation

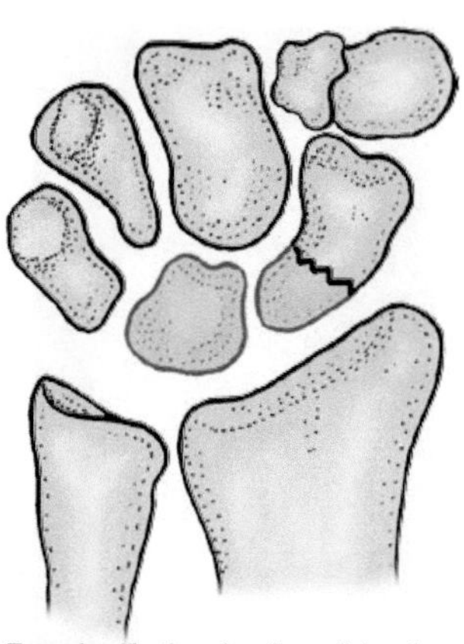

Jinpo Tang classification of perilunar dislocation
Type II: Fracture dislocation of large arc area.
Type IId: Trans-scaphoid lunate volar fracture dislocation

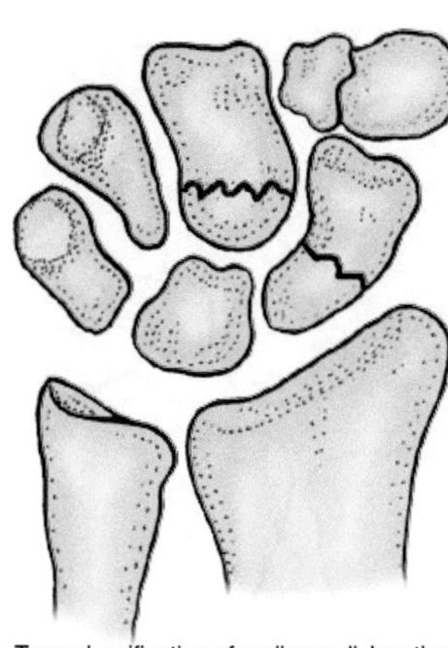

Jinpo Tang classification of perilunar dislocation
Type III: Variant type.
Type IIIc: Navicular-capurum syndrome

Rockwood Classification (1996, Fractures in Adults. 4th ed. Philadelphia: Lippincott-Raven Publishers)

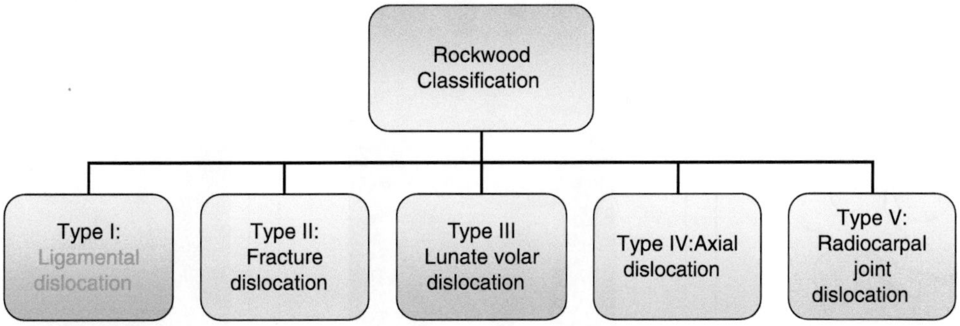

Type I: Ligamental dislocation.
Type II: Fracture dislocation.
Type III: Lunate volar dislocation.
Type IV: Axial dislocation.
Type V: Radiocarpal joint dislocation.

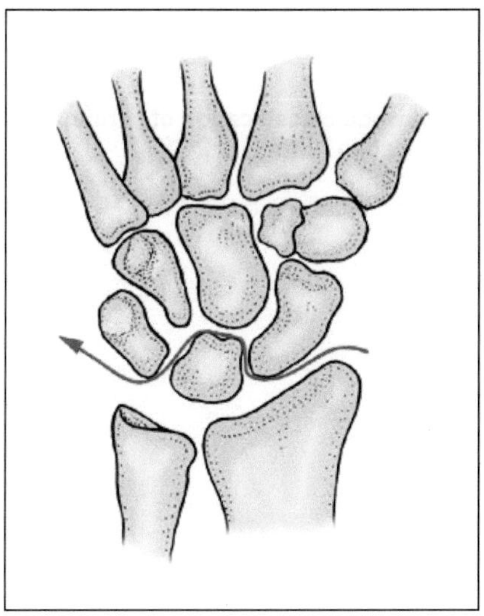

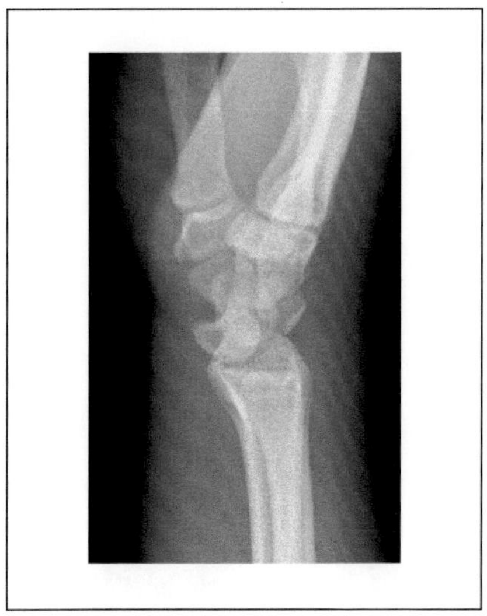

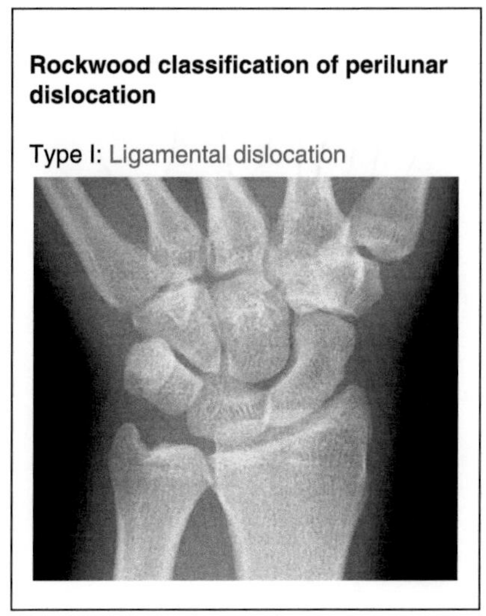

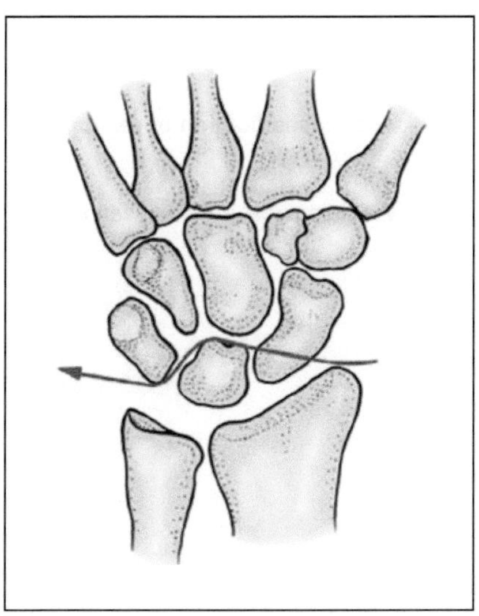

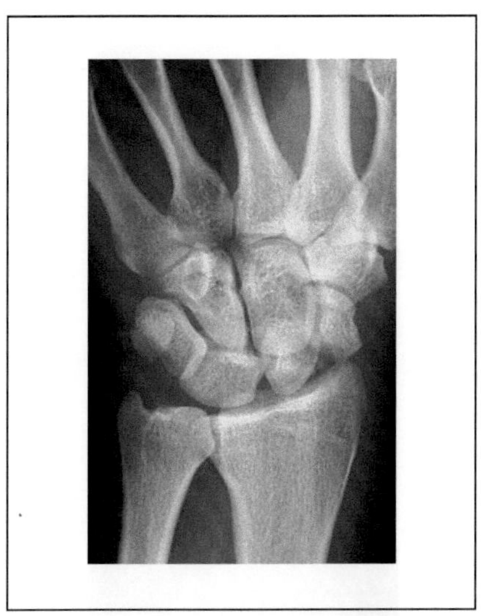

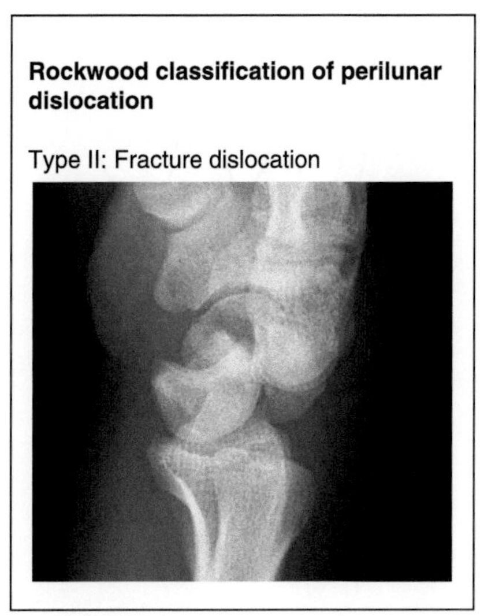

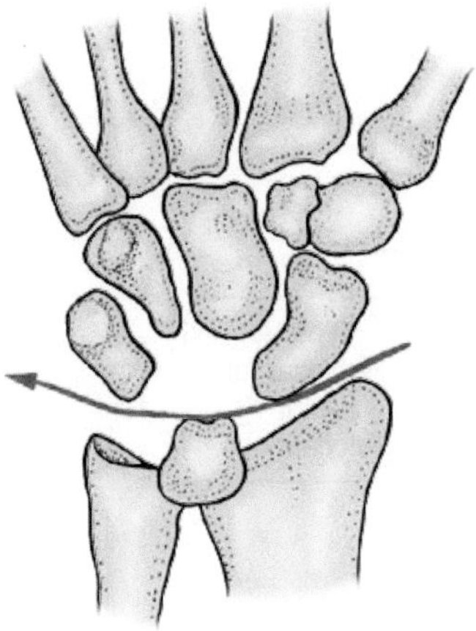

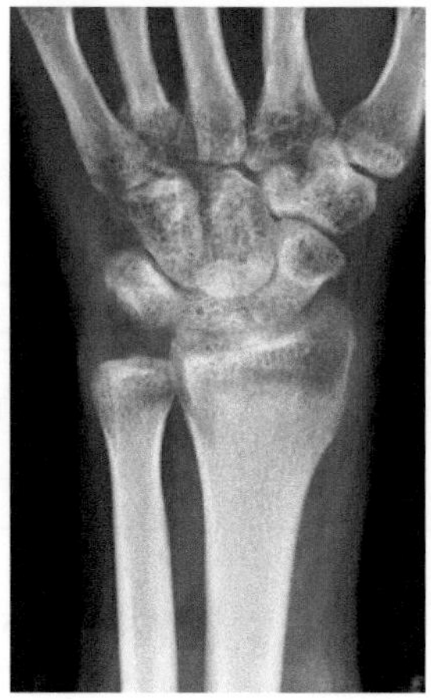

Rockwood classification of perilunar dislocation

Type III: Lunate volar dislocation

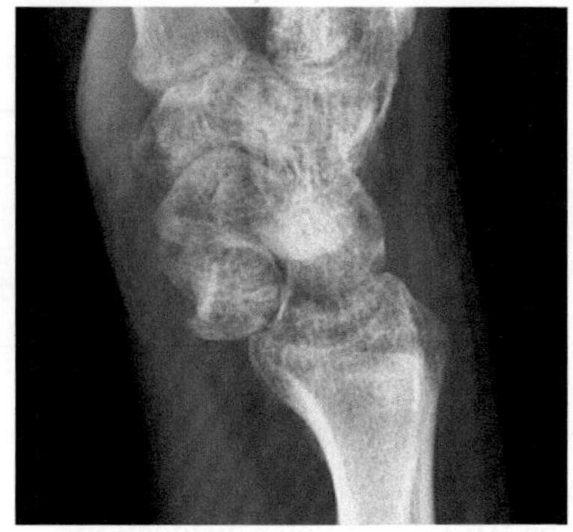

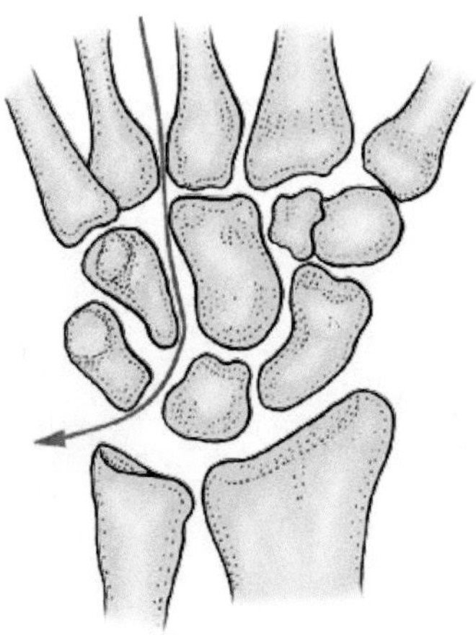

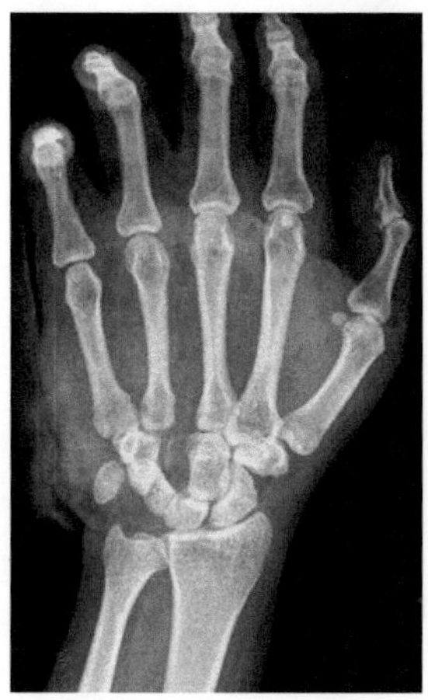

Rockwood classification of perilunar. dislocation

Type IV: Axial dislocation.

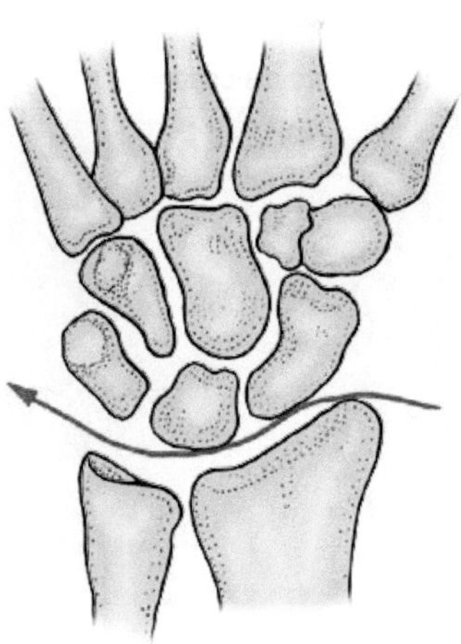

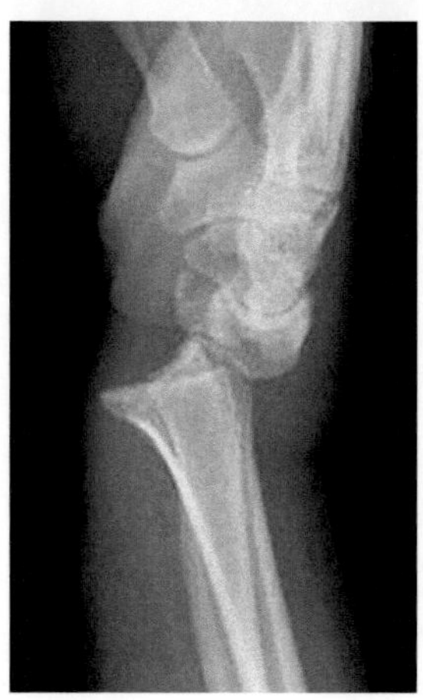

Rockwood classification of perilunar. dislocation

Type V: Radiocarpal joint dislocation.

5.3.3.3 Classification of Garcia-Elias of the Wrist Axial Injury and Dislocation (1989, J Hand Surg (Am), 14: 446–457)

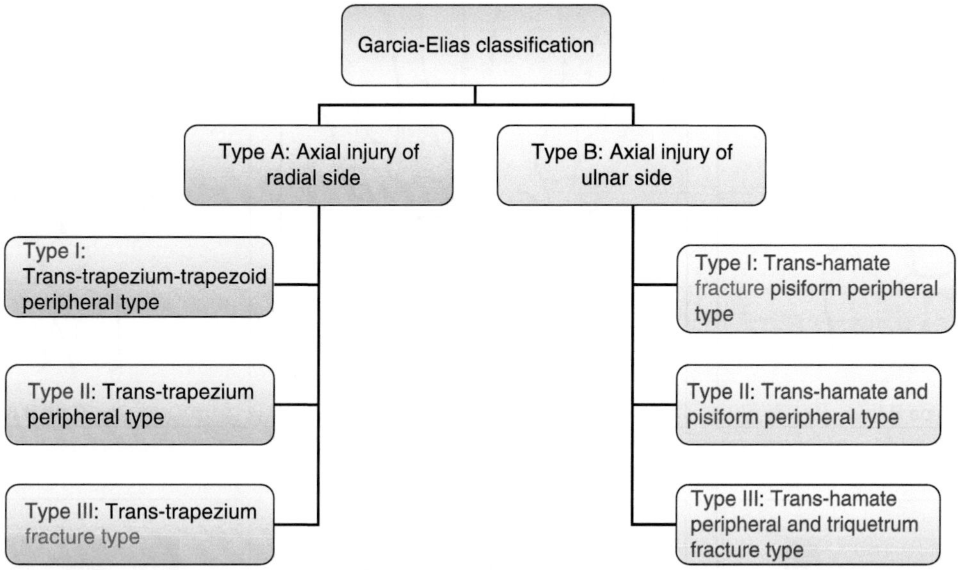

Type A: Axial injury of radial side (trans the trapezium and trapezoid).
- Type I: Trans-trapezium-trapezoid peripheral type.
- Type II: Trans-trapezium peripheral type.
- Type III: Trans-trapezium fracture type.

Type B: Axial injury of ulnar side (trans-hamate fracture, peril-hamate fracture, and triquetrum fracture type).
- Type I: Trans-hamate fracture pisiform peripheral type.
- Type II: Trans-hamate and pisiform peripheral type.
- Type III: Trans-hamate peripheral and triquetrum fracture type.

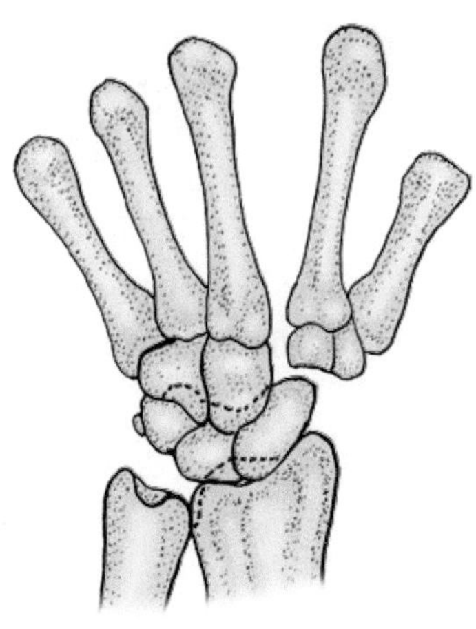
Type A I

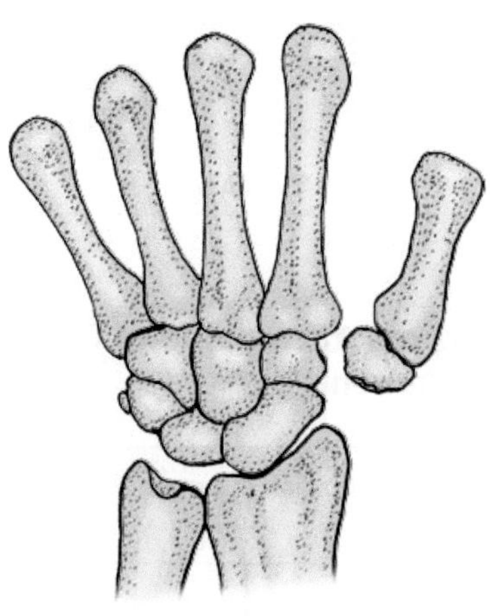
Type A II

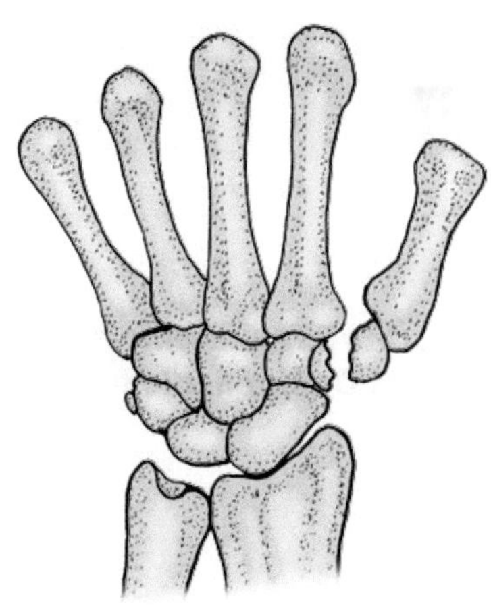
Type A III

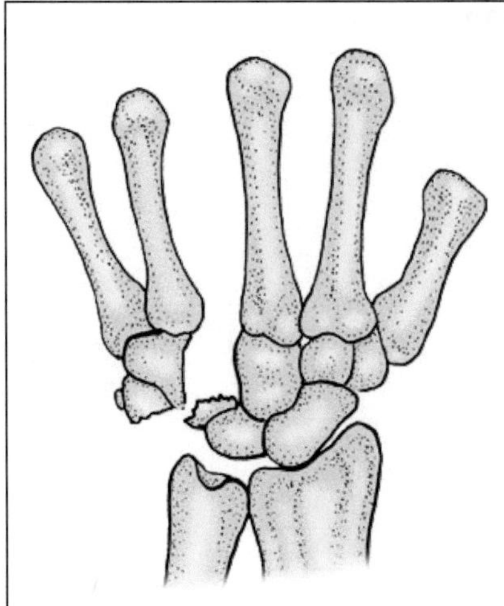

Type B I

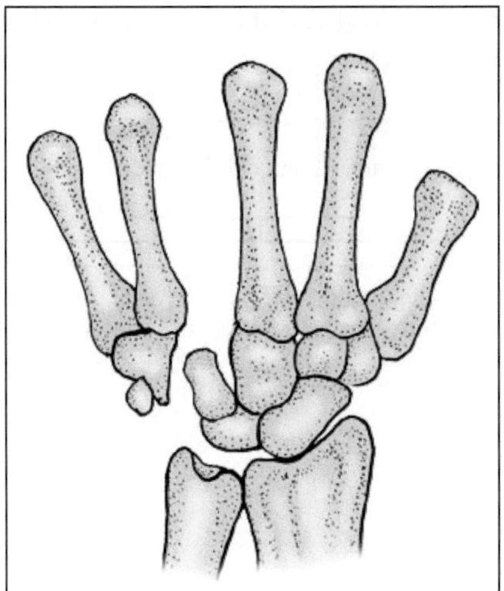

Type B II

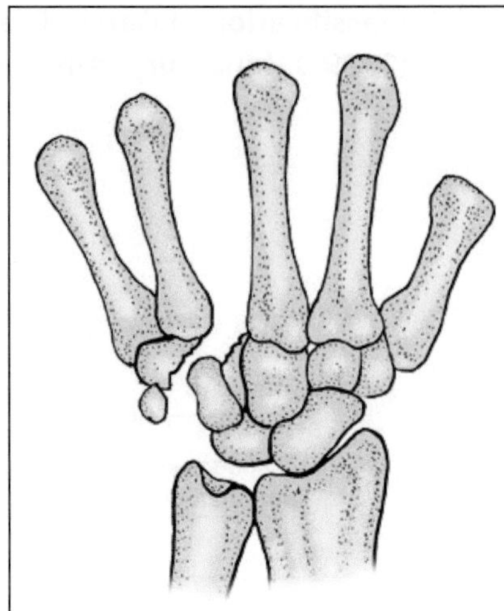

Type B III

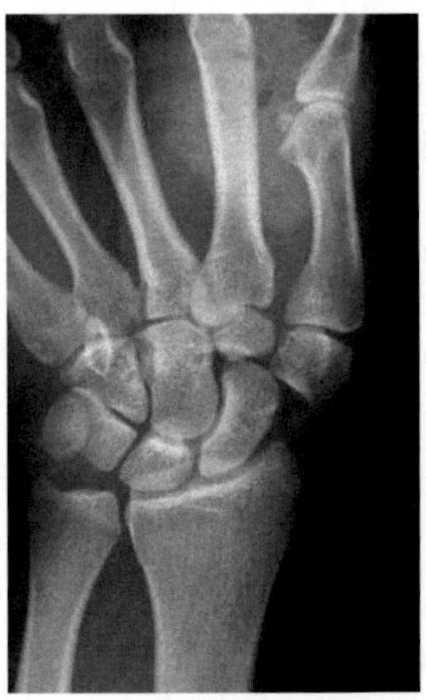

Type A II

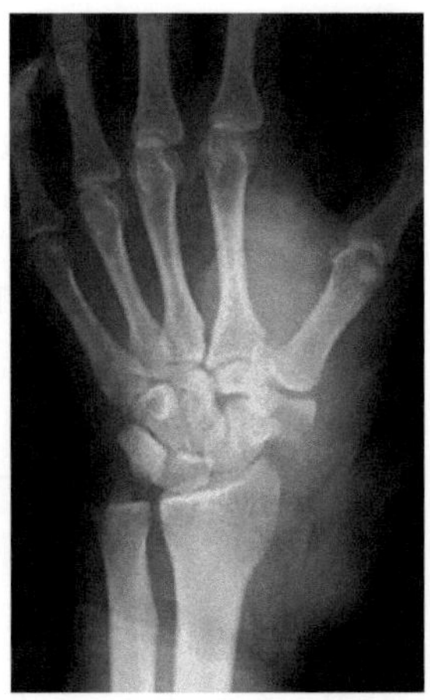

Type A III

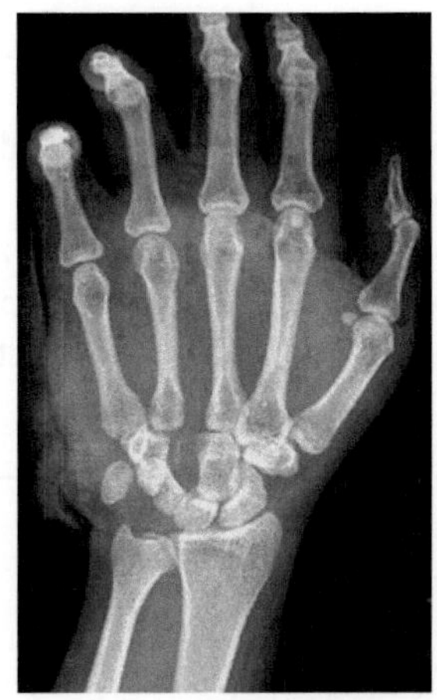

Type B II

5.3.4 AO/OTA Classification of the Carpometacarpal Joint Dislocation (2007 modified, Journal of Orthopaedic Trauma. 21 Supplement)

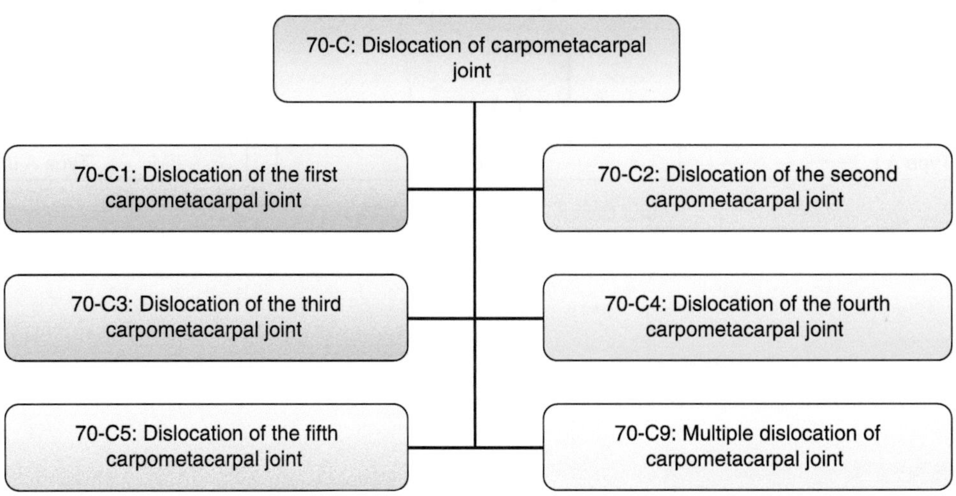

70-C: Dislocation of carpometacarpal joint, divided into:
70-C1: Dislocation of the first carpometacarpal joint.
70-C2: Dislocation of the second carpometacarpal joint.
70-C3: Dislocation of the third carpometacarpal joint.
70-C4: Dislocation of the fourth carpometacarpal joint.
70-C5: Dislocation of the fifth carpometacarpal joint.
70-C9: Multiple dislocation of carpometacarpal joint.

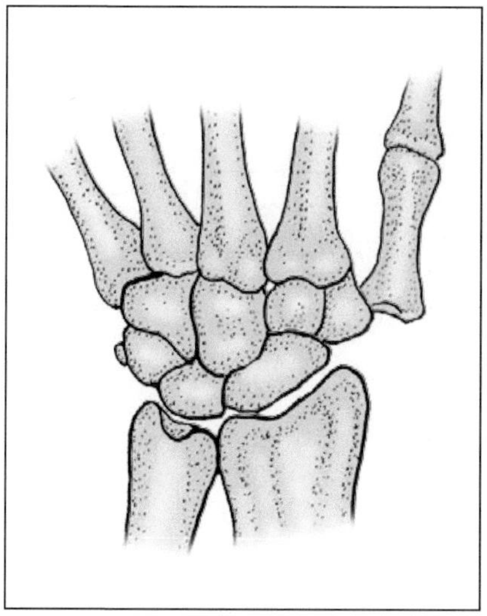

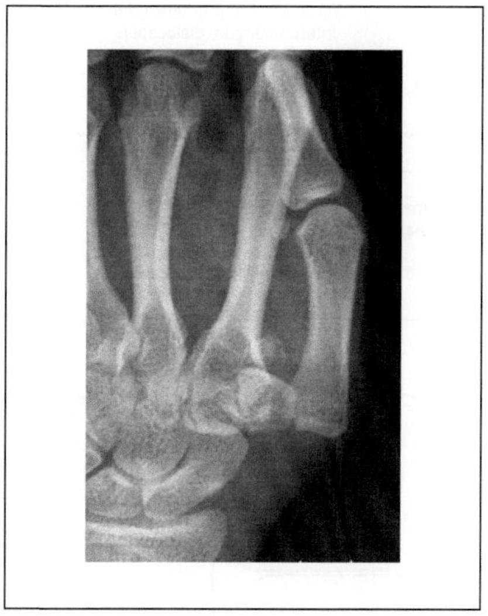

AO/OTA classification of the carpometacarpal joint dislocation

70-C: Dislocation of carpometacarpal joint.

C1 Dislocation of the first carpometacarpal joint

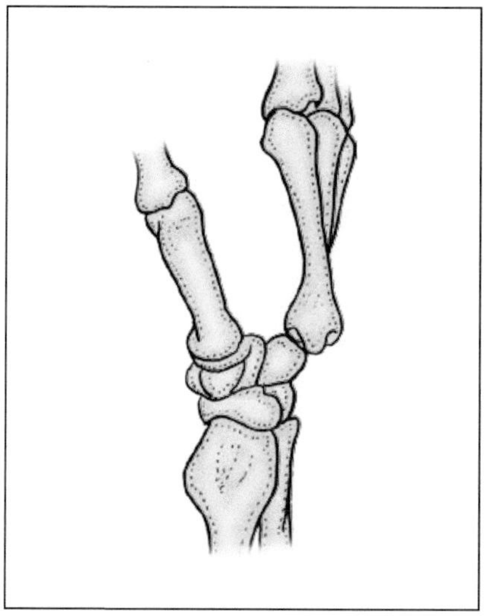

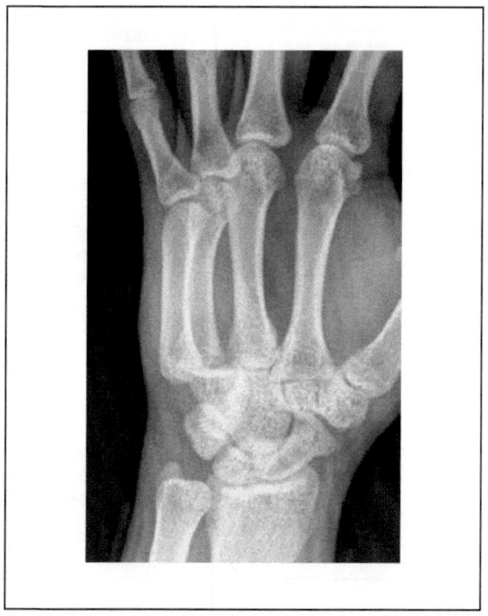

AO/OTA classification of the carpometacarpal joint dislocation

70-C: Dislocation of carpometacarpal joint.
70-C2: Dislocation of the second carpometacarpal joint.
70-C3: Dislocation of the third carpometacarpal joint.
70-C4: Dislocation of the fourth carpometacarpal joint.
70-C5: Dislocation of the fifth carpometacarpal joint

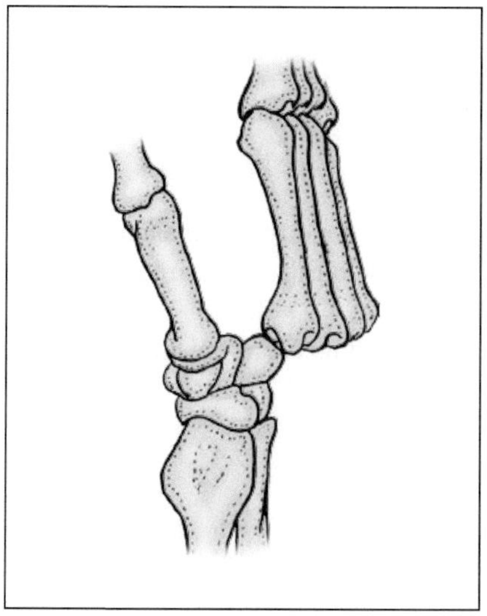

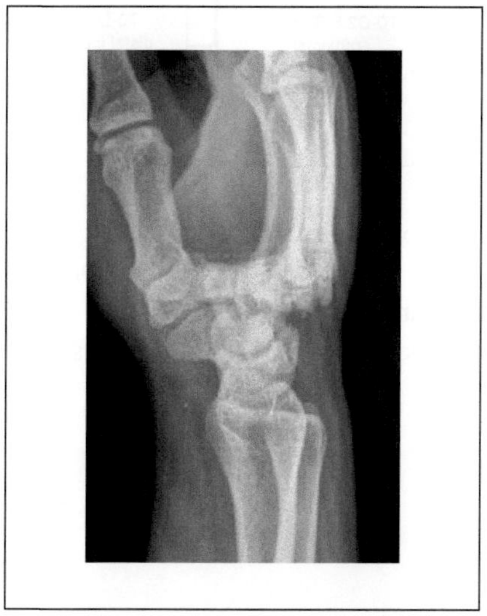

AO/OTA classification of dislocation of the carpometacarpal joint

70-C: Dislocation of carpometacarpal joint.

C9: Multiple dislocation of. carpometacarpal joint

5.3.5 Metacarpophalangeal, Interphalangeal Joint Dislocation

5.3.5.1 AO/OTA Classification (2007 revise, Journal of Orthopaedic Trauma. 21 Supplement)

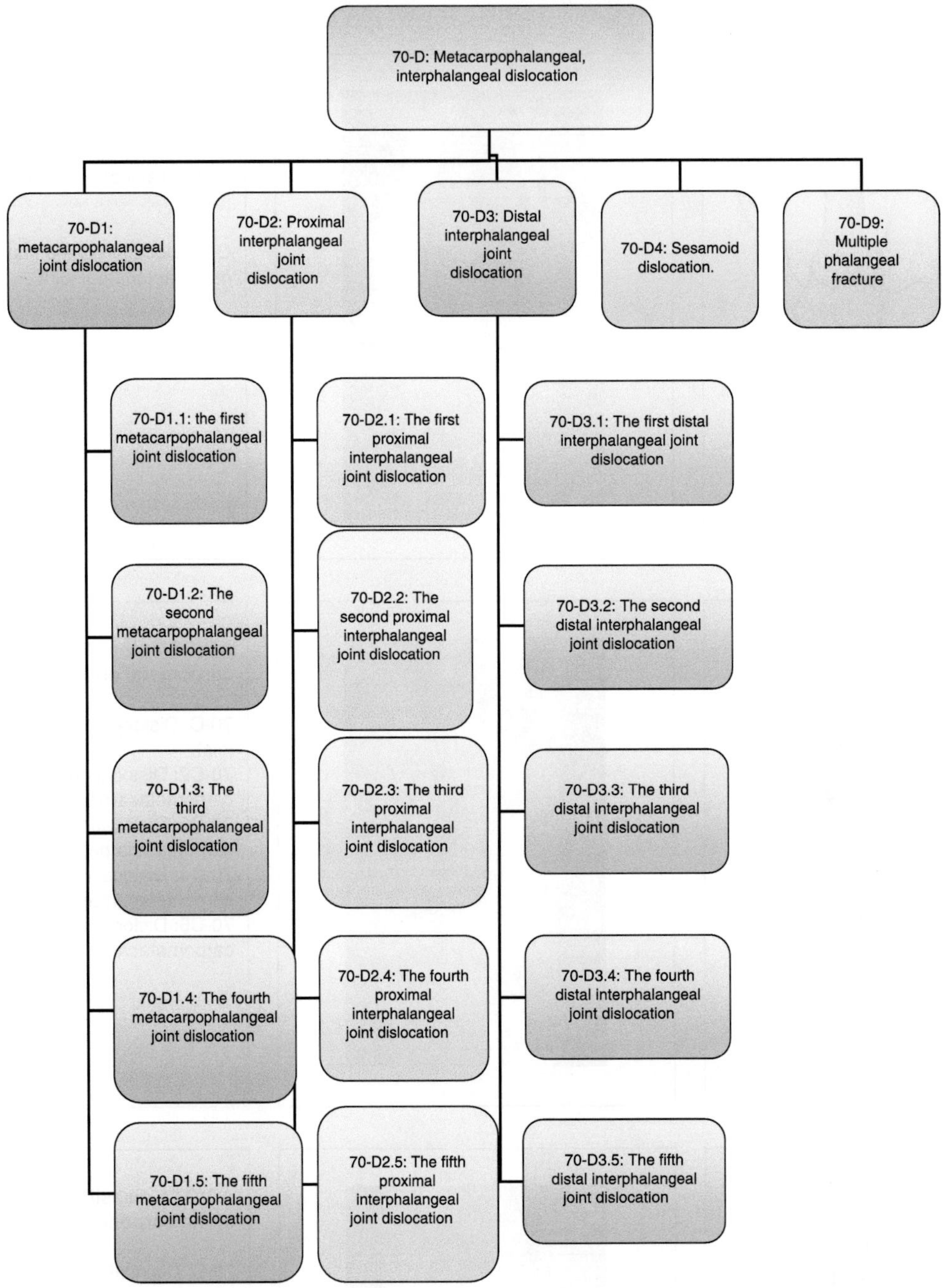

70-D1: Dislocation of metacarpophalangeal joint, further divided into:

- D1.1: Dislocation of the first metacarpophalangeal joint.
- D1.2: Dislocation of the second metacarpophalangeal joint.
- D1.3: Dislocation of the third metacarpophalangeal joint.
- D1.4: Dislocation of the fourth metacarpophalangeal joint.
- D1.5: Dislocation of the fifth metacarpophalangeal joint.

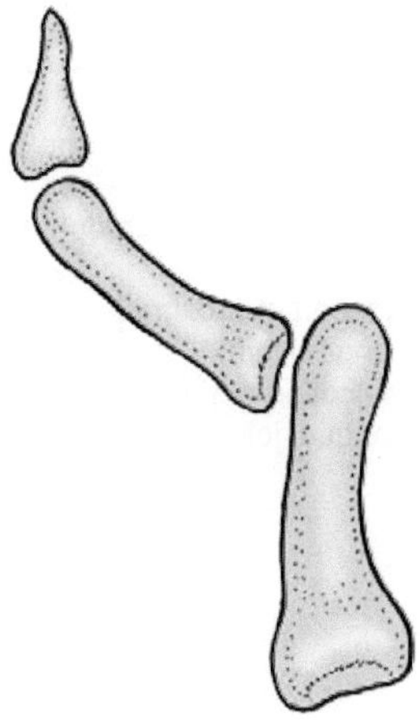

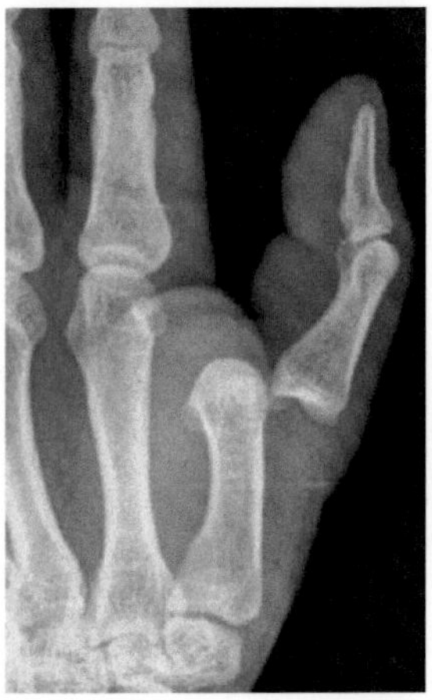

AO/OTA classification of the carpometacarpal joint dislocation

70-D: Metacarpophalangeal and interphalangealjoint dislocation

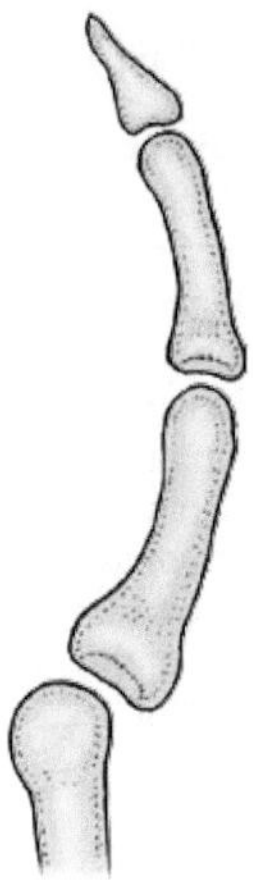

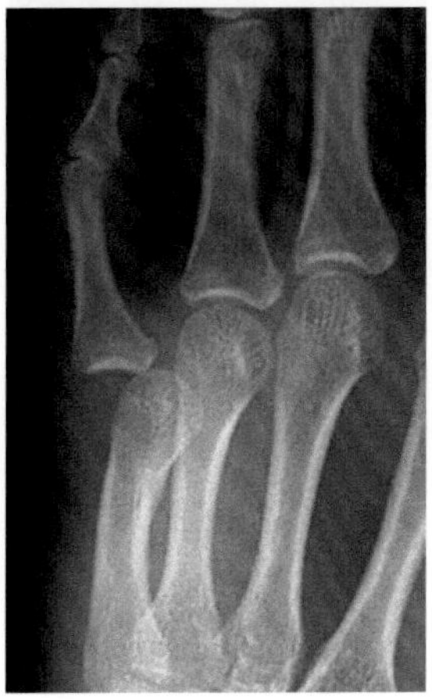

AO/OTA classification of the carpometacarpal joint dislocation

70-D: Metacarpophalangeal and interphalangealjoint dislocation.
D1: Dislocation of metacarpophalangeal joint.
D1.2: Dislocation of the second metacarpophalangeal joint.
D1.3: Dislocation of the third metacarpophalangeal joint.
D1.4: Dislocation of the forth metacarpophalangeal joint.
D1.5: Dislocation of the fifth metacarpophalangeal joint

70-D2: Dislocation of proximal interphalangeal joint, divided into:

D2.1: Dislocation of the first proximal interphalangeal joint.
D2.2: Dislocation of the second proximal interphalangeal joint.
D2.3: Dislocation of the third proximal interphalangeal joint.
D2.4: Dislocation of the fourth proximal interphalangeal joint.
D2.5: Dislocation of the fifth proximal interphalangeal joint.

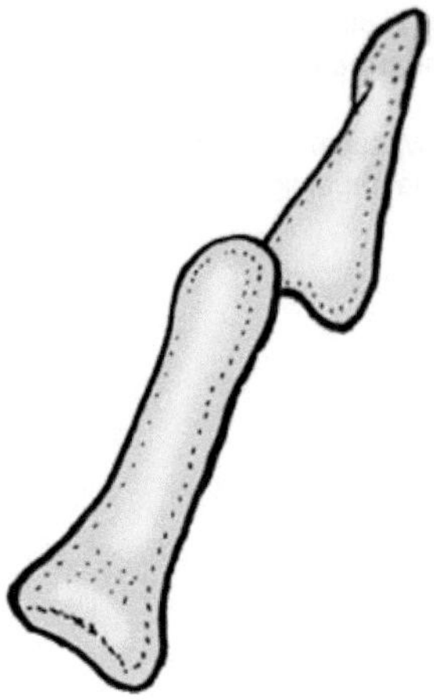

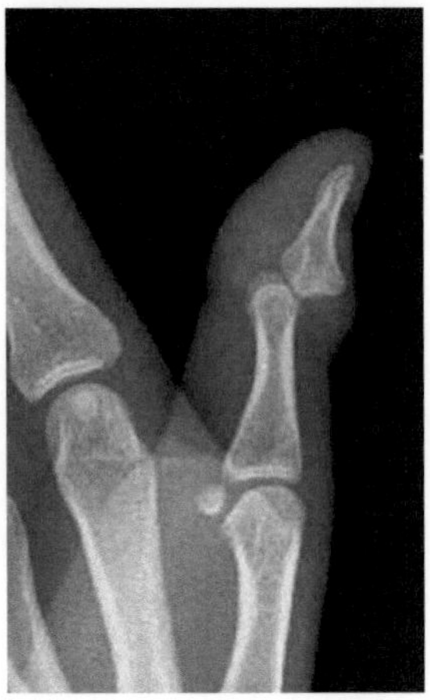

AO/OTA classification of the carpometacarpal joint dislocation

70-D: Metacarpophalangeal and interphalangeal joint dislocation.
D1: Dislocation of metacarpophalangeal joint.
D2: Dislocation of proximal interphalangeal joint.
D2.1: Dislocation of the first proximal interphalangeal joint

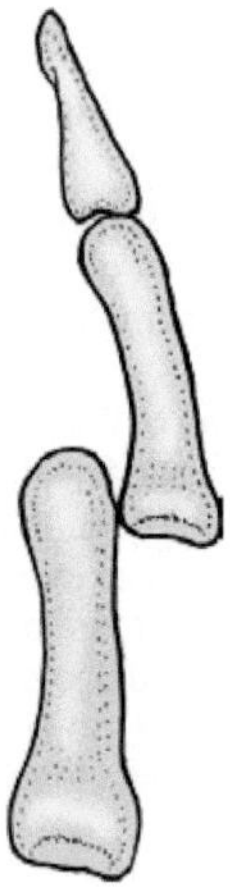

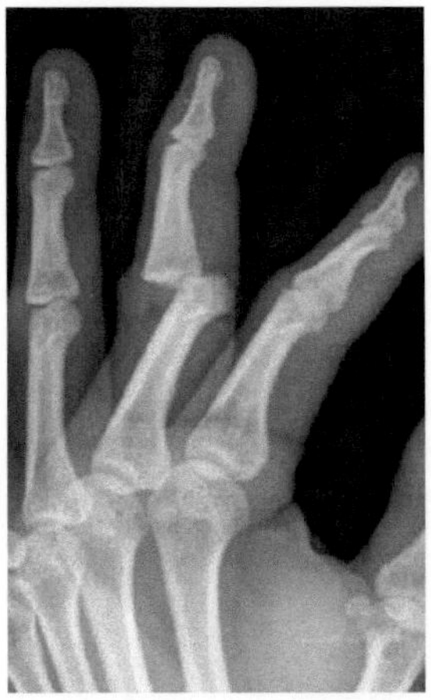

AO/OTA classification of the carpometacarpal joint dislocation

70-D: Metacarpophalangeal and interphalangeal joint dislocation.
D2: Dislocation of proximal interphalangeal joint.
D2.2: Dislocation of the second proximal interphalangeal joint.
D2.3: Dislocation of the third proximal interphalangeal joint.
D2.4: Dislocation of the fourth proximal interphalangeal joint.
D2.5: Dislocation of the fifth proximal interphalangeal joint

70-D3: Distal interphalangeal joint dislocation, further divided into:
- D3.2: The second distal interphalangeal joint dislocation.
- D3.3: The third distal interphalangeal joint dislocation.
- D3.4: The fourth distal interphalangeal joint dislocation.
- D3.5: The fifth distal interphalangeal joint dislocation.

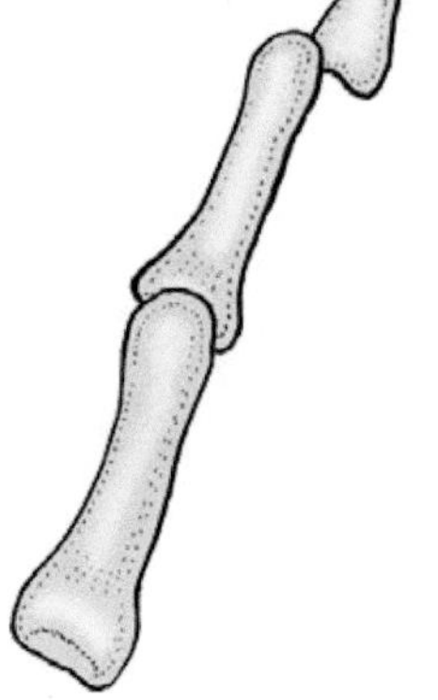

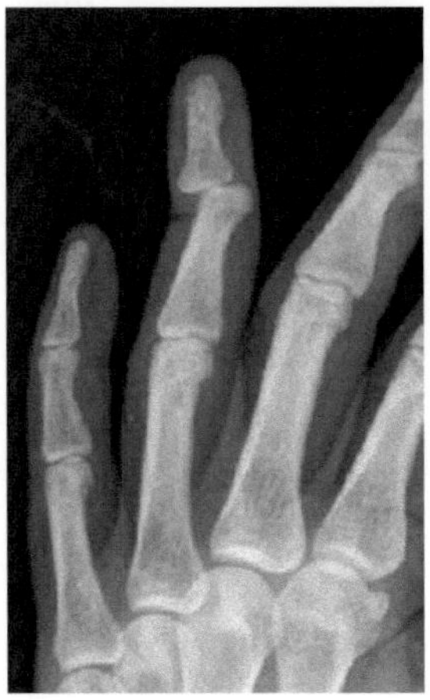

AO/OTA classification of the carpometacarpal joint dislocation

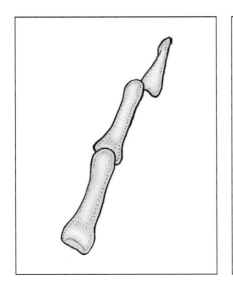

70-D: Metacarpophalangeal and interphalangeal joint dislocation.
D3: Distal interphalangealjoint dislocation.
D3.2: The second distal interphalangealjoint dislocation.
D3.3: The third distal interphalangeal joint dislocation.
D3.4: The fourth distal interphalangeal joint dislocation.
D3.5: The fifth distal interphalangeal joint dislocation

70-D4: Sesamoid dislocation.
70-D9: Multiple phalangeal fracture.

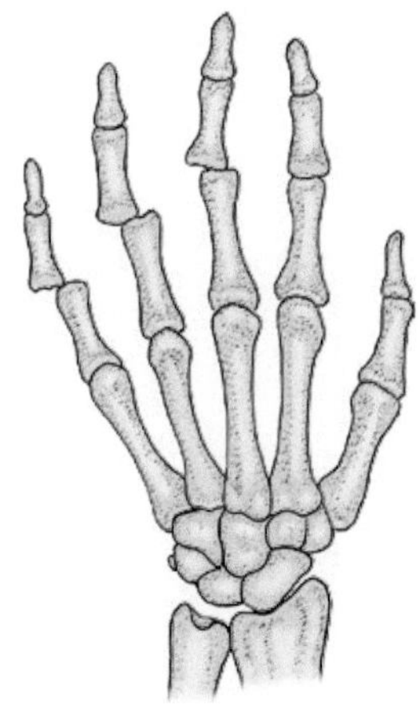

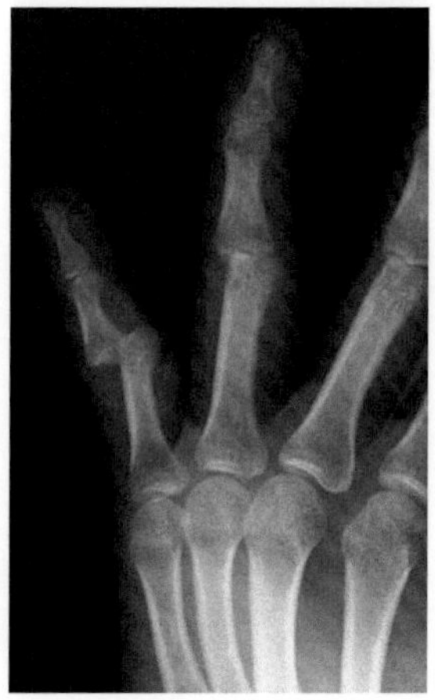

AO/OTA classification of the carpometacarpal joint dislocation

70-D: Metacarpophalangeal and interphalangeal joint dislocation.

D9: Multiple phalangeal fracture

5.3.5.2 Schenck Classification of the Proximal Interphalangeal Joint Dislocation (1994, Hand Clin, 10:179–185)

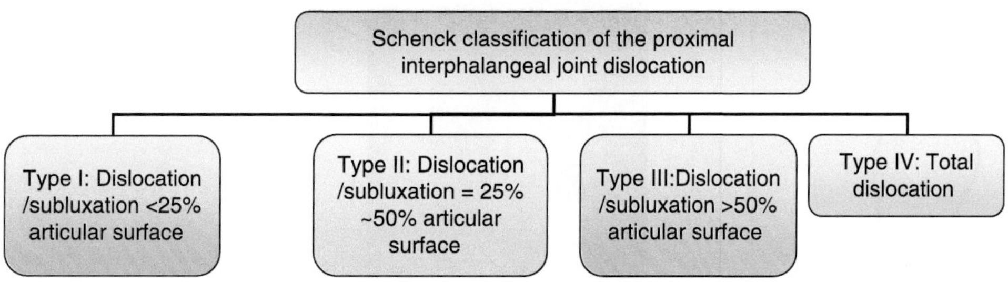

Evaluate according to the degree of joint dislocation percentage.

Type I: Dislocation/subluxation <25% articular surface.
Type II: Dislocation/subluxation = 25–50% articular surface.
Type III: Dislocation/subluxation >50% articular surface.
Type IV: Total

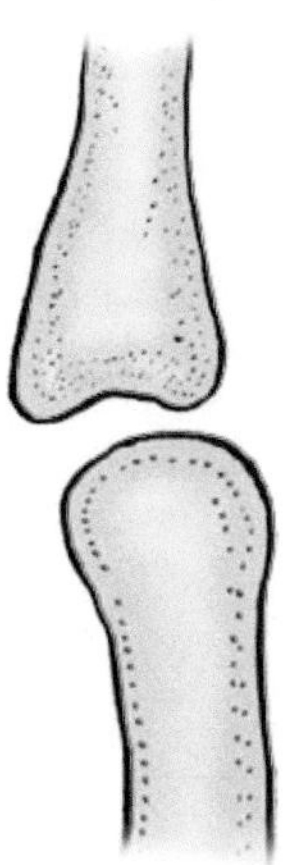

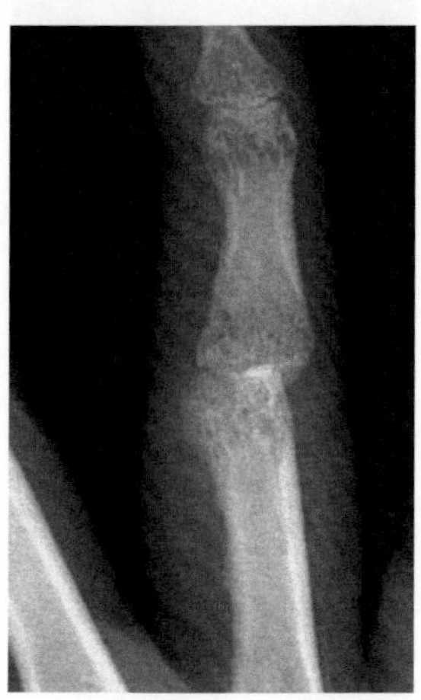

Schenck classification of the proximal interphalangeal joint dislocation

Type I: Dislocation/subluxation <25% articular surface

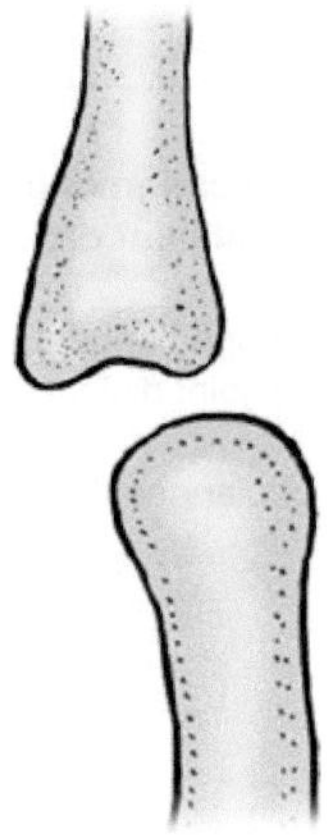

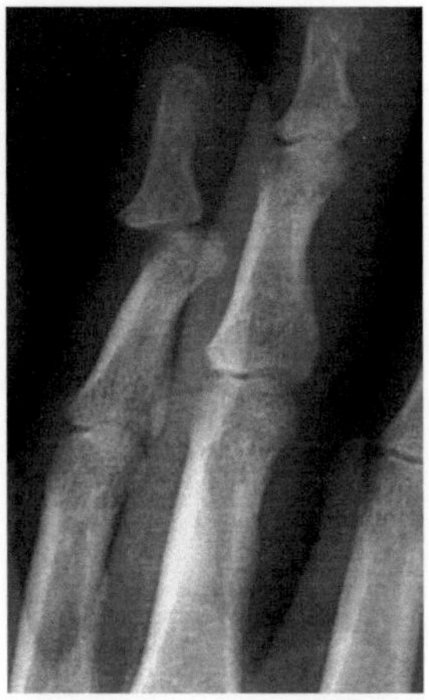

Schenck classification of the proximal interphalangeal joint dislocation

Type II: Dislocation/subluxation = 25% ~ 50% articular surface

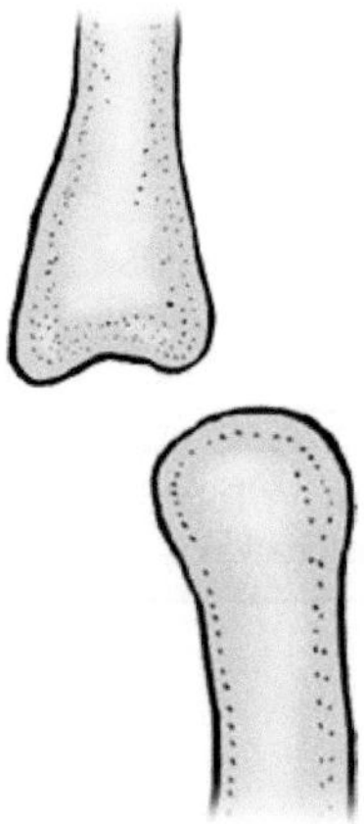

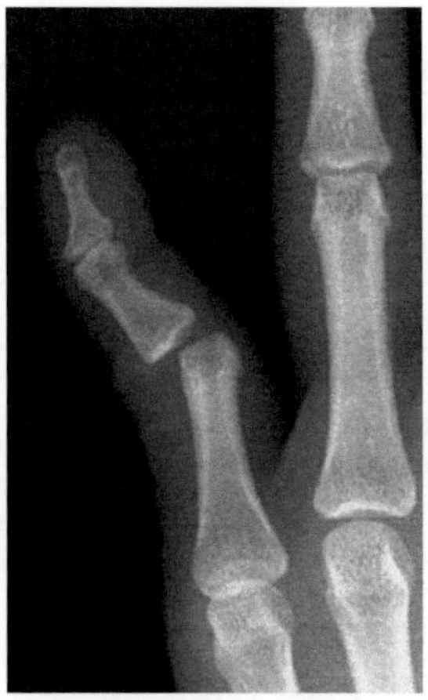

Schenck classification of the proximal interphalangeal joint dislocation

Type III: Dislocation/subluxation >50% articular surface

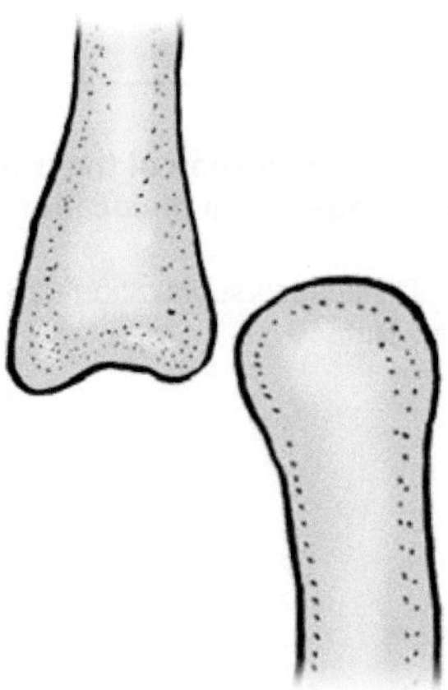

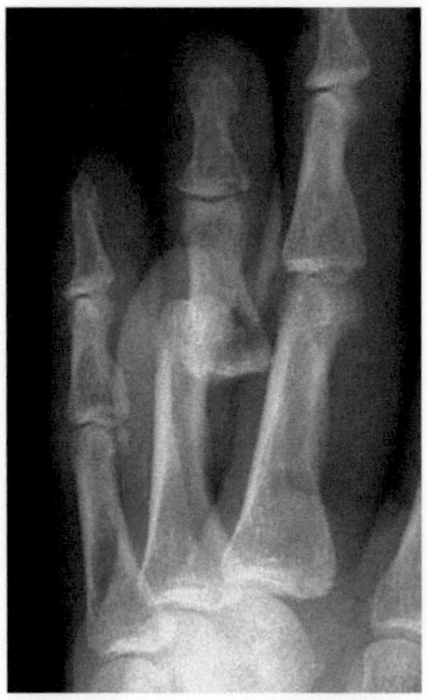

Schenck classification of the proximal interphalangeal joint dislocation

Type IV: Total dislocation

6 Classifications for Spine Fractures

Yingze Zhang and Wei Chen

6.1 Section 1 The Classification of Cervical Spine Fractures

6.1.1 The Classification of Upper Cervical Spine Fractures

The atlas fracture was first introduced by Cooper in 1822. Jefferson first proposed the injury mechanism and the classification in 1920. There are more than ten kinds of fracture classifications regarding upper cervical spine which can be found until now. Jefferson classification of atlas fractures, Anderson classification of odontoid fractures, and Levine–Edwards classification of hangman's fracture have showed the highest usage according to literature review's findings reported in recent 5 years.

6.1.1.1 The Classification of Atlas Fractures

Jefferson Classification (1920, Br J Surg, 7: 407–422)

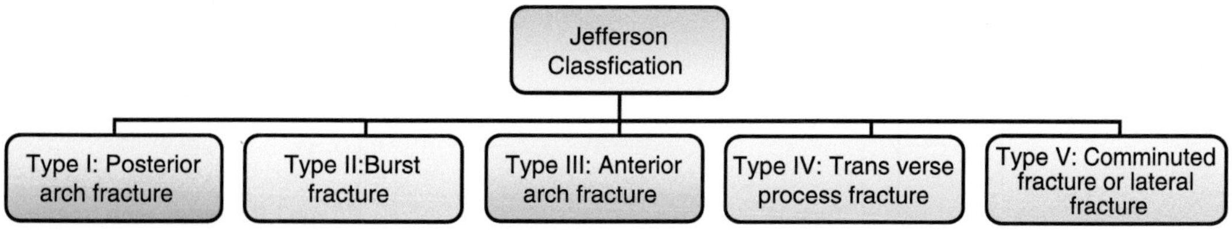

The reason is vertical force on cervical region.

Type I: Posterior arch fracture.
Type II: Burst fracture.
Type III: Anterior arch fracture.
Type IV: Transverse process fracture.
Type V: Comminuted fracture or lateral fracture.

Y. Zhang (✉) • W. Chen
Department of Orthopedics,
The Third Hospital of Hebei Medical University,
Shijiazhuang, China
e-mail: yzzhangdr@126.com, yzling_liu@163.com

Y. Zhang (ed.), *Clinical Classification in Orthopaedics Trauma*, https://doi.org/10.1007/978-981-10-6044-1_6

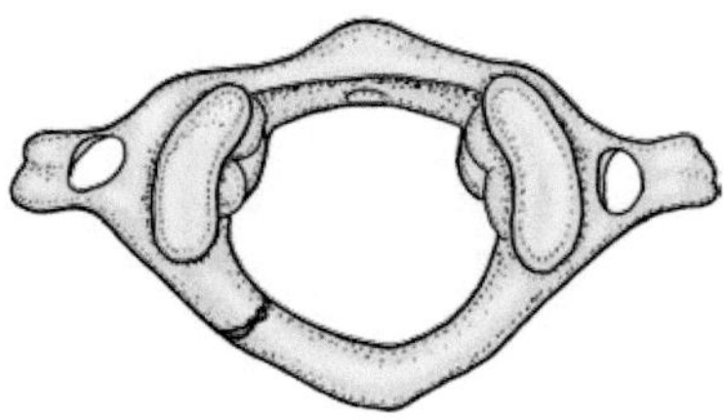

Type I

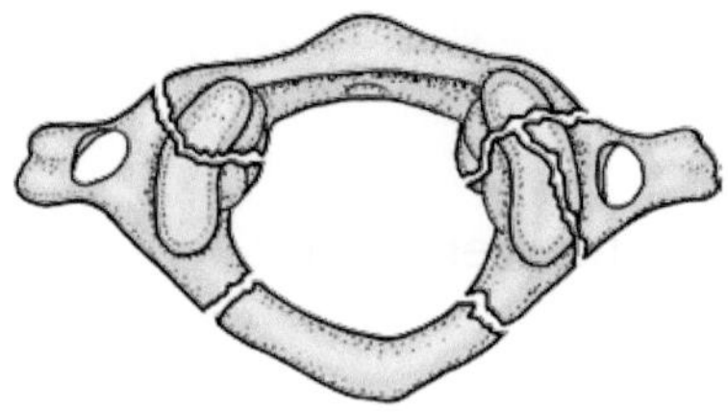

Type II

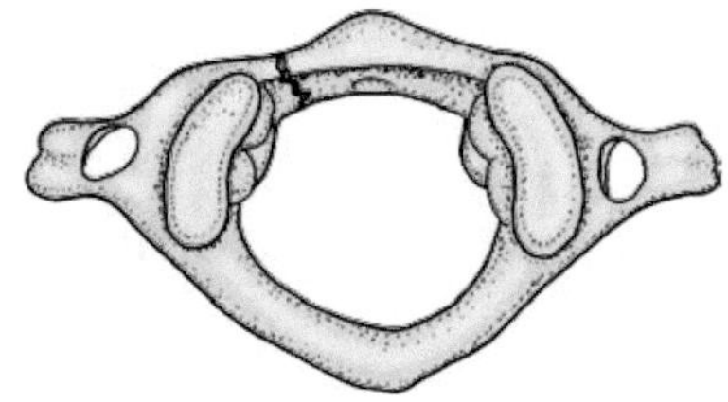

Type III

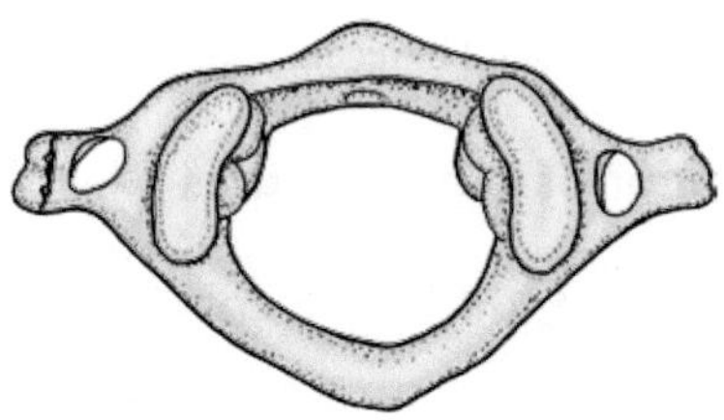

Type IV

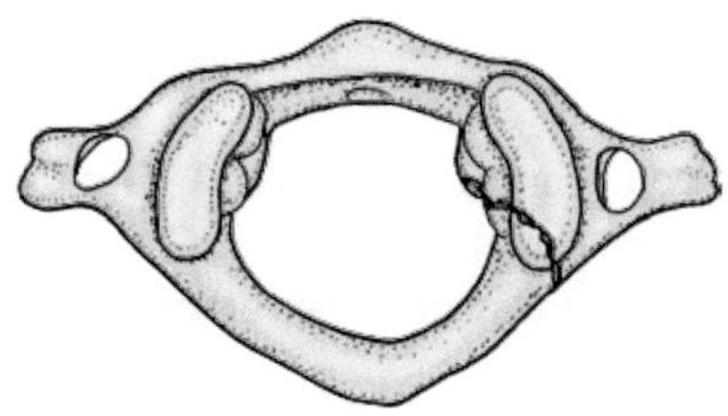

Type V

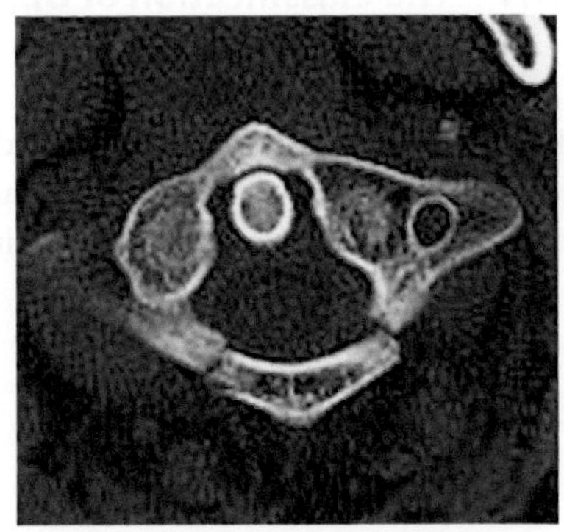

Type I: **Posterior arch fracture**

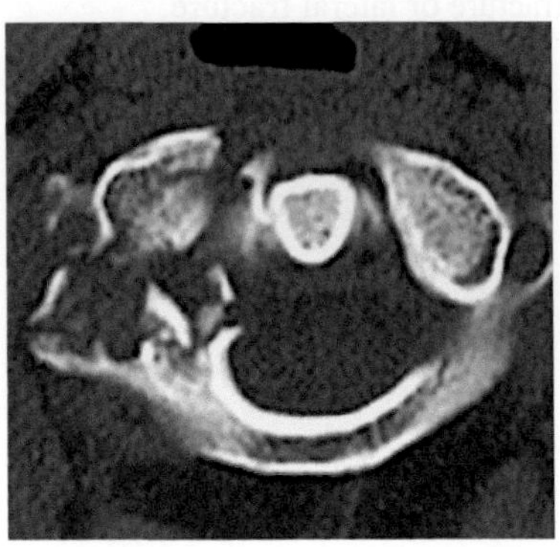

Type II: Burst fracture

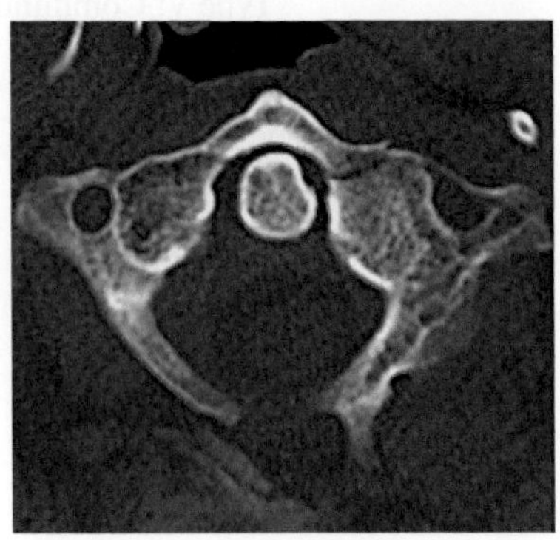

Type III: Anterior arch fracture

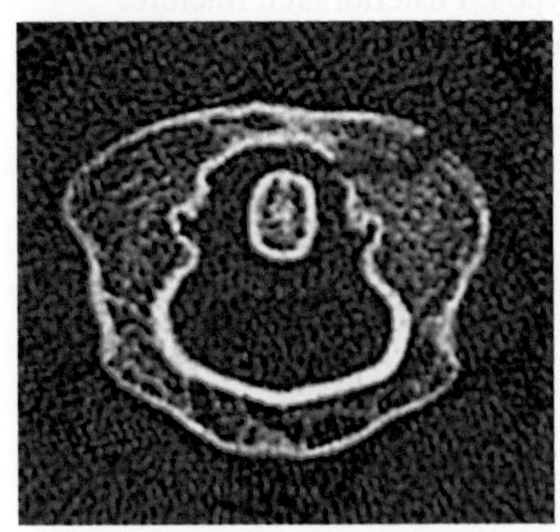

Type V: lateral fracture

Levine–Edwards Classification (1991, J Bone Joint Surg Am, 73(5): 680–91)

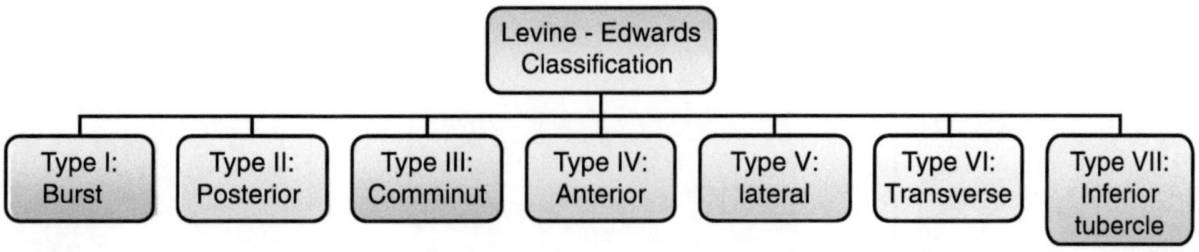

Type I: Burst fracture (Jefferson fracture), with two fractures on anterior arch and posterior arch, respectively, due to axial force.

Type II: Posterior arch fracture, with odontoid fracture and axis fracture due to hyperextension injury.

Type III: Comminuted fracture, due to axial force and flexural force, high risk of bone nonunion, poor prognosis.

Type IV: Anterior arch fracture, due to hyperextension injury.

Type V: Lateral fracture, due to axial force and flexural force.

Type VI: Transverse process fracture, due to avulsion injury.

Type VII: Inferior tubercle fracture, due to musculus longus colli avulsion injury.

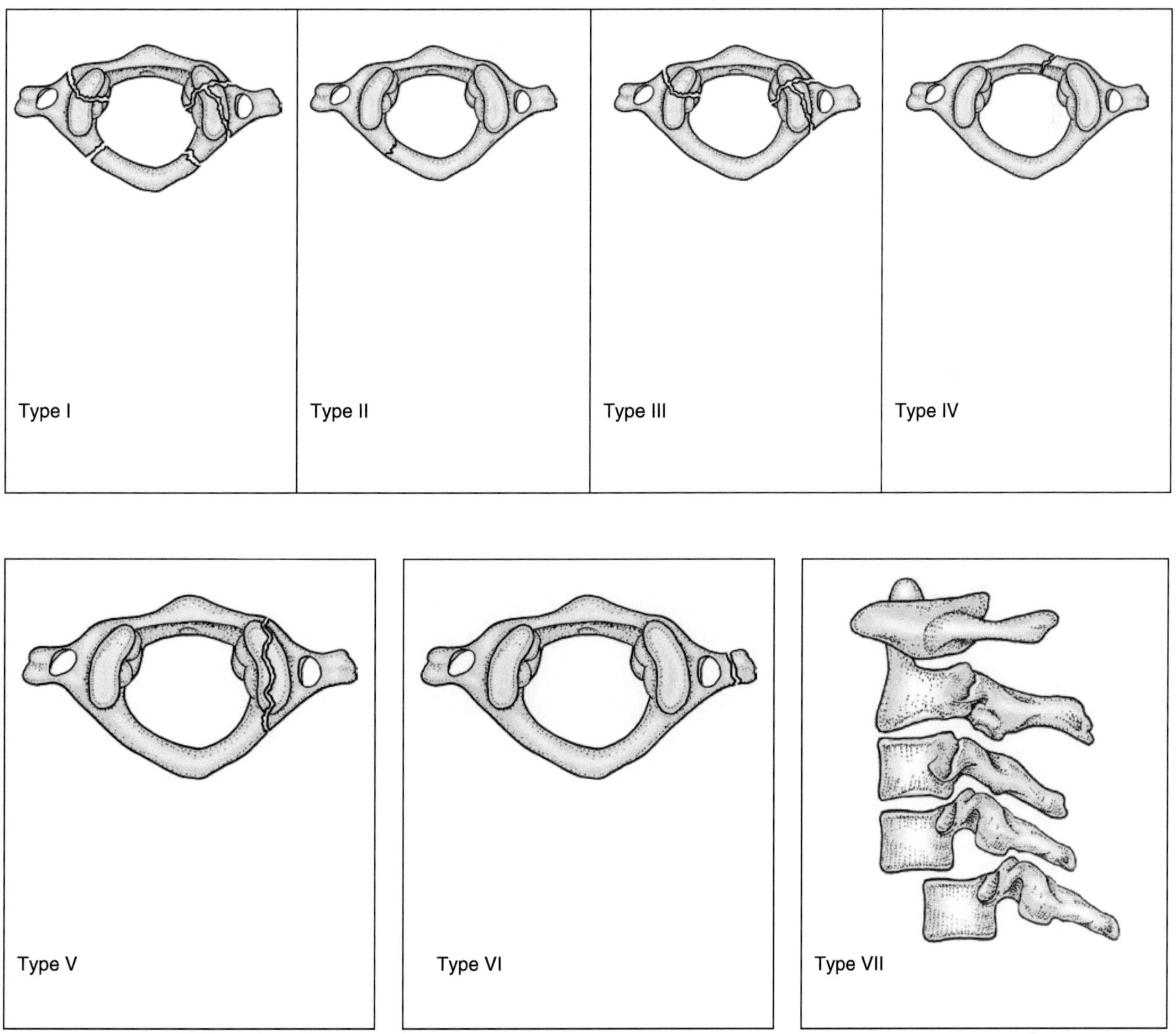

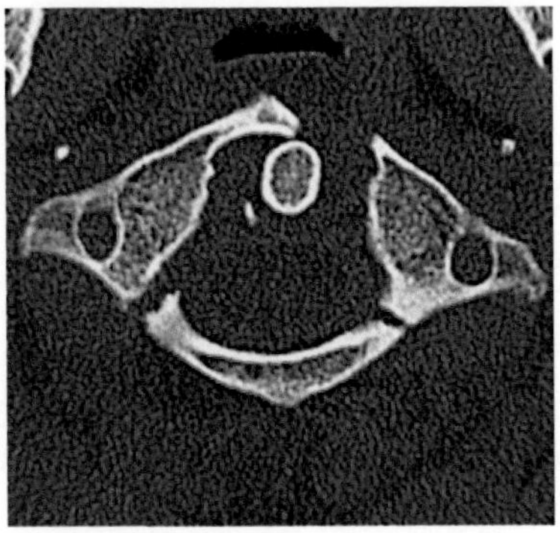

Type I: Burst fracture
(Jefferson fracture)

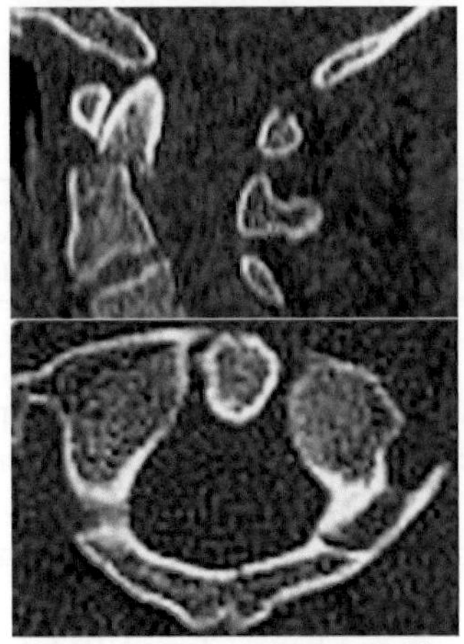

Type II: Posterior arch fracture, with odontoid fracture and axis fracture

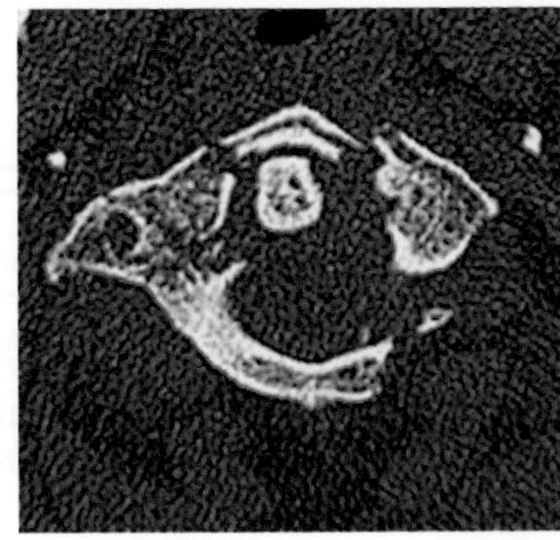

Type III: Comminuted fracture

AO/OTA Classification (2007, Journal of Orthopaedic Trauma. 21 Supplement)

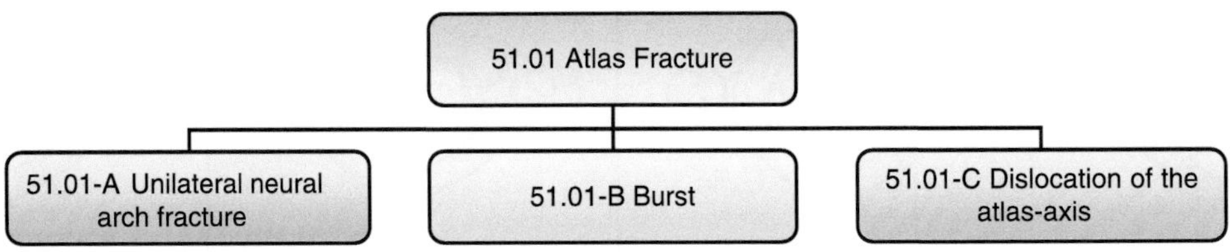

51. 01-A Unilateral neural arch fracture.
51. 01-B Burst.
51. 01-C Dislocation of the atlas-axis.

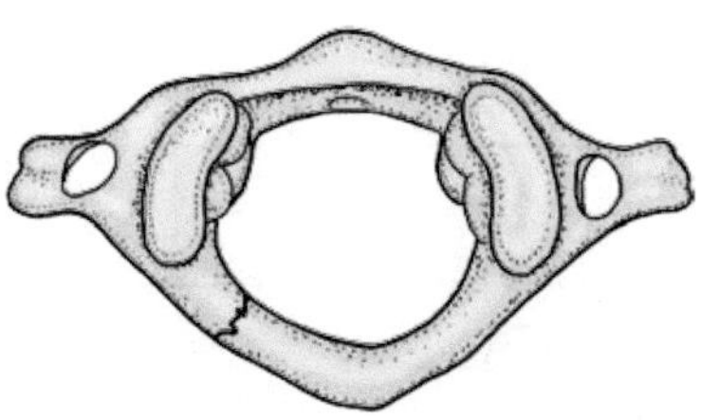

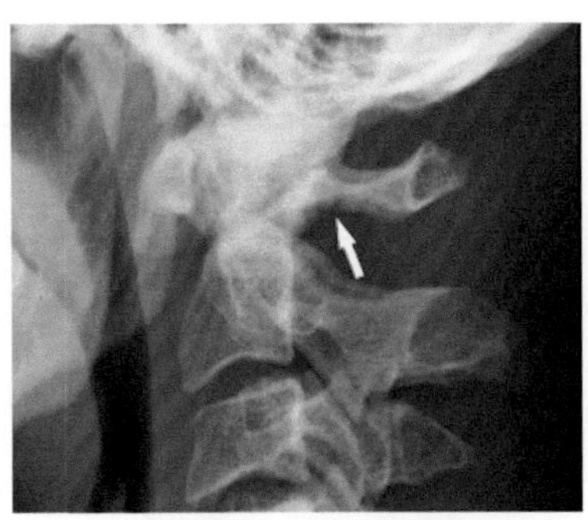

51 AO/OTA Classification of Cervical Spine Fractures

51.01 Atlas Fracture.
51. 01-A Unilateral neural arch fracture

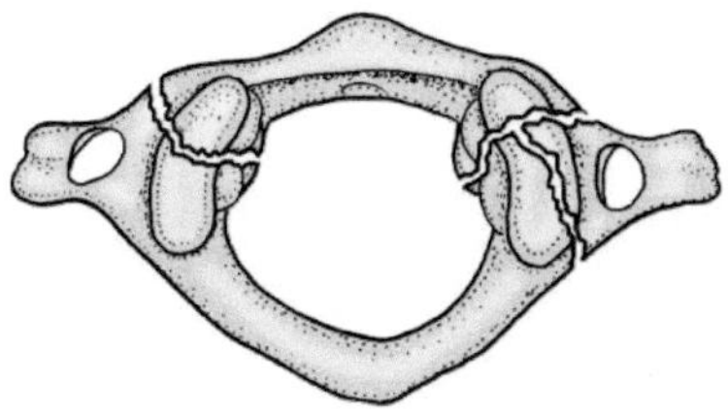

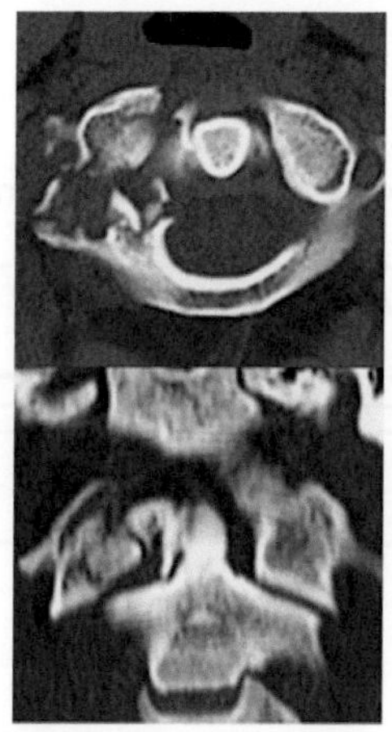

51 AO/OTA Classification of Cervical Spine Fractures

51.01 Atlas Fracture.
51.01-B Burst

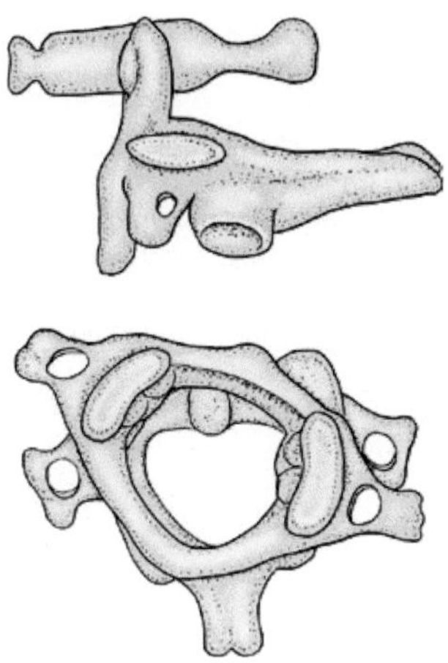

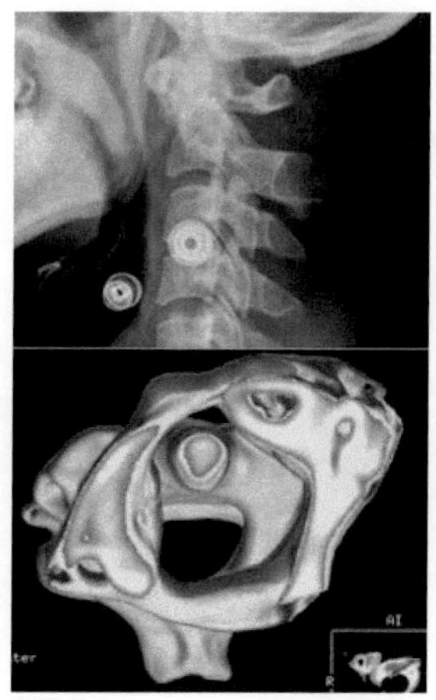

51 AO/OTA Classification of Cervical Spine Fractures

51.01 Atlas Fracture.
51. 01-C Dislocation of the atlas-axis

Landell Classification (1988, Spine, 13: 450–452)

There are three types:

Type I: Simple anterior or posterior arch fracture.
Type II: Burst fracture.
Type III: Lateral fracture.

Dickman Classification of Vertebral Transverse Ligament Damage (1996, Neurosurgery, 38: 44–50)

Type I: Transverse ligament tear without fracture.
Type II: Transverse ligament damage, with transverse ligament attachment avulsed fracture.

Levine–Edwards Classification of Craniocervical Region (1986, Orthop Clin North Am., 7: 31–44)

There are five types.

6.1.1.2 Classification of Axis Fractures

Classification of Odontoid Fractures

Anderson Classification of Odontoid Fractures (1974, J Bone Joint Surg (Am), 56: 1663–1674)

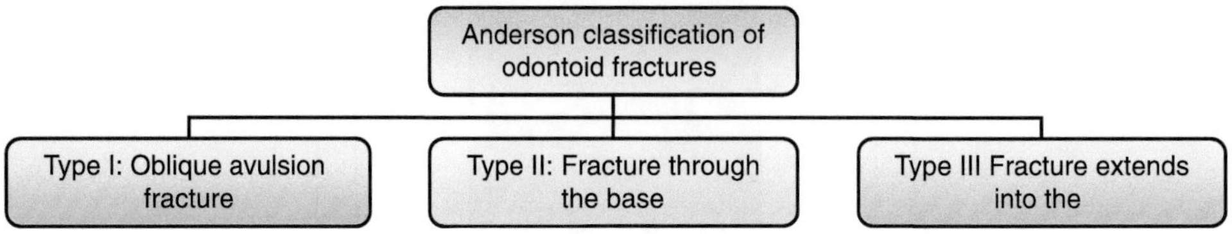

Type I: Oblique avulsion fracture of the tip of the dens. Fracture near the transverse ligament, belonging to the avulsion fracture of the ligament.

Type II: Fracture through the base of the odontoid process. Fracture through the base of the odontoid process. Blood supply is often compromised in this type and associated with a high rate of nonunion fractures.

Type III: Fracture extends into the vertebral body of C2.

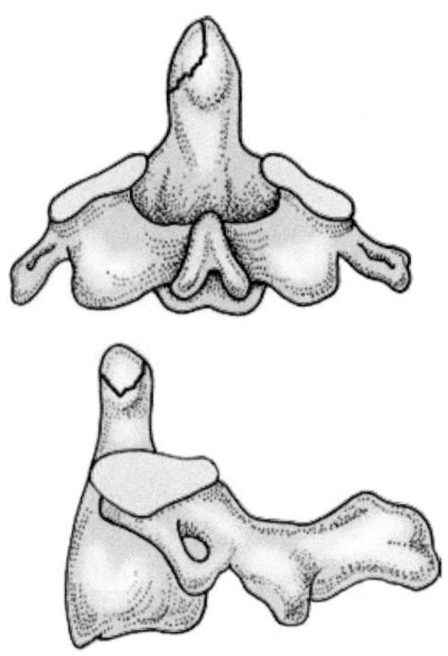

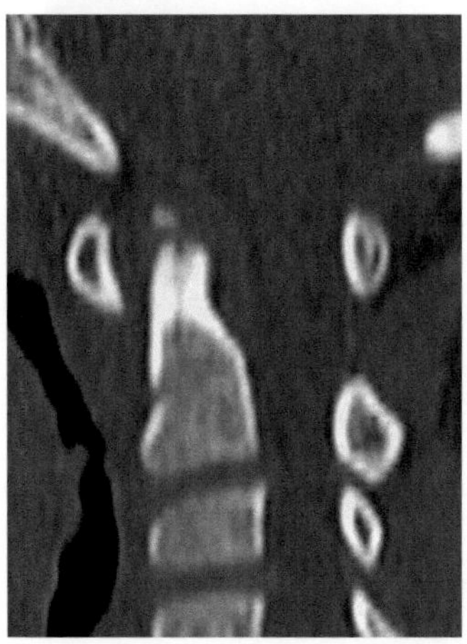

Anderson classification of odontoid fractures
Type I : Oblique avulsion fracture of the tip of the dens. Fracture near the transverse ligament, belonging to the avulsion fracture of the ligament

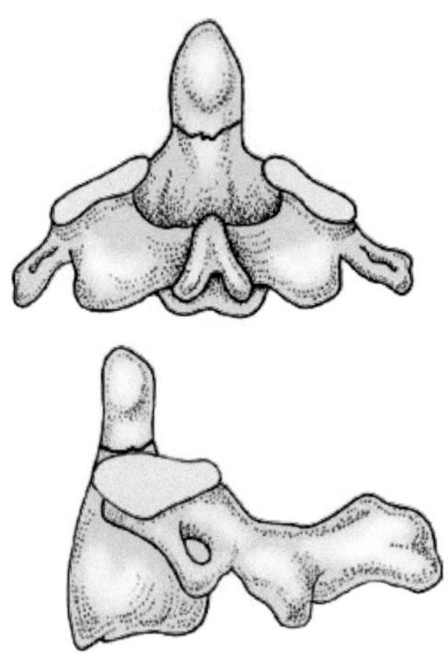

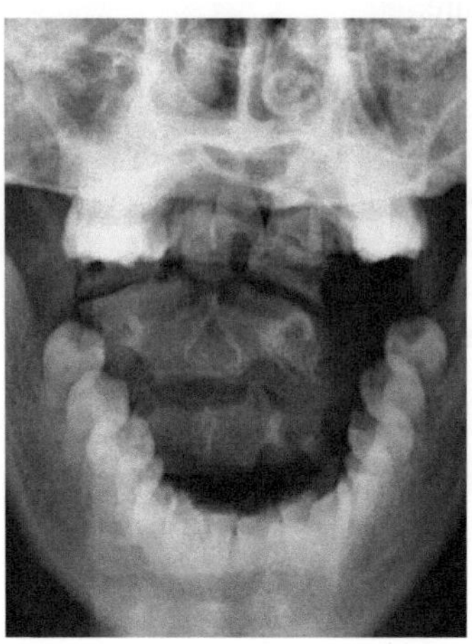

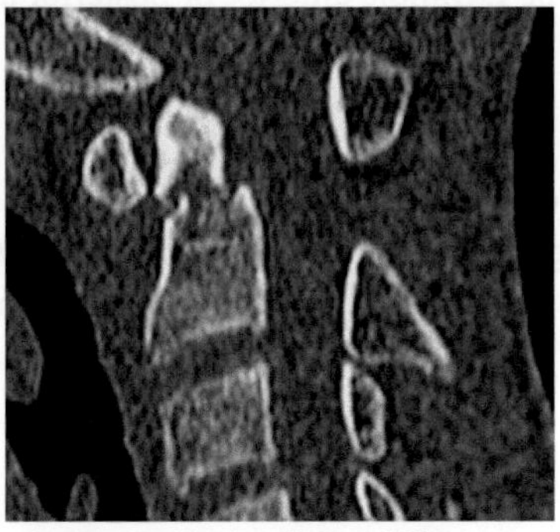

Anderson classification of odontoid fractures
Type II: Fracture through the base of t he odontoid process. Fracture through the base of the odontoid process. Blood supply is often compromised in this type and associated with a high rate of nonunion fractures.

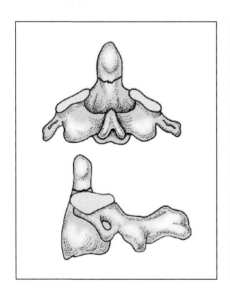

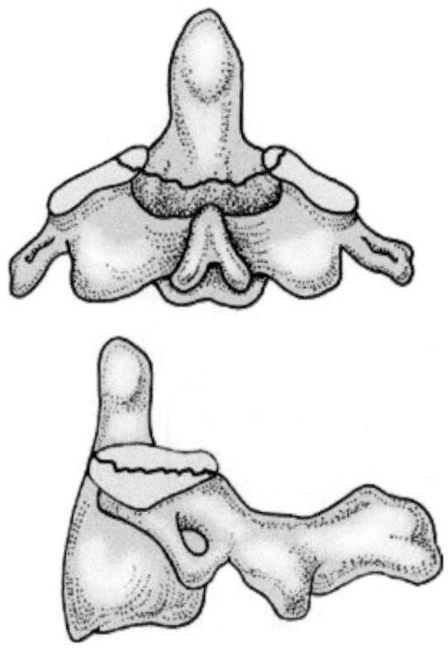

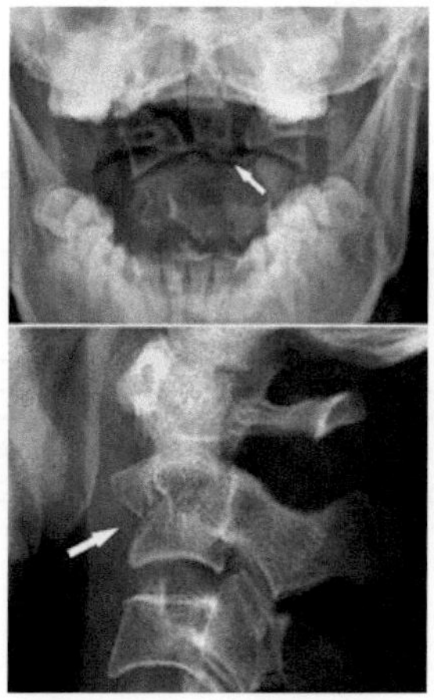

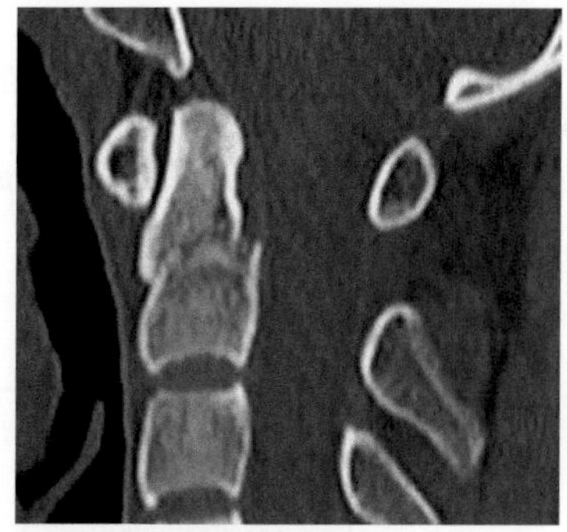

Anderson classification of odontoid fractures
Type III: Fracture extends into the vertebral body of C2

Schatzker Classification (1975, Clin Orthop Relat Res, 108: 127–137)

Schatzker was divided into two groups according to the fracture line above or below the collateral ligament.

Roy-Camille Classification (1973, Roy-Camille, De La Caffiniere JH, Saillant G. Traumatisme du rachis cervical uperieur C1 C2.1973, 51)

According to the lateral fracture line, the fracture is classified into three types.

Type I: OBAV (the fracture line inclined forward, obliquely downward and forward). The fracture line is tilted forward in the lateral position, and the typical displacement of the fracture is forward.

Type II: OBAR (the fracture line tilted backwards, obliquely downward and backward). The fracture line is tilted back to the side, and the typical displacement of the fracture is backward.

Type III: HTAL (fracture line level line). The fracture line is in lateral horizontal line, fractures can be moved forward or backward.

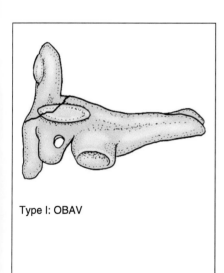

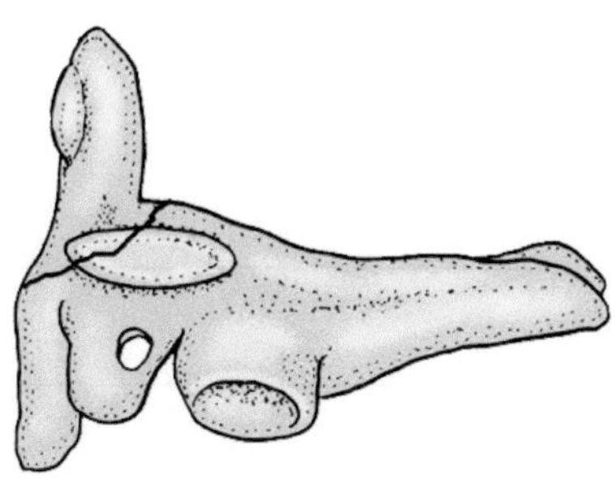

Type I: OBAV

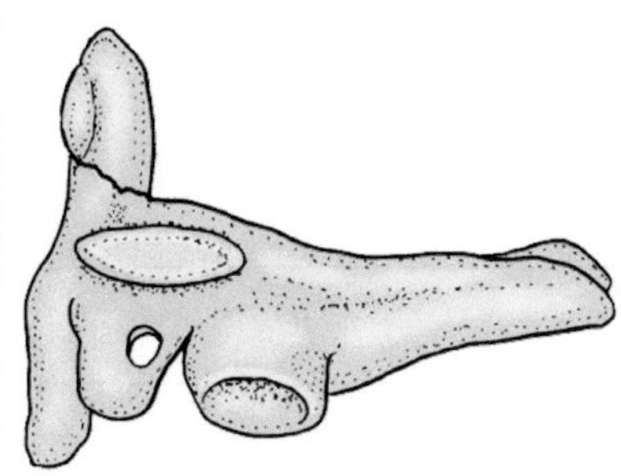

Type II: OBAR

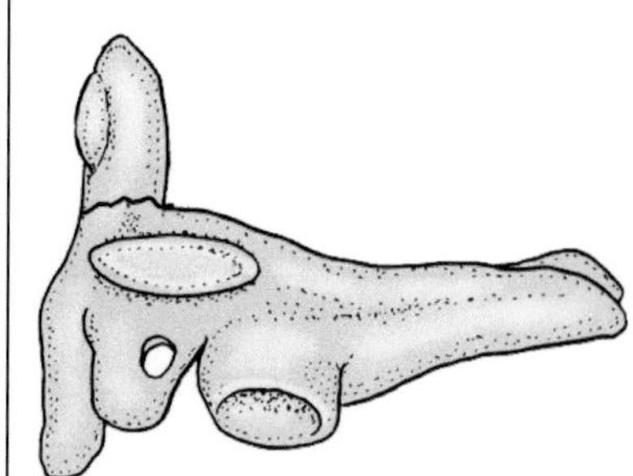

Type III: HTAL

Classification of Hangman's Fracture

Levine–Edwards Classification of Hangman's Fracture (1985, J Bone Joint Surg (Am), 67: 217–226)

The hangman's fracture consists of a bilateral pedicle or pars fracture involving the vertebral body of C2. Anterior subluxation or dislocation of the C2 vertebral body is associated with this fracture.

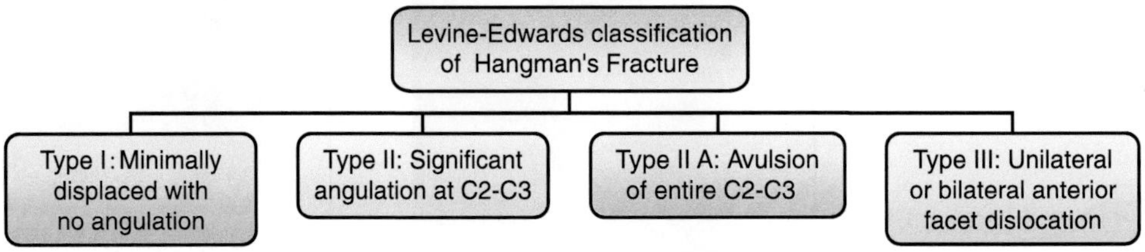

Type I: Minimally displaced with no angulation; translation <3 mm; stable.

Type II: Significant angulation at C2–C3; translation >3 mm; unstable; C2–C3 disk disrupted; subclassified into flexion, extension, and listhetic types.

Type II A: Avulsion of entire C2–C3 intervertebral disk in flexion, anterior longitudinal ligament intact; severe angulation; no translation; unstable due to flexion–distraction injury.

Type III: Unilateral or bilateral anterior facet dislocation of C2 on C3, due to extension injury; severe angulation, unstable.

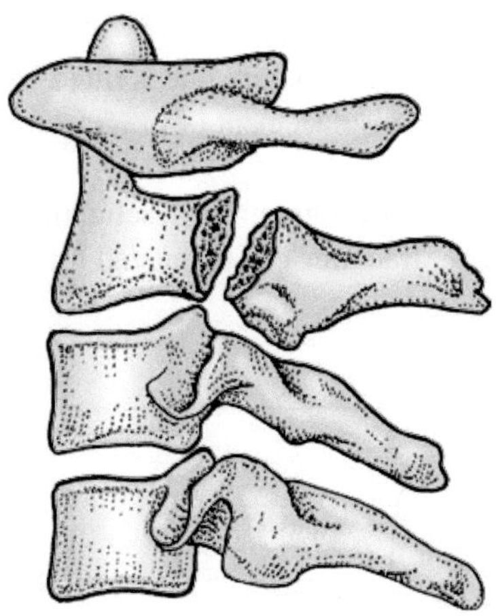

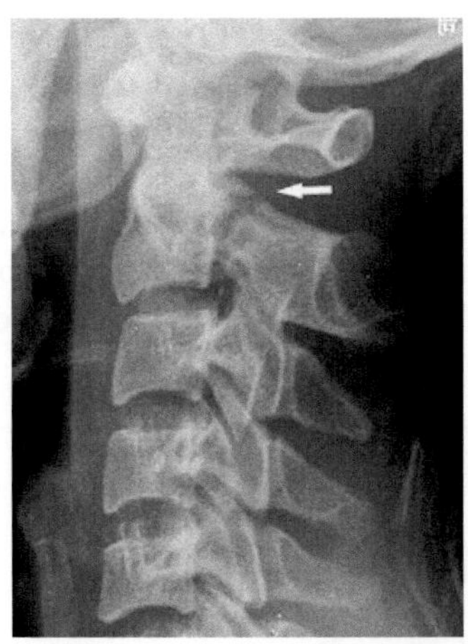

Levine–Edwards classification of hangman's fracture
Type I: Minimally displaced with no angulation; translation < 3 mm; stable

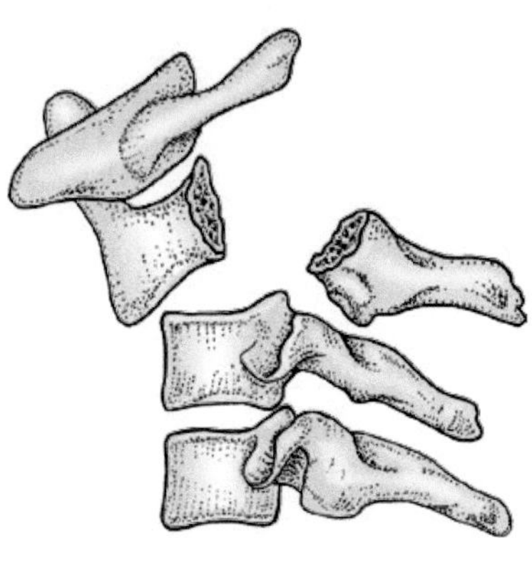

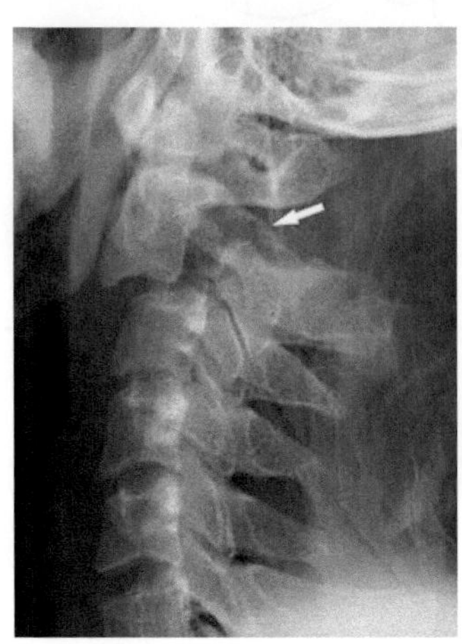

Levine–Edwards classification of hangman's fracture
Type II: Significant angulation at C2–C3; translation > 3 mm; unstable; C2–C3 disk disrupted; subclassified into flexion, extension, and listhetic types

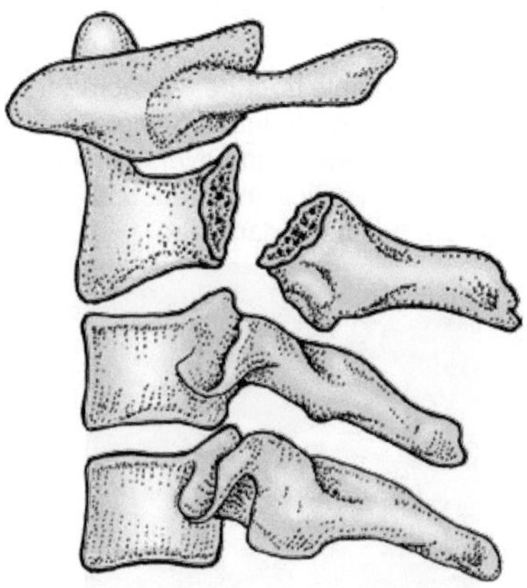

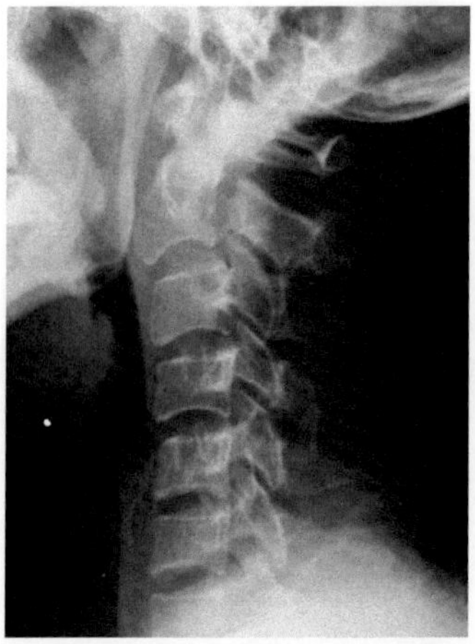

Levine–Edwards classification of hangman's fracture
Type III: Unilateral or bilateral anterior facet dislocation of C2 on C3, due to extension injury; severe angulation, unstable

Type I: Stable fracture, fracture line can be involved in any position of the arch with the first 2, 3 cervical interbody structure integrity.

Type II: Unstable fracture, vertebral flexion, or extension into the angle, or significantly forward transverse process, the first 2, 3 cervical intervertebral structure has been damaged.

Type III: Fracture and dislocation, the forward displacement of the vertebral body and with flexion, the first 2, 3 cervical facet joint dislocation and interlock.

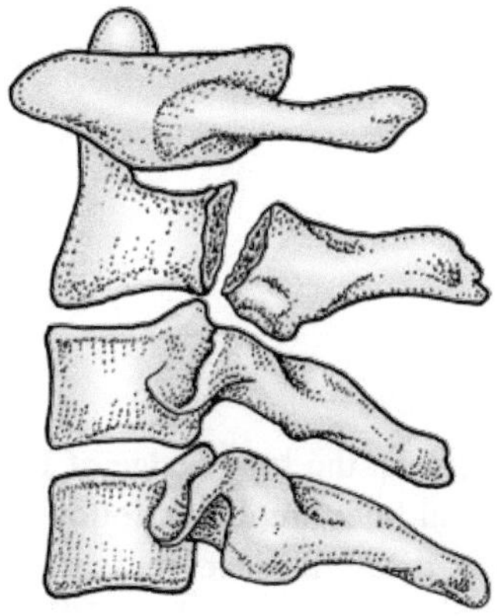

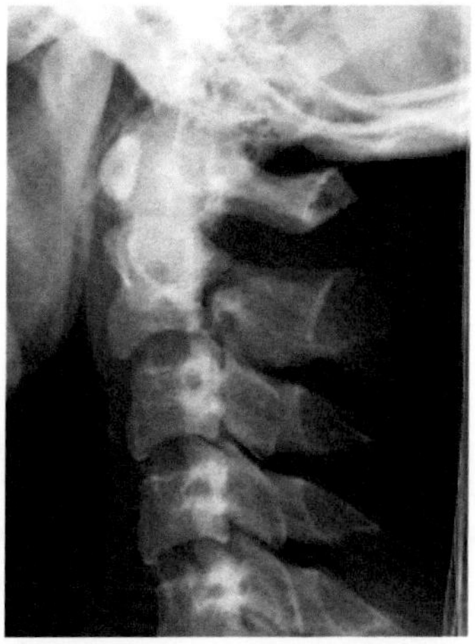

Effendi classification of Hangman fractures

Type I: Stable fracture, fracture line can be involved in any position of the arch with the first 2, 3 cervical interbody structure integrity

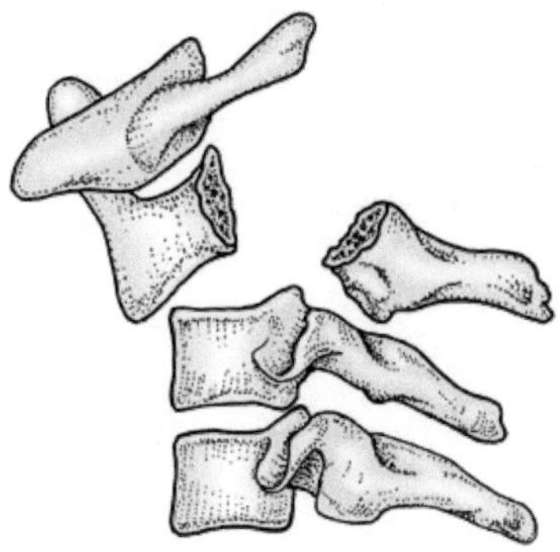

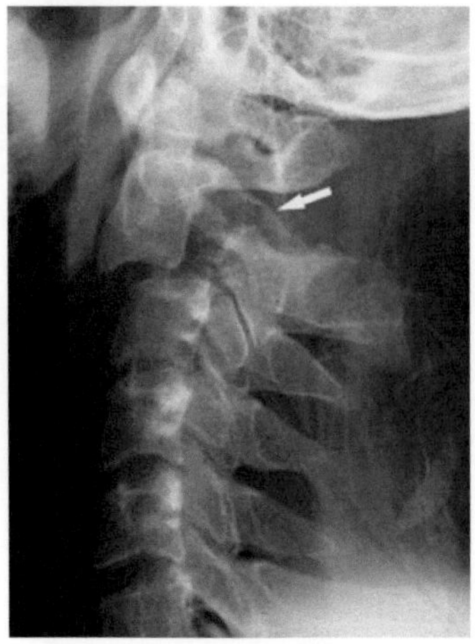

Effendi classification of Hangman fractures

Type II: Unstable fracture, vertebral flexion or extension into the angle, or significantly forward transverse process, the first 2, 3 cervical intervertebral structure has been damaged

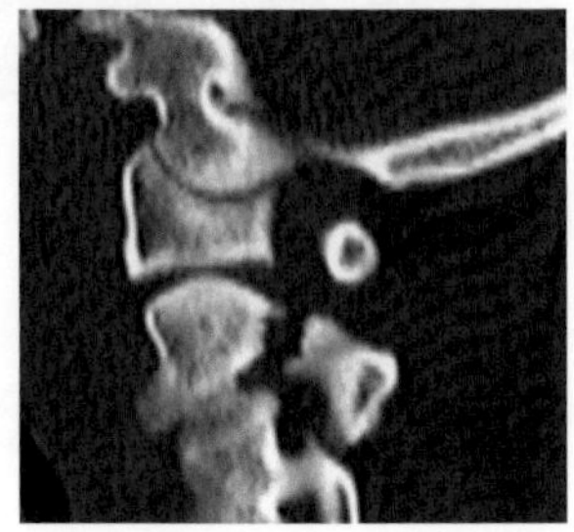

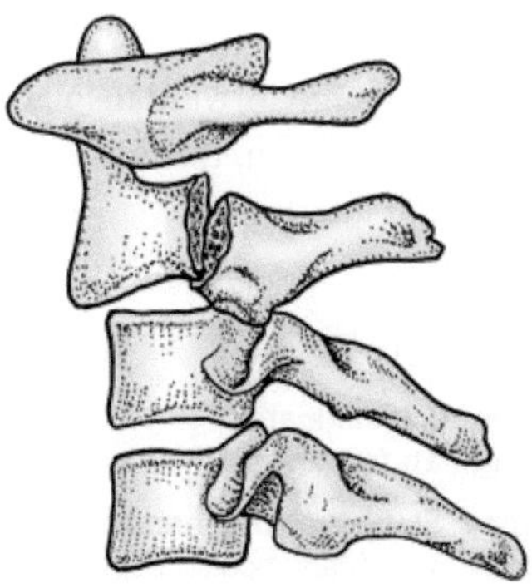

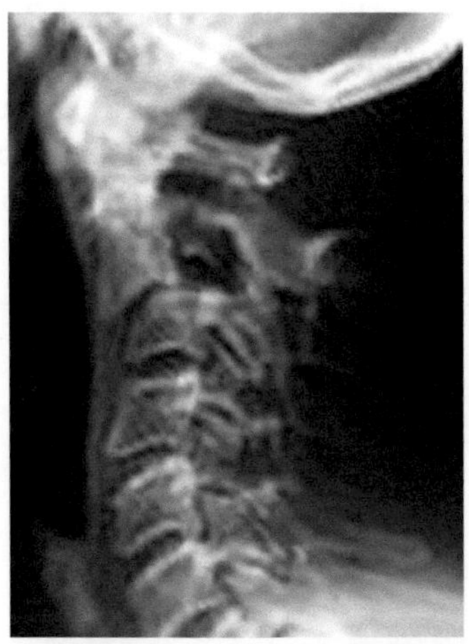

Effendi classification of Hangman fractures

Type III: Fracture and dislocation, the forward displacement of the vertebral body and with flexion, the first 2, 3 cervical facet joint dislocation and interlock

Francis Grade (1981, J Bone Joint Surg (Br), 63: 313–318)

Grade	Displacement	Angulation
Grade I stable	<3.5 mm	<11°
Grade II unstable	<3.5 mm	>11°
Grade III unstable	>3.5 mm or <1/2 vertebral width	<11°
Grade IV unstable	>3.5 mm or >1/2 vertebral width	>11°
Grade V	Rupture of intervertebral disc	

Displacement measurement: at the lower edge of lateral C2, C3 vertebral body, vertical lines are drawn followed by measurement of the two vertical distance measurement; Angulation: the two lines are drawn at the lateral C2, C3 vertebral body, respectively, whose angle is then measured.

Grade V fractures mean that the length of C2 vertebral body displacement exceeds half of that of the C3 vertebral body, or angular deformity has resulted in the fact that the height of at least one side of C2, C3 clearance is greater than that of the normal intervertebral disc.

AO/OTA Classification (2007, Journal of Orthopaedic Trauma. 21 Supplement)

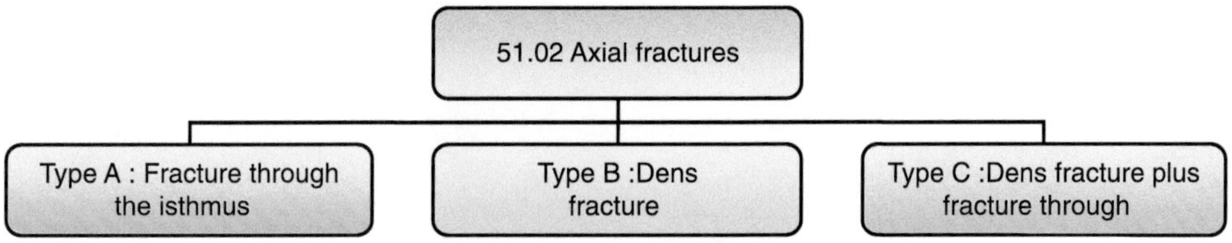

51.02-A Fracture through the isthmus.
51.02-B Dens fracture.
51.02-C Dens fracture plus fracture through the isthmus.

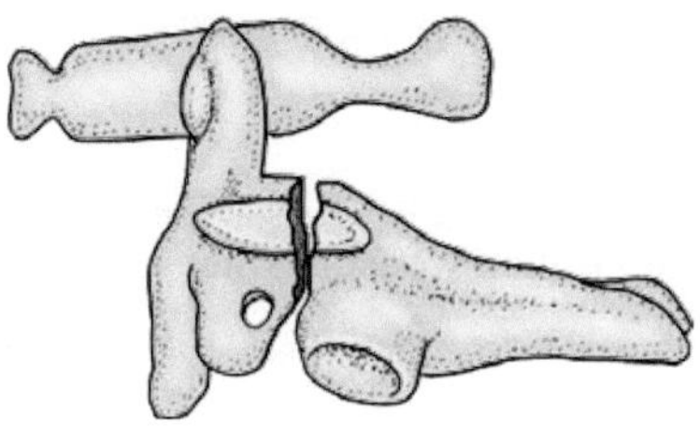

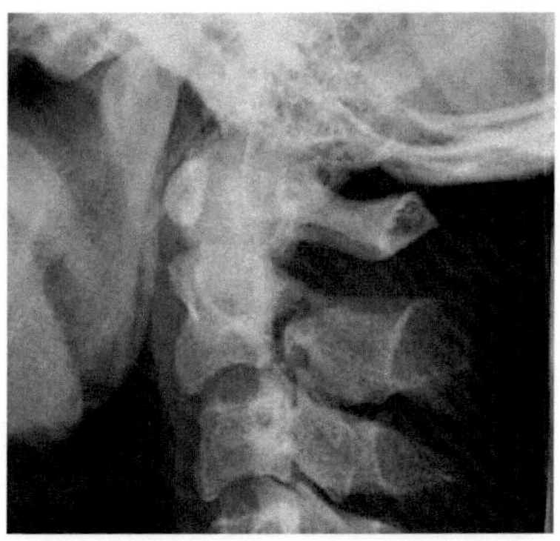

51 AO Classification of Cervical Spine Fractures
51.02 Axial fracture
Type A: Fracture through the isthmus

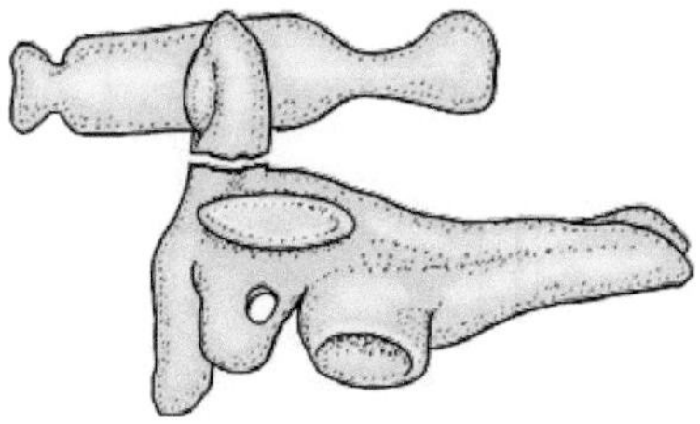

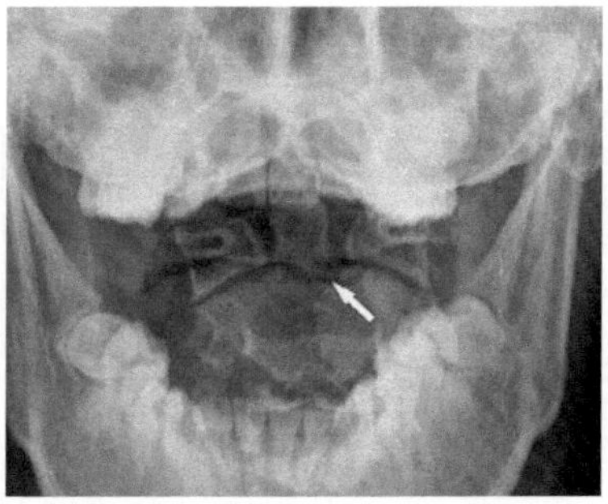

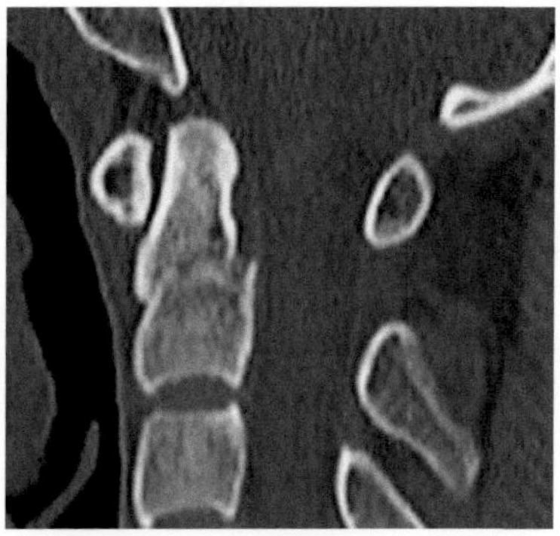

51 AO Classification of Cervical Spine Fractures
51.02 Axial fracture
Type B: Dens fracture

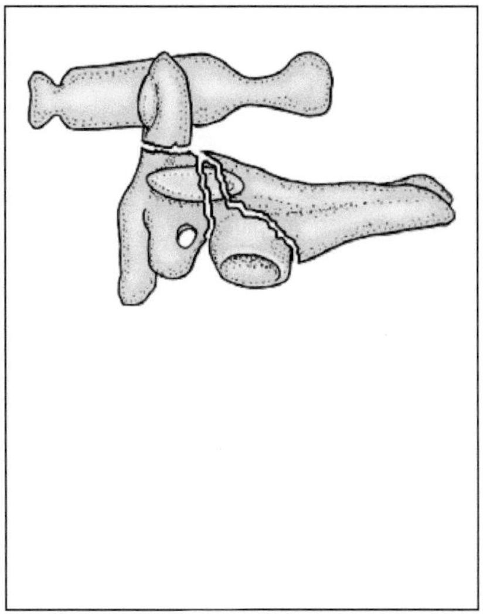

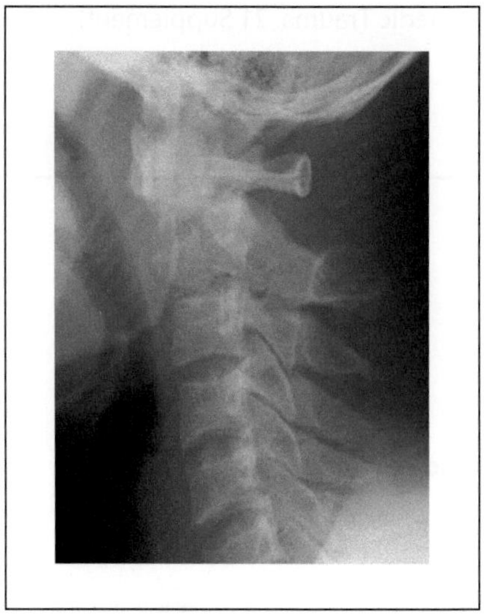

51 AO Classification of Cervical Spine Fractures
51.02 Axial fracture
Type C: Dens fracture plus fracture through the isthmus

Classification of Fractures of the Lower Cervical Spine

Lower cervical fractures include more than ten species, the most common type is Allen–Ferguson type. After reviewing the literature for 5 years, the Argenson classification, AO/OTA classification, and anatomical location were classified according to the usage rate.

Allen–Ferguson Classification (1982, Spine, 7: 1–27)

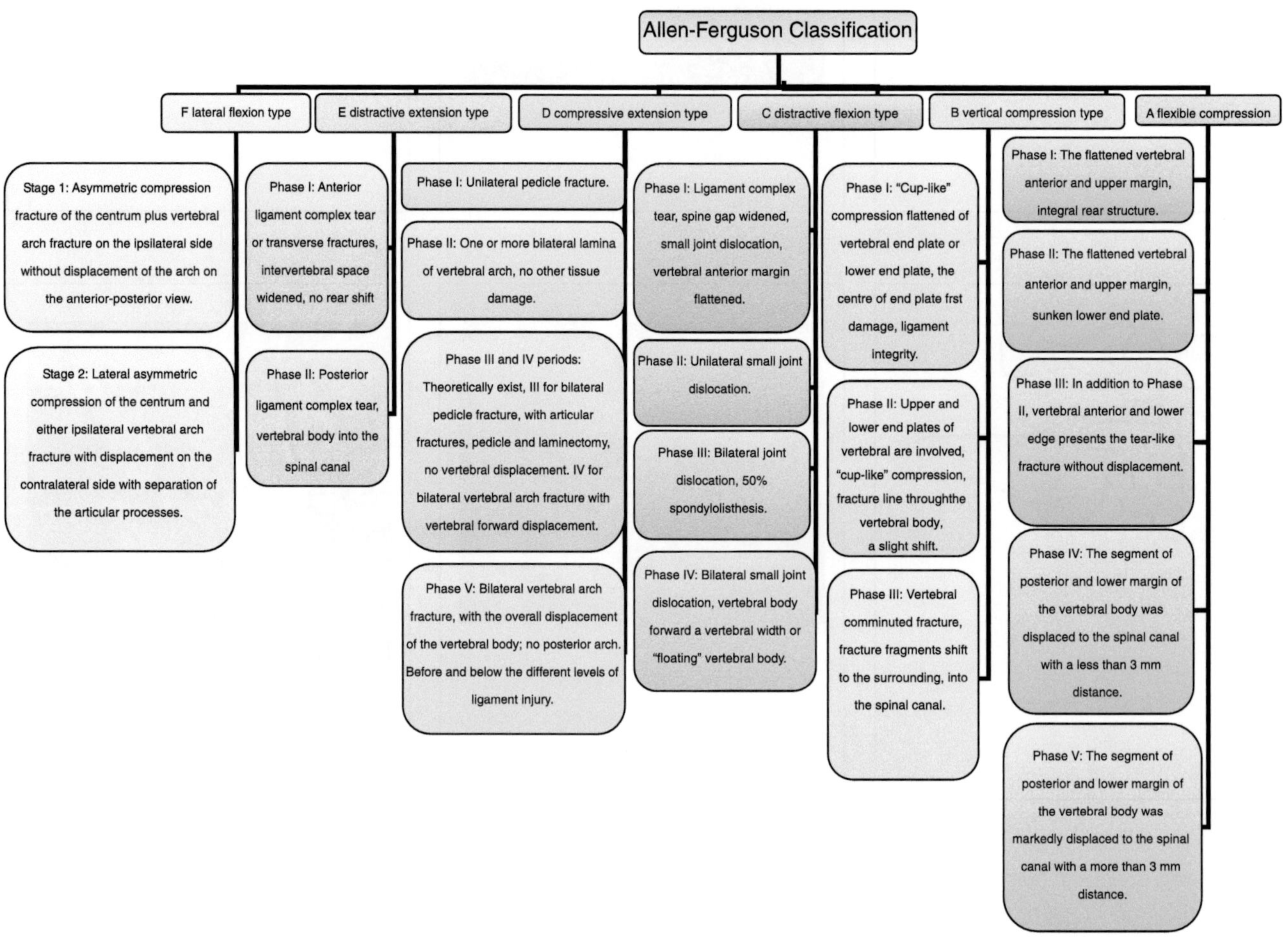

A flexible compression type:

Phase I: The flattened vertebral anterior and upper margin, integral rear structure.

Phase II: The flattened vertebral anterior and upper margin, sunken lower end plate.

Phase III: In addition to Phase II, vertebral anterior and lower edge presents the tear-like fracture without displacement.

Phase IV: The segment of posterior and lower margin of the vertebral body was displaced to the spinal canal with a less than 3 mm distance.

Phase V: The segment of posterior and lower margin of the vertebral body was markedly displaced to the spinal canal with a more than 3 mm distance; there are small joint dislocation, rupture of posterior longitudinal ligament and the rear of the ligament complex, accompanied with the widened spinous process space at corresponding injury segment.

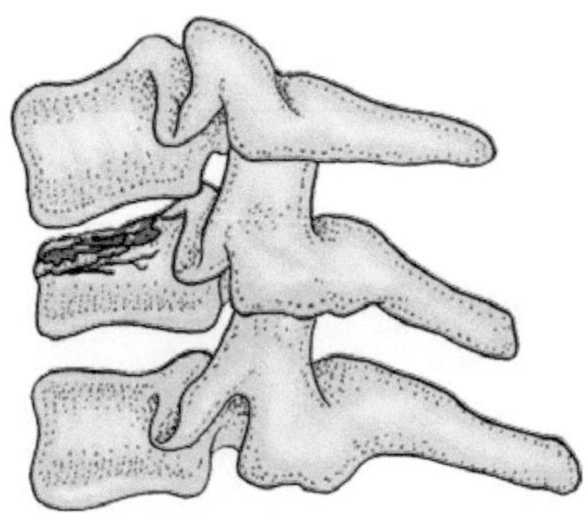

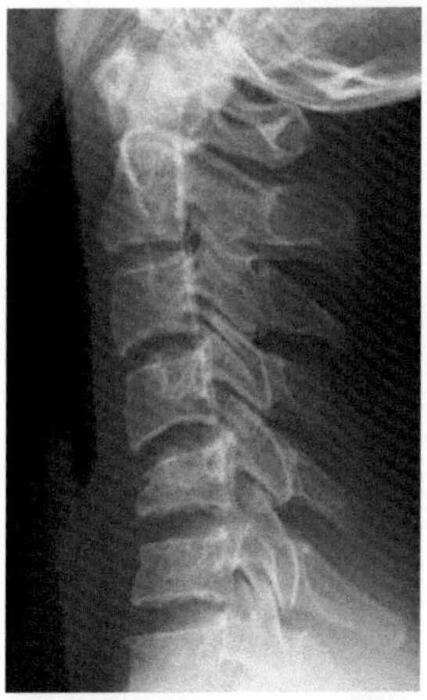

Allen Classification of Cervical Spine Fractures

A Flexible compression type:
Phase I: the flattened vertebral anterior and upper margin,
integral rear structure

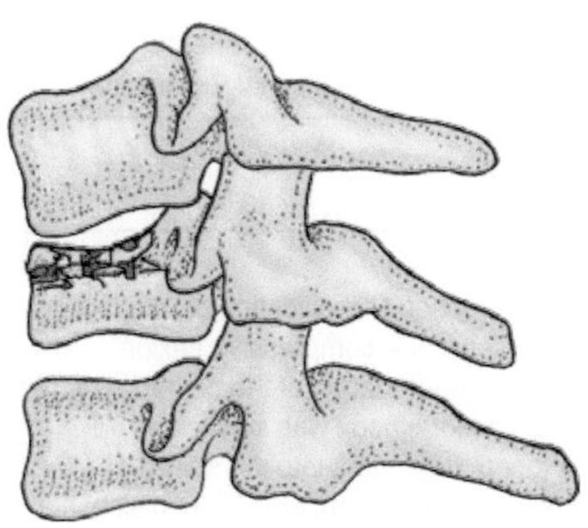

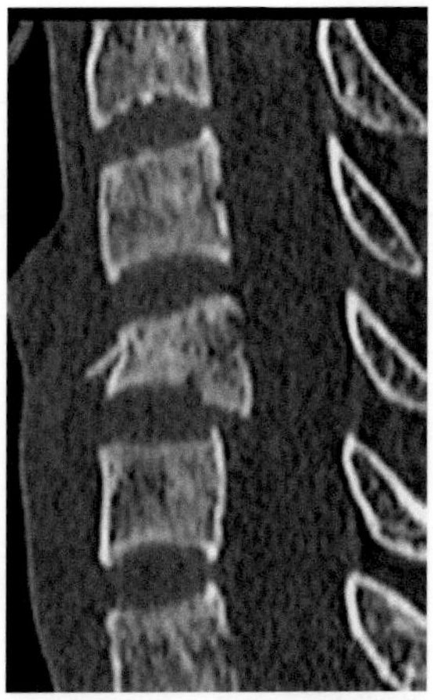

Allen Classification of Cervical Spine Fractures
A Flexible compression type:
Phase II: the flattened vertebral anterior and upper margin,
sunken lower end plate

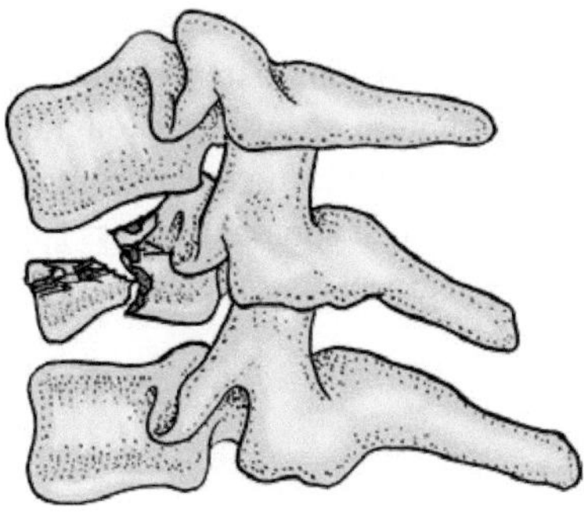

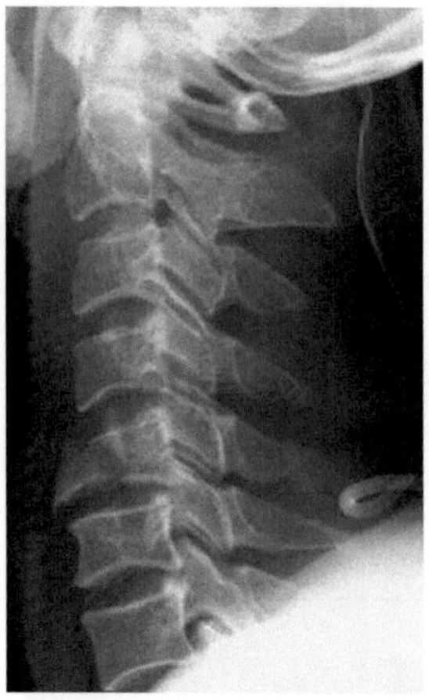

Allen Classification of Cervical Spine Fractures
A Flexible compression type:
Phase II I: In addition to Phase II, vertebral anterior and lower edge presents the tear-like fracture without displacement;

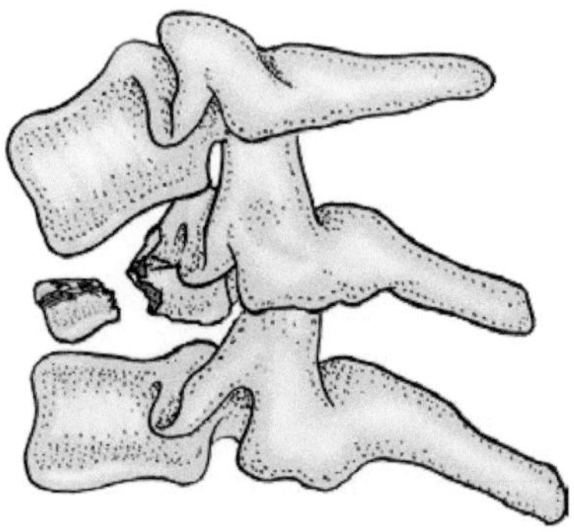

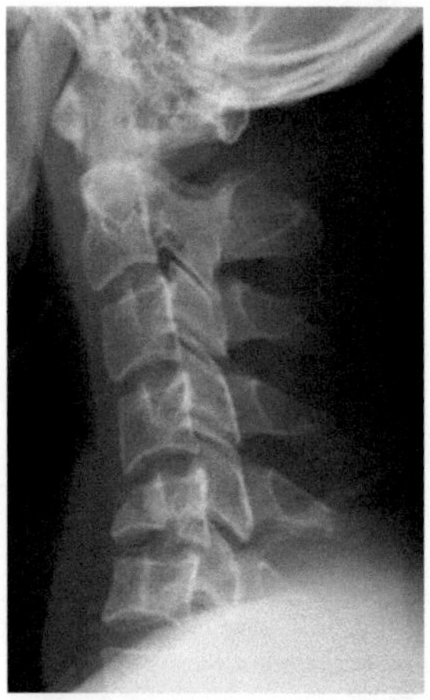

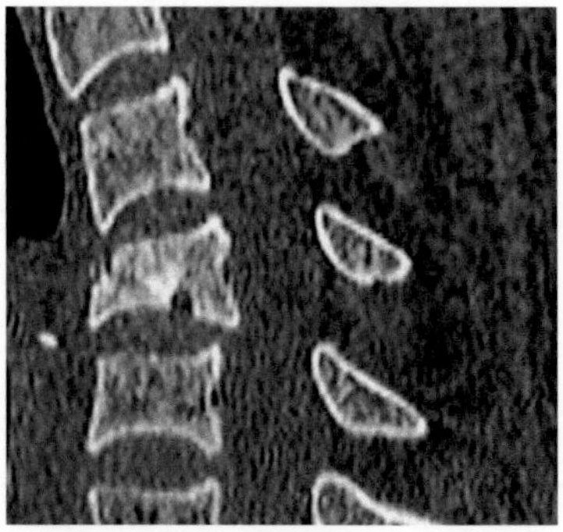

Allen Classification of Cervical Spine Fractures
A compressive flexion: IV stage:
the posterior margin of the vertebral body shift to the spinal canal, but less than 3mm

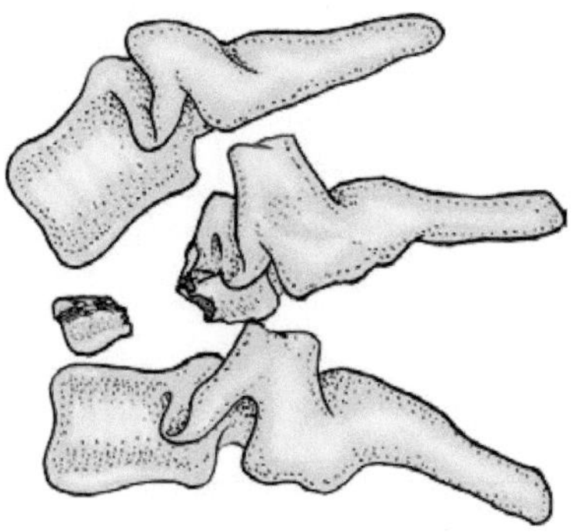

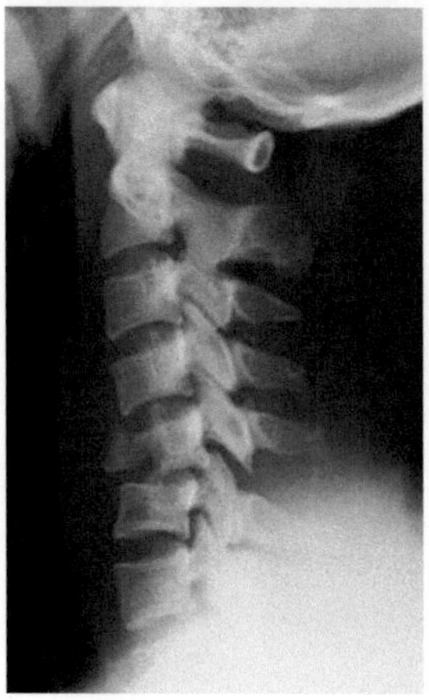

Allen–Ferguson Classification of Lower Cervical A compressive flexion
V: the posterior margin of the posterior margin of the vertebral body was significantly displaced, protruding into the spinal canal more than 3mm; small joint dislocation, posterior longitudinal ligament and the rear ligament complex rupture, the corresponding injury segment spinous process widened

B vertical compression:

Phase I: "Cup-like" compression flattened of vertebral end plate or lower end plate, the centre of end plate first damage, ligament integrity.

Phase II: Upper and lower end plates of vertebral are involved, "cup-like" compression, fracture line through the vertebral body, a slight shift.

Phase III: Vertebral comminuted fracture, fracture fragments shift to the surrounding, into the spinal canal.

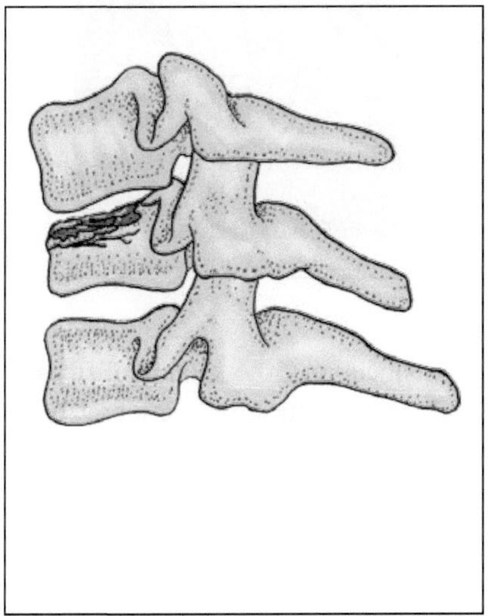

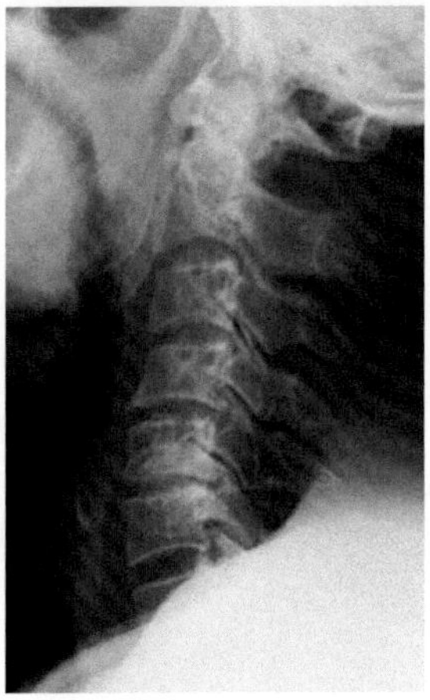

Allen–Ferguson Classification of Lower Cervical
B vertical compression:
Phase I: "cup-like" compression flattened of vertebral end plate or lower end plate, the center of end plate first damage, ligament integrity.

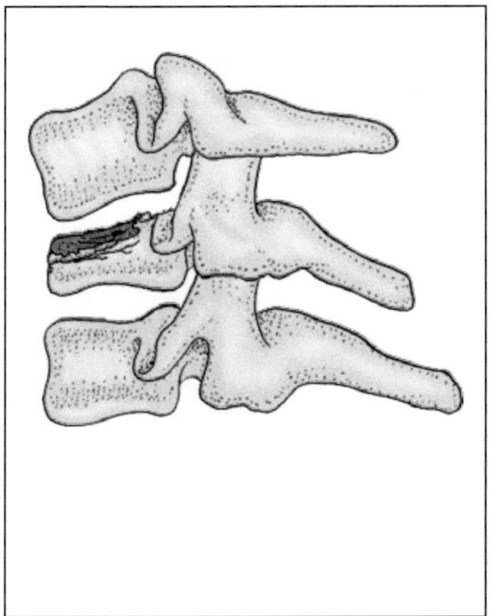

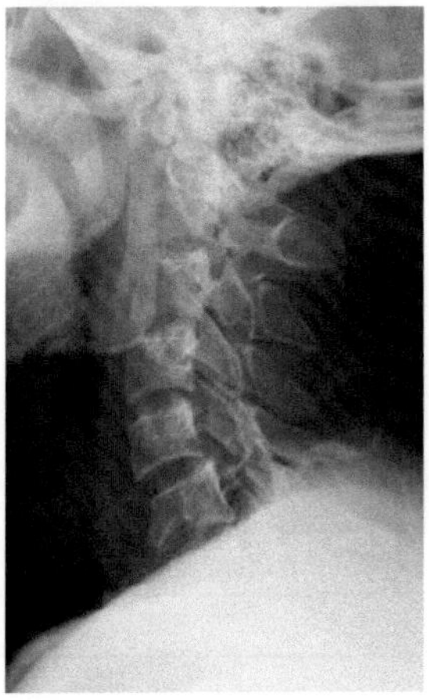

Allen–Ferguson Classification of Lower Cervical
B vertical compression:
Phase II: upper and lower end plates of vertebral are involved, "cup-like" compression, fracture line through the vertebral body, a slight shift.

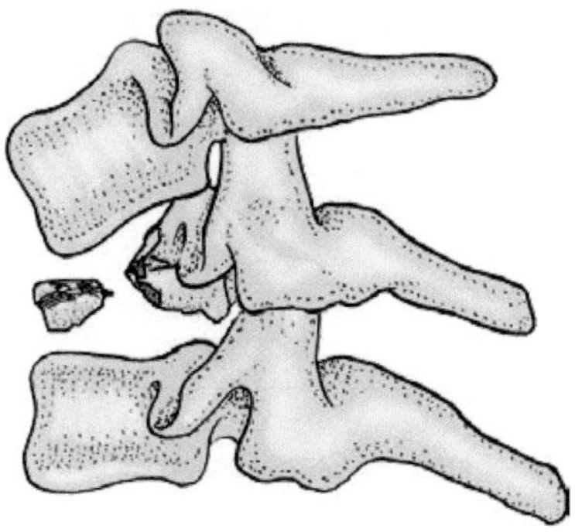

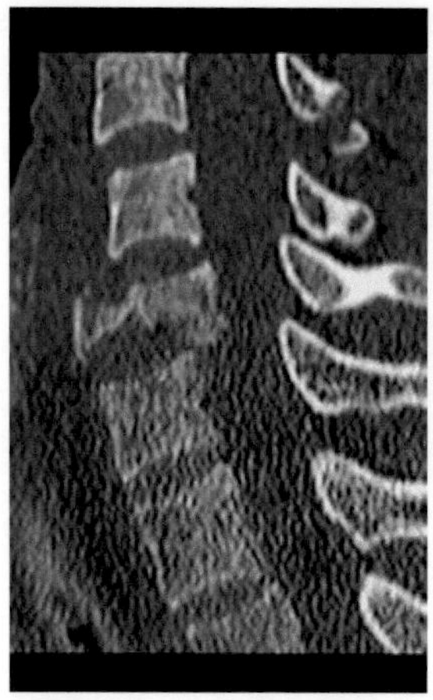

Allen–Ferguson Classification of Lower Cervical
B vertical compression:
III: vertebral comminuted fracture, fracture fragments shift to the surrounding, into the spinal canal.

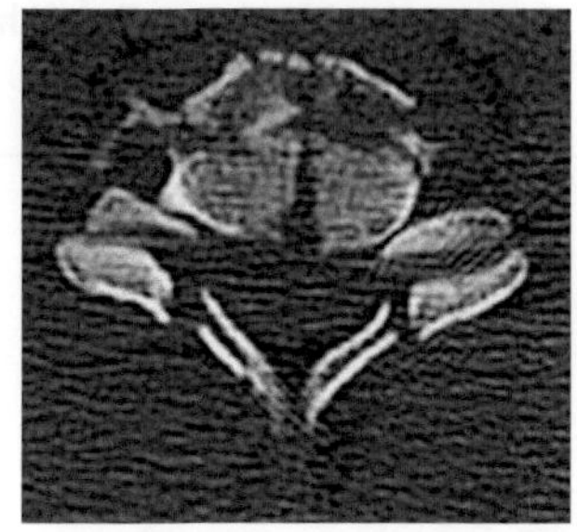

C distractive flexion

Phase I: Ligament complex tear, spine gap widened, small joint dislocation, vertebral anterior margin flattened.

Phase II: Unilateral small joint dislocation.

Phase III: Bilateral joint dislocation, 50% spondylolisthesis.

Phase IV: Bilateral small joint dislocation, vertebral body forward a vertebral width or "floating" vertebral body.

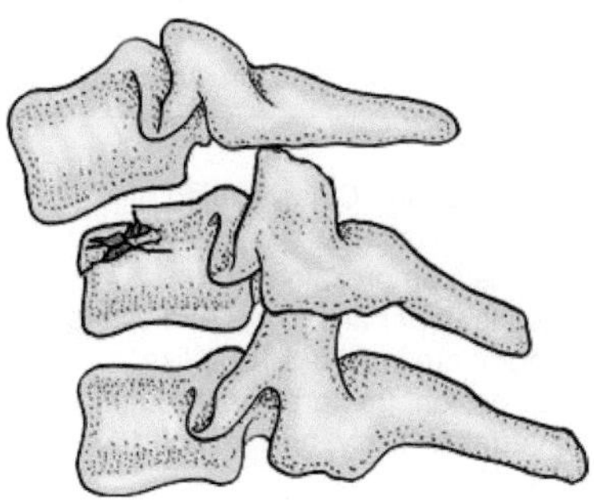

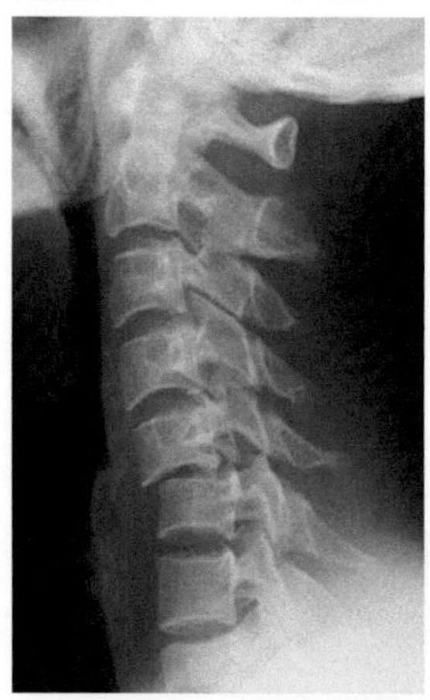

Allen–Ferguson Classification of Lower Cervical
C distractive flexion:
PhaseI: ligament complex tear, Spines gap widened, small joint dislocation, vertebral anterior margin flattened

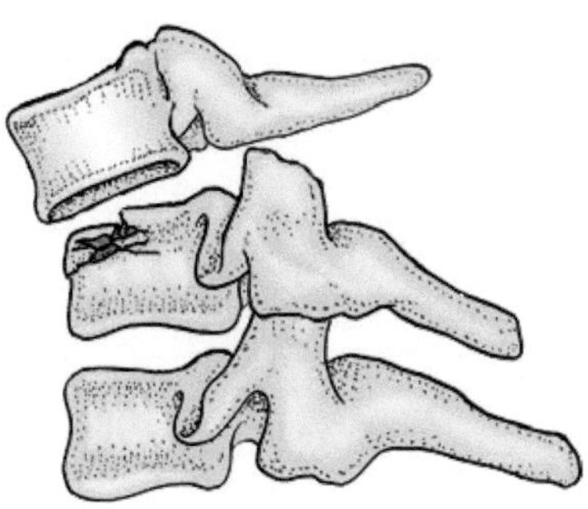

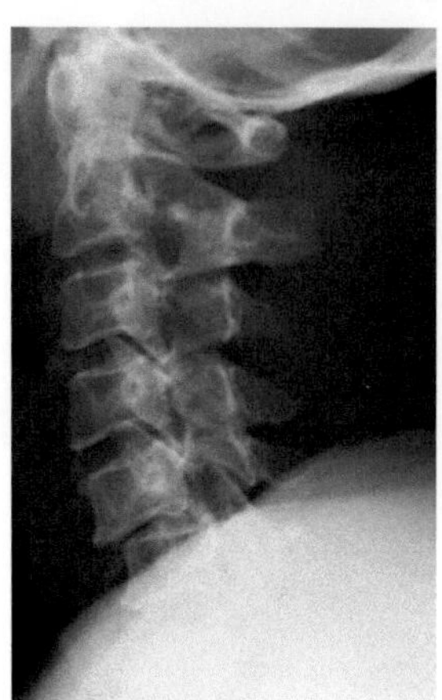

Allen–Ferguson Classification of Lower Cervical
C distractive flexion:
Phase II: unilateral small joint dislocation.

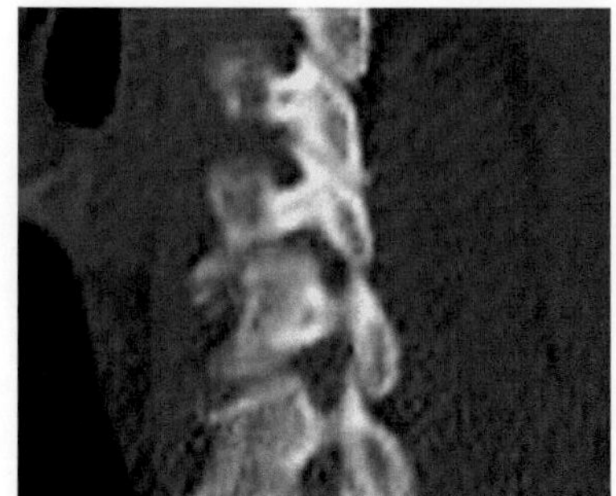

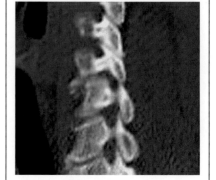

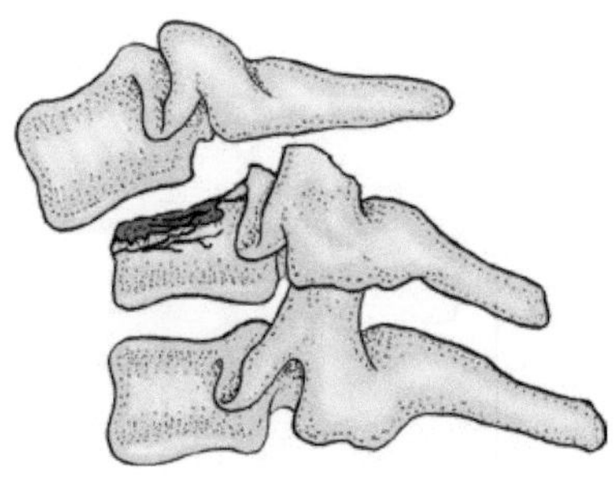

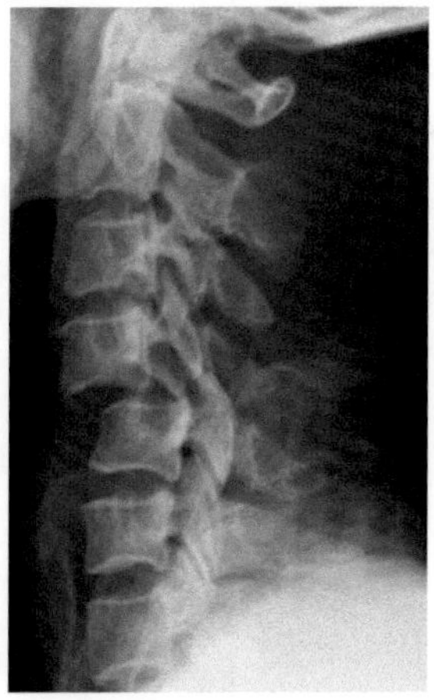

Allen–Ferguson Classification of Lower Cervical C distractive flexion: Phase III: bilateral joint dislocation, 50%spondylolisthesis .

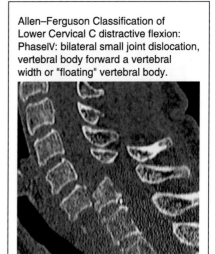

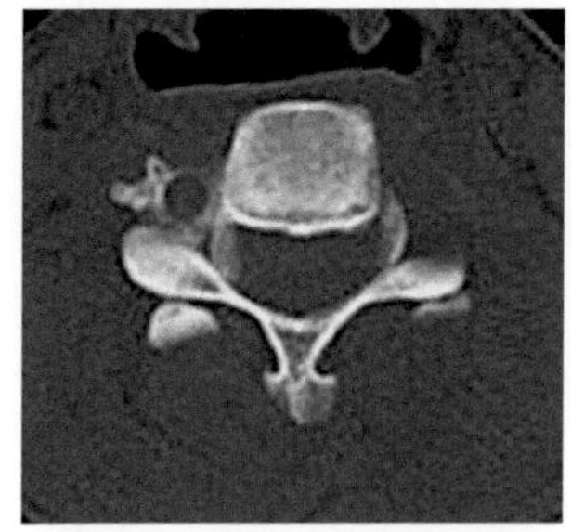

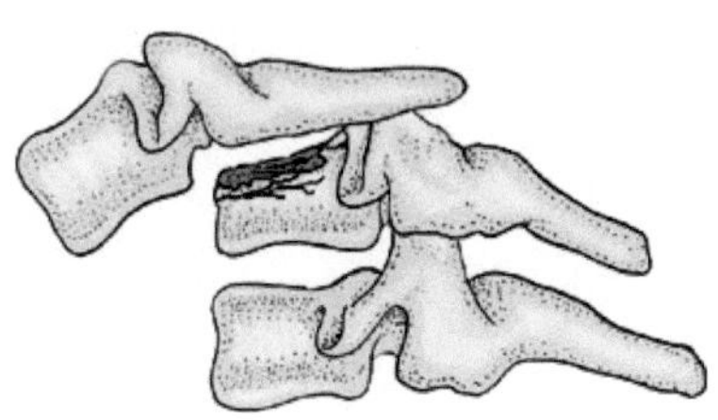

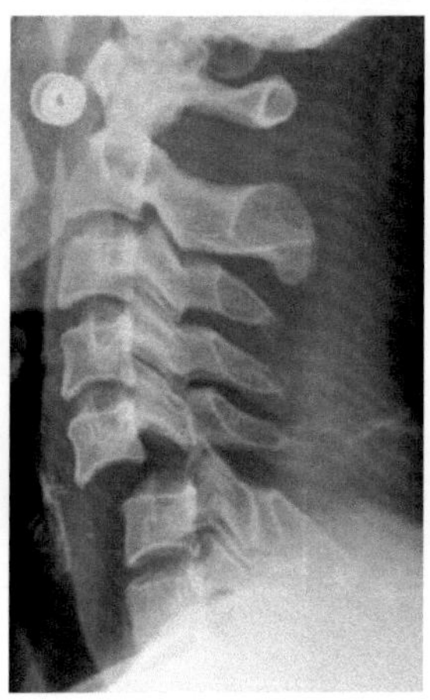

Allen–Ferguson Classification of Lower Cervical C distractive flexion: PhaseIV: bilateral small joint dislocation, vertebral body forward a vertebral width or "floating" vertebral body.

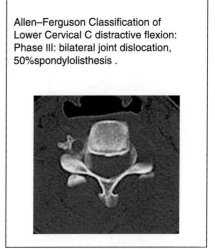

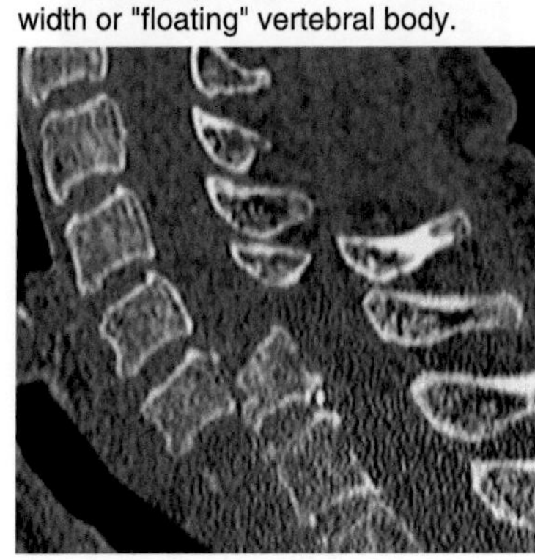

D compressive extension:

Phase I: Unilateral pedicle fracture.

Phase II: One or more bilateral lamina of vertebral arch, no other tissue damage.

Phase III and IV periods: Theoretically exist, III for bilateral pedicle fracture, with articular fractures, pedicle and laminectomy, no vertebral displacement. IV for bilateral vertebral arch fracture with vertebral forward displacement.

Phase V: Bilateral vertebral arch fracture, with the overall displacement of the vertebral body; no posterior arch. Before and below the different levels of ligament injury.

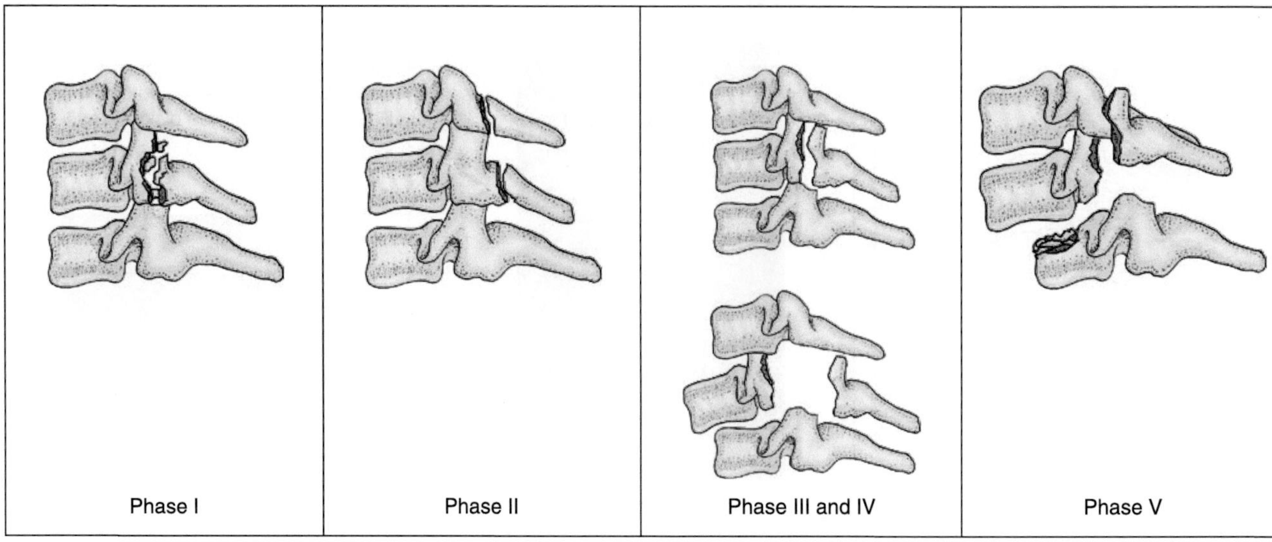

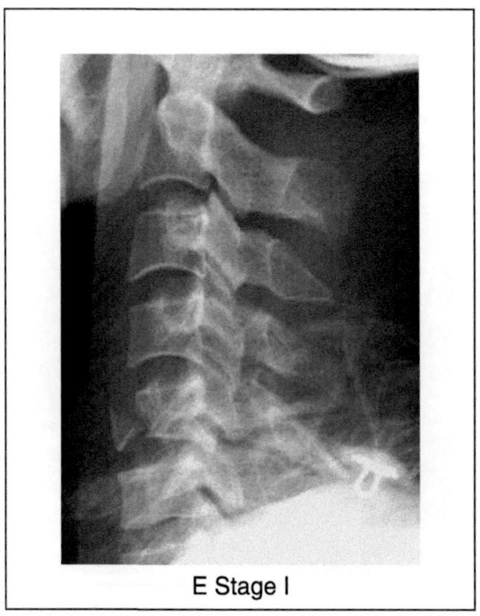

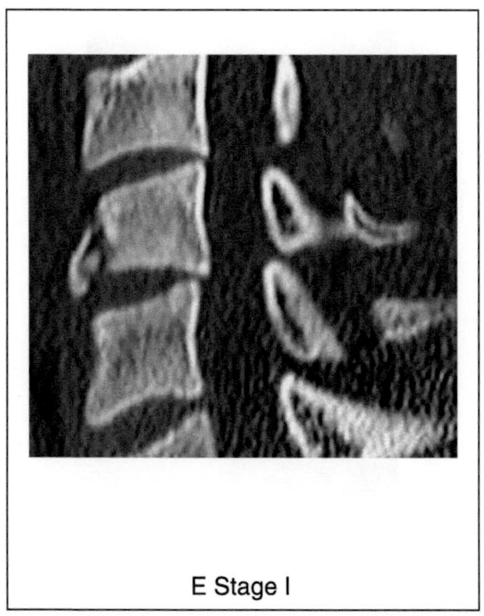

F lateral flexion:

Stage 1: Asymmetric compression fracture of the centrum plus vertebral arch fracture on the ipsilateral side without displacement of the arch on the anterior-posterior view.

Stage 2: Lateral asymmetric compression of the centrum and either ipsilateral vertebral arch fracture with displacement on the contralateral side with separation of the articular processes.

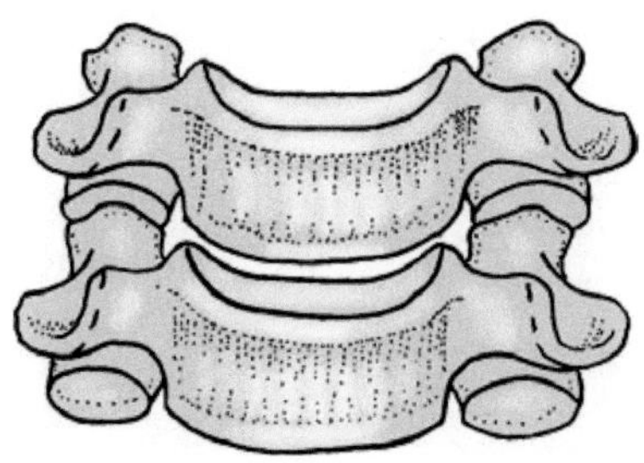

F Stage I

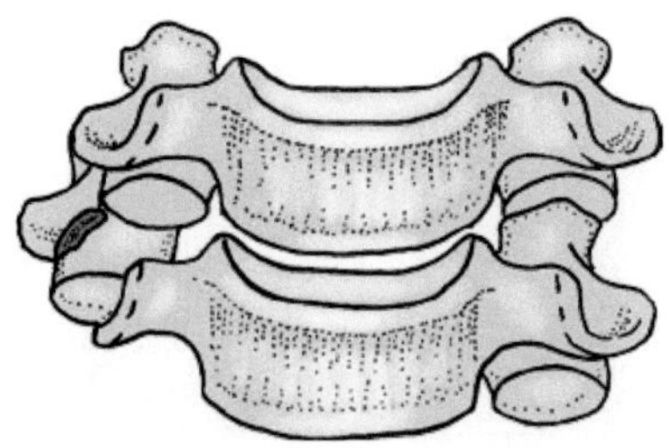

F Stage II

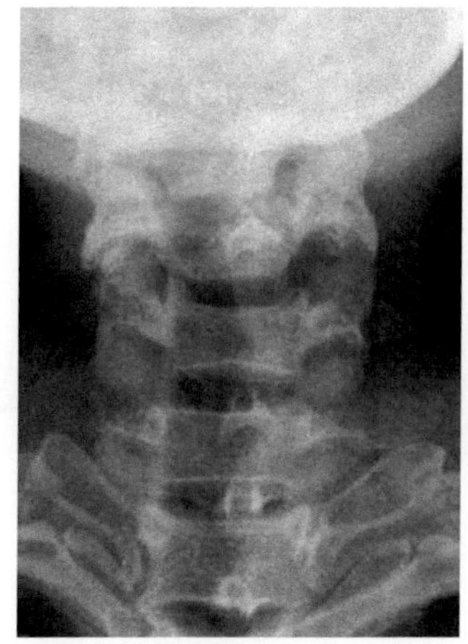

F Stage I

Argenson Classification (1997, Eur. J Orthop Surg. Traumatol, 7: 215–229)

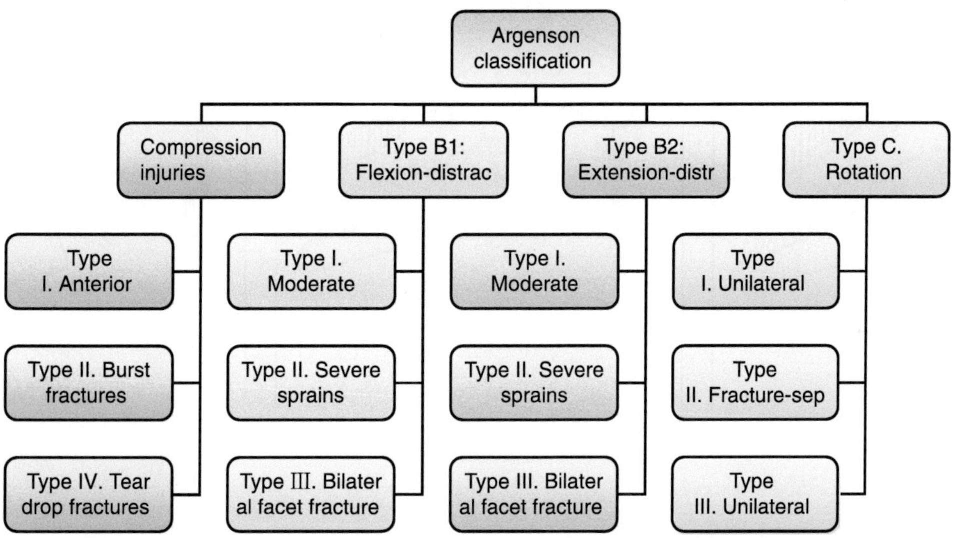

Type A: Compression injuries:
- I: Anterior wedge compression fractures.
- II: Burst fractures.
- III: Tear drop fractures.

Type B: Flexion–distraction injuries:
- I: Moderate sprains.
- II: Severe sprains.
- III: Bilateral facet fracture dislocations.

Type C: Rotation injuries:
- I: Unilateral facet fractures.
- II: Fracture-separation of the articular pillar.
- III: Unilateral facet dislocations.

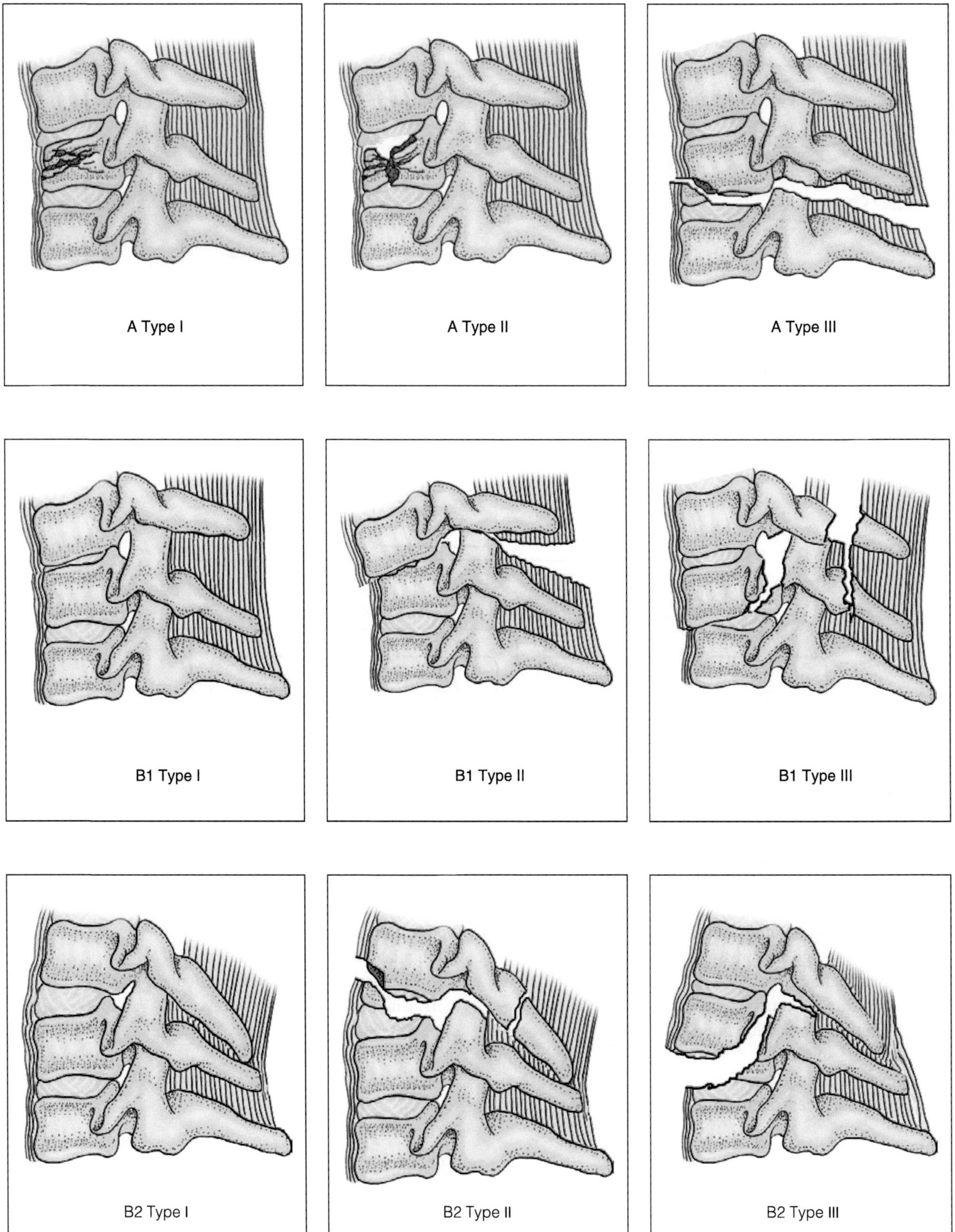
A Type I
A Type II
A Type III
B1 Type I
B1 Type II
B1 Type III
B2 Type I
B2 Type II
B2 Type III

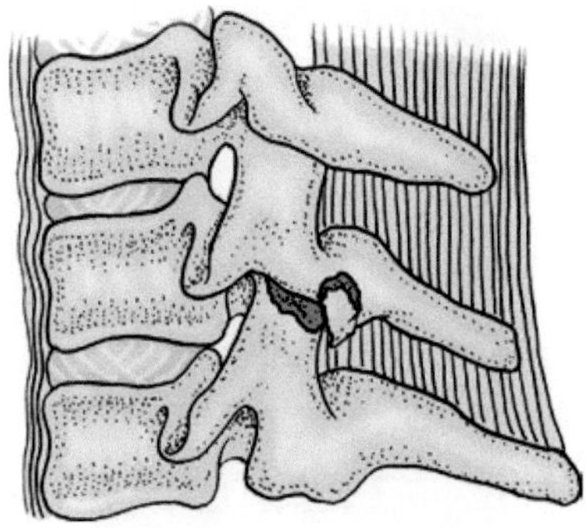

C Type I

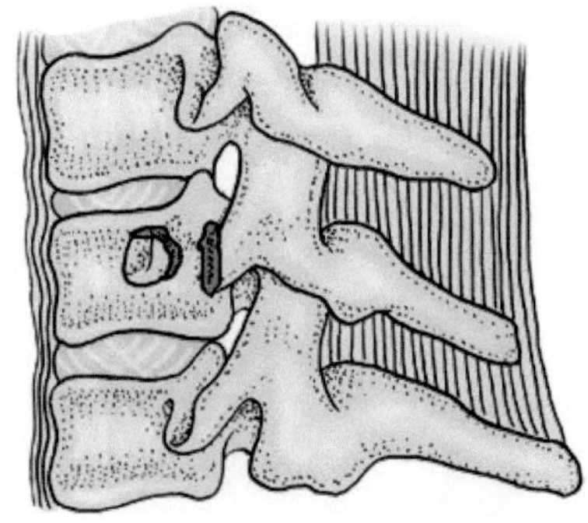

C Type II

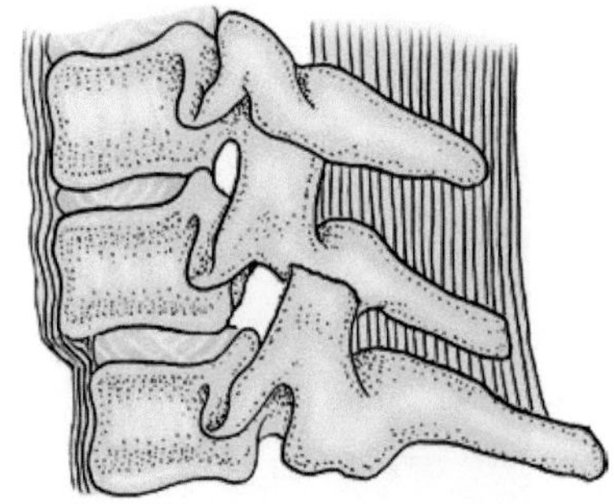

C Type III

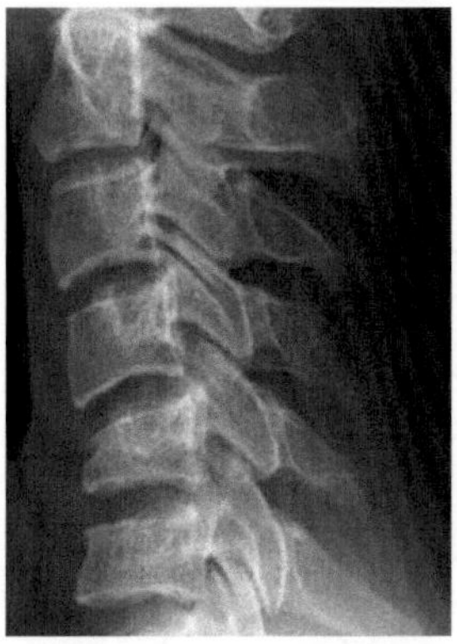

Type A Compression injuries
I Anterior wedge compression fractures

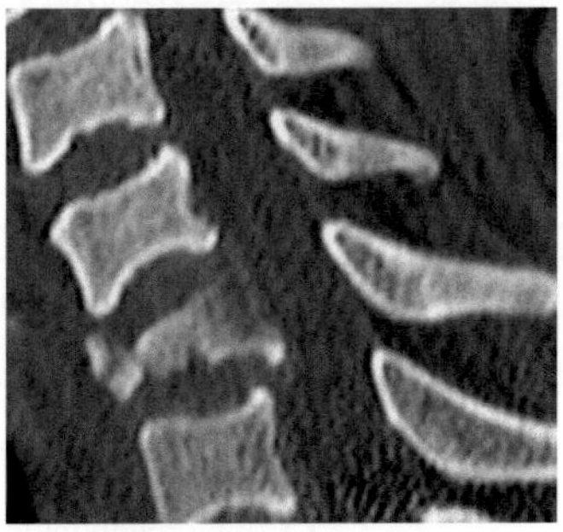

Type II Burst fractures

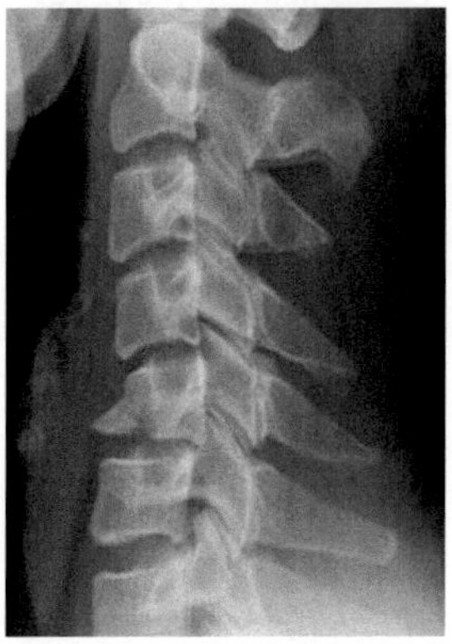

Type III Tear drop fractures

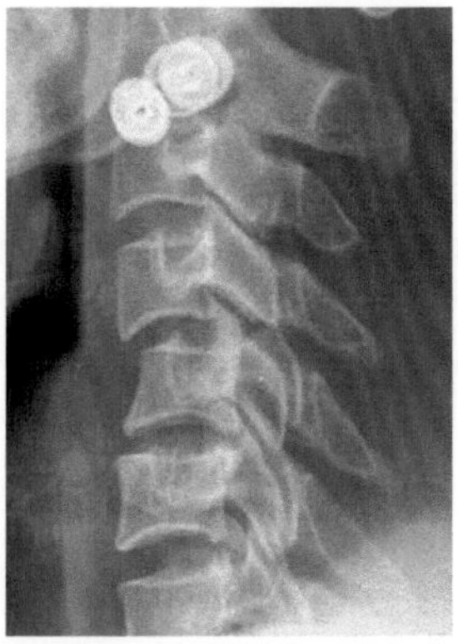

Type B1 Flexion-distraction injuries:
Type I. Moderate sprains

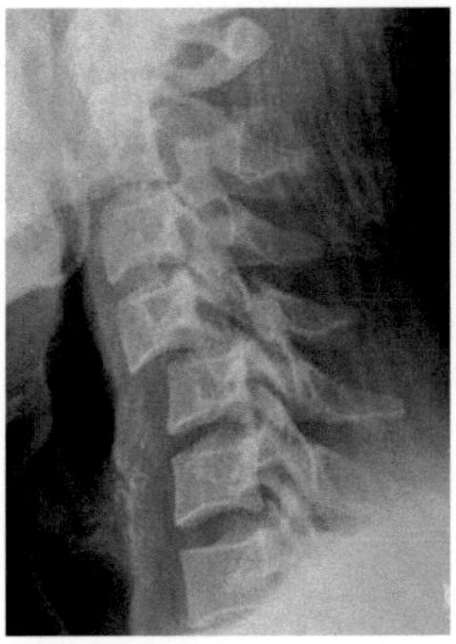

Type II. Severe sprains

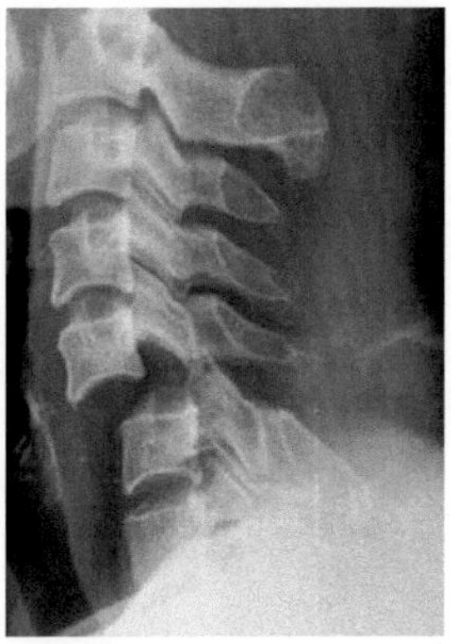

Type III.Bilateral facet fracture dislocations

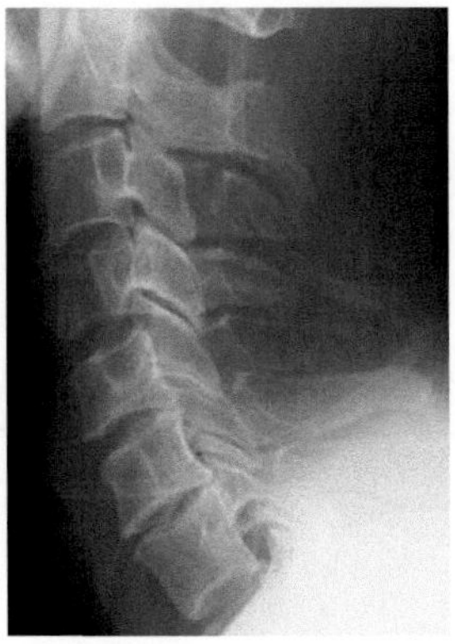

TypeB2: Extension-distraction injuries
Type I. Moderate sprains

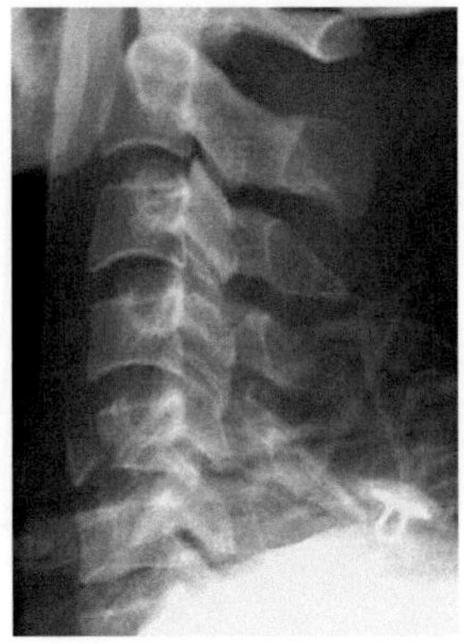

Type II. Severe sprains

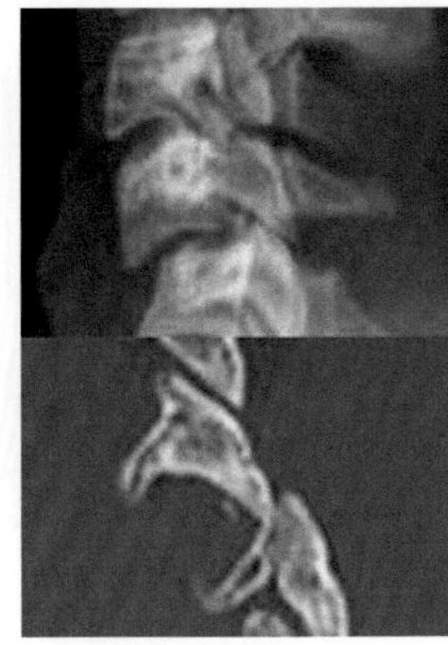

Type C Rotation injuries
Type III. Unilateral facet dislocations

AO/OTA Classification (2007 revised edition, Journal of Orthopaedic Trauma, 21 Supplement)

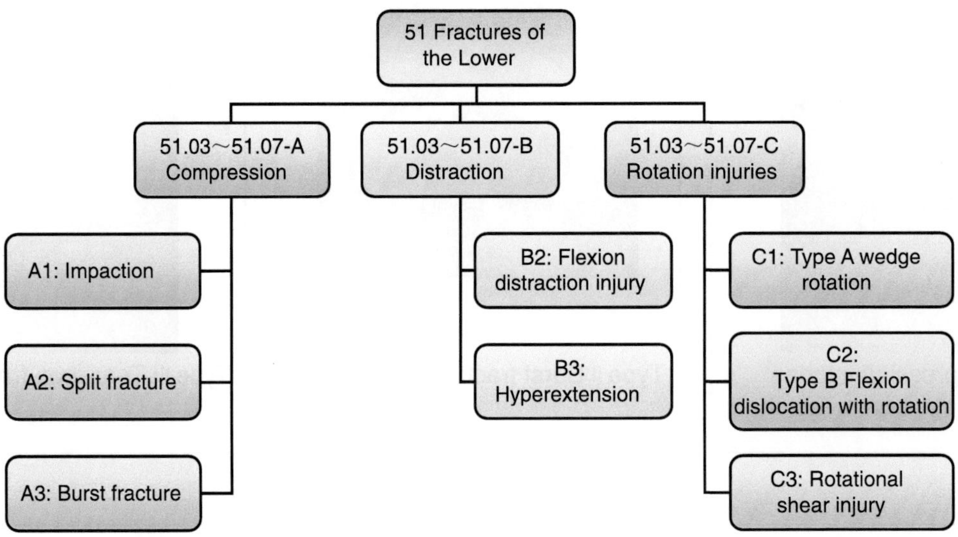

51.03–51.07-A: Compression fracture of the vertebral body:
- A1: Impaction fracture.
- A2: Split fracture.
- A3: Burst fracture.

51.03–51.07-B: Distraction injuries:
- B2: Flexion distraction injury, mainly bony structure distraction injury in the rear.
- B3: Hyperextension shear injury, anterior intervertebral disc distraction injury.

51.03–51.07-C: Rotation injuries:
- C1: Type A wedge rotation.
- C2: Type B Flexion dislocation with rotation.
- C3: Rotational shear injury (Holdsworth sliding fracture).

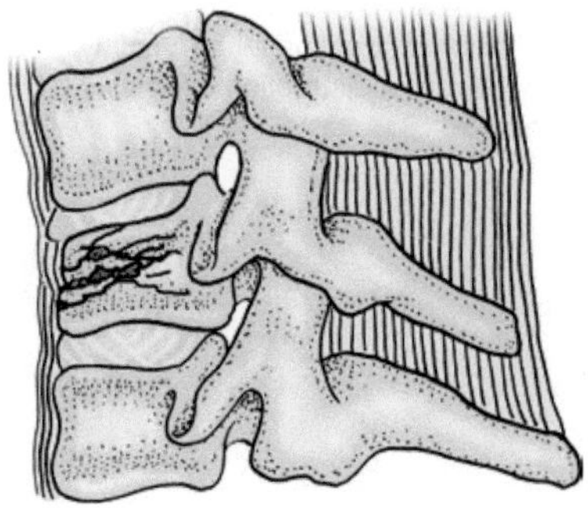

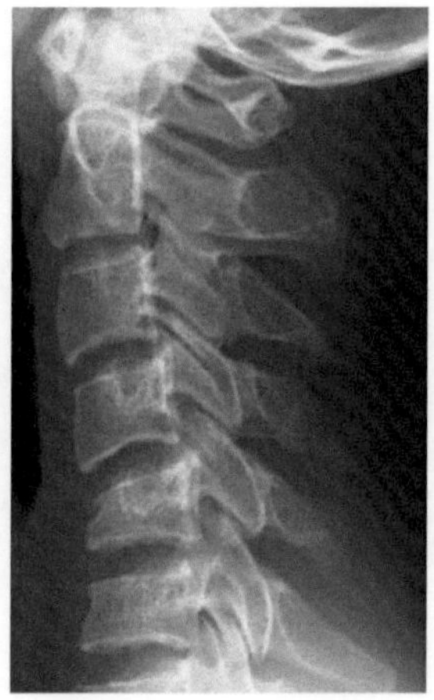

AO/OTA classification of lower cervical spine fractures

51.03~51.07-A Compression fracture of the vertebral body.
A1: Impaction fracture

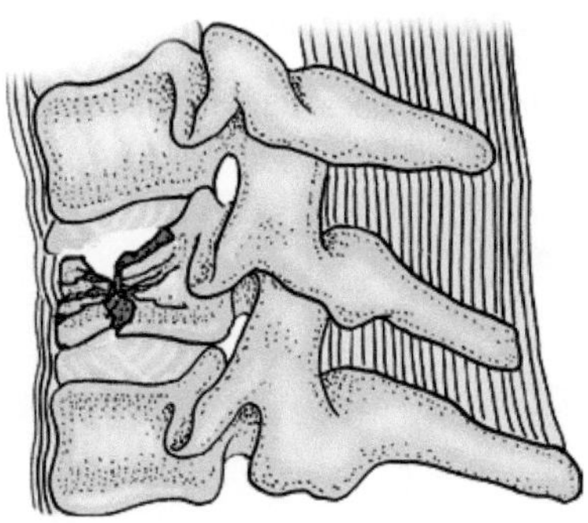

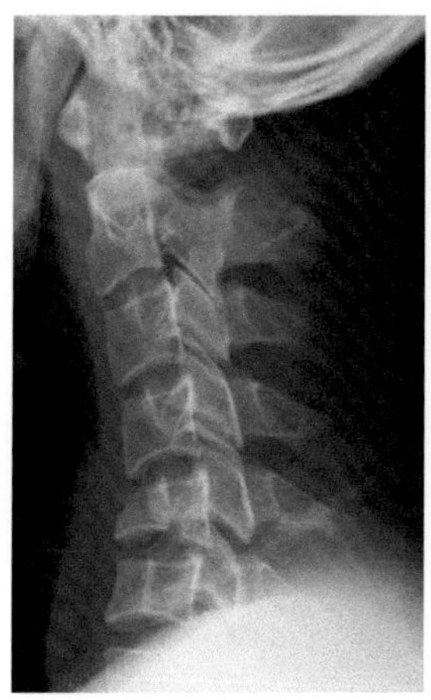

AO/OTA classification of lower cervical spine fractures
51.03~51.07-A Compression fracture of the vertebral body.
A2: Split fracture

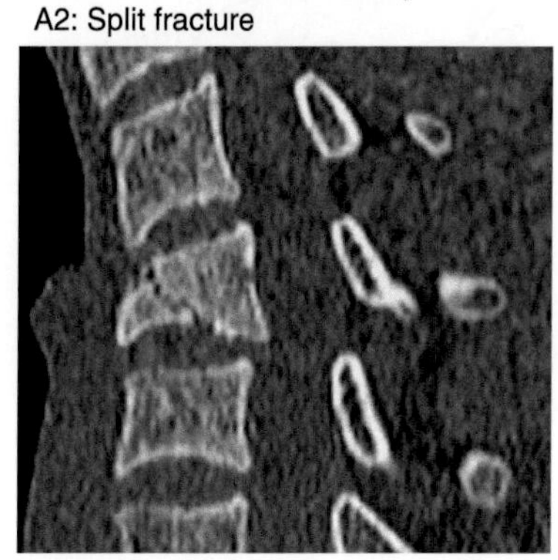

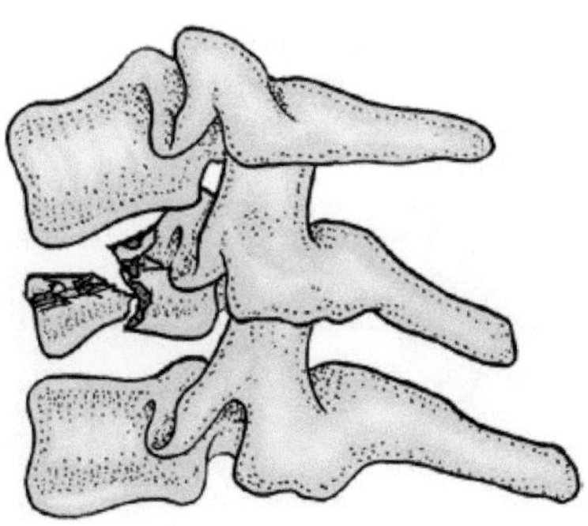

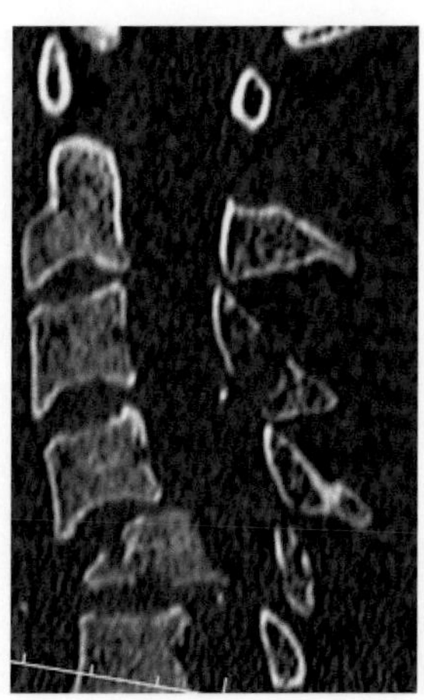

AO/OTA classification of lower cervical spine fractures
51.03~51.07-A Compression fracture of the vertebral body.
A3: Burst fracture

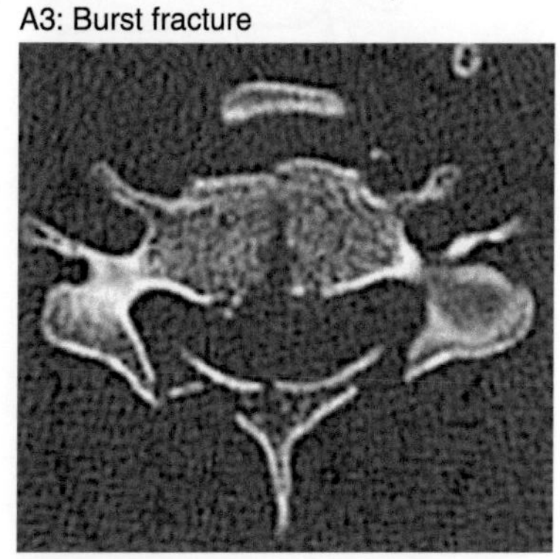

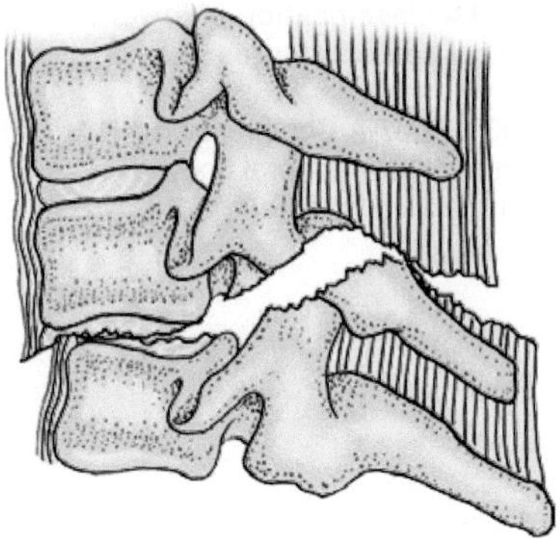

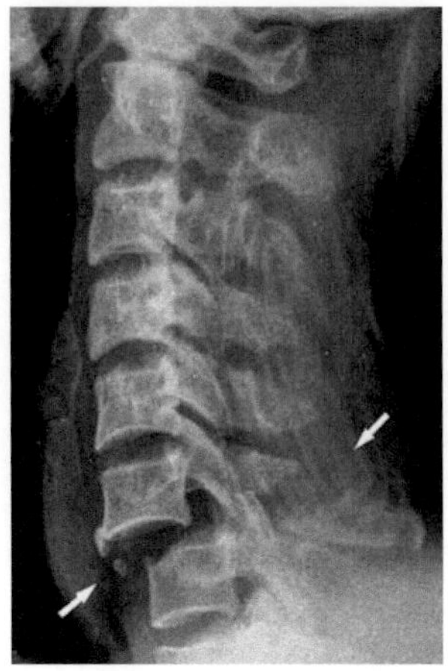

AO/OTA classification of lower cervical spine fractures
51.03~51.07-B Distraction injuries.
B2 Flexion distraction injury, mainly bony structure distraction injury in the rear

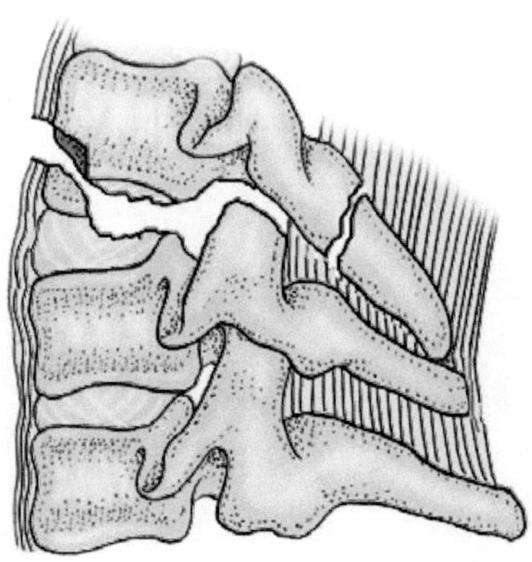

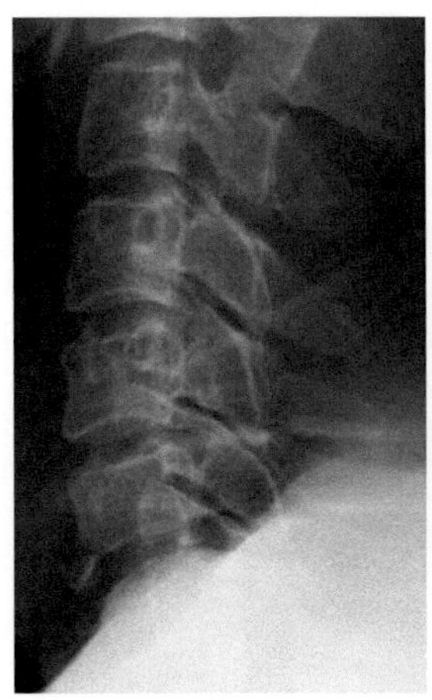

AO/OTA Classification
51.03~51.07-B
Distraction injuries. B3: stretched shear injury, anterior disc stretch injury

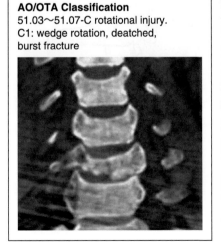

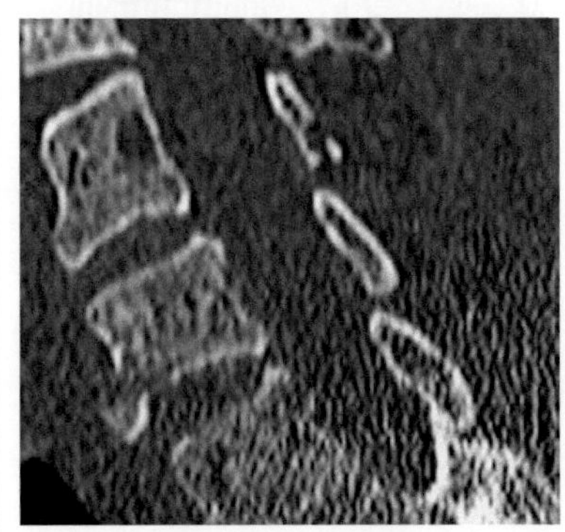

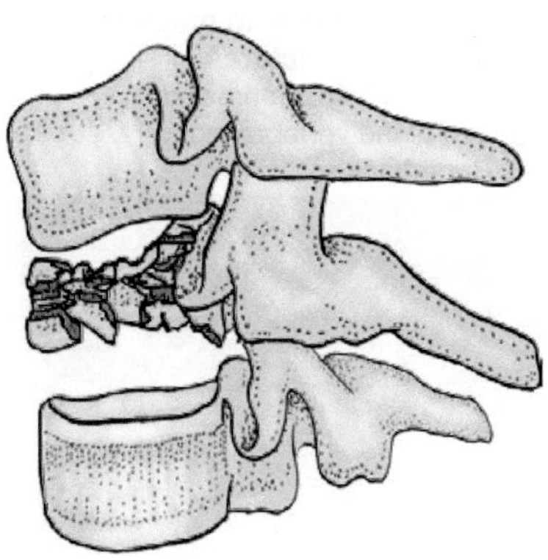

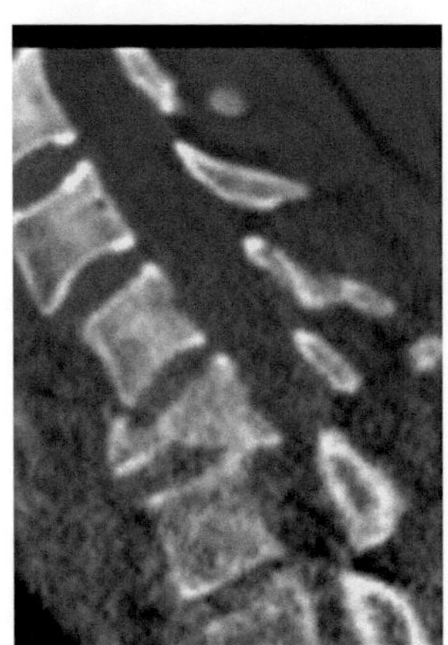

AO/OTA Classification
51.03~51.07-C rotational injury.
C1: wedge rotation, deatched, burst fracture

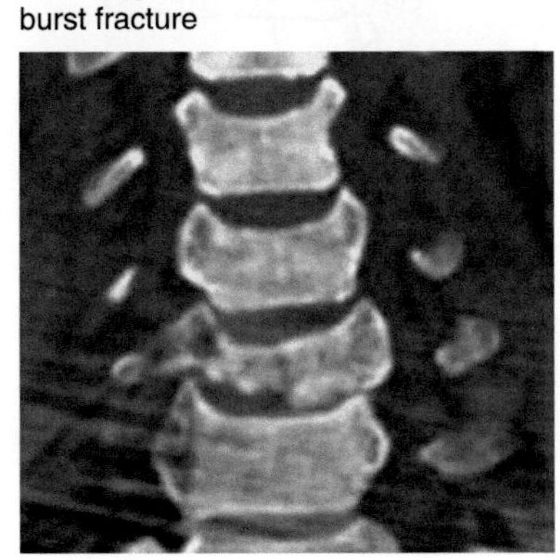

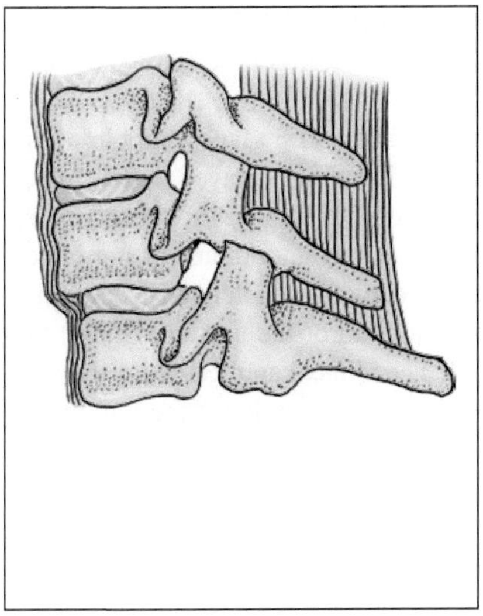

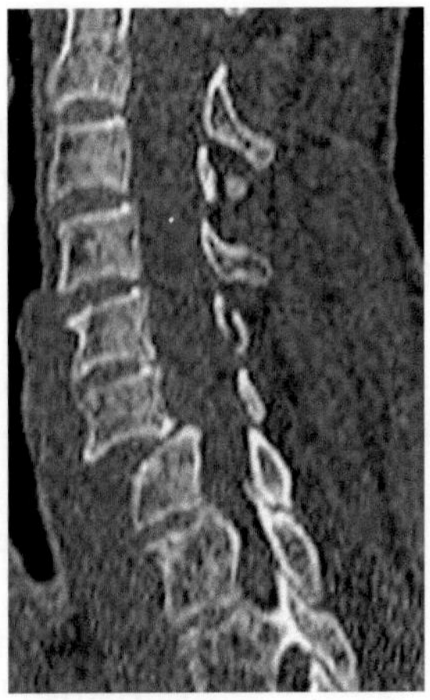

AO/OTA Classification
51.03~51.07-C rotational injury.
C2: Flexed subluxation with rotation

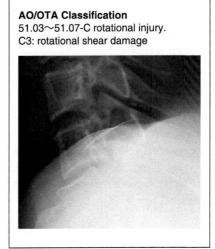

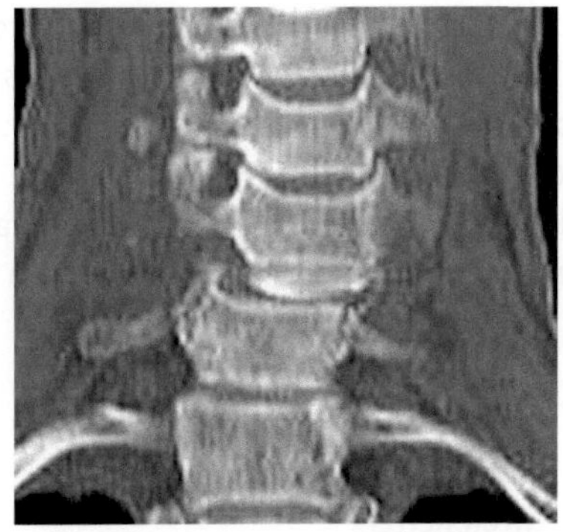

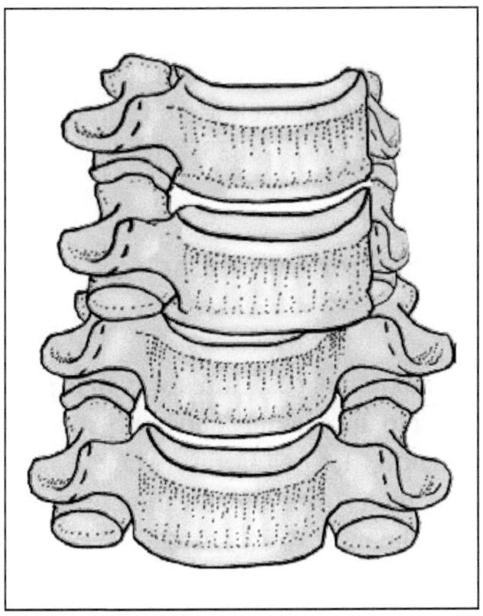

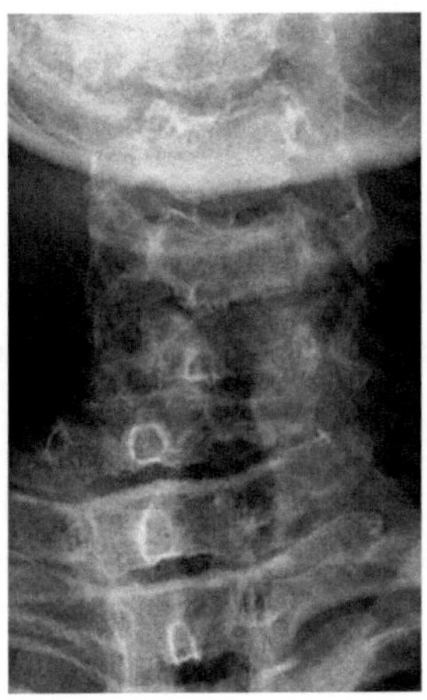

AO/OTA Classification
51.03~51.07-C rotational injury.
C3: rotational shear damage

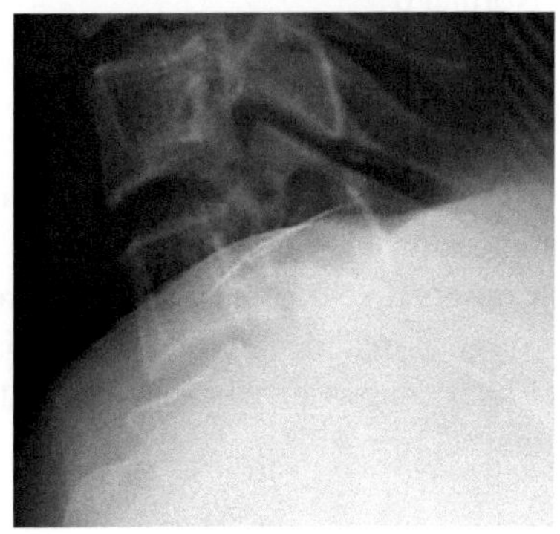

Lower Cervical Injury Classification According to Anatomy (1990, Philadelphia: JB Lippincott)

1. I: Posterior column injury:
   (a) Single posterior structural fractures:
   - Spinal process fracture.
   - Vertebral fracture.
     – Transverse process fracture

   (b) Posterior ligament injury:
   - Moderate ligament injury.
   - Severe ligament injury.

   (c) Traction injury with spinal cord injury
2. II: Fracture of the articular process:
   (a) Single articular process or pedicle fracture.
   (b) Unilateral articular process dislocation.
   - Articular process dislocation:
     – Articular process fracture with dislocation.
   - Lateral fragment detachment:

   (c) Bilateral articular process dislocation:
   - Bilateral articular process dislocation.
   - Bilateral articular process fracture with dislocation.
   - Bilateral articular facet fracture and dislocation with traumatic disc herniation.
     – Detached injury.
3. III: Anterior column injury:
   (a) Vertebral compression fractures.
   (b) Vertebral compression fractures with posterior ligament injury.
   (c) Traction injury of the intervertebral disc.
   (d) Stretched tear broken.
   (e) Traumatic slippage.
   (f) Stable burst fracture.
   (g) Unstable burst fracture.
   (h) Flexed tear fracture.

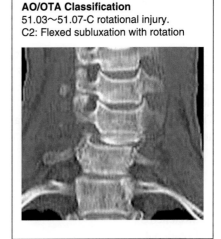

Magerl Classification (1994, Eur Spine J, 3: 184–201)
Magerl's classification to thoracolumbar fractures is also suitable for the subcervical spinal injury.

The Subcervical Injury Score System Proposed by Vaccaro [The Subaxial Cervical Spine Injury Classification System and Severity Scale (SLIC) Spine. 32 (23): 2620–2629, November 1, 2007]
The injury morphology, intervertebral disc ligament, and neurological condition are involved in this system.

Injury morphology
Normal 0
Compression 1
Burst 2
Stretched 3
Rotation 4
Intervertebral disc ligament
Intact 0
Suspicious injury 1
Rupture 2
Neurological condition
Normal 0
Neural root injury 1
Complete spinal cord injury 2
Incomplete spinal cord injury 3
Neurological dysfunction associated with persistent nerve compression +1
Conservative treatment if total score ≤3;
Surgical treatment if total score ≥5;
Either conservative or surgical treatment may be selected if total score = 4

Moore Proposed Subcervical Injury Modified Classification (Moore TA, Vaccaro AR, Anderson PA. Classification of Lower Cervical Spine Injuries. Spine, 2006, 31(11S): pp. S37–S43)
Moore modified the subcervical injury classification system in 2006, which divided the cervical spine into anterior column, posterior column, left column, and right column. Each part contained single injury and complicated injury.

Holdsworth Classification (Holdsworth F. Fractures, dislocations, and fracture-dislocations of the Spine. J Bone Joint Surg Am 1970;52: 1534–51)
All spinal injuries were divided into six types: simple wedge compression fractures, dislocation, delayed injury, burst fracture, and rotational dislocation with shear injury. Holdsworth divided the spine into anterior and posterior column. Stable and unstable fractures were defined according to the injury of posterior column. For the unstable injury, two columns were damaged. The clinical application of the classification is limited because it did not depict the importance of stability clearly.

Other Classification
1. Harris classification (1986, Orthop Clin North Am, 17: 15–30)
2. Anderson-Steinmann classification
3. Senegas classification

(Sénégas J, Vital JM, Barat M, Caille JM, Dabadie PH: Traumatismes du rachis cervical. Encycl. Med. Chir. (Paris, France), Appareil Locomoteur, 1987, 15825; A10: 9, 21.)

6.1.2 Classification of Thoracolumbar Fractures

The classification of thoracolumbar fractures was first proposed by Bohler according to the anatomy and injury mechanisms. Nicholl, Holdsworth, Louis, Denis, Magerl, and McCormac put forward their own classification. Magerl classification, AO type, is the most widely used.

6.1.2.1 AO/OTA/AO-Magerl Classification (2007, Journal of Orthopaedic Trauma. 21 Supplement. Presented by Magerl in 1994)

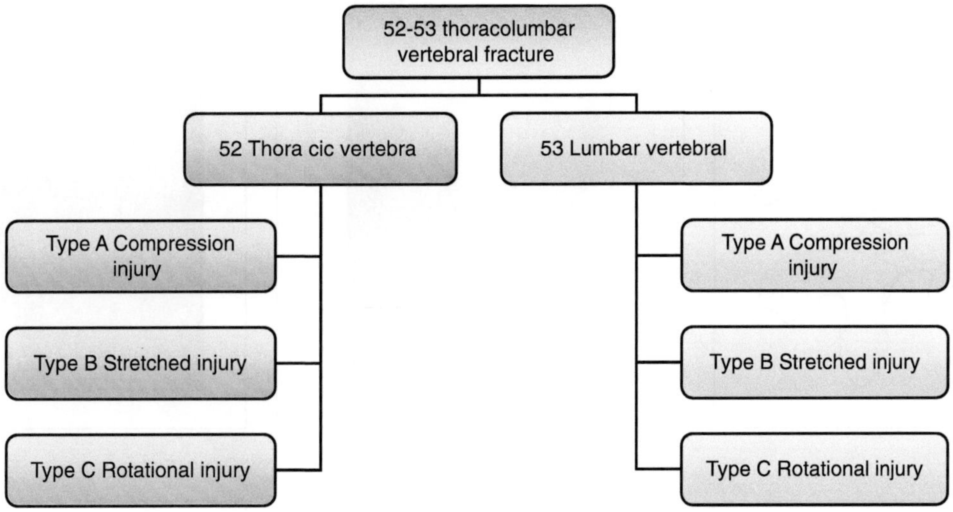

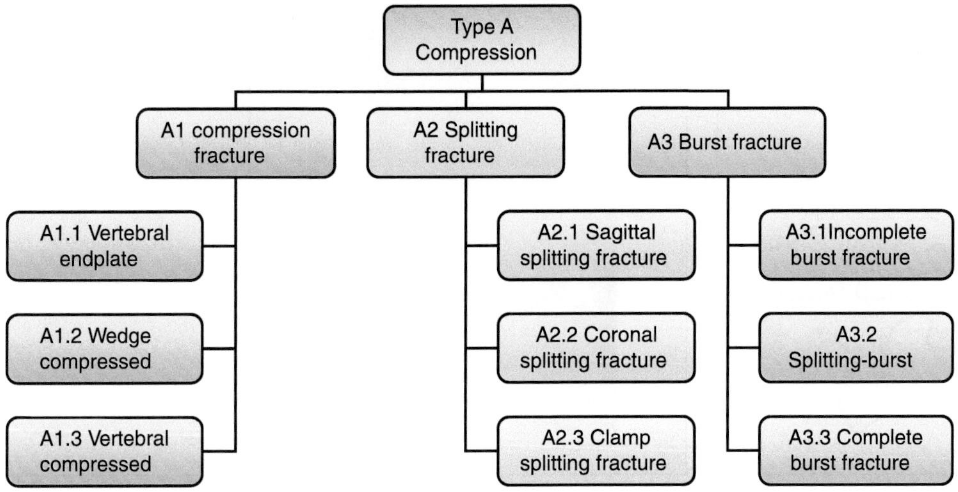

52–53 Type A: Thoracolumbar compressed fracture:
- A1: compressed fracture:
  - A1.1: Vertebral endplate compression fracture.
  - A1.2: Wedge compressed fracture.
  - A1.3: Vertebral compressed fracture
- A2: Splitting fracture:
  - A2.1: Sagittal splitting fracture.
  - A2.2: Coronal splitting fracture.
  - A2.3: Clamp splitting fracture
- A3: Burst fracture:
  - A3.1: Incomplete burst fracture.
  - A3.2: Splitting-burst fracture.
  - A3.3: Complete burst fracture

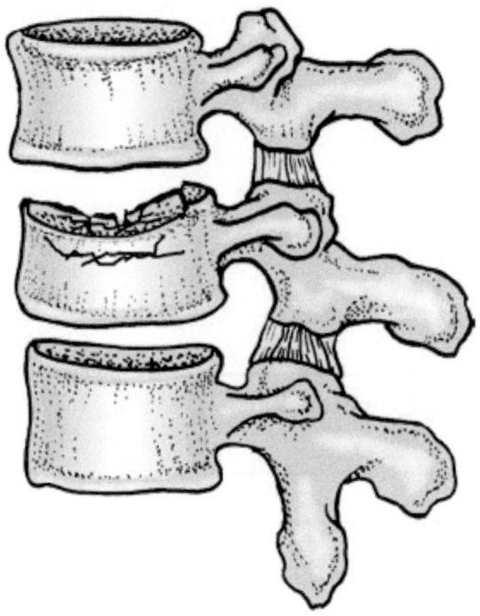

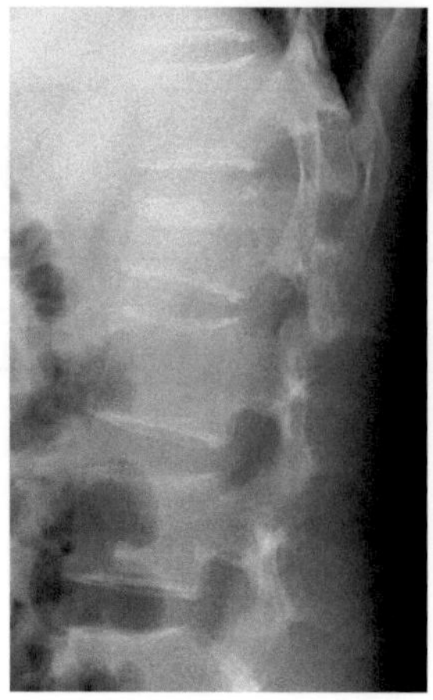

AO classification
Type A Thoracolumbar compressed fracture. A1 compressed fracture A1.1 Vertebral endplate compression fracture

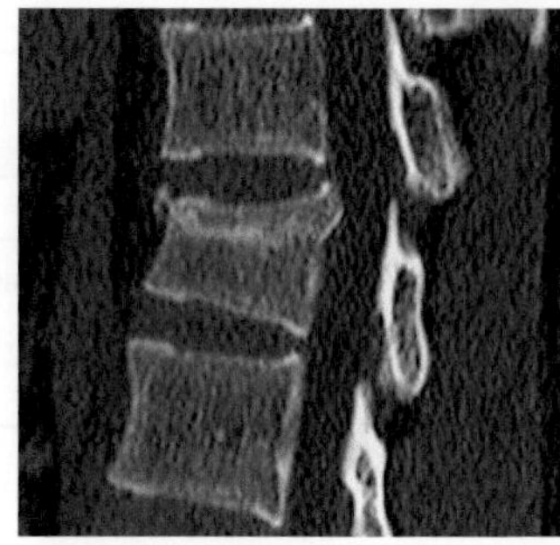

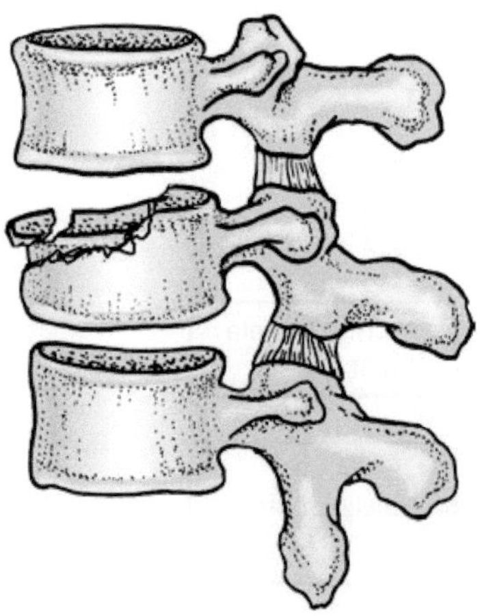

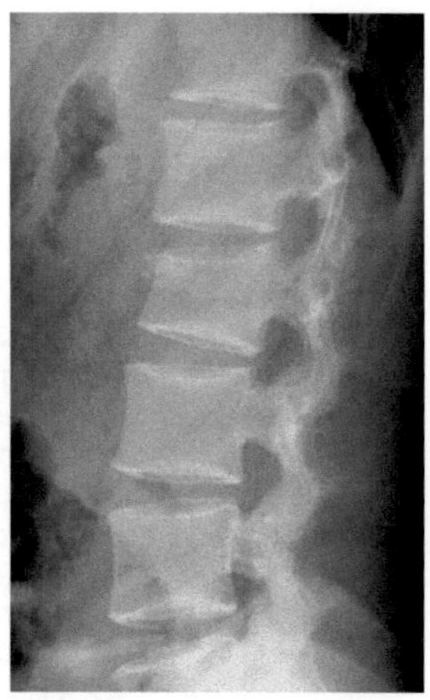

AO classification
Type A Thoracolumbar compressed fracture. A1 compressed fracture A1.2 Wedge compressed fracture

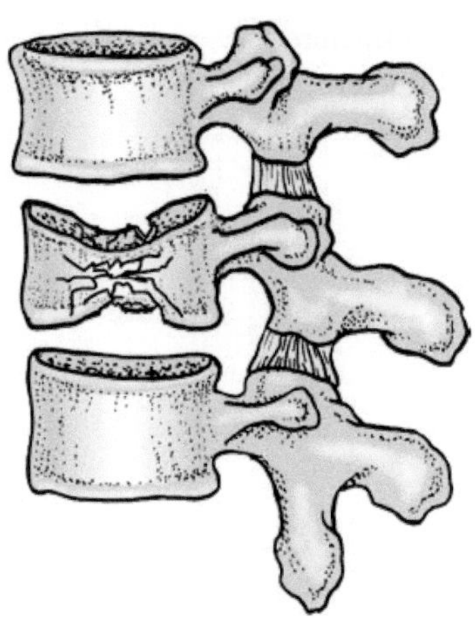

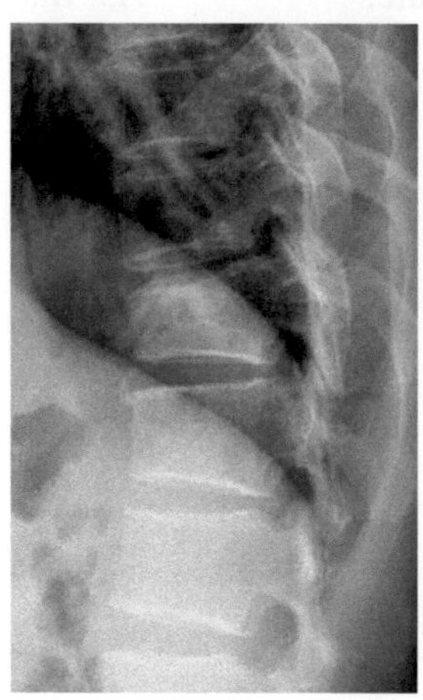

AO classification
Type A Thoracolumbar compressed fracture. A1 compressed fracture A1.3 Vertebral compressed fracture

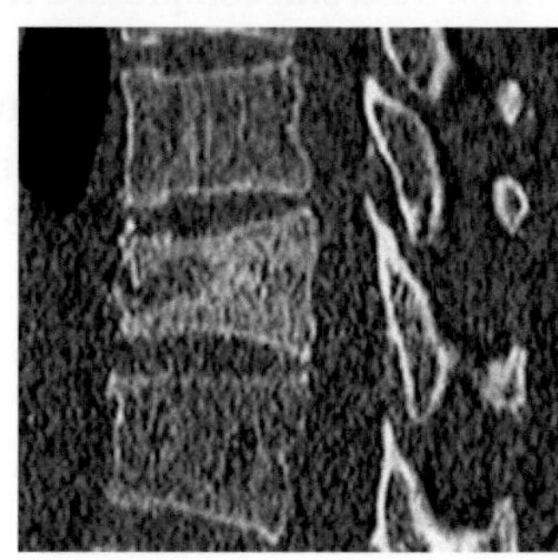

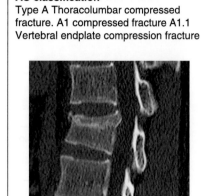

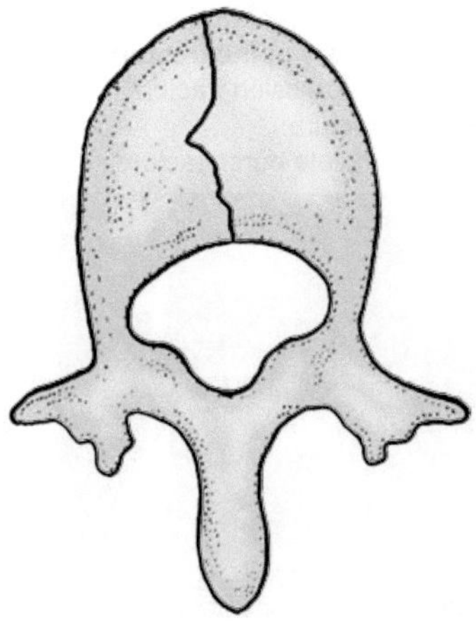

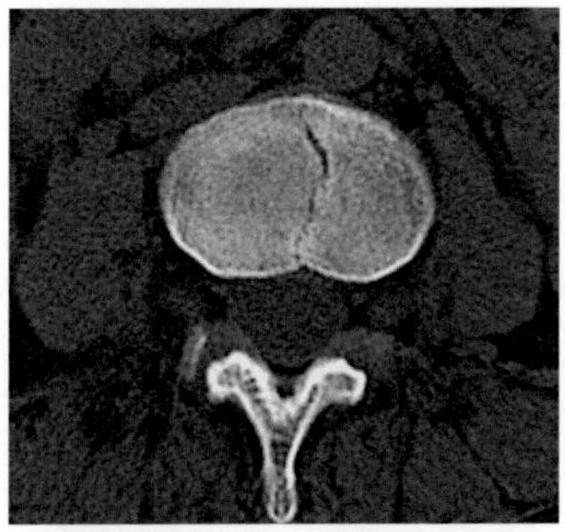

AO classification
Type A Thoracolumbar compressed fracture.
A2 Splitting fracture
A2.1 Sagittal splitting fracture

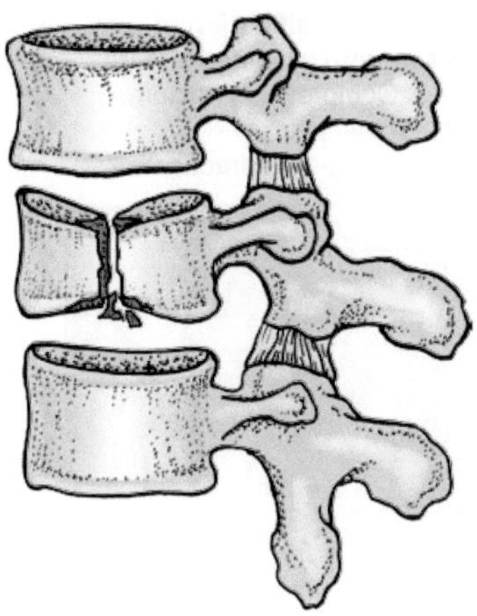

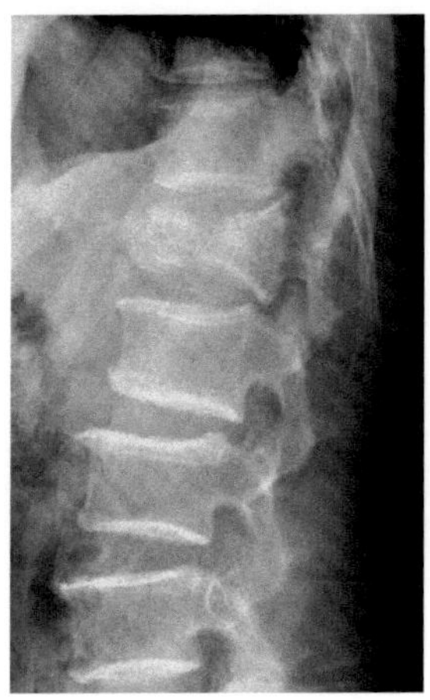

52-53 AO classification of thoracolumbar spine fracture
Type A Compression fracture.
A2 Splitting fracture:
A2.2 Coronal splitting fracture

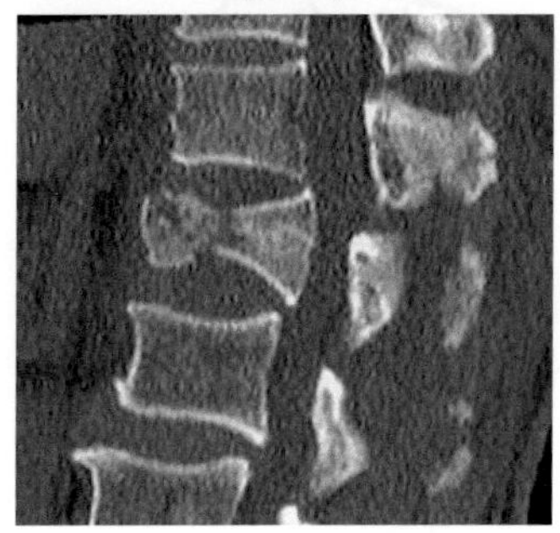

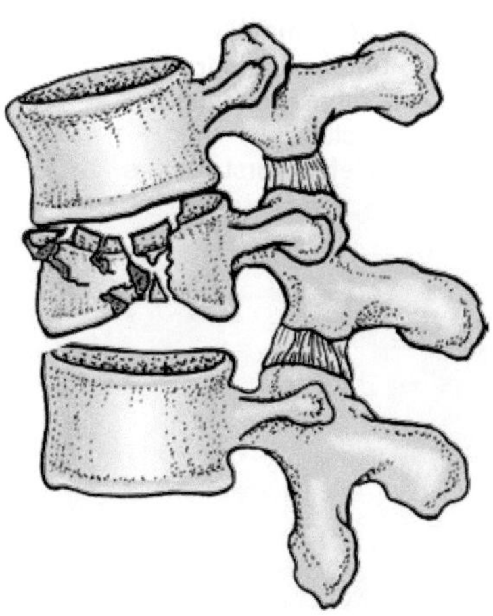

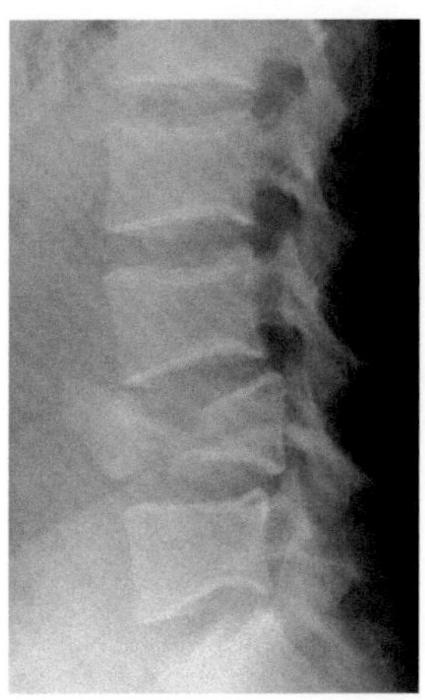

52-53 AO classification of thoracolumbar spine fracture
Type A Compression fracture.
A2 Splitting fracture:
A2.3 Clamp-like splitting fracture

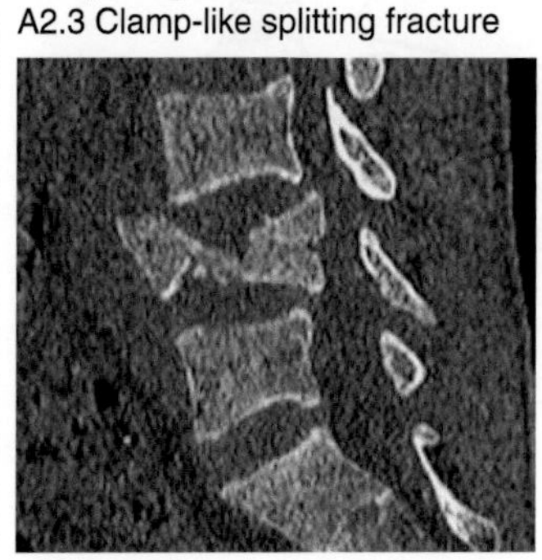

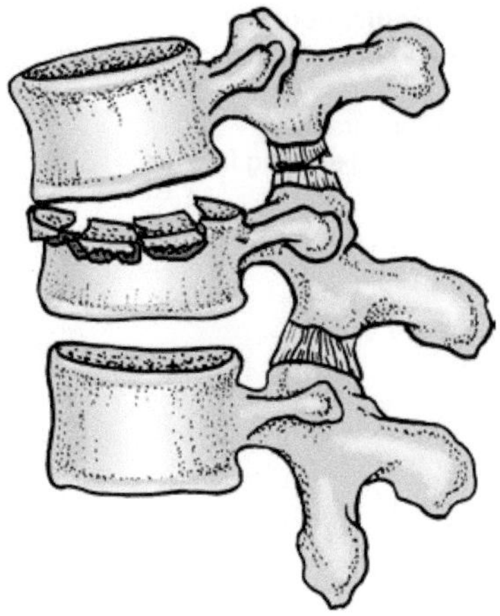

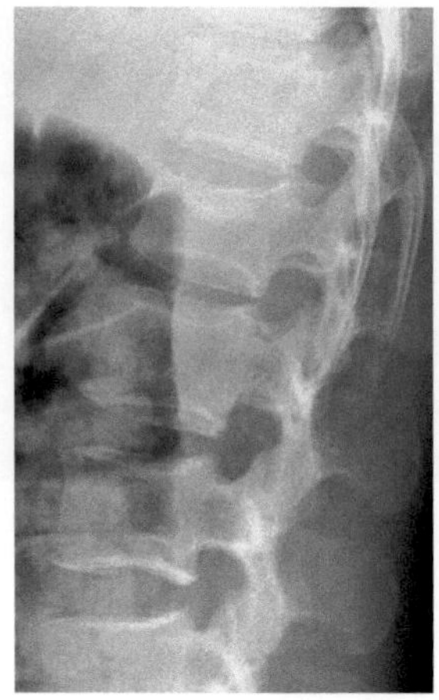

52-53 AO classification of thoracolumbar spine fracture
Type A Compression fracture.
A3 burst fracture:
A3.1 Incomplete burst fracture

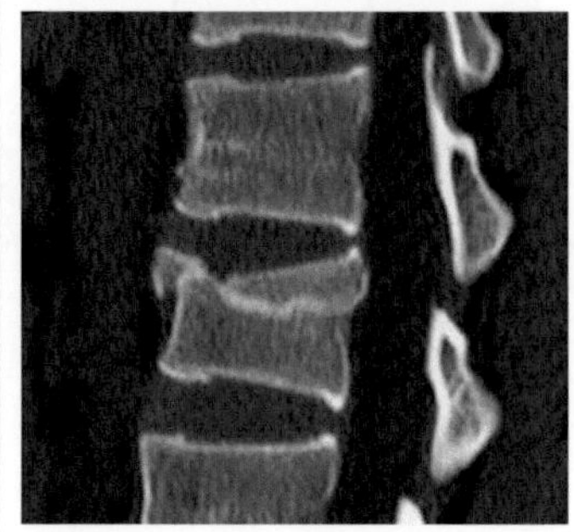

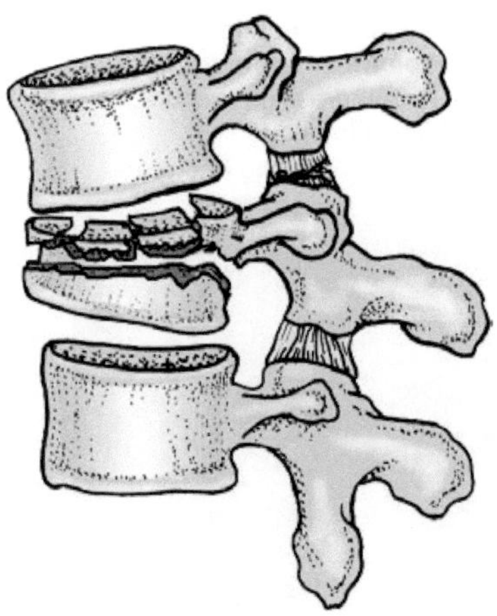

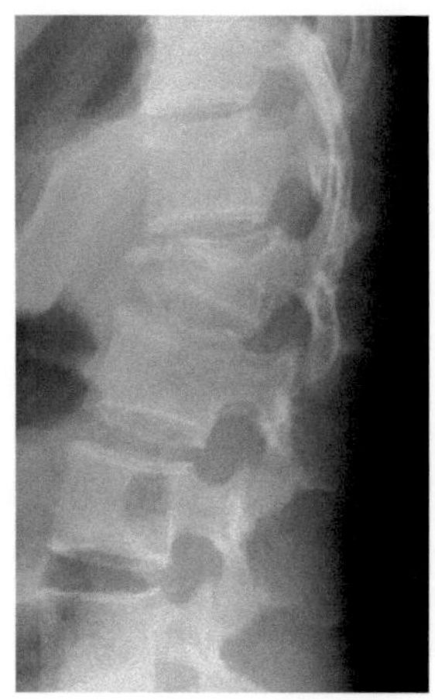

52-53 AO classification of thoracolumbar spine fracture
Type A Compression fracture.
A3 burst fracture:
A3.2 Splitting-burst fracture

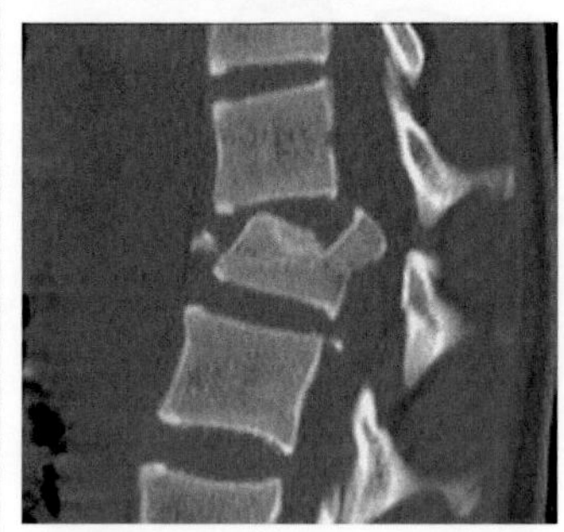

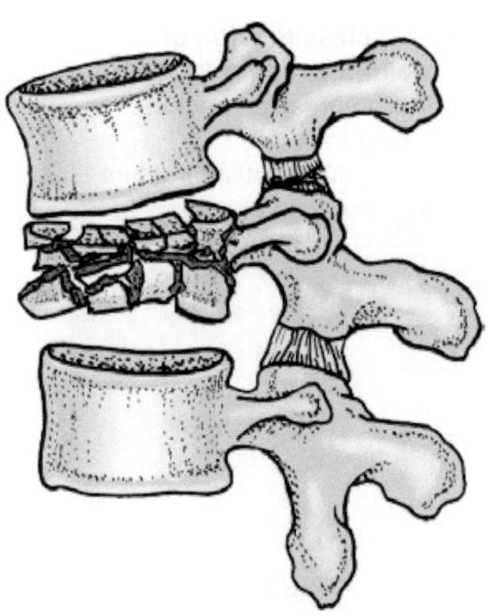

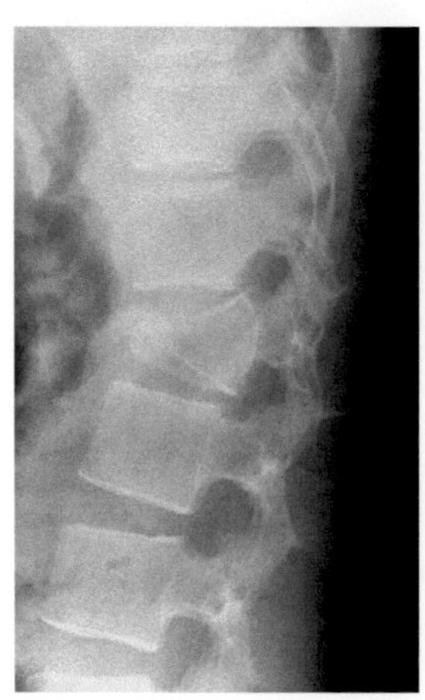

52-53 AO classification of thoracolumbar spine fracture
Type A Compression fracture.
A3 burst fracture:
A3.3 Completely burst fracture

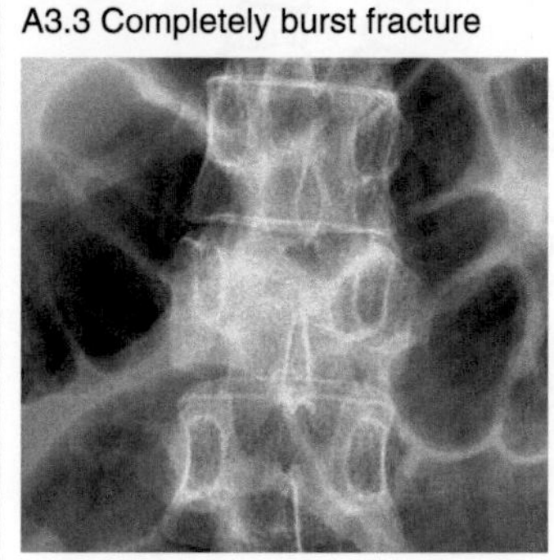

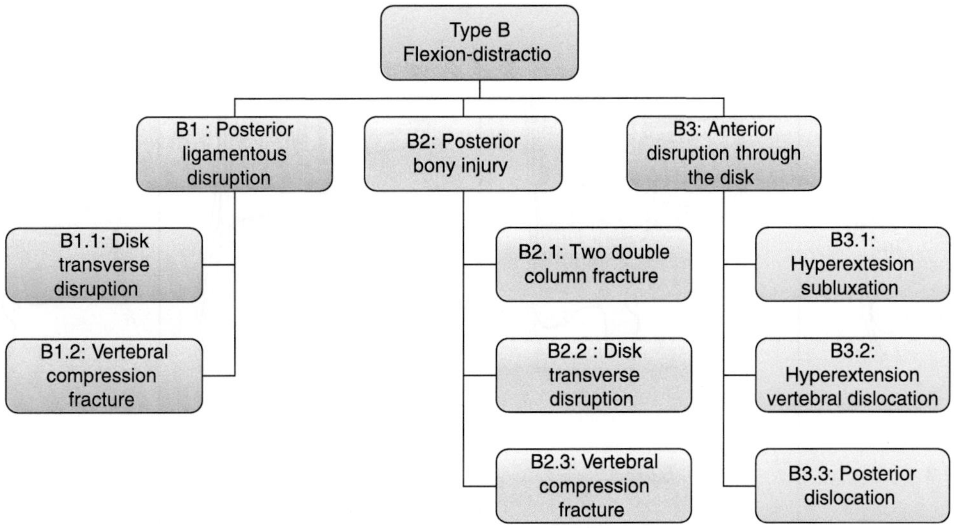

52–53 Type B: Thoracolumbar flexion–distraction injury.

52–53 B1: Posterior ligamentous disruption. Which is divided into:

B1.1: Disc transverse disruption.

B1.2: Vertebral compression fracture.

52–53 B2: Posterior bony injury:

B2.1: Two double-column fracture.

B2.2: Disc transverse disruption.

B2.3: Vertebral compression fracture.

52–53 B3: Anterior disruption through the disc:

B3.1: Hyperextension subluxation.

B3.2: Hyperextension vertebral dislocation.

B3.3: Posterior dislocation.

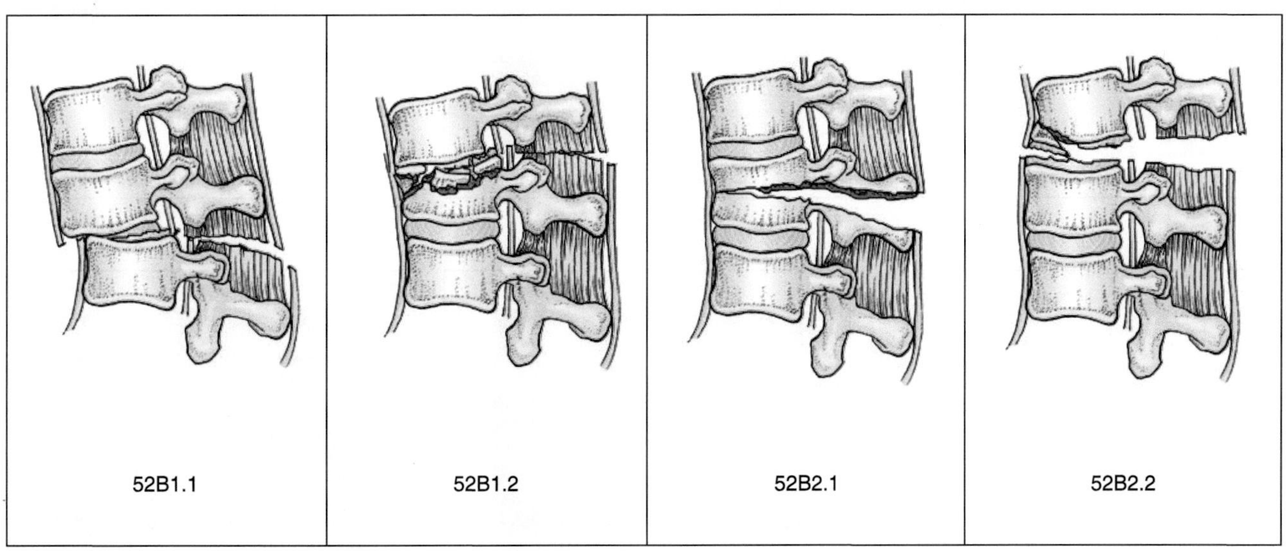

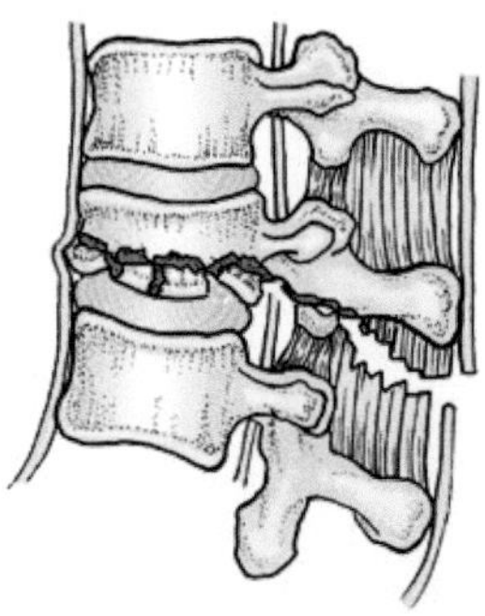

52B2.3

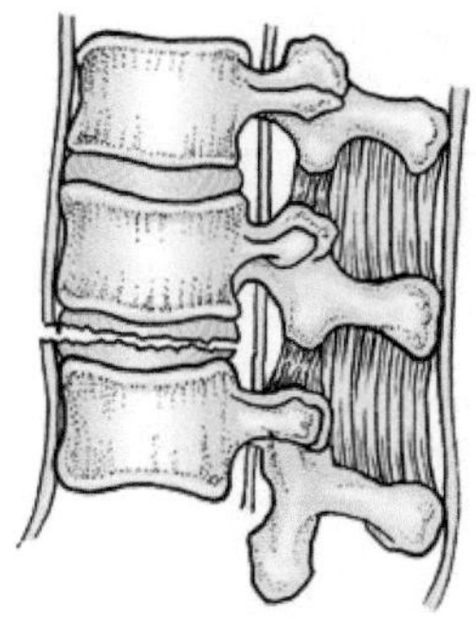

52B3.1

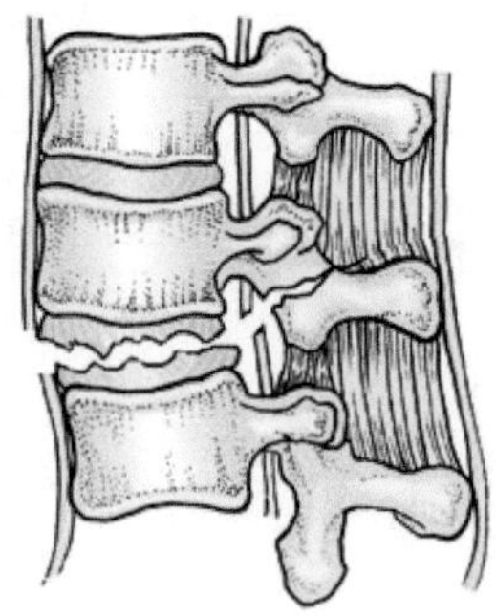

52B3.2

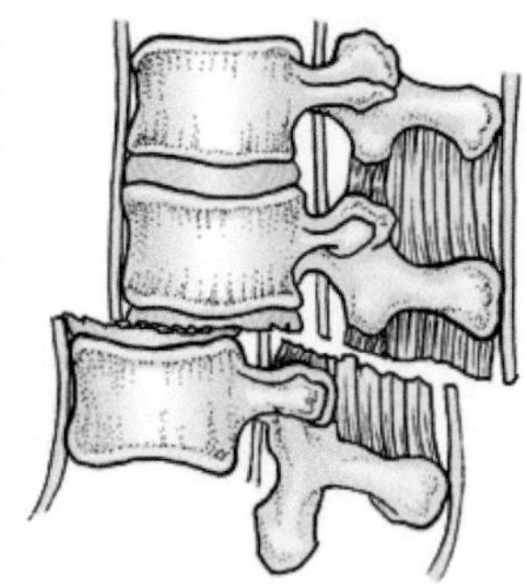

52B3.3

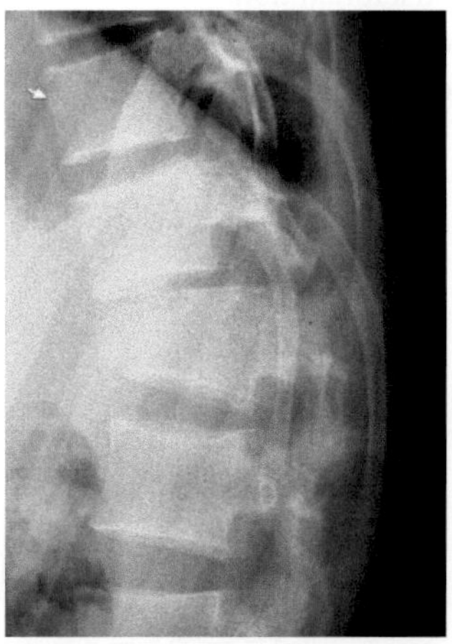

52-53 B1.2 Vertebral compression fracture

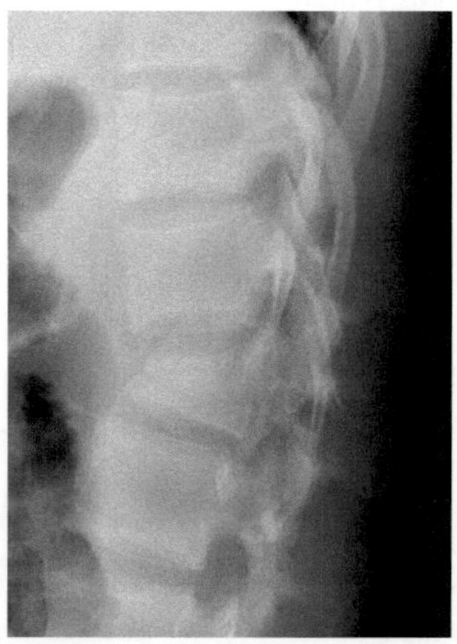

52-53 B2.1 Two double column fracture

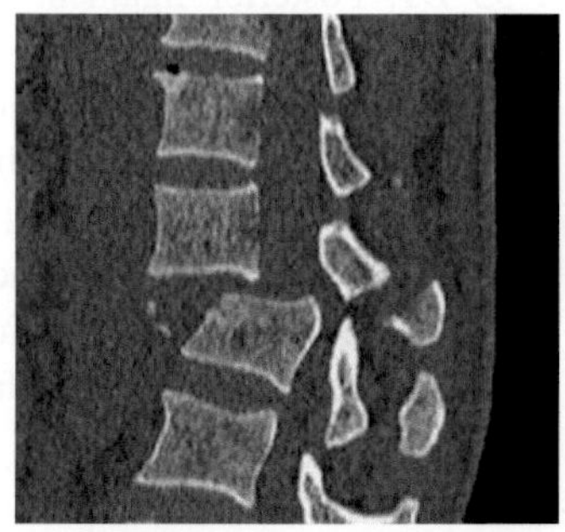

52-53 B2.2 Disk transverse disruption

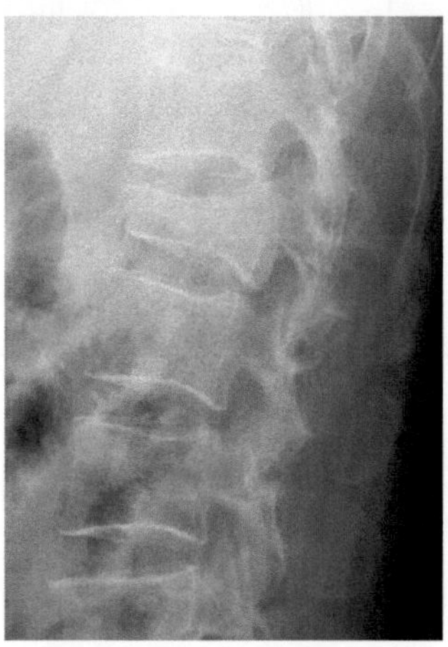

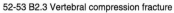

52-53 B2.3 Vertebral compression fracture

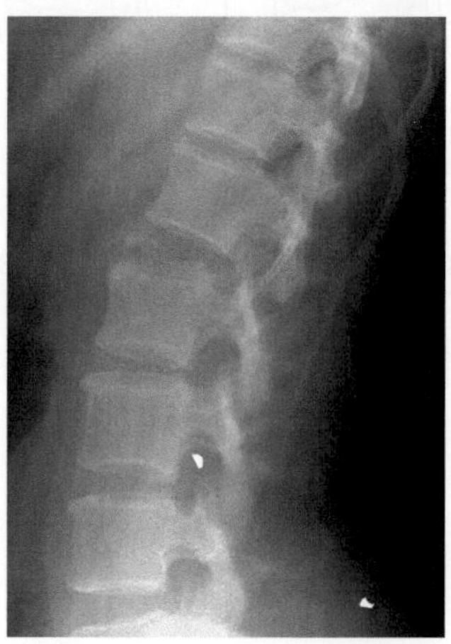

52-53 B3.1 Hyperextesion subluxation

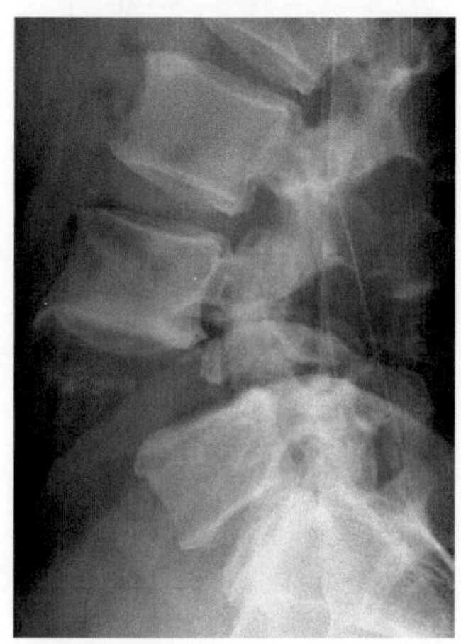

52-53 B3.2 Hyperextension vertebral dislocation

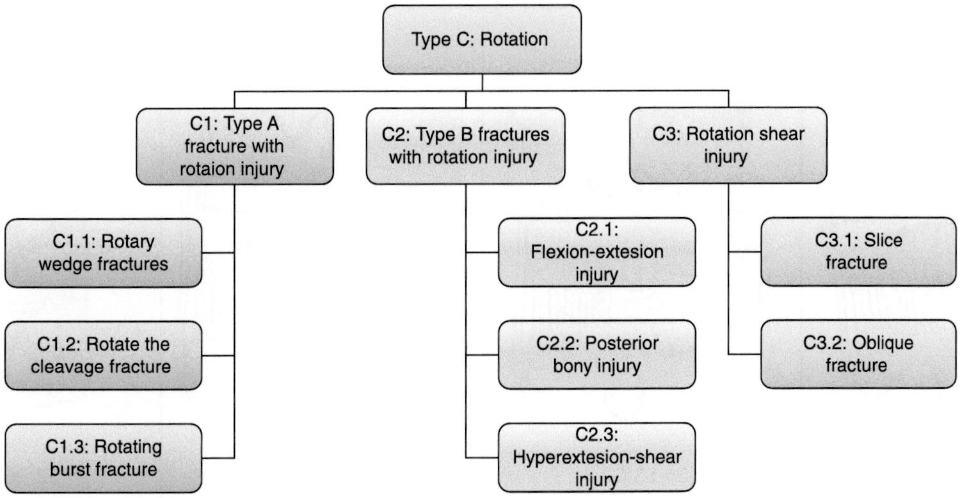

52–53 Type C: Thoracolumbar fracture rotation injury:

52–53 C1: Type A fracture with rotation injury. Which is divided into:

C1.1: Rotary wedge fracture.

C1.2: Rotating cleavage fracture.

C1.3: Rotating burst fracture.

52–53 C2: Type B fracture with rotation injury:

C2.1: Flexion-extension injury.

C2.2: Posterior bony injury.

C2.3: Hyperextension-shear injury.

52–53 C3: Rotation shear injury:

C3.1: Slice fracture.

C3.2: Oblique fracture.

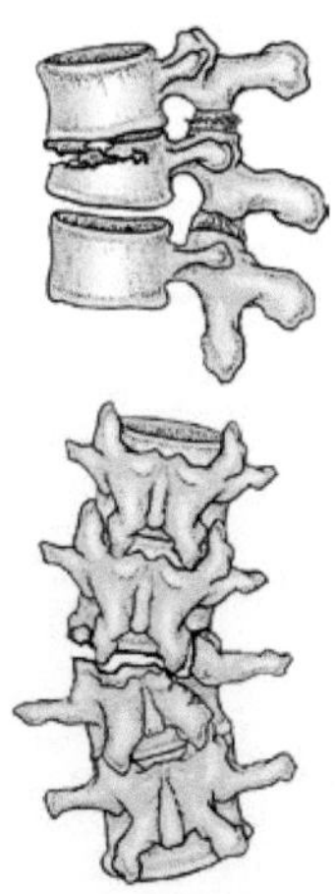
52～53 C1.1

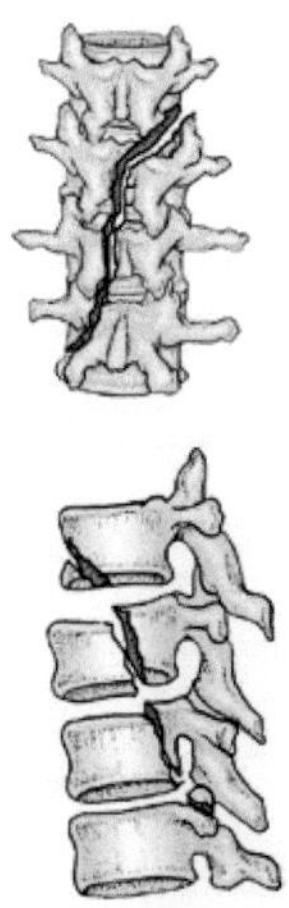
52～53 C1.2

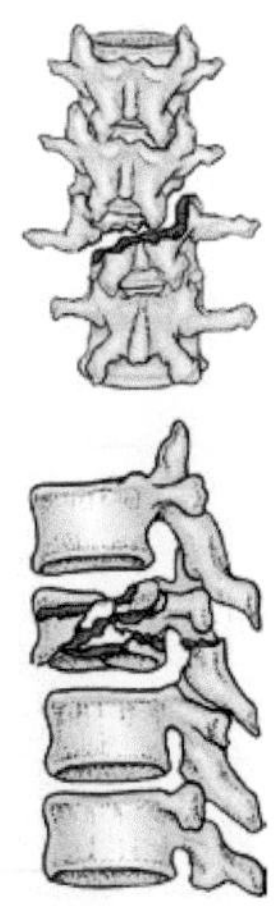
52～53 C1.3

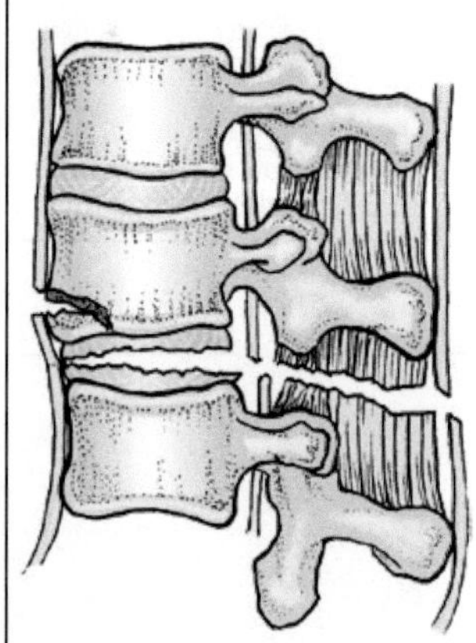
52～53 C2.1

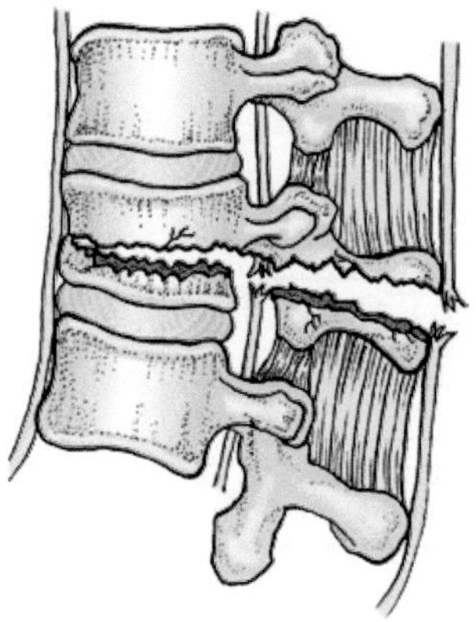

52～53 C2.2

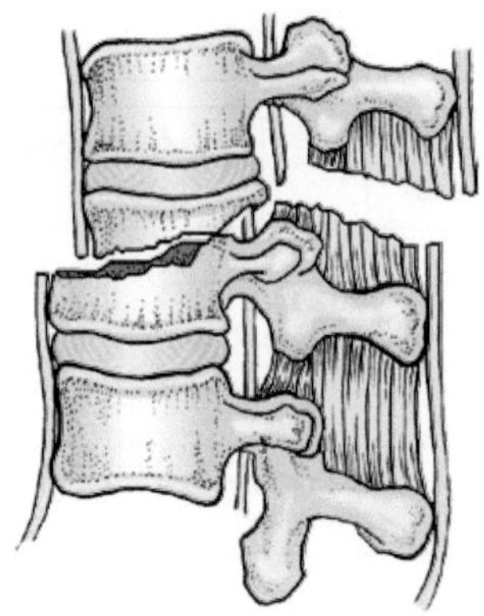

52～53 C2.3

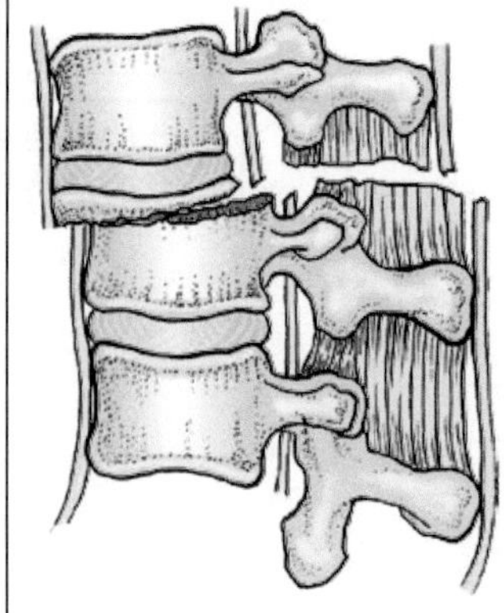

52～53 C3.1

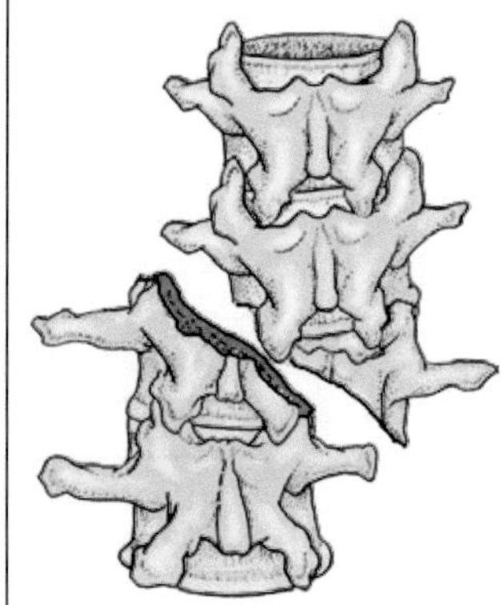

52～53 C3.2

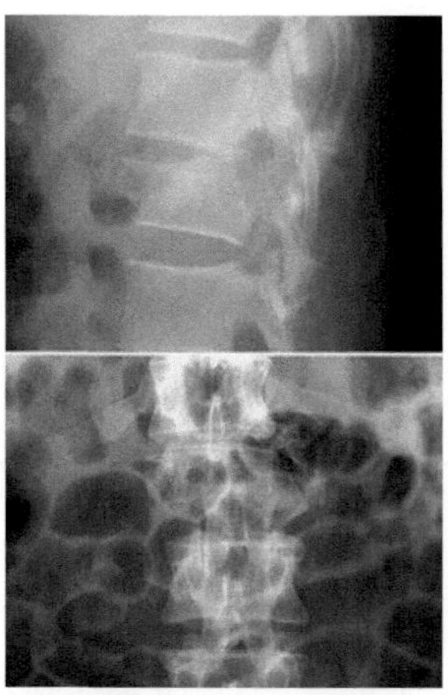

C1.1 Rotary wedge fracture

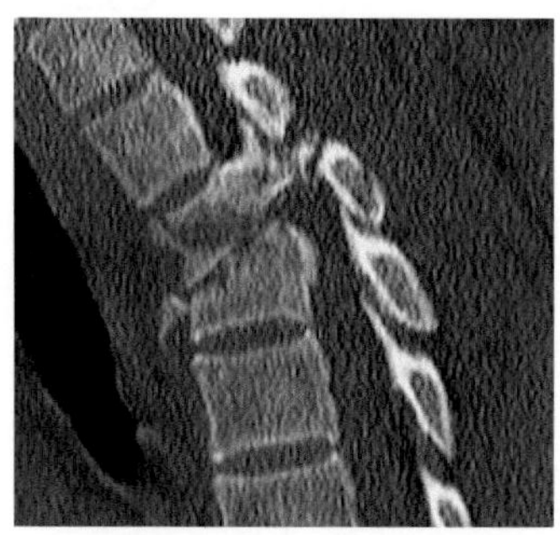

C1.3 rotating burst fracture

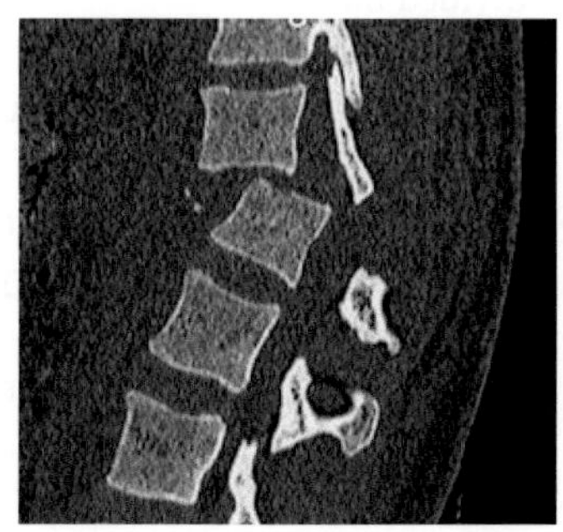

C2.1 Flexion-extesion injury

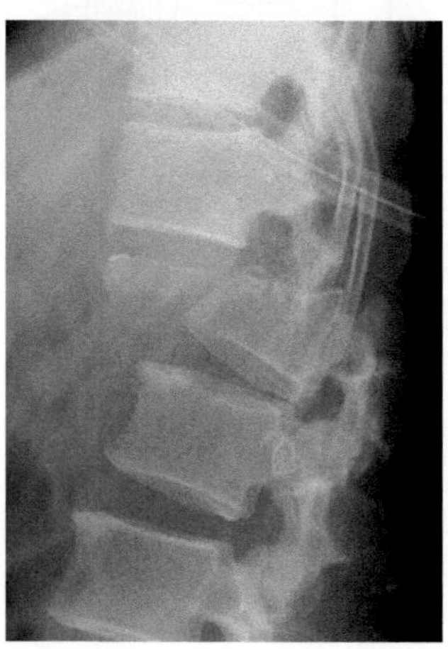

C2.3 Hyperextesion-shear injury

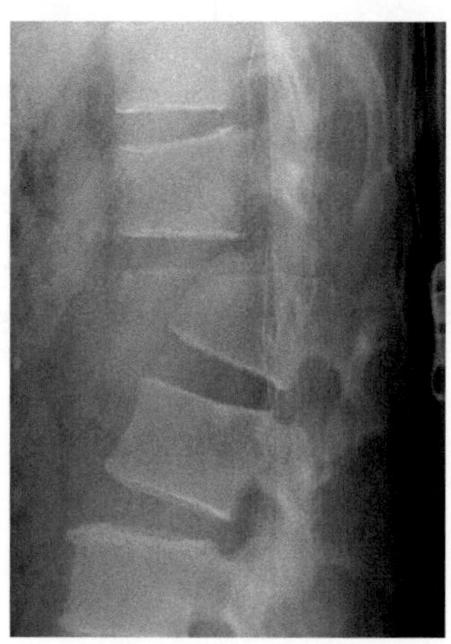

C3.1 Slice fracture

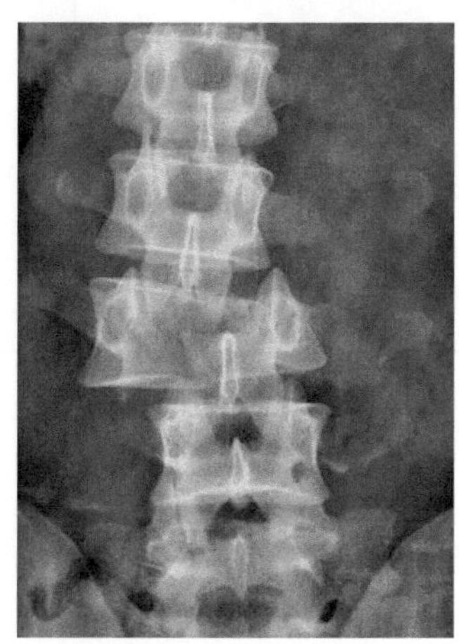

C3.2 Oblique fracture

6.1.2.2 Denis Classification (1988, Clin Orthop Relat Res, 227: 67–81)

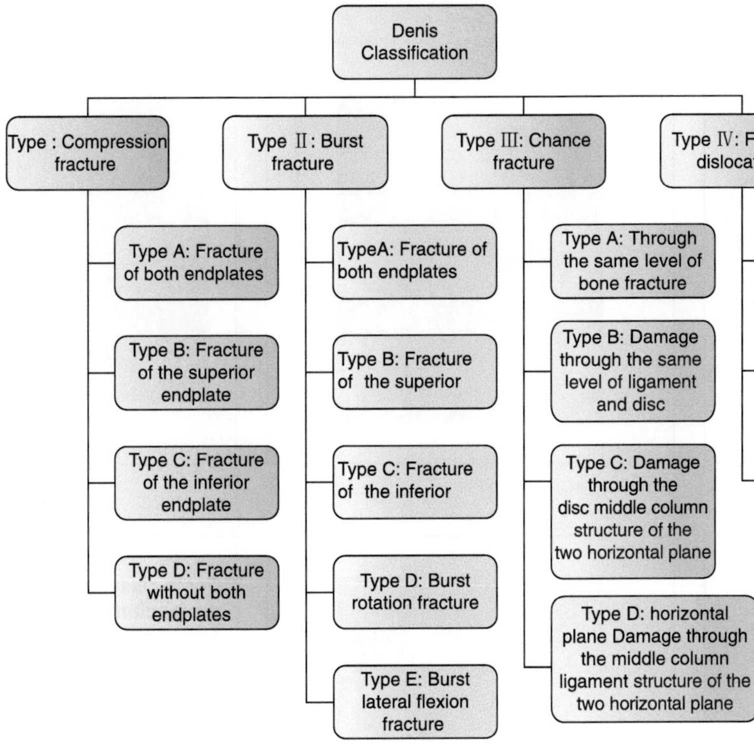

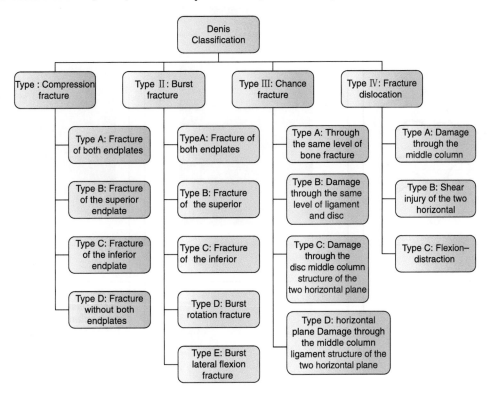

Denis divided fractures into **minor fractures** (including transverse processes, synapses, isthmus, spinous process fractures) and **severe fractures** (including compression fractures, burst fractures, harness-type injuries, fracture dislocations). The latter is divided into the following four types:

Type I compression fractures: According to the degree of involvement of the endplate further points:
Type A: Fracture of both endplates.
Type B: Fracture of the superior.
Type C: Fracture of the inferior.
Type D: Fracture without both endplates.

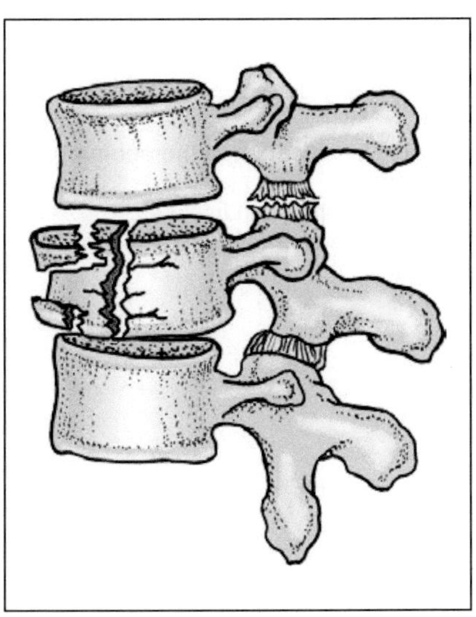

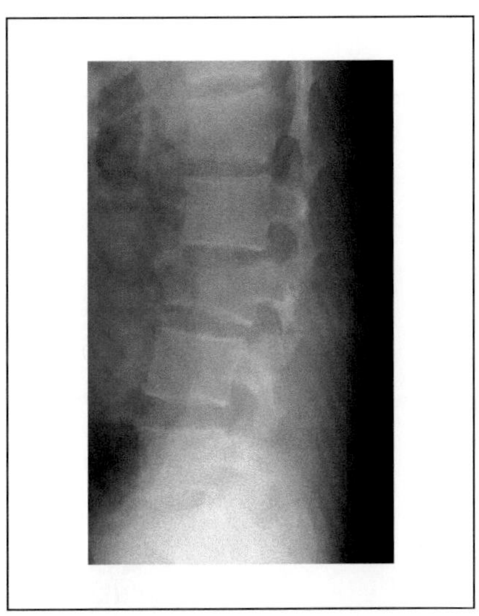

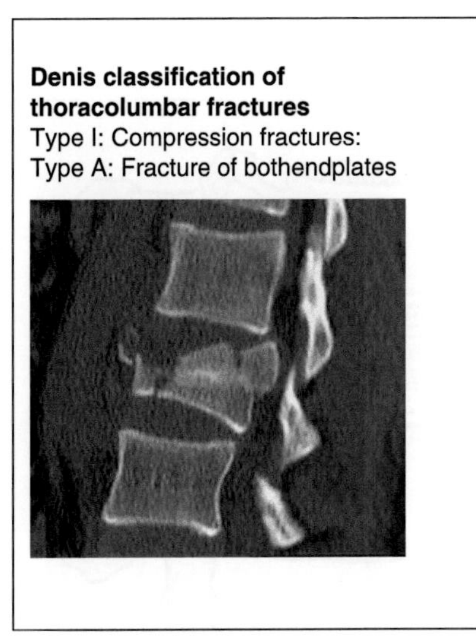

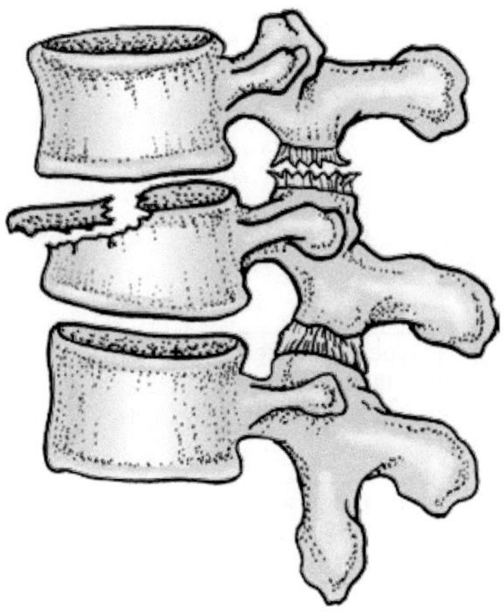

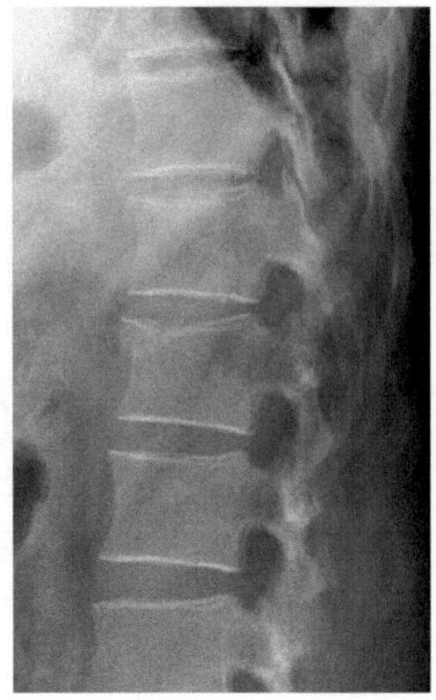

Denis classification of thoracolumbar fractures
Type I: Compression fractures:
Type B: Fracture of the superior

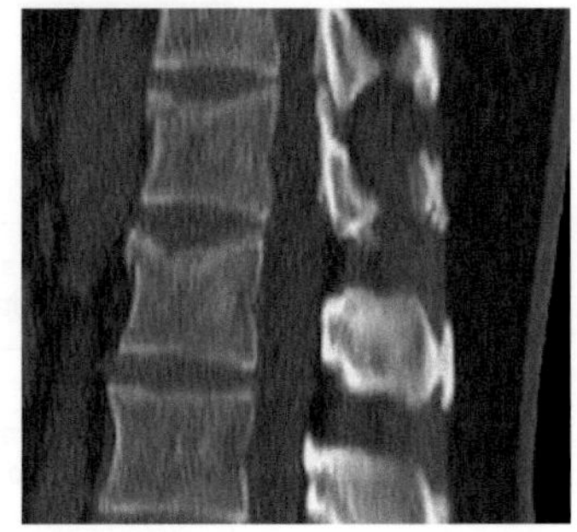

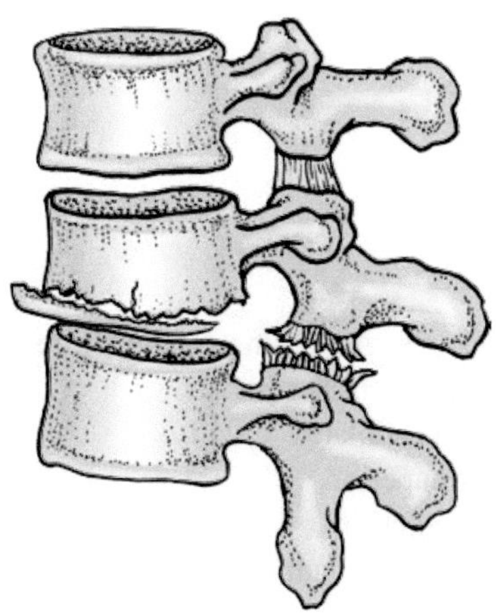

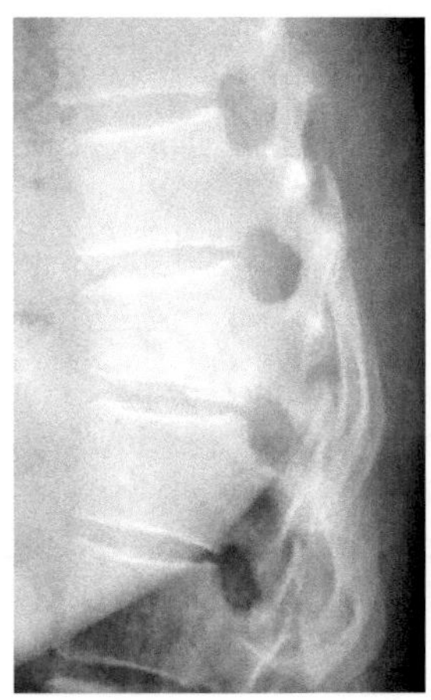

Denis classification of thoracolumbar fractures
Type I: Compression fractures:
Type C: Fracture of the inferior

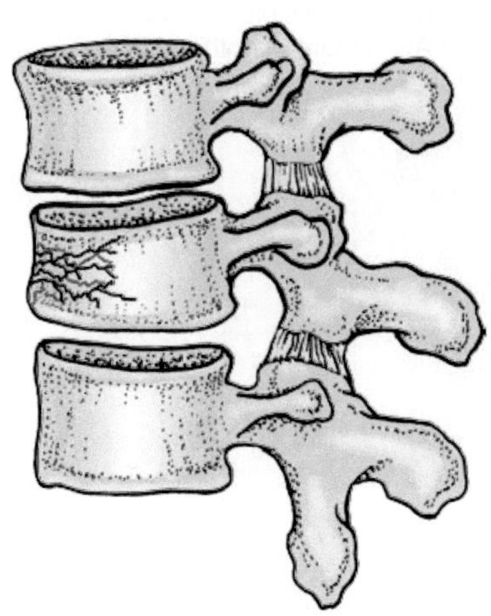

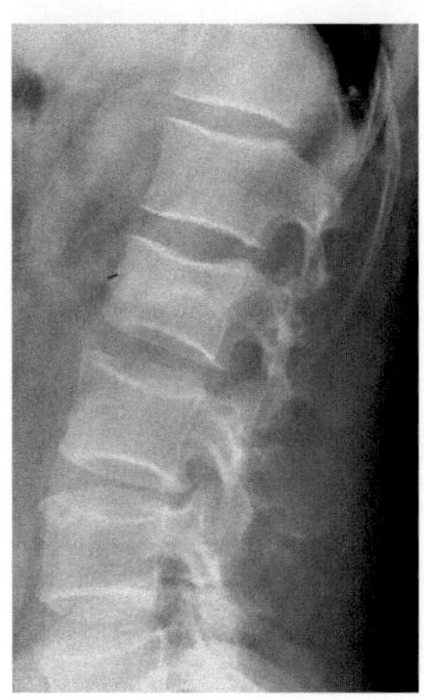

Denis classification of thoracolumbar fractures
Type I: Compression fractures:
Type D: Fracture without both endplates

Type II: Burst fracture:
- Type A: Fracture of both endplates.
- Type B: Fracture of the superior.
- Type C: Fracture of the inferior.
- Type D: Burst rotation fracture.
- Type E: Burst lateral flexion fracture.

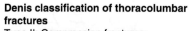

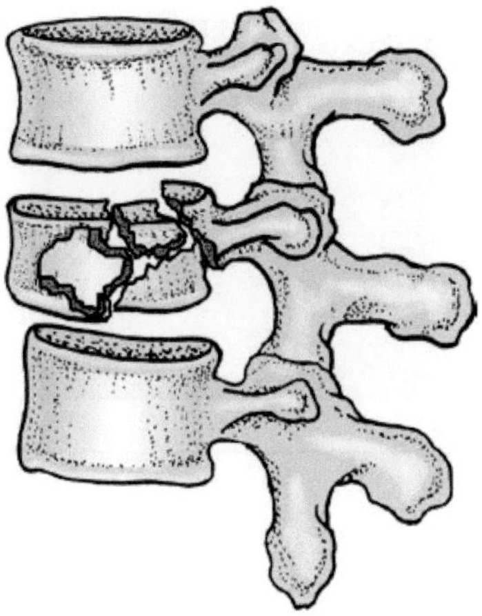

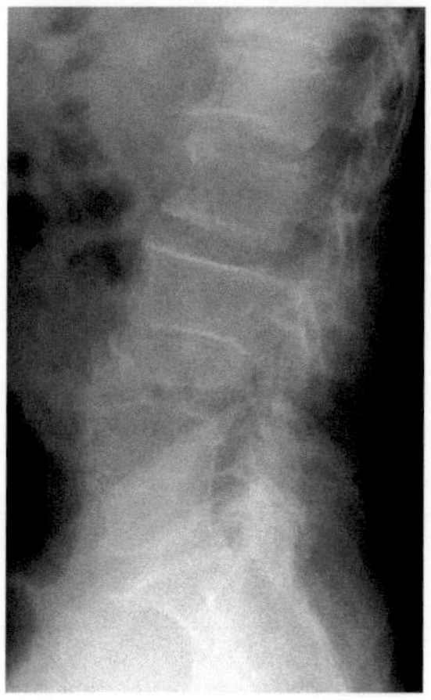

Denis classification of thoracolumbar fractures
Type II: Compression fractures:
Type A: Fracture of both endplates

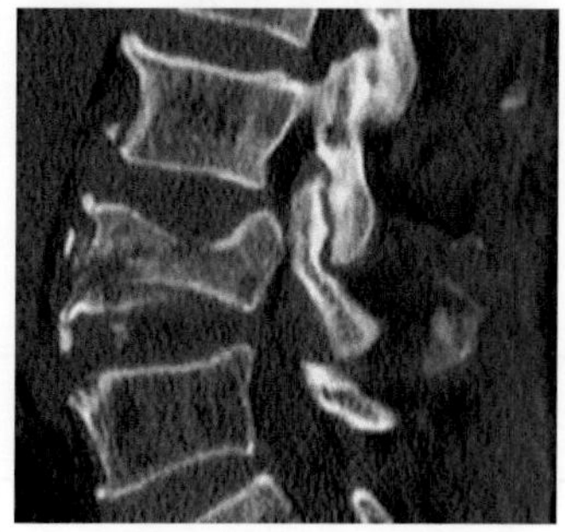

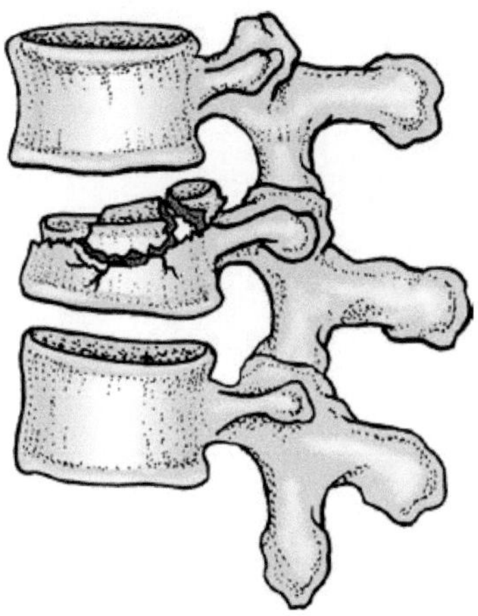

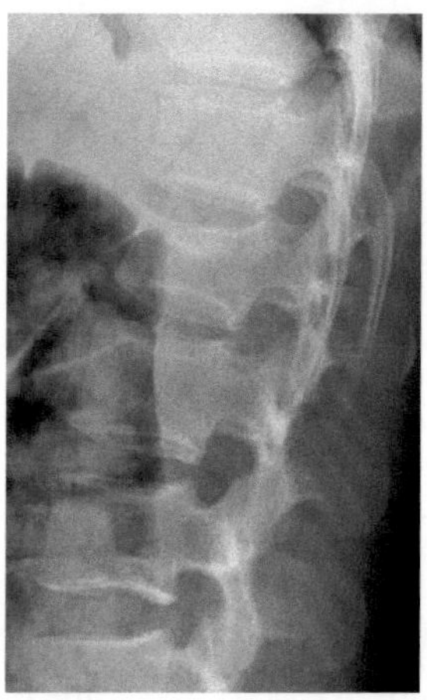

Denis classification of thoracolumbar fractures
Type II: Burst fracture:
Type B: Fracture of the superior

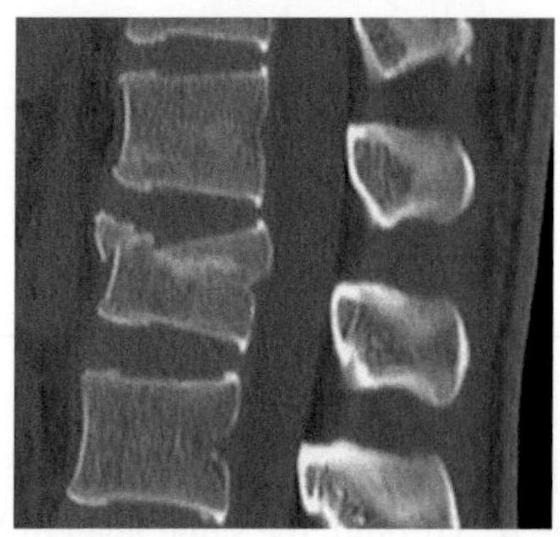

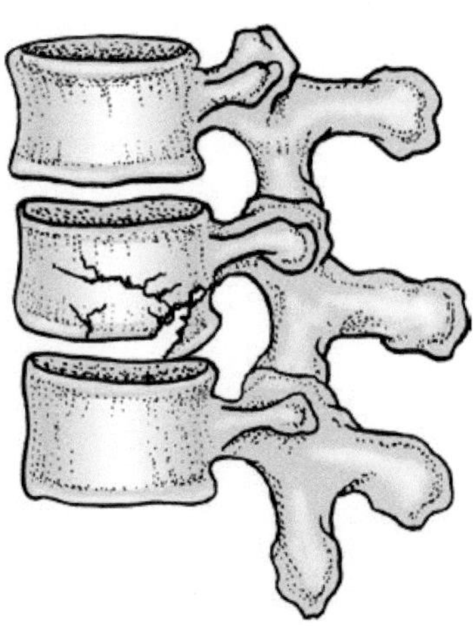

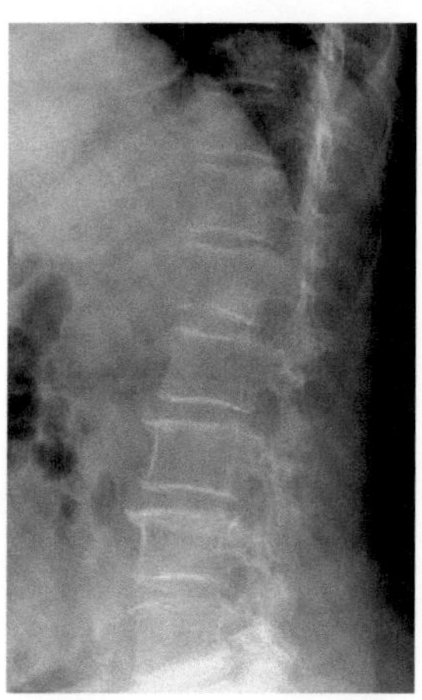

Denis classification of thoracolumbar fractures
Type II: Burst fracture:
Type C: Fracture of the inferior

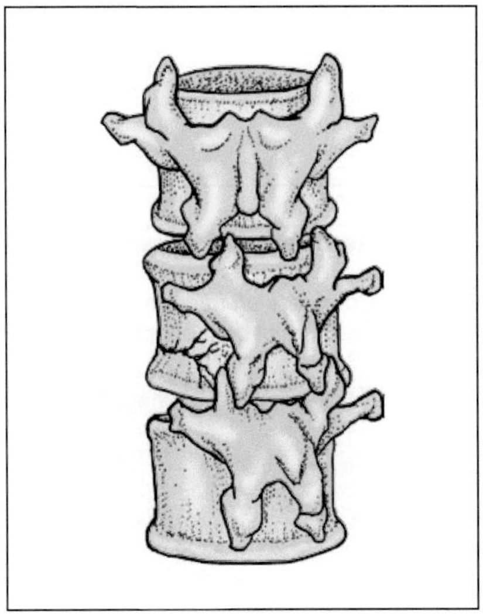

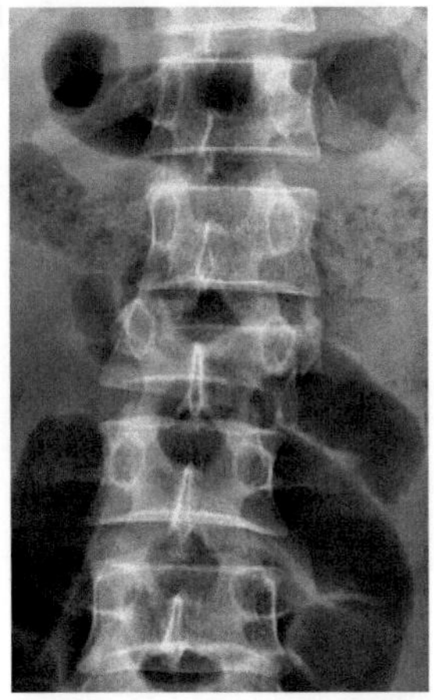

Denis classification of thoracolumbar fractures
Type II: Burst fracture:
Type D: Burst rotation fracture

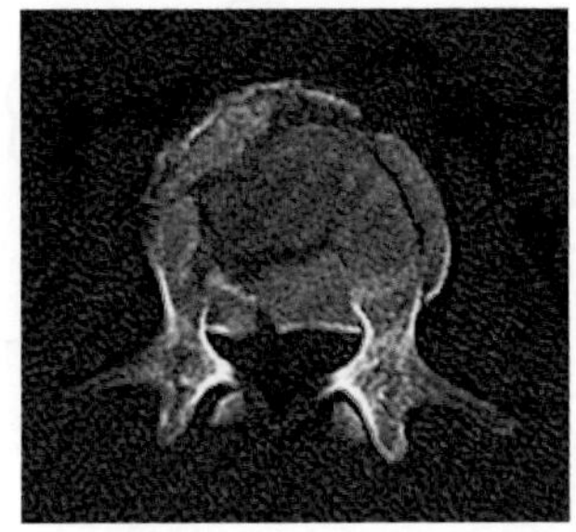

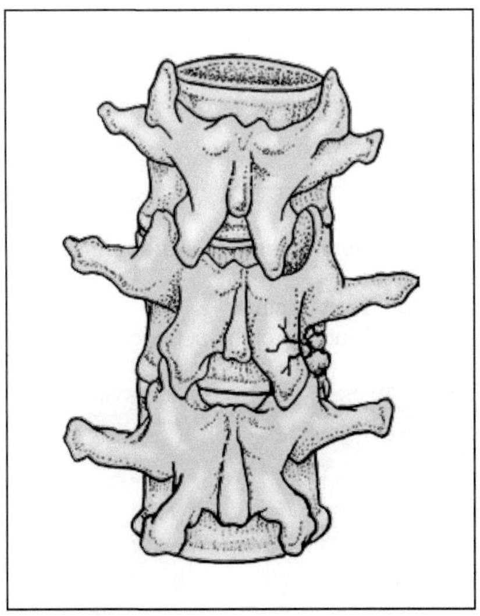

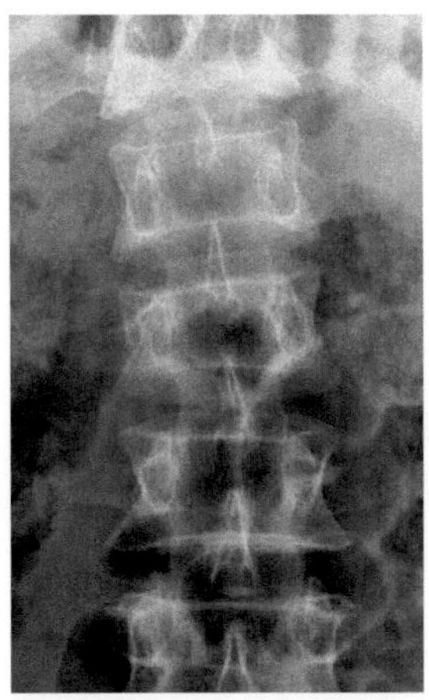

Denis classification of thoracolumbar fractures
Type II: Burst fracture:
Type E: Burst lateral flexion fracture

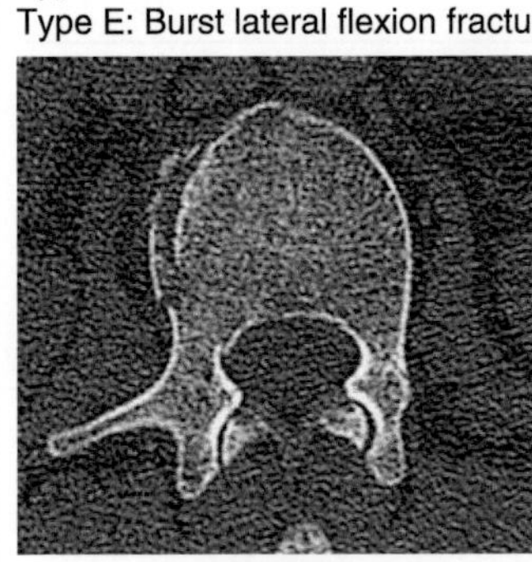

Type III: Chance fracture.

Type A: Through the same level of bone fracture.

Type B: Damage through the same level of ligament and disc.

Type C: Damage through the middle column structure of the two horizontal planes.

Type D: Damage through the middle column ligament structure of the two horizontal planes.

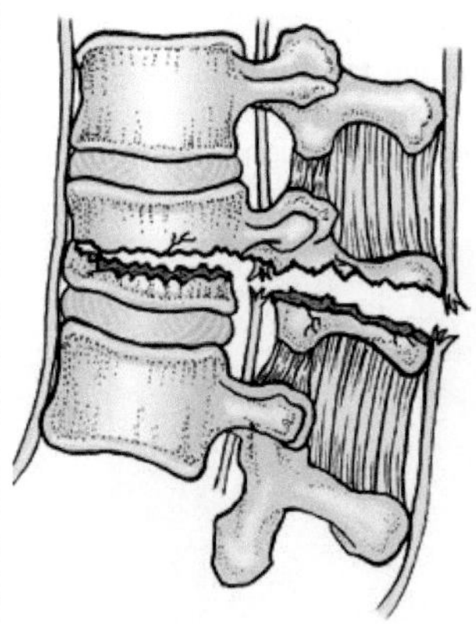

Type III A

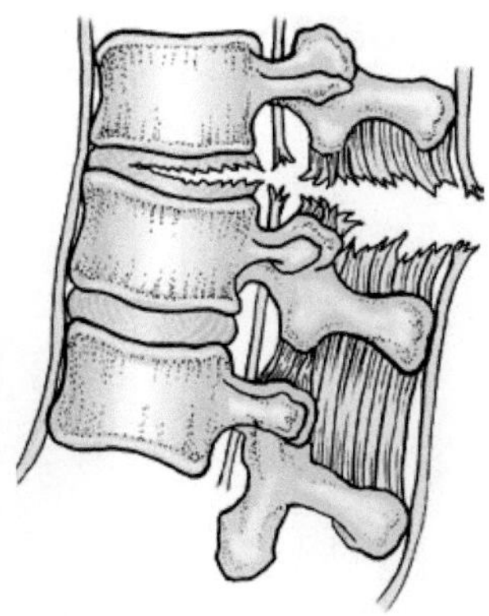

Type III B

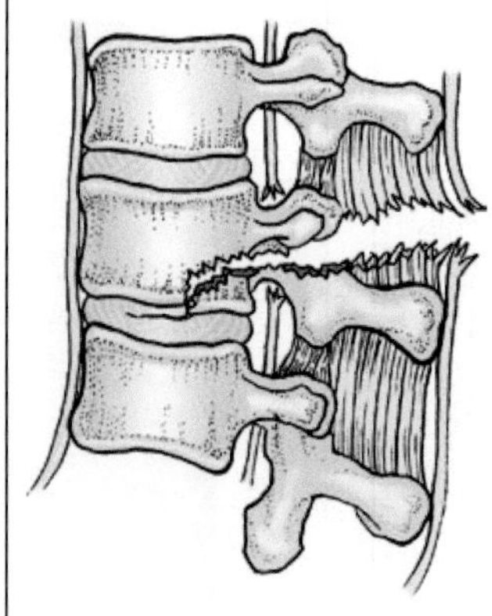

Type III C

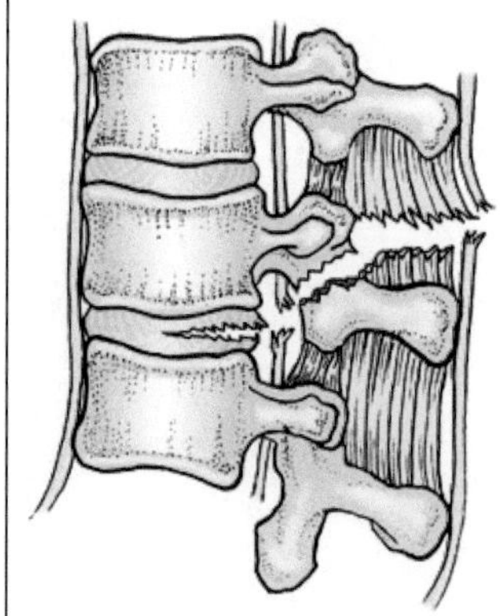

Type III D

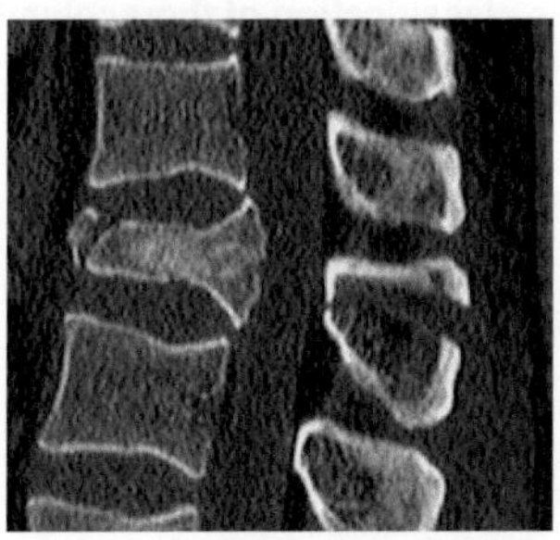

Type A: Through the same level of bone fracture (Chance Fracture)

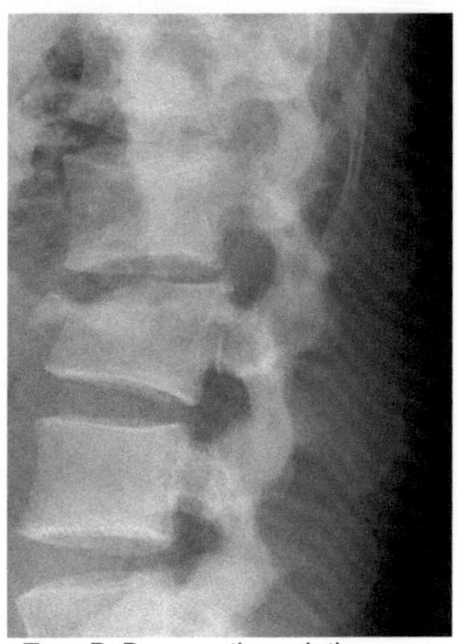

Type B: Damage through the same level of ligament and disc

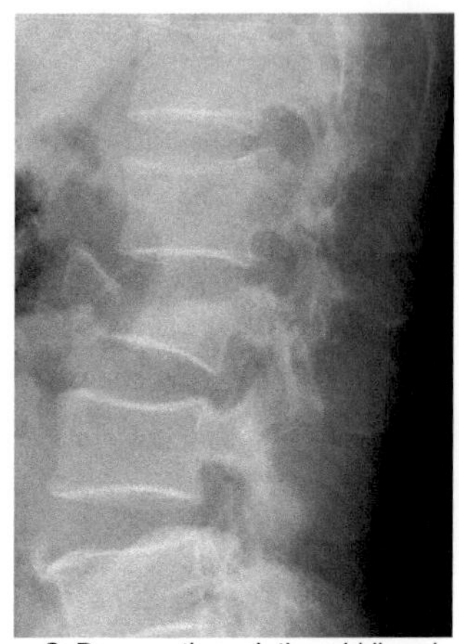

Type C: Damage through the middle column structure of the two horizontal plane

Type IV: Fracture dislocation.

Type A: Damage through the middle column.

Type B: Shear injury.

Type C: Flexion–distraction.

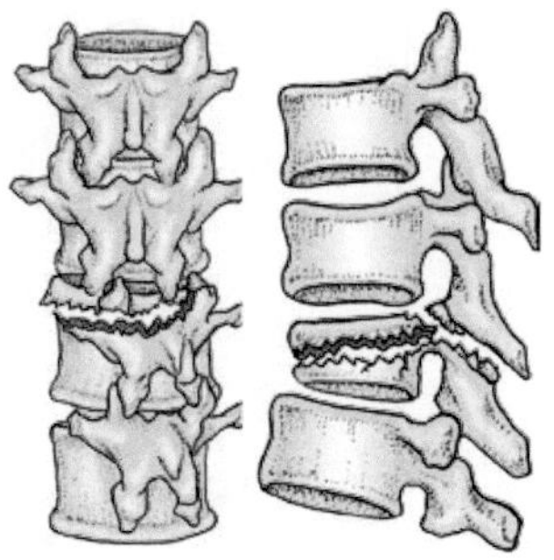

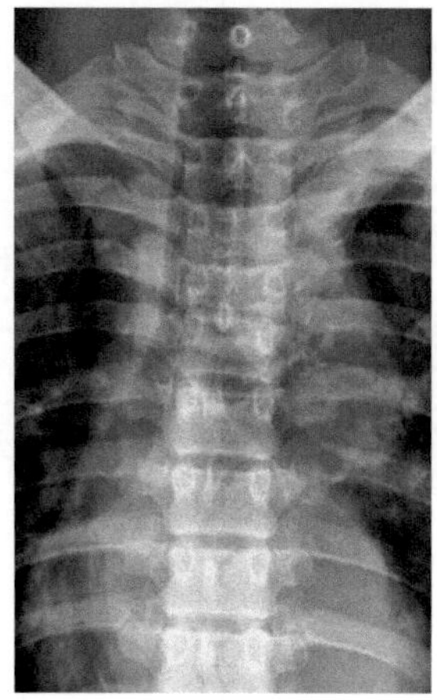

Denis classification of thoracolumbar fractures
Type IV: Fracture dislocation.
Type A: Damage through the middle column

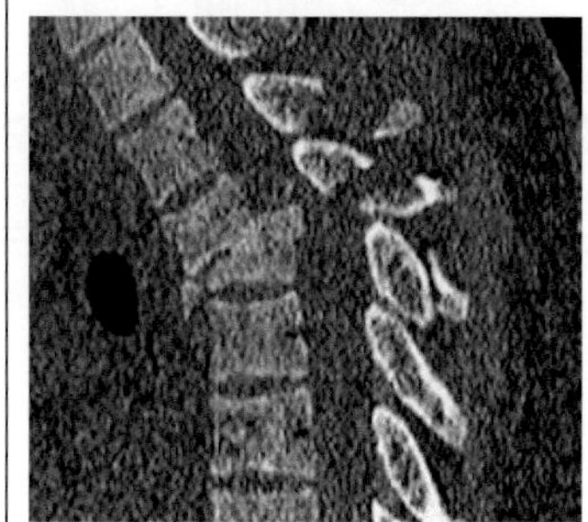

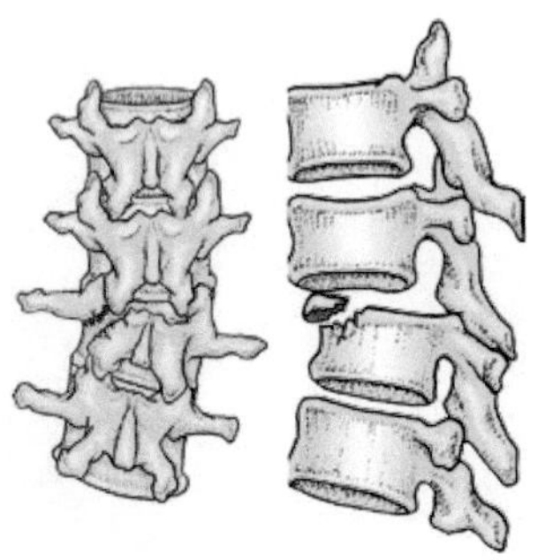

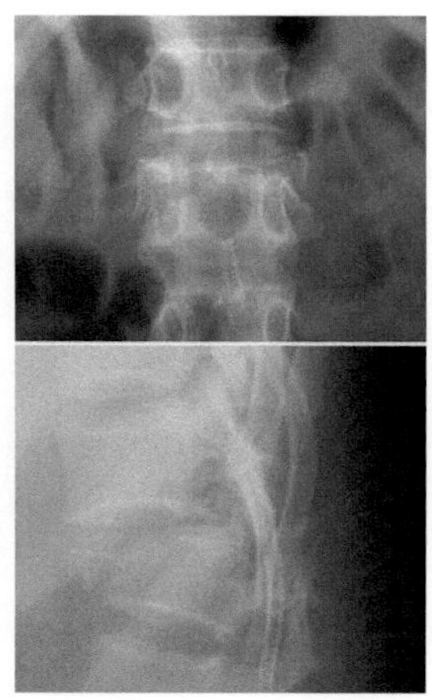

Denis classification of thoracolumbar fractures
Type IV: Fracture dislocation.
Type B: Shear injury

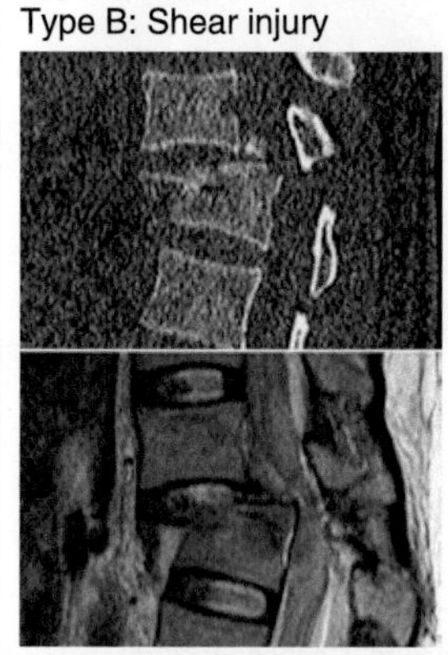

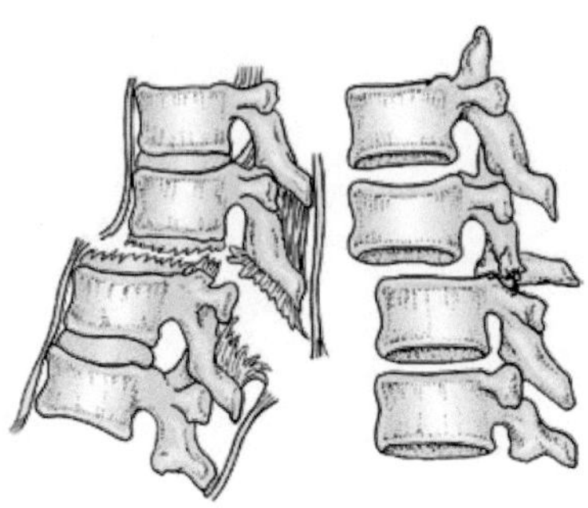

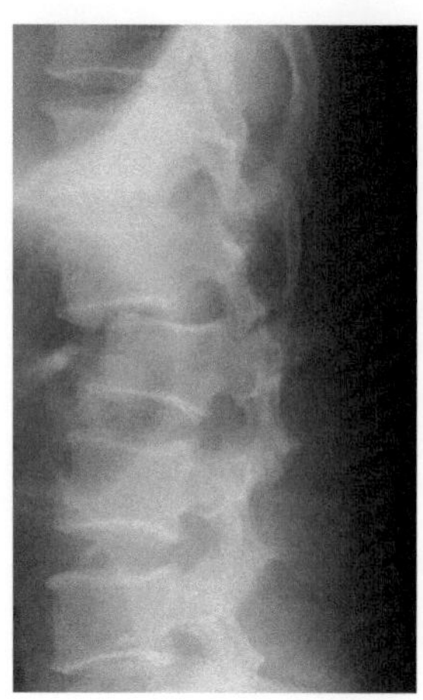

Denis classification of thoracolumbar fractures
Type IV: Fracture dislocation.
Type C: Flexion–distraction

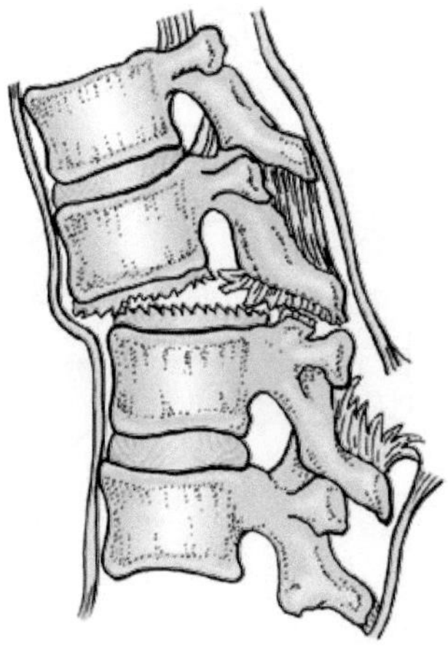

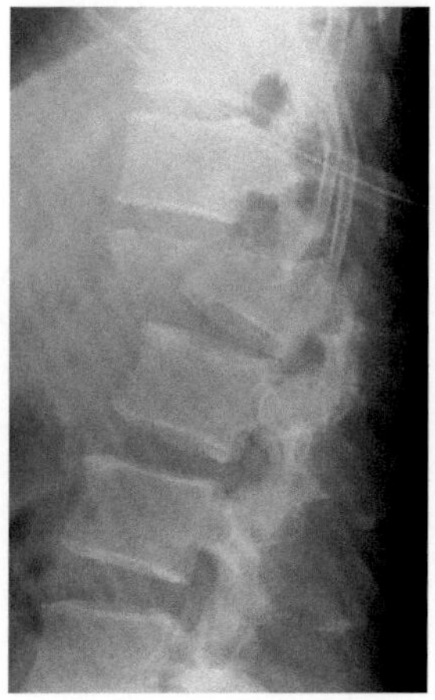

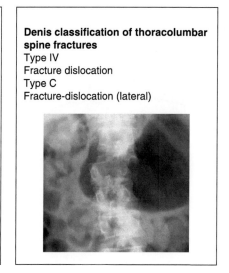

Denis classification of thoracolumbar spine fractures
Type IV
Fracture dislocation
Type C
Fracture-dislocation (lateral)

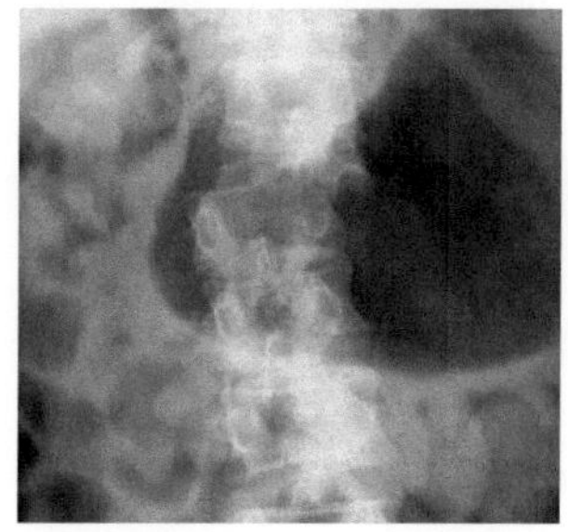

6.1.2.3 McAfee Classification (1983, J Bone Joint Surg Am, 65: 461–473)

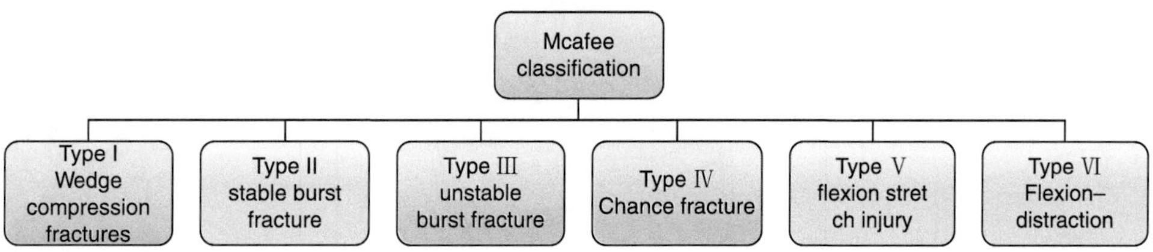

McAfee classification is divided into six types. Burst fracture is subdivided into stable and unstable fracture. Seat belt damage is subdivided into chance fracture and flexion–distraction.

Type I: Axial compression.
Type II: Stable burst fracture.
Type III: Unstable burst fracture.
Type IV: Chance fracture.
Type V: Flexion stretch injury.
Type VI: Flexion–distraction.

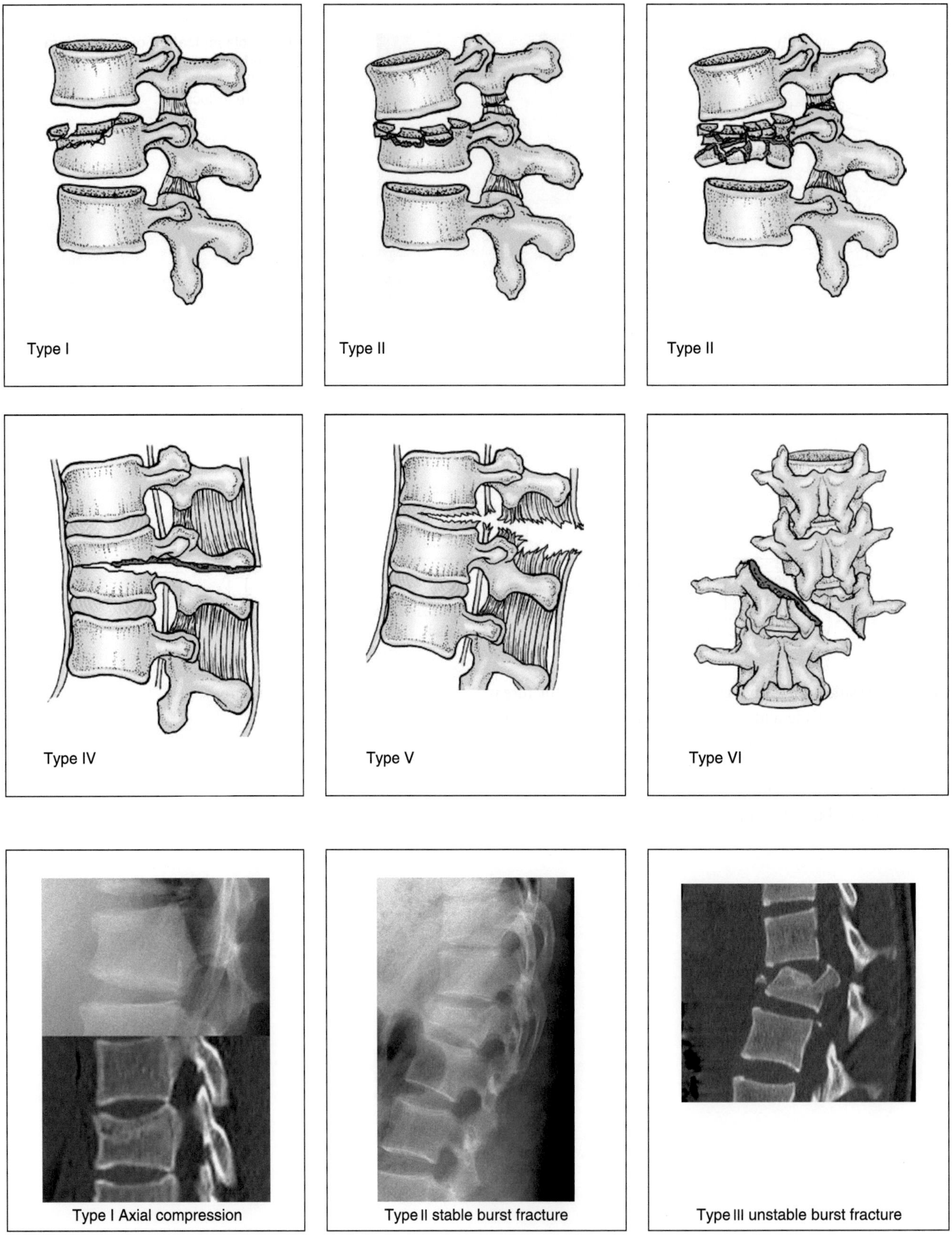
Type I
Type II
Type II
Type IV
Type V
Type VI
Type I Axial compression
Type II stable burst fracture
Type III unstable burst fracture

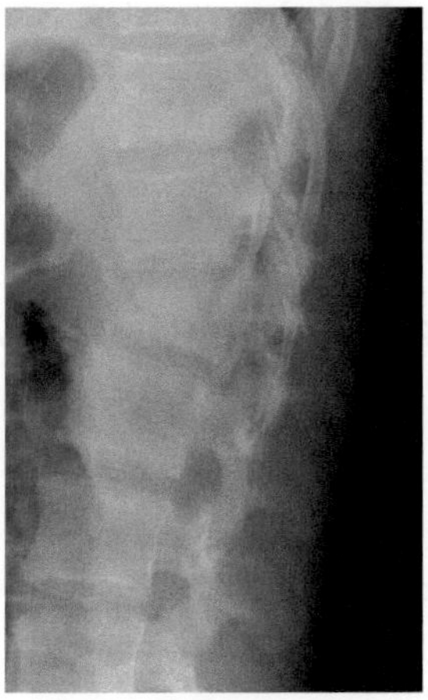

Type IV Chance fracture

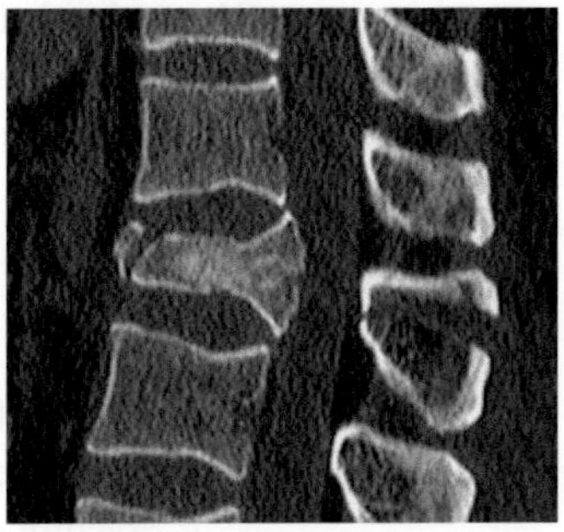

Type IV Chance fracture

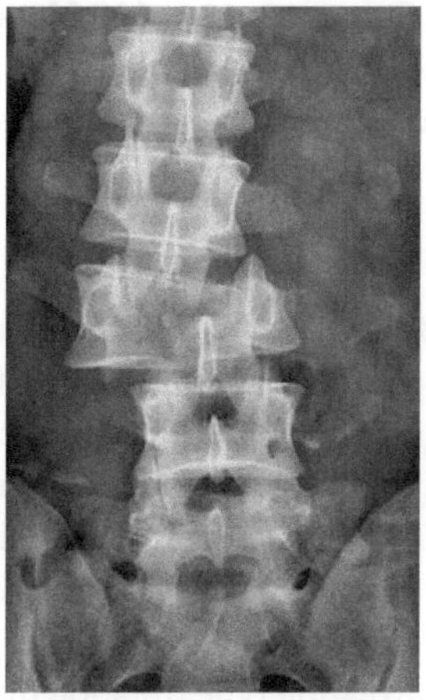

Type IV Flexion–distraction

6.1.2.4 Other Classifications of Spinal Fractures

Nicoll Classifications (1949, J Bone Joint Surg (Br), 31: 376–394)

There are four types, anterior wedge fracture, lateral wedge fracture, and vertebral arch fracture.

Estimate the stability according to the interspinous ligament completeness and the location of the fracture. Anterior wedge fracture, lateral wedge fracture, and vertebral plate fracture above L4 are the stable fractures. Interspinous ligament injury combined with subluxation/luxation fracture, vertebral arch fracture, or L4–5 vertebral plate fracture is the unstable fracture.

Holdsworth Classifications (1963, J Bone Joint Surg (Br), 45: 6–20)

Thoracolumbar fractures can be divided into stable fracture and unstable fracture according to the posterior column completeness. Stable fracture contains wedge compression fracture and compression burst fracture. Unstable fracture contains dislocation stretch fracture dislocation and rotation fracture dislocation.

Kelly-Whitesides Classifications (1977, Clin Orthop Relat Res, 128: 78–92)

Integrate thoracolumbar fractures are divided into two categories and seven types:

1. Type A stable fracture: Compression fracture and stable burst fracture.
2. Type B unstable fracture: Slice fracture, unstable burst fracture, flexion stretch fracture dislocation, and stretch fracture.

Ferguson–Allen Classification (1984, Clin Orthop Relat Res, 189: 77–88)

Thoracolumbar fractures were classified into eight types according to the injury mechanism.

1. Buckling compression type: Type I: The front pillar wedge is deformed and the post and post pillars remain intact. Type II: Vertebral posterior column injury combined with anterior column wedge deformation. Type III: Vertebral three-column injury.
2. Buckling separation type: Similar to chance fractures, including simple bony injury or ligament injury.
3. Lateral flexion type: Can be divided into unilateral front column, middle column injury, and in the unilateral front column and the middle column at the same time, with tension side vertebral rear structural damage.
4. Shift type.
5. Torsion buckling type.
6. Vertical compression type.
7. Stretch compression type.
8. Isolated type: Including individual articular processes, transverse processes, and pedicle isthmus fractures.

Magerl Typing (AO/Magerl type. 1994, Eur Spine J, 3: 184–201)

Thoracolumbar fractures are divided into three types by Magerl: (1) Type A: Vertebral compression categories: including crush fractures, splitting fractures, burst fractures. (2) Type B: Stretchable double-column fractures: including posterior column of ligament-based injury, bone-based posterior column injury, by the former intervertebral disc injury. (3) Type C: Rotational double-column injury: including type A fracture with rotation, type B fracture with rotation, and rotation-shear injury.

Gertzbein Comprehensive Classification (1994, Spine, 19: 626–628 Magerl typing was modified by Gertzbein)

Type A: Vertebral compression fractures.
- A1: Compression fractures.
- A2: Splitting fractures.
- A3: Burst fractures.

Type B: Vertebral distraction injury.
- B1: Rear through the ligament level.
- B2: Rear by bone level (chance fracture).
- B3: In front of the intervertebral disc type.

Type C: Combined injury with displacement.
- C1: Front and rear type (dislocation).
- C2: Side type (lateral shear).
- C3: Rotation type (rotation dislocation).

McCormack Classification (1994, Spine, 19: 1741–1744)

McCormack et al. developed a theory of the load sharing classification, which rates the fracture according to the severity of the anatomy of anterior and middle column, including the extent of the injured vertebra, dispersion of the fragments, and post-trauma kyphosis correction. There are 3 ° of every type: mild (1 pt.), moderate (2 pts), and severe (3 pts). More than 6 pts in total leads to the operation of posterior column reconstruction.

Vaccaro Classification (2005, Spine, 30: 2325–2333)

Vaccaro et al. proposed the concept of Thoracolumbar Injury Classification and Scoring System (THCS). In the system, there are three independent variables: (1) the morphology of injury as determined by reviewing the pattern of disruption on available imaging studies, (2) the integrity of the posterior ligamentous complex (PLC), and (3) the neurologic status of the patient. These three injury characteristics were thought to be largely independent predictors of clinical outcome. Within each of the three categories, subgroups were identified and arranged from least to most significant. A comprehensive severity score of three or less suggests a nonoperative injury, while a score of five or more suggests that surgical intervention may be considered. Injuries assigned a total score of four might be handled conservatively or surgically. The final classification according to the TLICS system combines the descriptors of injury morphometry, neurologic condition, and integrity of the posterior ligaments with the injury severity score. The general principles are as follows: (1) an incomplete neurologic injury generally requires an anterior procedure if neural compression from the anterior spinal elements is present following attempts at postural or open reduction; (2) PLC disruption generally requires a posterior procedure; and (3) a combined incomplete neurologic injury and PLC disruption generally requires a combined anterior and posterior procedure.

Wolter Classification

Wolter divided the spinal canal into three equal parts with the help of CT scan. This classification includes constriction of the spinal canal, whereby constriction of 1/3 is given the number 1, 2/3 the number 2, 3/3 the number 3, and no constriction 0.

Classification According to the Fracture Site (2002, Tao Tianzun, New Clinical Orthopaedics and Traumatology)

1. I: Fracture of vertebra body:
   (a) Anterior vertebral body fracture.
   (b) Simple flexion compression fracture of vertebral body.
   (c) Vertebral burst fracture.
   (d) Posterior vertebral body fracture
   (e) Chance fracture.
2. II: Spinal adnexal injuries:
   (a) Fracture of articular process.
   (b) Dislocation of articular process.
   (c) Isthmus fractures.
   (d) Fracture of transverse process.
   (e) Odontoid fracture
3. III: Intervertebral disc injury
4. IV: Spinal ligament injury

Shucheng Rao Classification

- Flexion compression fracture, which is classified into three types according to Ferguson–Allen classification.
- Burst fracture, which is classified into five types according to Denis classification.
- Distractive flexion injuries, which is classified according to A-C2 types in Gertzbein classification.
- Flexion rotation fracture dislocation, including intervertebral disc dislocation and "slice" fracture.
- Shear force-type dislocation.

Dadi King Classification

Dadi King use "class-type-subtype" system: (1) According to the damage mechanism and pathological morphology, it was divided into buck compression class (class A), vertical compression class (B class), and distraction (class C). (2) In each class according to its specific pathological morphology and the probability in clinical, they divided each class into A and B. Type A is the common injury clinically, and type B is rare. (3) According to the instability and the severity of the fracture each type is divided into three subtypes: Subtype 1 for the fracture type, consistent with the fracture of the most basic pathological features, without shift. Subtype 2 is subluxation type, combining with subluxation on the basis of fracture type. This subtype fractures are posterior deformity except for the subluxation caused by stretch and compression showing hyperextension deformity and the subluxation caused by lateral flexion and compression showing lateral distension. Subtype 3 for the dislocation type is multidirectional

Xuezhe Zhang Classification (1988)

According to the injury mechanism, the three-column theory and the spinal canal involvement he first proposed CT comprehensive diagnosis type. Classification method: according to the injury mechanism sub-C simple buckling compression fractures, B-burst fracture, S-belt fracture, F-fracture and dislocation fracture, and U-other types of fractures. According to the situation of three pillars, the A-front column, B-middle column, and C- later column are used, respectively. According to the degree of spinal canal involvement (WOLTER) to divide. When spinal stenosis is without stenosis, the index is 0. When spinal stenosis accounted for 1/3, the index is 1. When spinal stenosis accounted for 1/3–2/3 were 2; 2/3–total is 3.

Li Li Classification

Li Li according to the thoracolumbar burst fracture after the posterior column of the fracture of the spinal canal form of CT classification: Type A for fracture block into the spinal canal accounted for vertebral volume <30%. Type B for fracture block into the spinal canal accounted for vertebral volume 30–50%. Type B1 for fracture block which is relatively complete over the sagittal midline. B2 type for the fracture block single or multiple, located in the one side of the spinal canal, but didn't cross the sagittal midline of the spinal canal. C for the fracture block into the spinal canal volume >50%.

Multisegmental Spinal Fractures (Multiple-Level Spinal fracture M, SF)

At present, our country uses Tang Sanyuan (1992) classification method. Where the spine bone segment (except for spinous process and transverse process) two or more blocks that are multi-segmental spinal fractures. It is generally divided into adjacent type (I type) and non-adjacent type (II type).

- Type I (adjacent type): There is no normal segmental separation between the spine. Then according to the number of fractures it was divided into two subtypes:
  - IA: Adjacent two fractures.
  - IB: Adjacent to three or more segments of the fracture.
- Type II (non-adjacent type): There is at least one normal segment between the spine. There are three classification methods below:
  - Calenoff method: According to the anatomical site of the first and secondary spinal injury which is non-adjacent multisegmental, it was divided into A, B, and C types.
    - Type A: The first spine injury segment is in the C5–C7 levels, and secondary spinal injury happens in the T12 and lumbar spine levels.
    - Type B: The first spine injury segment is at the level of T12 and lumbar spine, and secondary spinal injury in the cervical spine level.
    - C type: The first spine injury segment is in the T12–L2 level, and secondary spinal injury segment in the L4–L5 levels.
  - Henderson method: According to the anatomical site and morbidity of the spine, non-adjacent multisegmental spinal injury is divided into five regions, C1–C3, C4–C7, T1–T10, T11–L2, and L3–L5. The structure is divided into severe damage and mild injury.
  - Tang Sanyuan method: From the anatomical point of view, according to bone structure units to type it was divided into three types:
    - II A: Refers to the interval of a normal segment and there are two fractures.
    - II B: Refers to the interval of two or more segments and there are two fractures.
    - II C: Refers to the interval of one or more than one normal segment, but there are three or more than three fractures.

Guangbai Zhang Classification

Guangbai Zhang classified the thoracolumbar vertebral fracture according to the three-column injury and the spinal canal occlusion based on Denis classification.

6.2 Segment 3 Sacrum Fracture Classification

Denis classification is the most widely used among all the sacrum fracture classification.

6.2.1 Denis Classification (1996, Philadelphia: Lippincott-Racen Publishers)

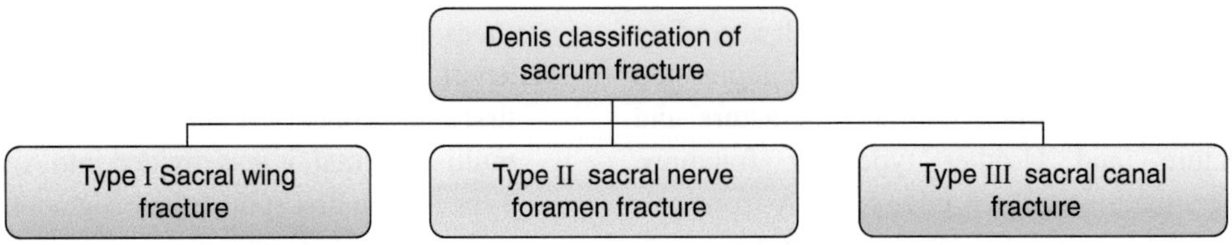

Denis divided sacrum into type I, II, and III, which is sacral wing fracture, sacral nerve foramen fracture, and sacral canal fracture.

Type I: Sacral wing fracture. Fracture line through the sacral wing without sacral foramen fracture and sacral canal fracture.

Type II: Sacral nerve foramen fracture. One or more sacral foramen fracture may be accompanied by sacral wing fracture. But without sacral canal fracture.

Type III: Sacral canal fracture. May be accompanied by sacral wing fracture or sacral foramen fracture. Sacral canal transverse fracture also belongs to this type which fracture line get through the above three areas at the same time.

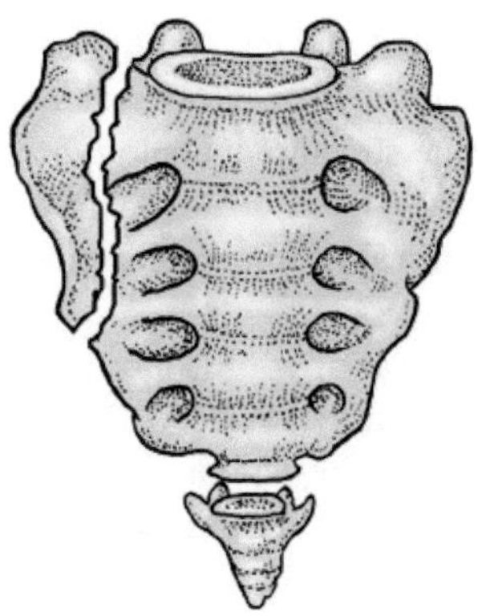

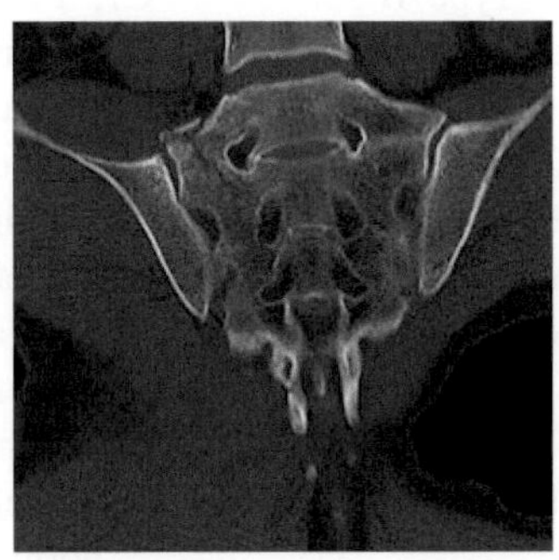

Denis classification of sacrum fracture
Type I: sacral wing fracture. Fracture line through the sacral wing without sacral foramen fracture and sacral canal fracture.

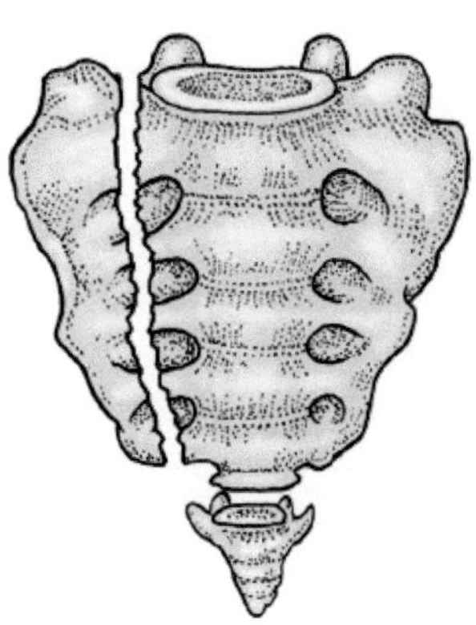

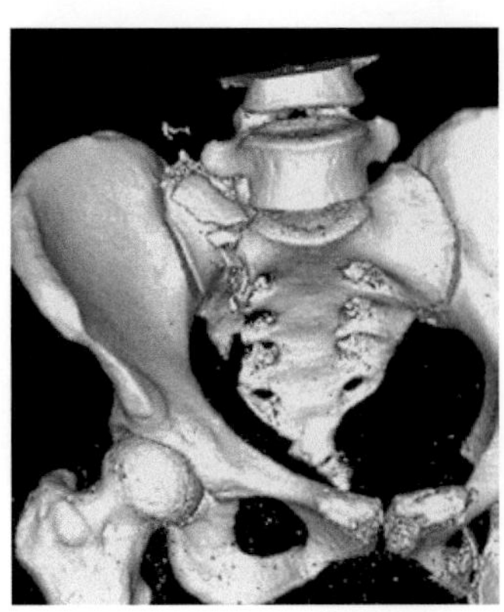

Denis classification of sacral fracture
Type II: fracture of neural foramina zone. Fractures involve one or several sacral foramina, and sometimes sacral ala, but do not enter the central sacral canal

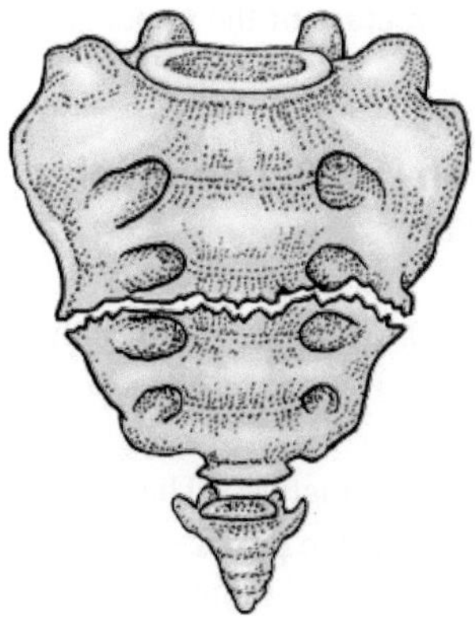

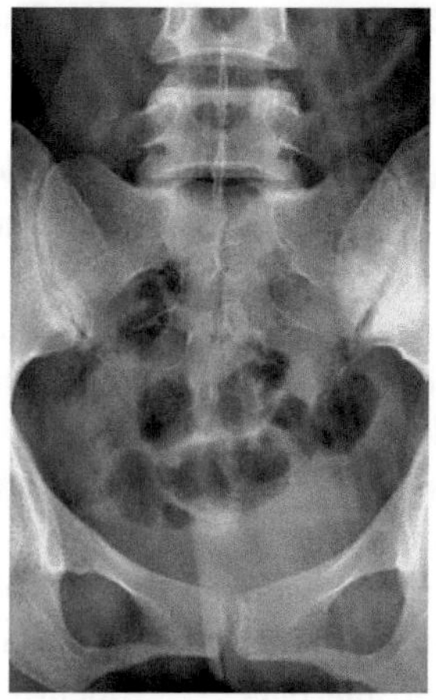

Denis classification of sacral fracture
Type III: fracture of the central sacral canal zone. Fractures occur through the central sacral canal. Fractures can involve the sacral ala and foramina zone, such as the transverse fracture that pass through those three zone

6.2.2 Rockwood Classification (1996, Fractures in Adult. 4th Ed. Philadelphia: Lippincott-Raven Publishers)

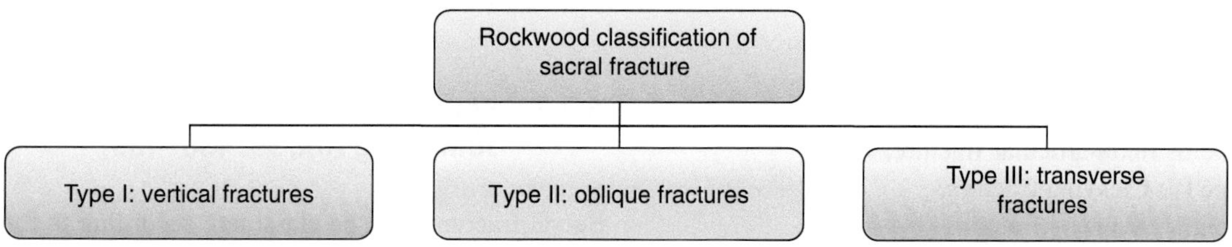

Type I: Vertical fractures
Type II: Oblique fractures
Type III: Transverse fractures

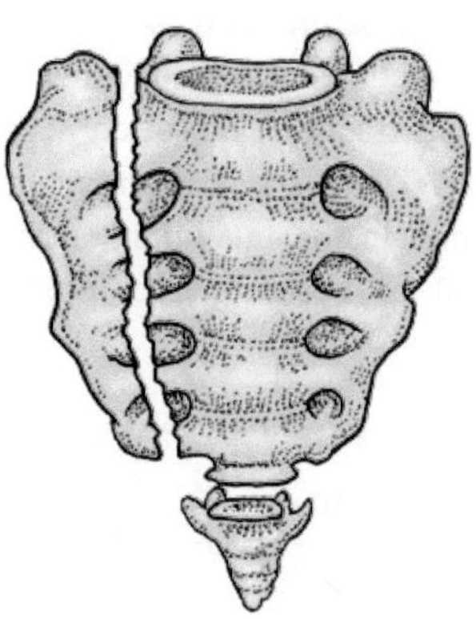

Type I: vertical fractures

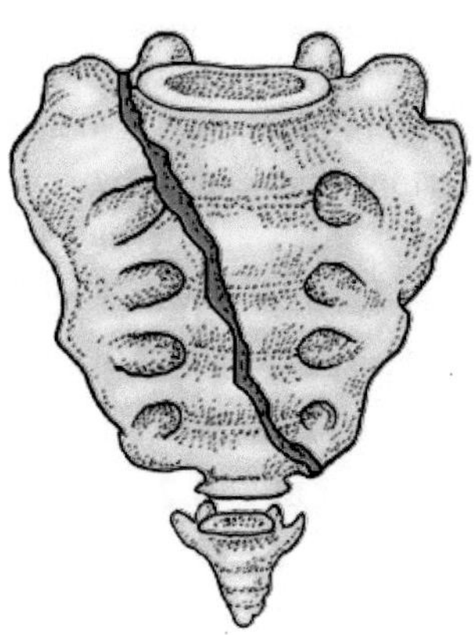

Type II: oblique fractures

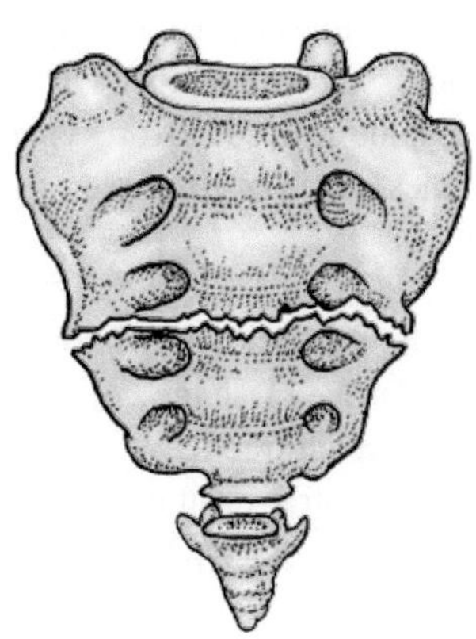

Type III: transverse fractures

6.2.3 Schmidek Classification (1984, Neurosurgery, 15: 735–746)

According to the trauma mechanism, Schmidek divided the sacral fracture into direct trauma and indirect trauma.

1. Direct trauma:
   (a) Penetrating injury: Gunshot wounds are the most common cause and are often complicated by extensive visceral damage. The fracture usually confined to the posterior pelvic ring that implies a stable structural condition of pelvic. This is a stable fracture.
   (b) Comminuted fractures: This fracture is caused by severe blunt trauma, and often involved sacral nerve roots.
   (c) Low transverse fracture: Direct blow onto the buttocks causes the fracture, and makes the distal segment move forward.
2. Indirect trauma: The majority of the sacral fractures are caused by indirect trauma.
   (a) High transverse fractures:
   - Type I: Sacral ala fracture.
   - Type II: Foramina zone fracture.
   - Type III: Sacral canal fracture.

   (b) Vertical fractures:
   - Type I: Lateral mass fracture.
   - Type II: Juxta-articular fracture.
   - Type III: Cleaving fracture.
   - Type IV: Avulsion fracture.

6.2.4 Roy Camille Classification (1985, Spine, 10: 838–845)

Roy Camille.et al. found that transverse fractures of the upper sacrum result from falls from a height and are usually associated with suicidal attempts by jumping, and named this injury suicidal jumper's fracture. The position of the lumbar spine in lordosis or kyphosis at the time of impact determines which of the three types of morbid anatomy will result:

Type I: Crooked fracture without displacement.
Type II: Crooked fracture with forward displacement.
Type III: Stretch fracture with backward displacement.
(Type IV: Neutral position fracture. Strange Vognsen et al. reported one case and named it Roy Camille IV).

6.2.5 Sabiston Classification (1986, J Trauma, 26: 1113–1115)

Type I: The sacral fracture which occurs in conjunction with a pelvic fracture.
Type II: The isolated sacral fracture of the lower segments.
Type III: The isolated sacral fracture of the upper segments.

6.2.6 Tile Classification (1988, J Bone Joint Surg Br, 70: 1–12)

Tile classified sacral fractures, associated with pelvic fractures, into three categories.

Type A (pure sacral or coccygeal fracture): The pelvic posterior ring was intact and so was the pelvic stability.
Type B: Rotational violence causes incomplete disruption and rotationally unstability of the pelvic ring: (B1) "open-book"-type injury, (B2) lateral compression and internal rotation injury, which crush the front part of sacram and cause compression fractures with contralateral or bilateral fractures of the pubic bone, (B3) bilateral "open-book"-type injury or internal rotation injury.
Type C: Completely breaking of unilateral or bilateral pelvic ring, with rotational and vertical unstability.

6.2.7 Fountain Classification (1977, J Bone Joint Surg Am, 59: 486–489)

Sacral fractures can be classified, according to the shape of the fracture line, into two categories: (1) transverse fracture and (2) longitudinal fracture.

6.2.8 Gibbons Classification (1990, J Neurosurg, 72: 889–893)

Gibbons classified Denis III fracture into two categories: longitudinal and transverse fractures. The injury mechanism is not the same. Longitudinal fractures are often accompanied by severe pelvic injury. Transverse fractures can exist independently, more common in the fall injury and traffic injuries, often accompanied by severe nerve injury, also known as jumper's fracture.

6.2.9 Montana Classification (1986, Radiology, 161: 499–503)

Montana, et al. devised this sacral fracture classification according to CT scan.

6.3 Classification of Spinal Dislocation

6.3.1 Classification of Atlanto-occipital Dislocation

According to the position of the occipital bone relative to the atlas, there are three types:

Type I: The most common, the occipital condyle, has anterior dislocation relative to the atlas.

Type II: The atlas has longitudinal separation with occipital.

Type III: The occipital condylar has posterior dislocation relative to the atlas.

6.3.1.1 Atlanto-axial Dislocation

6.3.1.2 Fielding Classification (1977, J Bone Joint Surg (Am), 59: 37–44)

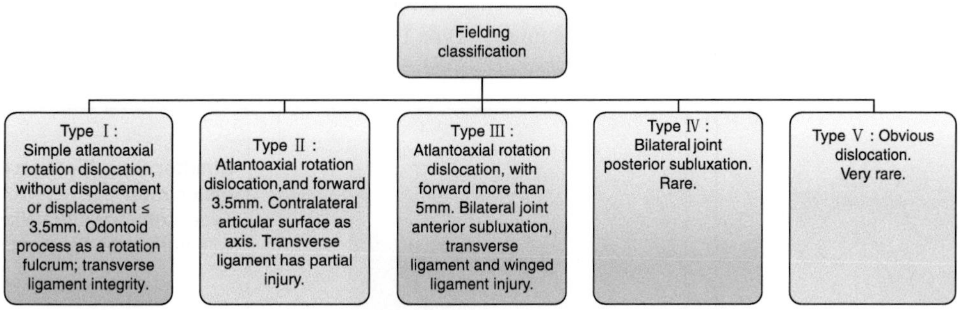

Type I: Simple atlanto-axial rotation dislocation, without displacement or displacement ≤3.5 mm. Odontoid process as a rotation fulcrum; transverse ligament integrity.

Type II: Atlanto-axial rotation dislocation, and forward 3.5 mm. Contralateral articular surface as axis. Transverse ligament has partial injury.

Type III: Atlanto-axial rotation dislocation, with forward more than 5 mm. Bilateral joint anterior subluxation, transverse ligament, and winged ligament injury.

Type IV: Bilateral joint posterior subluxation. Rare.

Type V: Obvious dislocation. Very rare.

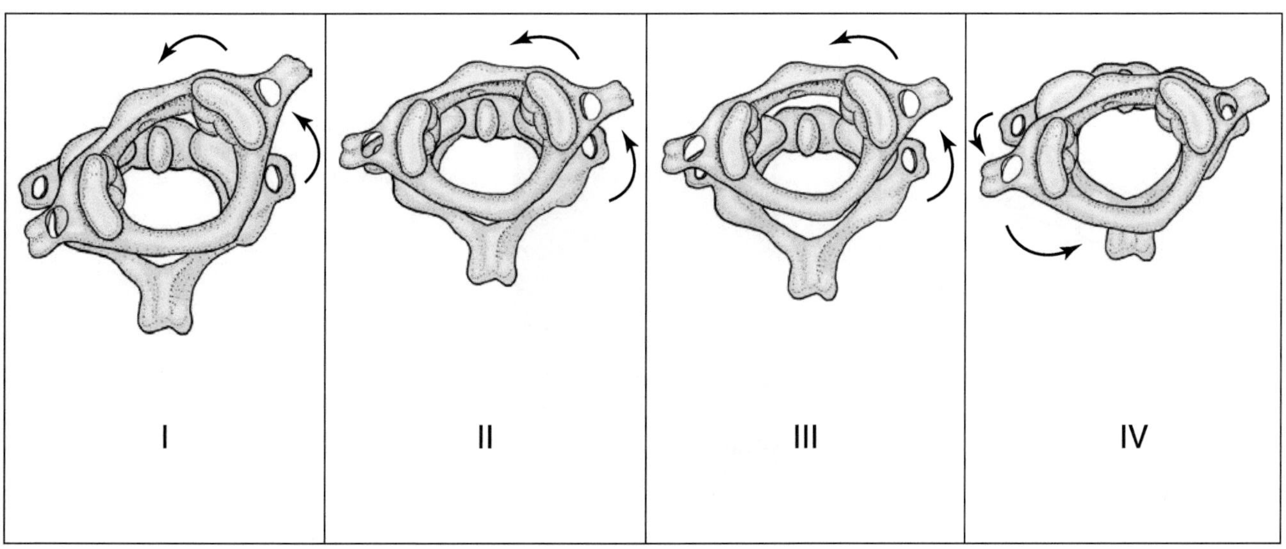

6.3.1.3 Stauffer Classification (1991, Philadelphia: JB Lippincott Co., 1014)

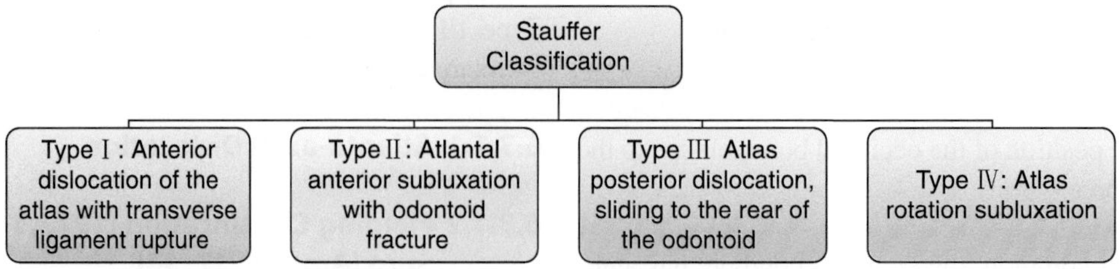

Type I: Anterior dislocation of the atlas with transverse ligament rupture.

Type II: Atlantal anterior subluxation with odontoid fracture.

Type III: Atlas posterior dislocation, sliding to the rear of the odontoid.

Type IV: Atlas rotation subluxation.

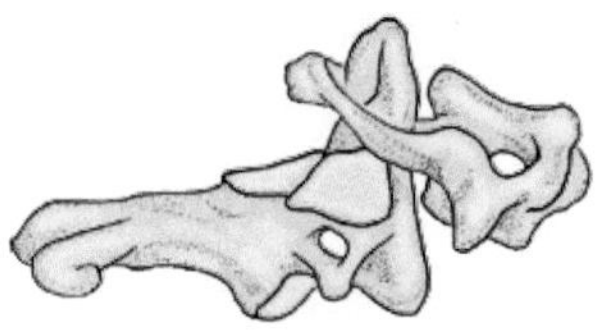

P1

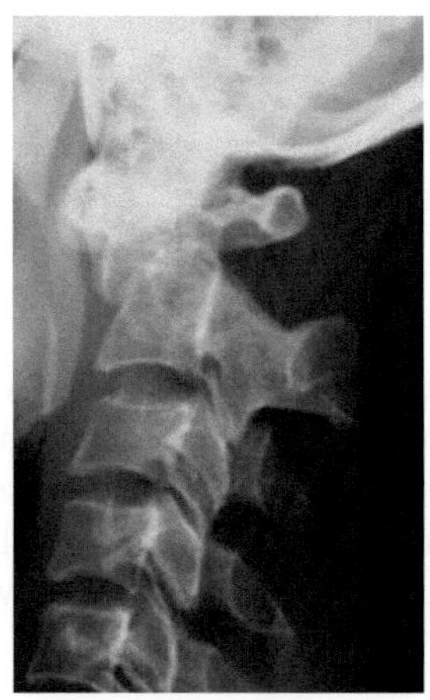

Stauffer Classification of atlantoaxial dislocation
Type I: Anterior dislocation of the atlas with transverse ligament rupture

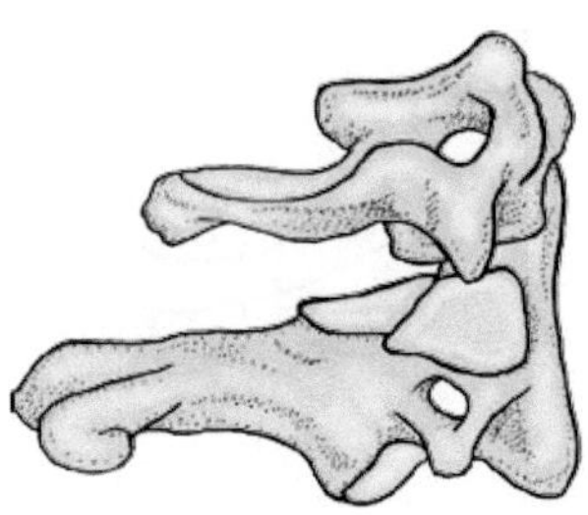

684633

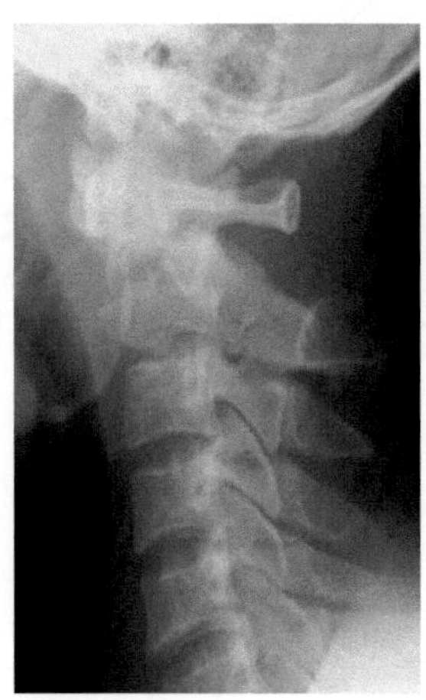

Stauffer Classification of atlantoaxial dislocation
Type II: Atlantal anterior subluxation with odontoid fracture

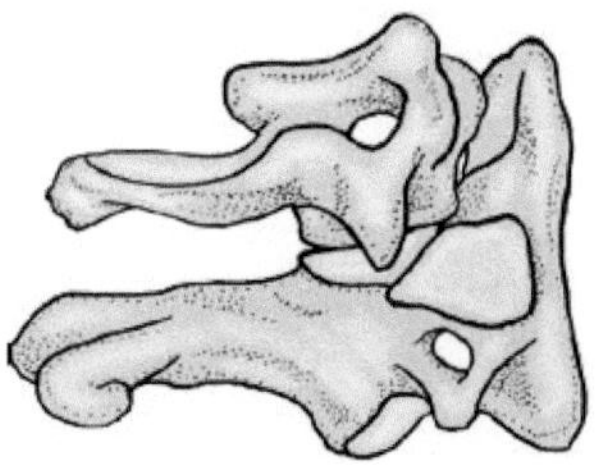

16B1

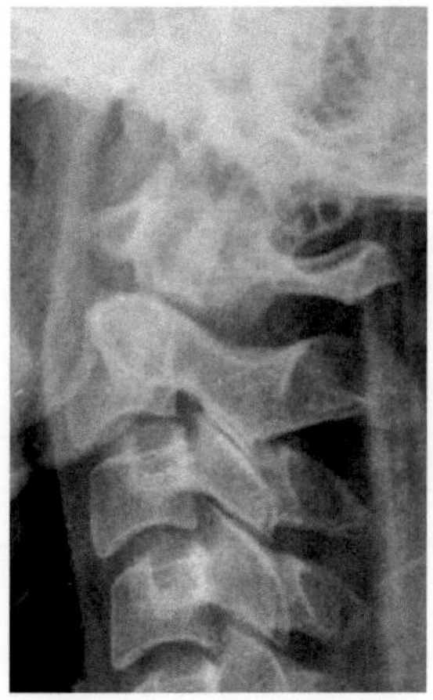

Stauffer Classification of atlantoaxial dislocation
Type III: Atlas posterior dislocation, sliding to the rear of the odontoid

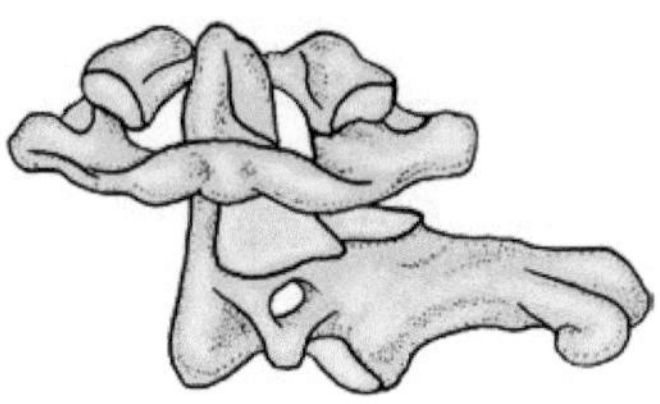

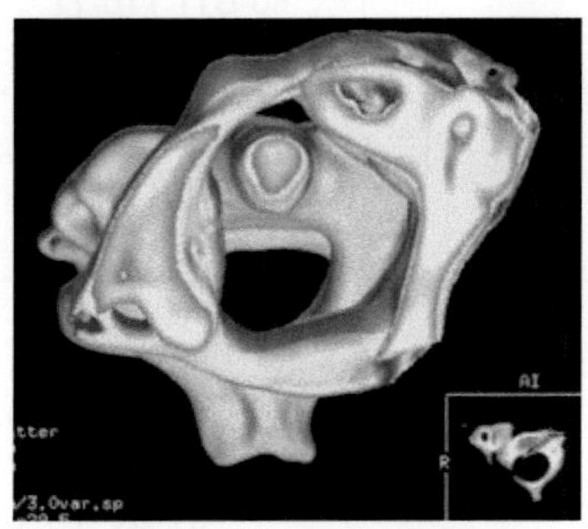

Stauffer Classification of atlantoaxial dislocation
Type IV: Atlas rotation subluxation

6.3.2 Levine Classification of Cervical Unilateral Fracture and Dislocation (1992, Spine, 17: 447–454)

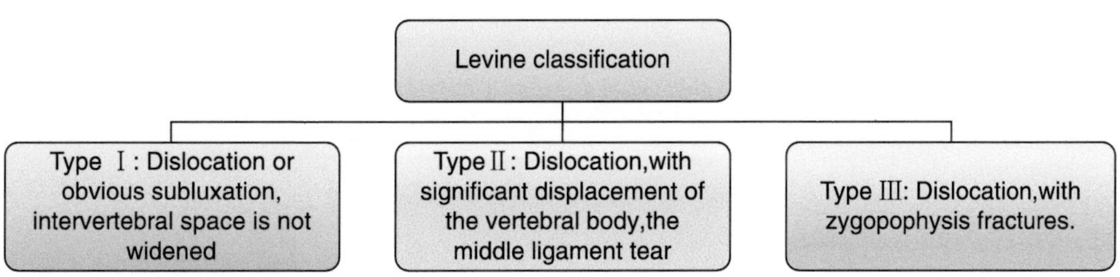

Type I: Dislocation or obvious subluxation, intervertebral space is not widened.
Type II: Dislocation, with significant displacement of the vertebral body, the middle ligament tear.
Type III: Dislocation, with zygopophysis fractures.

6.3.3 AO/OTA Classification (2007, Journal of Orthopaedic Trauma. 21 Supplement)

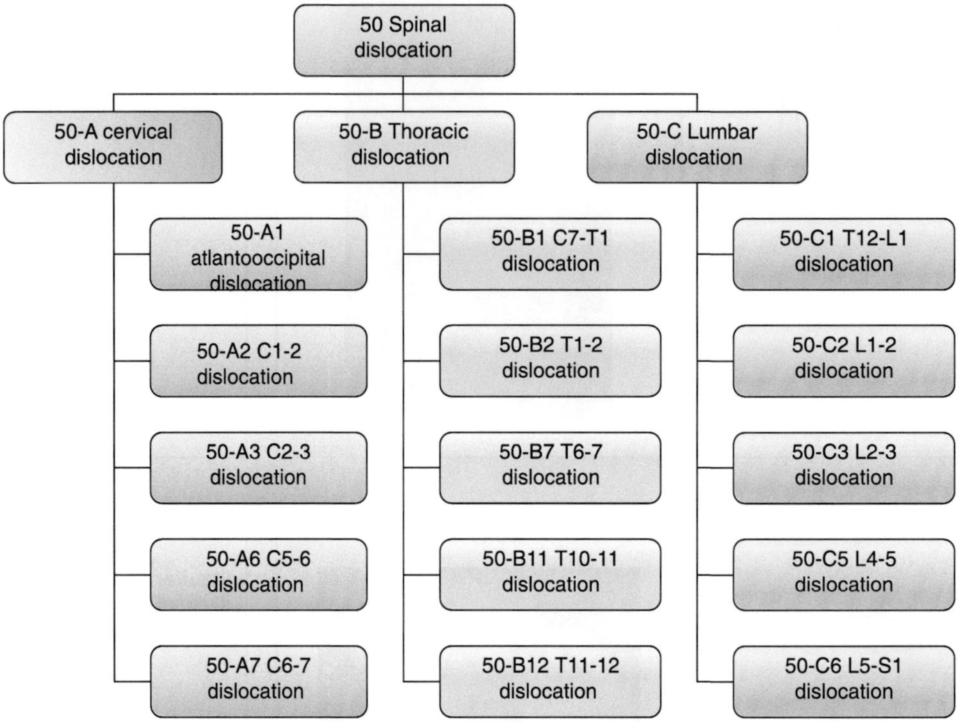

50-A Cervical dislocation

50-A1: Atlanto-occipital:
50-A2 C1-2: Dislocation.
50-A3 C2-3: Dislocation.
50-A4 C3-4: Dislocation.
50-A5 C4-5: Dislocation.
50-A6 C5-6: Dislocation.
50-A7 C6-7: Dislocation.

50-B Thoracic dislocation

50-B1 C7-T1: Dislocation.
50-B2 T1-2: Dislocation.
50-B3 T2-3: Dislocation.
50-B4 T3-4: Dislocation.
50-B5 T4-5: Dislocation.
50-B6 T5-6: Dislocation.
50-B7 T6-7: Dislocation.
50-B8 T7-8: Dislocation.
50-B9 T8-9: Dislocation.
50-B10 T9-10: Dislocation.
50-B11 T10-11: Dislocation.
50-B12 T11-12: Dislocation.

50-C Lumbar dislocation

50-C1 T12-L1: Dislocation.
50-C2 L1-2: Dislocation.
50-C3 L2-3: Dislocation.
50-C4 L3-4: Dislocation.
50-C5 L4-5: Dislocation.
50-C6 L5-S1: Dislocation.

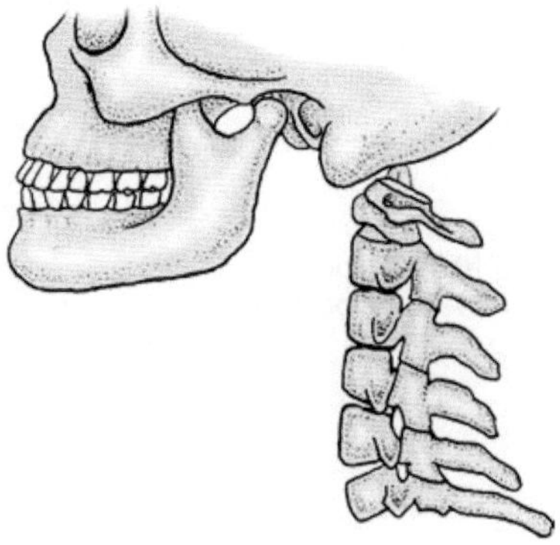

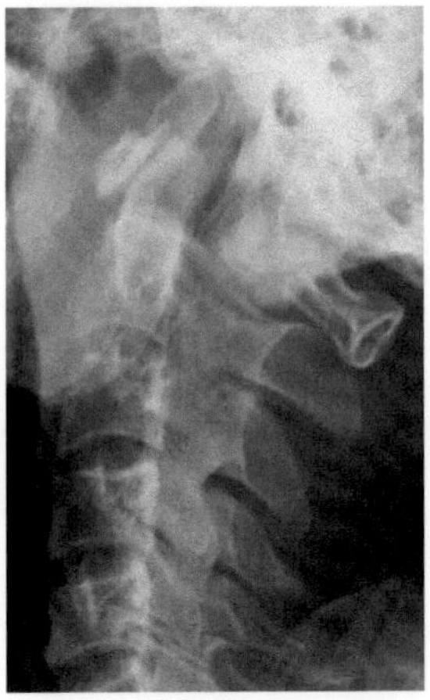

AO/OTA Classification
50-A cervical dislocation:
A1 Atlanto occipital dislocation

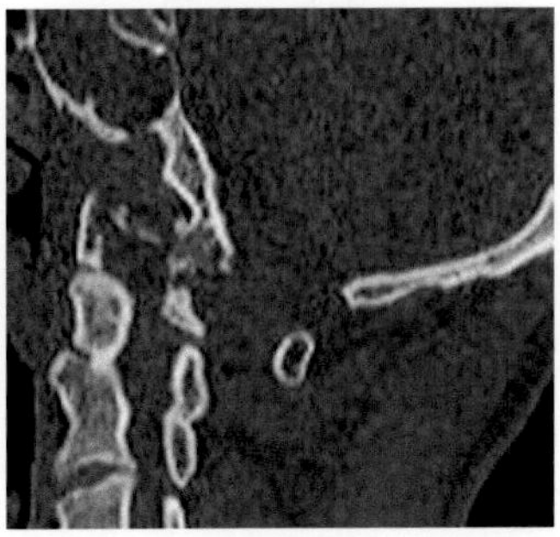

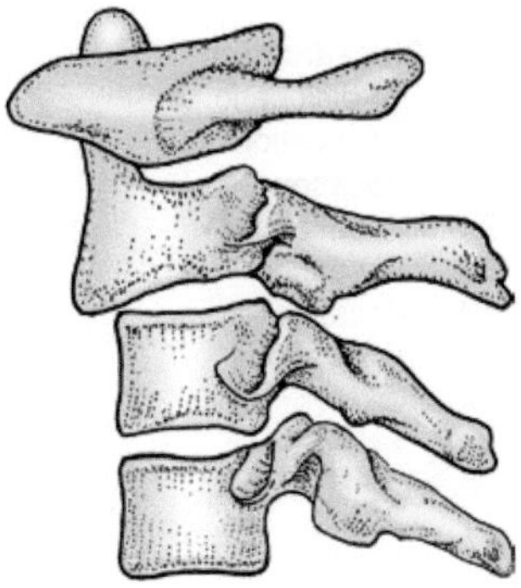

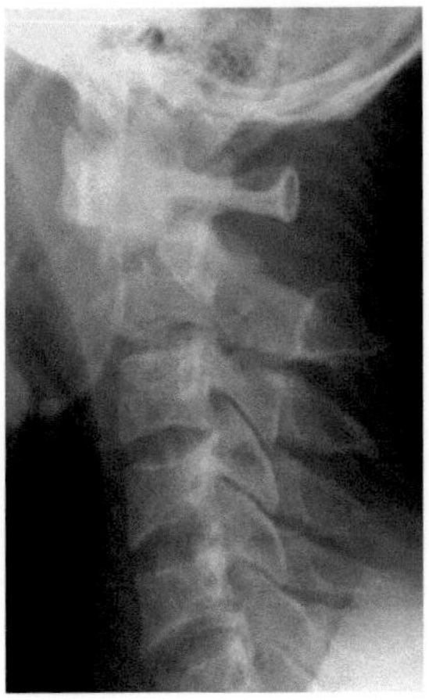

AO/OTA Classification
50-A cervical dislocation
A2 Atlantoaxial dislocation

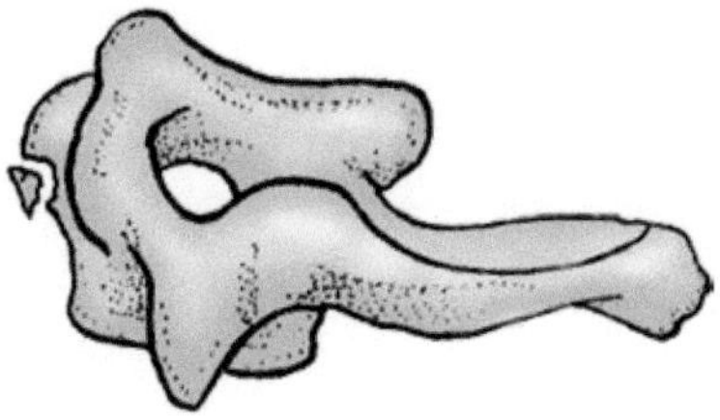

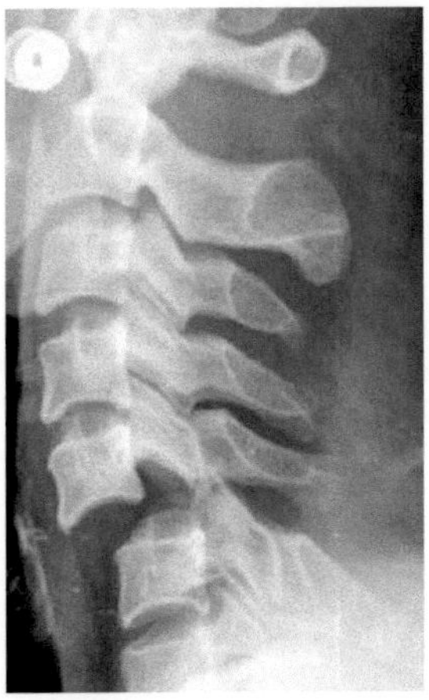

AO/OTA Classification
50-A cervical dislocation
A3 C2-3 dislocation
A4 C3-4 dislocation
A5 C4-5 dislocation
A6 C5-6 dislocation
A7 C6-7 dislocation

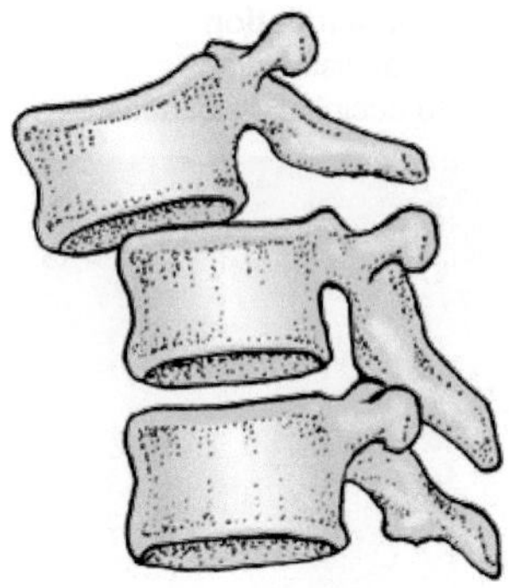

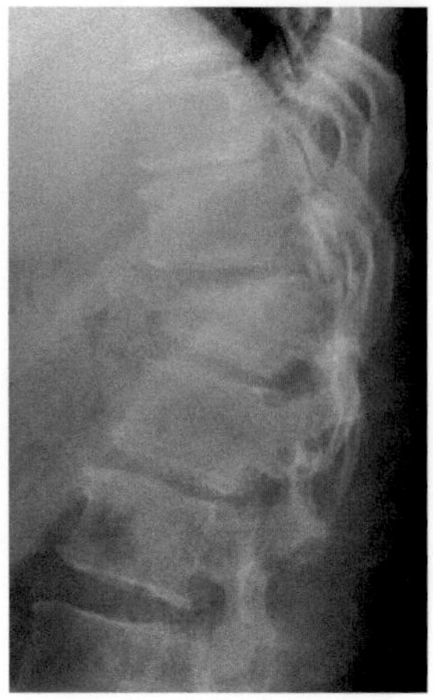

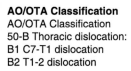

AO/OTA Classification
AO/OTA Classification
50-B Thoracic dislocation:
B1 C7-T1 dislocation
B2 T1-2 dislocation
.
.
.
B11 T10-11 dislocation
B12 T11-12 dislocation

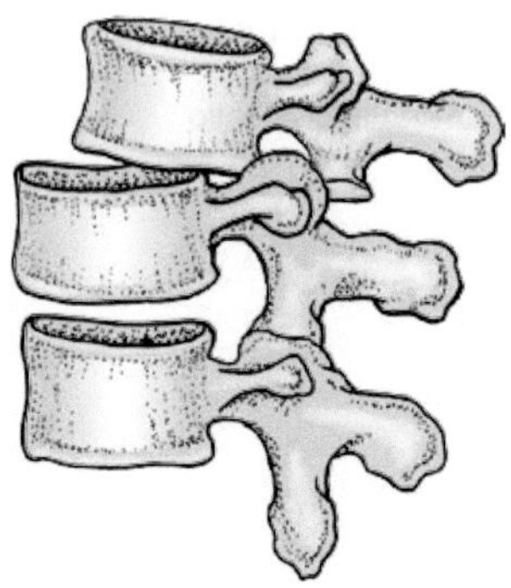

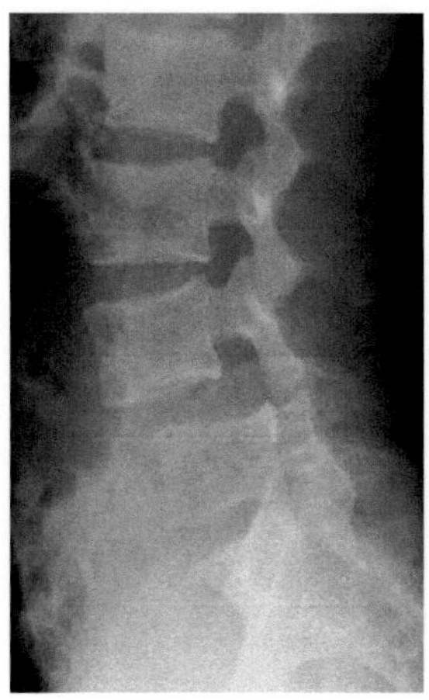

AO/OTA Classification
50-C Lumbar dislocation:
C1 T12-L1 dislocation
C2 T1-2 dislocation
C3 T2-3 dislocation
C4 T3-4 dislocation
C5 T4-5 dislocation
C6 T5-S1 dislocation

7 Classification of Pelvic Ring Fracture and Dislocation

Yingze Zhang and Zhiyong Hou

7.1 Classification of Pelvic Ring Fracture

The classification for pelvic ring fractures was established by Pennal and Tile (1980, Clin Orthop, 151:12–23), based on the stability of a posterior lesion, its direction, and the nature of the force involved. Young and Burgess developed and established their own classification to describe pelvic ring fractures. There are many types of pelvic fracture classification, 5 years at the most recent literature reports, utilization rate of Tile classification, Young—Bergess classification, AO/OTA classification, etc.

7.1.1 Tile Classification (1988, J Bone Joint Surg (Br), 70:1–12)

Type A: Stable:
- A1: Avulsion fracture, without disruption of the pelvic ring.
- A2: Pure iliac wing fracture with minimal displacement.
- A3: Transverse sacral or coccygeal fracture.

Type B: Rotationally unstable but vertically stable:
- B1: "Open-book"-type injury.
- B2: Lateral compression; ipsilateral.
- B3: Lateral compression; contralateral ("bucket-handle" type).

Type C: Rotationally and vertically unstable:
- C1: Unilateral injury.
- C2: Bilateral injury, ipsilateral vertically unstable, contralateral rotationally unstable.
- Type C3: Bilateral type C injury, involving an acetabular fracture.

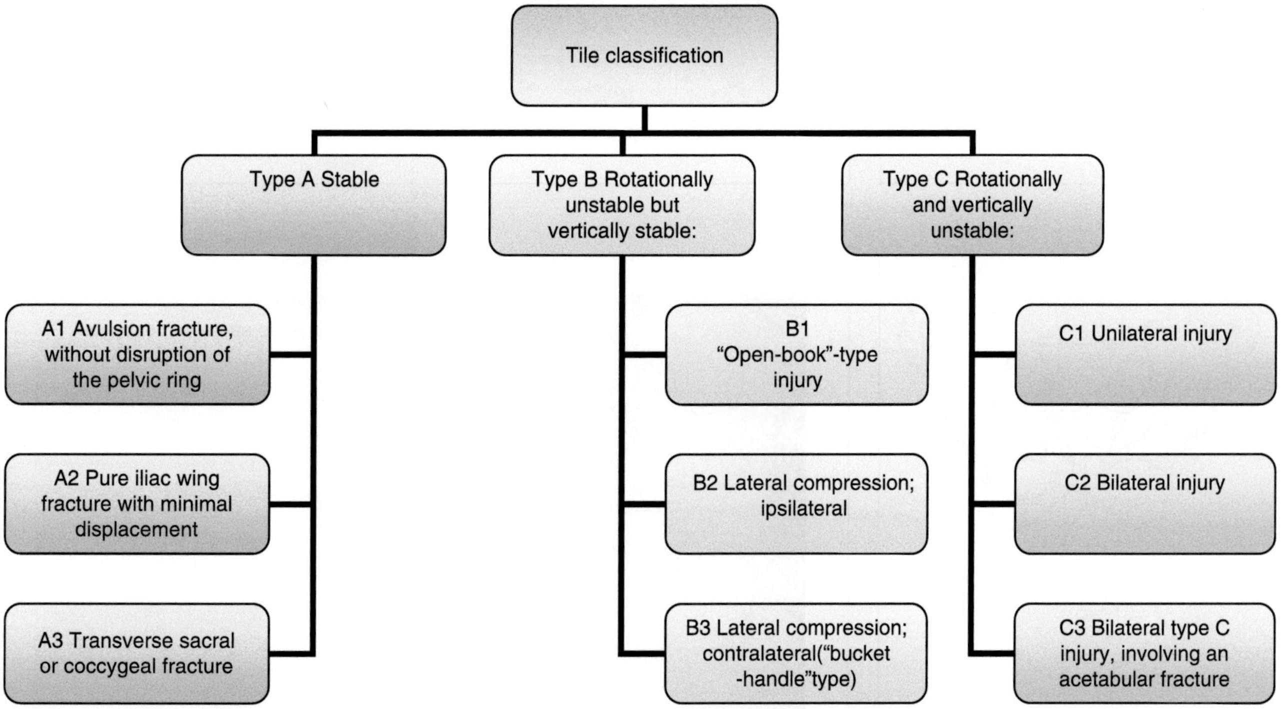

Y. Zhang (✉) • Z. Hou
Department of Orthopedics, The Third Hospital of Hebei Medical University, Shijiazhuang, China
e-mail: yzzhangdr@126.com, yzling_liu@163.com

Y. Zhang (ed.), *Clinical Classification in Orthopaedics Trauma*, https://doi.org/10.1007/978-981-10-6044-1_7

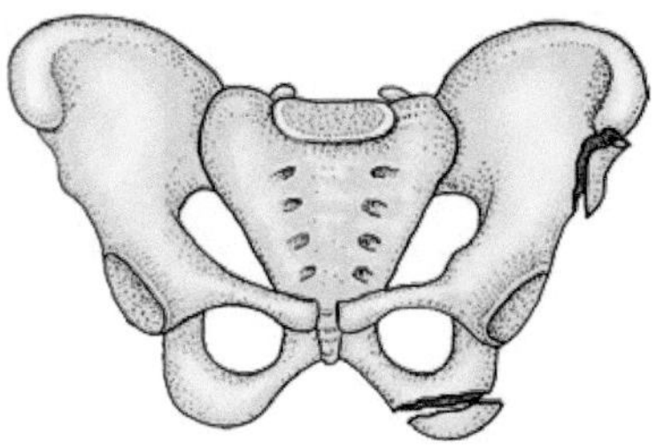

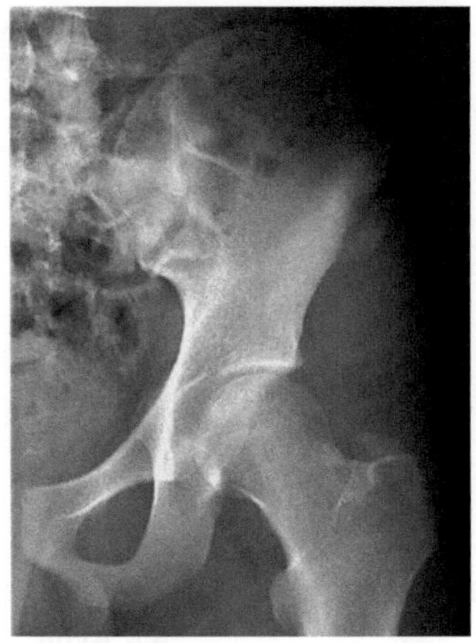

Type A Stable:
A1: Avulsion fracture, without disruption of the pelvic ring

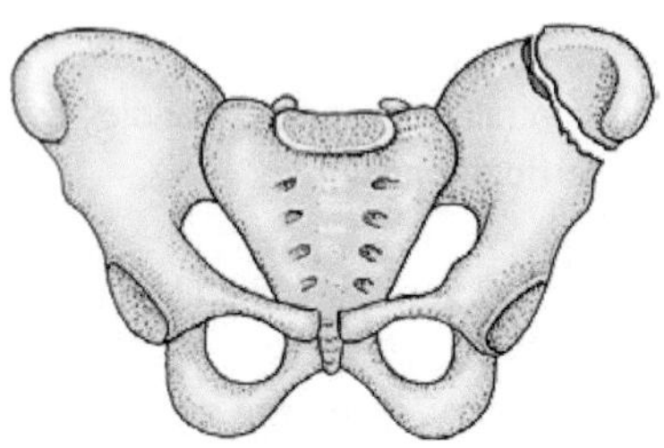

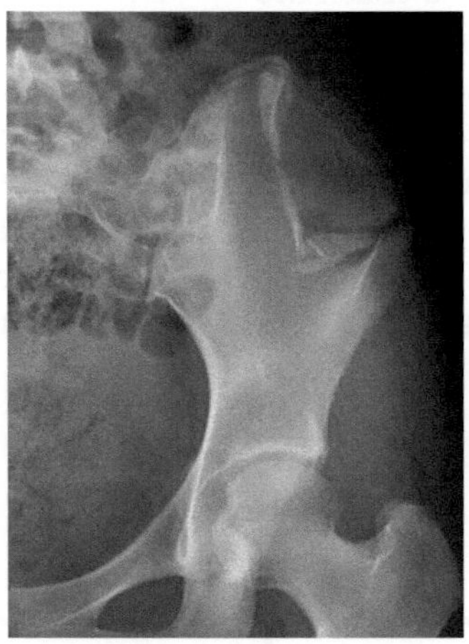

Type A Stable:
A2: Pure iliac wing fracture with minimal displacement

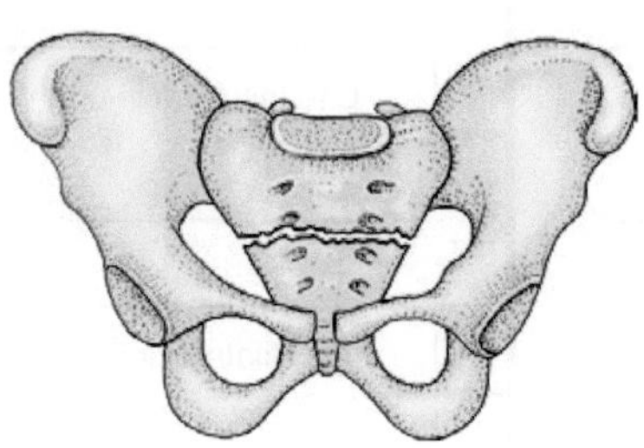

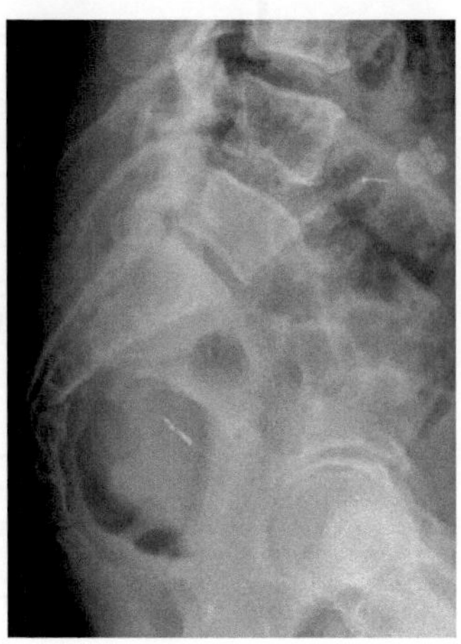

Type A Stable:
A3: Transverse sacral or coccygeal fracture

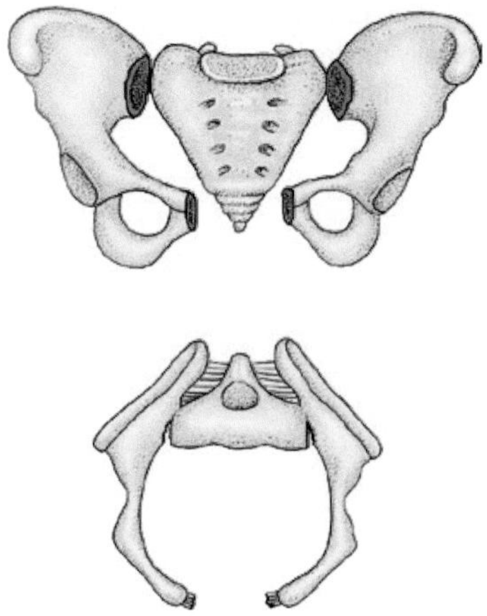

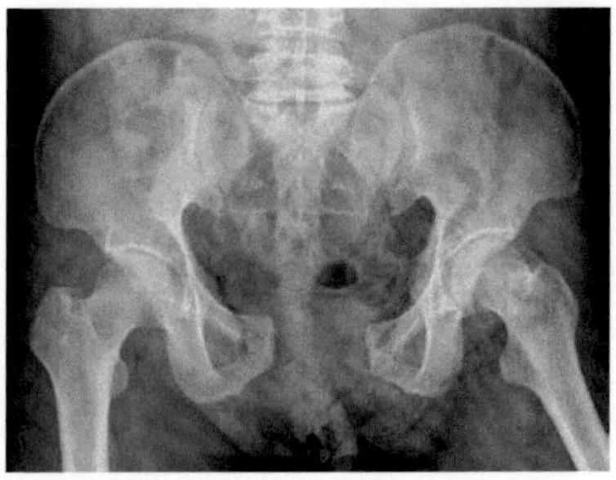

Type B Rotationally unstable but vertically stable:
B1: “Open-book”-type injury

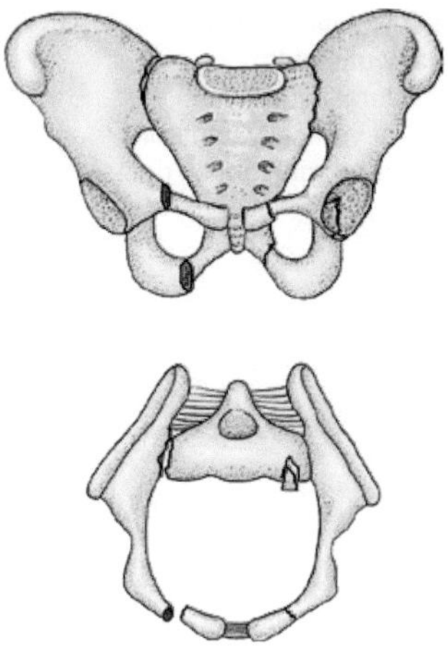

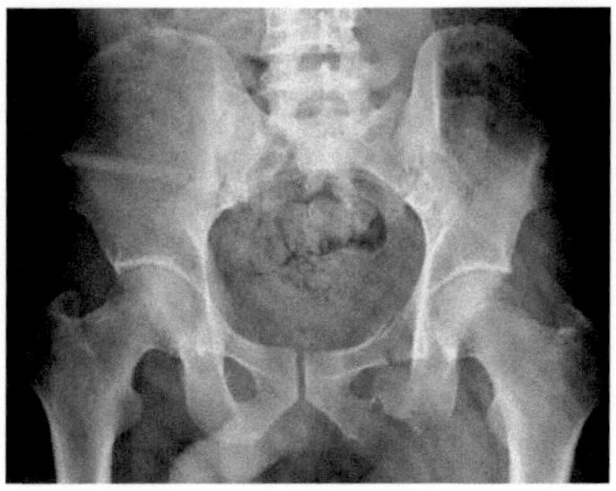

Type B Rotationally unstable but vertically stable:
B2: Lateral compression; ipsilateral

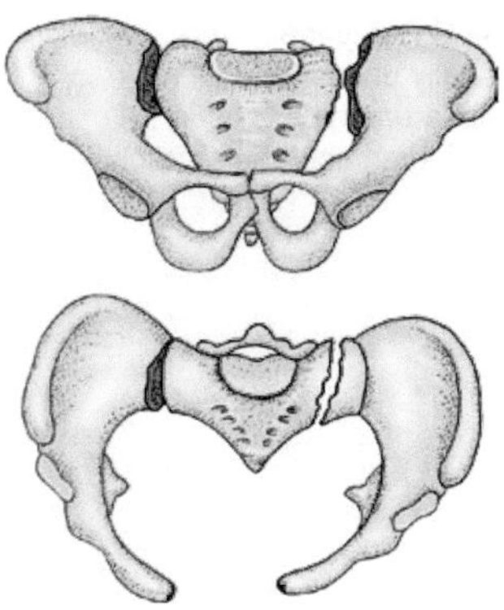

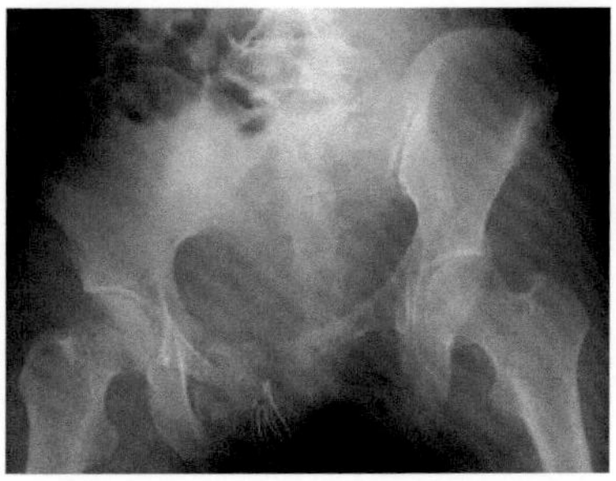

Type B Rotationally unstable but vertically stable:
B3: Lateral compression.
contralateral(“bucket-handle” type)

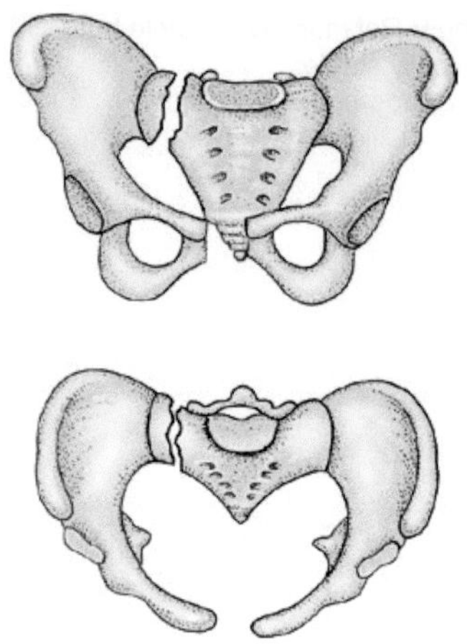

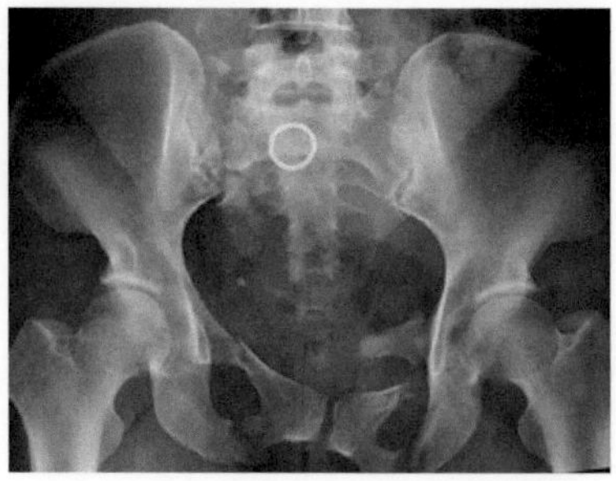

Type C Rotationally and
vertically unstable:
C1: Unilateral injury

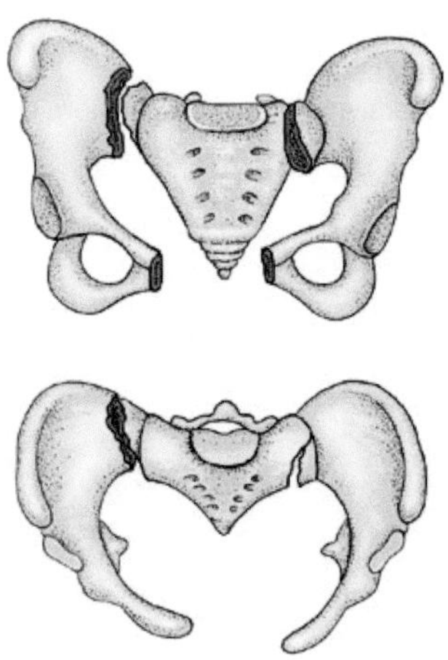

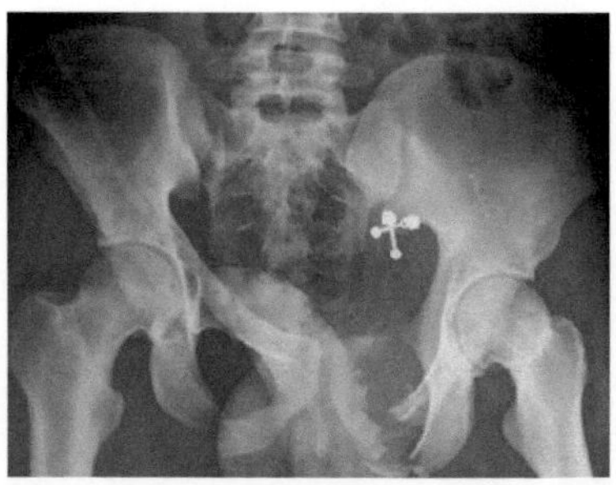

Type C Rotationally and
vertically unstable:
C2: Bilateral injury,
ipsilateral vertically unstable,
contralateral rotationally unstable

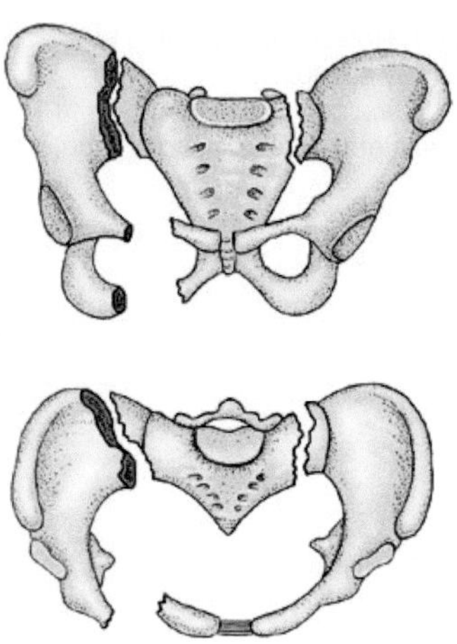

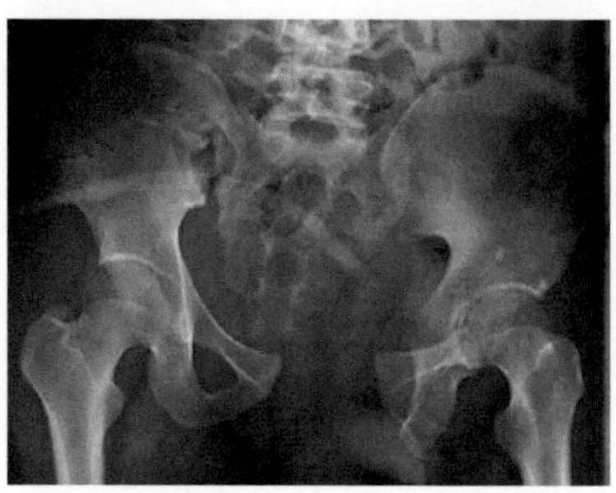

Type C Rotationally and
vertically unstable:
C3: Bilateral type C injury,
involving an acetabular fracture

7.1.2 Young-Burgess Classification (1987, Radiological Management of Pelvic Ring Fractures. Baltimore, Urban & Schwarzenberg)

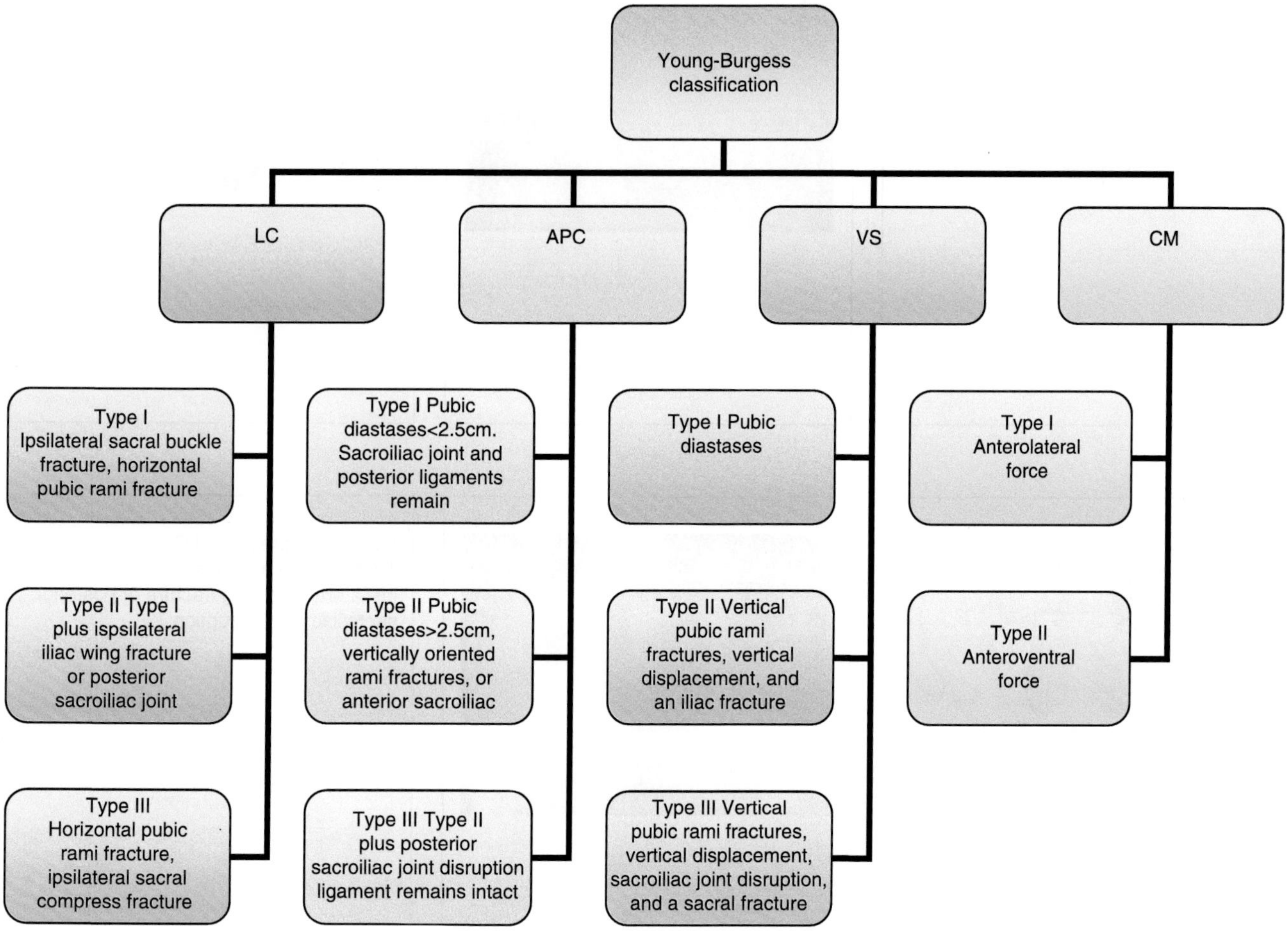

Lateral compression (LC):

- Type LC-I: Ipsilateral sacral buckle fracture, horizontal pubic rami fracture; stable.
- Type LC-II: Type I plus ipsilateral iliac wing fracture or posterior sacroiliac joint disruption.
- Type LC-III: Type I or II plus contralateral pubic rami fracture or disruption of the sacrotuberous and/or sacrospinous ligament. "Open-book" (type-APC)

Anteroposterior compression (APC):

- Type APC-I: Pubic diastases <2.5 cm. Sacroiliac joint and posterior ligaments remain intact, and stability is maintained.
- Type APC-II: Pubic diastases >2.5 cm, vertically oriented rami fractures, or anterior sacroiliac joint disruption, posterior sacroiliac joint ligament remains intact.
- Type APC-III: Type II plus posterior sacroiliac joint disruption.

Vertical shear (VS):

- Type VS-I: Pubic diastases.
- Type VS-II: Vertical pubic rami fractures, vertical displacement, and an iliac fracture.
- Type VS-III: Vertical pubic rami fractures, vertical displacement, sacroiliac joint disruption, and a sacral fracture.

Combined mechanism (CM):

- Type CM-IA: Anterolateral force.
- Type CM-IIA: Anterovertical force.

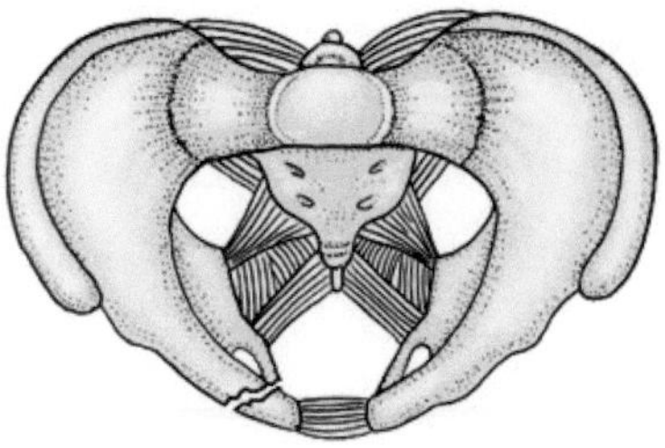

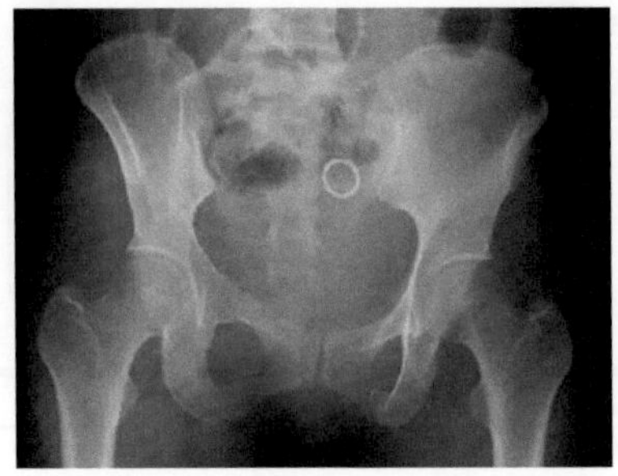

Lateral compression (LC):
Type LC-II ipsilateral
sacral buckle fracture,
horizontal pubic rami fracture; stable

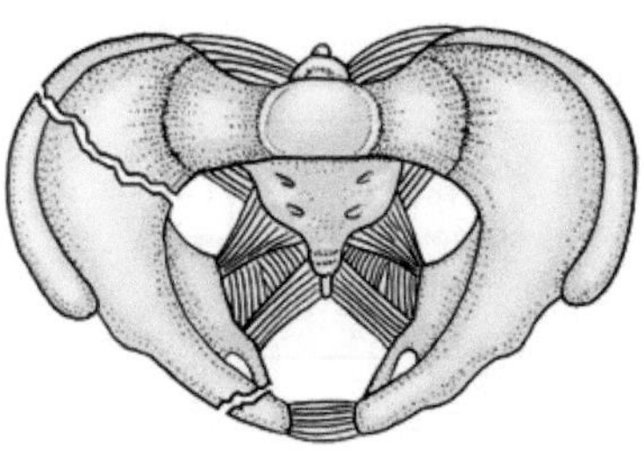

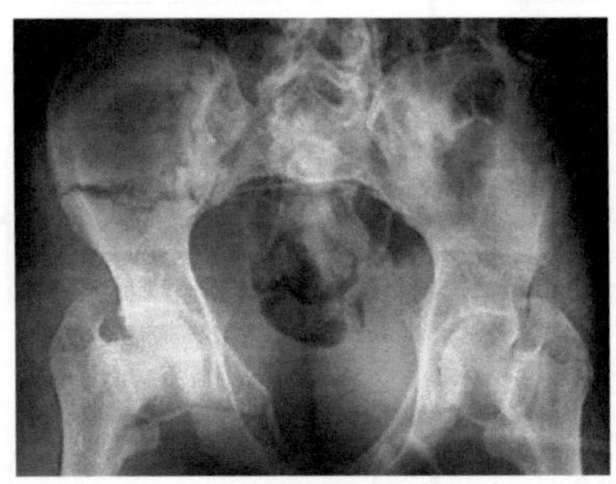

Lateral compression (LC):
Type LC-II Type I plus
ipsilateral iliac wing fracture or posterior
sacroiliac joint disruption

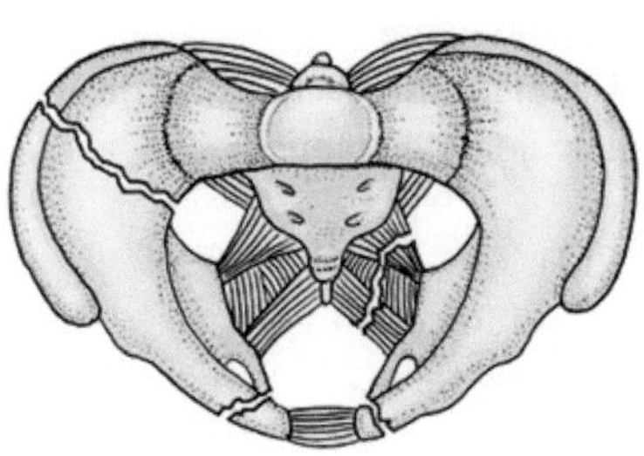

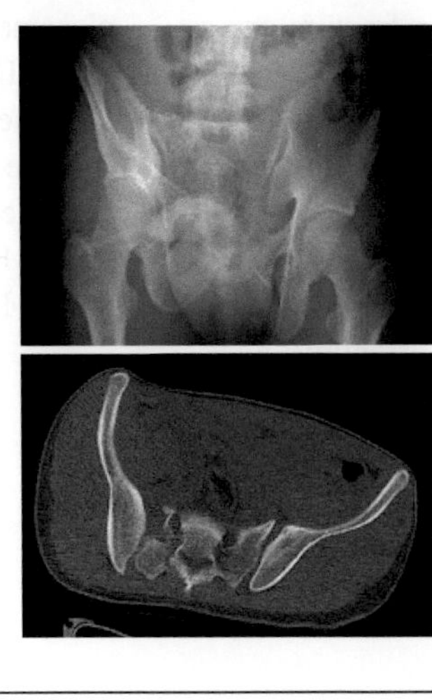

Lateral compression (LC):
Type LC-III Type I or II
plus contralateral pubic
rami fracture or disruption
of the sacrotuberous and/or
sacrospinous ligament.
"Open-book" (type-APC)

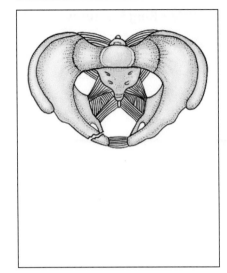

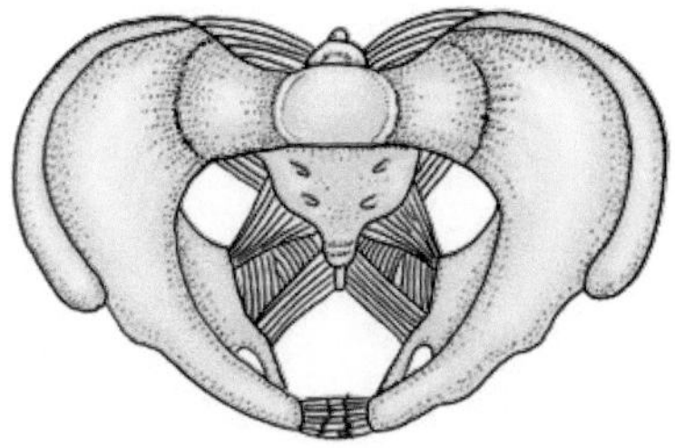

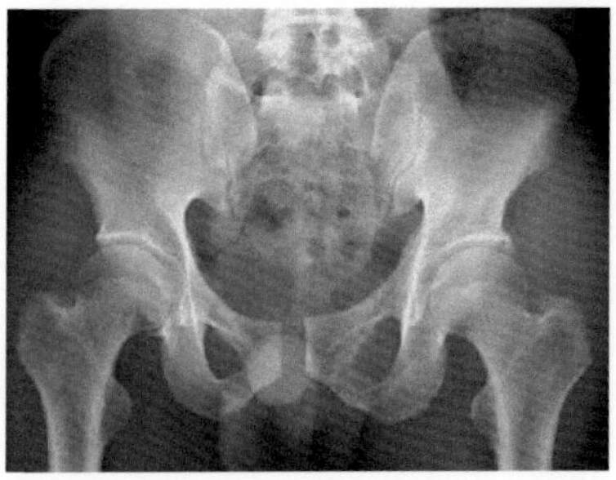

Anteroposterior compression (APC):
Type APC-I Pubic
diastases<2.5cm.
Sacroiliac joint and posterior
ligaments remain intact, and stability is
maintained

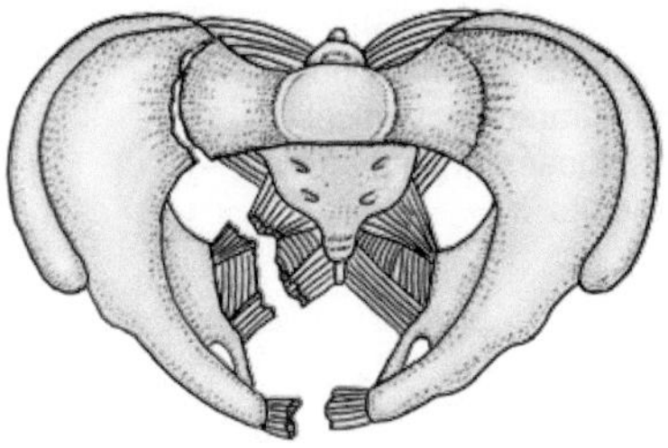

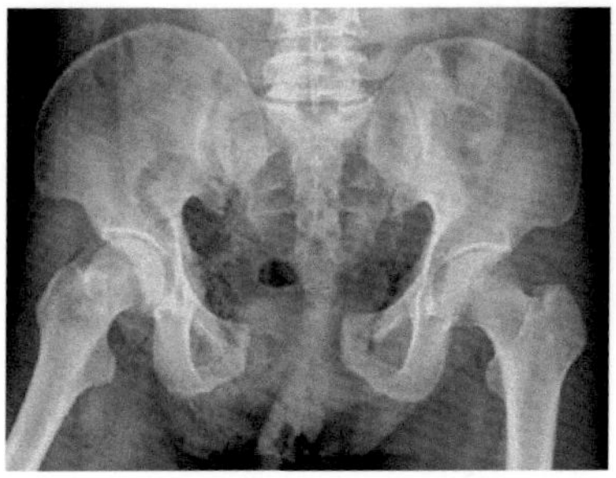

Anteroposterior compression (APC):
Type APC-II Pubic
diastases>2.5cm,
vertically oriented rami fractures,
or anterior sacroiliac joint disruption,
posterior sacroiliac joint
ligament remains intact

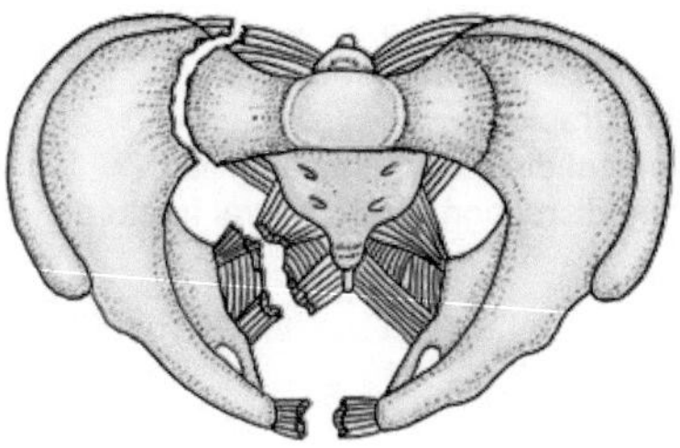

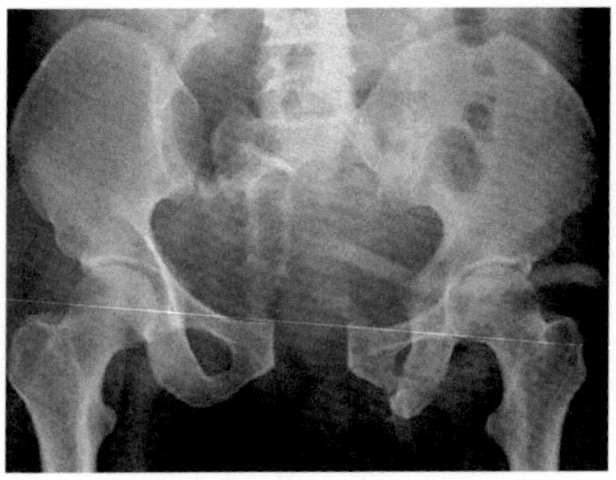

Anteroposterior compression (APC):
Type APC-III Type II plus
posterior sacroiliac joint disruption

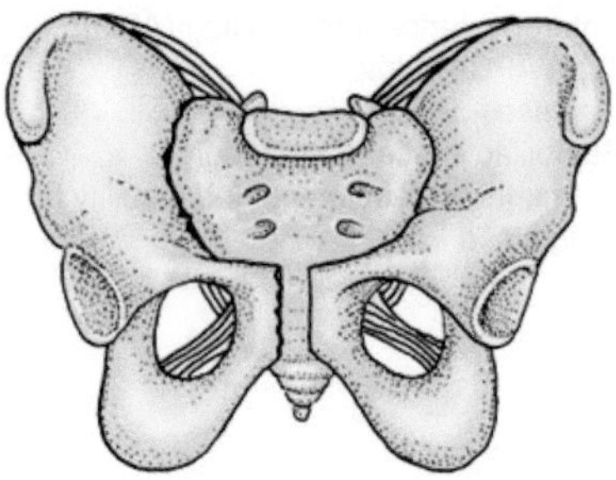

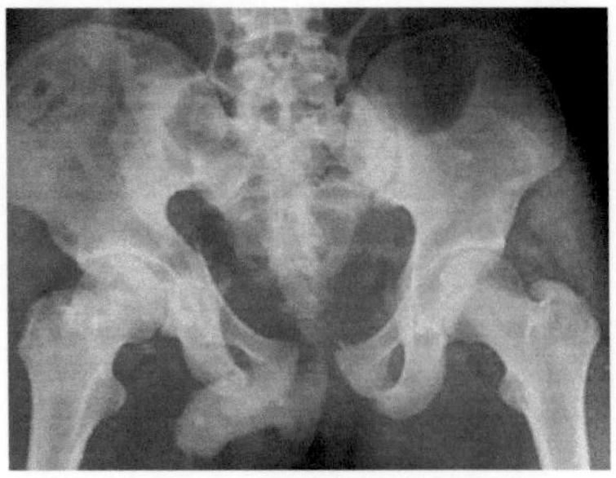

Vertical shear (VS):
Type VS-I Pubic diastases

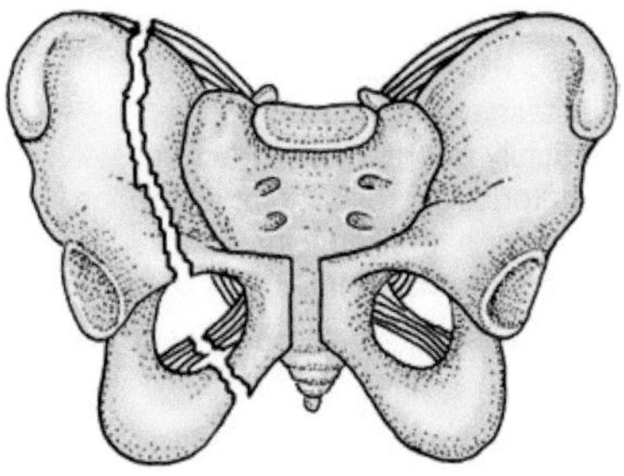

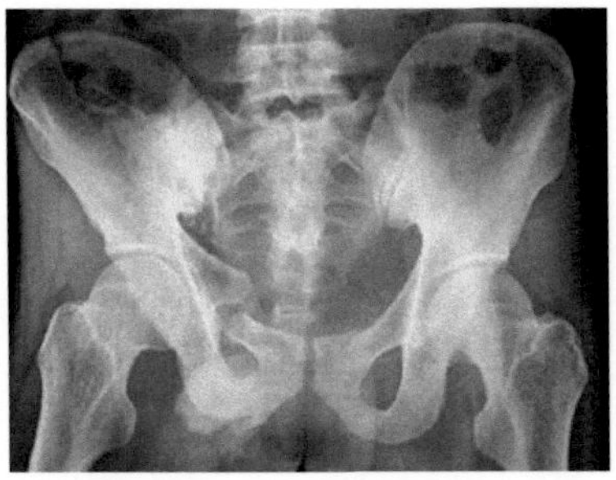

Vertical shear (VS):
Type VS-II Vertical pubic rami fractures, vertical displacement, and an iliac fracture

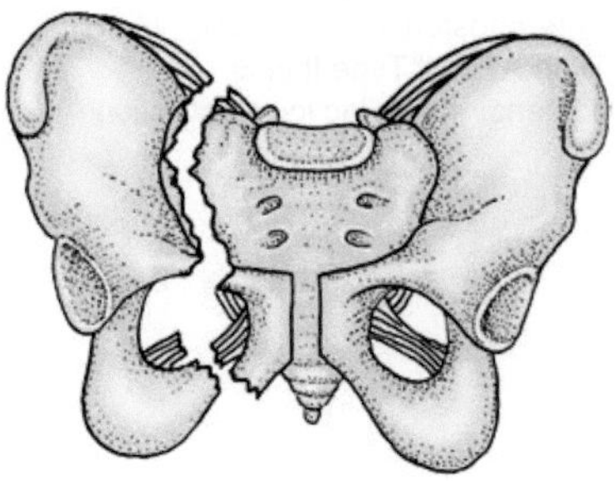

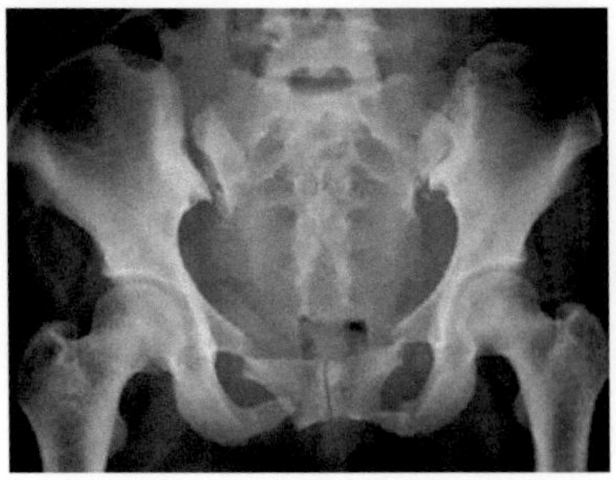

Vertical shear (VS):
Type VS-III Vertical pubic rami fractures,
vertical displacement,sacroiliac joint disruption, and a sacral fracture

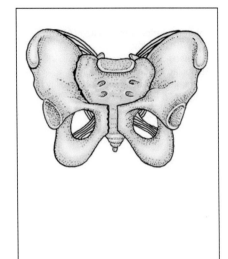

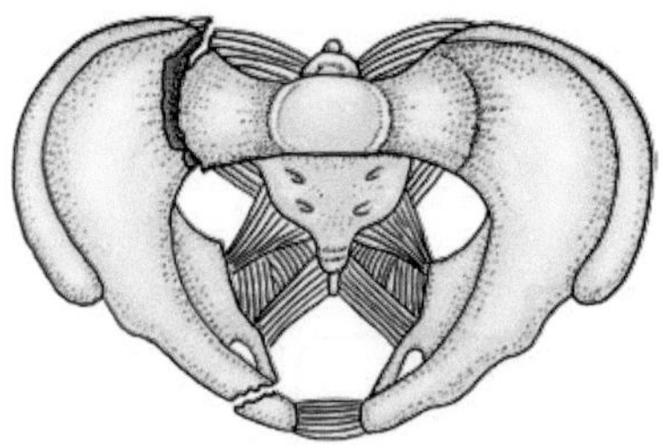

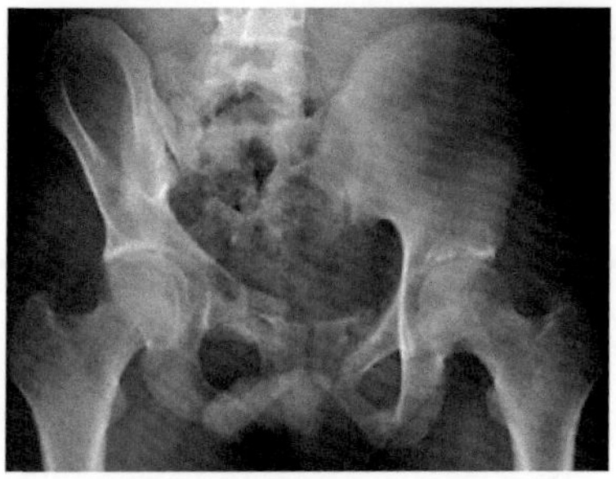

Combined mechanism
(CM):
Type CM-I Anterolateral force

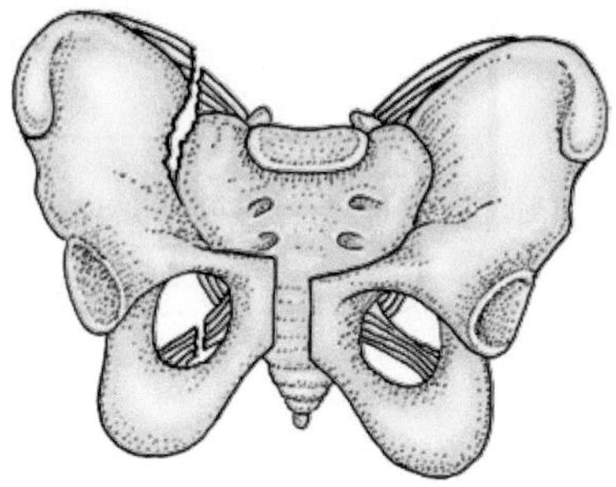

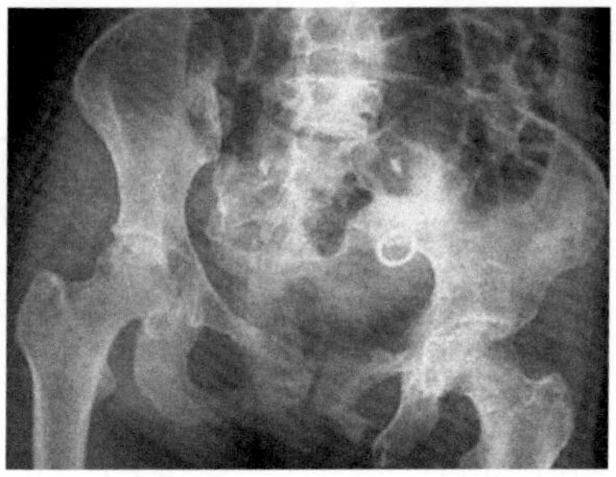

Combined mechanism
(CM):
Type CM-II
Anterovertical force

7.1.3 AO/OTA Classification (Journal of Orthopaedic Trauma, 21 Supplement)

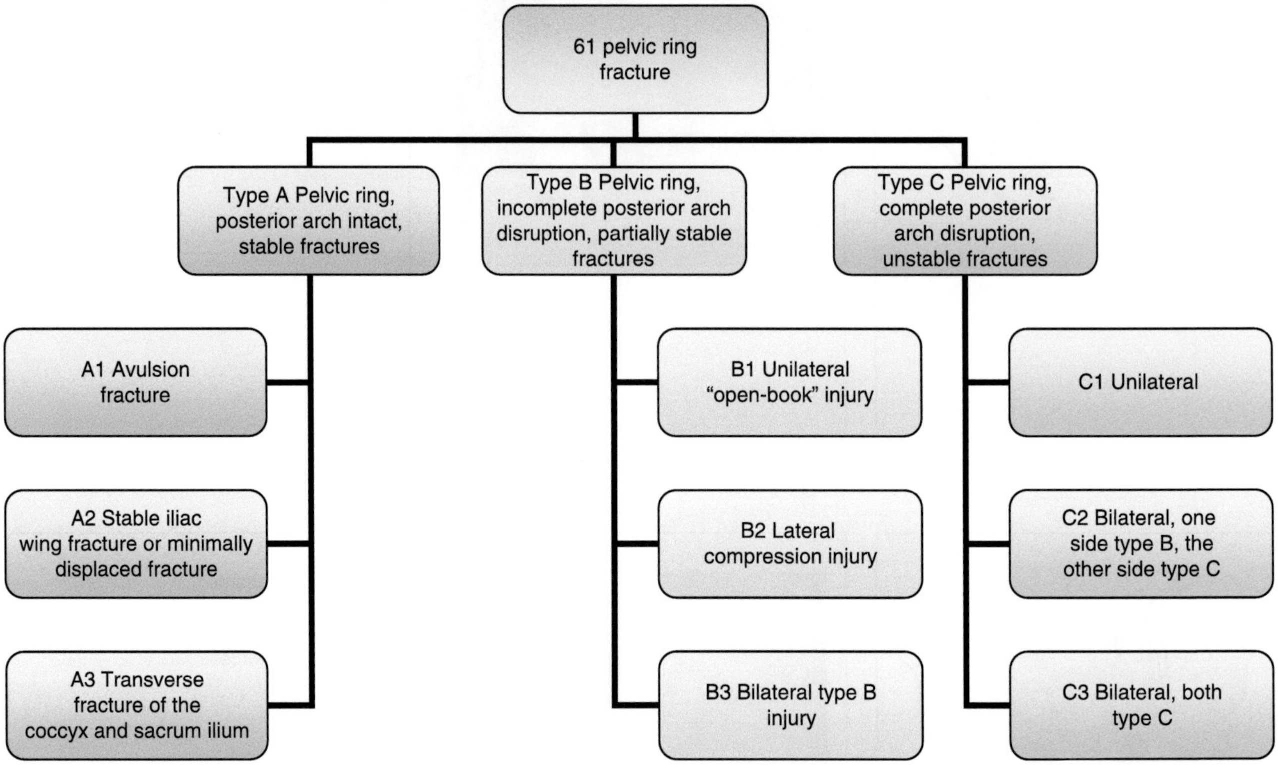

61-A Pelvic ring, posterior arch intact, stable fractures
- A1: Avulsion fracture:
  - A1.1: Fracture involving the anterior superior iliac spine, anterior inferior iliac spine, or pubic spine.
  - A1.2: Iliac crest.
  - A1.3: Ischial tuberosity.
- A2: Stable iliac wing fracture or minimally displaced fracture of the pelvic ring, as a result of a direct blow to the ilium:
  - A2.1: Iliac wing fracture, with one or more fragments.
  - A2.2: Unilateral pubic rami fracture.
  - A2.3: Bilateral pubic rami fracture.
- A3: Transverse fracture of the coccyx and sacrum:
  - A3.1: Sacrococcygeal dislocation.
  - A3.2: Non-displaced sacral fracture.
  - A3.3: Displaced sacral fracture.

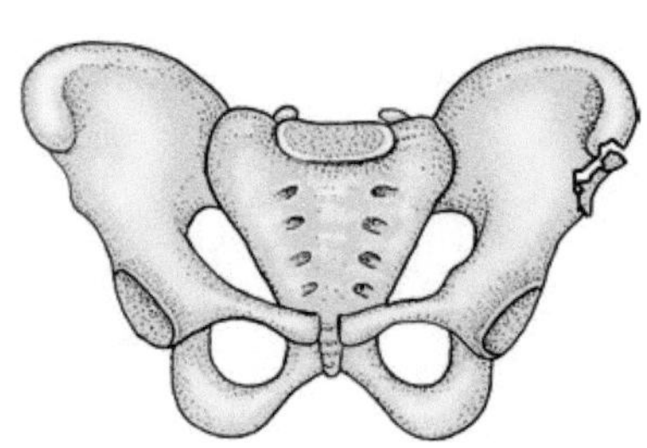

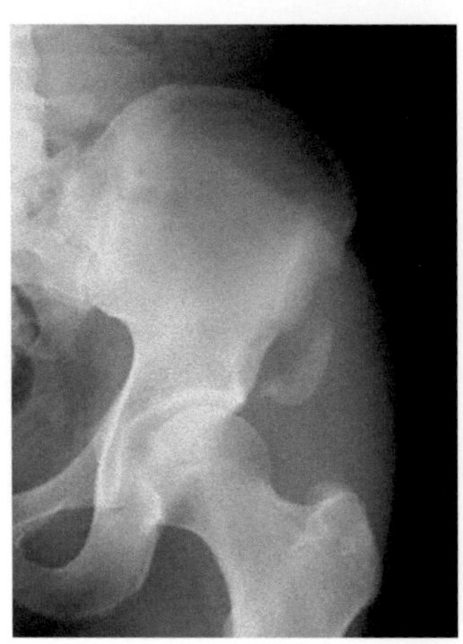

61-A Pelvic ring, posterior arch intact, stable fractures
A1: Avulsion fracture
A1.1: Fracture involving the anterior superior iliac spine, anterior inferior iliac spine, or pubic spine

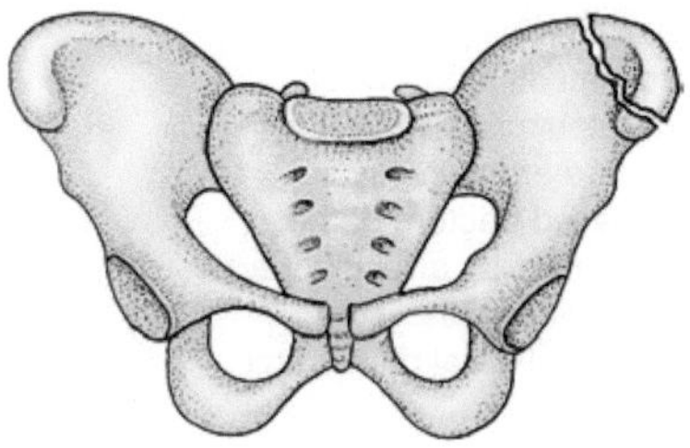

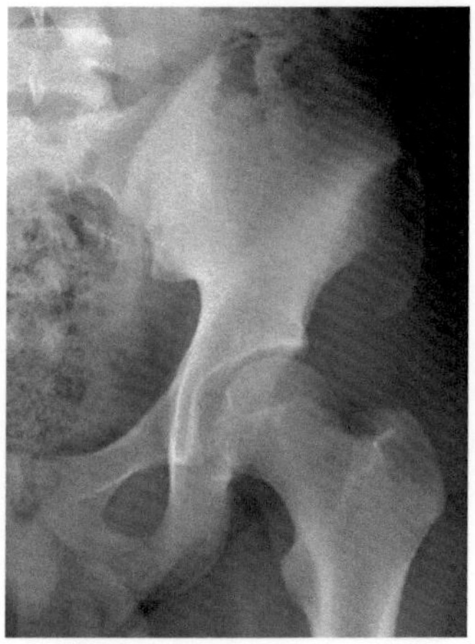

61-A Pelvic ring, posterior arch intact, stable fractures
A1: Avulsion fracture
A1.2: Iliac crest

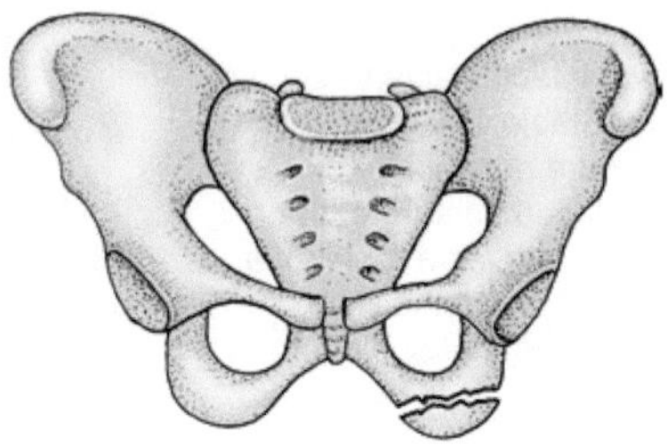

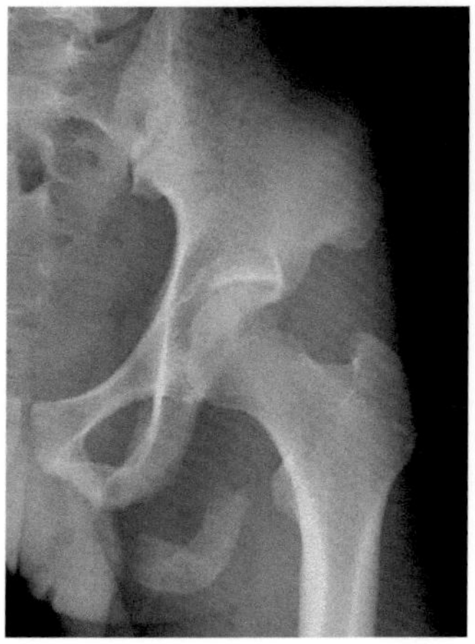

61-A Pelvic ring, posterior arch intact, stable fractures
A1: Avulsion fracture
A1.3: Ischial tuberosity

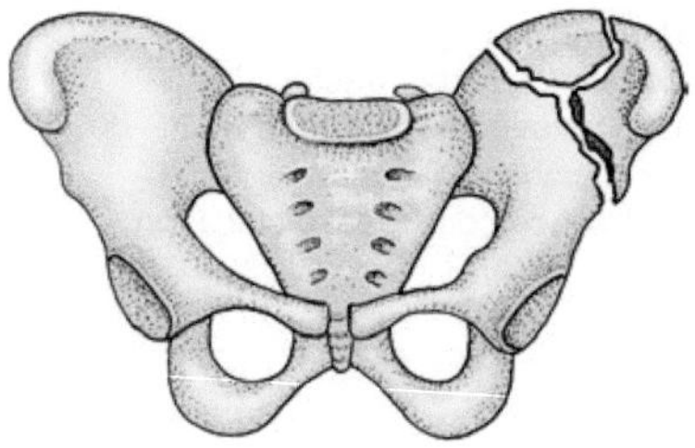

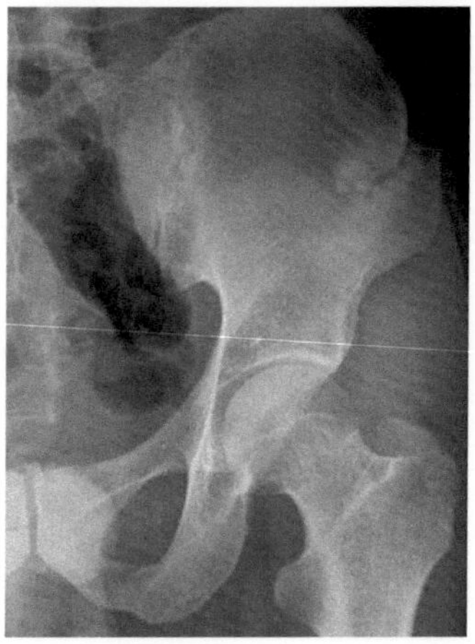

61-A Pelvic ring, posterior arch intact, stable fractures
A2: Stable iliac wing fracture or minimally displaced fracture of the pelvic ring, as a result of a direct blow to the ilium
A2.1: Iliac wing fracture, with one or more fragments

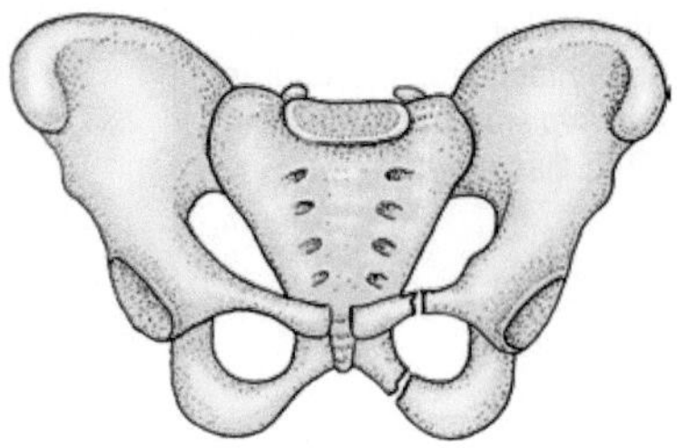

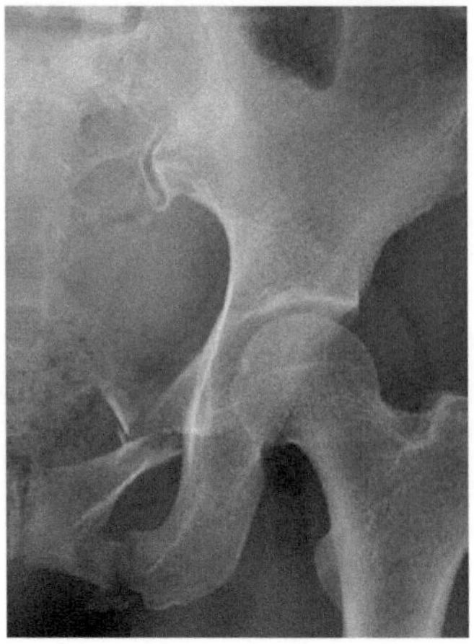

61-A Pelvic ring, posterior arch intact, stable fractures
A2: Stable iliac wing fracture or minimally displaced fracture of the pelvic ring, as a result of a direct blow to the ilium
A2.2: Unilateral pubic rami fracture

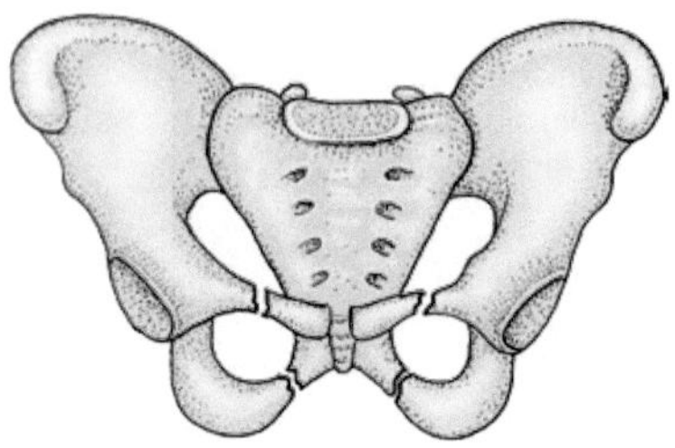

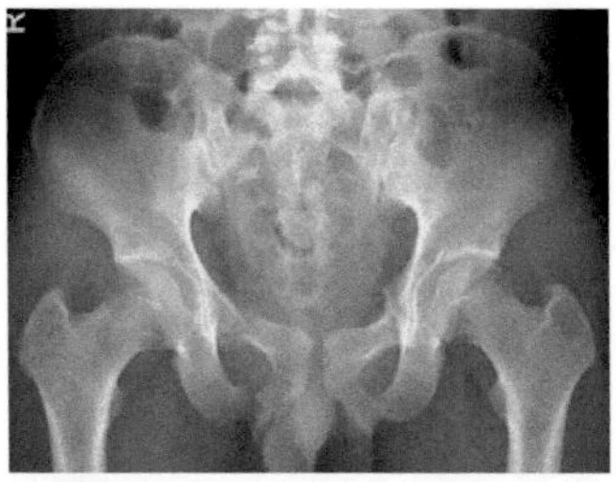

61-A Pelvic ring, posterior arch intact, stable fractures
A2: Stable iliac wing fracture or minimally displaced fracture of the pelvic ring, as a result of a direct blow to the ilium
A2.3: Bilateral pubic rami fracture

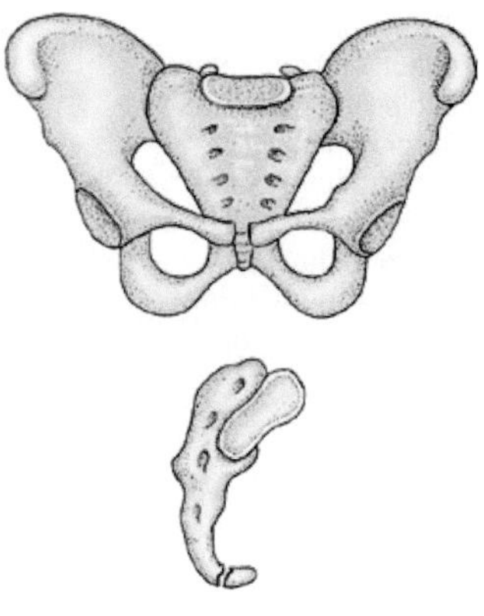

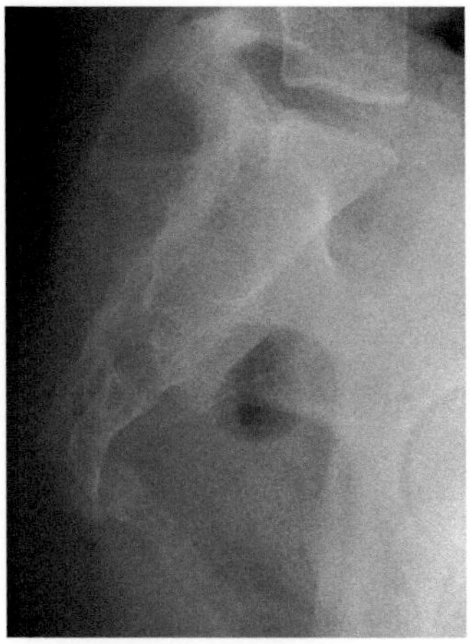

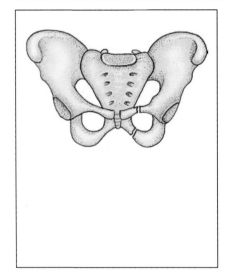

61-A Pelvic ring, posterior arch intact, stable fractures
A3: Transverse fracture of the coccyx and sacrum
A3.1: Sacrococcygeal dislocation

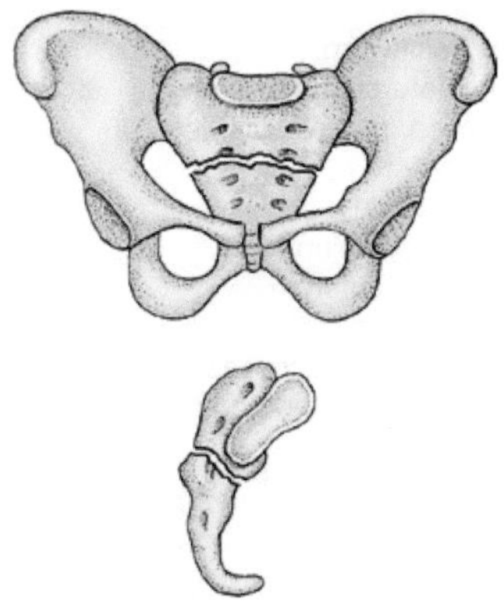

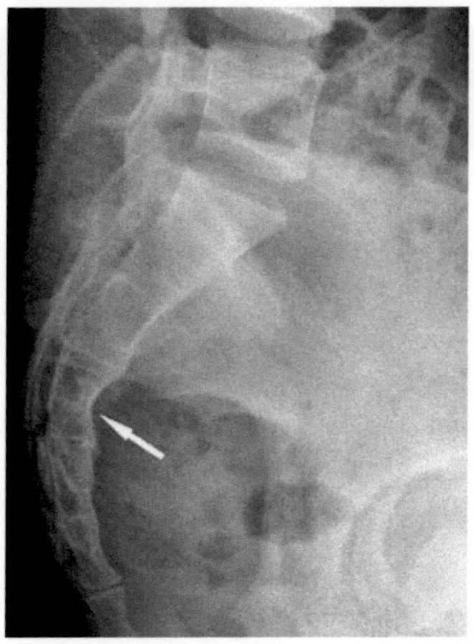

61-A Pelvic ring, posterior arch intact, stable fractures
A3: Transverse fracture of the coccyx and sacrum
A3.2: Nondisplaced sacral fracture

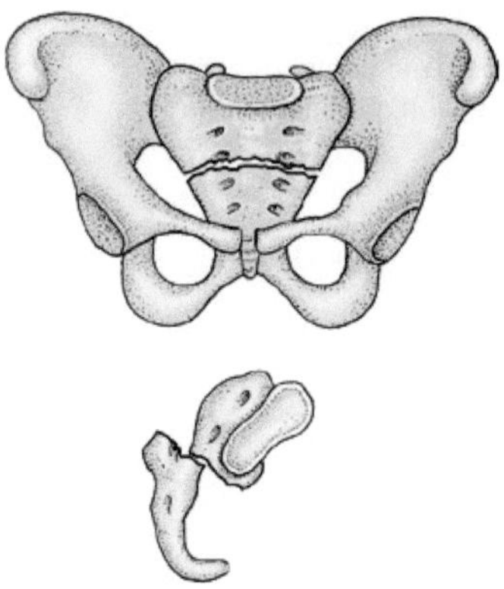

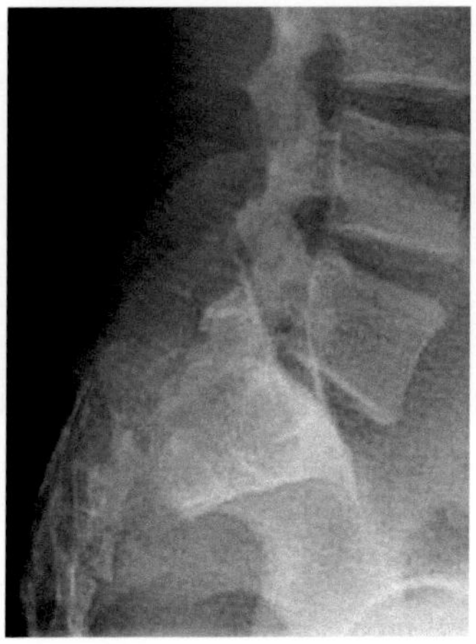

61-A Pelvic ring, posterior arch intact, stable fractures
A3: Transverse fracture of the coccyx and sacrum
A3.3: Displaced sacral fracture

61-B: Pelvic ring, incomplete posterior arch disruption, partially stable fractures:

- B1: Unilateral "open-book" injury (external rotational instability):
  - B1.1: Anterior sacroiliac joint disruption and A injury.
  - B1.2: Sacral fracture and A injury.
- B2: Lateral compression injury (internal rotational instability):
  - B2.1: Ipsilateral, anterior sacral buckle fracture, and A injury.
  - B2.2: Contralateral, partial sacroiliac joint fracture/subluxation (bucket-handle) and A injury.
  - B2.3: Incomplete posterior iliac fracture and A injury.
- B3: Bilateral type B injury:
  - B3.1: Bilateral type B1 injury.
  - B3.2: One side type B1 injury, the other side type B2 injury.
  - B3.3: Bilateral type B2 injury.

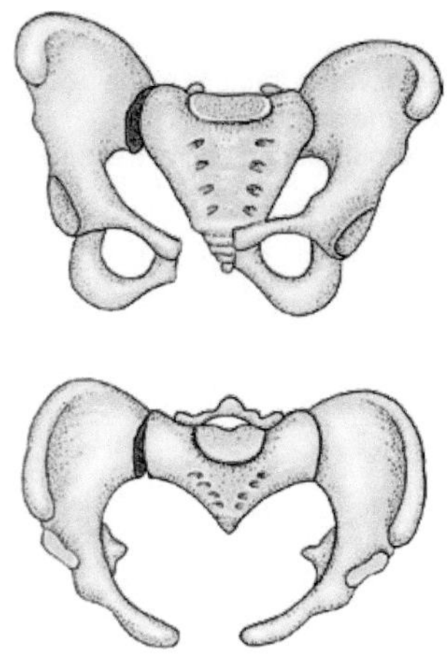

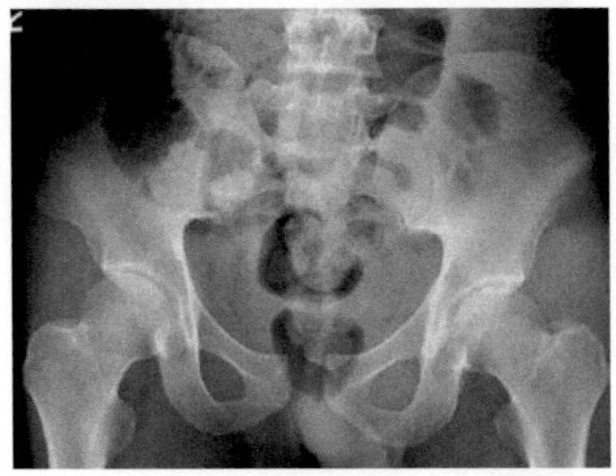

61-B Pelvic ring, incomplete posterior arch disruption, partially stable fractures
B1: Unilateral "open-book" injury (external rotational instability)
B1.1: Anterior sacroiliac joint disruption and A injury

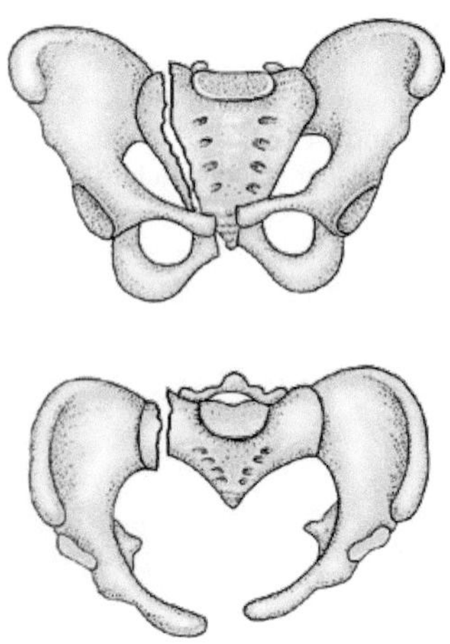

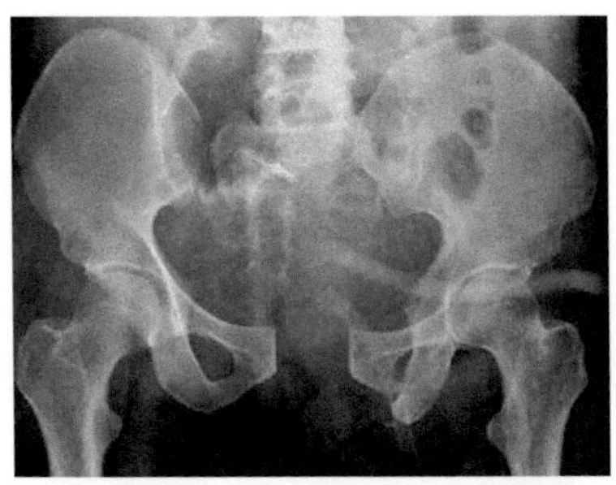

61-B Pelvic ring, incomplete posterior arch disruption, partially stable fractures
B1: Unilateral "open-book" injury (external rotational instability)
B1.2: Sacral fracture and A injury

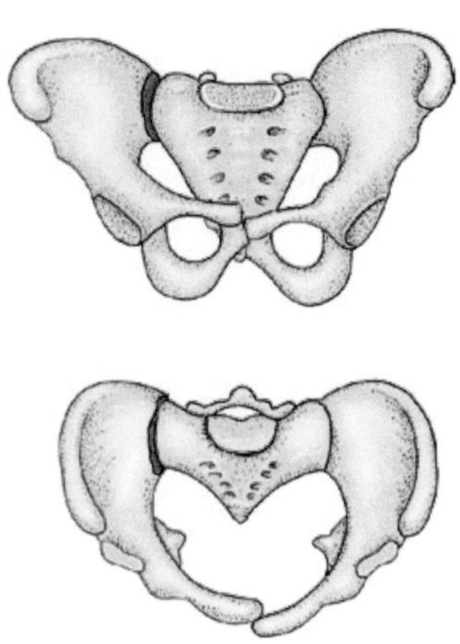

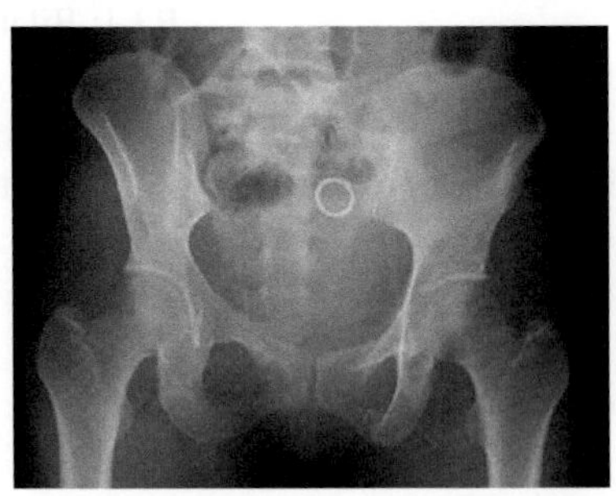

61-B Pelvic ring, incomplete posterior arch disruption, partially stable fractures
B2: Lateral compression injury(internal rotational instability)
B2.1: Ipsilateral, anterior sacral buckle fracture and A injury

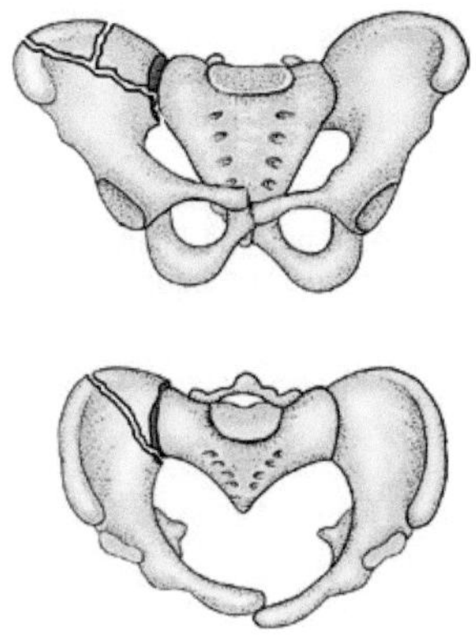

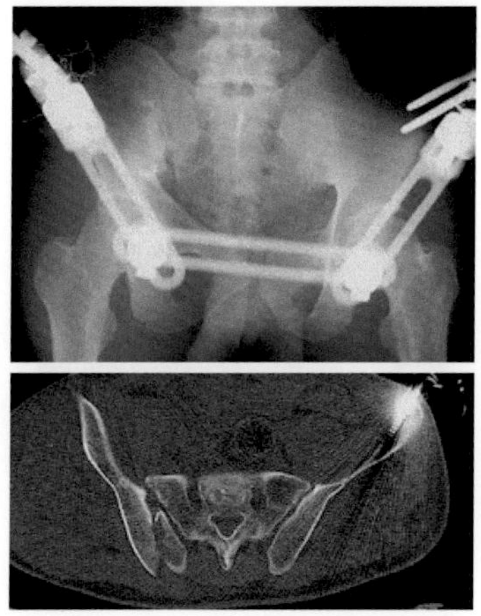

61-B Pelvic ring, incomplete posterior arch disruption, partially stable fractures
B2: Lateral compression injury (internal rotational instability)
B2.2: Contralateral, partial sacroiliac joint fracture/subluxation (bucket-handle) and A injury

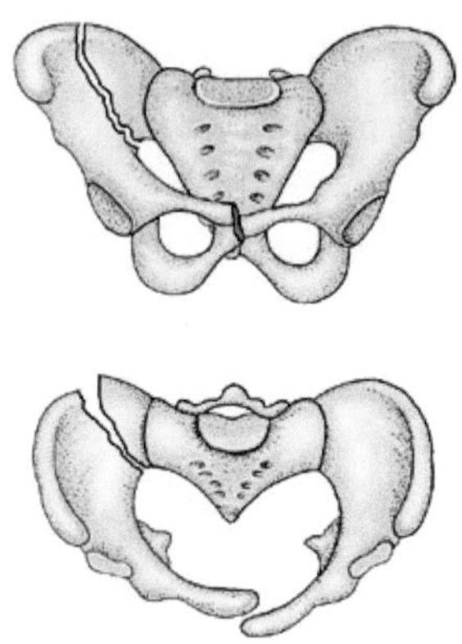

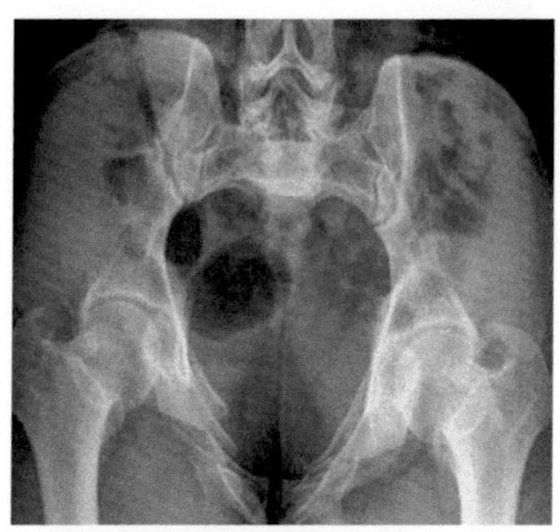

61-B Pelvic ring, incomplete posterior arch disruption, partially stable fractures
B2: Lateral compression injury(internal rotational instability)
B2.3: Incomplete posterior iliac fracture and A injury

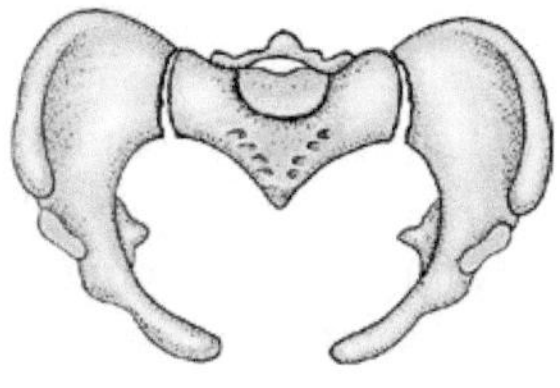

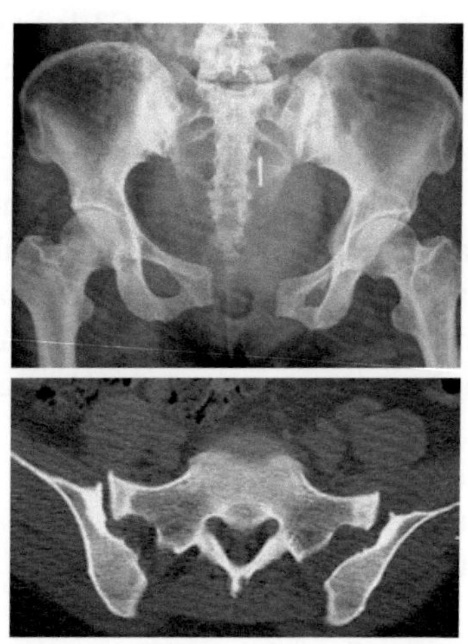

61-B Pelvic ring, incomplete posterior arch disruption, partially stable fractures
B3: Bilateral type B injury
B3.1: Bilateral type B1 injury

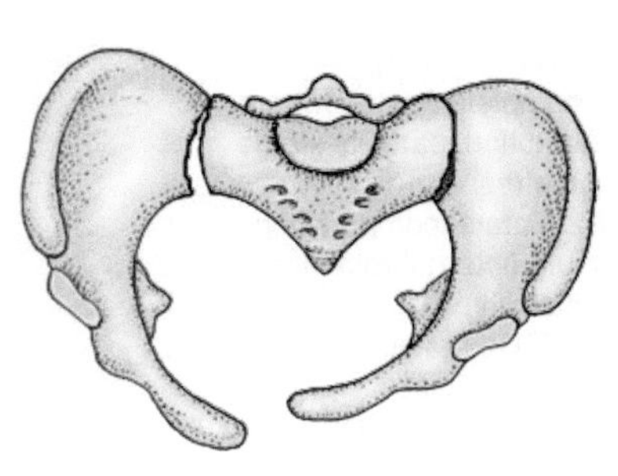

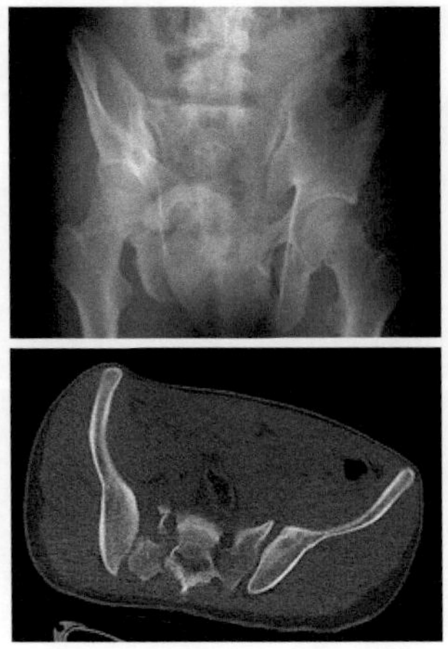

61-B Pelvic ring, incomplete posterior arch disruption, partially stable fractures
B3: Bilateral type B injury
B3.2: One side type B1 injury, the other side type B2 injury

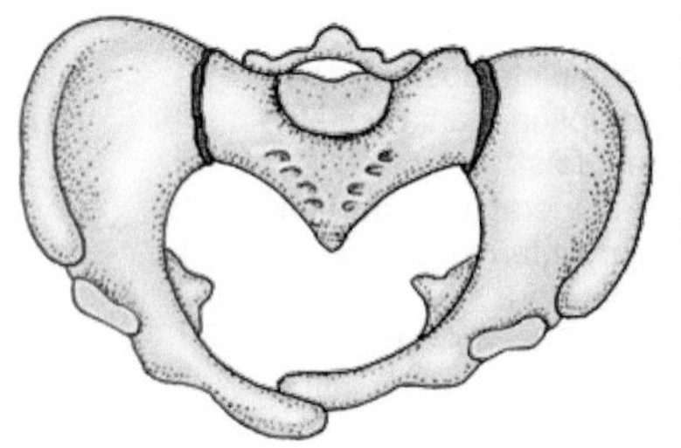

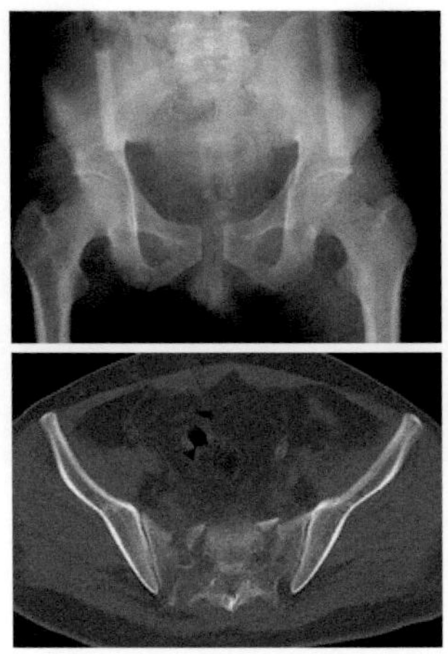

61-B Pelvic ring, incomplete posterior arch disruption, partially stable fractures
B3: Bilateral type B injury
B3.3: Bilateral type B2 injury

61-C: Pelvic ring, complete posterior arch disruption, unstable fractures:
- C1: Unilateral:
  - C1.1: Fracture of ilium and A injury.
  - C1.2: Sacroiliac dislocation or fracture dislocation and A injury.
  - C1.3: Fracture of the sacrum (lateral, medial, or through the sacral foramina) and A injury.
- C2: Bilateral, one side type B, the other side type C:
  - C2.1: Ipsilateral C1 lesion through the ilium, contralateral B1 or B2 injury, and A injury.
  - C2.2: Ipsilateral C1 lesion through the sacroiliac joint (transiliac fracture dislocation, pure dislocation, transsacral fracture dislocation), contralateral B1 or B2 injury, and A injury.
  - C2.3: Ipsilateral C1 lesion through the sacrum (lateral, medial, or through the sacral foramina) contralateral B1 or B2 injury and A injury.
- C3: Bilateral, both type C:
  - C3.1: Extrasacral on both sides (ilium, transiliac sacroiliac joint fracture/dislocation, transsacral sacroiliac joint fracture/dislocation, sacroiliac joint dislocation).
  - C3.2: One side C1 lesion through the sacrum (lateral, medial, or through the sacral foramina), the other side extrasacral lesion and A injury.
  - C3.3: Sacral lesion on both sides (lateral, medial, or through the sacral foramina) and A injury.

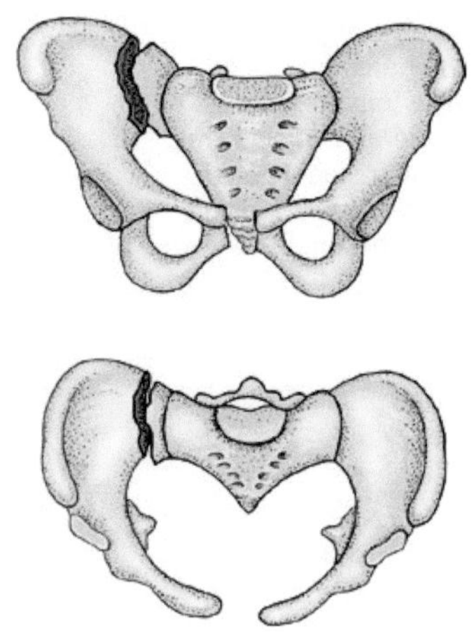

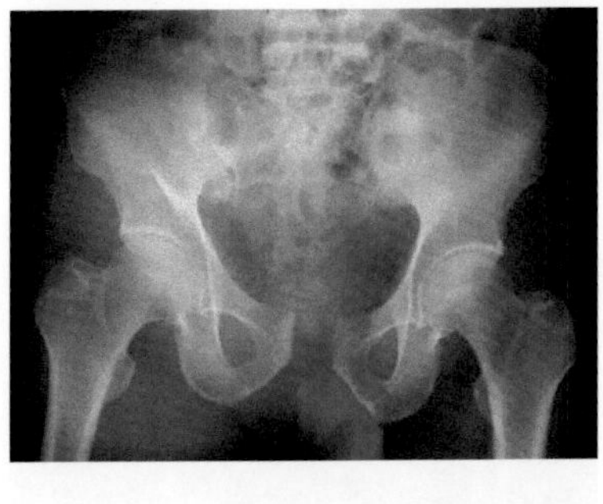

61-C Pelvic ring,
complete posterior arch
disruption,
unstable fractures
C1: Unilateral
C1.1: Fracture of ilium and
A injury

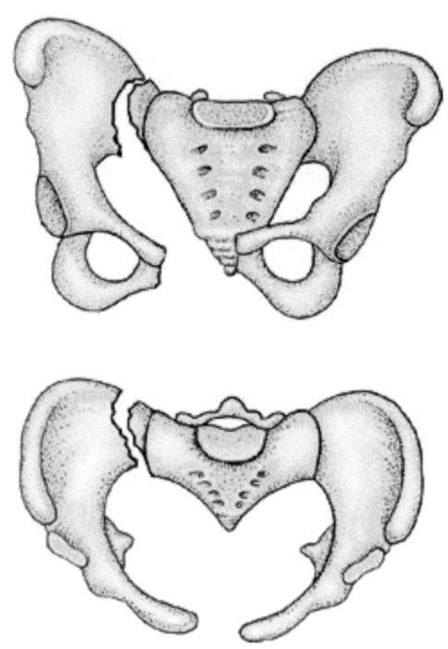

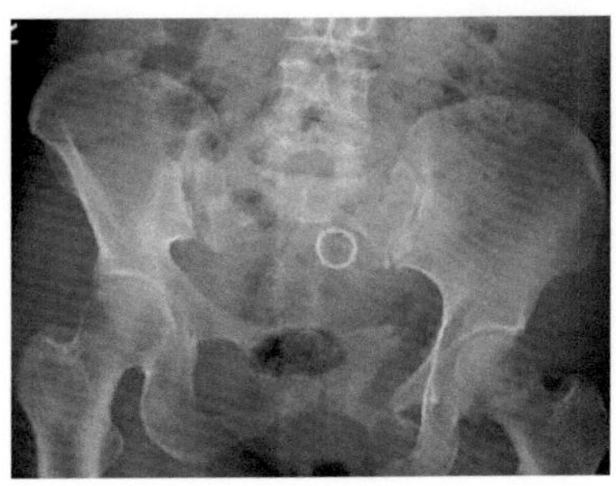

61-C Pelvic ring,
complete posterior arch
disruption,
unstable fractures
C1: Unilateral
C1.2: Sacroiliac dislocation
or fracture dislocation and
A injury

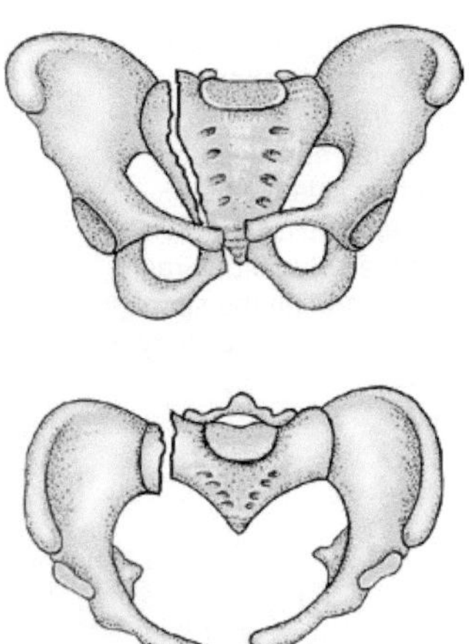

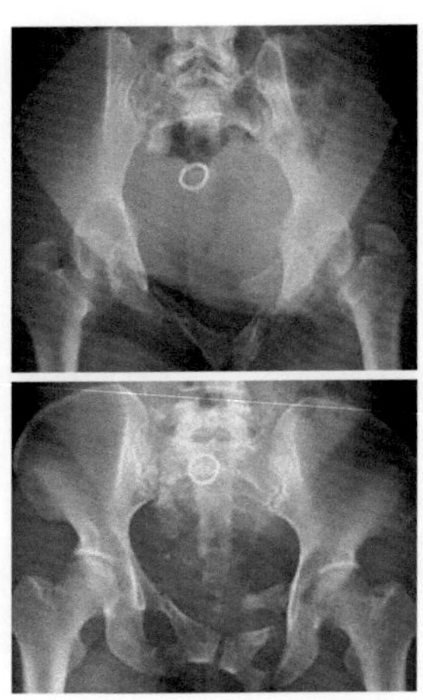

61-C Pelvic ring,
complete posterior arch disruption,
unstable fractures
C1: Unilateral
C1.3: Fracture of the
sacrum (lateral, medial, or
through the sacral
foramina) and A injury

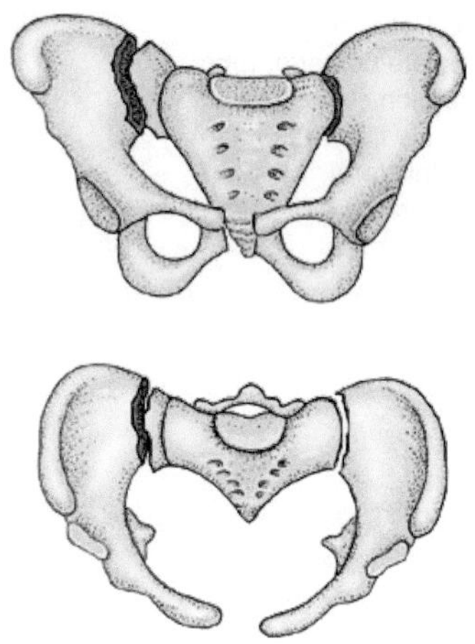

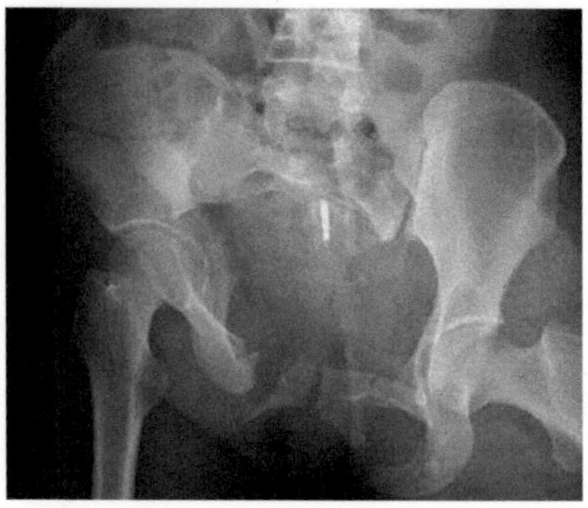

61-C Pelvic ring,complete posterior arch disruption, unstable fractures
C2: Bilateral, one side type B, the other side type C
C2.1: Ipsilateral C1 lesion through the ilium, contralateral B1 or B2 injury and A injury

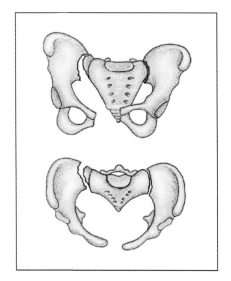

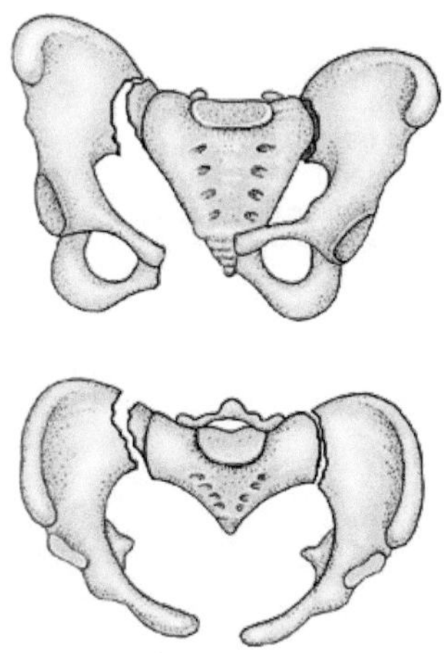

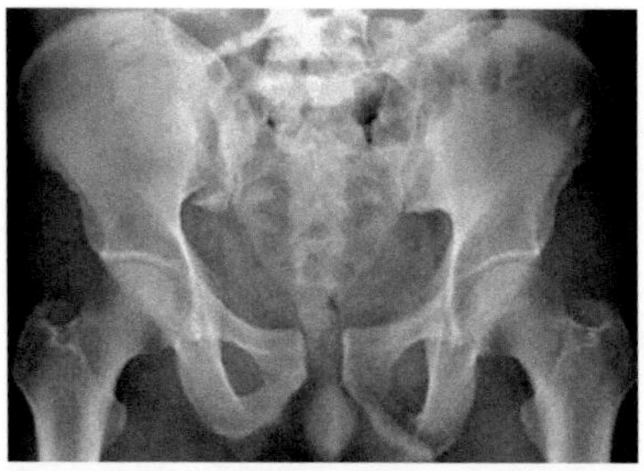

61-C Pelvic ring, complete posterior arch disruption, unstable fractures
C2: Bilateral, one side type B, the other side type C
C2.2: Ipsilateral C1 lesion through the sacroiliac joint (transiliac fracture dislocation, pure dislocation, transsacral fracture dislocation), contralateral B1 or B2 injury and A injury

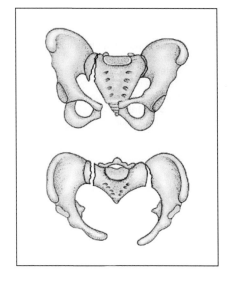

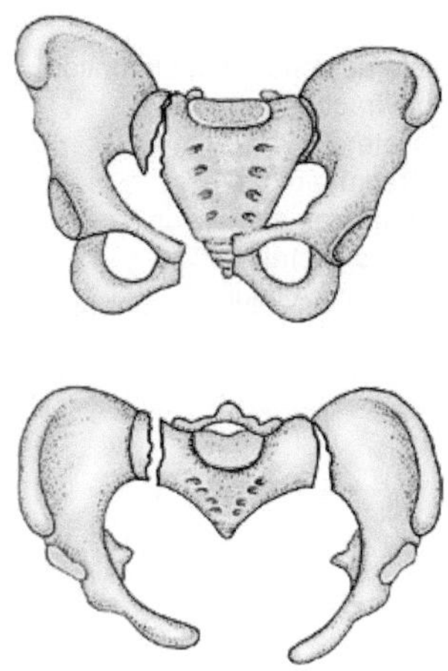

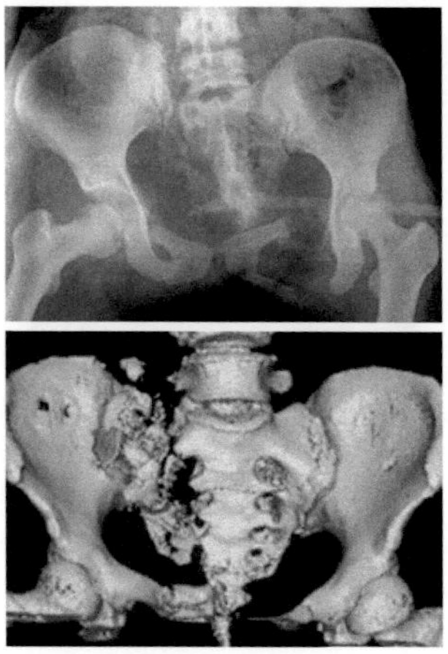

61-C Pelvic ring, complete posterior arch disruption, unstable fractures
C2: Bilateral, one side type B, the other side type C
C2.3: Ipsilateral C1 lesion through the sacrum (lateral, medial, or through the sacral foramina) contralateral B1 or B2 injury and A injury

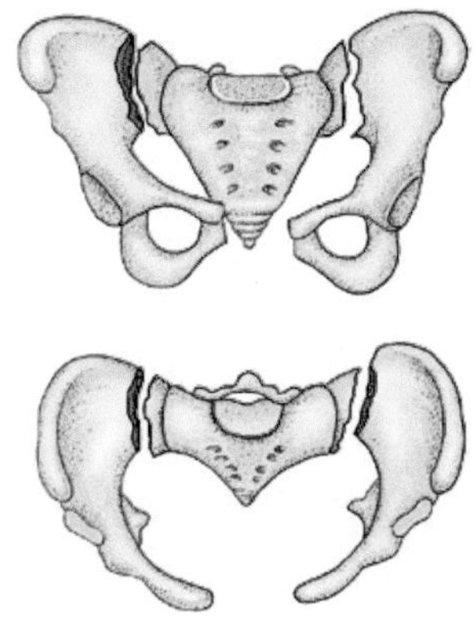

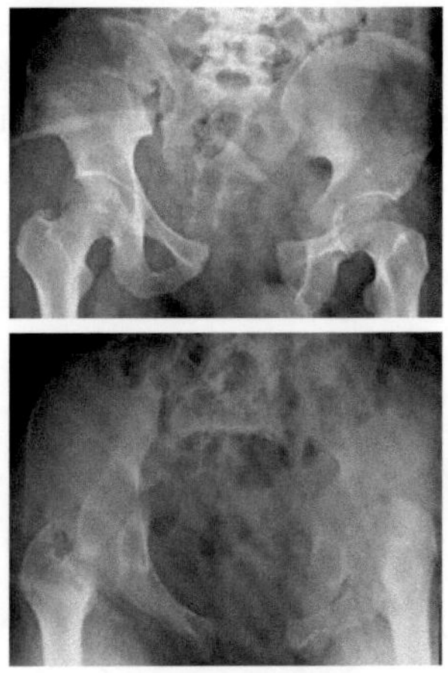

61-C Pelvic ring, complete
posterior arch disruption,
unstable fractures
C3: Bilateral, both type C
C3.1: Extrasacral on both
sides (ilium,transiliac sacroiliac
joint fracture/dislocation,
trans-sacral sacroiliac joint
fracture/dislocation,
Sacroiliac joint dislocation)

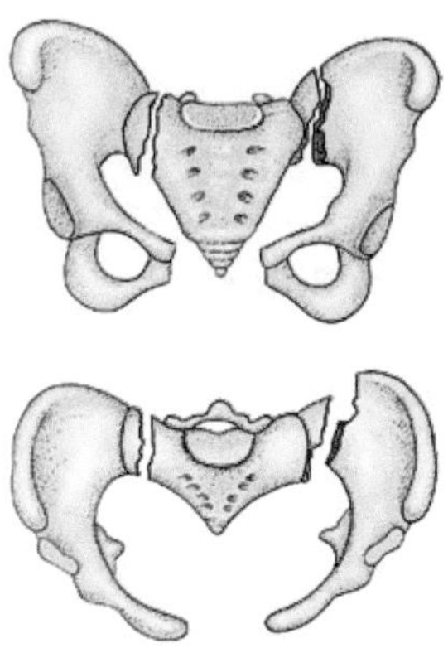

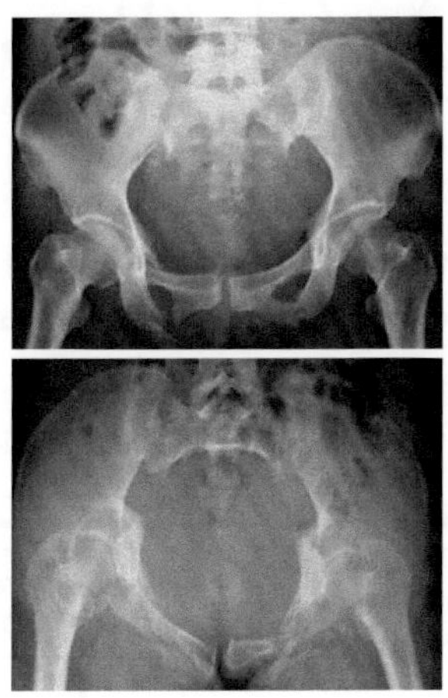

61-C Pelvic ring, complete
posterior arch disruption,
unstable fractures
C3: Bilateral, both type C
C3.2: One side C1 lesion
through the sacrum
(lateral,medial or through the
sacral foramina), the other
side extrasacral lesion and A injury

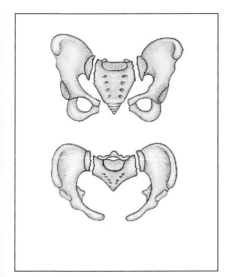

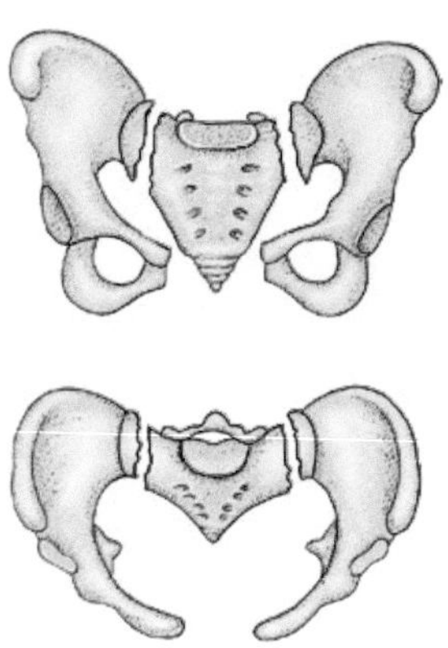

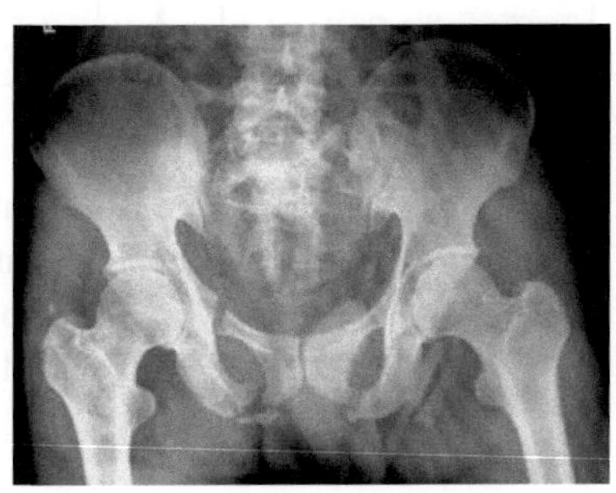

61-C Pelvic ring, complete
posterior arch disruption,
unstable fractures
C3: Bilateral, both type C
C3.3: Sacral lesion on both
sides (lateral, medial, or
through the sacral foramina) and A injury

7.1.4 Letournel Classification (1980, Clin Orthop, Relat Res, 151: 81–106)

Type A: Iliac wing fracture.
Type B: Iliac and partial sacroiliac joint fracture.
Type C: The sacral fracture.
Type D: Unilateral sacral fracture.
Type E: Sacroiliac joint fracture and dislocation.
Type F: Acetabulum fracture.
Type G: Pubic rami fracture.
Type H: Ischial fracture.
Type I: Pubic diastasis.

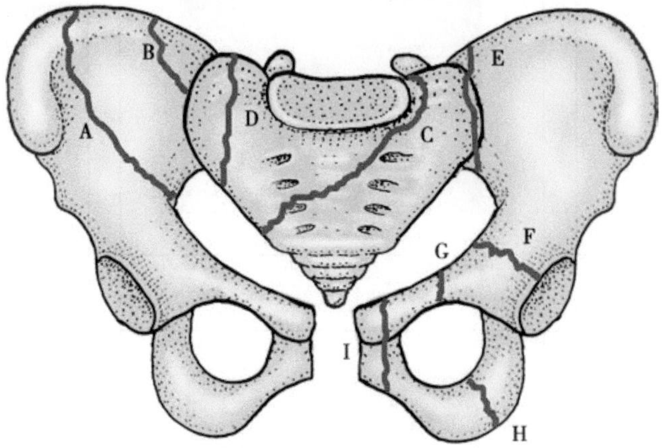

7.1.5 Pennal Classification (1961, Fractures of the pelvis (motion picture). Park Ridge, IL: American Academy of Orthopaedic Surgeons Film Library, 1961)

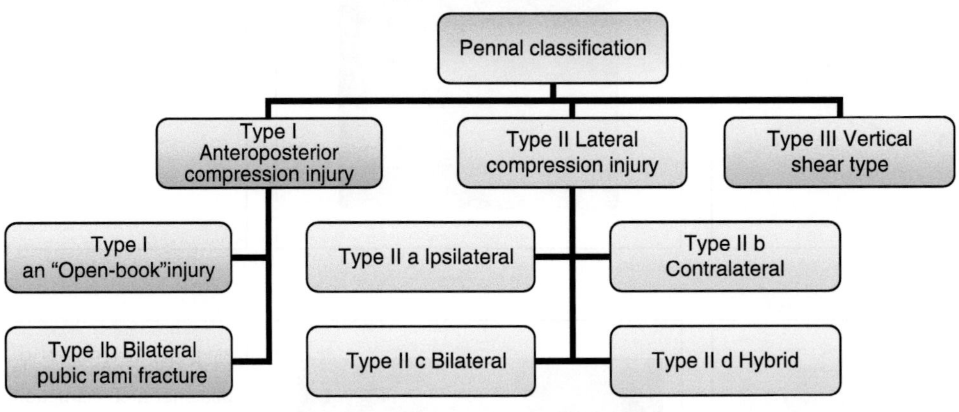

Type I: Anteroposterior compression injury:
- Type Ia: "Open-book" injury.
- Type Ib: Bilateral pubic rami fracture.

Type II: Lateral compression injury:
- Type IIa: Ipsilateral.
- Type IIb: Contralateral.
- Type IIc: Bilateral.
- Type IId: Hybrid.

Type III: Vertical shear type

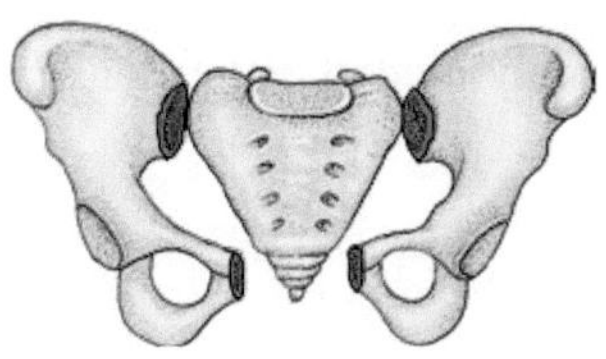

Type I a

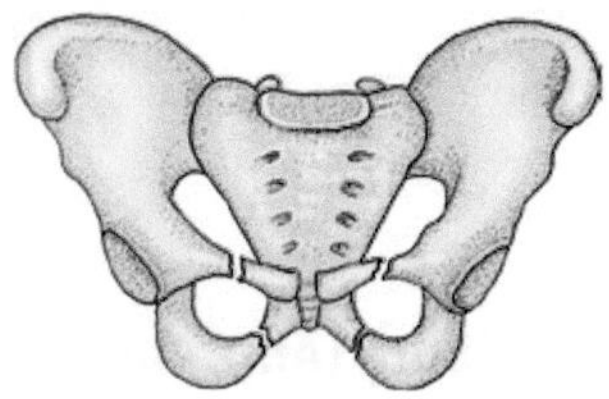

Type I b

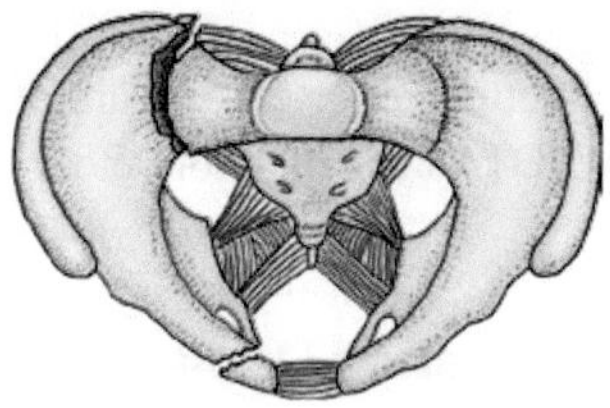

Type II a

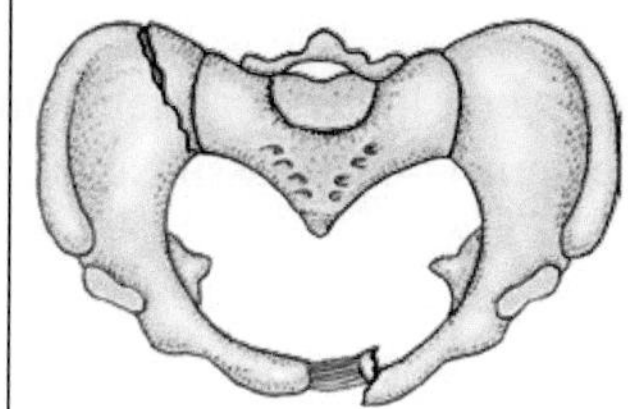

Type II b

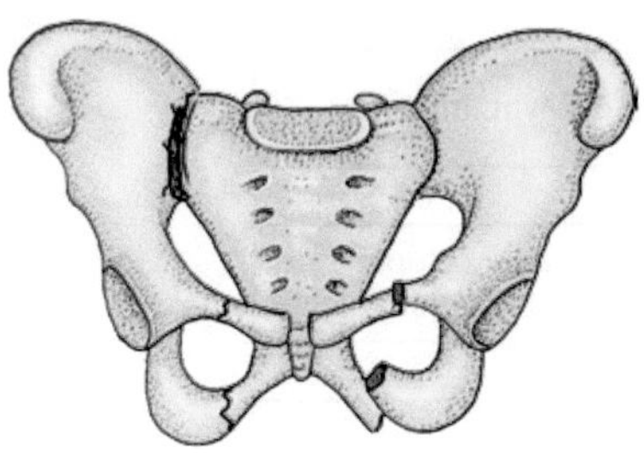

Type IIc

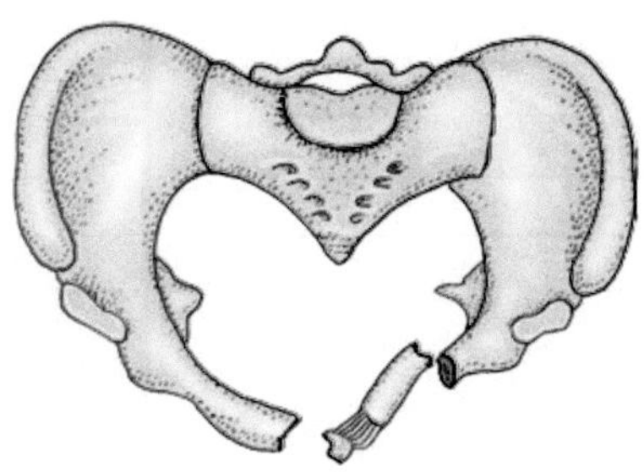

Type IId

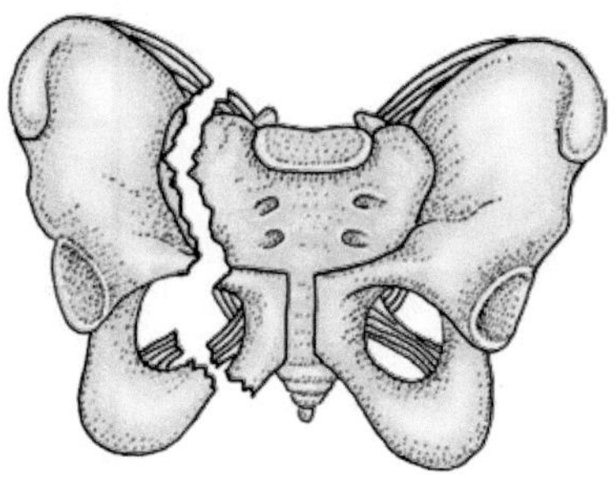

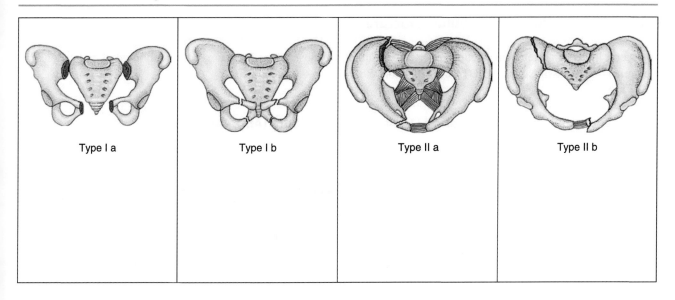

Type III

7.2 Classification of Acetabulum Fracture

In several kinds of acetabulum fracture reported 5 years at the most recent literature, commonly used classifications are Letournel-Judet classification, AO/OTA classification, etc.

7.2.1 Letournel-Judet Classification (1964, J Bone Joint Surg (Am), 46:1615)

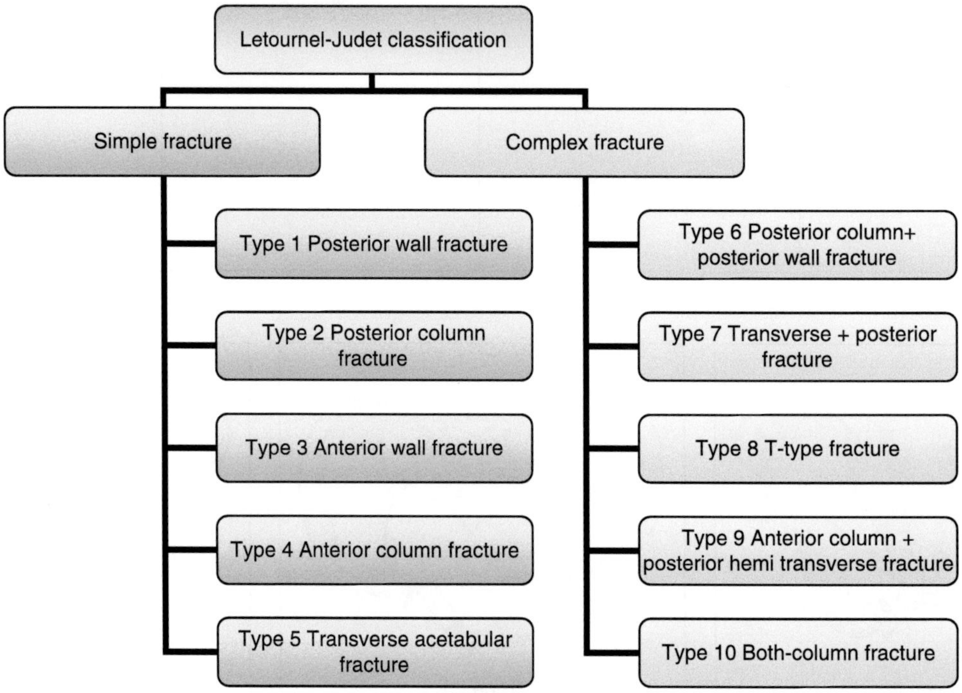

Simple fracture:
Type 1: Posterior wall fracture.
Type 2: Posterior column fracture.
Type 3: Anterior wall fracture.
Type 4: Anterior column fracture.
Type 5: Transverse acetabular fracture.

Complex fracture:
Type 6: Posterior column + posterior wall fracture.
Type 7: Transverse + posterior fracture.
Type 8: T-type fracture.
Type 9: Anterior column + posterior hemitransverse fracture.
Type 10: Both column fracture.

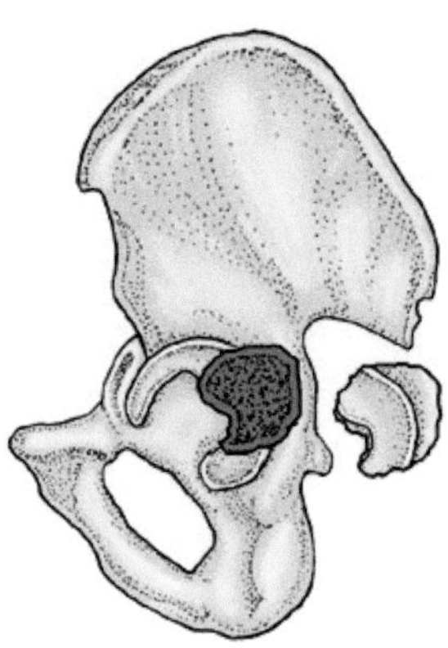

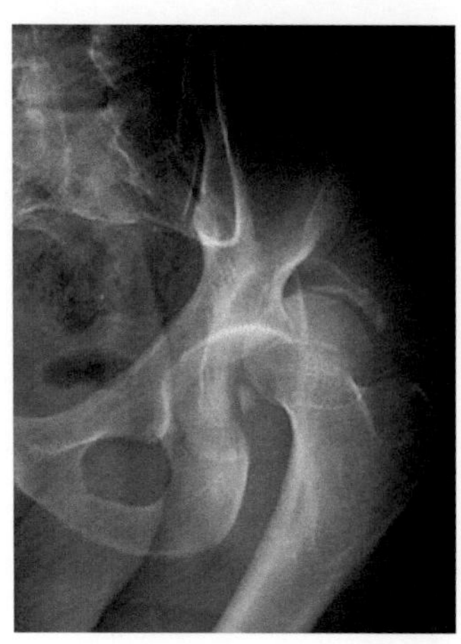

Simple fracture
Type 1: Posterior wall fracture

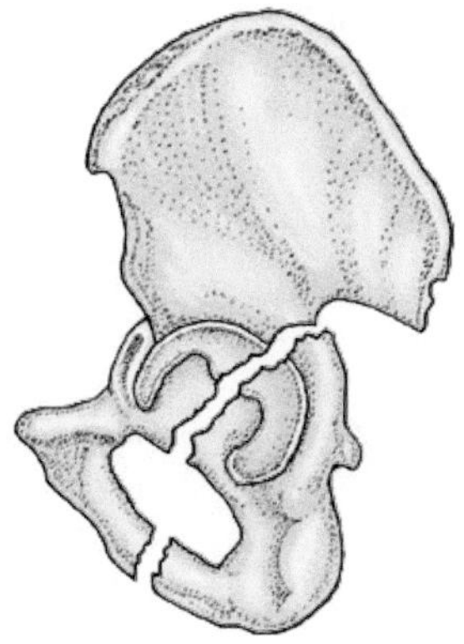

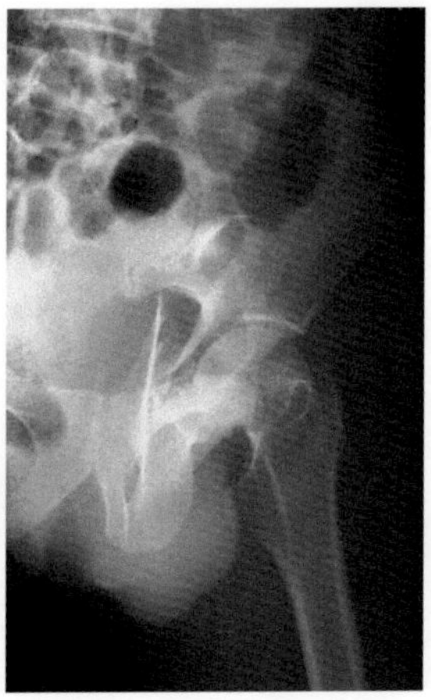

Simple fracture
Type 2: Posterior column fracture

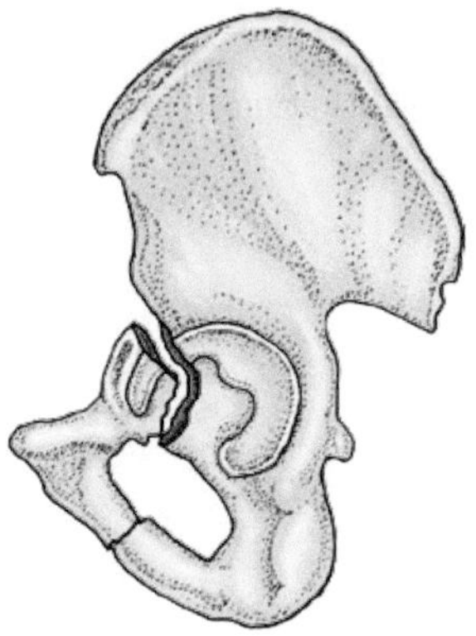

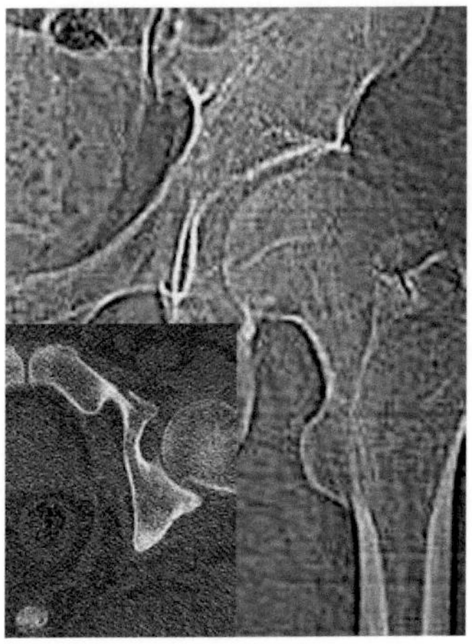

Simple fracture
Type 3: Anterior wall fracture

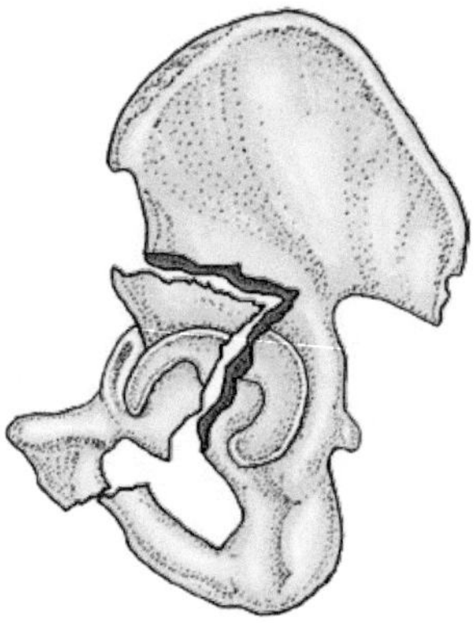

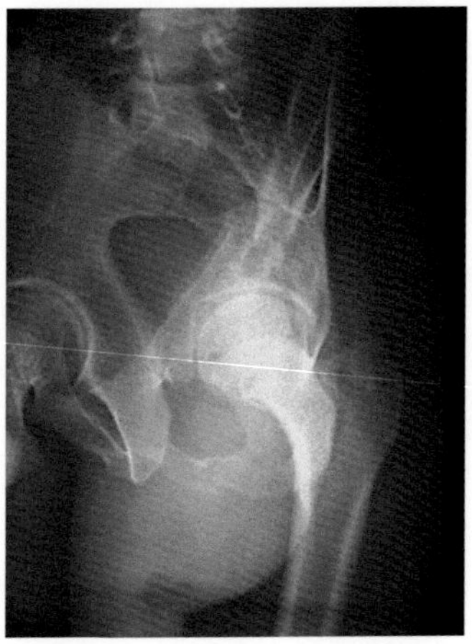

Simple fracture
Type 4: Anterior column fracture

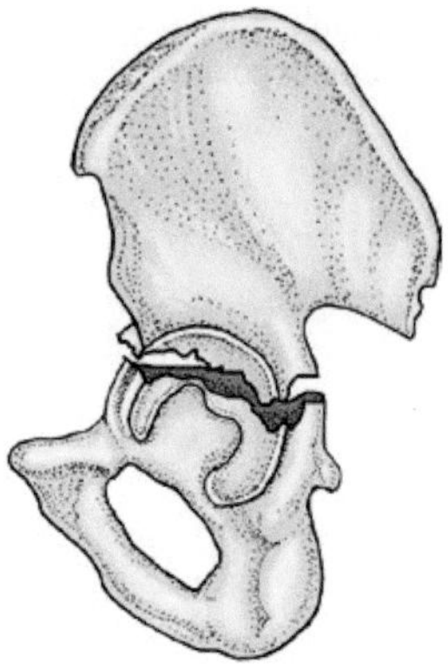

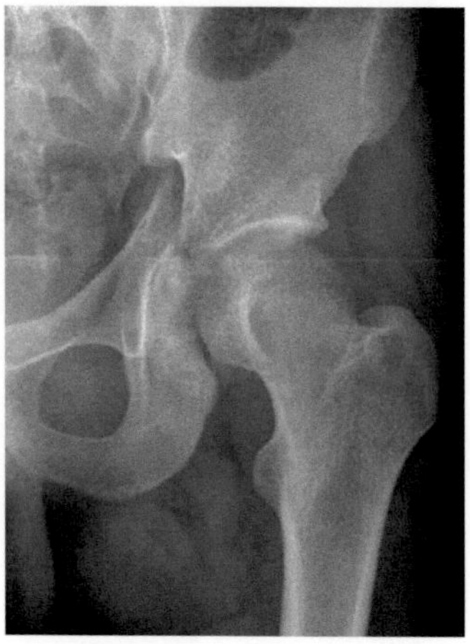

Simple fracture
Type 5: Transverse acetabular fracture

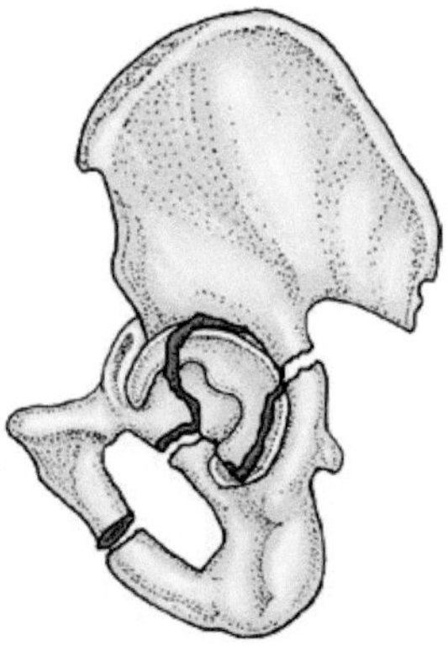

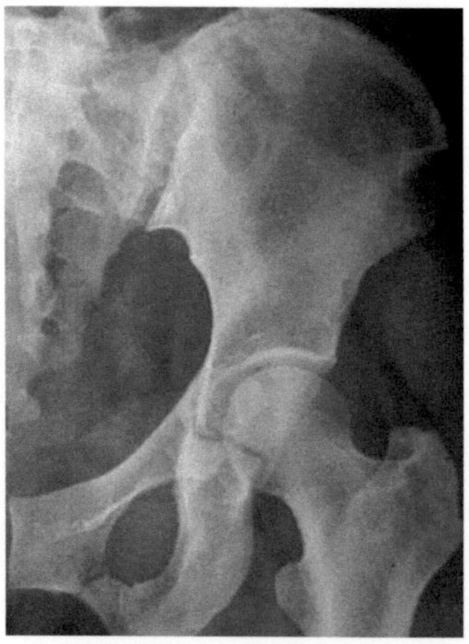

Complex fracture
Type 6: Posterior column+ posterior wall fracture

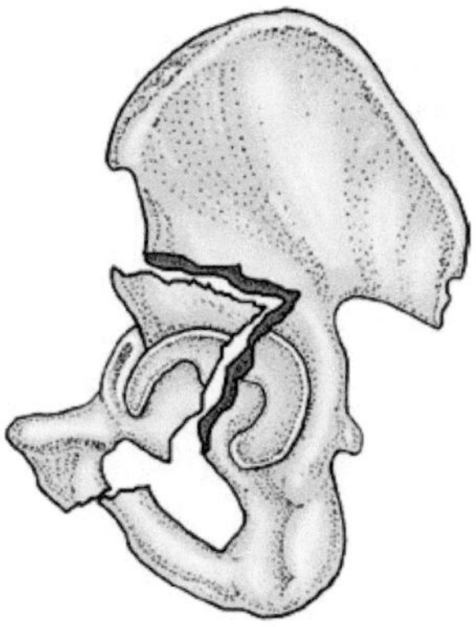

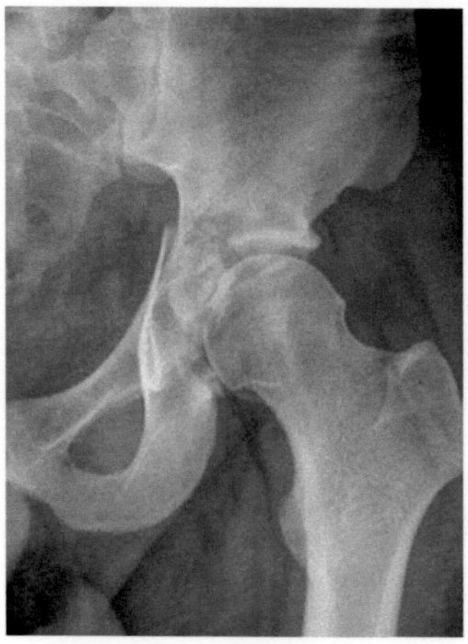

Complex fracture
Type 7: Transverse + posterior fracture

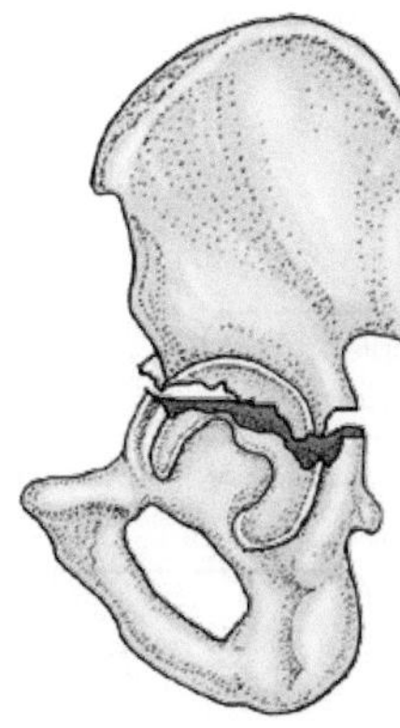

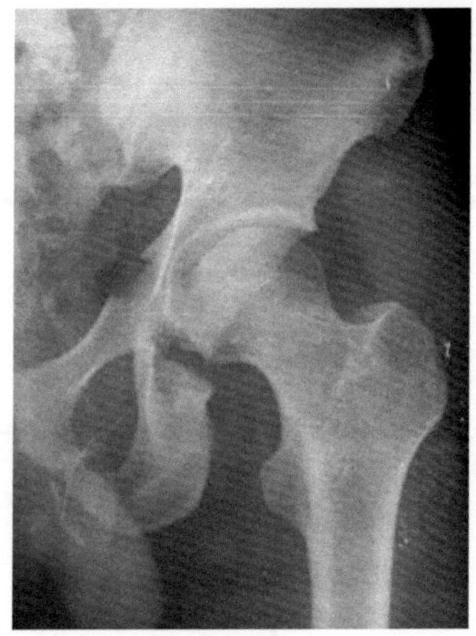

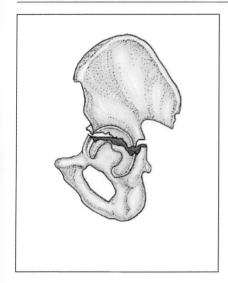

Complex fracture
Type 8: T-type fracture

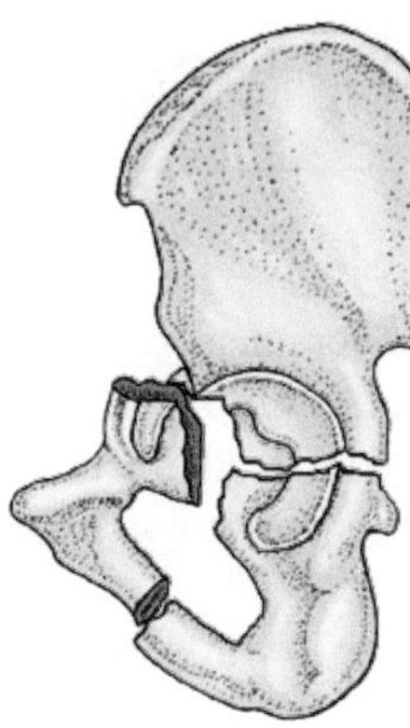

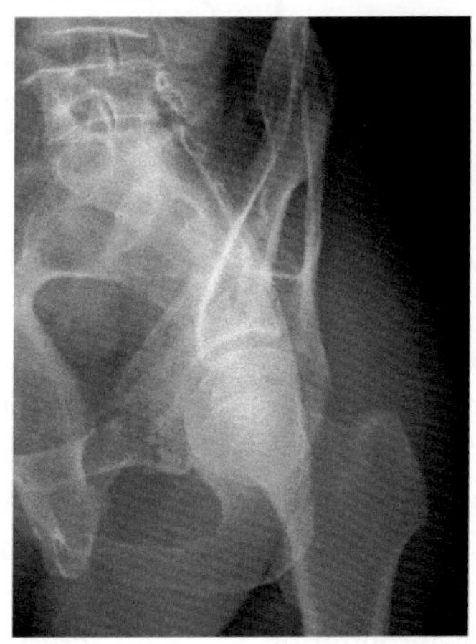

Complex fracture
Type 9: Anterior column +
posterior hemitransverse fracture

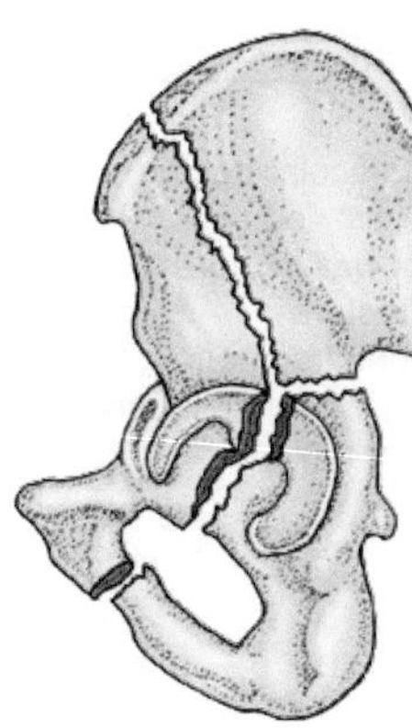

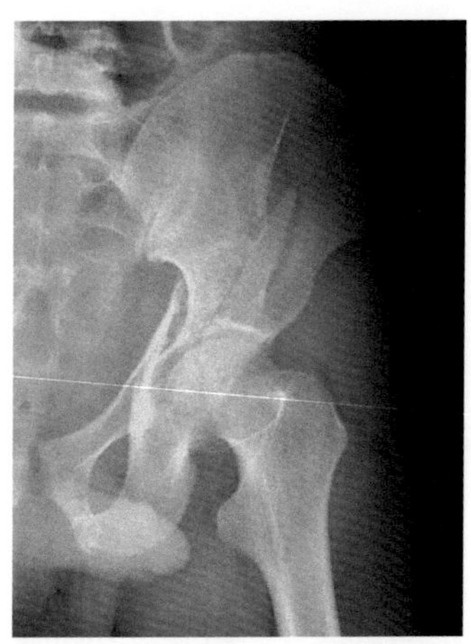

Complex fracture
Type 10: Both-column fracture

7.2.2 AO/OTA Classification (Journal of Orthopaedic Trauma, 21 Supplement)

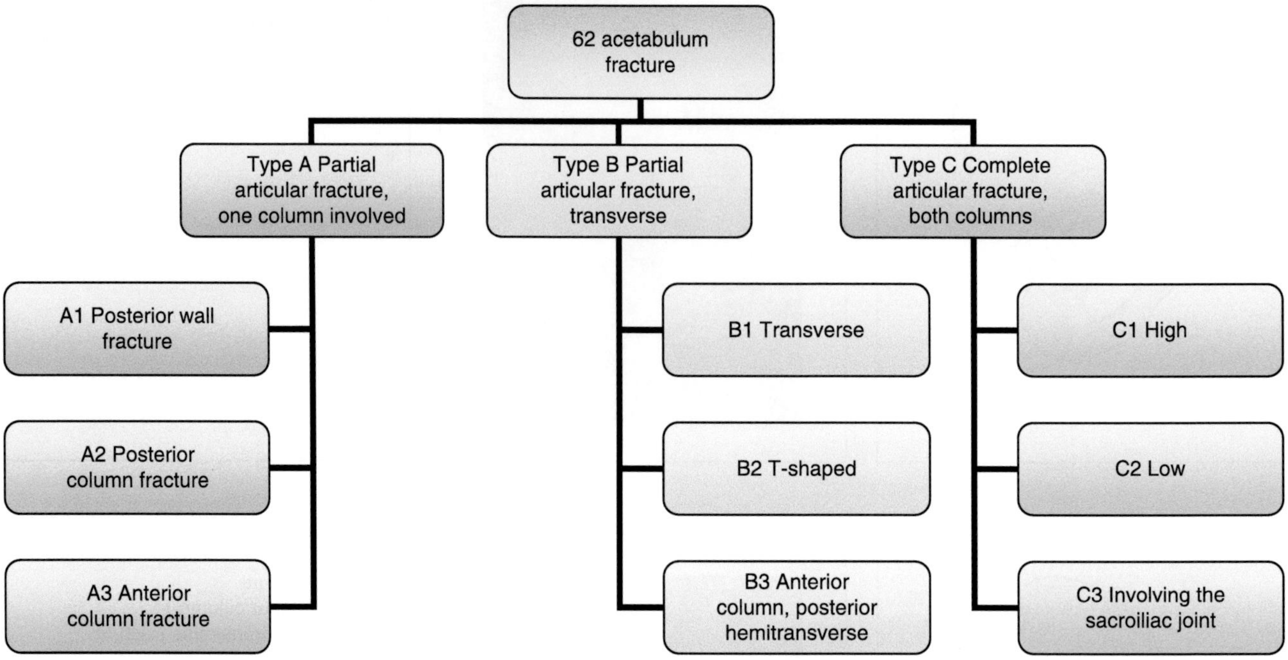

62-A: Partial articular fracture, one column involved

A1: Posterior wall fracture:

A1.1: Pure fracture dislocation, one fragment in the posterior, posterosuperior, or posteroinferior region.

A1.2: Pure fracture dislocation, multifragmentary in the posterior, posterosuperior, or posteroinferior region.

A1.3: Fracture dislocation, with marginal impaction in the posterior, posterosuperior, or posteroinferior region.

A2: Posterior column fracture:

A2.1: Through the ischium.

A2.2: Through the obturator foramen (preserving the tear drop or involving the tear drop).

A2.3: Associated with posterior wall fracture in the posterior, posterosuperior, or posteroinferior region.

A3: Anterior column fracture:

A3.1: Anterior wall fracture, with one or more fragments.

A3.2: Anterior column fracture, high fracture to iliac crest, with one or more fragments.

A3.3: Anterior column fracture, low fracture to anterior border, with one or more fragments.

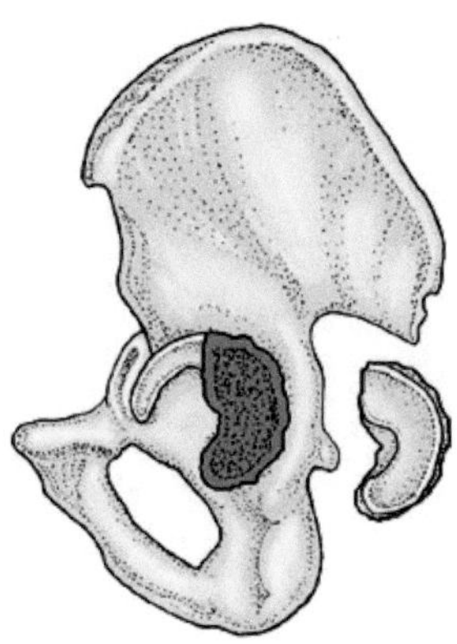

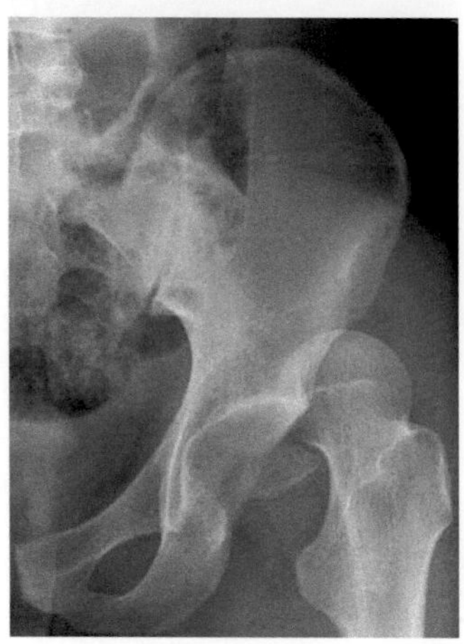

62-A Partial articular fracture, one column involved
A1: Posterior wall fracture
A1.1: Pure fracture dislocation, one fragment in the posterior, posterosuperior, or posteroinferior region

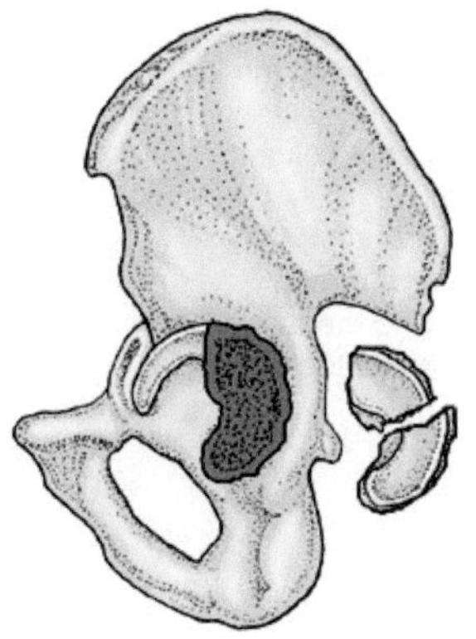

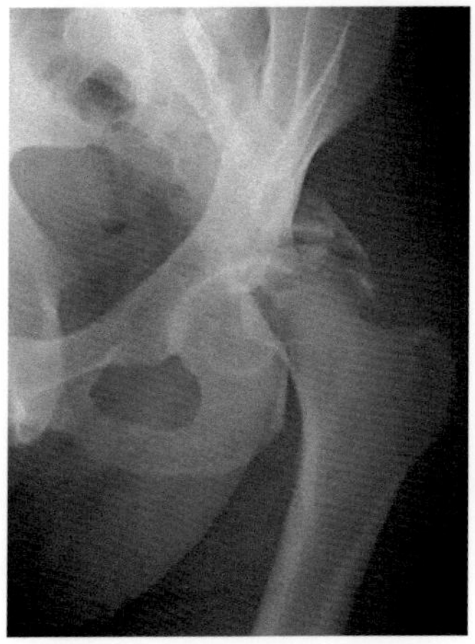

62-A Partial articular fracture,one column involved
A1: Posterior wall fracture
A1.2: Pure fracture dislocation, multifragmentary in the posterior, posterosuperior, or posteroinferior region

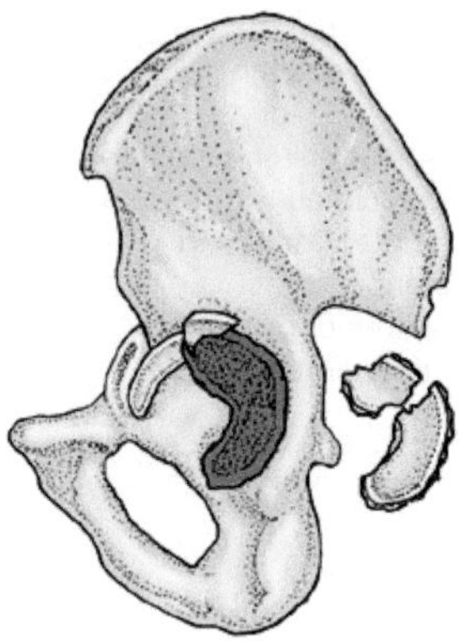

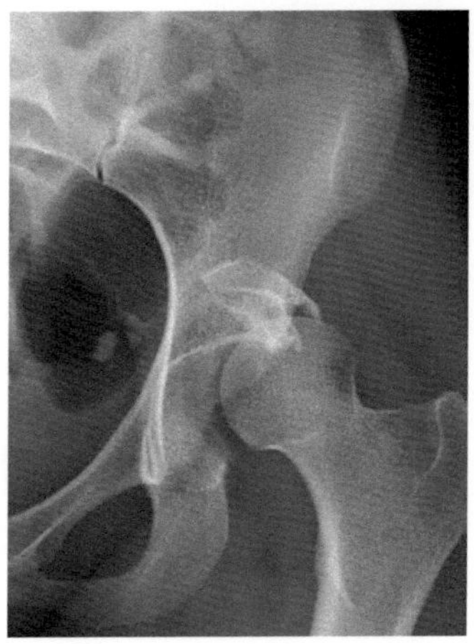

62-A Partial articular fracture, one column involved
A1: Posterior wall fracture
A1.3: Fracture dislocation, with marginal impaction in the posterior, posteriosuperior,or posteroinferior region

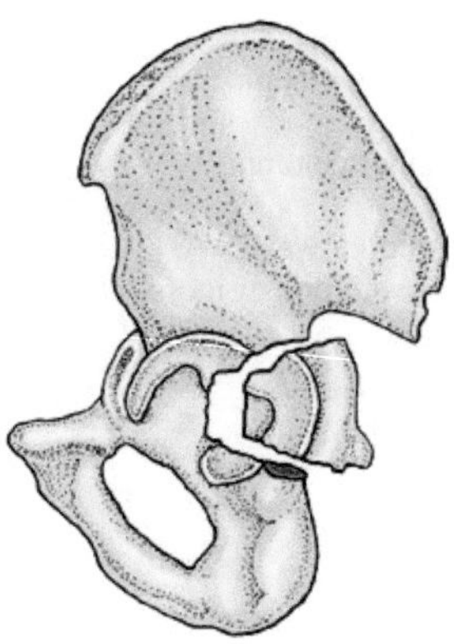

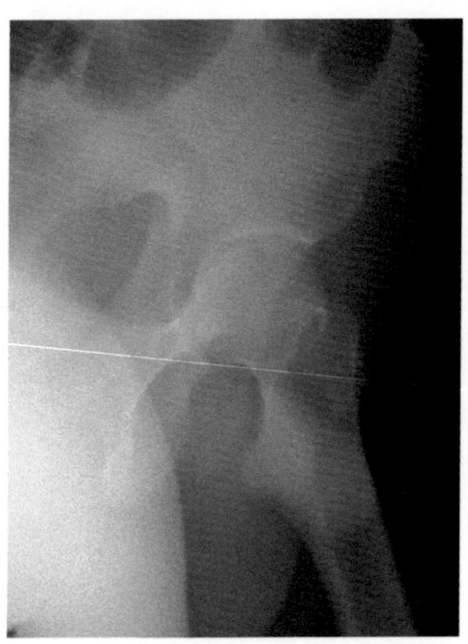

62-A Partial articular fracture, one column involved
A2: Posterior column fracture
A2.1: Through the ischium

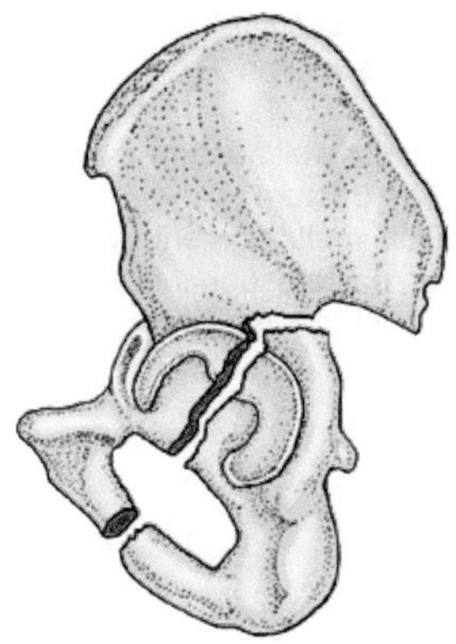

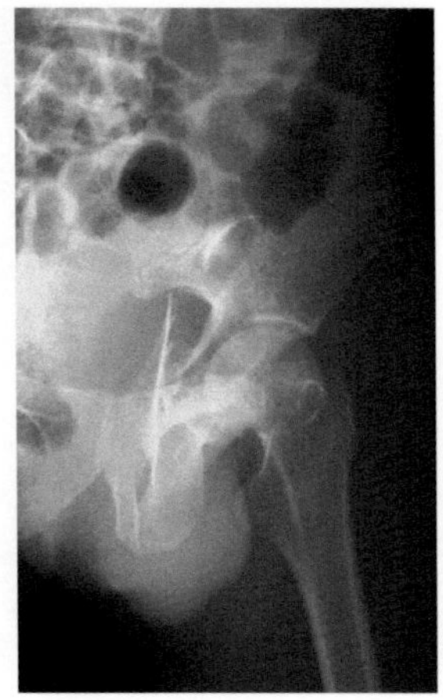

62-A Partial articular fracture, one column involved
A2: Posterior column fracture
A2.2: Through the obturator foramen (preserving the tear drop or involving the tear drop)

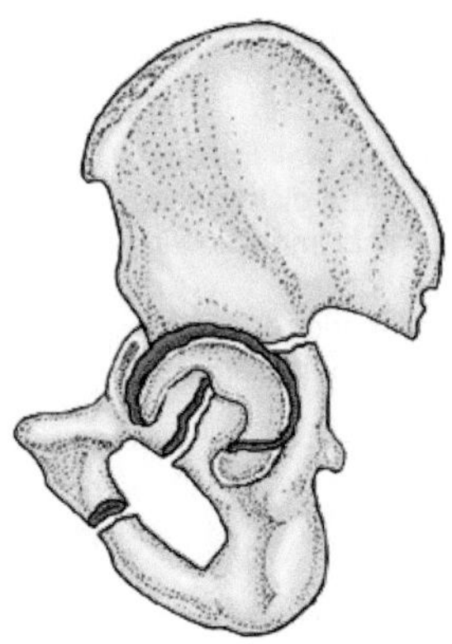

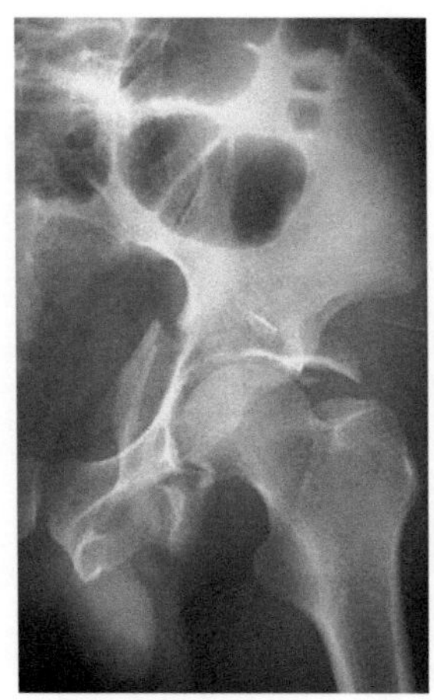

62-A Partial articular fracture, one column involved
A2: Posterior column fracture
A2.3: Associated with posterior wall fracture in the posterior, posterosuperior or posteroinferior region

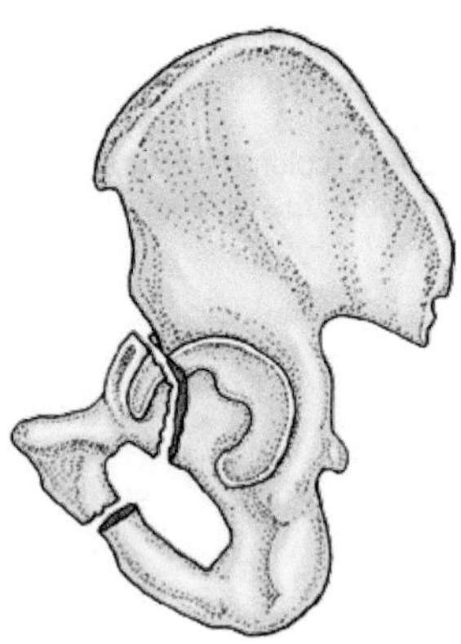

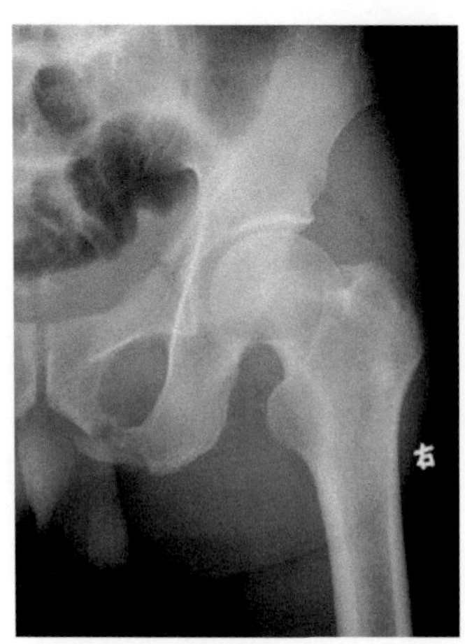

62-A Partial articular fracture, one column involved
A3: Anterior column fracture
A3.1: Anterior wall fracture, with one or more fragments

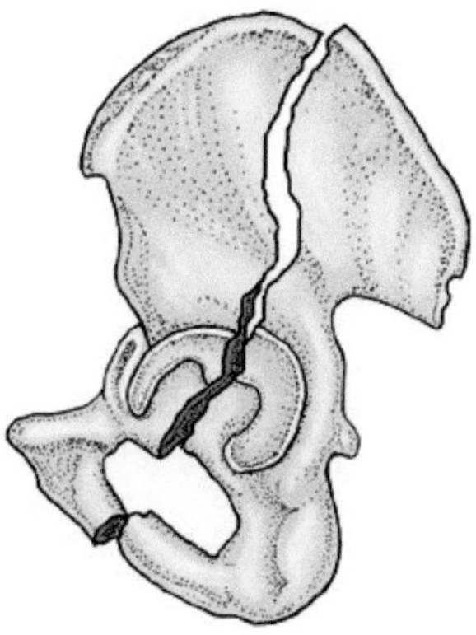

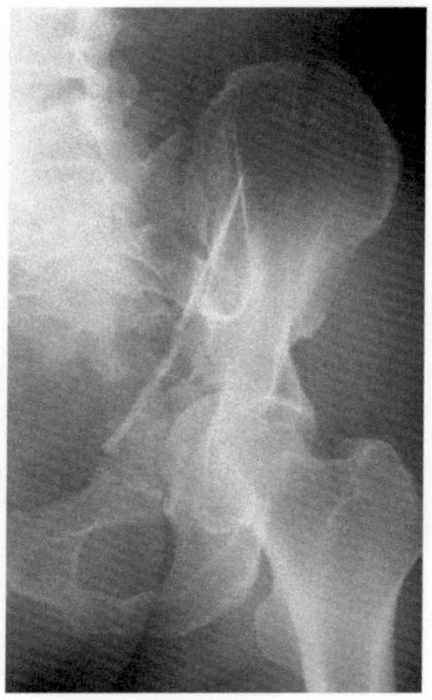

62-A Partial articular fracture, one column involved
A3: Anterior column fracture
A3.2: Anterior column fracture, high fracture to iliac crest, with one or more fragments

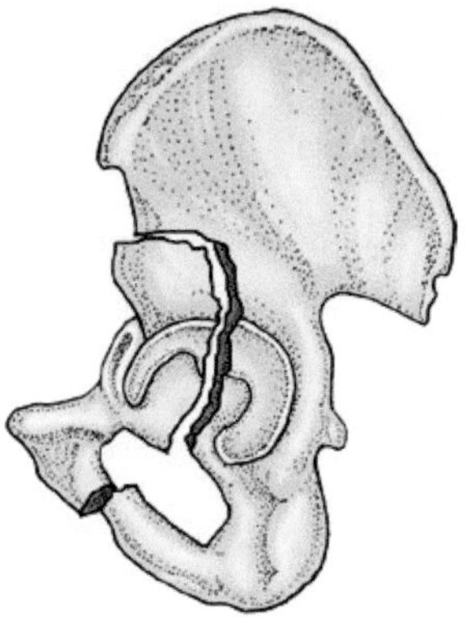

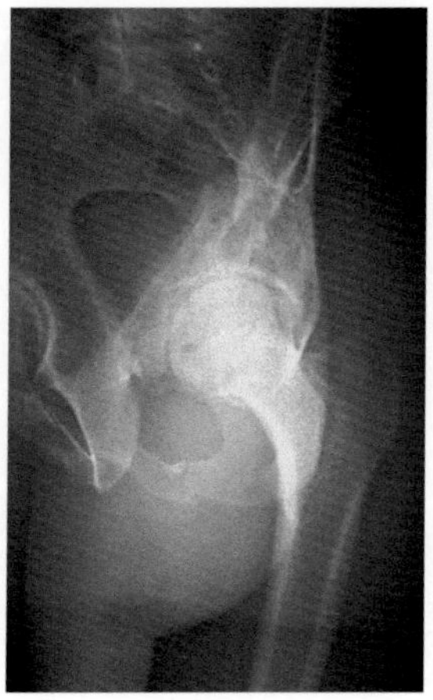

62-A Partial articular fracture,one column involved
A3: Anterior column fracture
A3.3: Anterior column fracture, low fracture to anterior border, with one or more fragments

62-B: Partial articular fracture, transverse:
- B1: Transverse:
  - B1.1: Infratectal.
  - B1.2: Juxtatectal.
  - B1.3: Transtectal.
- B2: T-shaped:
  - B2.1: Infratectal fracture (stem posterior, stem through obturator foramen, stem anterior).
  - B2.2: Juxtatectal fracture (stem posterior, stem through obturator foramen, stem anterior).
  - B2.3: Transtectal fracture (stem posterior, stem through obturator foramen, stem anterior).
- B3: Anterior column, posterior hemitransverse:
  - B3.1: Anterior wall.
  - B3.2: Anterior column high.
  - B3.3: Anterior column low.

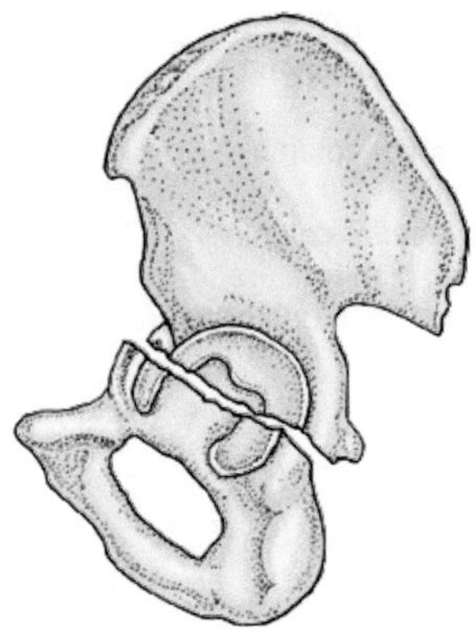

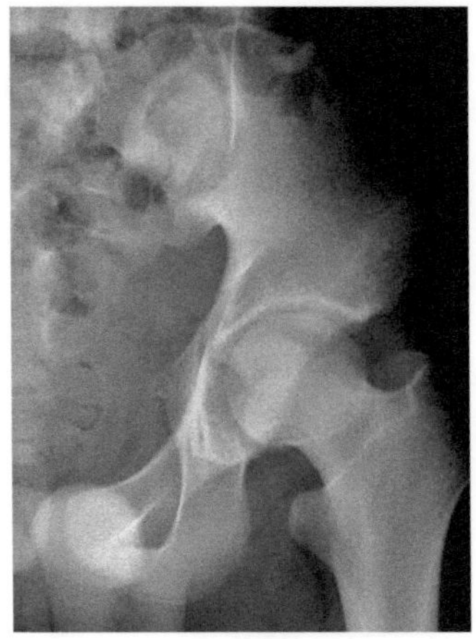

62-B Partial articular fracture,transverse
B1: Transverse
B1.1: Infratectal

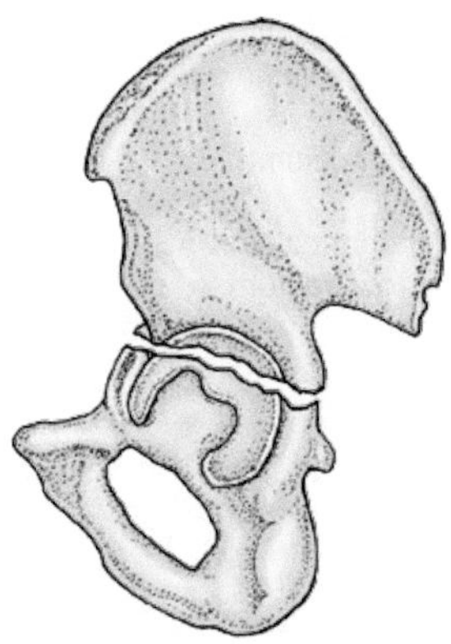

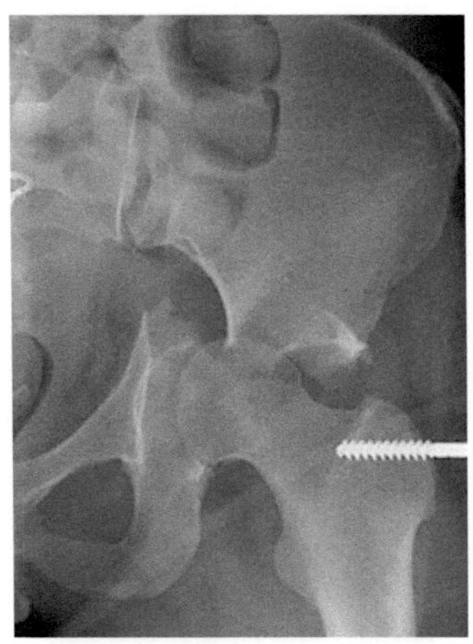

62-B Partial articular fracture, transverse
B1: Transverse
B1.2 :Juxtatectal

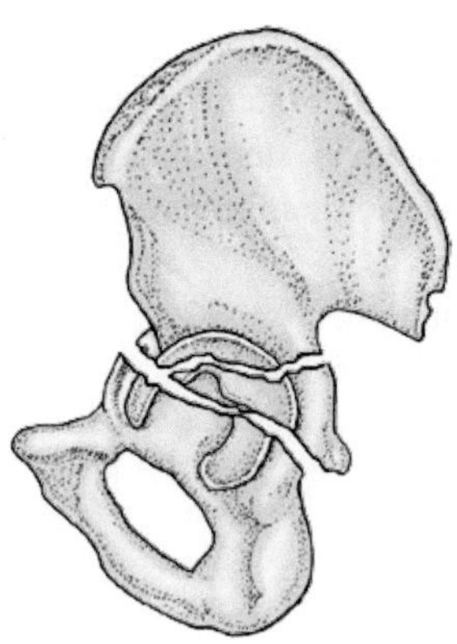

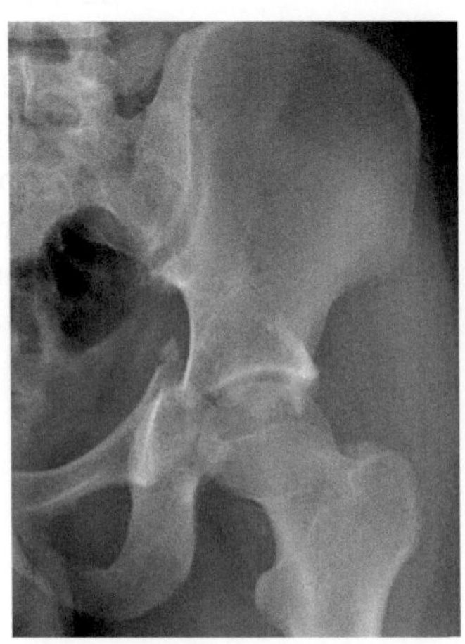

62-B Partial articular fracture, transverse
B1: Transverse
B1.3: Transtectal

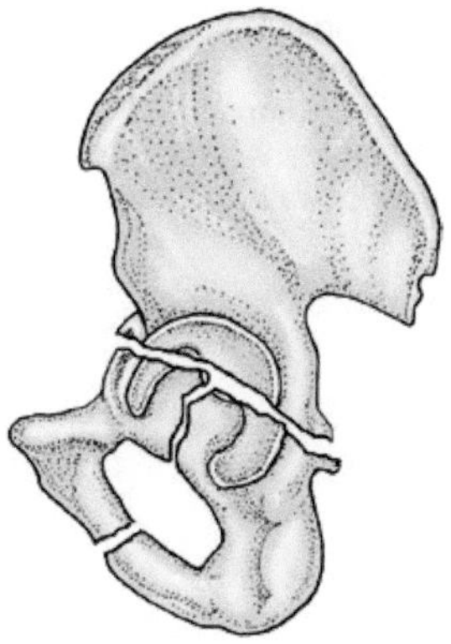

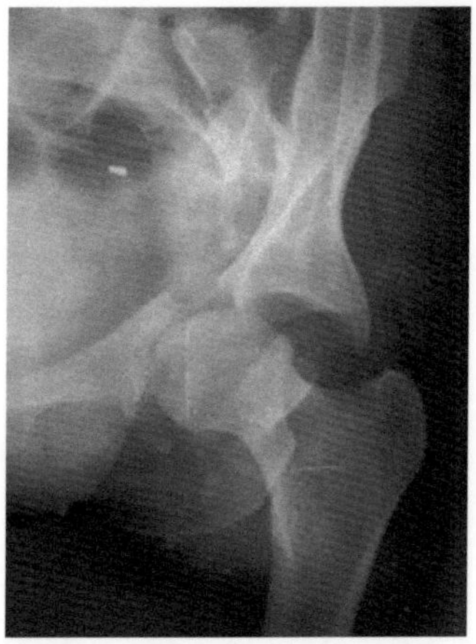

62-B Partial articular fracture, transverse
B2: T-shaped
B2.1: Infratectal fracture (stem posterior, stem through obturator foramen, stem anterior)

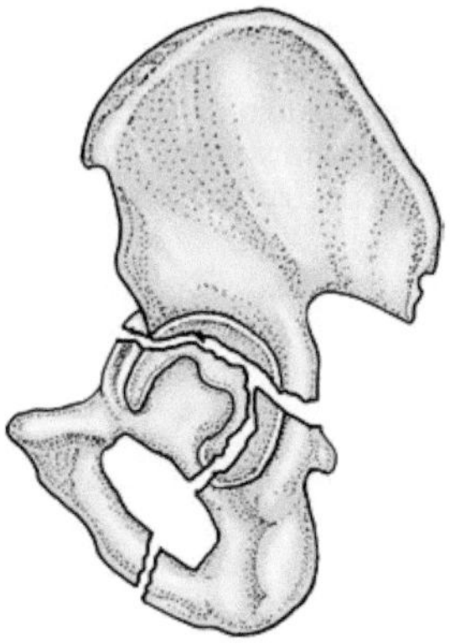

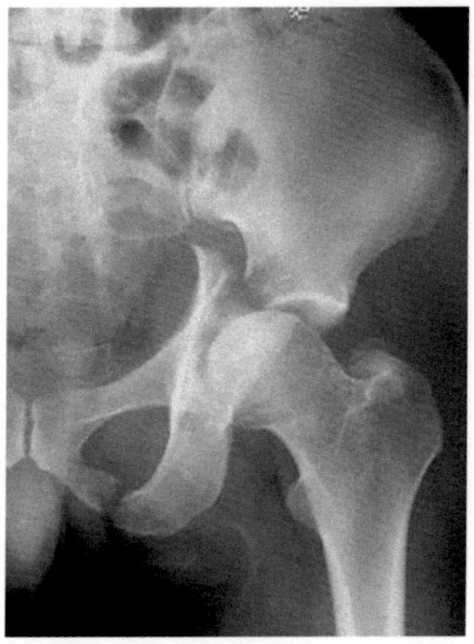

62-B Partial articular fracture, transverse
B2: T-shaped
B2.2: Juxtatectal fracture (stem posterior, stem through obturator foramen, stem anterior)

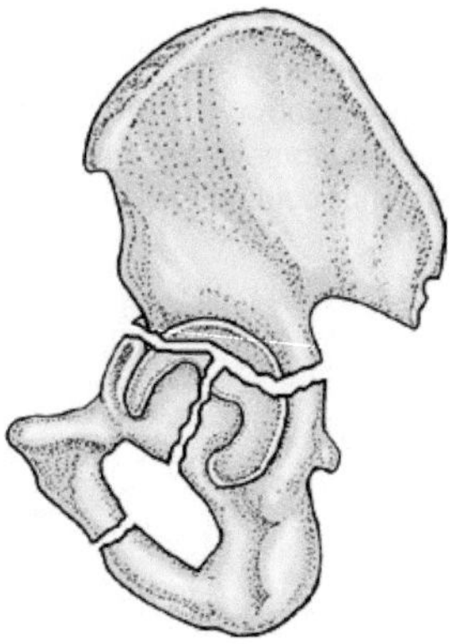

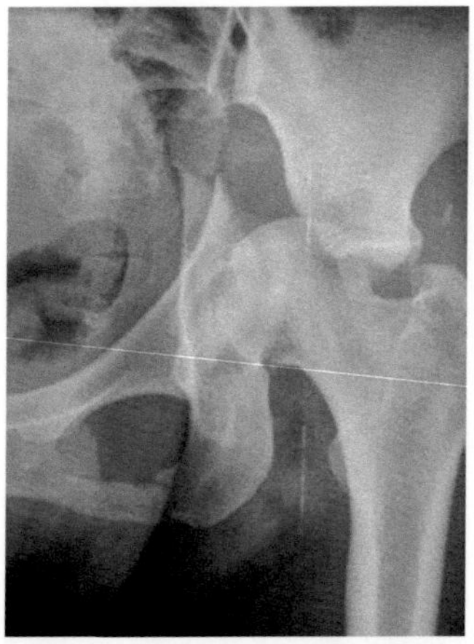

62-B Partial articular fracture, transverse
B2: T-shaped
B2.3: Transtectal fracture (stem posterior, stem through obturator foramen, stem anterior)

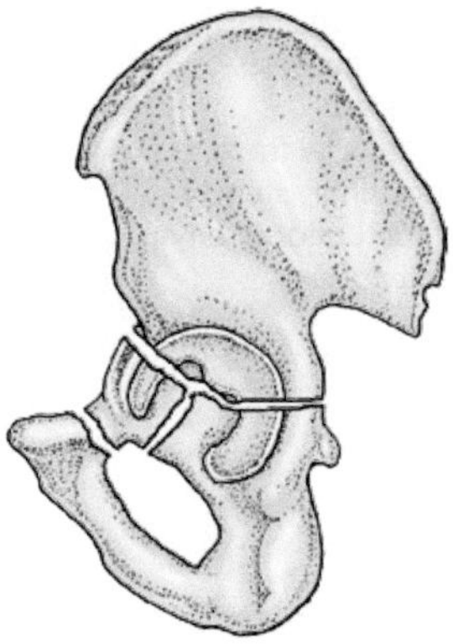

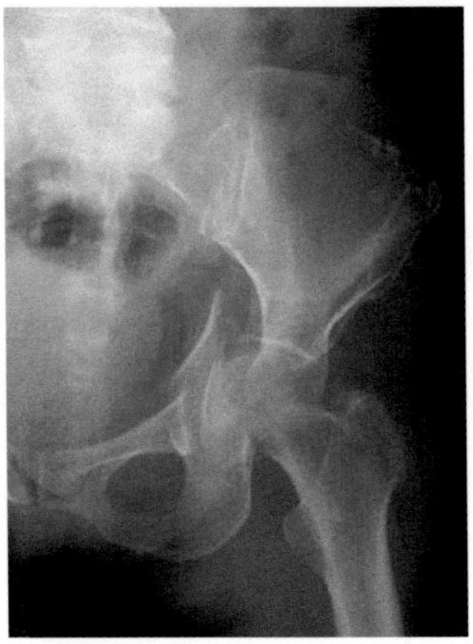

62-B Partial articular fracture, transverse
B3: Anterior column, posterior hemitransverse
B3.1: Anterior wall

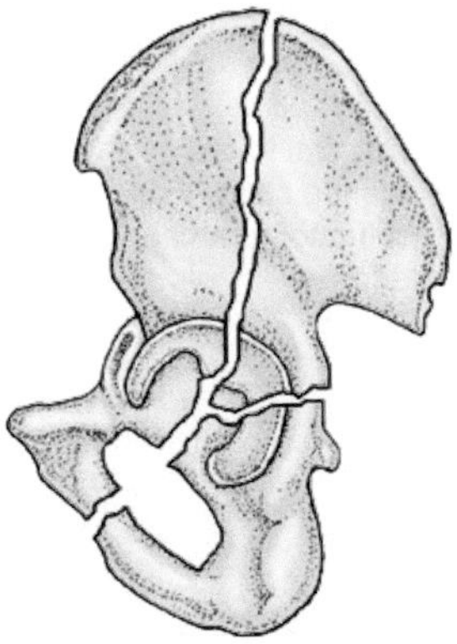

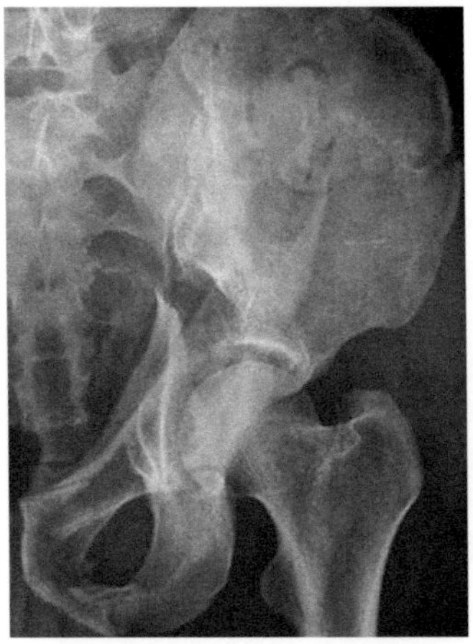

62-B Partial articular fracture, transverse
B3: Anterior column, posterior hemitransverse
B3.2: Anterior column high

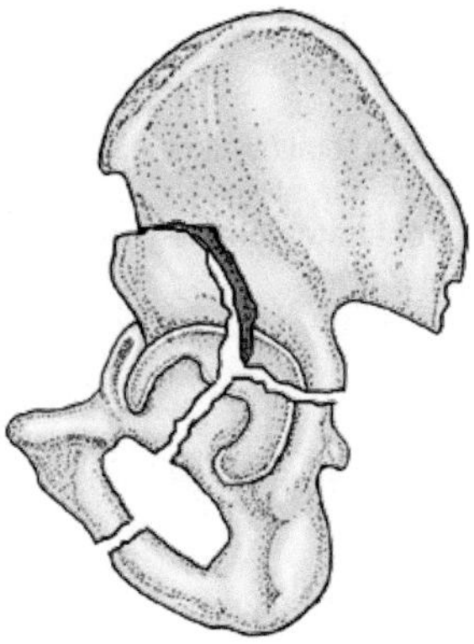

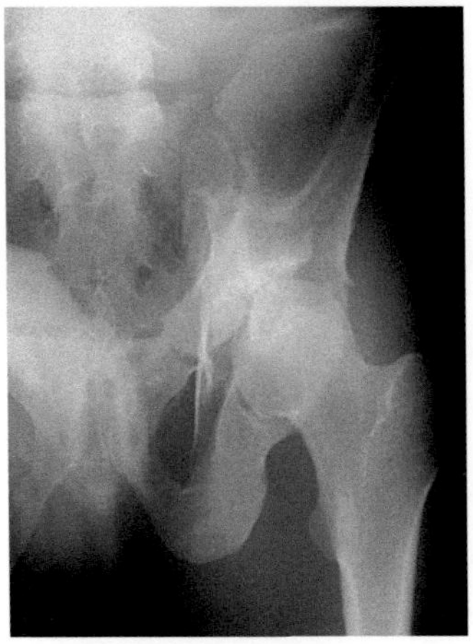

62-B Partial articular fracture, transverse
B3: Anterior column, posterior hemitransverse
B3.3: Anterior column low

62-C: Complete articular fracture, both columns
- C1: High:
  - C1.1: Both columns simple.
  - C1.2: Posterior column simple, anterior column multifragmentary.
  - C1.3: Posterior column and posterior wall.
- C2: Low:
  - C2.1: Both columns simple.
  - C2.2: Posterior column simple, anterior column multifragmentary.
  - C2.3: Posterior column and posterior wall.
- C3: Involving the sacroiliac joint:
  - C3.1: Anterior wall (anterior column high/low, simple; high/low multifragmentary).
  - C3.2: Posterior column multifragmentary, anterior column high.
  - C3.3: Posterior column multifragmentary, anterior column low.

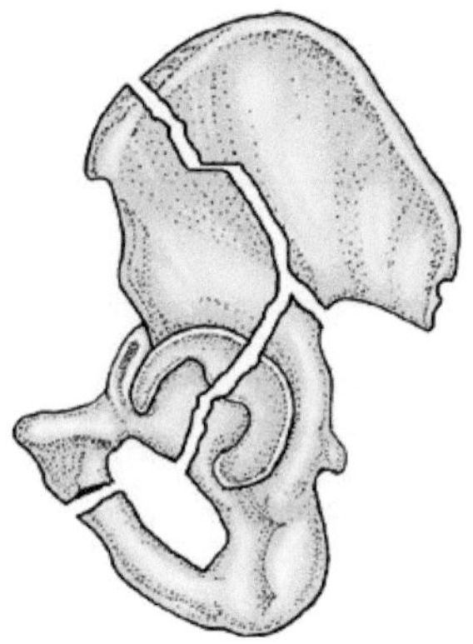

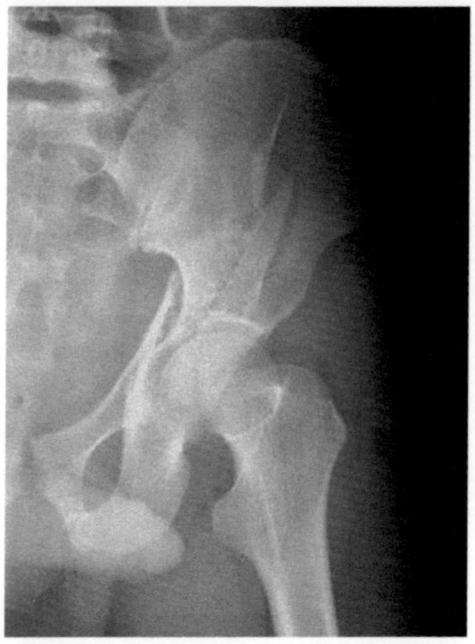

62-C Complete articular fracture, both columns
C1: High
C1.1: Both columns simple

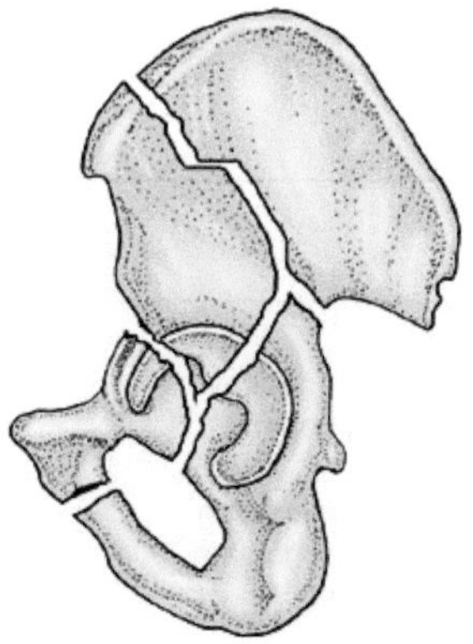

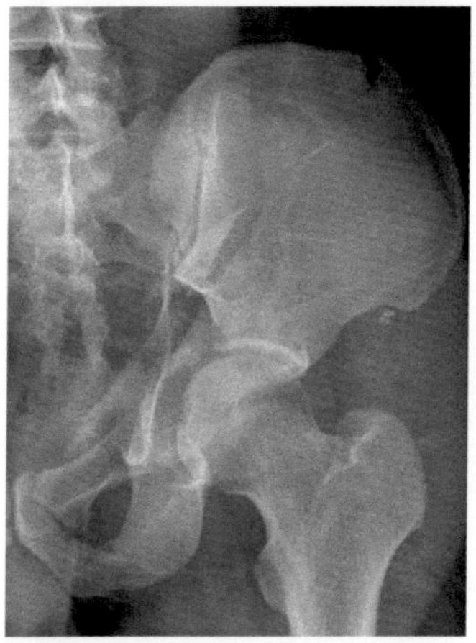

62-C Complete articular fracture, both columns
C1: High
C1.2: Posterior column simple, anterior column multifragmentary

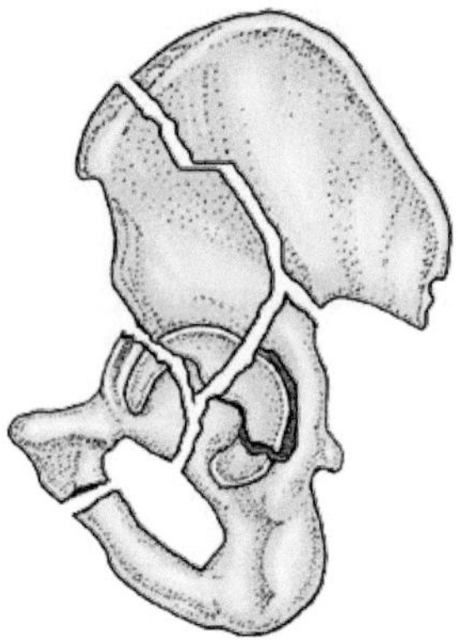

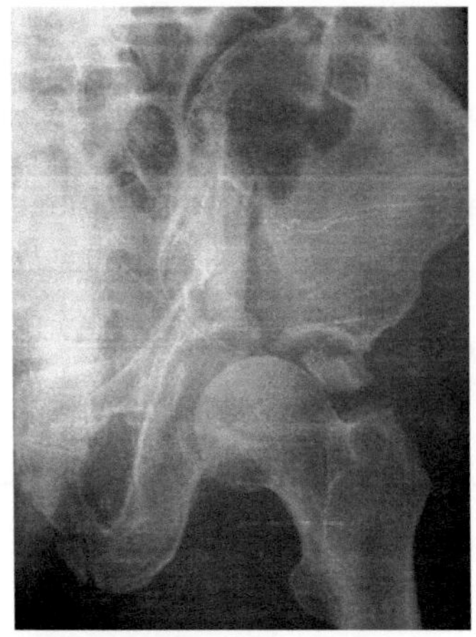

62-C Complete articular fracture, both columns
C1: High
C1.3: Posterior column and posterior wall

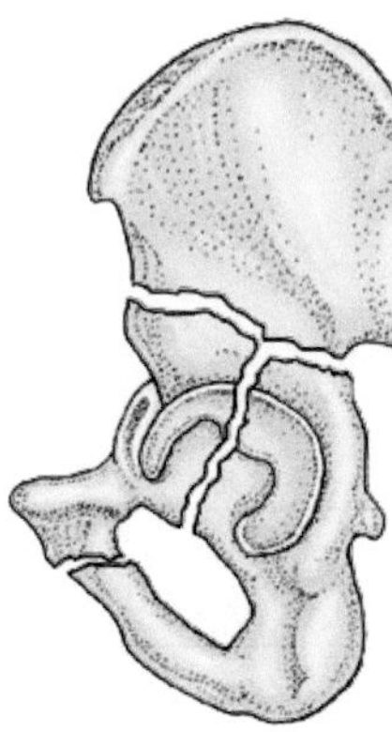

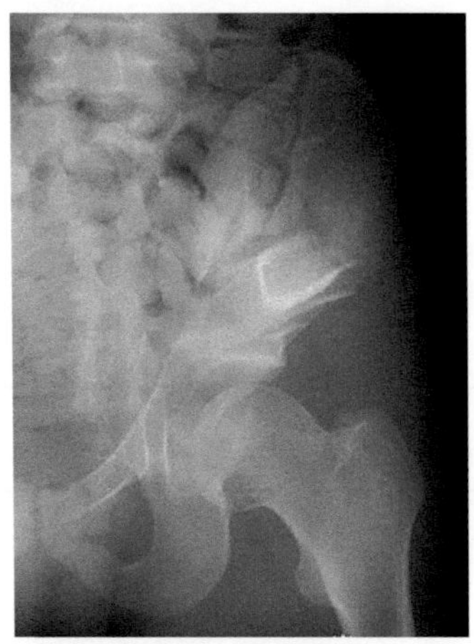

62-C Complete articular fracture, both columns
C2: Low
C2.1: Both columns simple

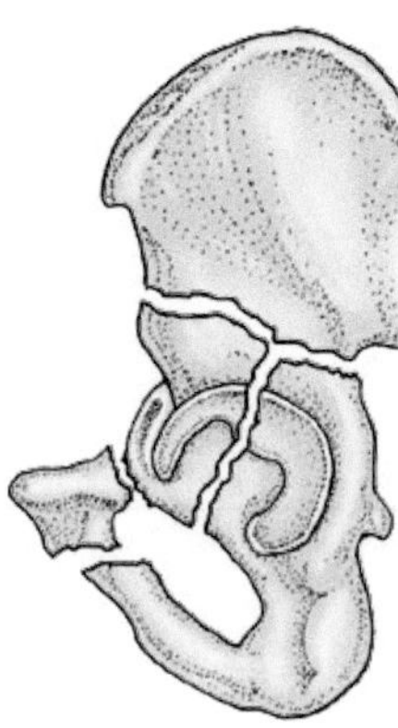

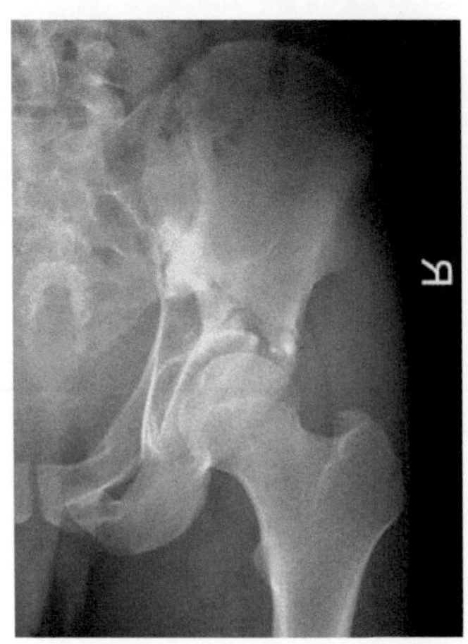

62-C Complete articular fracture, both columns
C2: Low
C2.2: Posterior column simple, anterior column multifragmentary

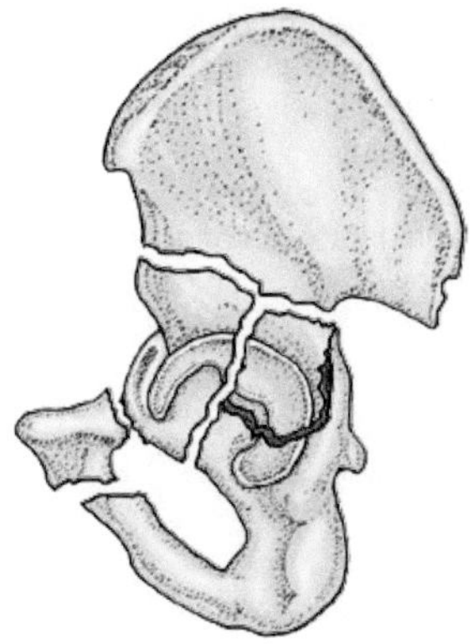

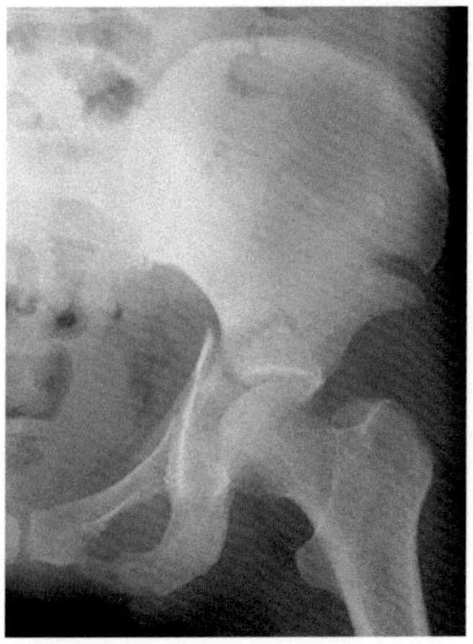

62-C Complete articular fracture, both columns
C2: Low
C2.3: Posterior column and posterior wall

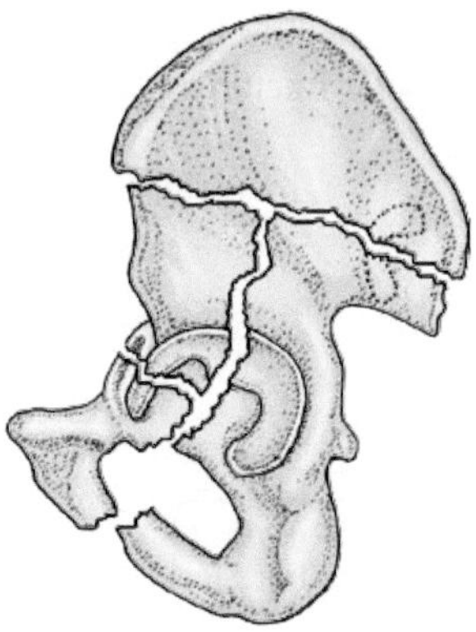

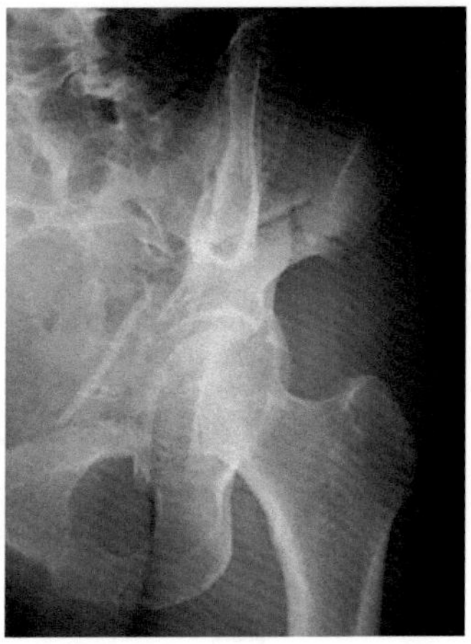

62-C Complete articular fracture, both columns
C3: Involving the sacroiliac joint
C3.1: Anterior wall (anterior column high/low, simple; high/low multifragmentary)

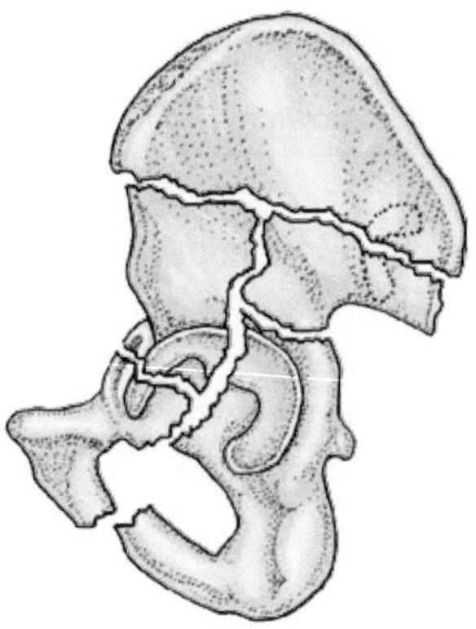

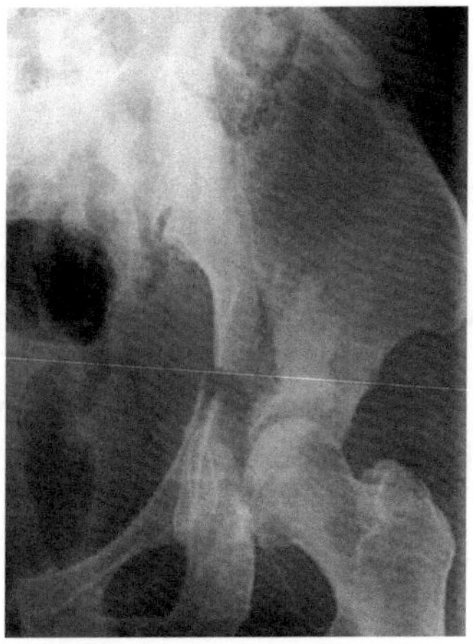

62-C Complete articular fracture, both columns
C3: Involving the sacroiliac joint
C3.2: Posterior column multifragmentary, anterior column high

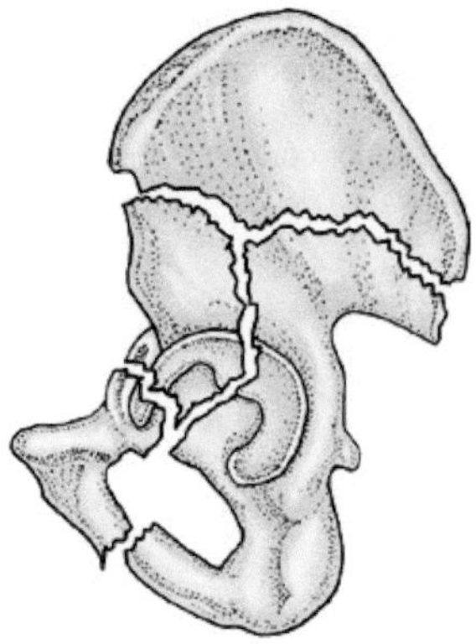

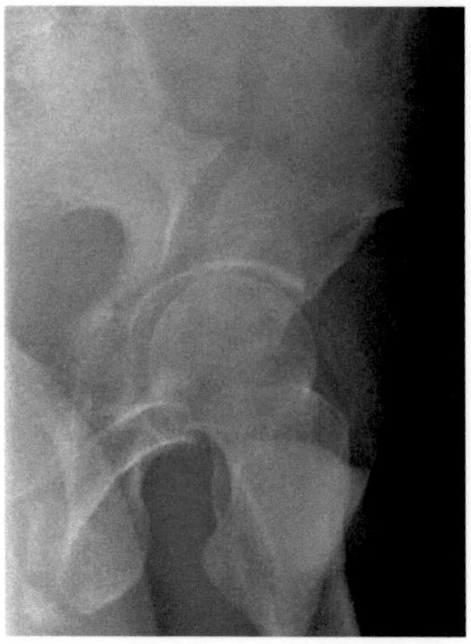

62-C Complete articular fracture, both columns
C3: Involving the sacroiliac joint
C3.3: Posterior column multifragmentary, anterior column low

7.2.3 Marvin Tile Classification

Acetabulum fractures are divided into displaced acetabular fractures and non-displaced acetabular fractures.

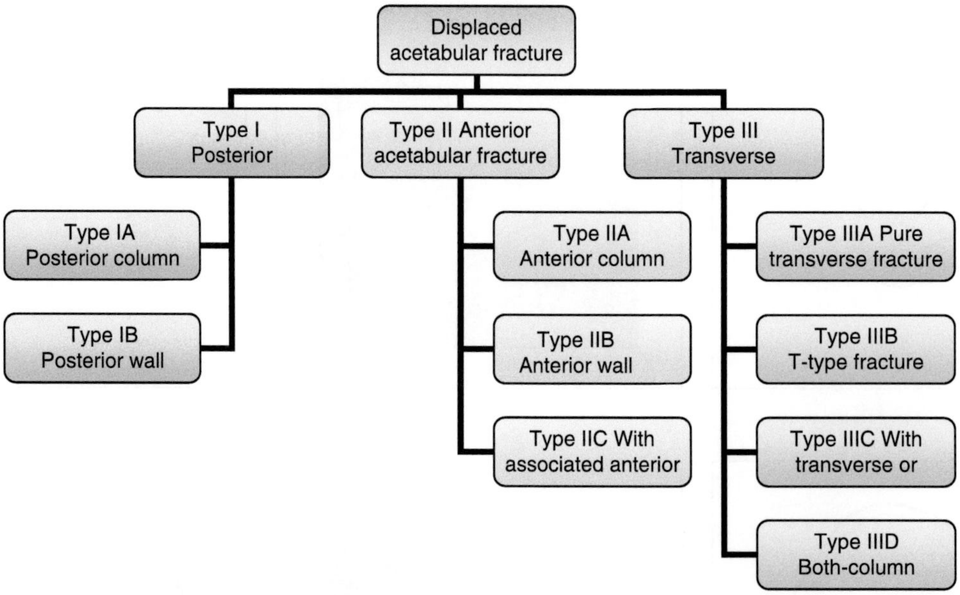

Displaced acetabular fracture

Type I: Posterior acetabular fracture with or without posterior dislocation:
- Type IA: Posterior column fracture.
- Type IB: Posterior wall fracture, with associated posterior column or transverse fracture.

Type II: Anterior acetabular fracture with or without anterior dislocation:
- Type IIA: Anterior column fracture.
- Type IIB: Anterior wall fracture.
- Type IIC: With associated anterior or transverse fracture.

Type III: Transverse fracture with or without central dislocation of the hip:
- Type IIIA: Pure transverse fracture.
- Type IIIB: T-type fracture.
- Type IIIC: With transverse or acetabular wall fracture.
- Type IIID: Both column fracture.

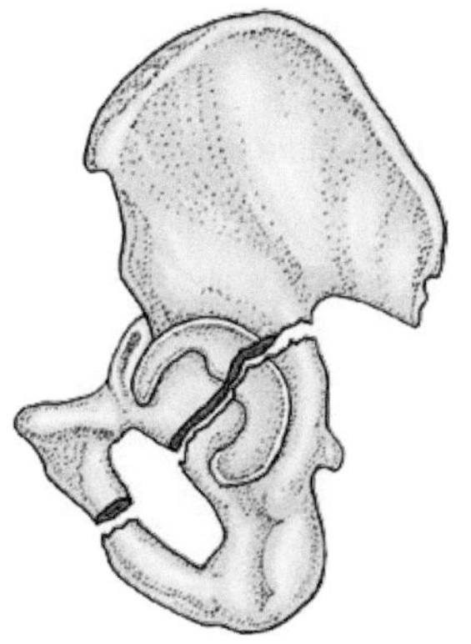

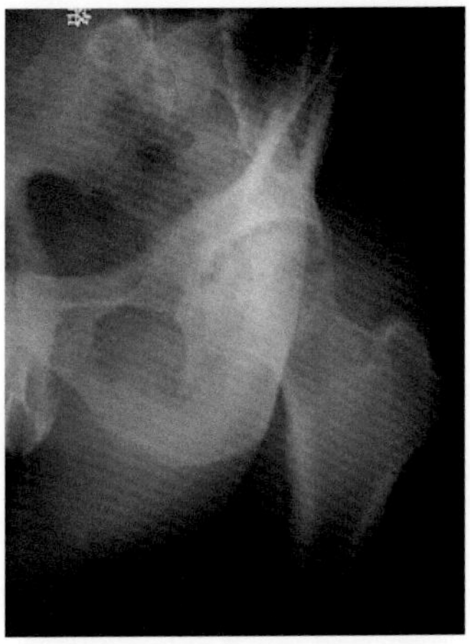

Displaced acetabular fracture:
Type I: Posterior acetabular fracture with or without posterior dislocation
Type IA: Posterior column fracture

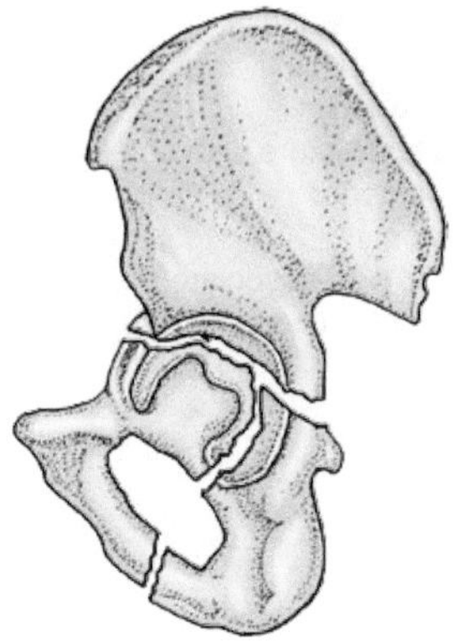

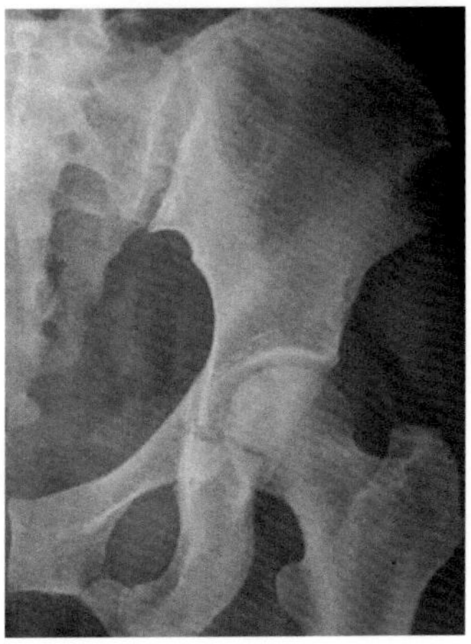

Displaced acetabular fracture:
Type I: Posterior acetabular fracture with or without posterior dislocation
Type I B: Posterior wall fracture, with associated posterior column or transverse fracture

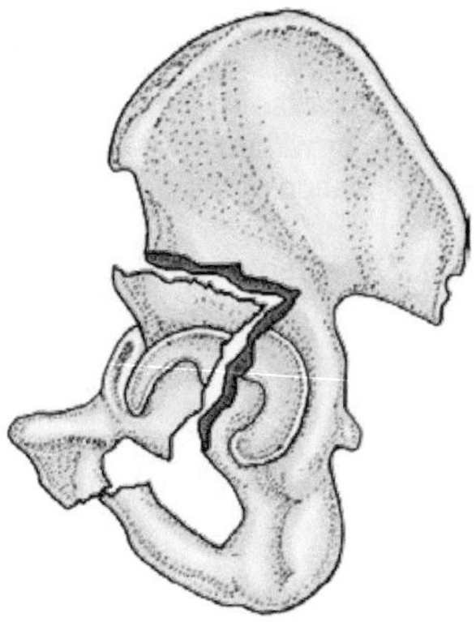

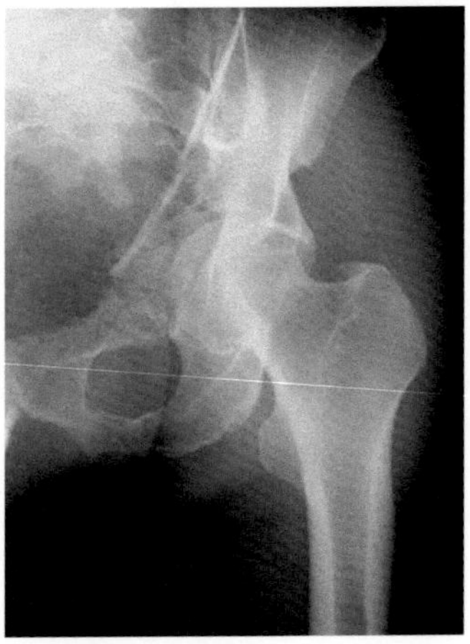

Displaced acetabular fracture:
Type II: Anterior acetabular fracture with or without anterior dislocation
Type IIA: Anterior column fracture

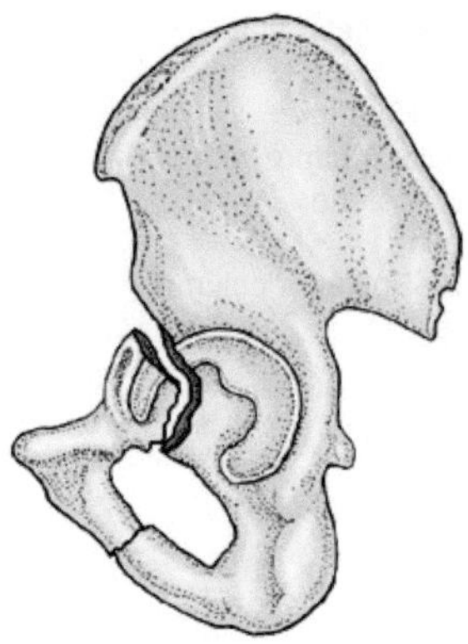

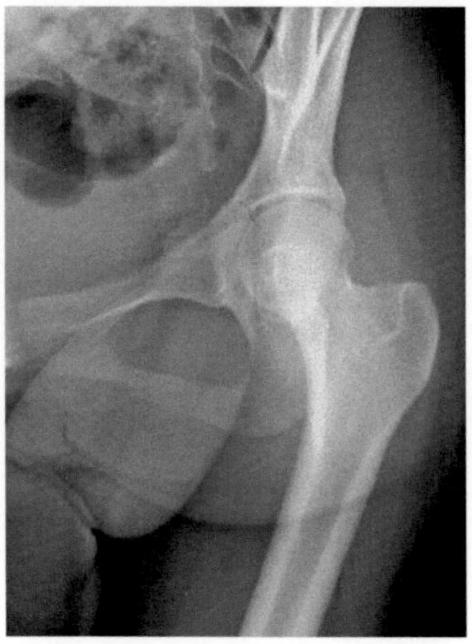

Displaced acetabular fracture:
Type II: Anterior acetabular fracture with or without anterior dislocation
Type IIB: Anterior wall fracture

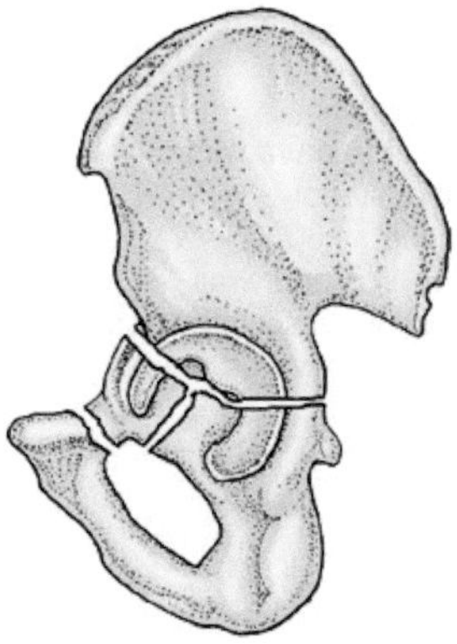

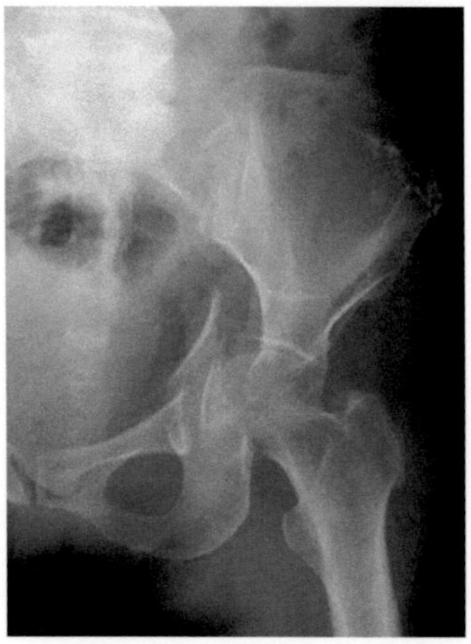

Displaced acetabular fracture:
Type II: Anterior acetabular fracture with or without anterior dislocation
Type IIC: With associated anterior or transverse fracture

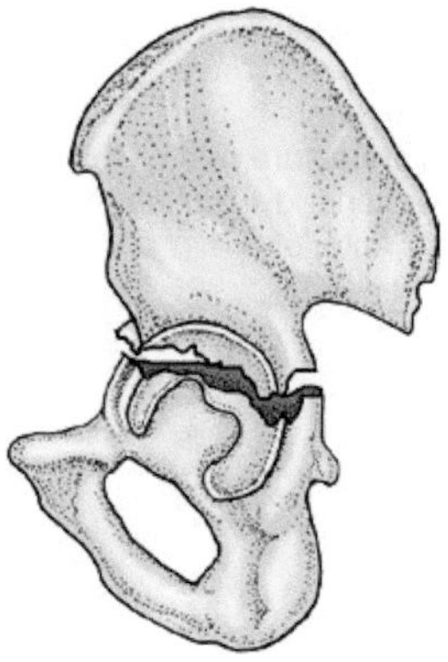

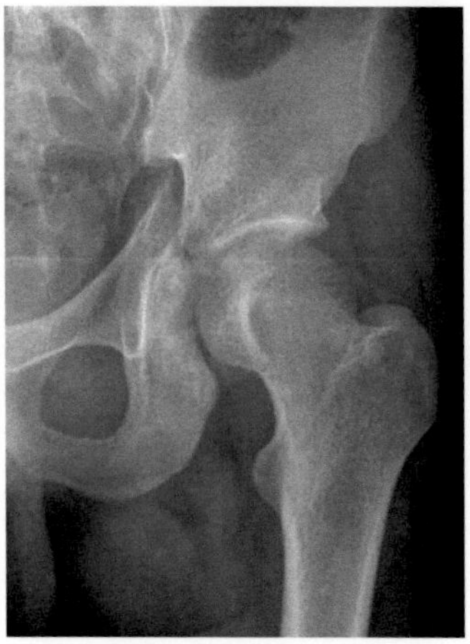

Displaced acetabular fracture:
Type III: Transverse fracture with or without central dislocation of the hip
Type IIIA: Pure transverse fracture

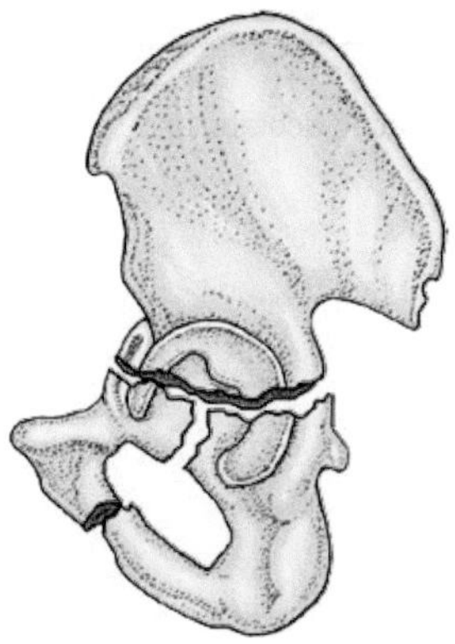

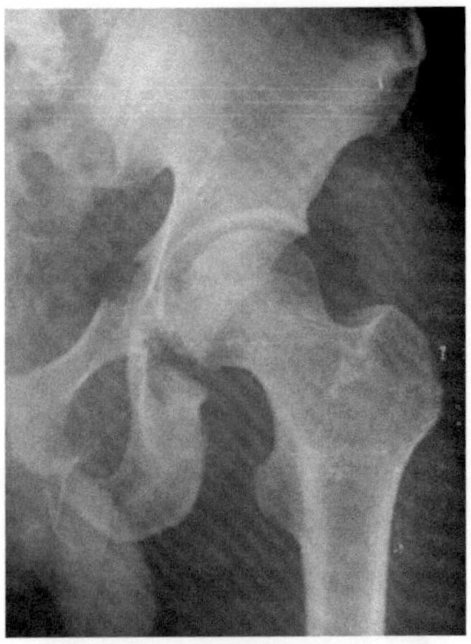

Displaced acetabular fracture:
Type III: Transverse fracture with or without central dislocation of the hip
Type IIIB: T-type fracture

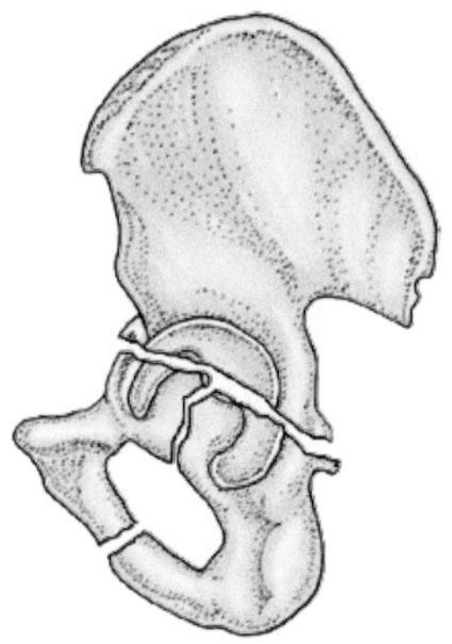

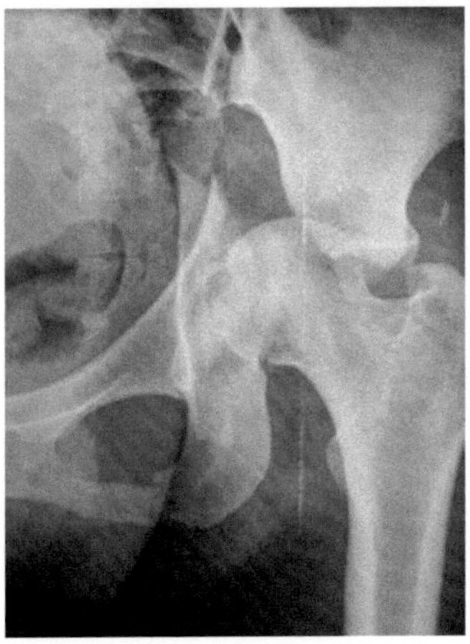

Displaced acetabular fracture:
Type III: Transverse fracture with or without central dislocation of the hip
Type IIIC: With transverse or acetabular wall fracture

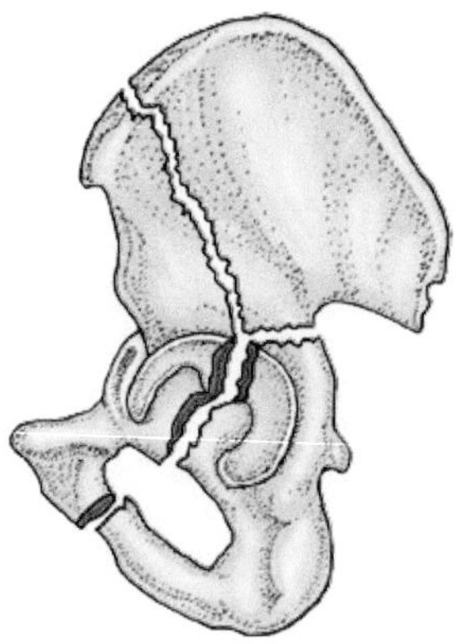

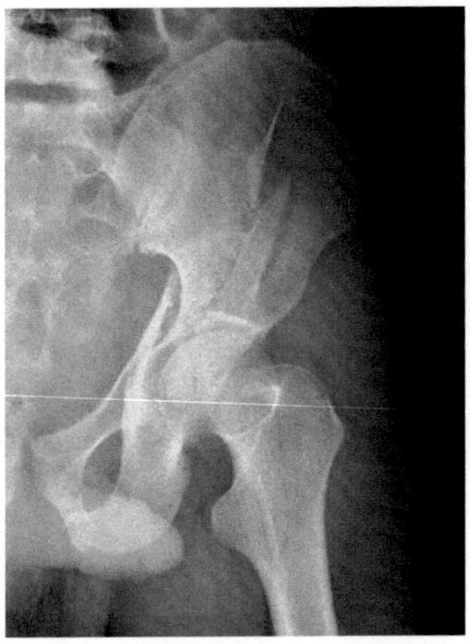

Displaced acetabular fracture:
Type III: Transverse fracture with or without central dislocation of the hip
Type III D: Both-column fracture

Non-displaced acetabular fracture

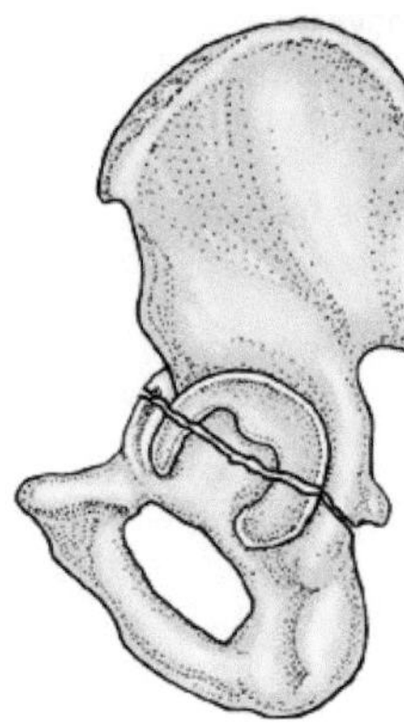

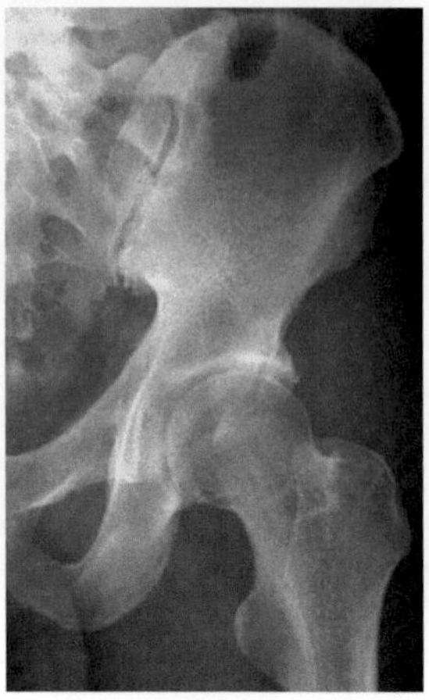

Nondisplaced acetabular fracture

7.3 Classification of Pelvic Dislocation

7.3.1 AO/OTA Classification

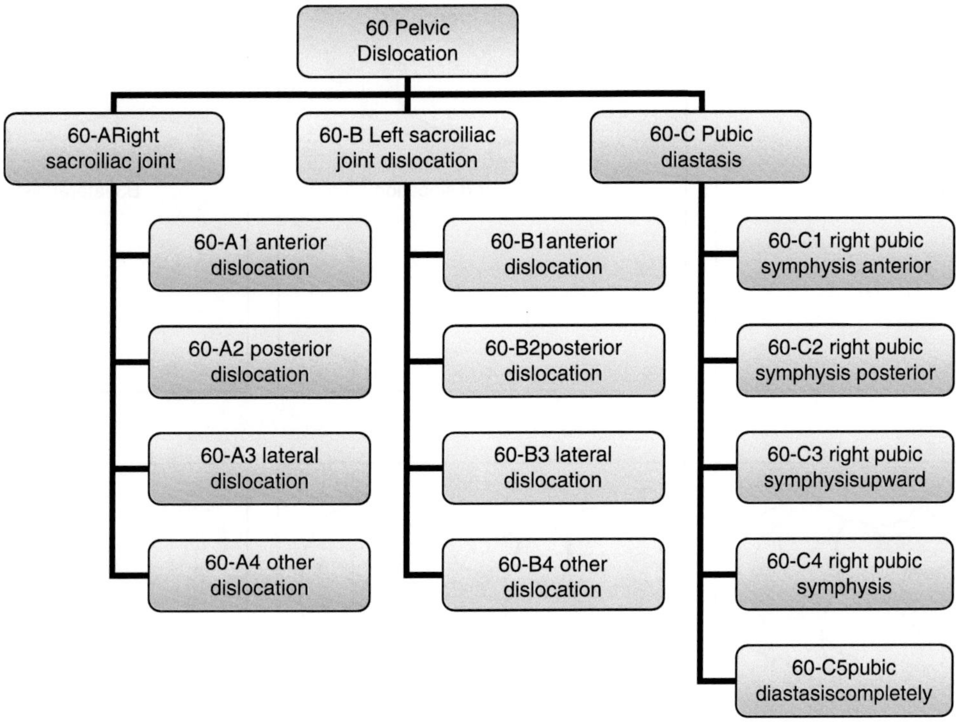

60 Pelvic dislocation:
- 60-A: Right sacroiliac joint dislocation:
  - 60-A1: Anterior dislocation.
  - 60-A2: Posterior dislocation.
  - 60-A3: Lateral dislocation.
  - 60-A4: Other dislocation.
- 60-B: Left sacroiliac joint dislocation:
  - 60-B1: Anterior dislocation.
  - 60-B2: Posterior dislocation.
  - 60-B3: Lateral dislocation.
  - 60-B4: Other dislocation.
- 60-C: Pubic diastasis:
  - 60-C1: Right pubic symphysis anterior dislocation.
  - 60-C2: Right pubic symphysis posterior dislocation.
  - 60-C3: Right pubic symphysis upward dislocation.
  - 60-C4: Right pubic symphysis downward dislocation.
  - 60-C5: Pubic diastasis completely.

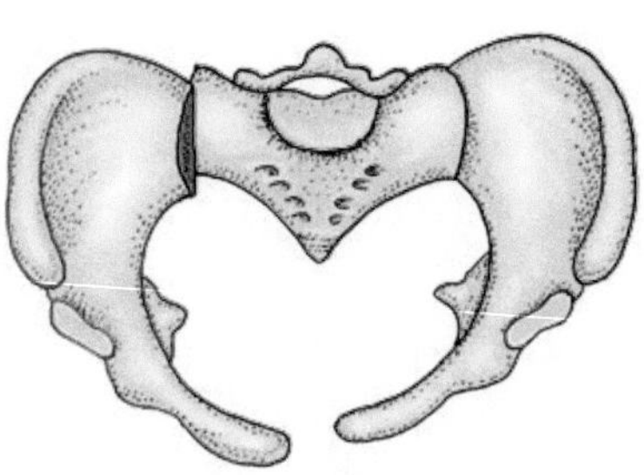
A1 anterior dislocation

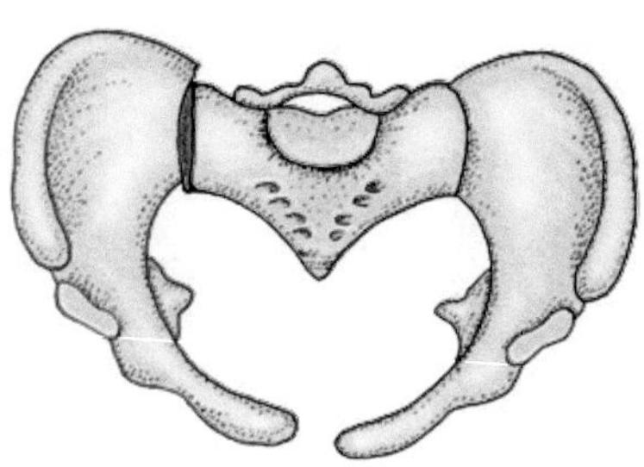
A2 posterior dislocation

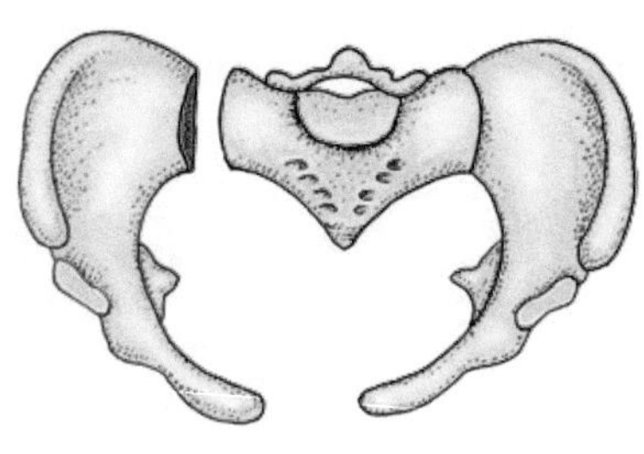
A3 lateral dislocation

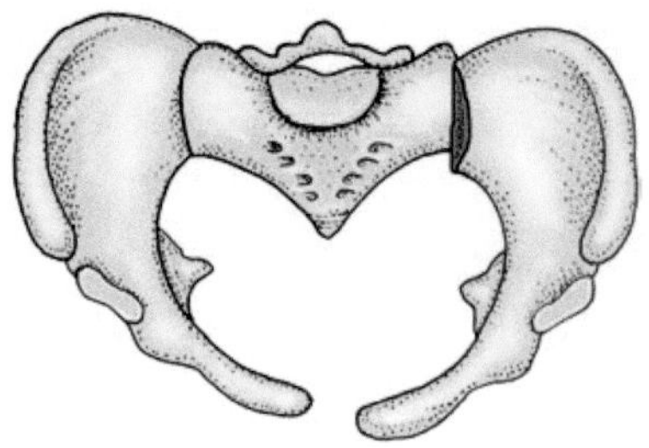

B1anterior dislocation

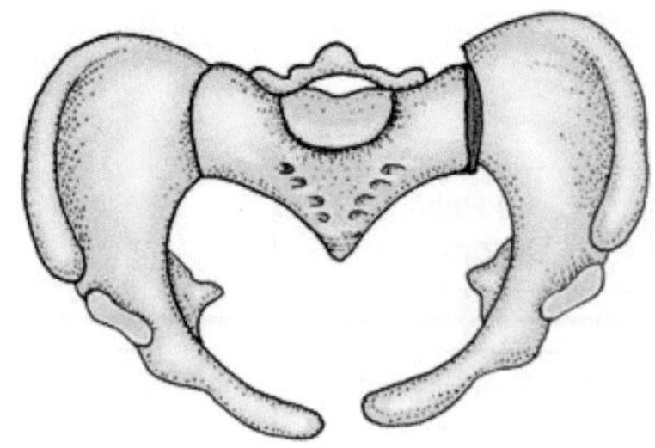

B2 posterior dislocation

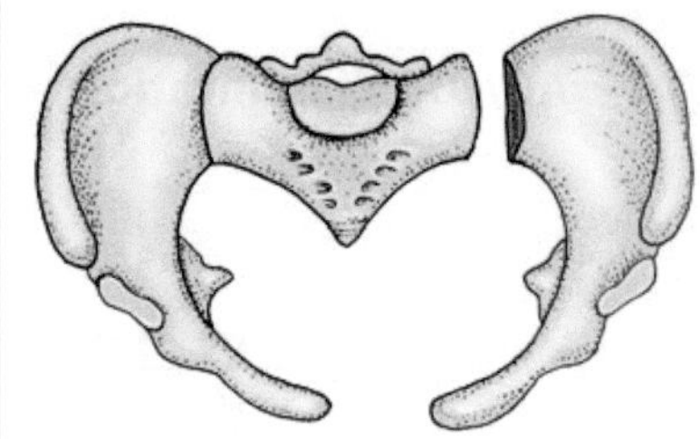

B3 lateral dislocation

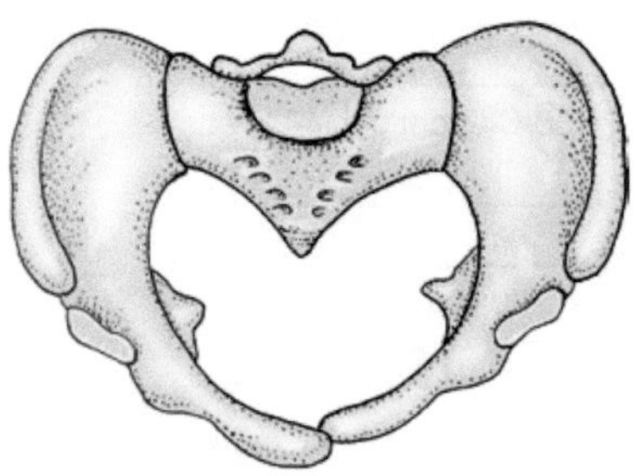

C1 right pubic symphysis
anterior dislocation

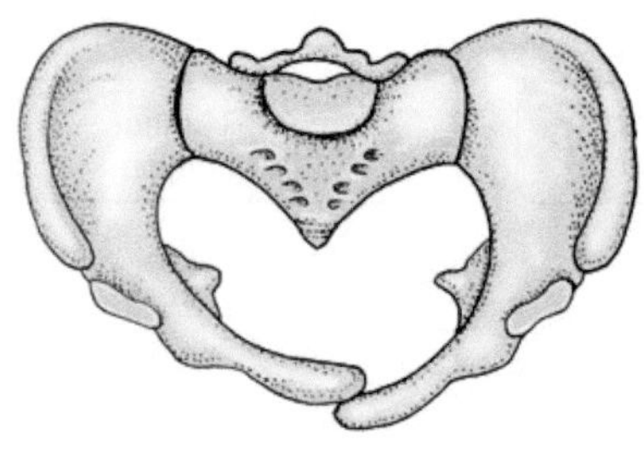

C2 right pubic symphysis
posterior dislocation

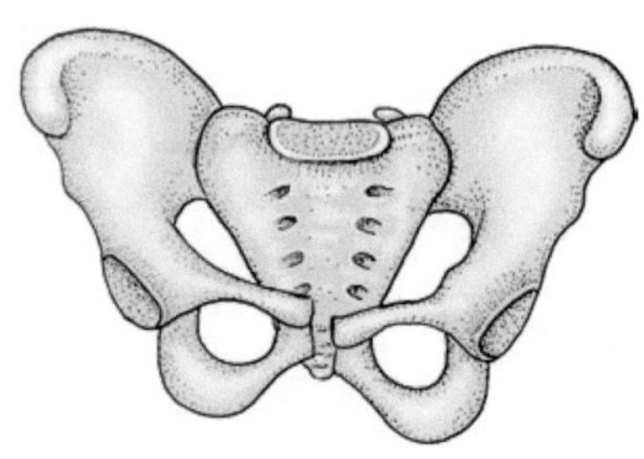

C3 right pubic symphysis
upward dislocation

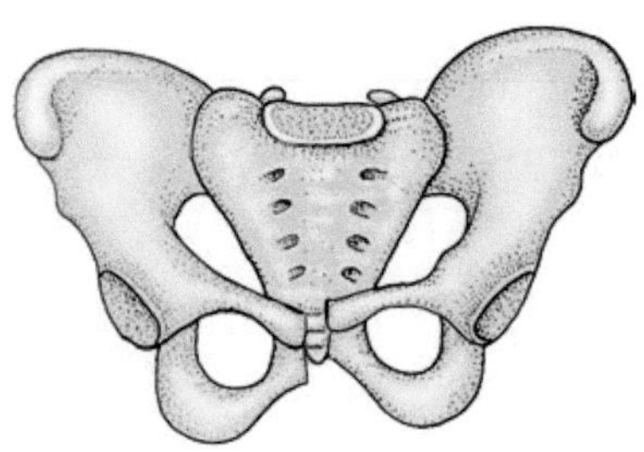

C4 right pubic symphysis
downward dislocation

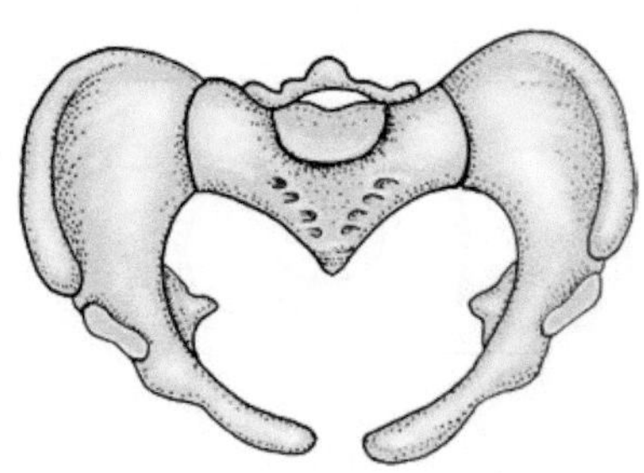

C5 Pubic diastasis
completely

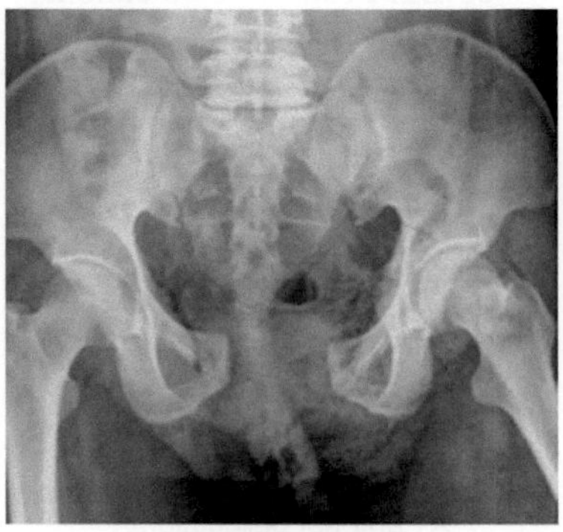

C5 Pubic diastasis
completely

Classification of Femoral Fractures

8

Yingze Zhang and Yanbin Zhu

8.1 Proximal Femur Fractures

8.1.1 Femoral Head Fractures

Pipkin proposed a classification system for femoral head fractures in 1957 for the first time. So far, there are nearly ten kinds of classification that can be found. According to the last 5 years' literature reported, Pipkin was the most useful classification followed by AO/OTA and Brumbaek classification.

8.1.1.1 Pipkin Classification (1957, Acta Chir Belg, 3: 130–135;1957, J Bone Joint Surg (Am), 39: 1027–1042, 1197)

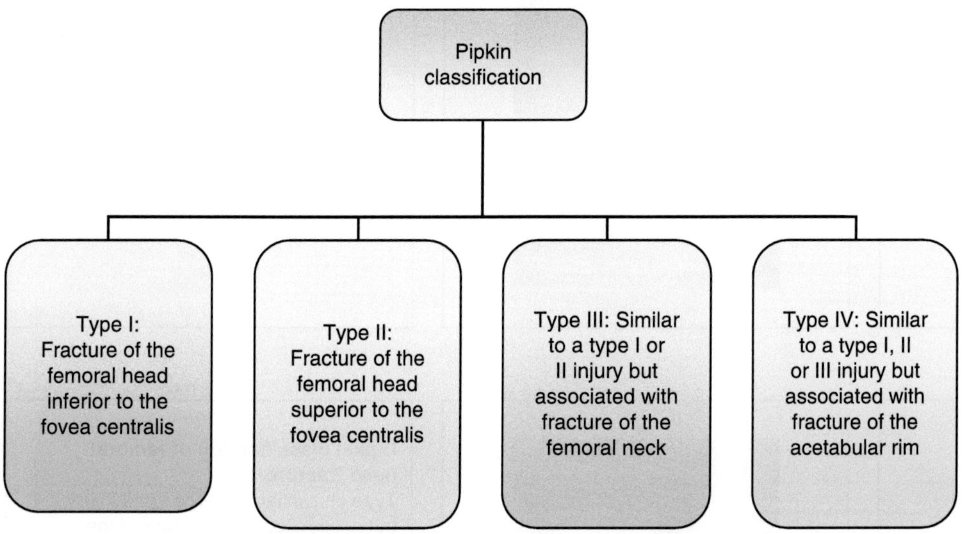

Pipkin proposed a classification system for femoral head fracture to divide the Thompson-Epstein's type V (femoral head fracture in association with posterior dislocation, seen in Chapter Dislocation) of the hip into four subtypes.

Type I: Posterior dislocation of the hip with fracture of the femoral head inferior to the fovea centralis.

Type II: Posterior dislocation of the hip with fracture of the femoral head superior to the fovea centralis.

Type III: Similar to a type I or II injury but associated with fracture of the femoral neck.

Type IV: Similar to a type I or II injury but associated with fracture of the acetabular rim.

Y. Zhang (✉) • Y. Zhu
Department of Orthopedics,
The Third Hospital of Hebei Medical University,
Shijiazhuang, China
e-mail: yzzhangdr@126.com, yzling_liu@163.com

Y. Zhang (ed.), *Clinical Classification in Orthopaedics Trauma*, https://doi.org/10.1007/978-981-10-6044-1_8

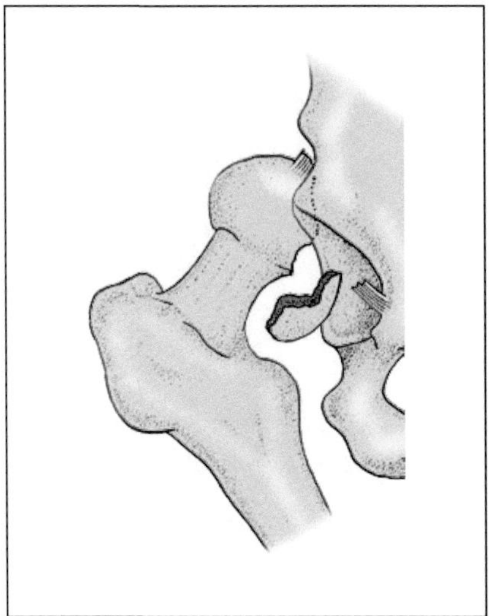

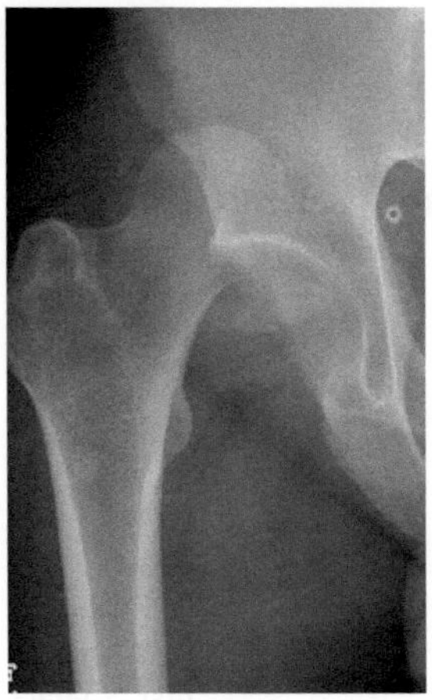

Pipkin classification of femoral head fracture.
Type I: posterior dislocation of the hip with fracture of the femoral head inferior to the fovea centralis

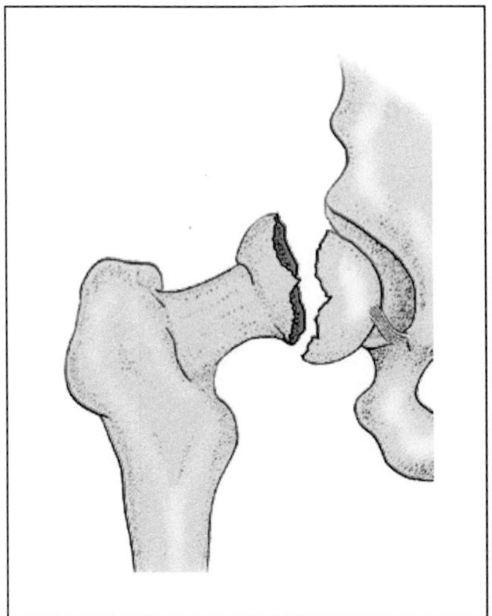

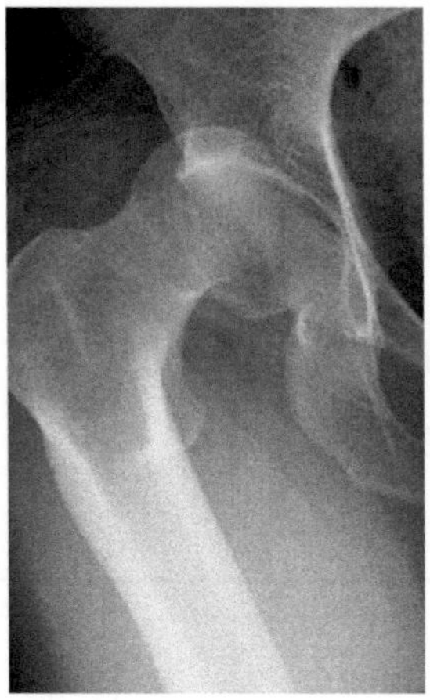

Pipkin classification of femoral head fracture.
Type II: posteriordislocation of the hip with fracture of the femoral head superior to the fovea centralis

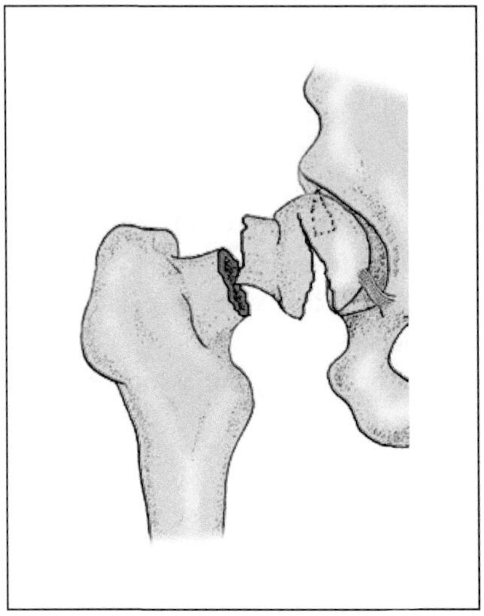

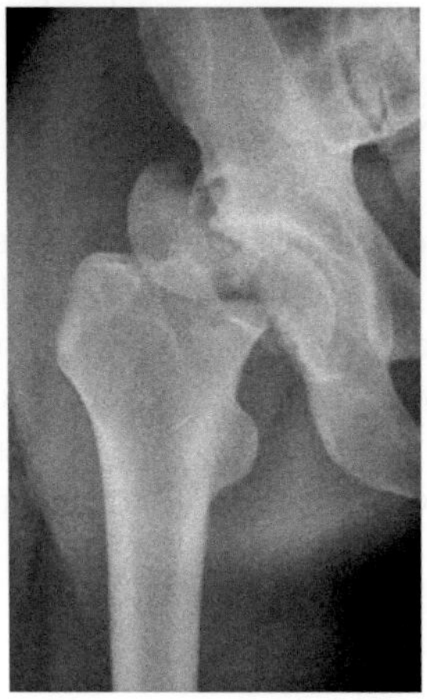

Pipkin classification of femoral head fracture.
Type III: similar to a type I or II injury but associated with fracture of the femoral neck

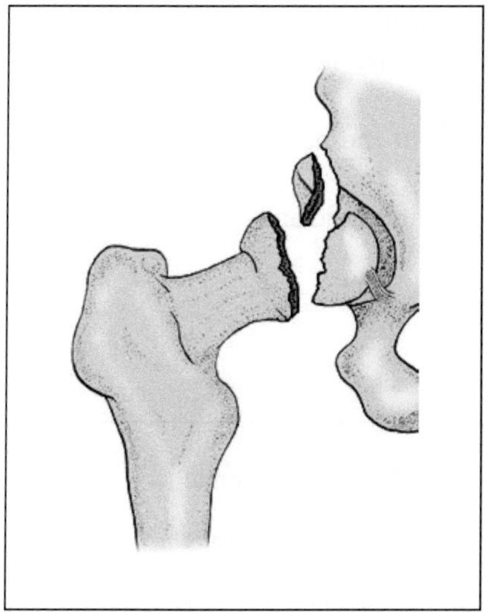

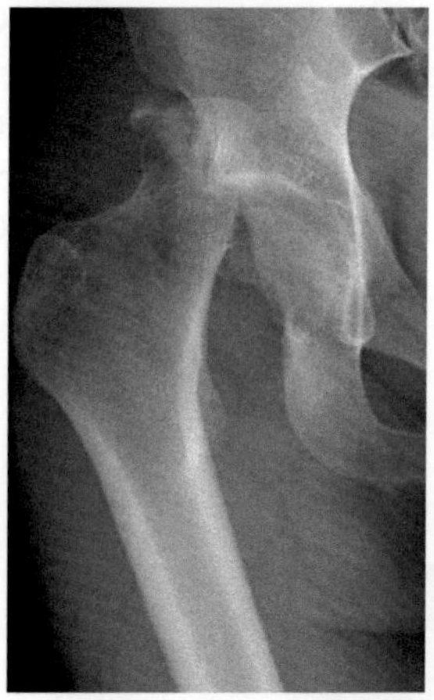

Pipkin classification of femoral head fracture.
Type IV: similar to a type I, II or III injury but associated with fracture of the acetabular rim

8.1.1.2 AO/OTA Classification (2007 revised edition, Journal of Orthopaedic Trauma, 21 supplement. Muller's diaphyseal fracture AO classification was originally published in the 1980s)

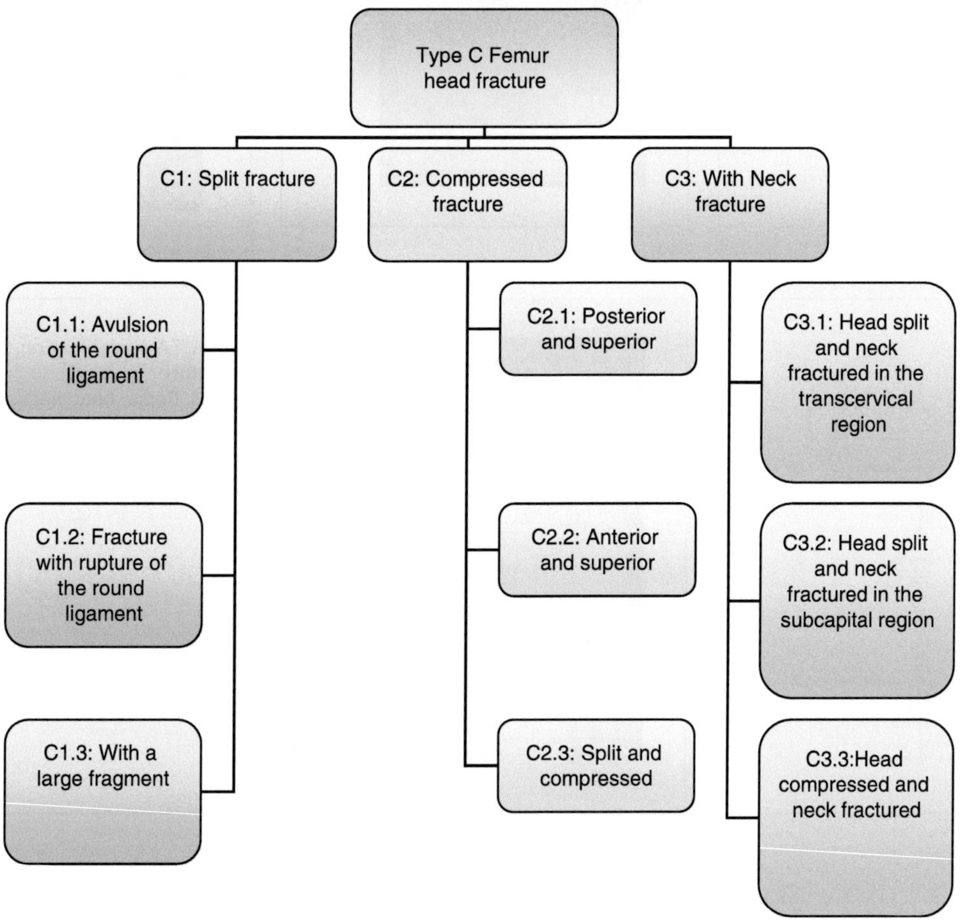

Type C: Femur head fracture:
- Type C1: Split fracture:
  - Type C1.1: Avulsion of the round ligament.
  - Type C1.2: Fracture with rupture of the round ligament.
  - Type C1.3: With a large fragment.
- Type C2: With compression:
  - Type C2.1: Posterior and superior.
  - Type C2.2: Anterior and superior.
  - Type C2.3: Split and compressed.

Type C3: With neck fracture:
- Type C3.1: Head split and neck fractured in the transcervical region.
- Type C3.2: Head split and neck fractured in the subcapital region.
- Type C3.3: Head compressed and neck fractured.

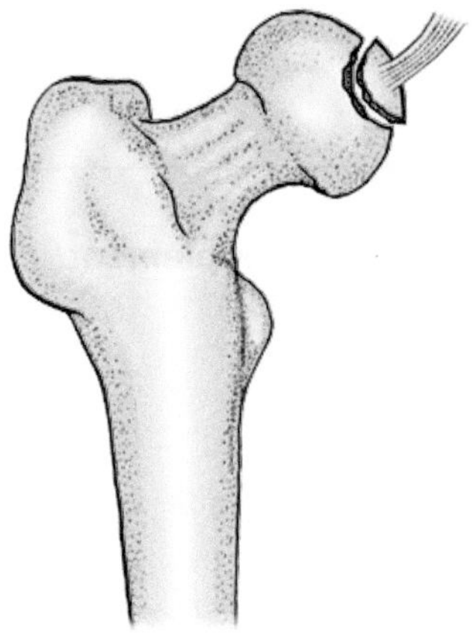

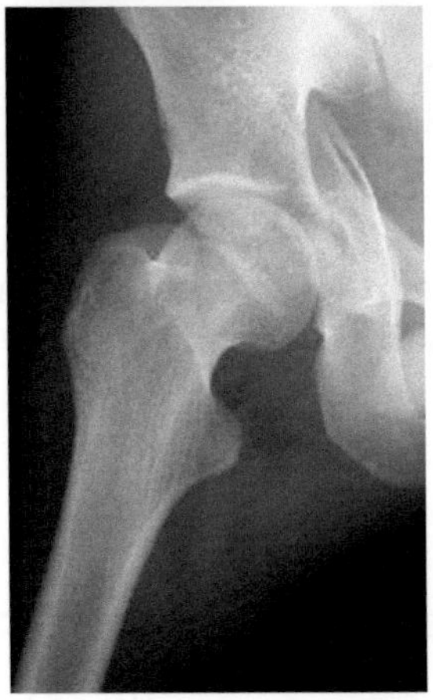

AO/OTA classification of Femur fracture
31-C: Femur head fracture.
C1: Split fracture
C1.1: Avulsion of the round ligament

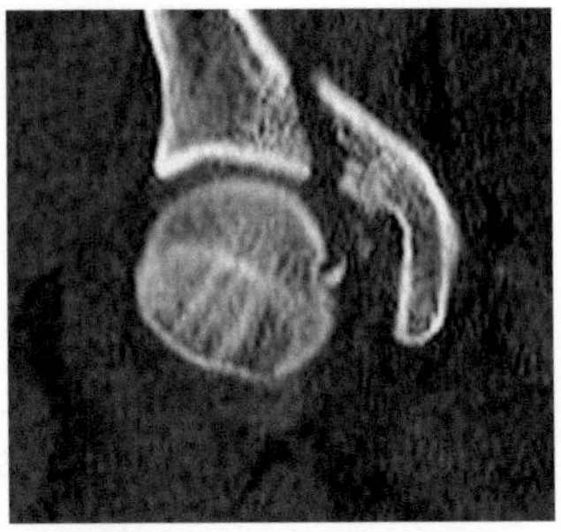

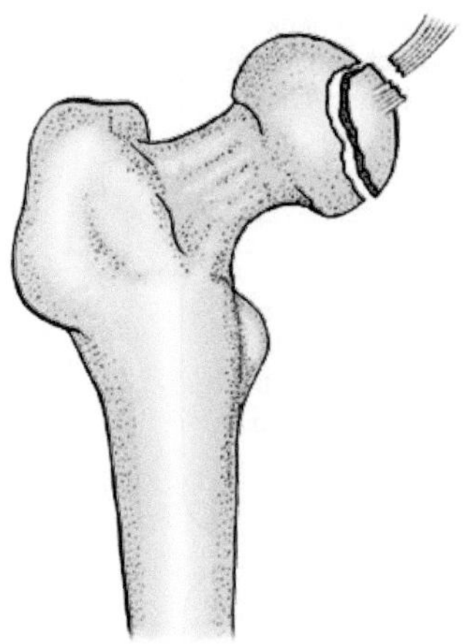

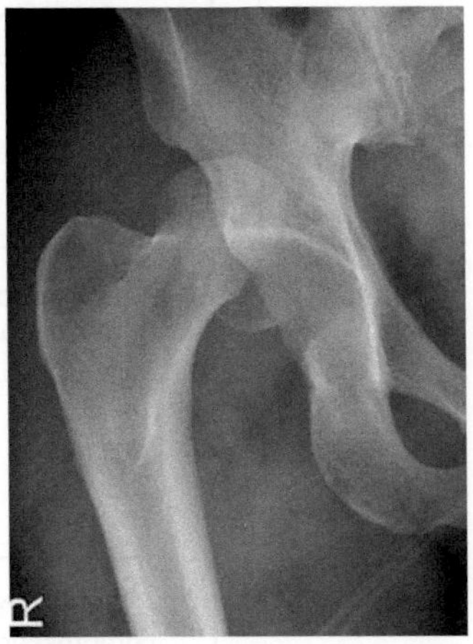

AO/OTA classification of Femur fracture
31-C: Femur head fracture.
C1: Split fracture
C1.2: Fracture with rupture of the round ligament

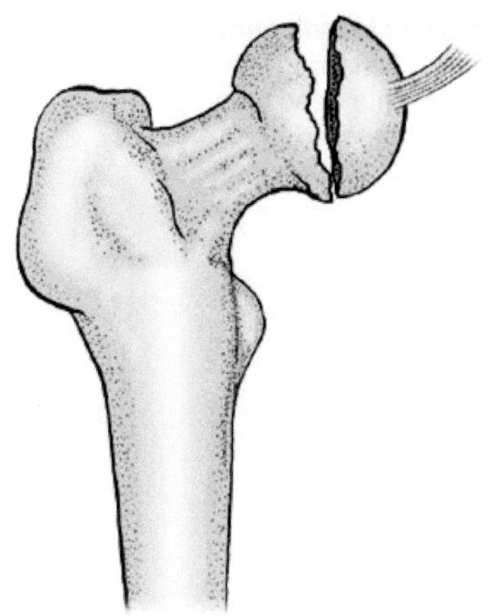

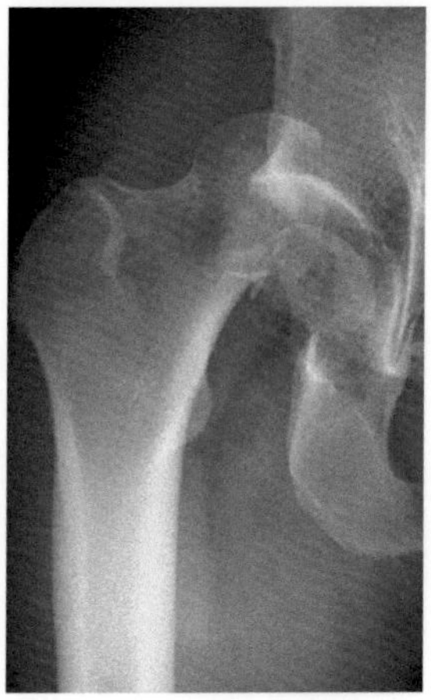

AO/OTA classification of Femur fracture
31-C: Femur head fracture.
C1: Split fracture
C1.3: With a large fragment

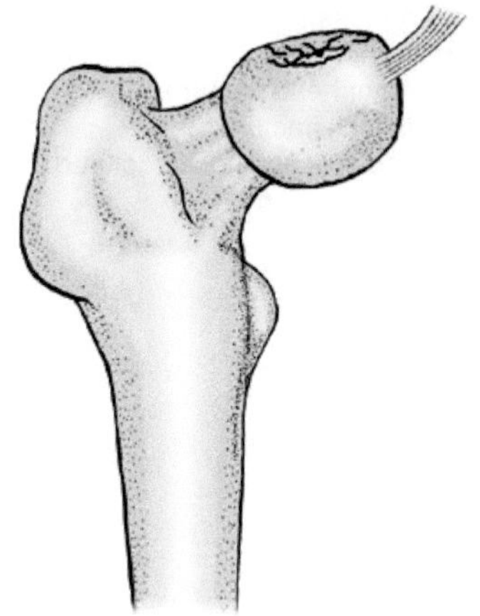

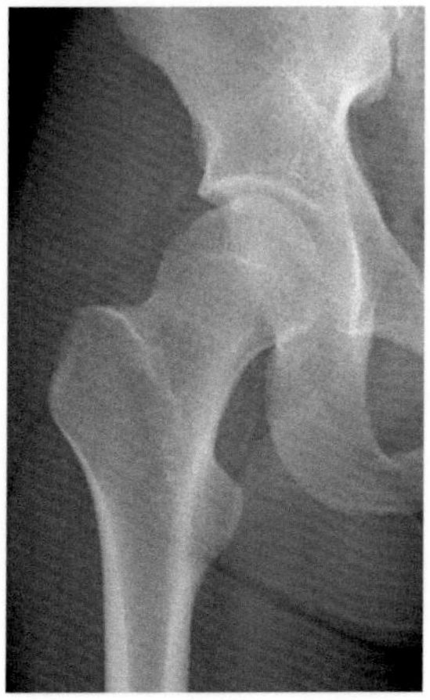

AO/OTA classification of Femur fracture
31-C: Femur head fracture.
C2: Compressed
C2.1: Posterior and superior

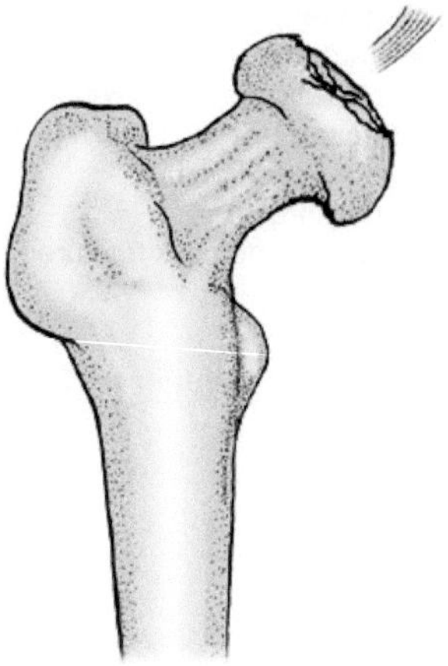

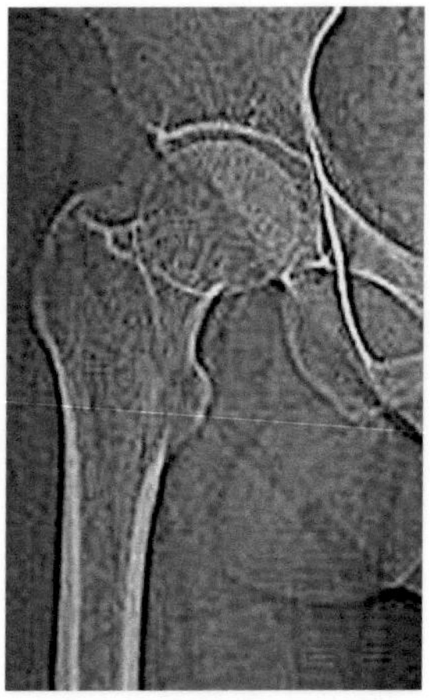

AO/OTA classification of proximal femoral fracture
31-C: Femur head fracture.
C2: Compressed
C2.2: Anterior and superior

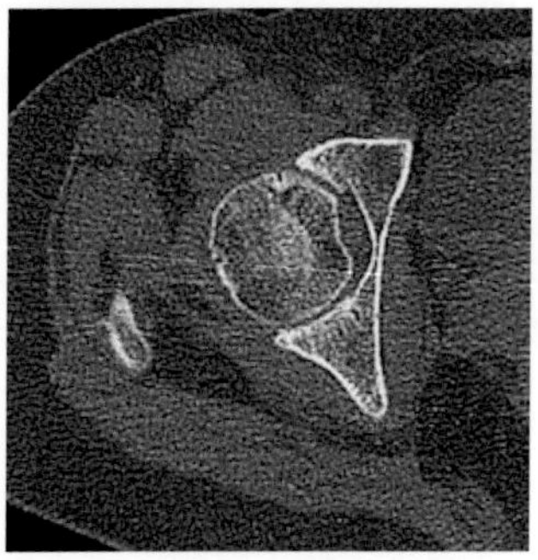

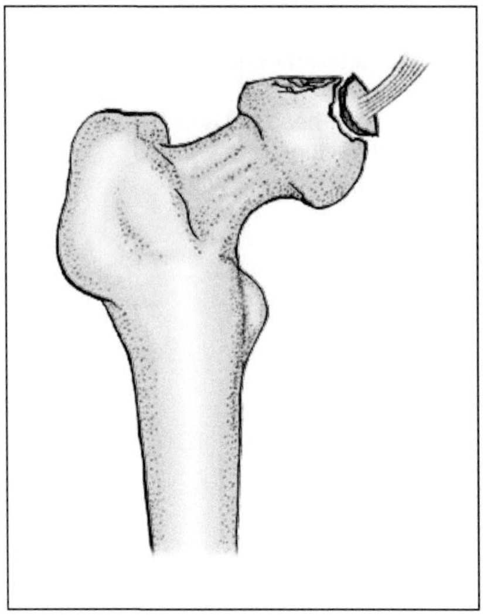

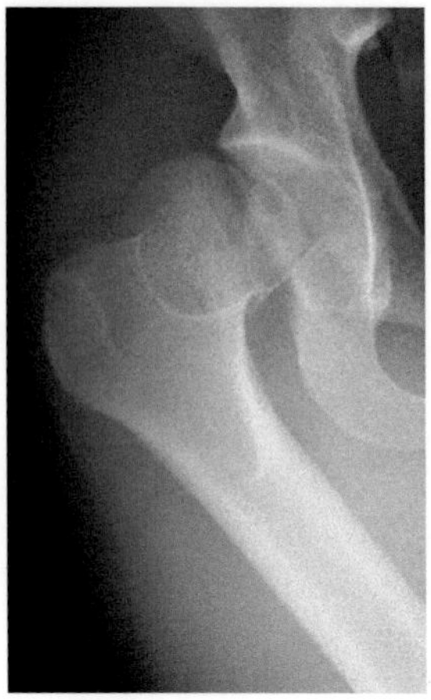

AO/OTA classification of proximal femoral fracture
31-C: Femur head fracture.
C2: Compressed
C2.3: Split and compressed

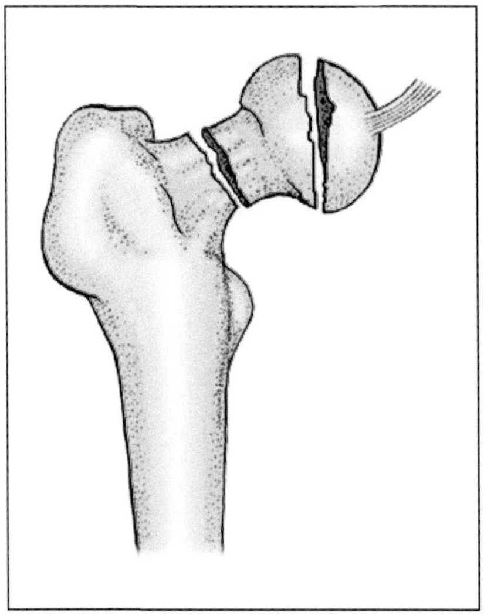

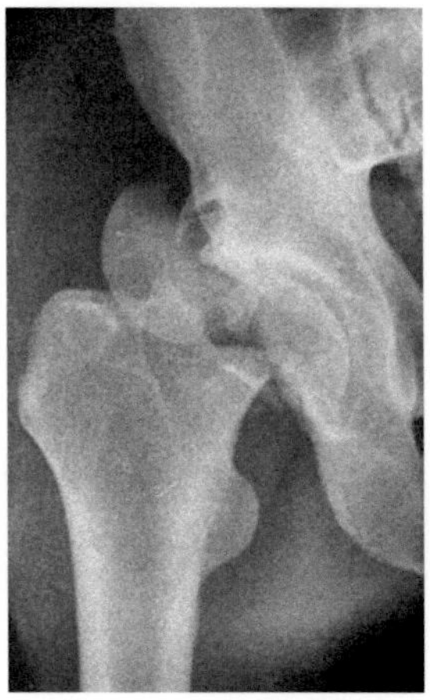

AO/OTA classification of proximal femoral fracture
31-C: Femur head fracture.
C3: With neck fracture
C3.1: head split and neck fractured in transcervical region

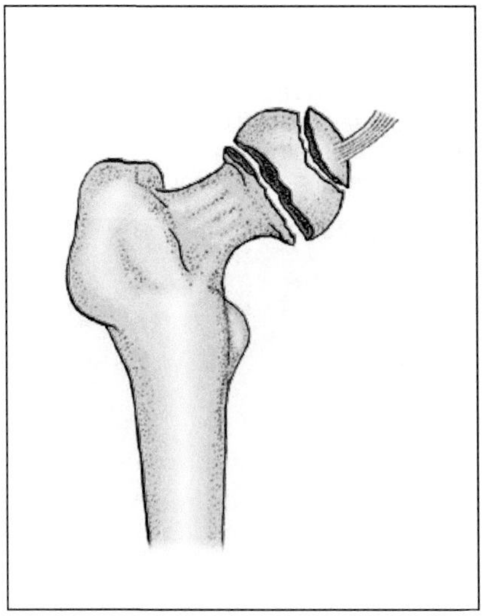

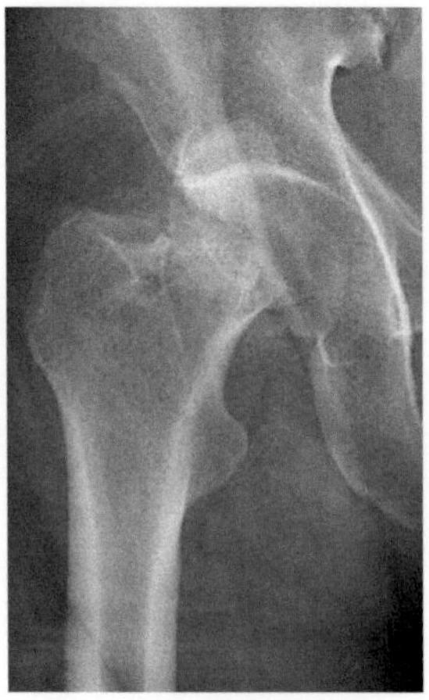

AO/OTA classification of proximal femoral fracture
AO/OTA classification of proximal femoral fracture
31-C: Femur head fracture.
C3: With neck fracture
C3.2: head split and neck fractured in subcapital region

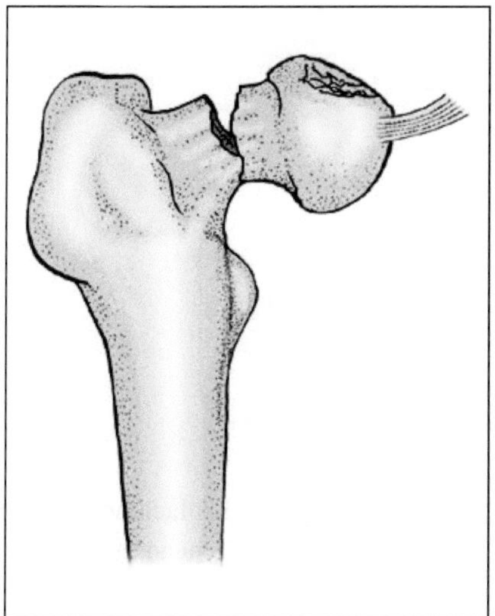

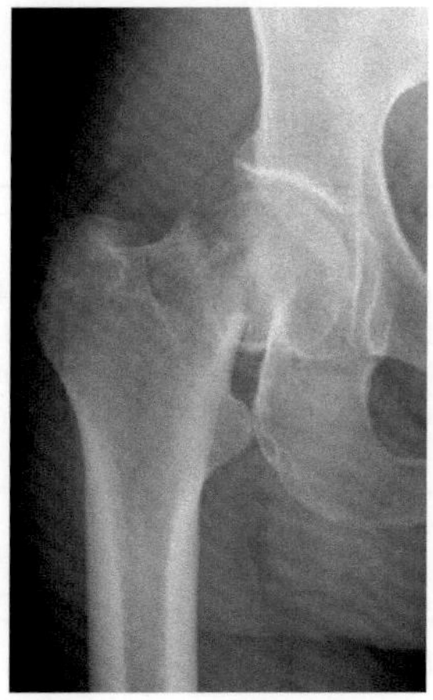

AO/OTA classification of proximal femoral fracture
31-C: Femur head fracture.
C3: With neck fracture
C3.3: Head compressed and neck fractured

8.1.1.3 Brumback Classification (1987, Fractures of the femoral head. In: The Hip Society, editor. Proceeding of the hip Society, 1986 Mf. St. Louis: Mosby, 1987: 181–206)

Type I: Posterior dislocation of hip with fracture of upper part of the femoral head.
Type II: Posterior dislocation of hip with fracture of lower part of the femoral head.
Type II: Anterior or posterior dislocation of hip with fracture of femoral neck.
Type IV: Anterior or posterior dislocation of hip with fracture of proximal femur.
Type V: Fractures of the femoral head with central dislocation.

Although this classification system is more improved than Pipkin classification system, it is still unable to effectively cover the different types of the fracture of femoral head, and is not mainly based on fracture of femoral head, so is rarely mentioned in the clinical.

8.1.1.4 Yoon Classification (2001, Acta Orthop Scand, 72: 348–353)

Yoon classification is modified for Pipkin classification. Femoral fractures can be classified into four types.

Type I: A small fragment of the head distal to the fovea centralis. The fragment(s) was/were too small to be fixed with screws.
Type II: A larger fragment of the head distal to the fovea centralis.
Type III: A large fragment of the head proximal to the fovea centralis.
Type IV: Comminuted fracture.

8.1.1.5 Matejka Classification (2002, Acta Chir Orthop Traumatol Cech, 4: 219–228)

Matejka subdivided Pipkin type IV into four subtypes.

Type A: Chondral fracture of the head.
Type B: Osteochondral fracture of the head.
Type C: Compression of the head.
Type D: Fragment of the head exceeding 1 cm.

8.1.1.6 Giebel Classification

Type I: Fracture without dislocation:
  Type Ia: Compression of the head.
  Type Ib: Comminuted fracture.
Type II: Fracture with hip dislocation:
  Type IIa: Fracture with anterior dislocation.
  Type IIb: Fracture with posterior dislocation.

8.1.2 Classification of Femoral Neck Fractures

Femoral neck fracture classification was put forward by Abraham Colles (Irish surgeon) for the first time in 1818. Now there are still more than ten kinds of classification systems. According to the literature in the last 5 years, Garden classification was used most frequently, followed by AO/OTA classification, classifications according to the anatomic site, and Pauwels classification.

8.1.2.1 Garden Classification (1961, J Bone Joint Surg (Br), 43: 647–663)

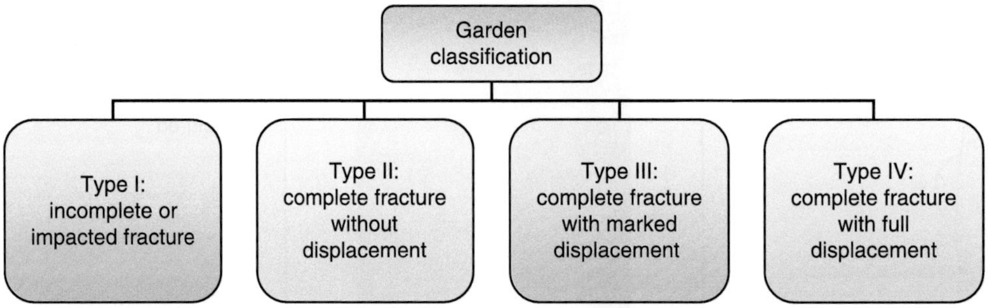

Type I: Incomplete or impacted fracture of the neck.

Type II: Complete fracture without displacement in anterior or lateral direction.

Type III: Complete fracture with partial displacement. The direction of bone trabecula in femoral head is not inconsistent with that of acetabulum.

Type IV: Complete fracture with full displacement. The direction of bone trabecula in femoral head is parallel with that of acetabulum.

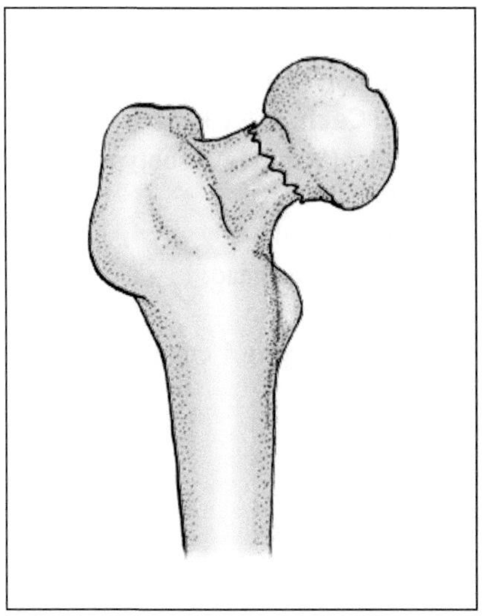

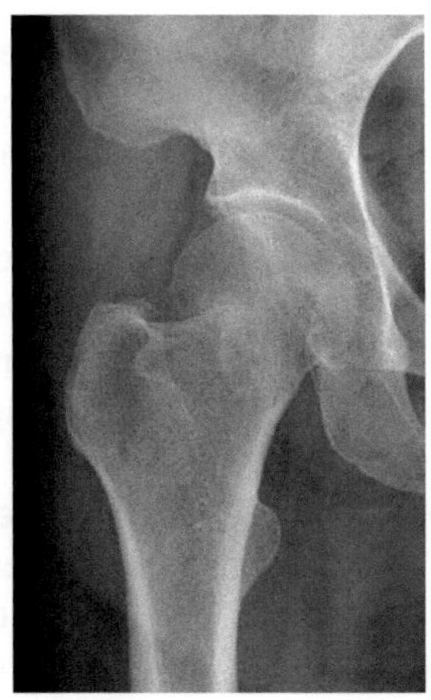

Garden classification of femoral neck fractures
Type I: Incomplete or impacted fracture

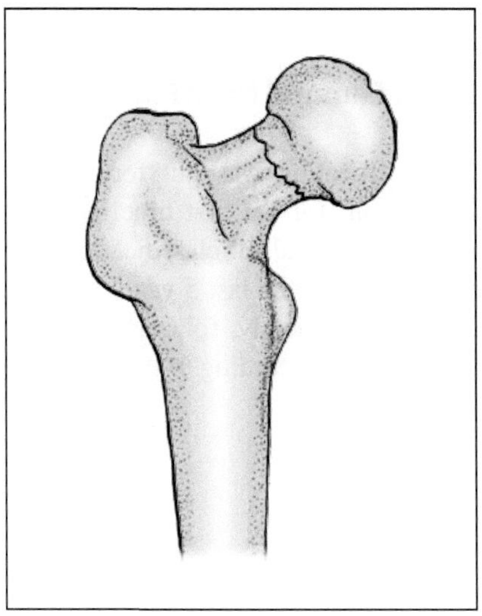

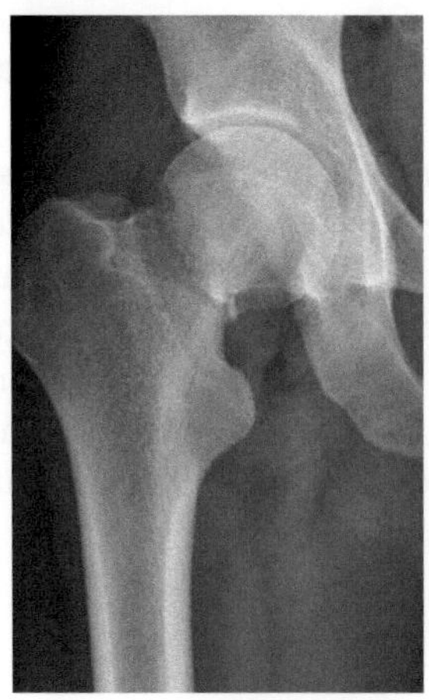

Garden classification of femoral neck fractures
Type II: Complete fracture without displacement

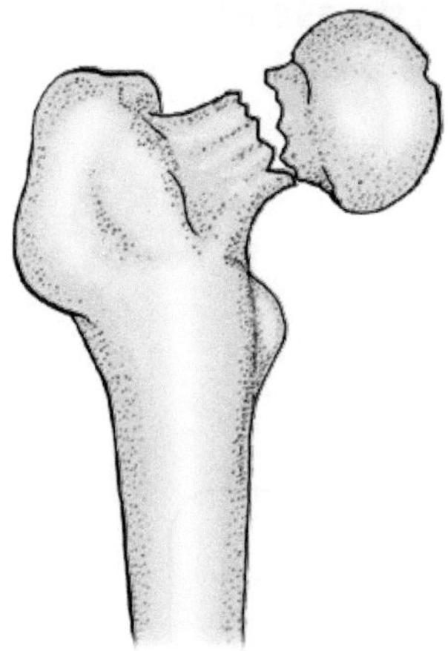

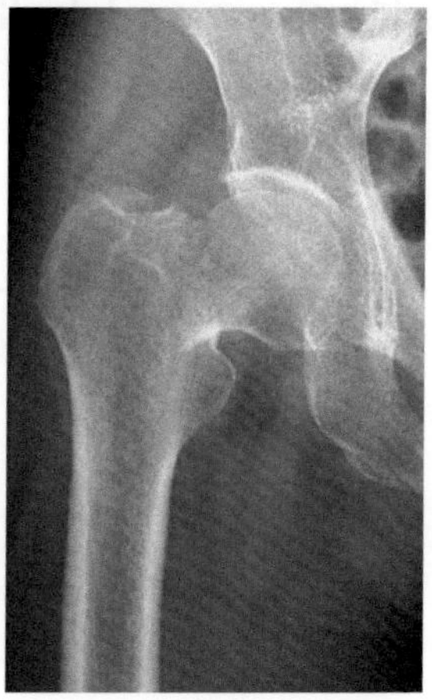

Garden classification of femoral neck fractures

Type III: Complete fracture with partial displacement. The direction of bone trabecula in femoral head is not inconsistent with that of acetabulum.

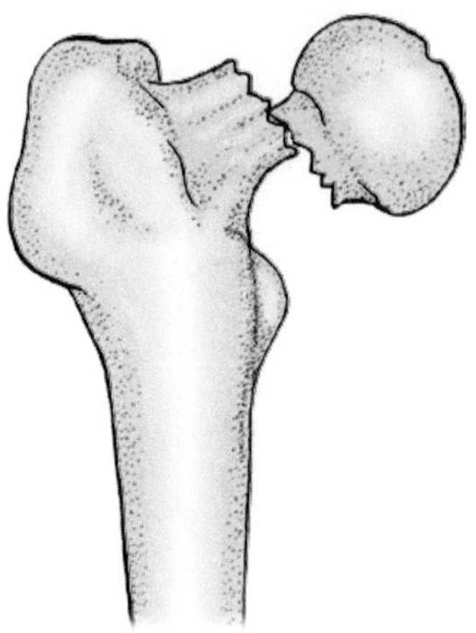

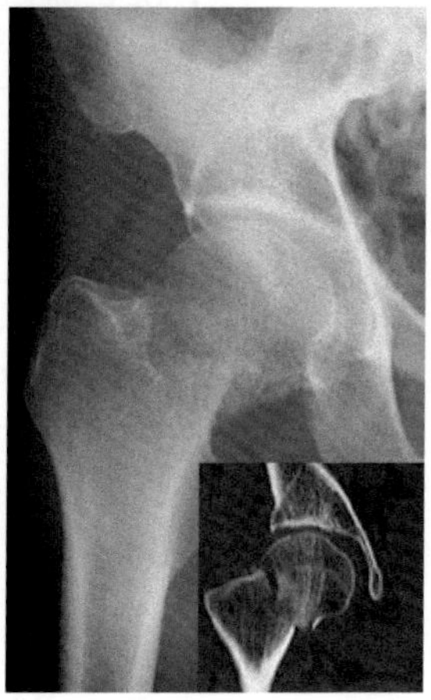

Garden classification of femoral neck fractures

Type IV: Complete fracture with full displacement. The direction of bone trabecula in femoral head is parallel with that of acetabulum.

8.1.2.2 AO/OTA Classification (2007 Revised Edition, Journal of Orthopaedic Trauma, 21 supplement. Muller's long bone fracture AO classification was originally published in the 1980s)

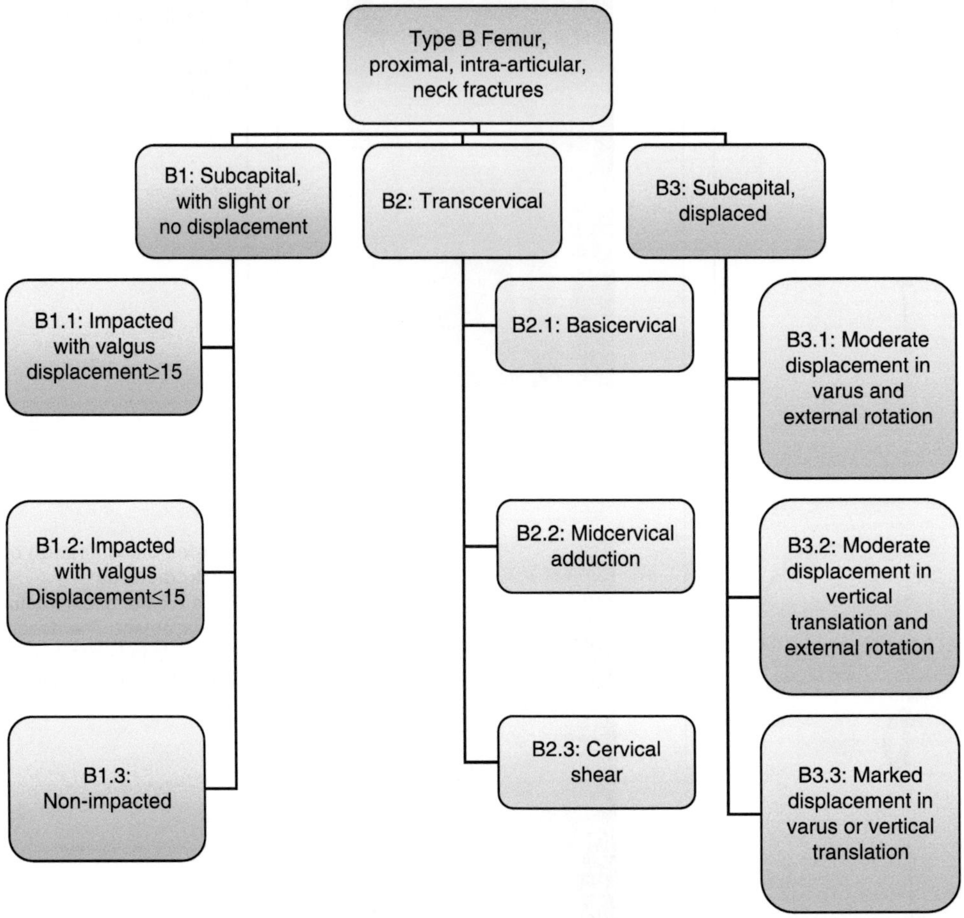

Type B: Femur, proximal, intra-articular, neck fractures:
- Type B1: Subcapital, with slight or no displacement:
  - Type B1.1: Impacted with valgus displacement ≥15°.
  - Type B1.2: Impacted with valgus displacement 15°.
  - Type B1.3: Non-impacted.
- Type B2: Transcervical, with minimal displacement:
  - Type B2.1: Basicervical.
  - Type B2.2: Midcervical adduction.
  - Type B2.3: Cervical shear.
- Type B3: Subcapital, displaced without impaction:
  - Type B3.1: Moderate displacement in varus and external rotation.
  - Type B3.2: Moderate displacement in vertical translation and external rotation.
  - Type B3.3: Marked displacement in varus or vertical translation.

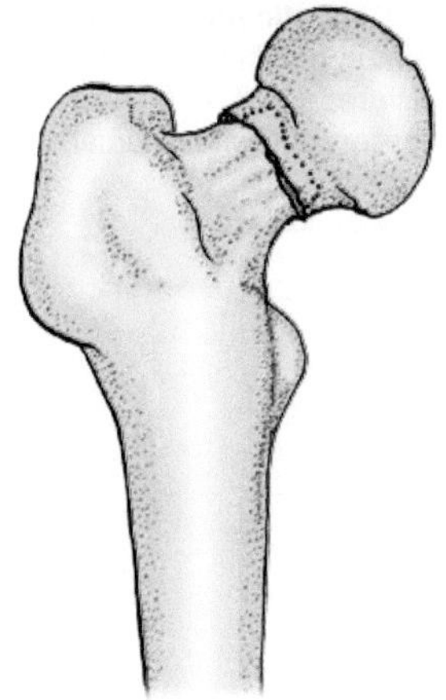

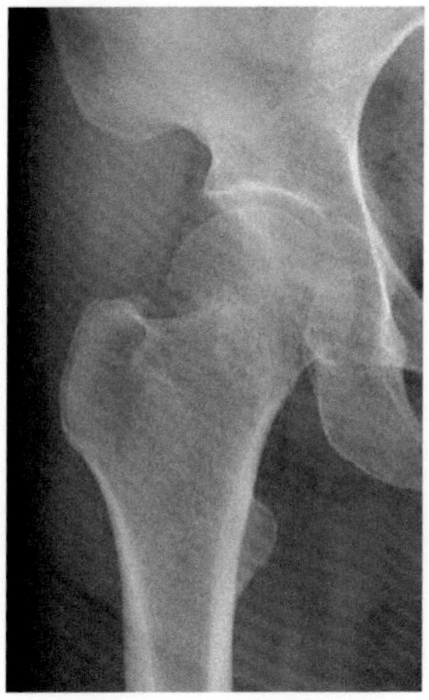

AO/OTA Classification of femur
31-B: Femur, proximal, intra-articular, neck fractures.
B1: Subcapital, with slight or no displacement
B1.1: Impacted with valgus displacement≥15°

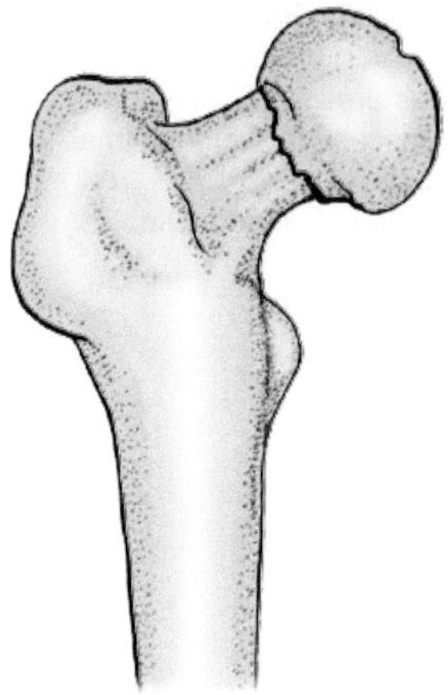

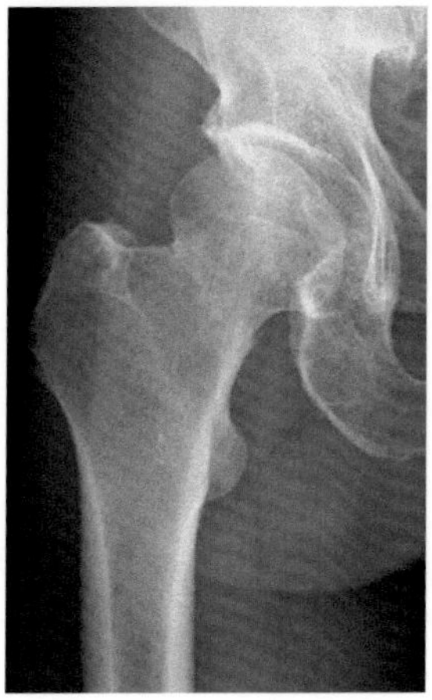

AO/OTA Classification of femur
31-B: Femur, proximal, intra-articular, neck fractures.
B1: Subcapital, with slight or no displacement
B1.2: Impacted with valgus displacement≤15°

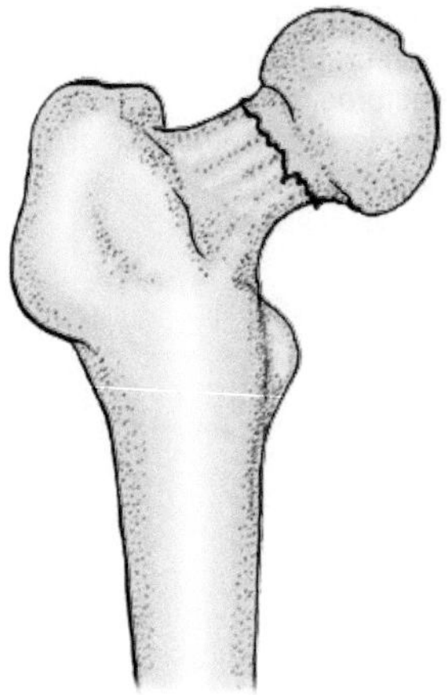

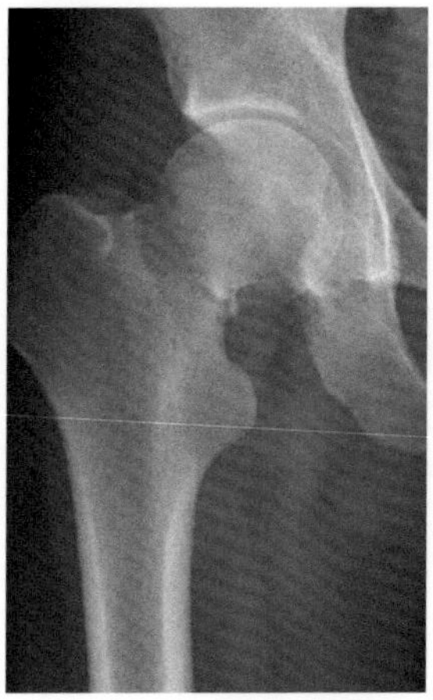

AO/OTA Classification of femur
31-B: Femur, proximal, intra-articular, neck fractures
B1: Subcapital, with slight or no displacement
B1.3: Non-impacted

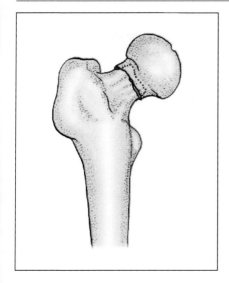

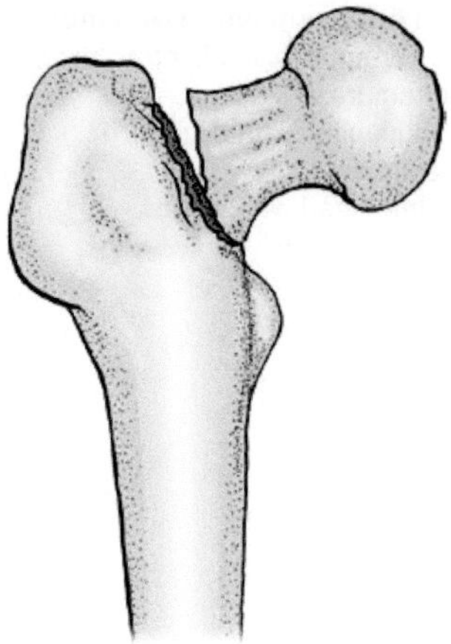

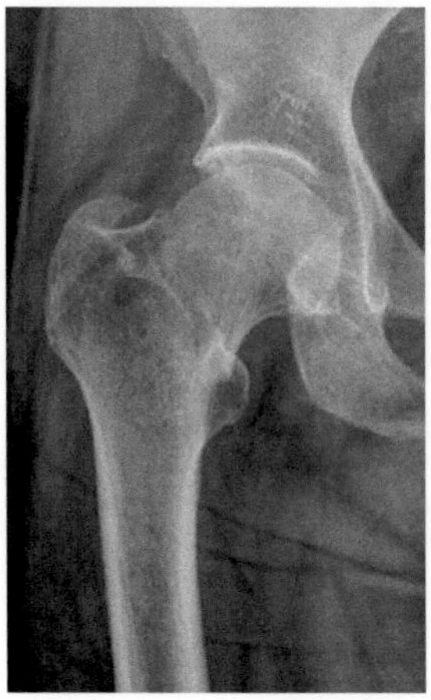

AO/OTA Classification of femur
31-B: Femur, proximal, intra-articular, neck fractures.
B2: Transcervical, with minimal displacement
B2.1: Basicervical

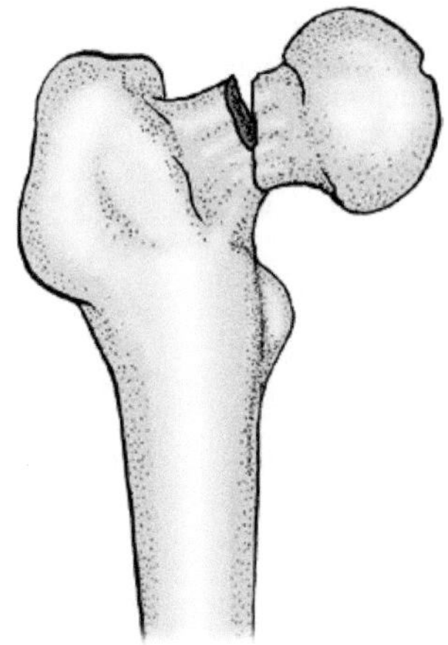

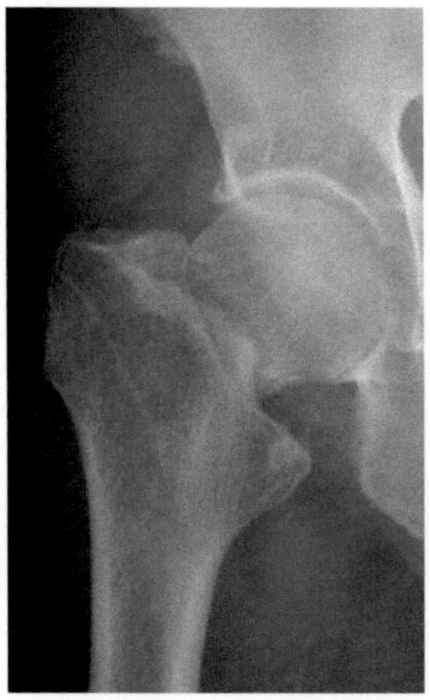

AO/OTA Classification of femur
31-B: Femur, proximal, intra-articular, neck fractures.
B2: Transcervical, with minimal displacement
B2.2: Midcervical adduction

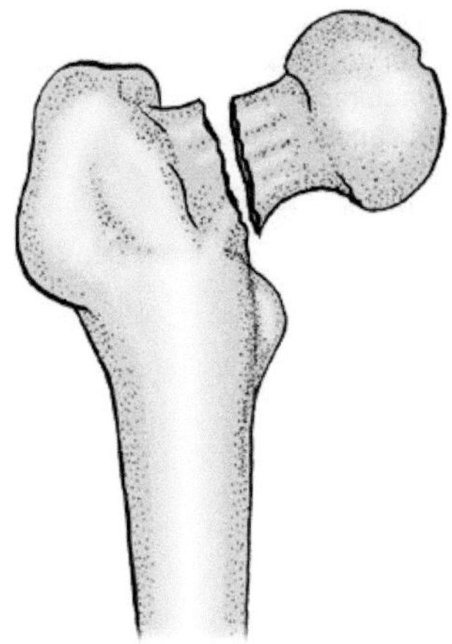

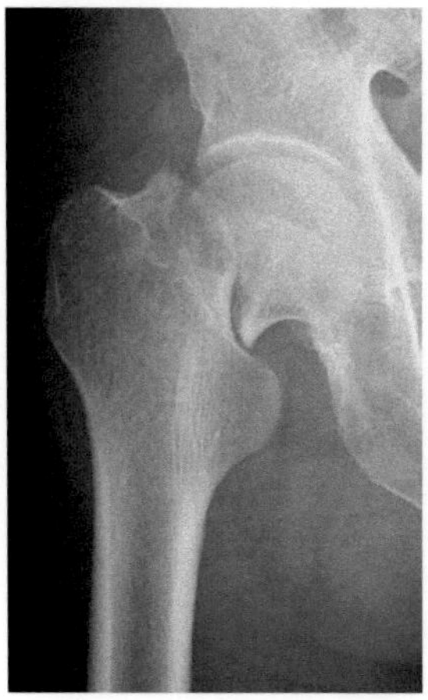

AO/OTA Classification of femur
31-B: Femur, proximal, intra-articular, neck fractures.
B2: Transcervical, with minimal displacement
B2.3: Cervical shear

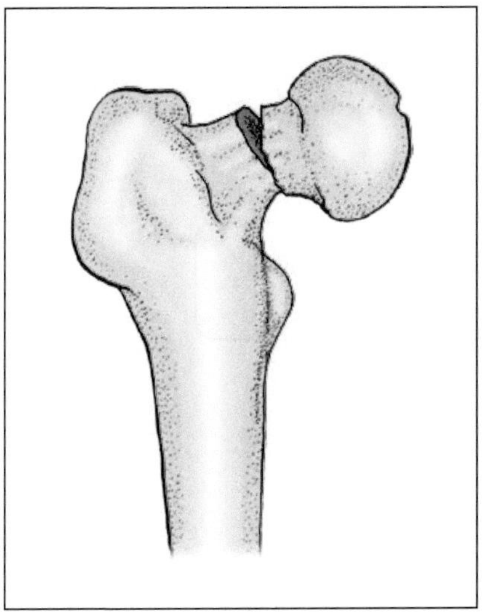

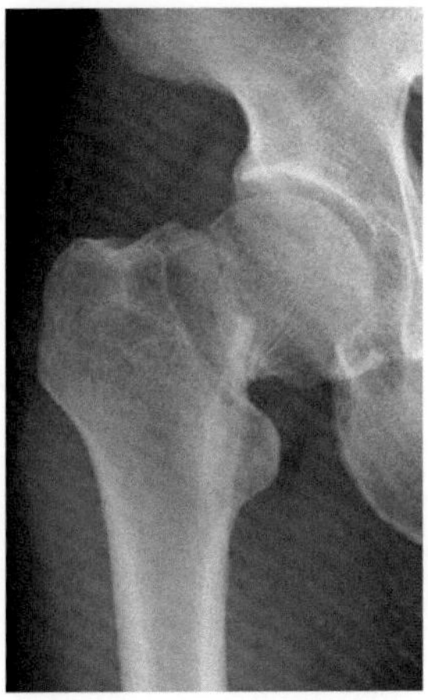

AO/OTA Classification of femur
31-B: Femur, proximal, intra-articular, neck fractures.
B3: Subcapital, displaced without impaction
B3.1: Moderate displacement in varus and external rotation

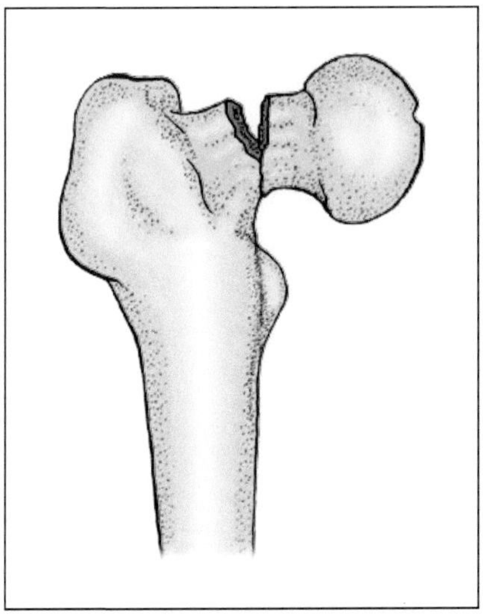

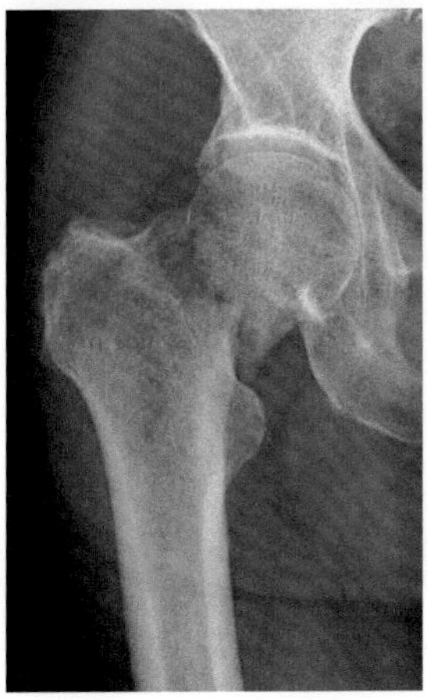

AO/OTA Classification of femur
31-B: Femur, proximal, intra-articular, neck fractures.
B3: Subcapital, displaced without impaction
B3.2: Moderate displacement in vertical translation and external rotation

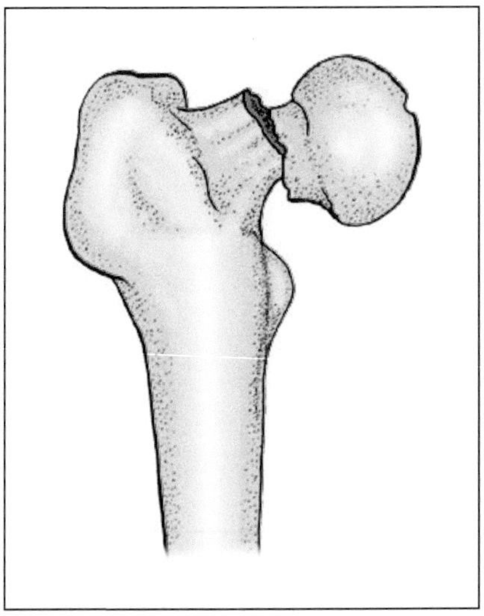

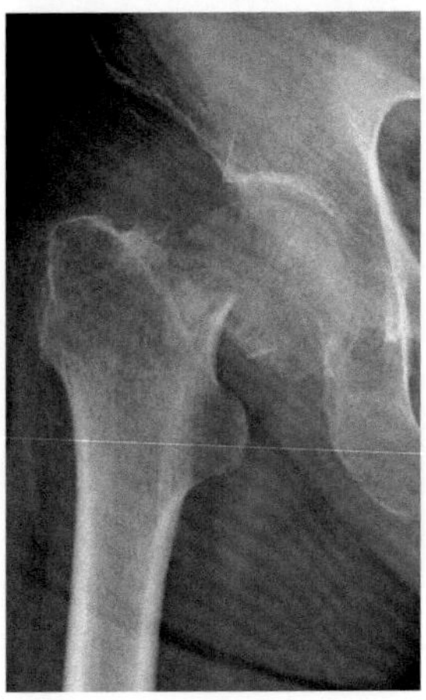

AO/OTA Classification of femur
31-B: Femur, proximal, intra-articular, neck fractures.
B3: Subcapital, displaced without impaction
B3.3: Marked displacement in varus or vertical translation

8.1.2.3 Classification Based on Anatomic Sites (Rockwood, 1984)

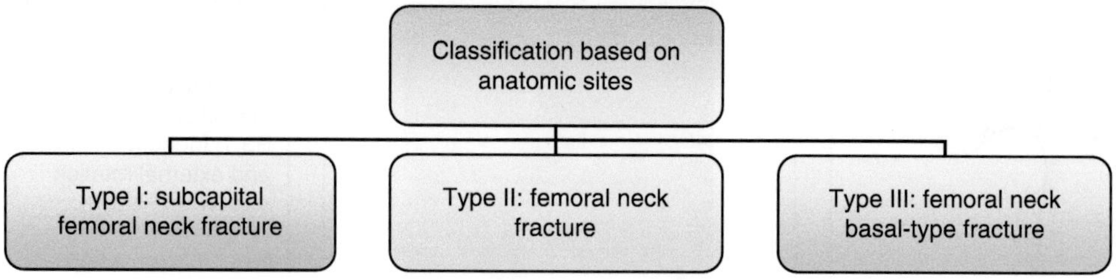

Type I: Subcapital femoral neck fracture.
Type II: Femoral neck fracture.
Type III: Basicervical fracture.

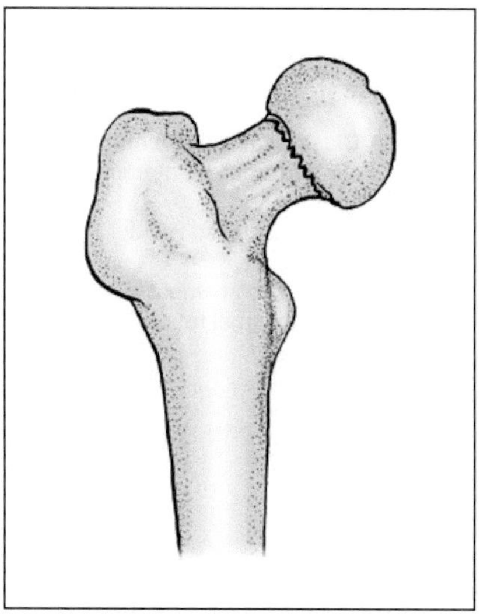

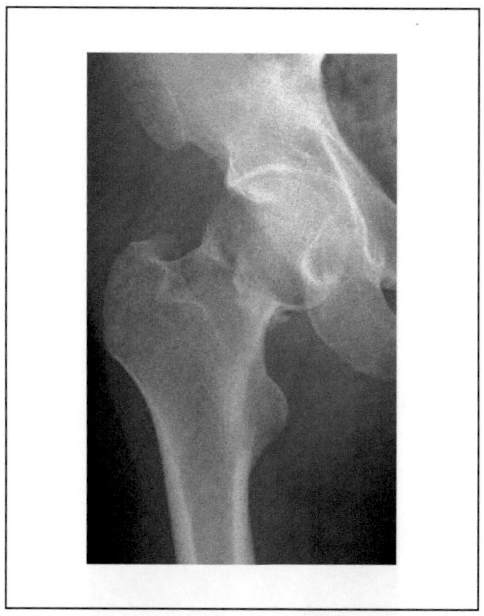

Anatomical classification:
Type I: subcapital femoral neck fracture

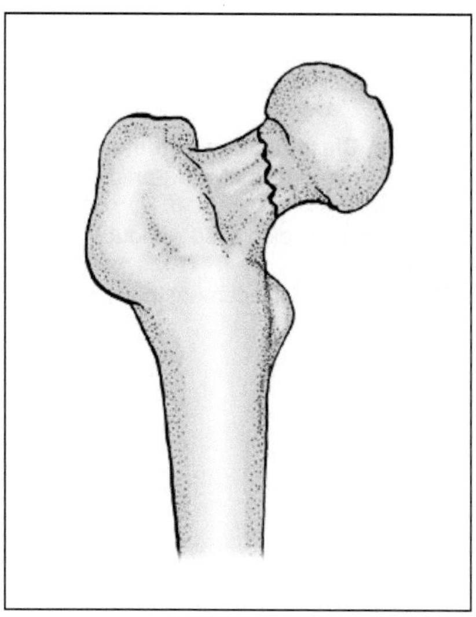

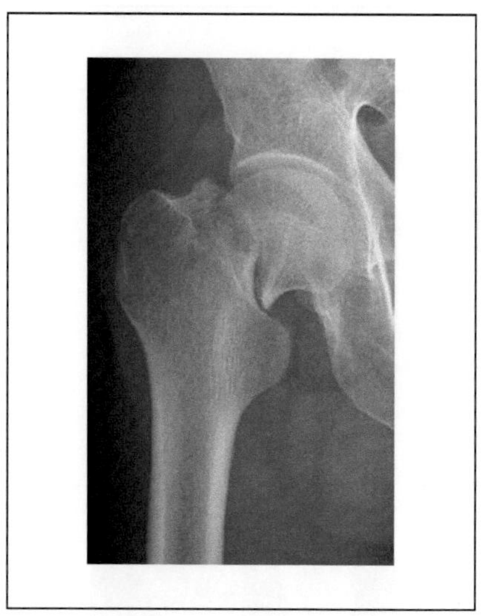

Anatomical classification
Type II: Femoral neck fracture

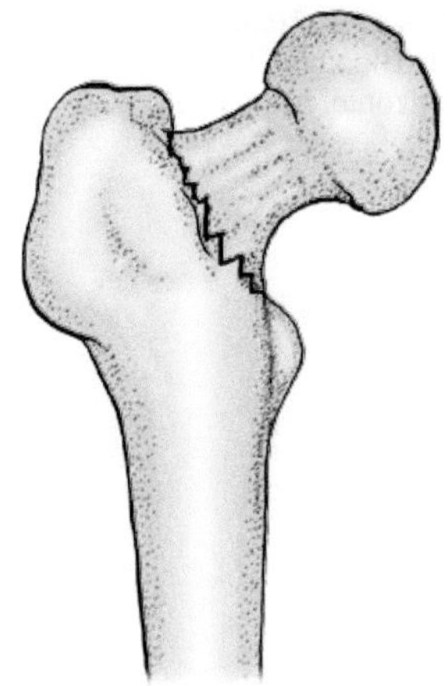

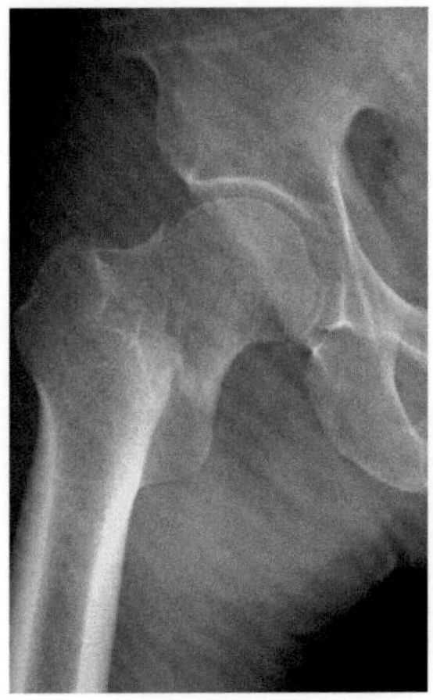

Anatomical classification
Type III: basicervical fracture

8.1.2.4 Pauwels Classification (1935, Stuttgart, Beilageheft zur Zeitschrift fur Orthopaedische Chirurgie, Ferdinand Enke)

Pauwels proposed a classification method in 1935, based on the angle of fracture line and the anterior superior iliac spine connection (Pauwels angle).

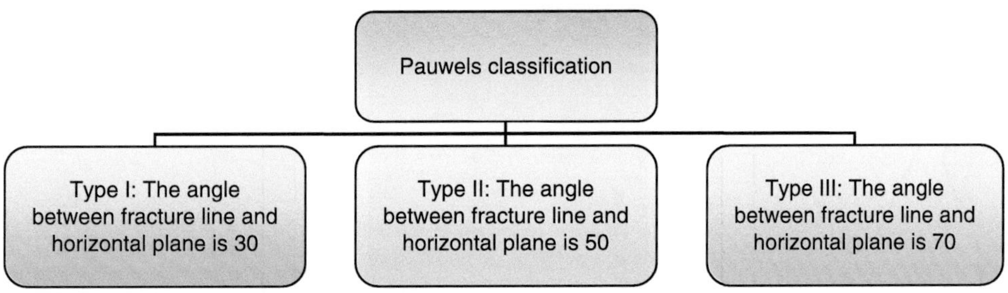

Type I: The angle between fracture line and horizontal plane is 30.
Type II: The angle between fracture line and horizontal plane is 50.
Type III: The angle between fracture line and horizontal plane is 70.

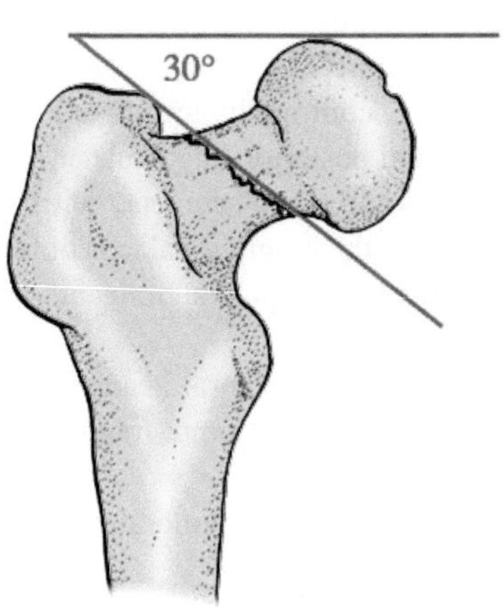

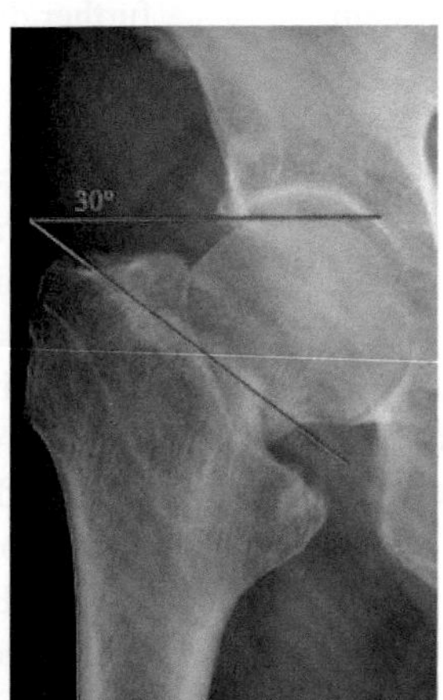

Pauwels classification
Type I: The angle between fracture line and horizontal plane is 30

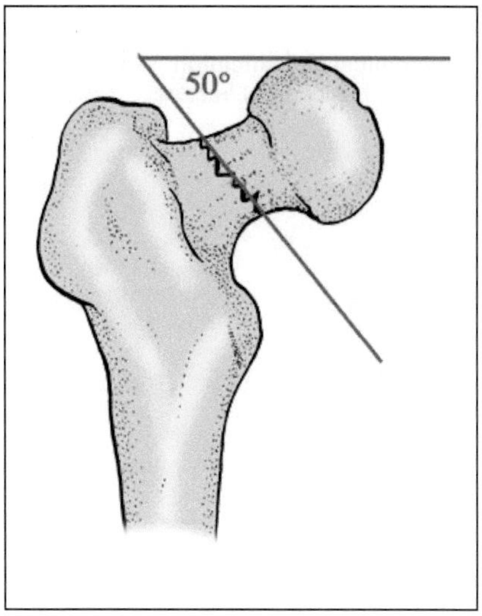

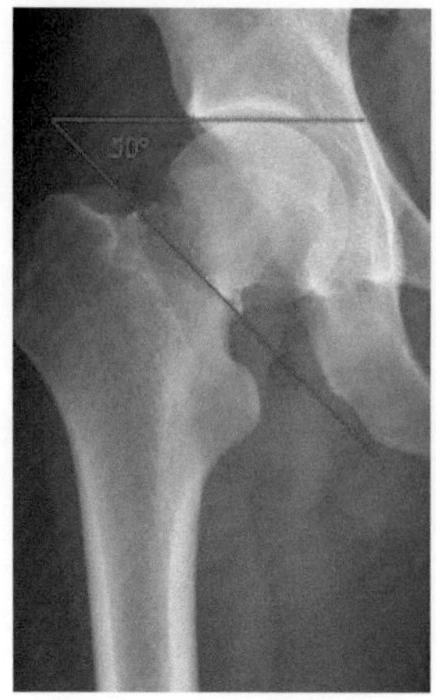

Pauwels classification
Type II: The angle between fracture line and horizontal plane is 50

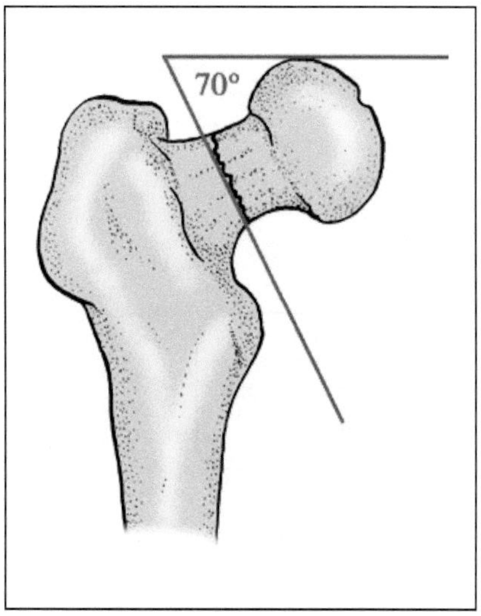

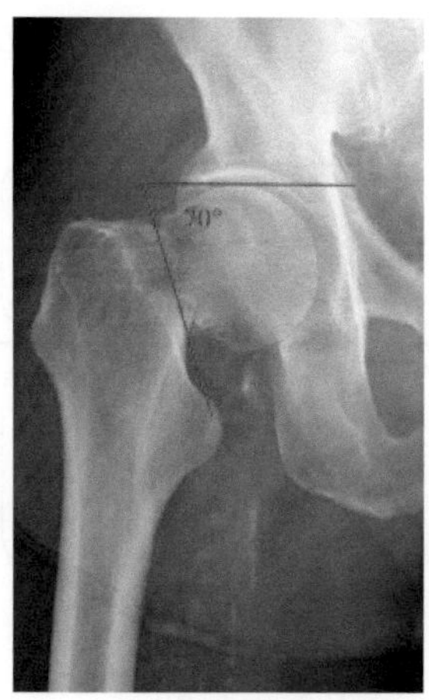

Pauwels classification
Type III: The angle between fracture line and horizontal plane is 70

8.1.2.5 Binyao Mao Classification (1992)

According to the anatomical sites of the fracture, Mao added a head-neck type to the traditional classification system.

Type I: Subcapital femoral neck fracture.
Type II: Head-neck femoral neck fracture.
Type III: Transcervical femoral neck fracture.
Type IV: Basicervical femoral neck fracture.

8.1.2.6 Linton Classification (1944)

According to the angle of femoral longitudinal axis perpendicular to fracture line (Linton angle), femoral neck fracture is divided into three types:

Type I: Linton angle <30°, stable fracture.
Type II: Linton angle between 30°and 50°, less stable.
Type III: Linton angle >50°, unstable fracture.

8.1.2.7 Yingze Zhang' CT Classification (2010)

Type I: Complete fracture without displacement, which is further divided into two subtypes.
- Type IA: Non-impacted fracture.
- Type IB: Impacted fracture, commonly accompanied by femoral head rotation and posterior fragments at.

Type II: Transverse fracture with displacement, with the fracture line perpendicular to the longitudinal axis of femoral neck and fracture displacement is significant. This type is divided into three subtypes.
- Type II A: Non-impacted and the femoral head was displaced posterior and rotated, with bone fragments at the posterior.
- Type II B: Impacted fracture, and the femoral head was displaced posterior and rotated.
- Type II C: Fracture separation.

Type III: Oblique displaced fracture with cortical bone fragment medial-inferior the femoral head. Fracture was displaced significantly. This type is further divided into two subtypes.

Type IIIA: Non-impacted fracture with femoral head post-inferior displaced, commonly accompanied with the rotation of the femoral head and the fragments at the posterior.

Type III B: Impacted fracture.

Type IV: Comminuted fracture with more than two bone fragments.

8.1.3 Classification of Femoral Trochanteric Fracture

Evans and Boyd, and Griffin, proposed the classification systems of femoral intertrochanteric fracture in 1949. There are a dozen types of classification systems. According to citation frequency in the recent 5 years' literature, AO classification was the first, followed by Evans-Jensen classification and Evans classification.

8.1.3.1 AO/OTA Classification (2007 Revised Edition, Journal of Orthopaedic Trauma, 21 supplement. Muller' AO classification of long bone fractures, firstly published in the 1980s)

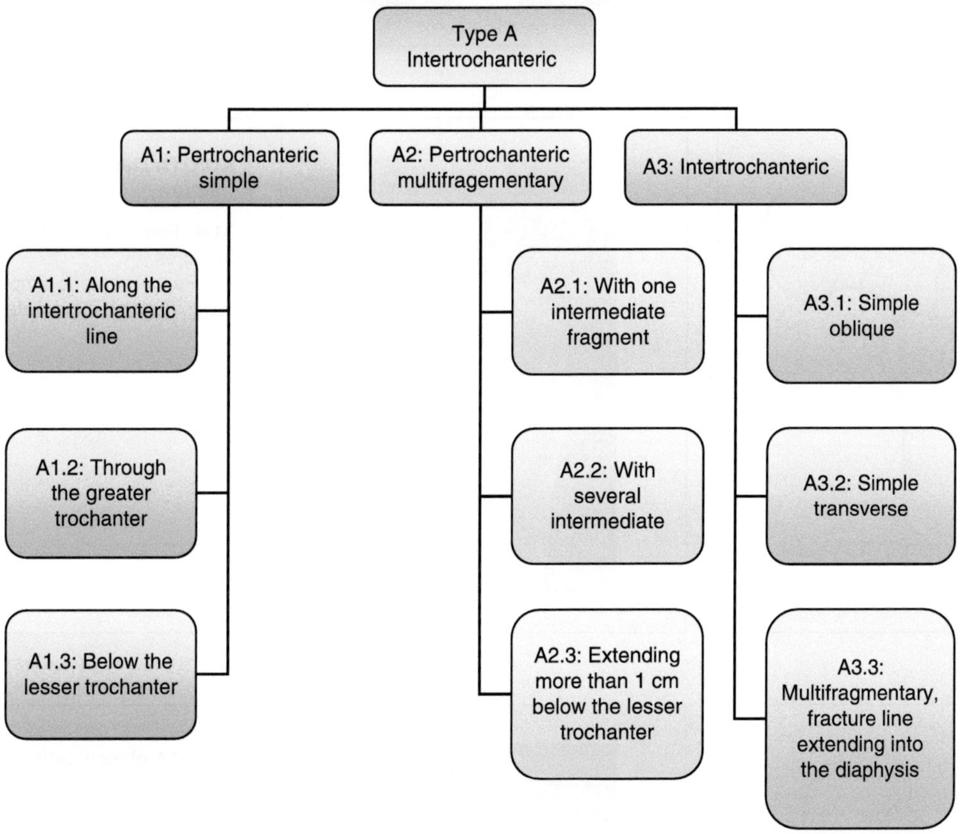

Type A: Intertrochanteric fracture:

Type A1: Pertrochanteric simple:

Type A1.1: Along the intertrochanteric line.

Type A1.2: Through the greater trochanter.

Type A1.3: Below the lesser trochanter.

Type A2: Pertrochanteric multifragmentary:

Type A2.1: With one intermediate fragment.

Type A2.2: With several intermediate fragments.

Type A2.3: Extending more than 1 cm below the lesser trochanter.

Type A3: Intertrochanteric:

Type A3.1: Simple oblique.

Type A3.2: Simple transverse.

Type A3.3: Multifragmentary, fracture line.

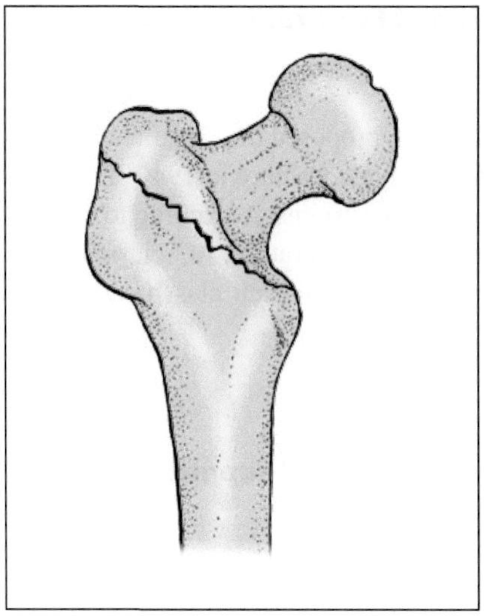

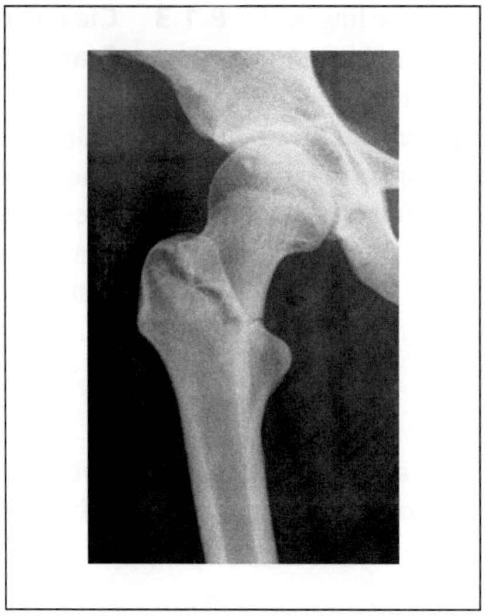

AO/OTA classification for femur fracture

31-A: Femur, proximal, trochanteric fractures.
A1: Pertrochanteric simple
A1.1: Along the intertrochanteric line

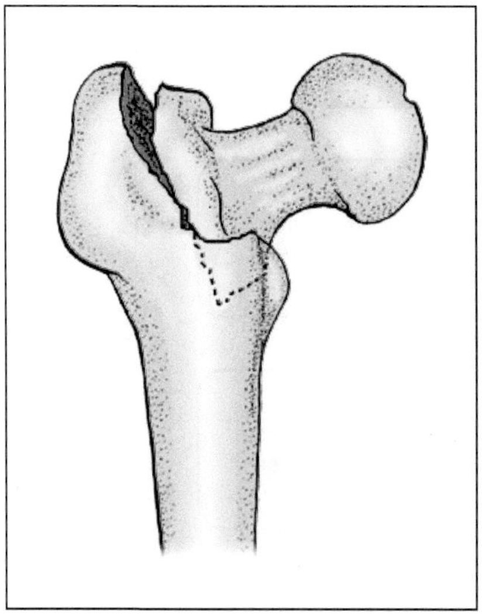

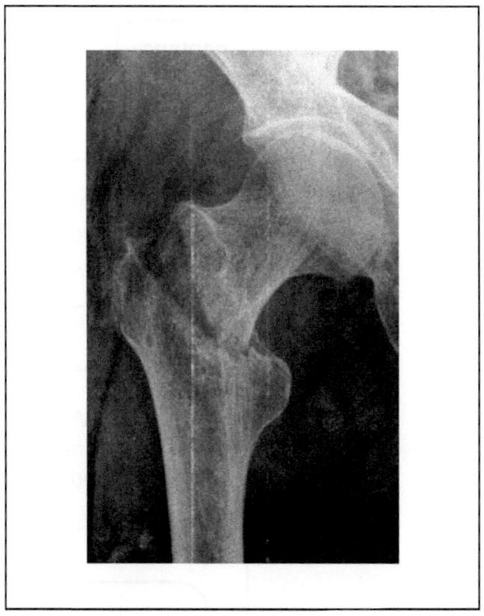

AO/OTA classification for femur fracture

31-A: Femur, proximal, trochanteric fractures.
A1: Pertrochanteric simple
A1.2: Through the greater trochanter

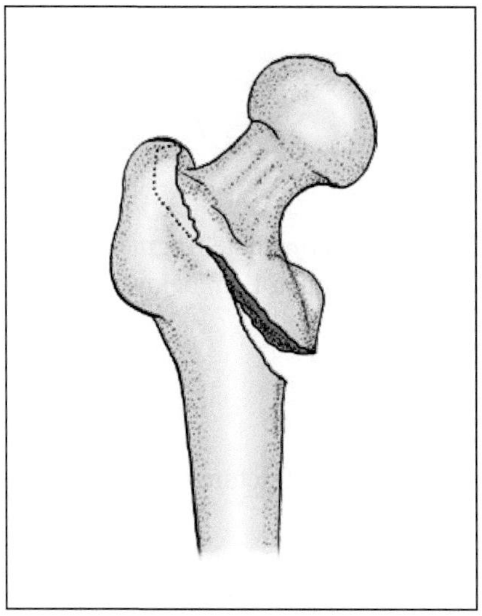

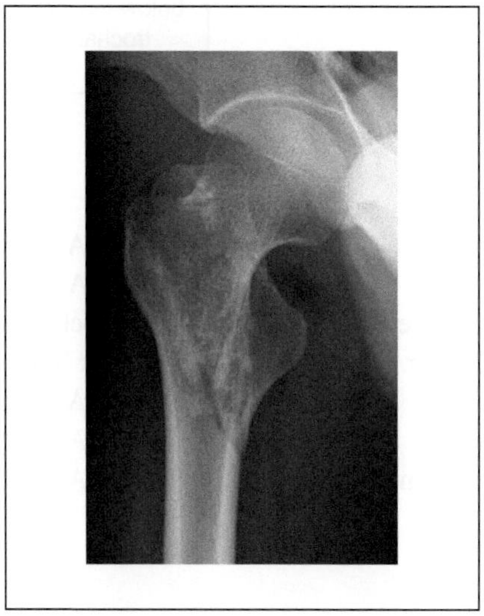

AO/OTA classification for femur fracture

31-A: Femur, proximal, trochanteric fractures.
A1: Pertrochanteric simple
A1.3: Below the lesser trochanter

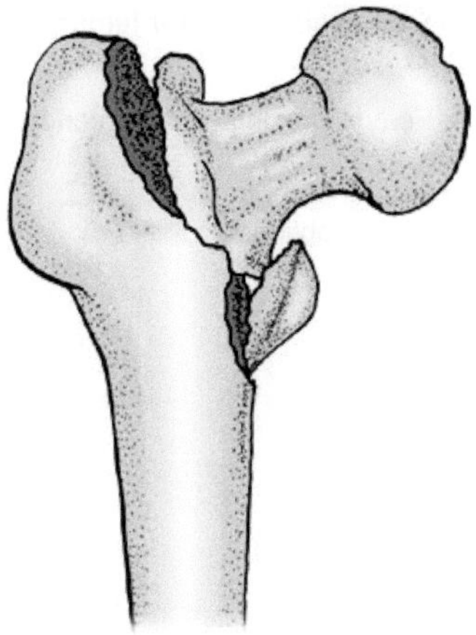

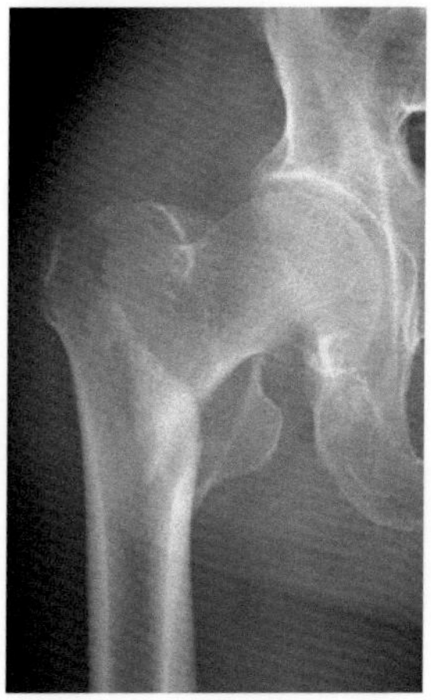

AO/OTA classification for femur fracture

31-A: Femur, proximal, trochanteric fractures.
A2: Pertrochanteric multifragmentary
A2.1: With one intermediate fragment

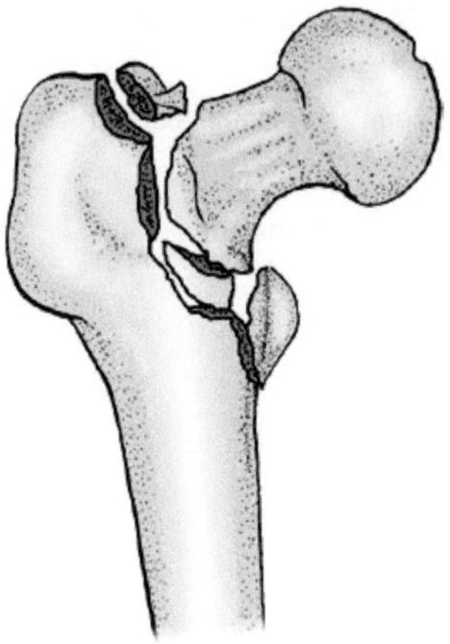

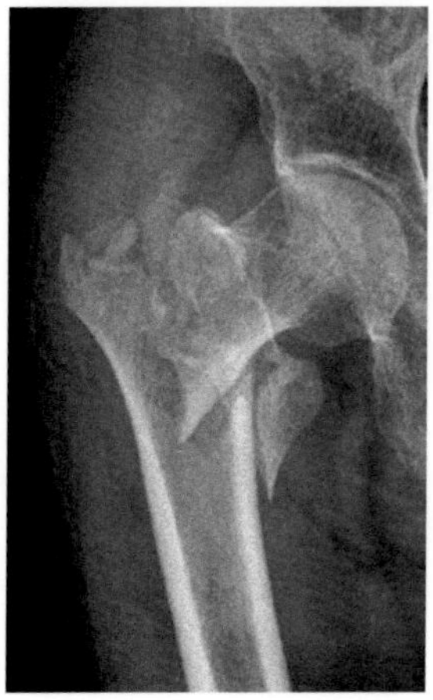

AO/OTA classification for femur fracture

31-A: Femur, proximal, trochanteric fractures.
A2: Pertrochanteric multifragmentary
A2.2: With several intermediate fragments

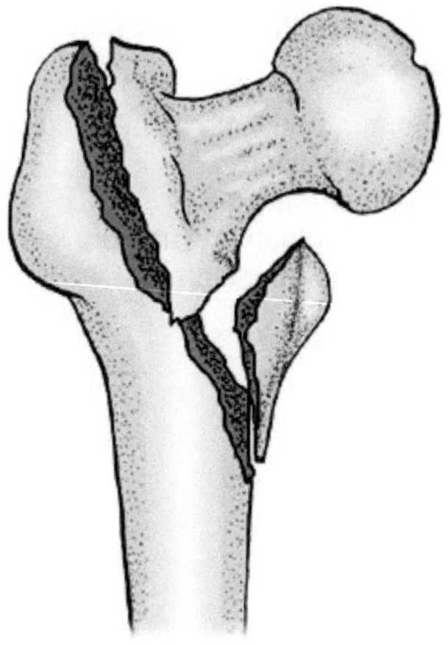

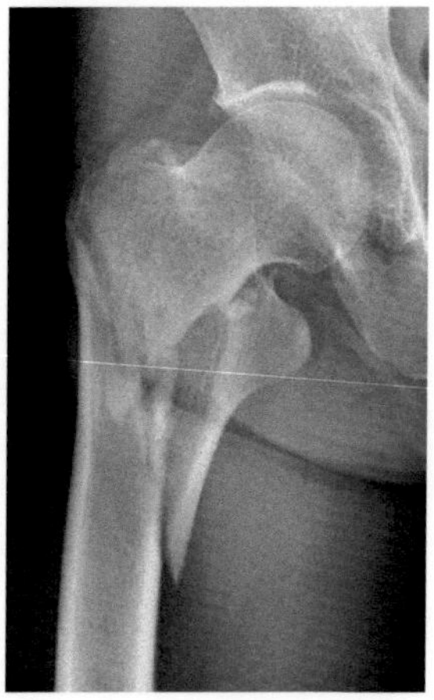

AO/OTA classification for femur fracture

31-A: Femur, proximal, trochanteric fractures.
A2: Pertrochanteric multifragmentary
A2.3: Extending more than 1 cm below the lesser trochanter

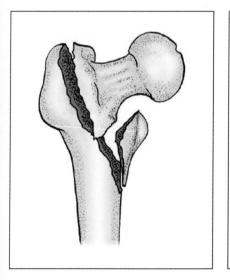

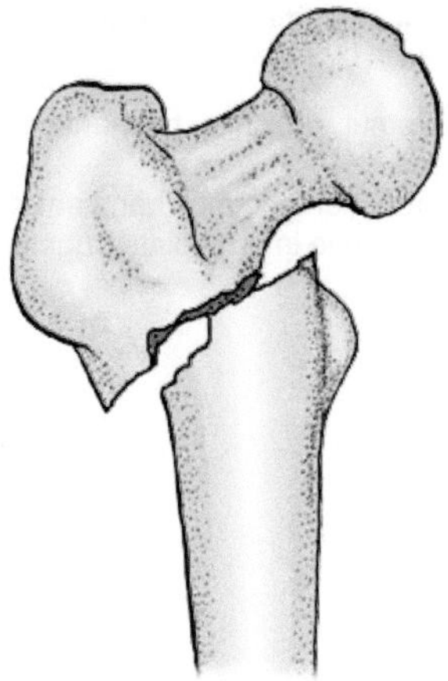

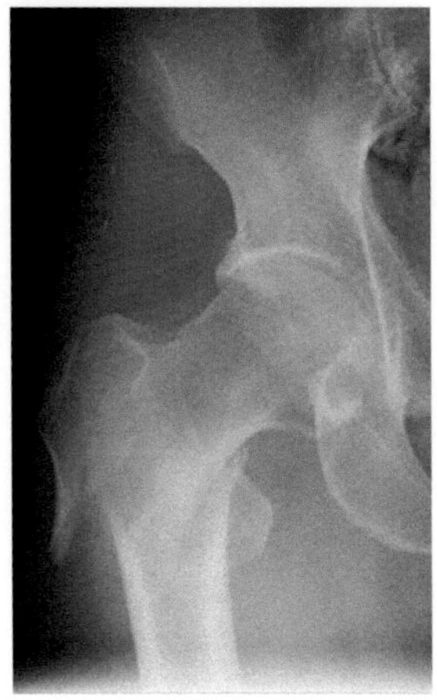

AO/OTA classification for femur fracture

31-A: Femur, proximal, trochanteric fractures.
A3: Intertrochanteric
A3.1: Simple oblique

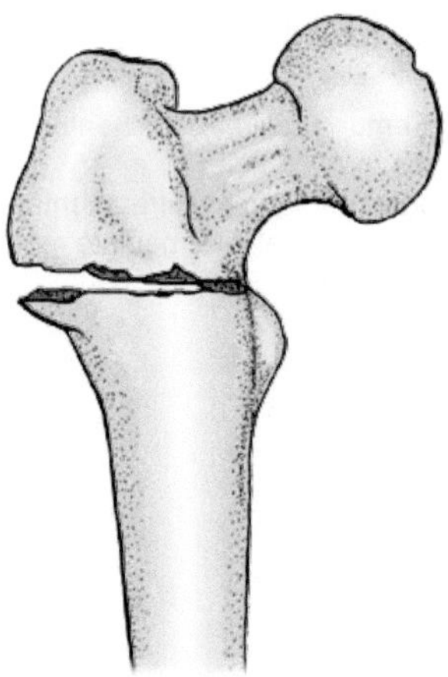

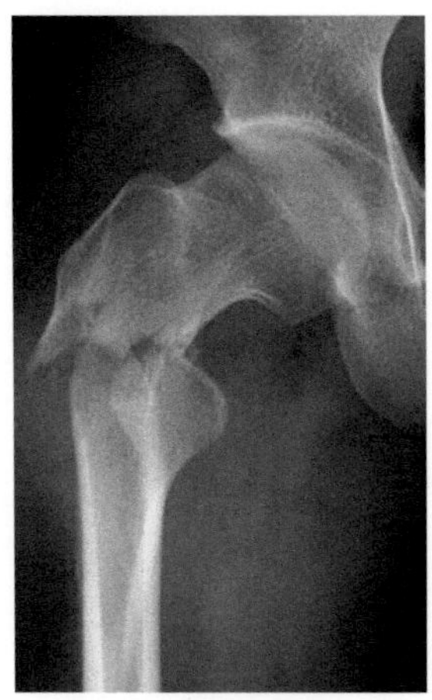

AO/OTA classification for femur fracture

31-A Femur, proximal, extra-articular, trochanteric fractures.
A3: Intertrochanteric
A3.2: Simple transverse

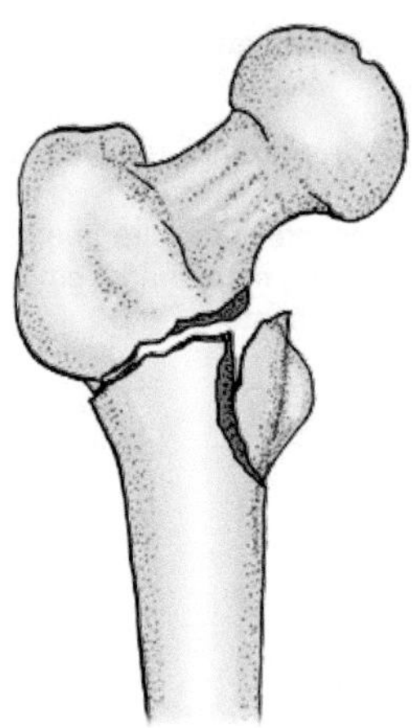

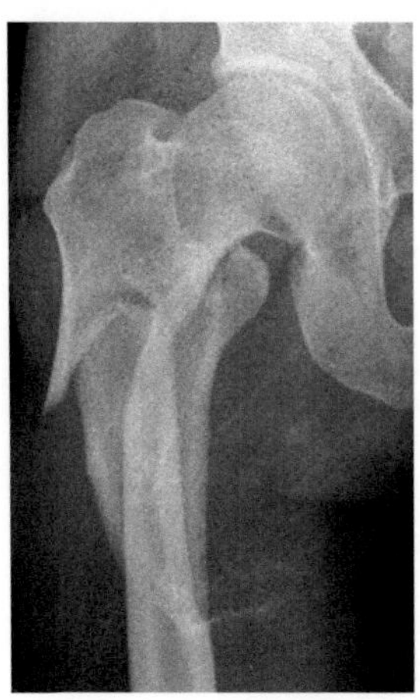

AO/OTA classification for femur fracture

31-A Femur, proximal, extra-articular, trochanteric fractures.
A3: Intertrochanteric
A3.3: Multifragmentary, fracture line extending into the diaphysis

8.1.3.2 Evans-Jensen Classification (1975, Acta Orthop Scand, 46: 795–803)

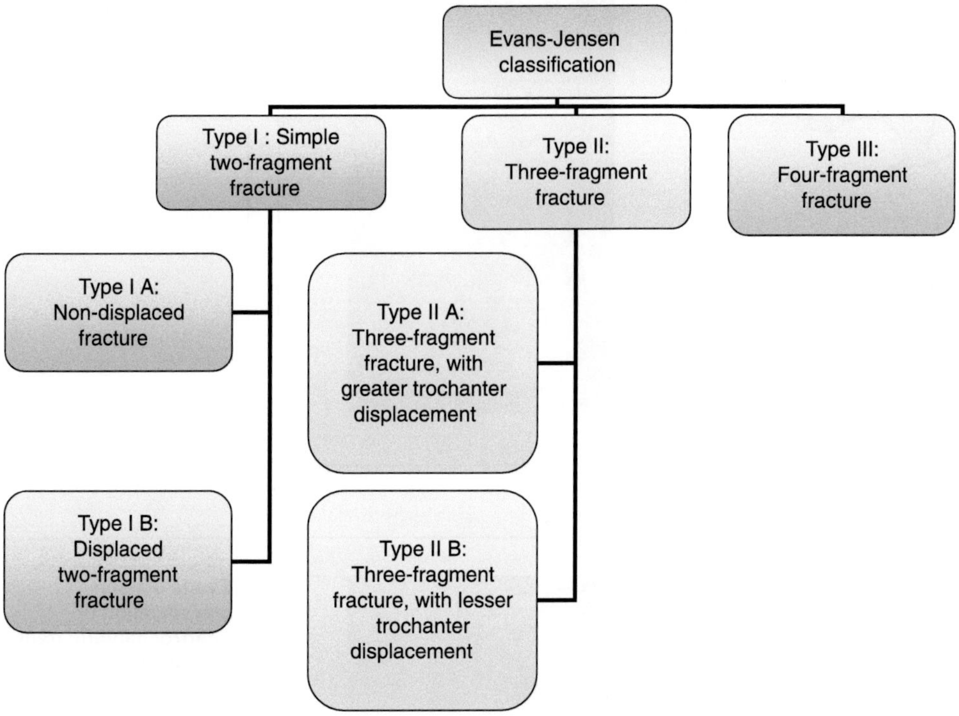

In 1975, Jensen and Michaelsen classified intertrochanteric fractures into three types modifying Evans classifying system.

Type I: Simple fracture (two-fragment fracture):
- Type IA: Non-displaced fracture.
- Type IB: Displaced fracture (two-fragment fracture).

Type II: Three-fragment fracture:
- Type IIA: Three-fragmentary fracture without posterolateral support.
- Type IIB: Three-fragmentary fracture without medial support.

Type III: Four-fragmentary fracture.

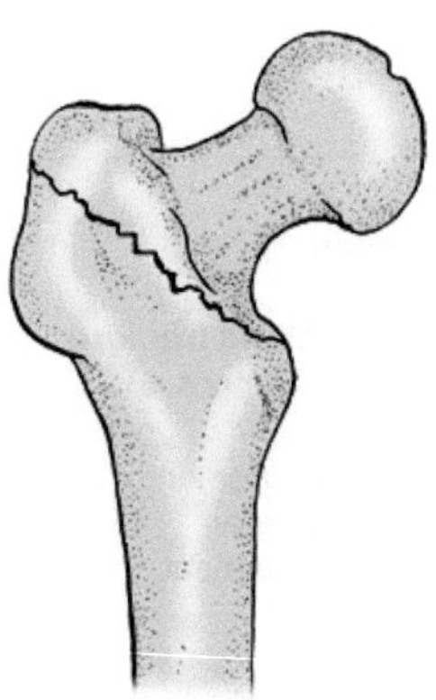

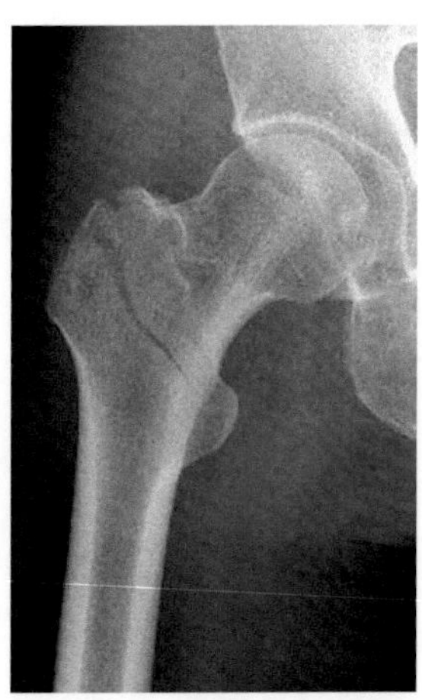

Evans-Jensen classification of intertrochanteric fracture
Type I : Simple fracture
Type I A : Undisplaced 2-fragment fracture

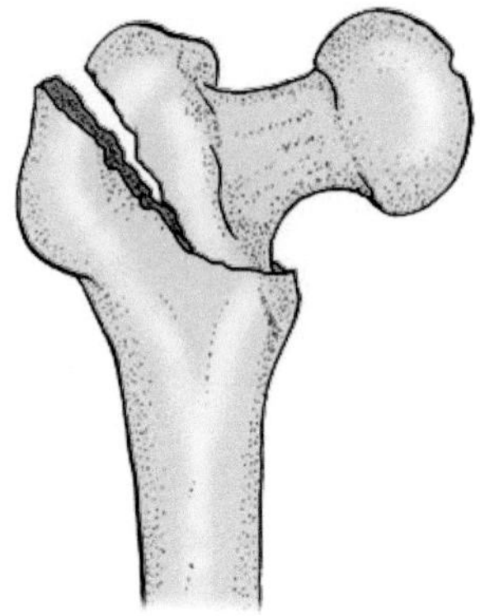

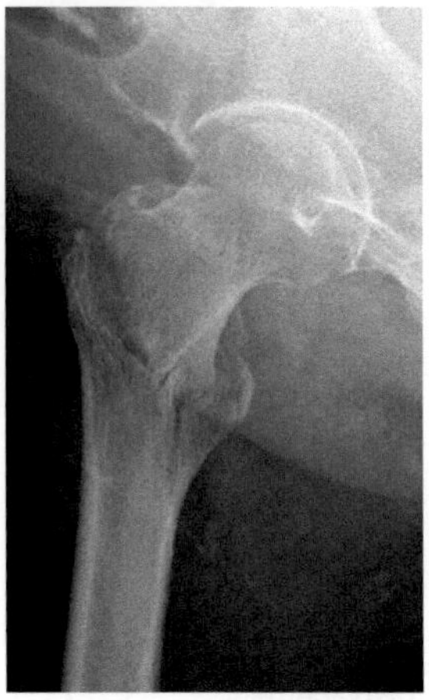

Evans-Jensen classification of intertrochanteric fracture
Type I : Simple fracture
Type I B : two-fragment displaced fractures

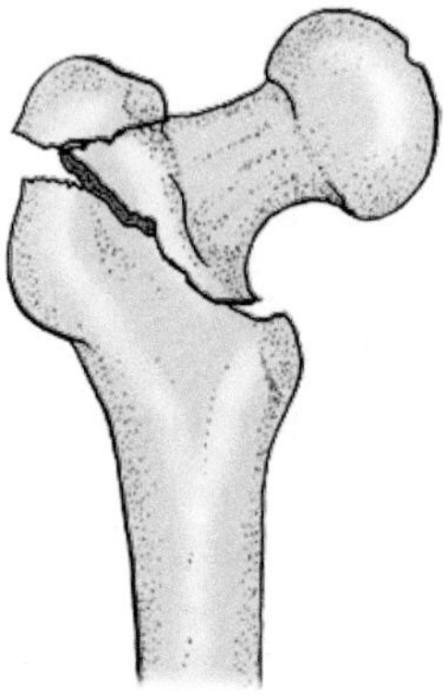

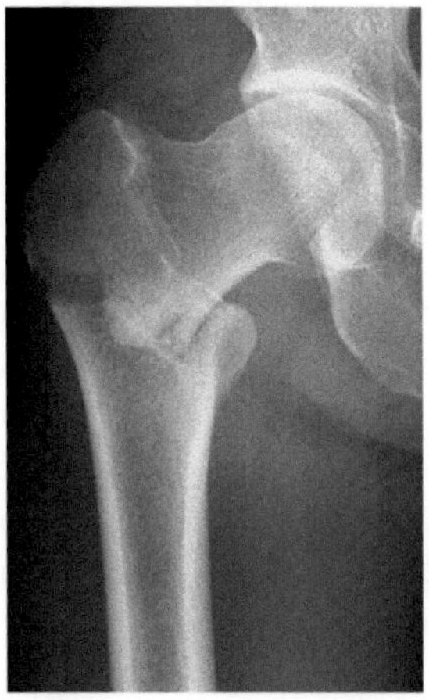

Evans-Jensen classification of intertrochanteric fracture
Type II : three-fragment fractures
Type I A : three-fragment fractures with greater trochanter displacement

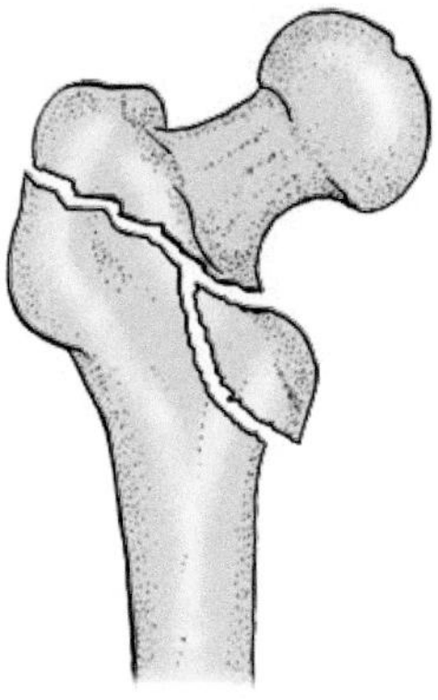

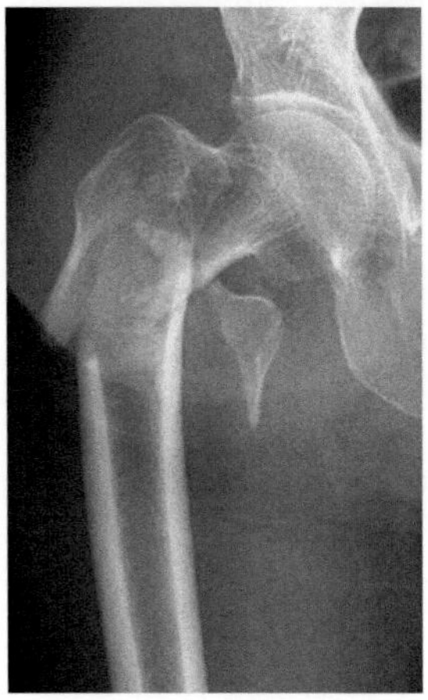

Evans-Jensen classification of intertrochanteric fracture
Type II: three-fragment fractures
Type II B: three-fragment fractures with greater trochanter displacement

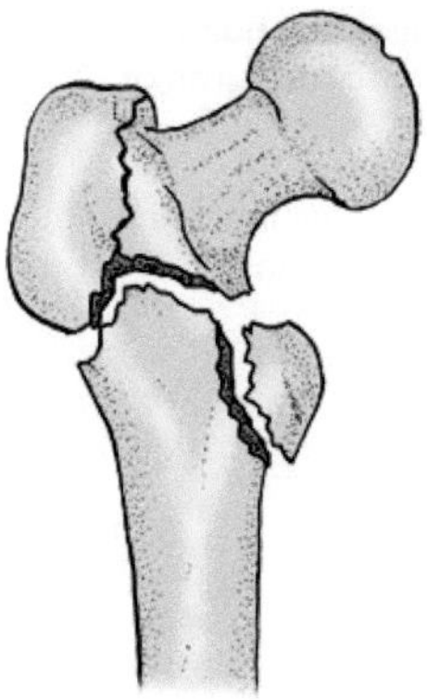

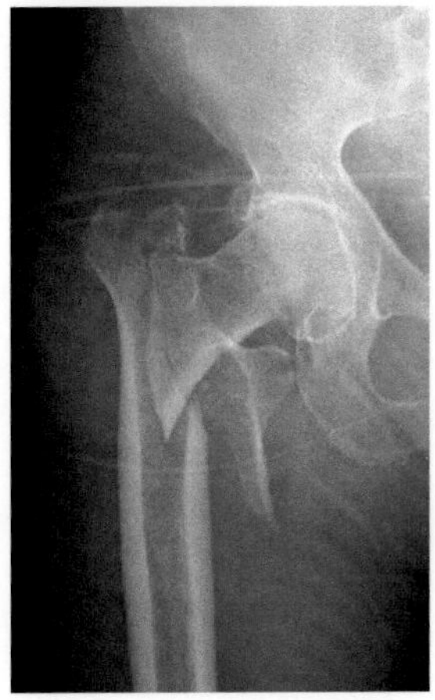

Evans-Jensen classification of intertrochanteric fracture
Type III: four-fragment fractures involving lesser and greater trochanter

8.1.3.3 Evans Classifications (1949, J Bone Joint Surg (Br), 31: 190–203)

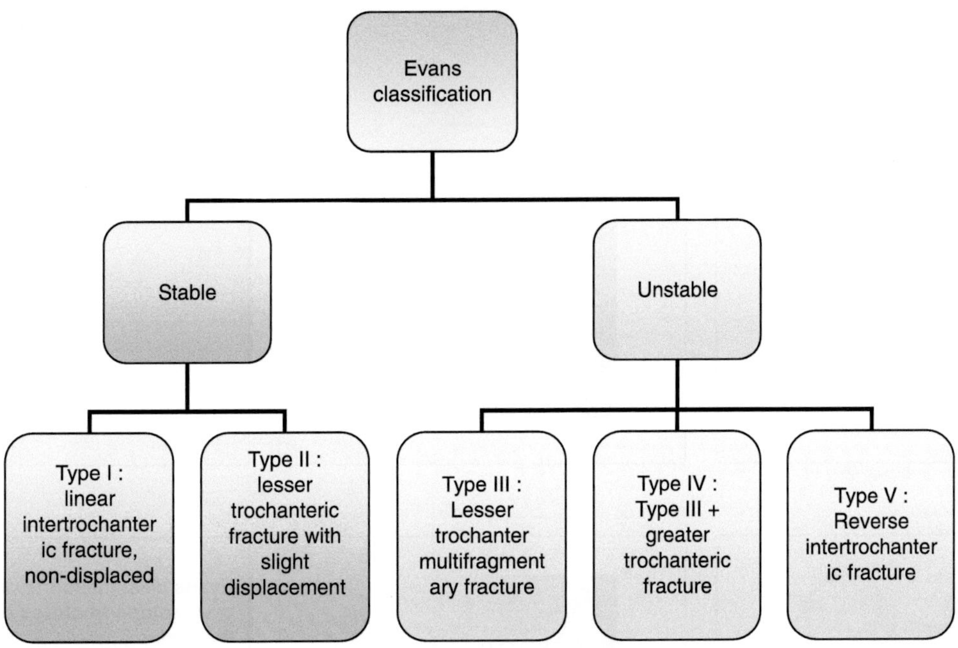

Type I: Linear non-displaced intertrochanteric fracture, stable.

Type II: Lesser trochanteric fracture with slight displacement but could be reduced, medial cortexes support with each other, stable.

Type III: Lesser trochanter multifragmentary fracture, displaced and unreduced, without medial cortex support, unstable.

Type IV: Type III + greater trochanteric fracture, unstable.

Type V: Reverse intertrochanteric fracture, unstable.

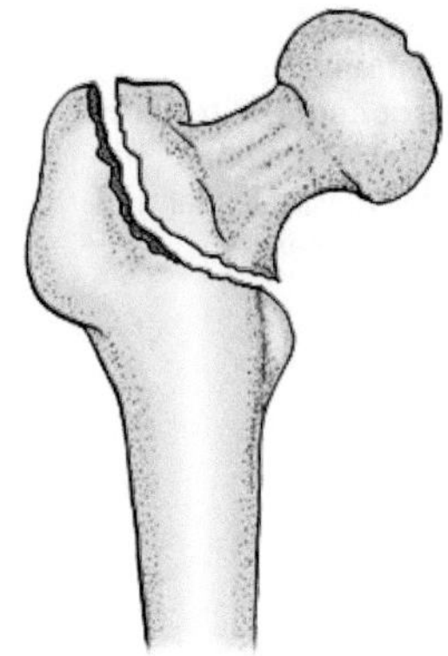

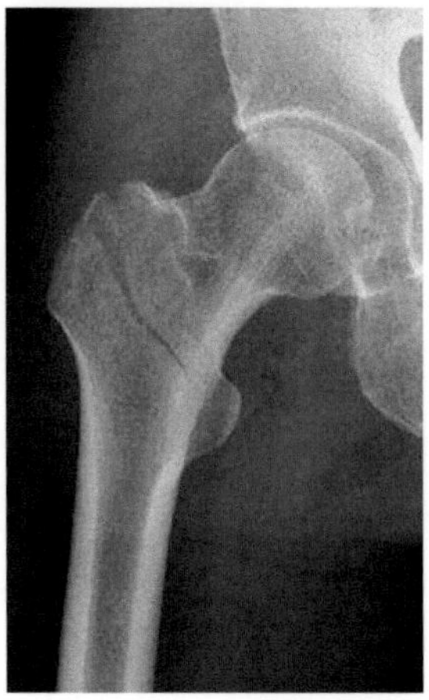

Evans classifications of trochanteric fractures of the femur
Type I: Linear intertrochanteric fracture, non-displaced, stable.

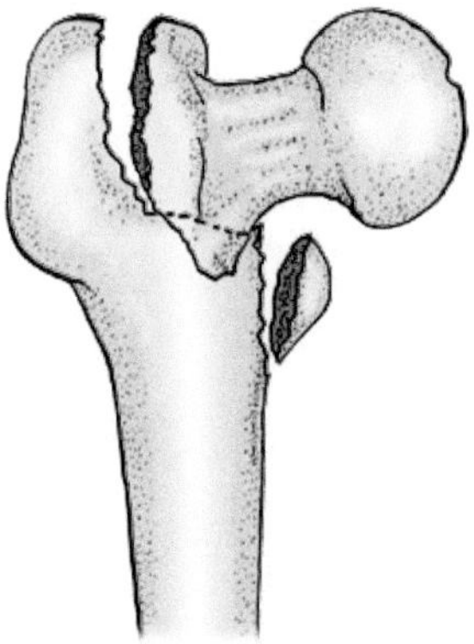

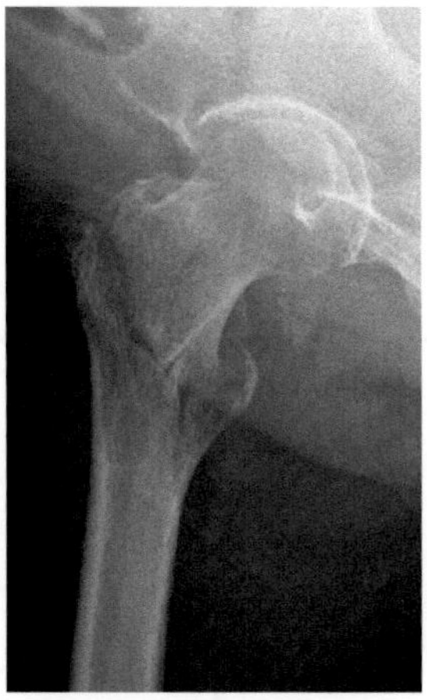

Evans classifications of trochanteric fractures of the femur
Type II: Lesser trochanteric fracture with slight displacement but could be reduced, medial cortexes support with each other, stable.

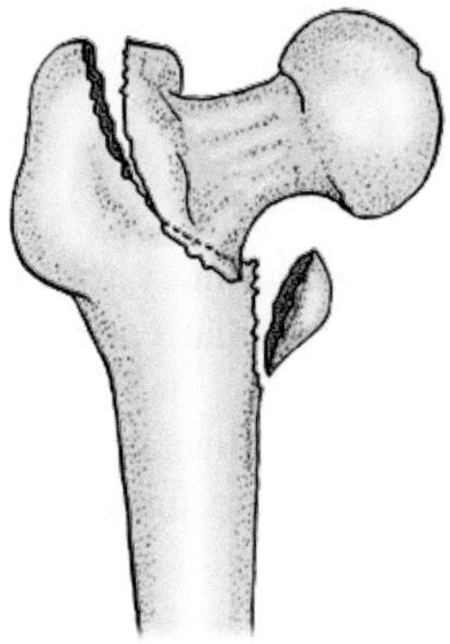

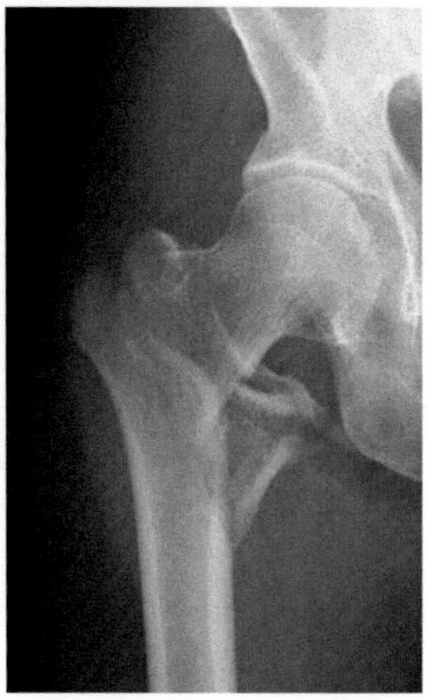

Evans classifications of trochanteric fractures of the femur
Type III: Lesser trochanter multifragmentary fracture, displaced and unreduced, without medial cortex support, unstable.

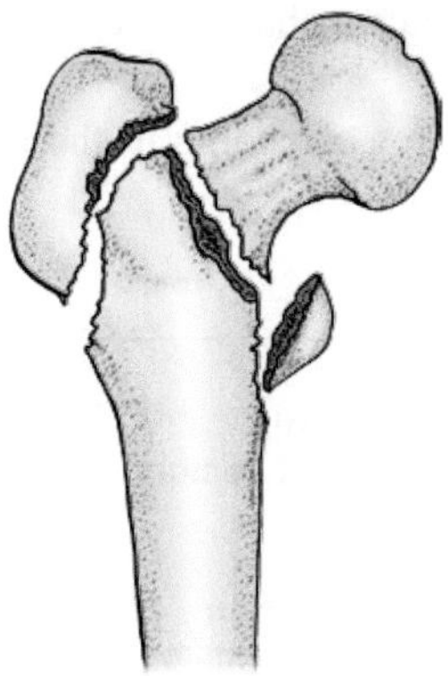

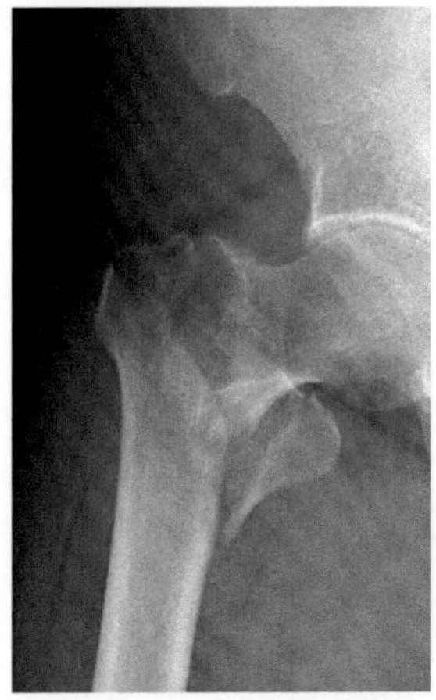

Evans classifications of trochanteric fractures of the femur
Type IV: Type III + greater trochanteric fracture, unstable.

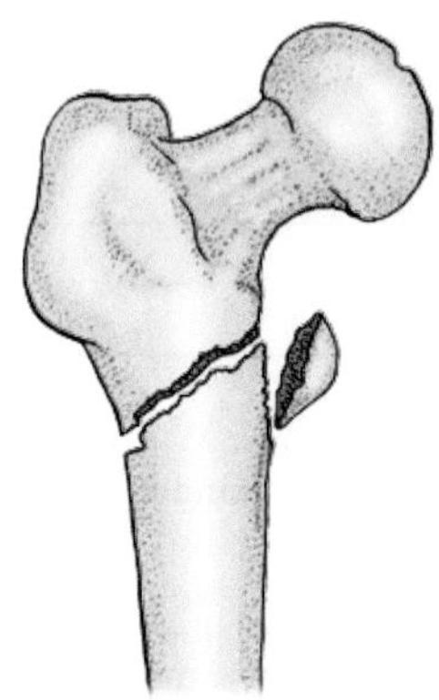

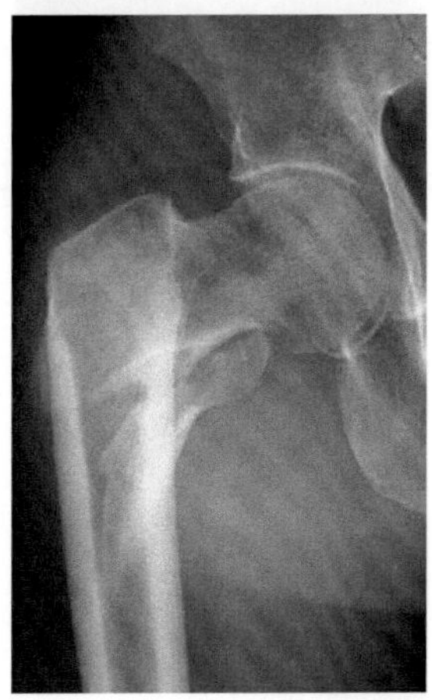

Evans classifications of trochanteric fractures of the femur
Type V: Reverse intertrochanteric fracture with fracture line running upward and inward. extends above the lesser trochanter, unstable.

8.1.3.4 Boyd-Griffin Classifications (1949, Arch Surg, 58: 853–866)

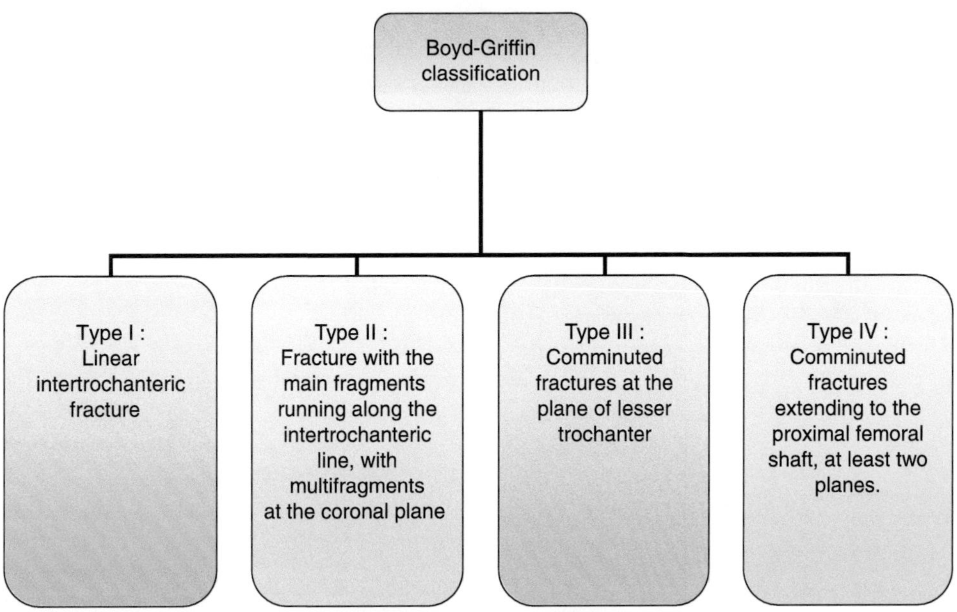

Type I: Simple linear intertrochanteric fracture, stable and easily be reducible.

Type II: Fracture with the main fragments running along the intertrochanteric line, with multifragments at the coronal plane.

Type III: Comminuted fractures at the plane of lesser trochanter, extending to the intertrochanteric region (reverse oblique).

Type IV: Comminuted fractures extending to the proximal femoral shaft, at least two planes.

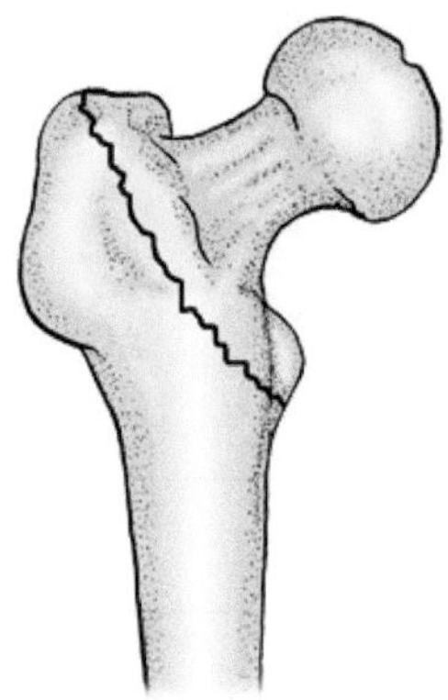

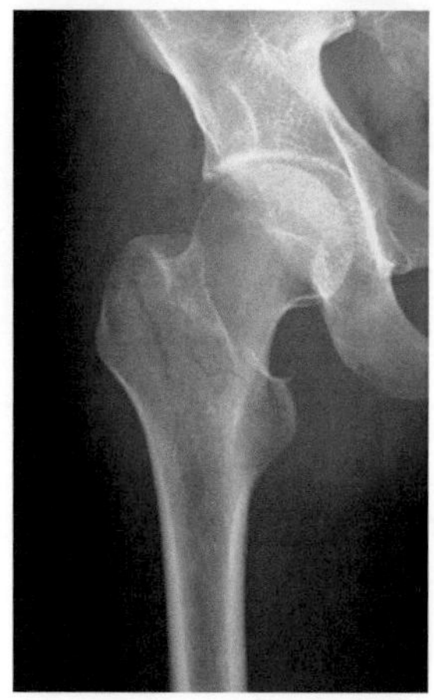

The Boyd - Griffin Classification of Femoral Intertrochanteric Fractures

Type I : Simple Linear intertrochanteric fracture, stable and easily be reducible.

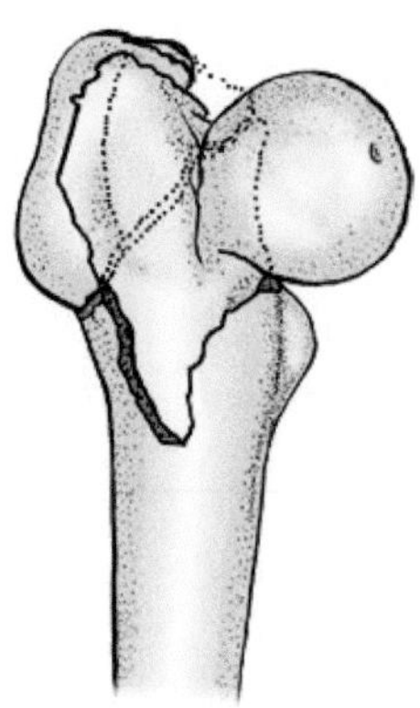

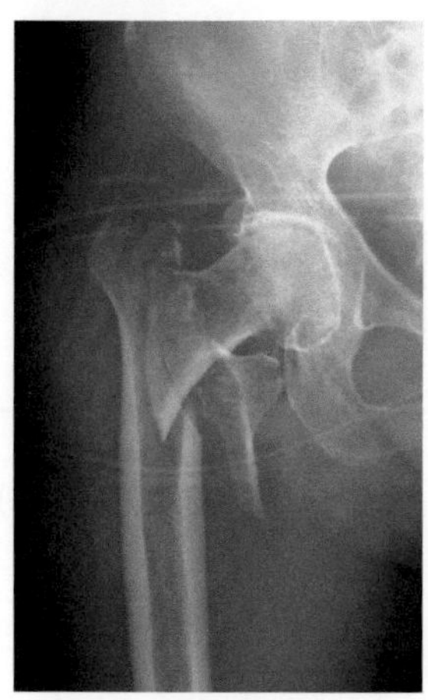

The Boyd - Griffin Classification of Femoral Intertrochanteric Fractures

Type II: Fracture with the main fragments running along the intertrochanteric line, with multifragments at the coronal plane.

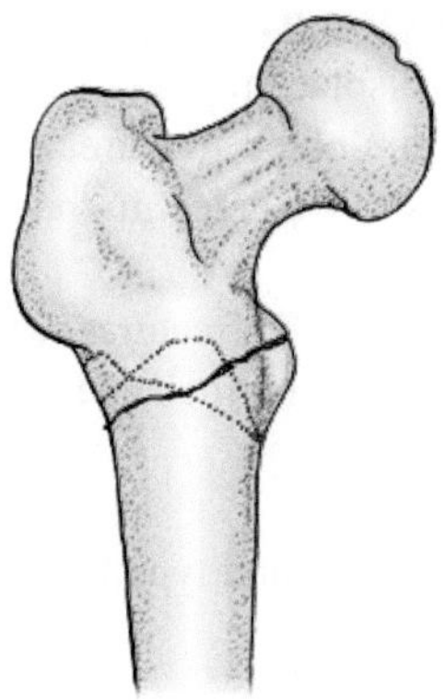

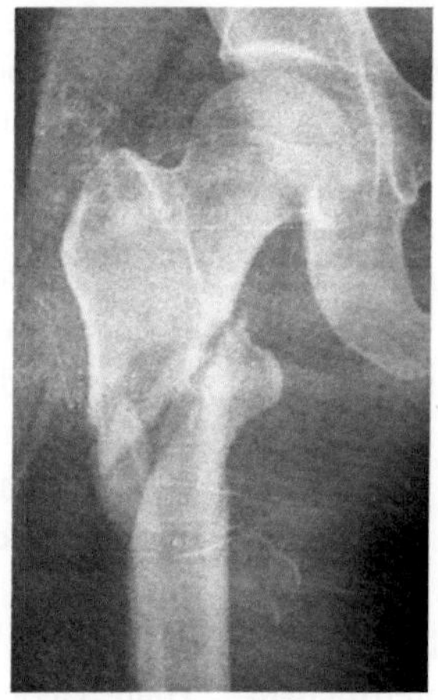

The Boyd - Griffin Classification of Femoral Intertrochanteric Fractures
Type III: Comminuted fractures at the plane of lesser trochanter, extending to the intertrochanteric region (reverse oblique).

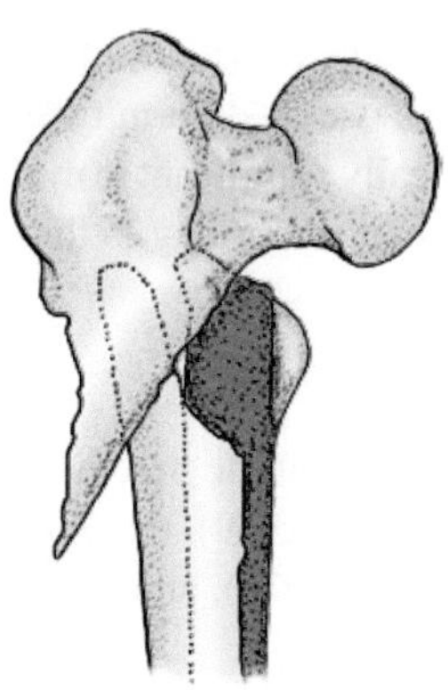

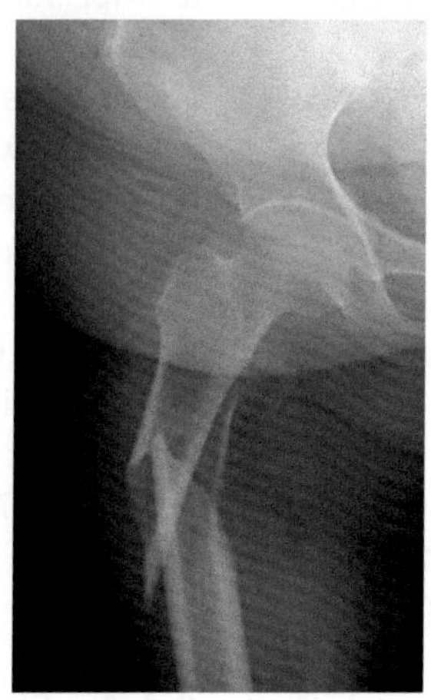

The Boyd - Griffin Classification of Femoral Intertrochanteric Fractures
Type IV: Comminuted fractures extending to the proximal femoral shaft, at least two planes.

8.1.3.5 Kyle Classification (Kyle-Gustilo Classification, 1979)

Modified Boyd-Griffin classification.

Type I: Non-displaced fracture, stable.

Type II: Fracture with displacement, with small pieces of fragments at the lesser trochanter and proximal fracture segment varus, stable.

Type III: Fracture with displacement, with post-medial comminuted fragments and greater trochanter fracture, proximal fracture segment was varus, instable.

Type IV: Comminuted fractures of intertrochanteric and post-medial cortex, with subtrochanteric fracture, unstable.

8.1.3.6 Tronzo Classification (1973)

Type I: Incomplete intertrochanteric fractures which can be anatomically reduced by traction method.

Type II: Non-comminuted fracture of the two trochanters, with or without displacement, can be reduced through traction, often to achieve anatomical reduction.

Type III: Comminuted fracture, accompanied by larger bone pieces of the lesser trochanter, the fracture line leading to instability of the tip of the femoral neck.

Type IV: Unstable loose comminuted trochanteric fractures, with posterior wall rupture, femoral neck medial displacement.

Type V: Reversed oblique fracture of trochanter (the oblique line from the supra-medial to the inferolateral side).

8.1.3.7 Ramadier Classification (1956, widely used in France)

Type A: Femoral basicervical-intertrochanteric fracture.
Type B: Simple pertrochanteric fracture.
Type C: Complex pertrochanteric fracture.
Type D: Pertrochanteric fracture with valgus displacement.
Type E: Pertrochanteric fracture with intertrochanteric fracture line.
Type F: Intertrochanteric fractures involving the shaft.
Type G: Subtrochanteric fracture.

8.1.3.8 Lu Shibi Classification (1989)

Lu Shibi divided the intertrochanteric fractures into stable type and unstable type. Stable intertrochanteric fracture is a linear fracture; the fracture line runs along the intertrochanter line, without comminuted fragments. Unstable intertrochanteric fractures include lesser trochanteric fractures, great trochanteric rear fractures, fractures with more than three fragments, subtrochanteric fractures involving the trochanteric area, etc.

8.1.3.9 Classification of Tianjin Hospital

Four types

Type I: Syn-intertrochanteric fracture.
Type II: Syn-intertrochanteric comminuted fracture.
Type III: Reversed intertrochanteric fracture.
Type IV: Subtrochanteric fracture.

Type II fracture is the most common and most unstable type; the incidence of coxa vara is the highest and most severe. Type I is the most stable type. The incidence of fractures of type III and IV is low, accounting for about 15% of intertrochanteric fractures. The stability of the two types is between type I and II.

8.1.3.10 Huang Gongyi Classification

Huang Gongyi divided the fractures into four types and two kinds, referring to Kyle and Evans Classifications.

Type I: Fracture line from the greater trochanter to the lesser trochanter, the lesser trochanter is not completely separated.
Type II: Fracture line from the greater trochanter to the lesser trochanter, accompanied by avulsion separation of the lesser trochanter and varus displacement.
Type III. Intertrochanteric comminuted fracture, with more than four fracture fragments, bone defect in the posterior or medial wall, and displacement.
Type IV: Intertrochanteric comminuted fractures, with transverse or oblique fractures of the subtrochanteric area and varying degrees of displacement.

Type I and II are stable fractures, and type III and IV are unstable fractures.

8.1.3.11 Wang Yicong Classification

Wang Yicong considers that the original state of the fracture is the more important basis. Fracture with varus deformity immediately after trauma is unstable, and the more severe the original varus deformity, the greater the possibility of leftover varus deformity after treatment. On the contrary, those who are without original hip varus is the stable type, and the possibility of residual varus deformity is greatly reduced. It will be more practically significant to evaluate the prognosis and guide the treatment according to this classification method.

8.1.3.12 Other Classifications

Other classifications of intertrochanteric fractures include the Decoulx-Lavarde classification (1969), the Ender classification (1970), the Deburge type (1976), and the Briot type (1980).

8.1.4 Classification of Femoral Shaft Fracture

Regarding femoral shaft fractures (including subtrochanteric fracture), more than ten classifications can be found. According to the citation frequency in the last 5 years' literature, AO/OTA classification was the most commonly used one, followed by Winquist-Hansen classification and classification according to anatomic sites.

Due to its special location, there is a separate classification for the subtrochanteric fractures, which is described at the end of this section.

8.1.4.1 AO/OTA Classification (2007 Revised Edition, Journal of Orthopaedic Trauma, 21 supplement. Muller's AO classification of long bone fracture, originally published in the 1980s)

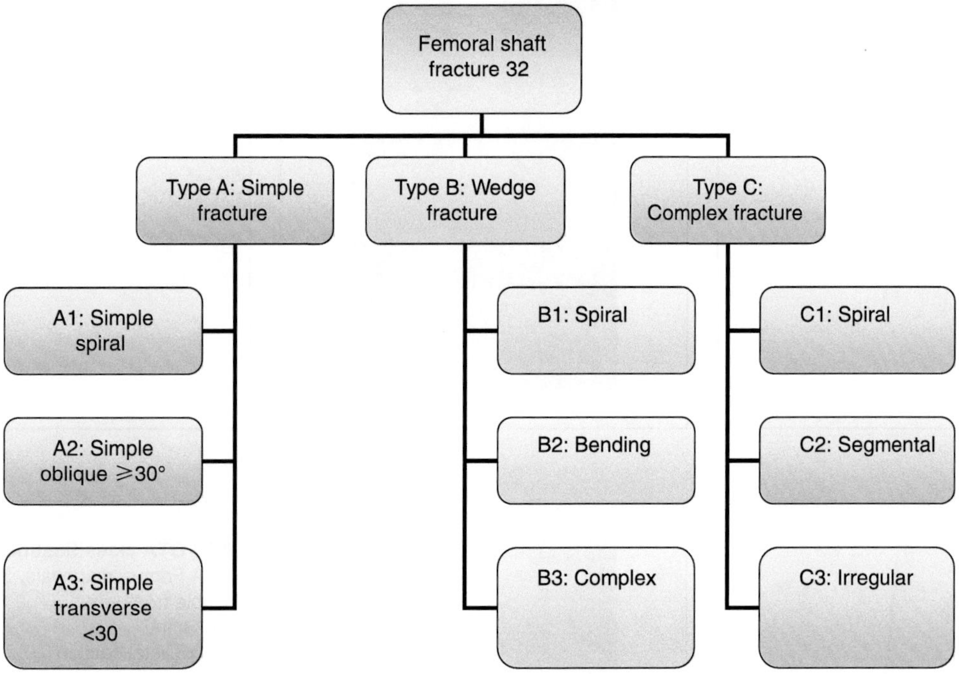

Type A: Simple fracture:

- Type A1: Simple spiral fracture. This is divided into three types.
  - Type A1.1: Subtrochanteric section.
  - Type A1.2: Middle section.
  - Type A1.3: Distal section.
- Type A2: Simple oblique ≥30°. This is divided into three types.
  - Type A2.1: Subtrochanteric section.
  - Type A2.2: Middle section.
  - Type A2.3: Distal section.
- Type A3: Simple transverse <30°. This is divided into three types.
  - Type A3.1: Subtrochanteric section.
  - Type A3.2: Middle section.
  - Type A3.3: Distal section.

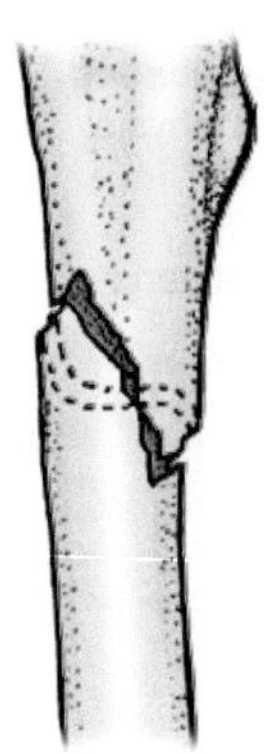

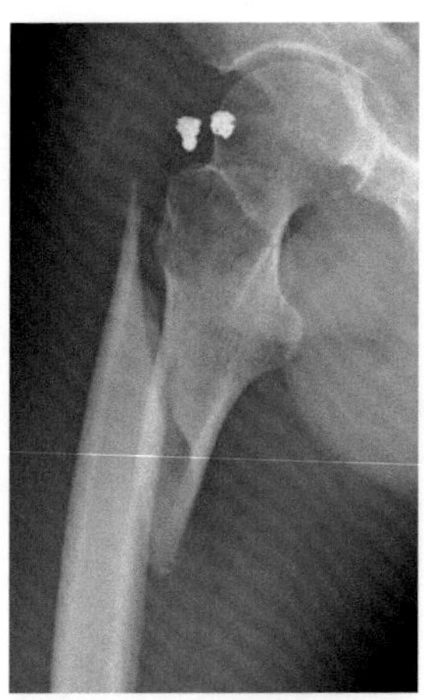

AO / OTA classification of femoral fracture
Type 32-A Simple femoral shaft fracture.
A1: simple spiral fracture
A1.1: subtrochanteric section

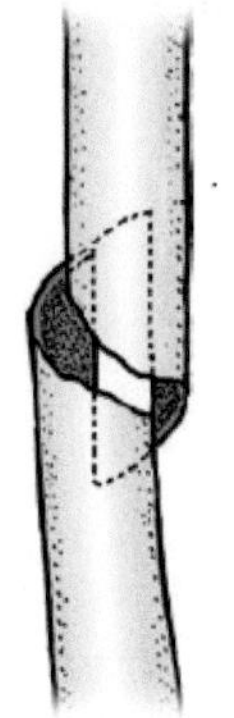

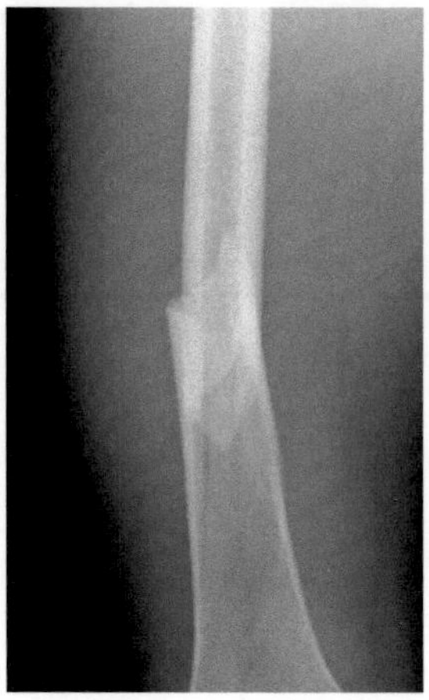

AO / OTA classification
32-A Femur, diaphysis, simple fractures.
A1: Spiral
A1.2: Middle section

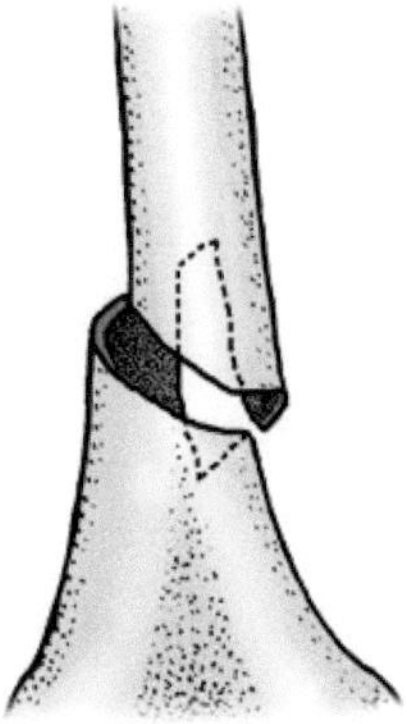

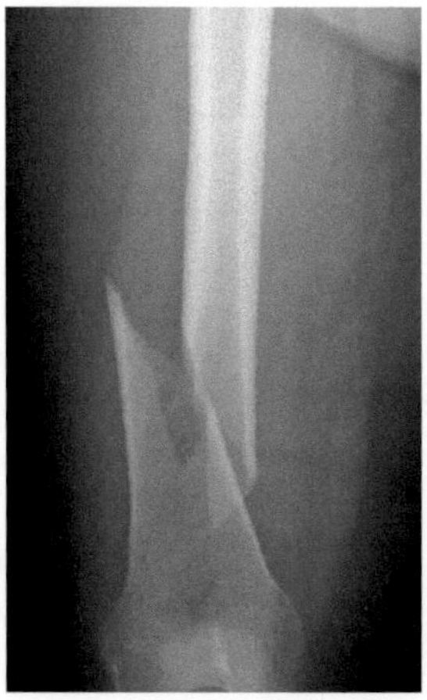

AO / OTA classification
32-A Femur, diaphysis, simple fractures.
A1: Spiral
A1.3: Distal section

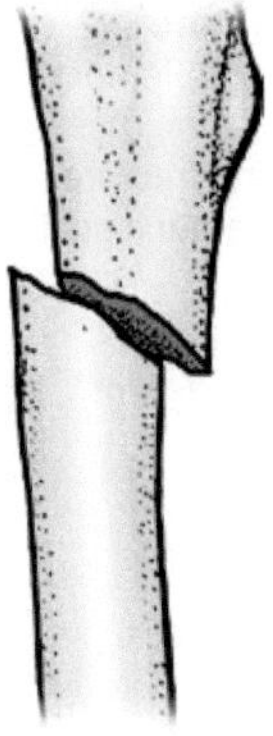

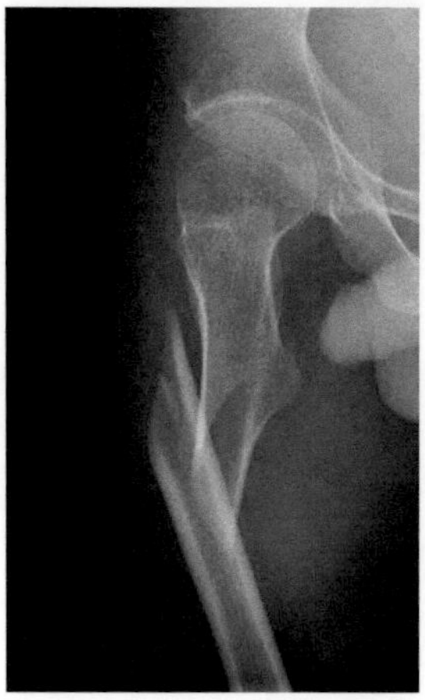

AO/OTA Classification
32-A Femur, diaphysis, simple fractures.
A2: Oblique (≥ 30°)
A2.1: Subtrochanteric section

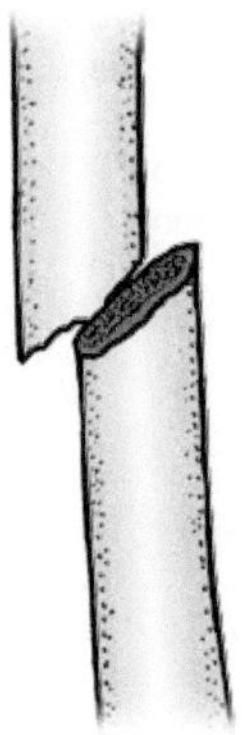

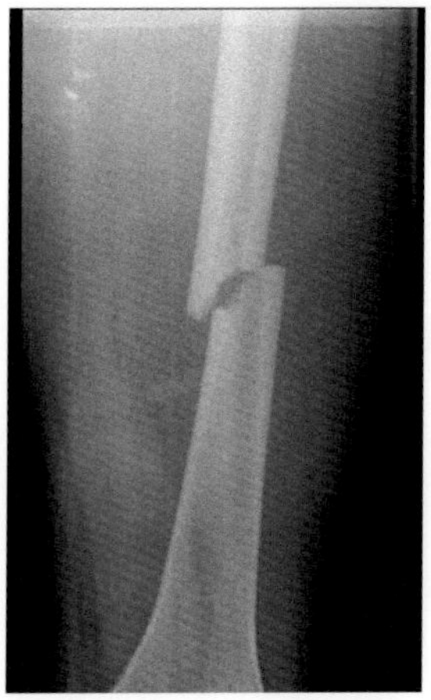

AO/OTA Classification
32-A Femur, diaphysis, simple fractures.
A2: Oblique (≥ 30°)
A2.1: Middle section

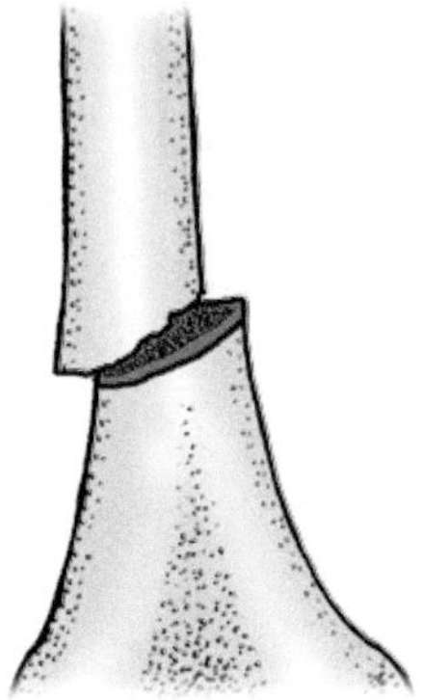

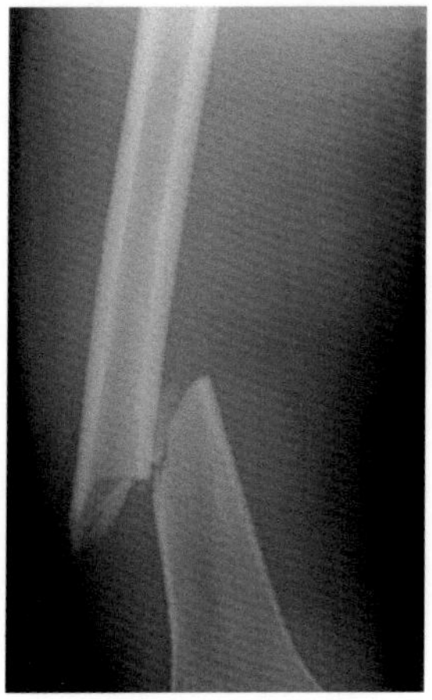

AO/OTA Classification
32-A Femur, diaphysis, simple fractures.
A2: Oblique (≥ 30°)
A2.1: Distal section

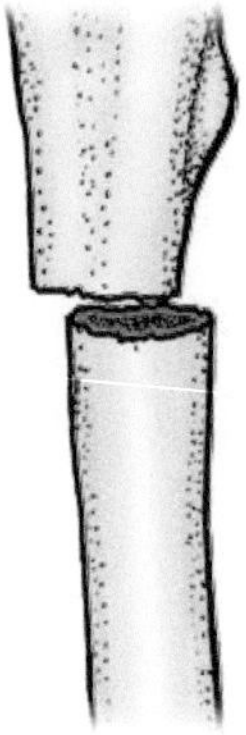

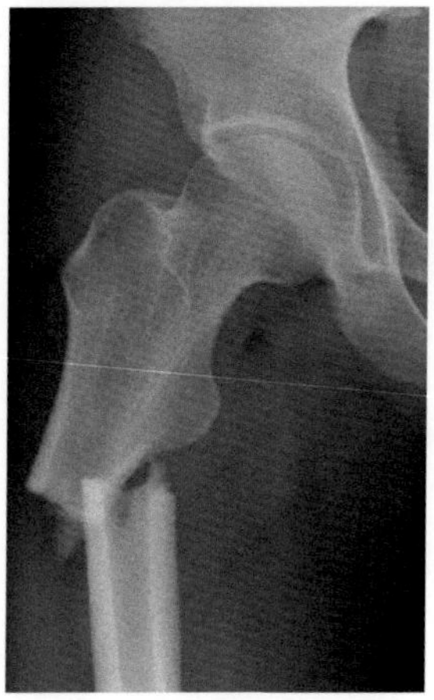

AO/OTA Classification
32-A Femur, diaphysis, simple fractures.
A3 Transverse (≤ 30°)
A3.1: Subtrochanteric section

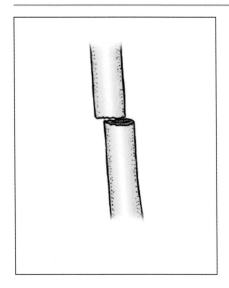

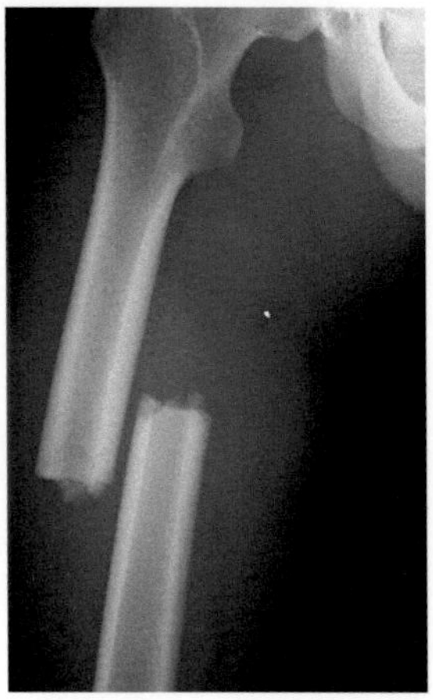

AO/OTA Classification
32-A Femur, diaphysis, simple fractures.
A3 Transverse (≤ 30°)
A3.2: Middle section

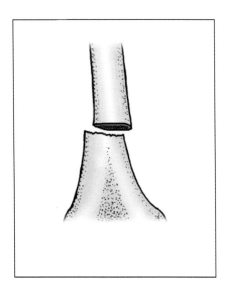

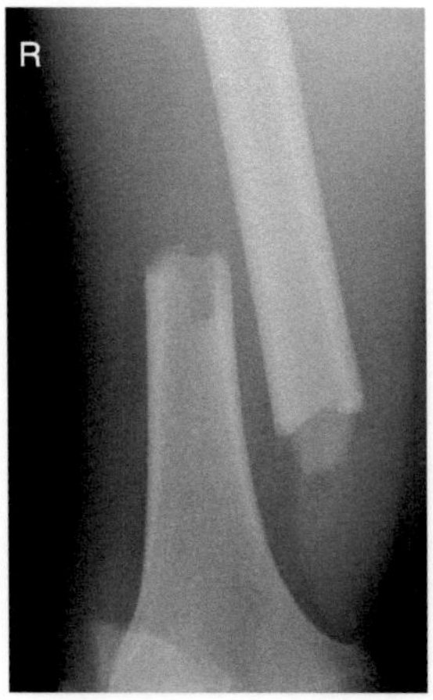

AO/OTA Classification
32-A Femur, diaphysis, simple fractures.
A3 Transverse (≤ 30°)
A3.3: Distal section

32-B: Femur, diaphysis, wedge fractures
- B1: Spiral:
  - B1.1: Subtrochanteric section.
  - B1.2: Middle section.
  - B1.3: Distal section.
- B2: Bending:
  - B2.1: Subtrochanteric section.
  - B2.2: Middle section.
  - B2.3: Distal section.
- B3: Complex:
  - B3.1: Subtrochanteric section.
  - B3.2: Middle section.
  - B3.3: Distal section.

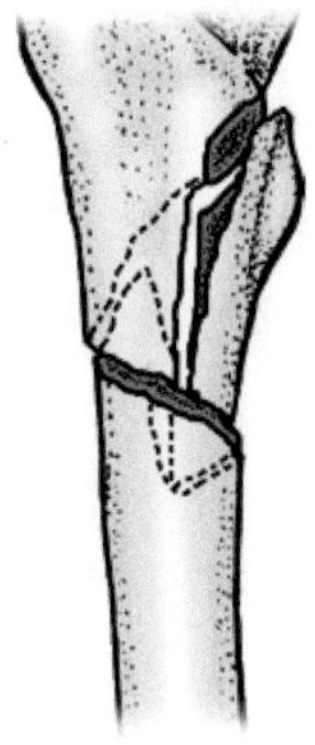

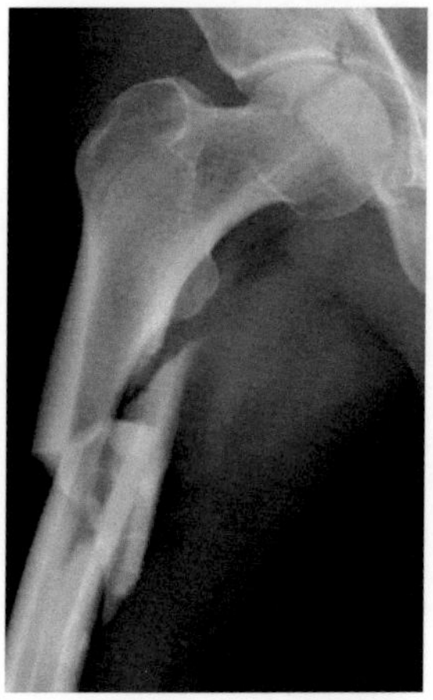

AO/OTA Classification
32-B: Femur, diaphysis, wedge fractures.
B1: Spiral
B1.1: Subtrochanteric section

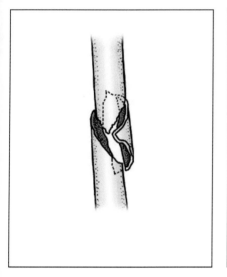

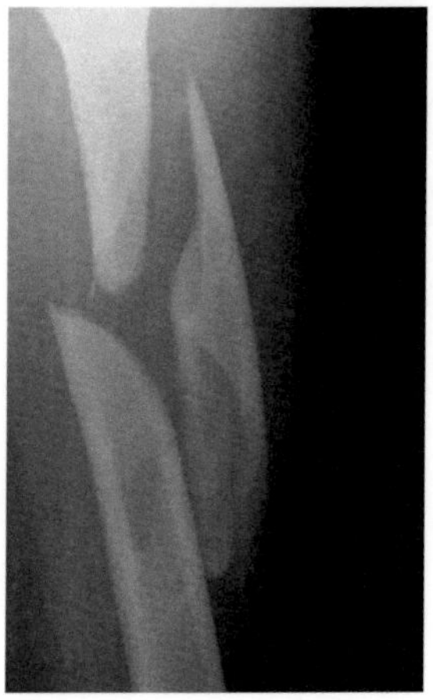

AO/OTA Classification
32-B: Femur, diaphysis, wedge fractures.
B1: Spiral
B1.2: Middle section

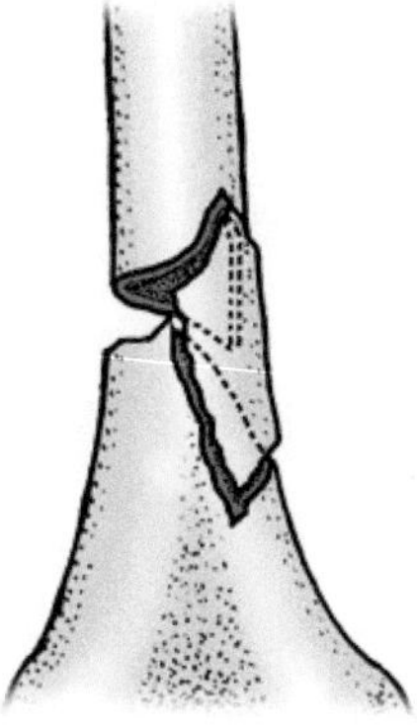

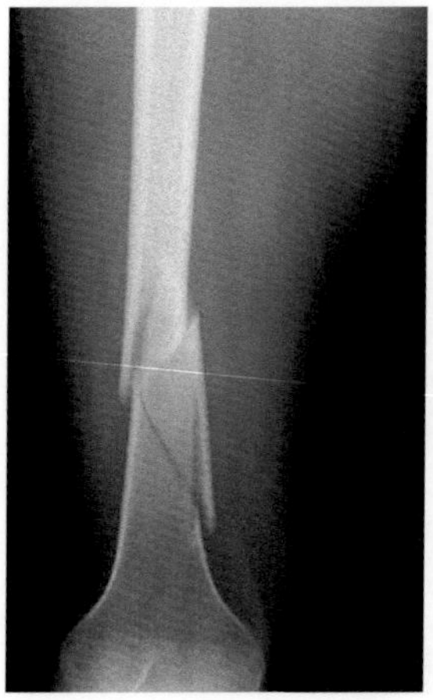

AO/OTA Classification
32-B: Femur, diaphysis, wedge fractures.
B1: Spiral
B1.3: Distal section

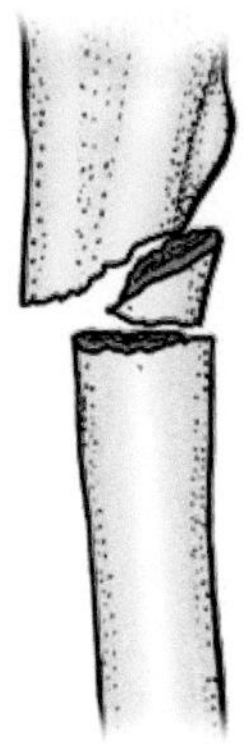

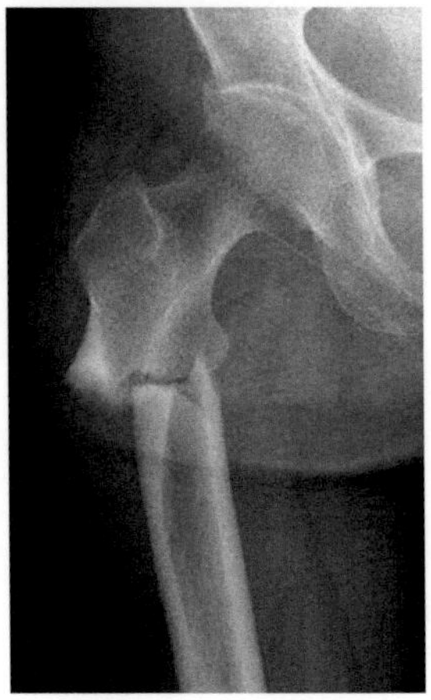

AO/OTA Classification
32-B: Femur, diaphysis, wedge fractures.
B2: Bending
B2.1: Subtrochanteric section

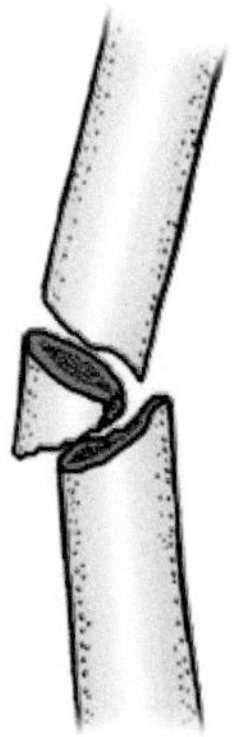

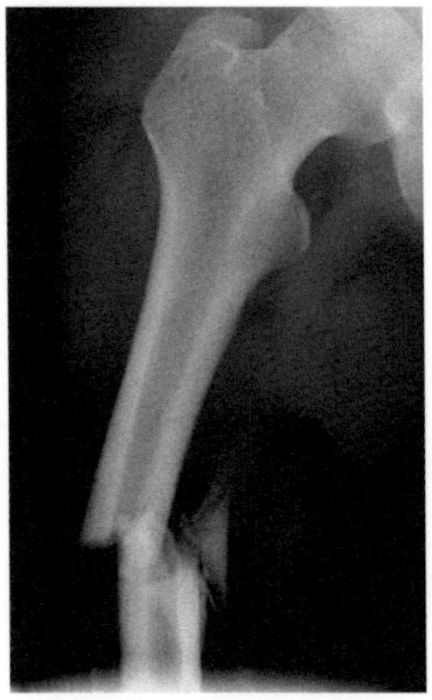

AO/OTA Classification
32-B: Femur, diaphysis, wedge fractures.
B2: Bending
B2.2: Middle section

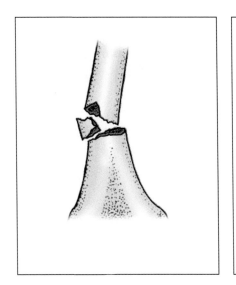

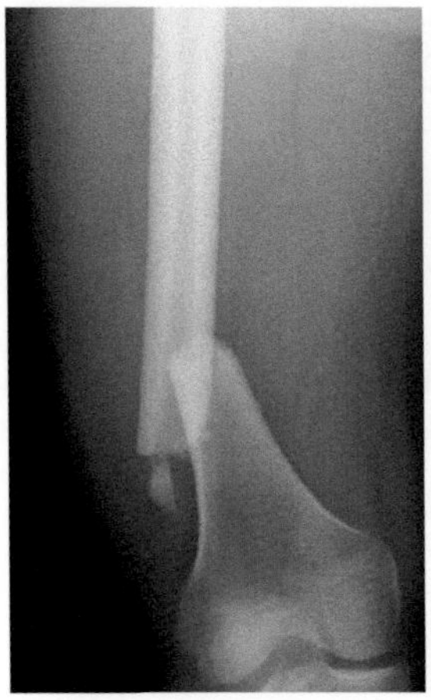

AO/OTA Classification
32-B: Femur, diaphysis, wedge fractures.
B2: Bending
B2.3: Distal section

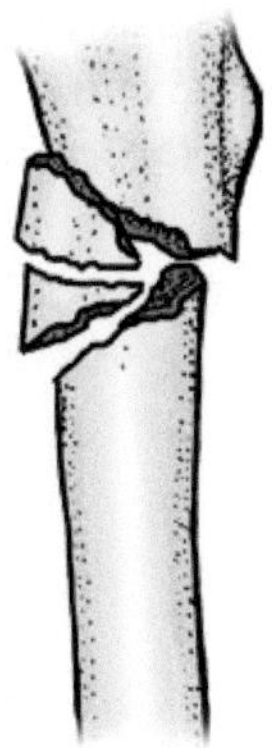

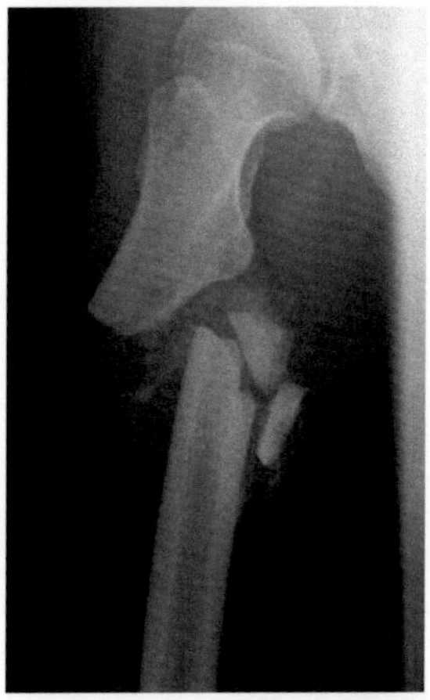

AO/OTA Classification
32-B: Femur, diaphysis, wedge fractures.
B3: Complex
B3.1: Subtrochanteric section

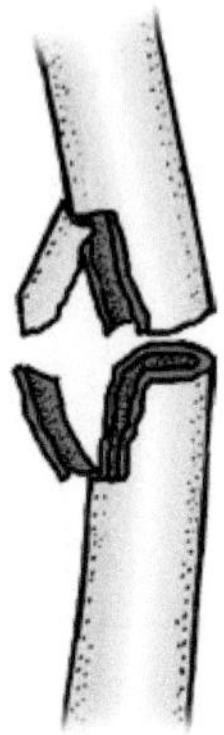

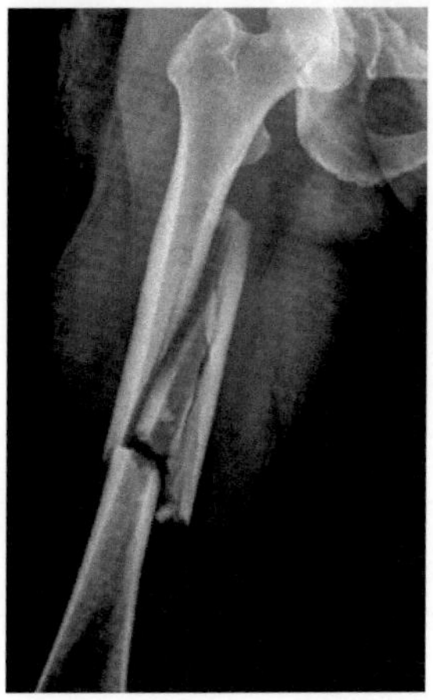

AO/OTA Classification
32-B: Femur, diaphysis, wedge fractures.
B3: Complex
B3.2: Middle section

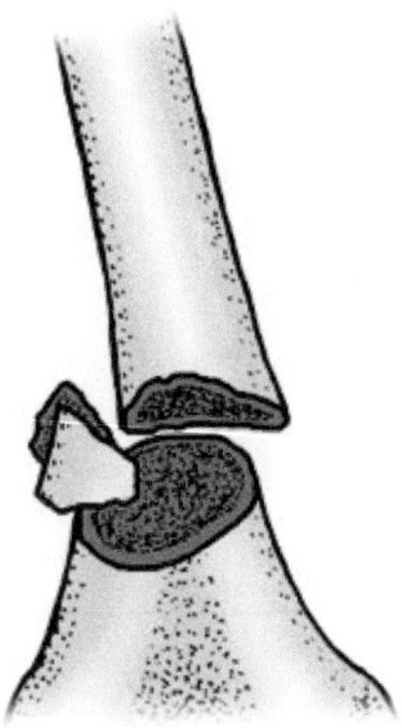

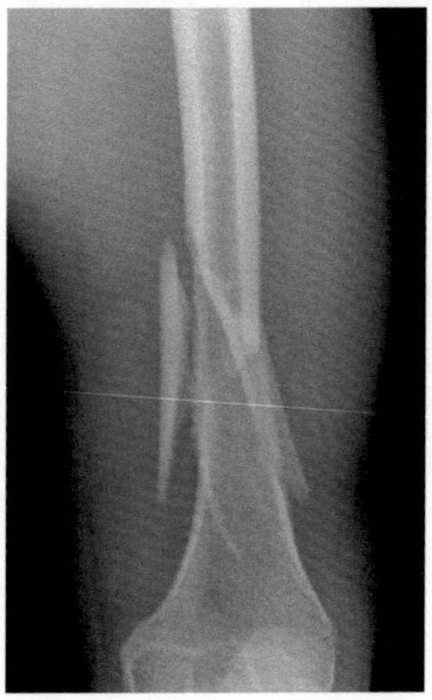

AO/OTA Classification
32-B: Femur, diaphysis, wedge fractures.
B3: Complex
B3.3: Distal section

32-C: Femur, diaphysis, complex fractures:
- C1: Spiral:
  - C1.1: With two intermediate fragments.
  - C1.2: With three intermediate fragments.
  - C1.3: With more than three intermediate fragments.
- C2: Segmental:
  - C2.1: With one intermediate segmental fragment.
  - C2.2: With one intermediate segmental fragment with an additional wedge fragment.
  - C2.3: With two or more intermediate segmental fragments.
- C3: Irregular:
  - C3.1: With two or three intermediate fragments.
  - C3.2: With limited shattering (<5 cm).
  - C3.3: With extensive shattering ($\geq$5 cm).

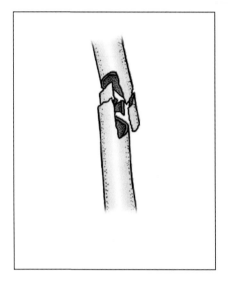

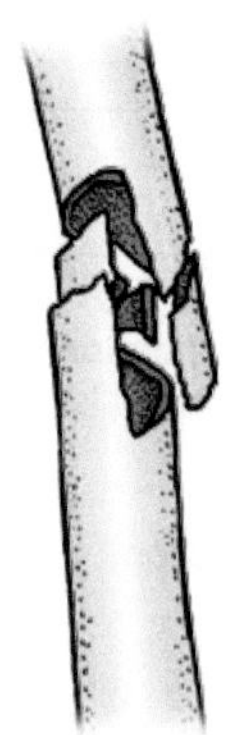

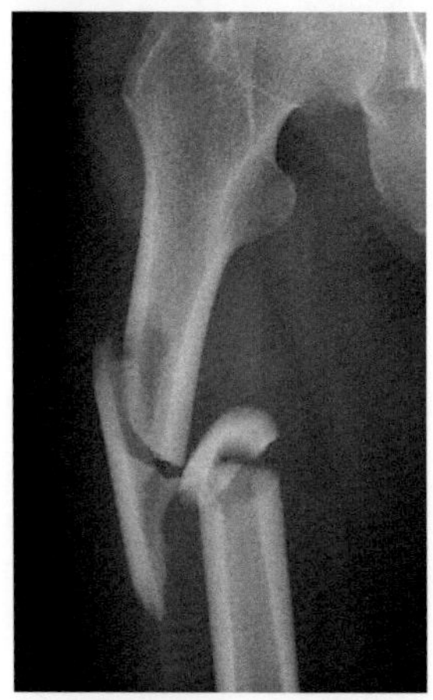

AO/OTA Classification
32-C: Femur, diaphysis, complex fractures.
C1: Spiral
C1.1: with two intermediate fragments

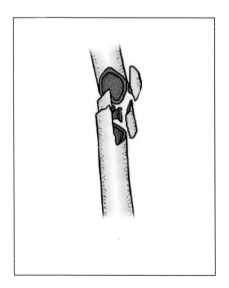

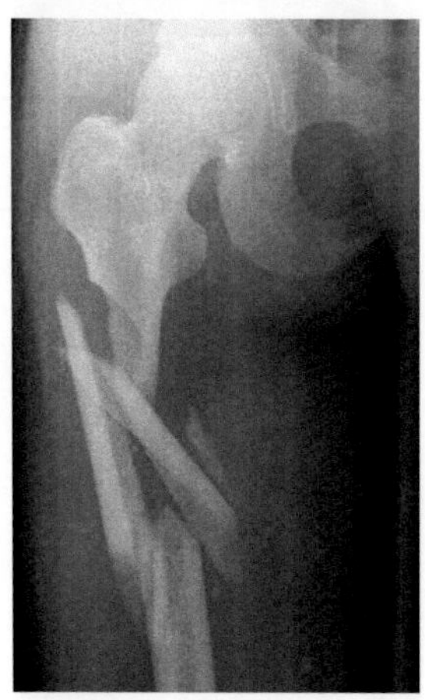

AO/OTA Classification
32-C: Femur, diaphysis, complex fractures.
C1: Spiral
C1.2: with three intermediate fragments

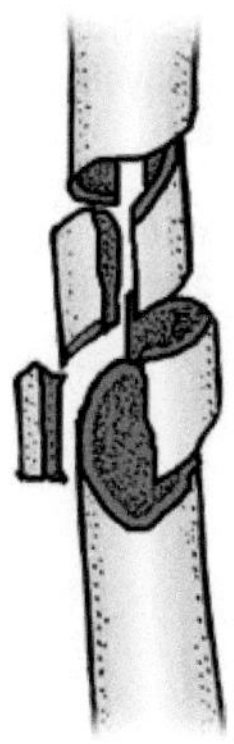

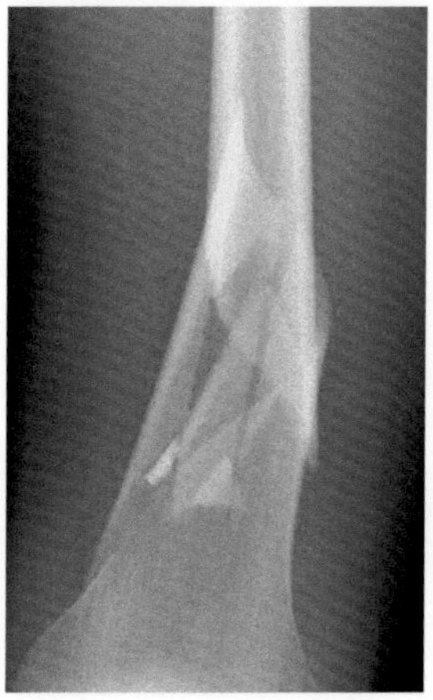

AO/OTA Classification
32-C: Femur, diaphysis, complex fractures.
C1: Spiral
C1.2: with more than three intermediate fragments

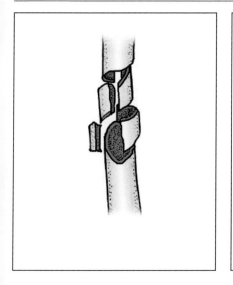

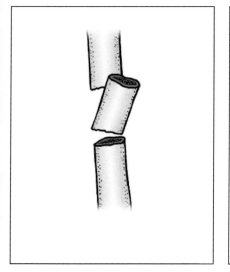

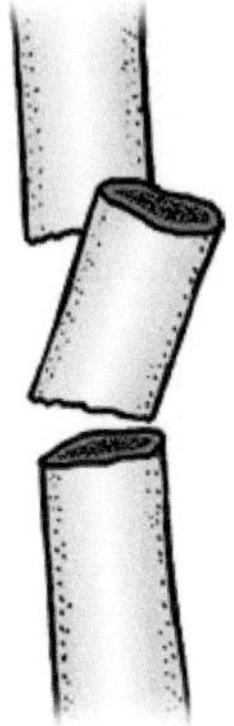

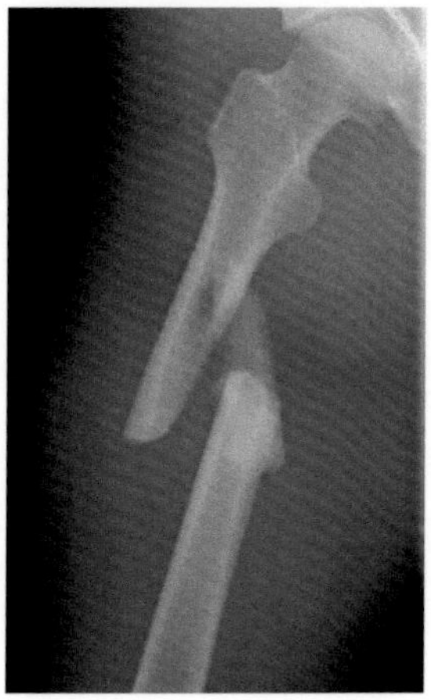

AO/OTA Classification
32-C: Femur, diaphysis, complex fractures.
C2: Segmental
C2.1: With one intermediate segmental fragment

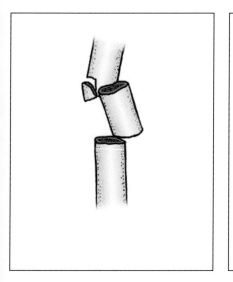

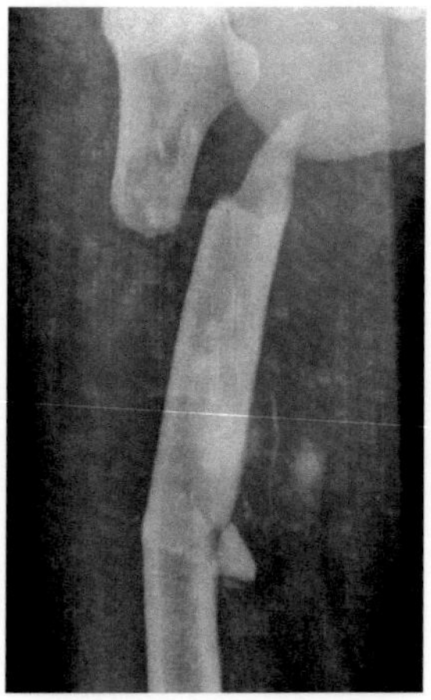

AO/OTA Classification
32-C: Femur, diaphysis, complex fractures.
C2: segmental
C2.2: with one intermediate segmental fragment with an additional wedge fragment

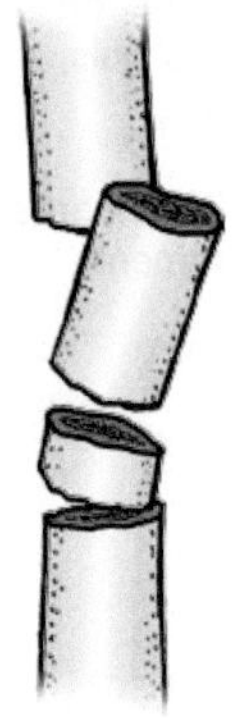

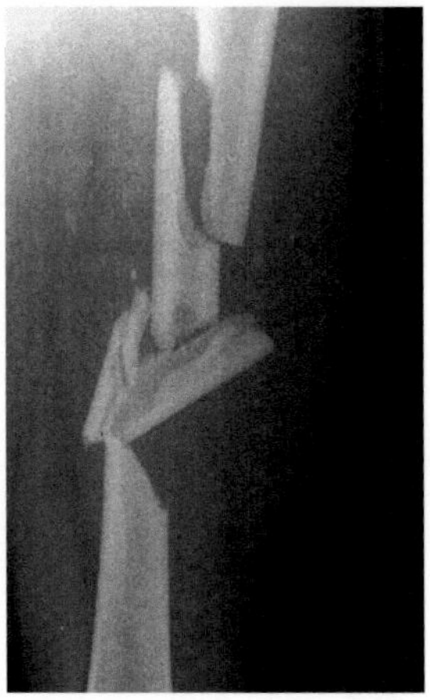

AO/OTA Classification
32-C: Femur, diaphysis, complex fractures.
C2: segmental
C2.3: with 2 or more intermediate segmental fracture

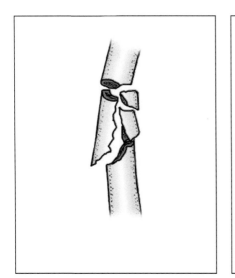

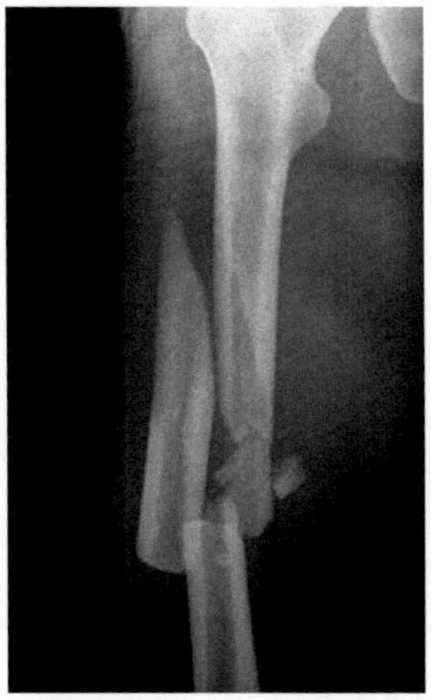

AO/OTA Classification
32-C: Femur, diaphysis, complex fractures.
C3: irregular
C3.1: with two or three intermediate fragments

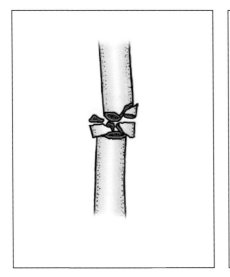

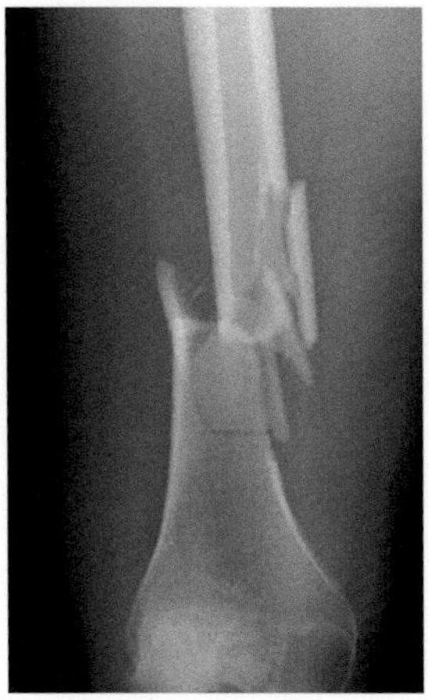

AO/OTA Classification
32-C: Femur, diaphysis, complex fractures.
C3: irregular
C3.2: with limited shattering(<5cm)

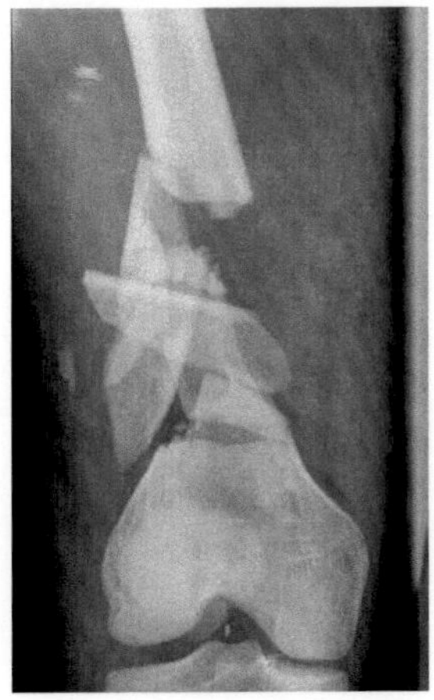

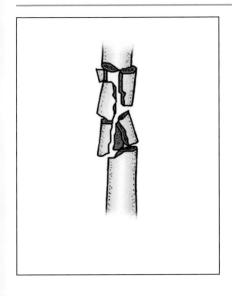

AO/OTA Classification
32-C: Femur, diaphysis, complex fractures.
C3: irregular
C3.3: with extensive shattering(≥5cm)

8.1.4.2 Winquist-Hansen Classification (1980, Orthop Clin 11:633–648)

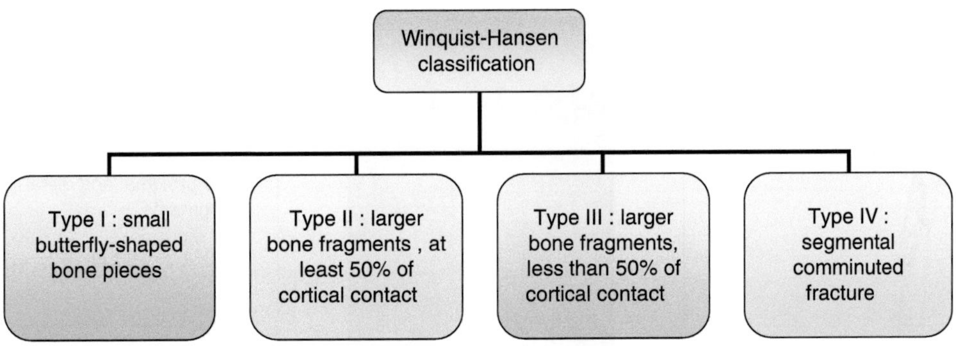

According to the degree of fracture of the fracture type. For the choice of locking nail has a guiding significance.

Type I: Small butterfly-shaped pieces of bone, with no influence on fracture stability.
Type II: Larger pieces of bone fragments, the proximal and distal segments have more than 50% of cortical contact.
Type III: Larger bone fragments, with less than 50% of cortical contact of the proximal and distal segments.
Type IV: Segmental comminuted fracture, with no cortical contact of the proximal and distal segments.

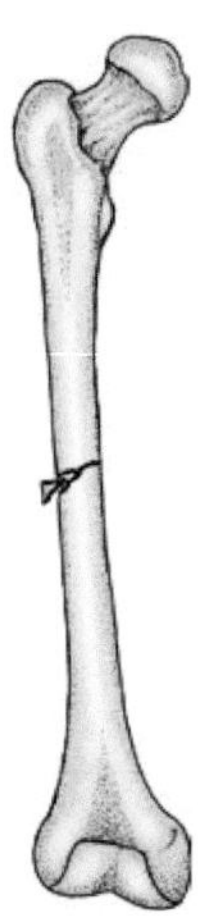

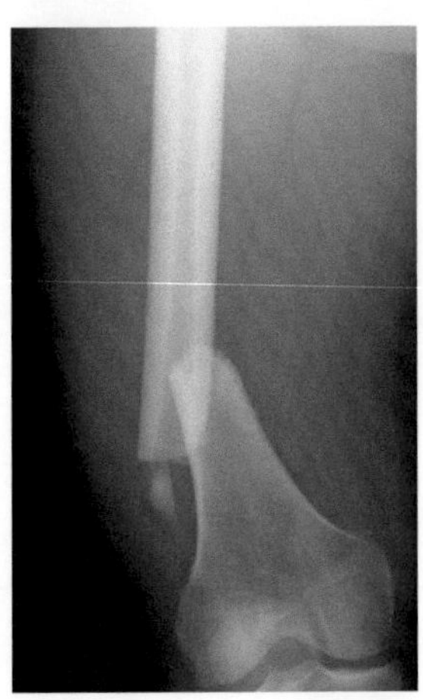

The Winquist - Hansen Classification of Femoral Shaft Fracture
Type I : small butterfly-shaped pieces of bone, with no influence on fracture stability.

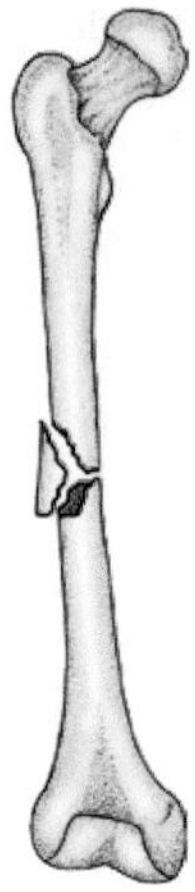

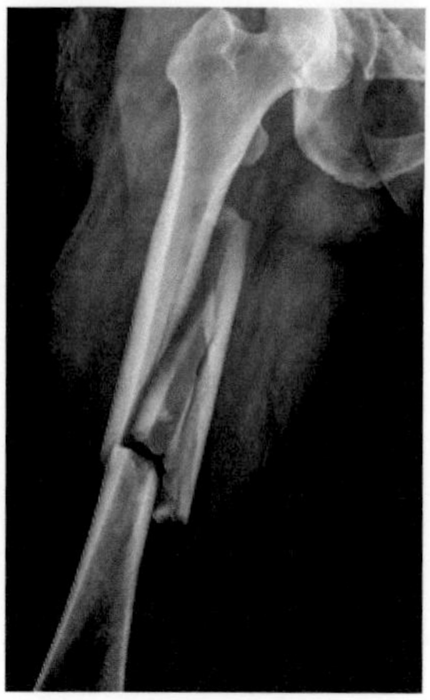

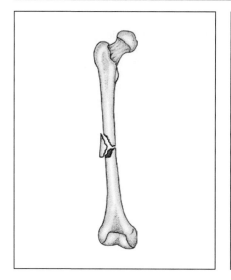

The Winquist - Hansen Classification of Femoral Shaft Fracture
Type II: larger pieces of bone fragments, the proximal and distal segments have more than 50% of cortical contact.

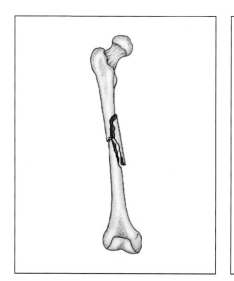

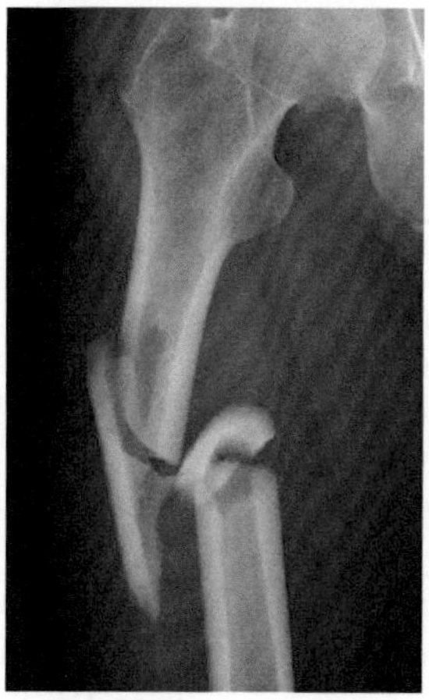

The Wiquist - Hansen Classification of Femoral Shaft Fracture
Type III: larger bone fragments, with less than 50% of cortical contact of the proximal and distal segments.

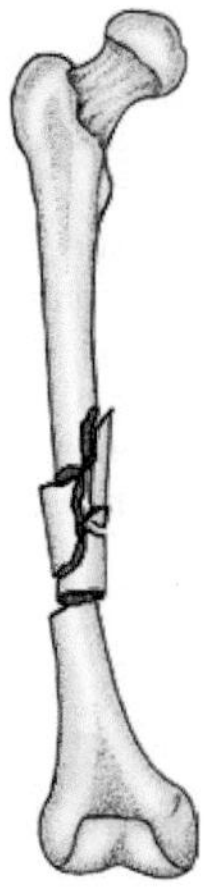

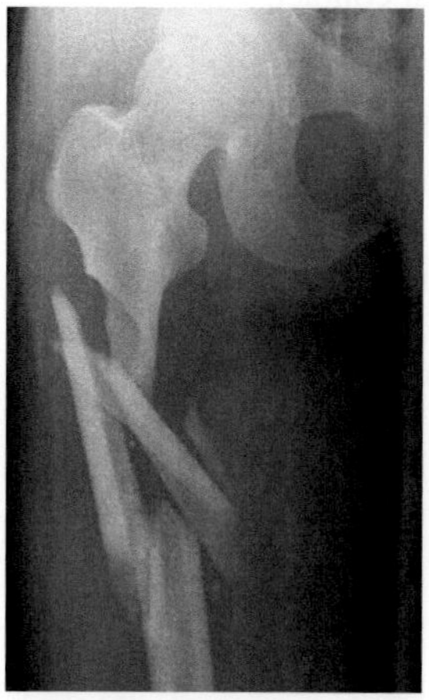

The Winquist - Hansen Classification of Femoral Shaft Fracture
Type IV: Segmental comminuted fracture, with no cortical contact of the proximal and distal segment

8.1.4.3 Classification According to the Anatomical Sites

According to the anatomical sites, femoral fracture is divided into three types: the proximal 1/3 femoral shaft fracture, the middle 1/3 femoral shaft fracture, and the distal 1/3 of femoral shaft fractures.

8.1.4.4 Classification According to Fracture Line Configuration

According to the fracture line configuration, femoral fracture can be divided into transverse fractures, oblique fractures, spiral fractures, and comminuted fractures.

8.1.4.5 Classification According to the Type of Soft-Tissue Integrity

According to the integrity of soft tissue surrounding the fracture sites, closed fractures and open fractures were divided.

8.1.4.6 Classification of the Subtrochanter Fracture of the Femur

Watson proposed the individual classification for subtrochanter fracture of the femur for the first time in 1964. So far, there are about ten kinds of classification for subtrochanter fracture of the femur available from the literature. Based on the citation frequency in literature in the past 5 years, Fielding classification, Seinsheimer classification, and Russell-Taylor classification were the first three kinds in order.

Fielding Classification (1966, Surg Gynecol Obstet, 122: 555–560)

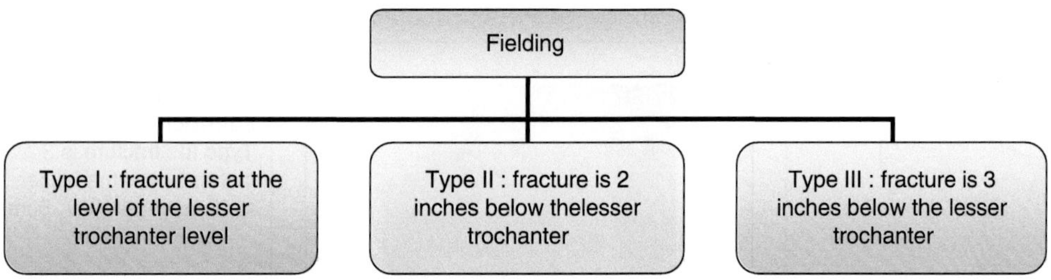

Type I: Fracture is at the level of the lesser trochanter level.
Type II: Fracture is 2 in. below the lesser trochanter (about 5 cm).
Type III: Fracture is 3 in. below the lesser trochanter (about 7.5 cm).

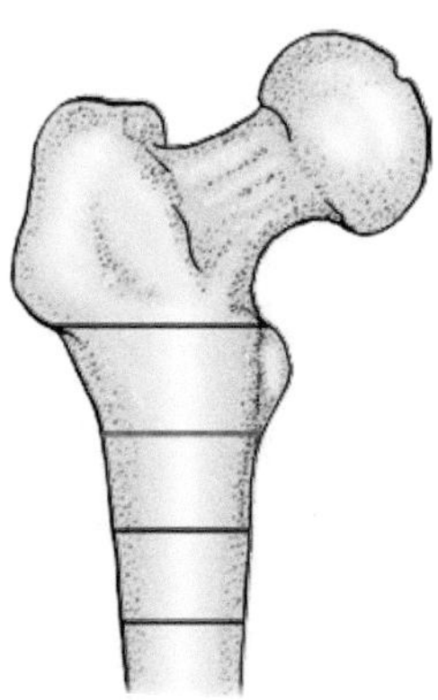

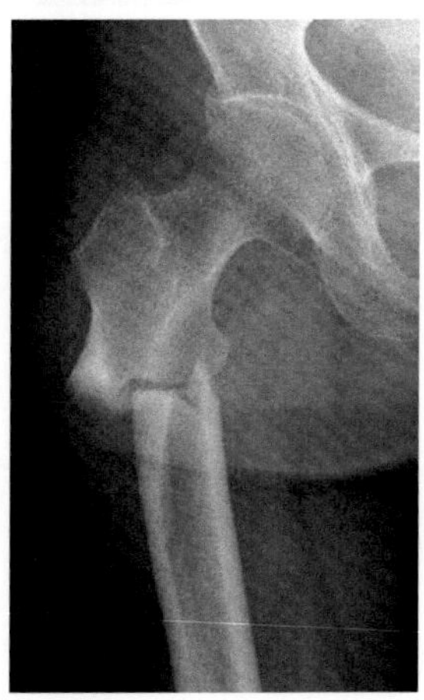

Fielding classification of sub - trochanteric fractures
Type I : fracture is at the level of the lesser trochanter level

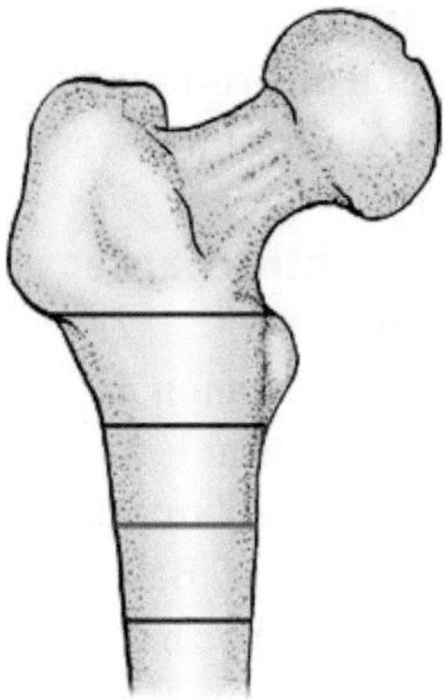

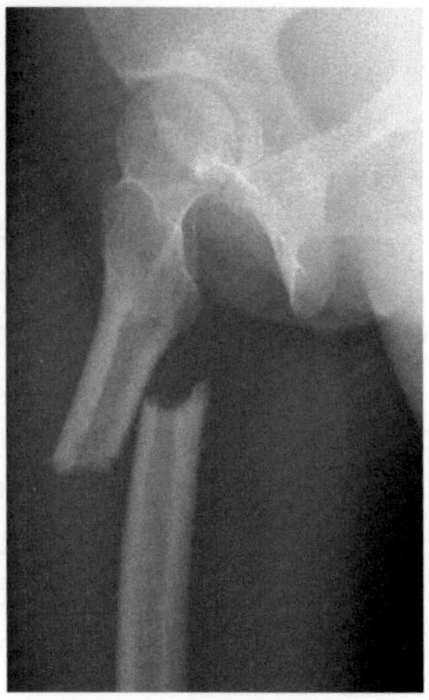

Fielding classification of subtrochanteric fractures
Type II: fracture is 2 inches below the lesser trochanter (about 5cm)

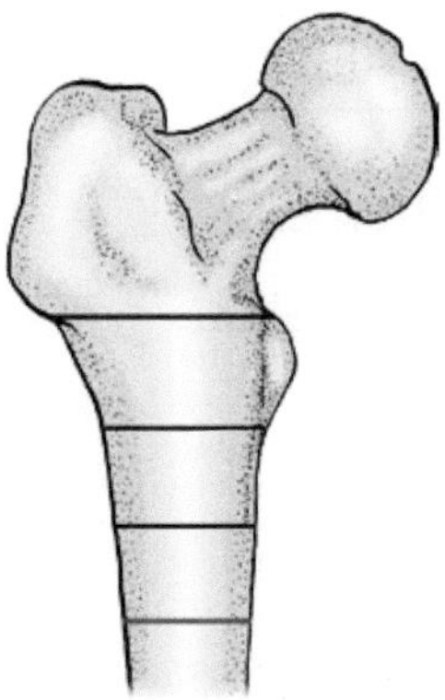

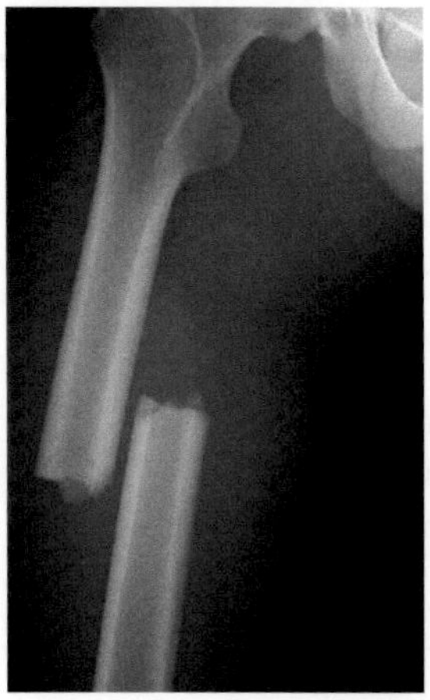

Fielding classification of subtrochanteric fractures
Type III : fracture is 3 inches below the lesser trochanter (about 7. 5cm).

Seinsheimer Classification (1978, J Bone Joint Surg (Am), 60: 300–306)

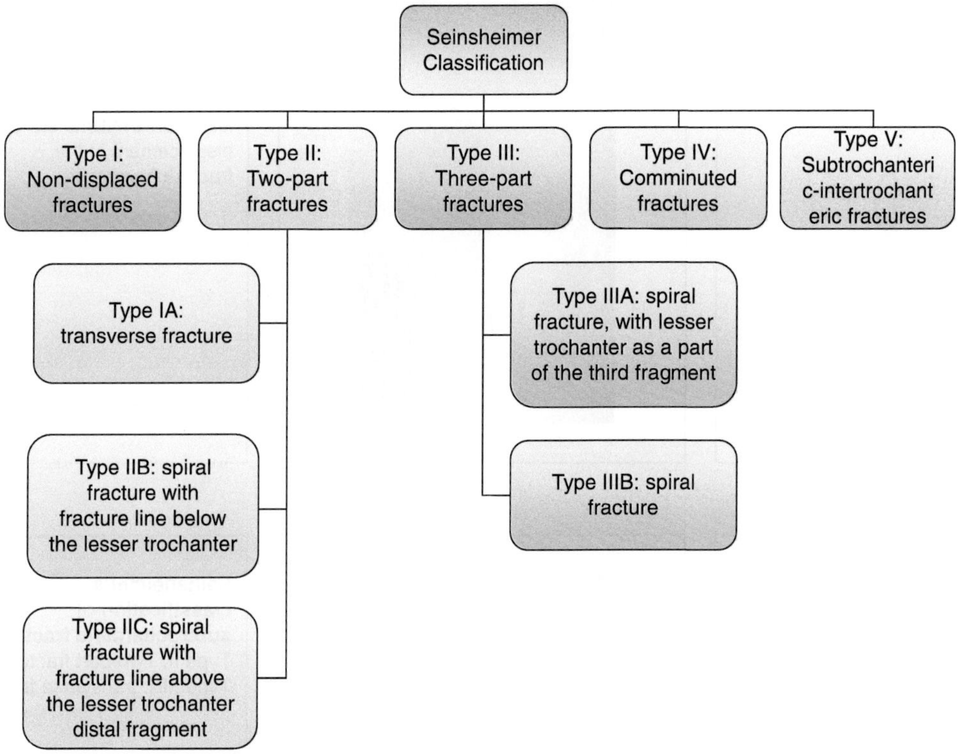

Type I: Non-displaced fractures or one with less than 2 mm of displacement.

Type II: Two-part fractures:

- Type IIA: Transverse fracture.
- Type IIB: Spiral fracture with the fracture line below the lesser trochanter.
- Type IIC: Spiral configuration with the fracture line above the lesser trochanter.

Type III: Three-part fractures:

- Type IIIA: Spiral fracture in which the lesser trochanter is part of the third fragment, which has an inferior spike of cortex of varying length.
- Type IIIB: Fracture of the proximal one-third of the femur with the third part a butterfly fragment.

Type IV: Comminuted fractures with four or more fragments.

Type V: Subtrochanteric-intertrochanteric fractures: any subtrochanteric fracture with extension through the greater trochanter.

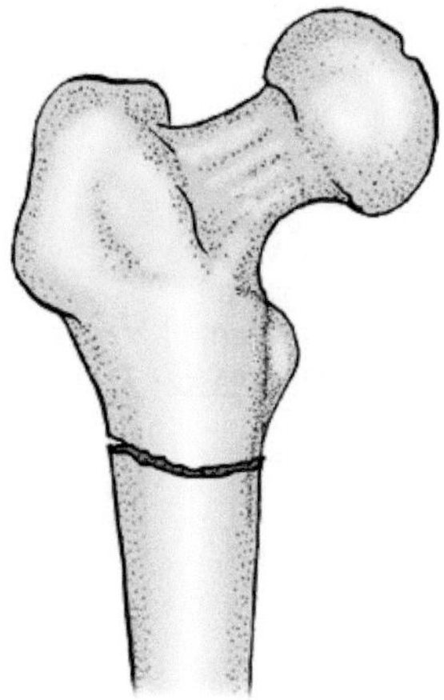

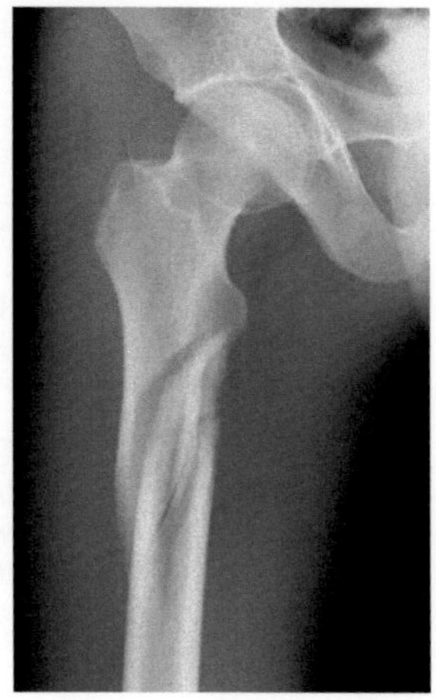

Seinsheimer's classification of subtrochanteric fractures
Type I: Non-displaced fractures: any fracture with less than 2 millimeters of displacement of the fracture fragments

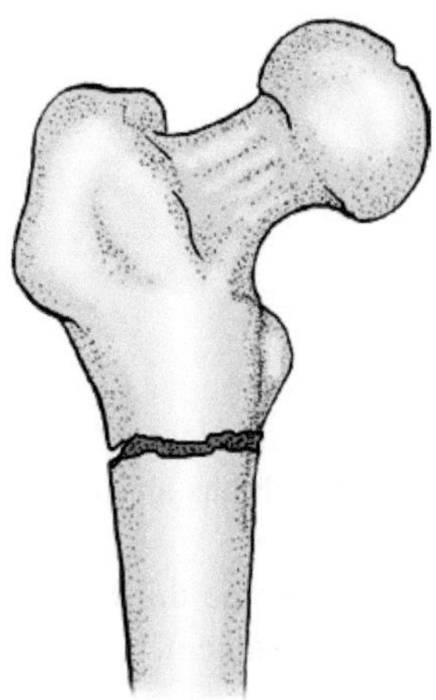

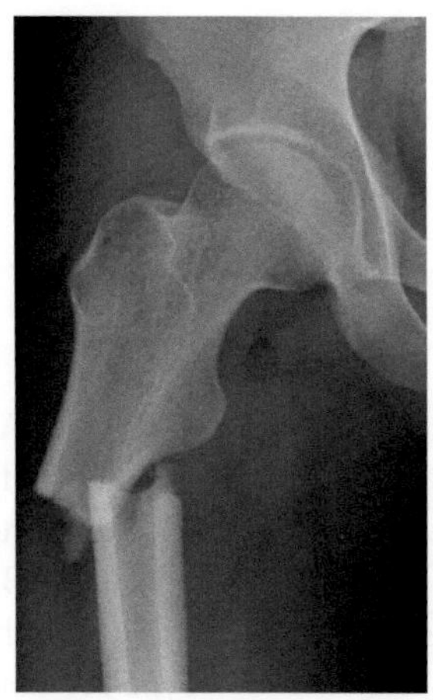

Seinsheimer's classification of subtrochanteric fractures
Type II: Two-part fractures.
Type IIIA: transverse fracture

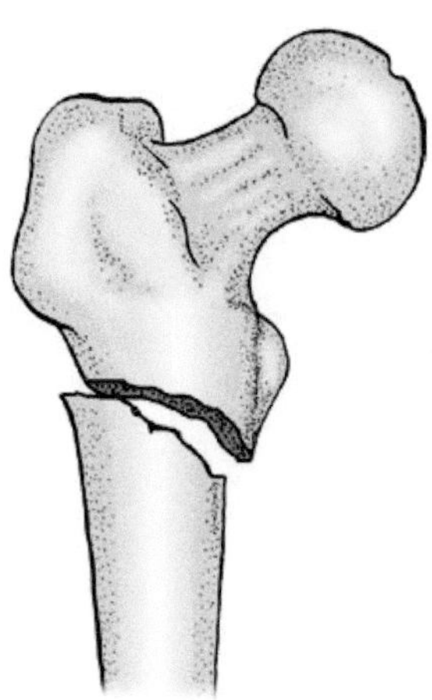

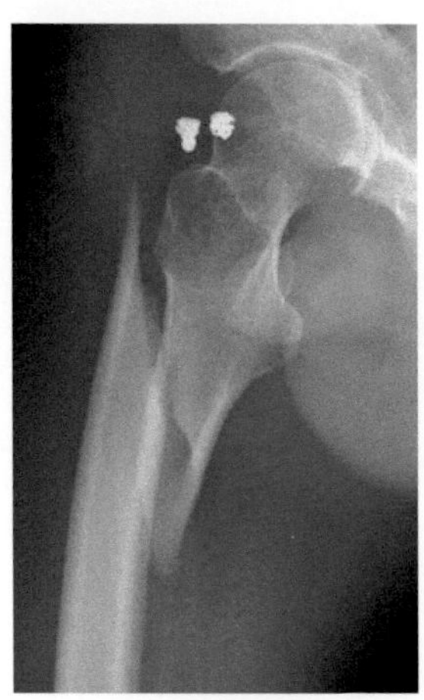

Seinsheimer's classification of subtrochanteric fractures
Type II: Two-part fractures.
Type IIB: spiral fracture with the fracture line below the lesser trochanter

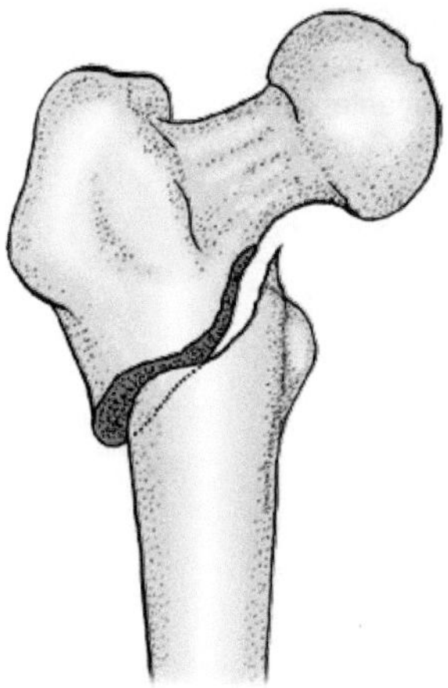

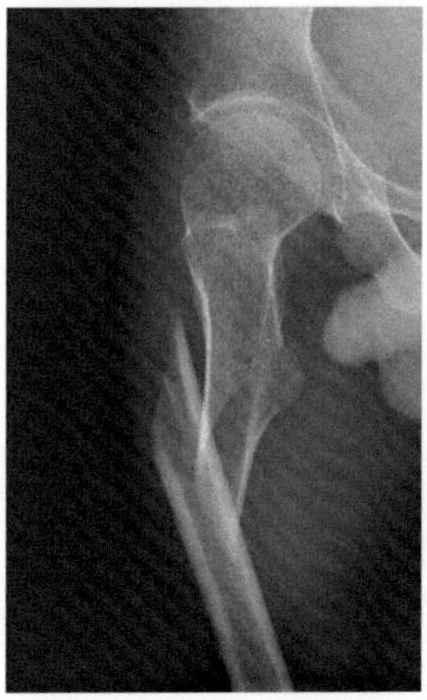

Seinsheimer's classification of subtrochanteric fractures
Type II: Two-part fractures.
Type IIC: spiral fracture with the fracture line above the lesser trochanter.

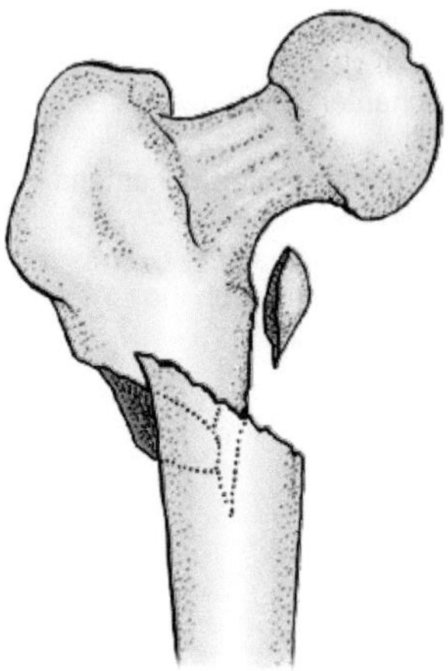

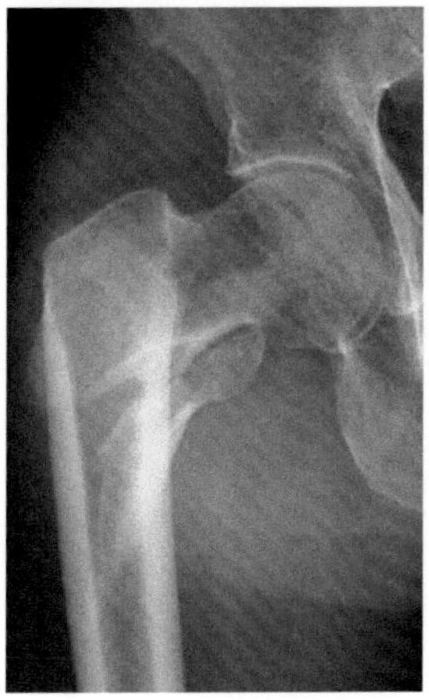

Seinsheimer's classification of subtrochanteric fractures
Type III: Three-part fractures.
Type IIIA: spiral fracture in which the lesser trochanter is part of the third fragment, which has an inferior spike of cortex of varying length

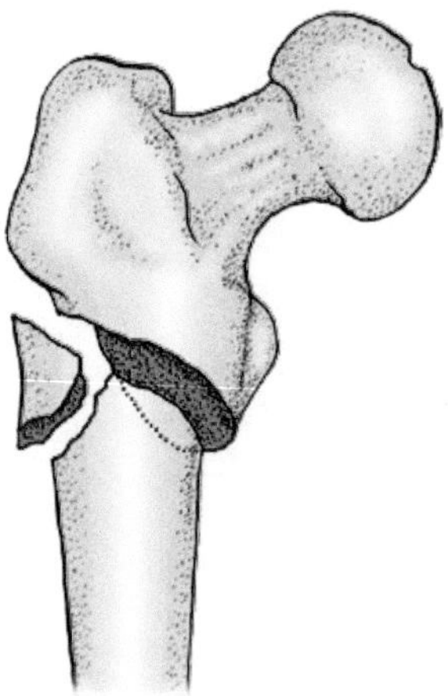

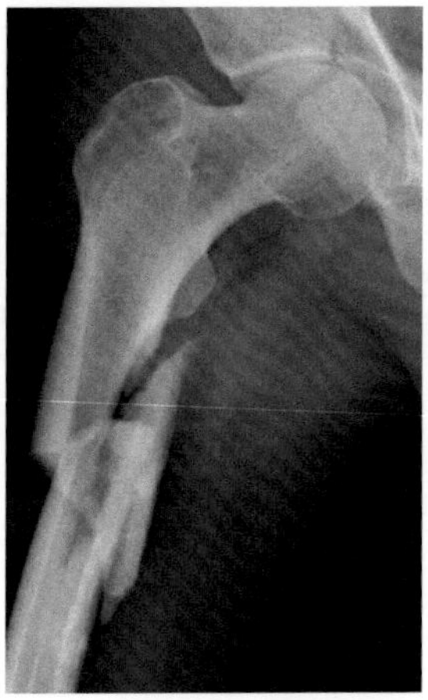

Seinsheimer's classification of subtrochanteric fractures
Type III: Three-part fractures.
Type IIIB: fracture of the proximal one third of the femur with the third part a butterfly fragment

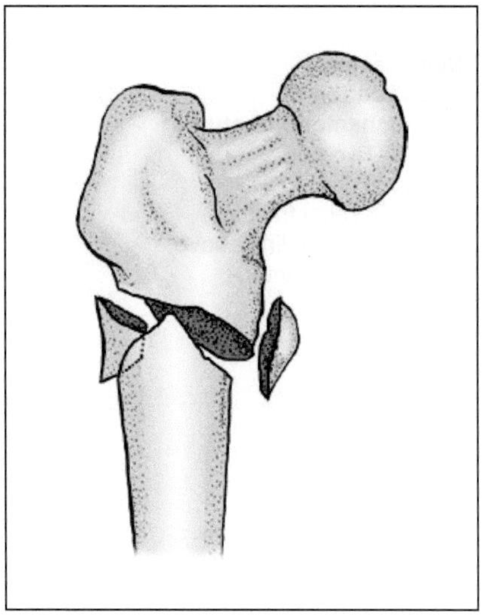

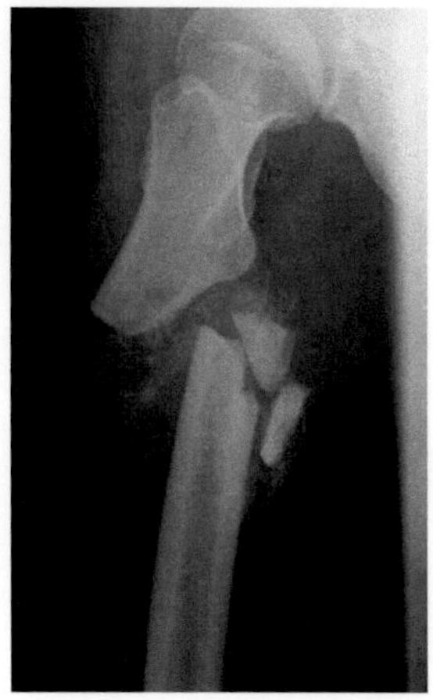

Seinsheimer's classification of subtrochanteric fractures
Type IV: Comminuted fractures: 4 or more fragments

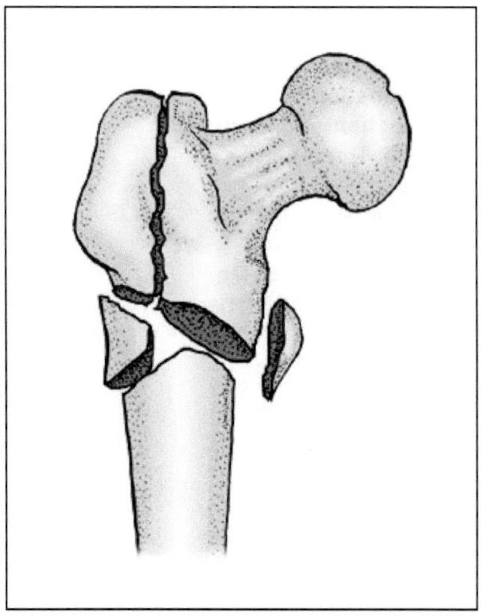

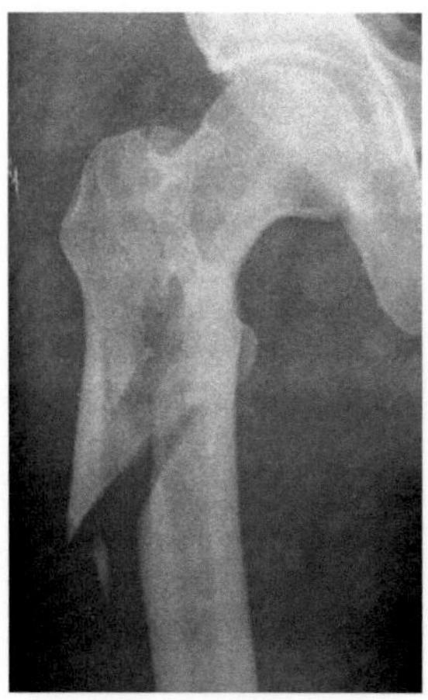

Seinsheimer's classification of subtrochanteric fractures
Type V: Subtrochanteric-intertrochanteric fractures: any subtrochanteric fracture with extension through the greater trochanter

Russell-Taylor Classification (1985, Memphis: Richards Medical Co)

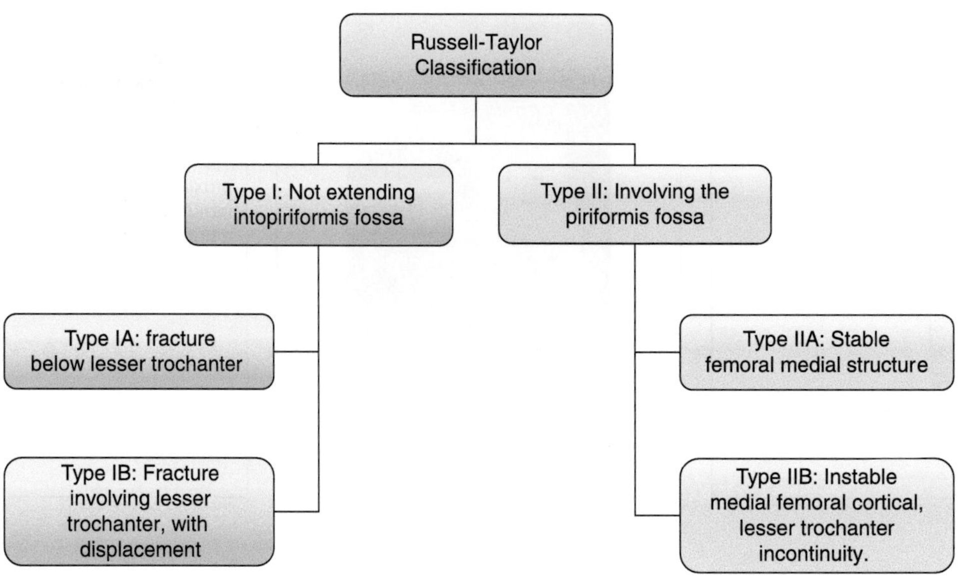

Type I: Fractures not extending into piriformis fossa:

Type IA: Fracture below lesser trochanter.

Type IB: Fracture involving lesser trochanter, with displacement.

Type II: Fracture involving piriformis fossa:

Type IIA: Stable medial structures of femur.

Type IIB: Instable medial femoral cortical, severe multi-fragmentary fracture, lesser trochanter in continuity.

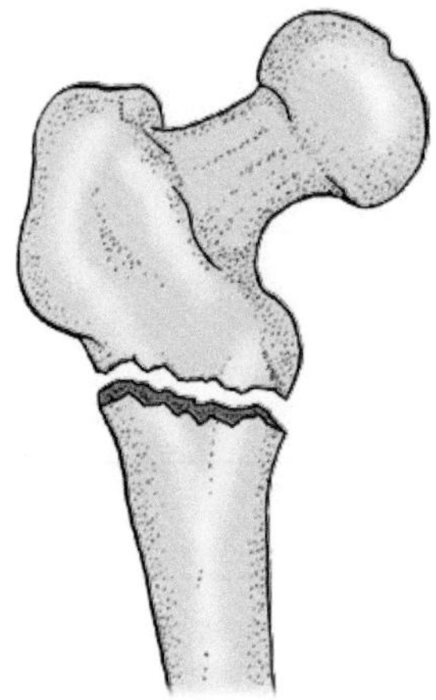

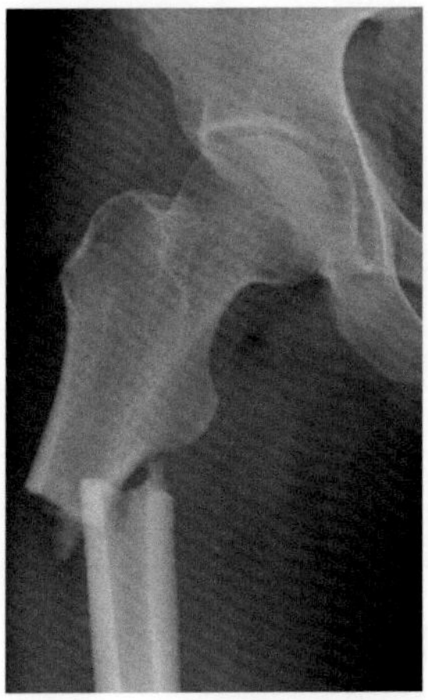

Russell-Taylor classification of subtrochanteric fractures
Type I: Not extending the piriformis fossa.
Type IA: fracture below lesser trochanter

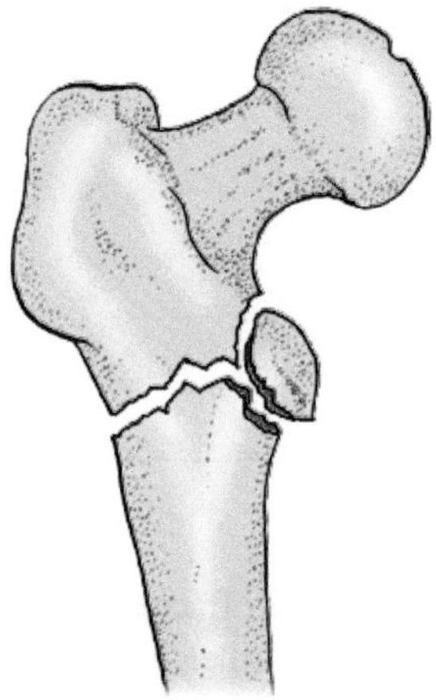

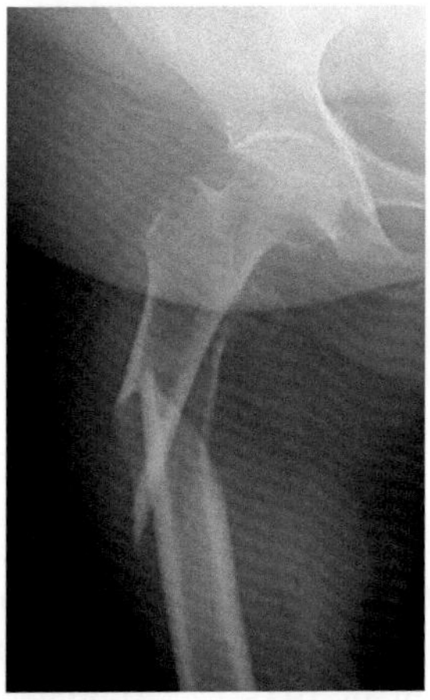

Russell-Taylor classification of subtrochanteric fractures
Type I: Not extending the piriformis fossa.
Type IB: lesser trochanter, diastatic

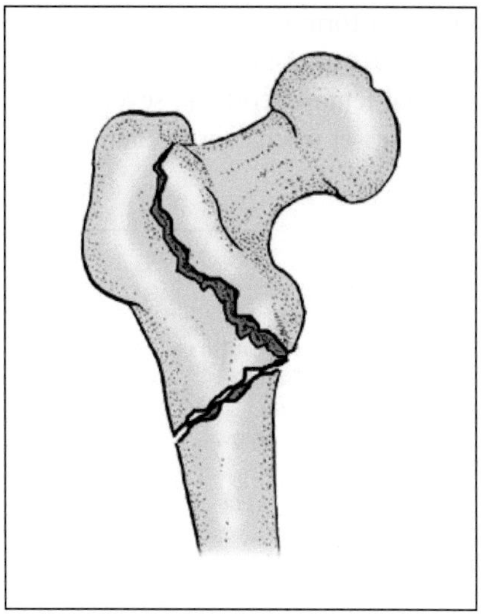

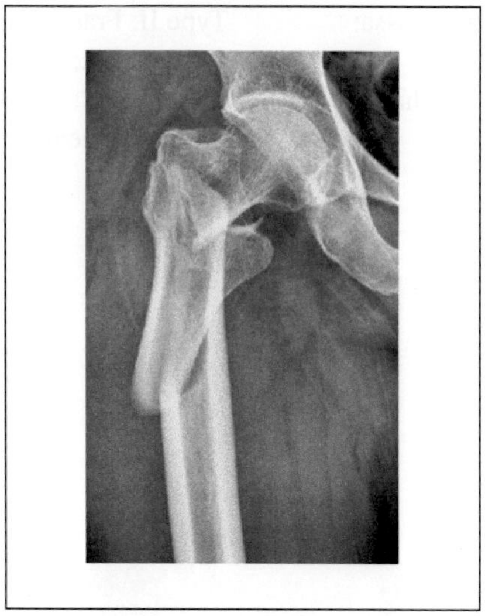

Russell-Taylor classification of subtrochanteric fractures
Type II: Involving the piriformis fossa.
Type IIA: stable femoral medial structure

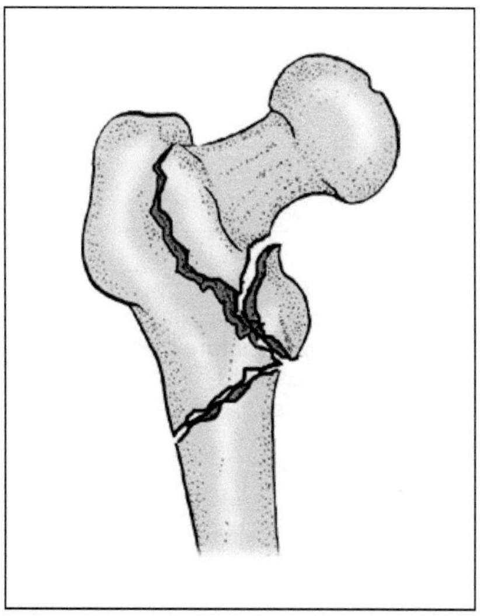

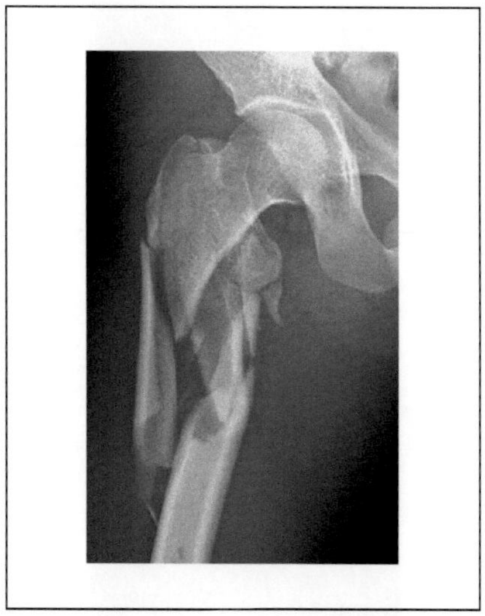

Russell-Taylor classification of subtrochanteric fractures
Type II: Involving the piriformis fossa.
Type IIB: medial femoral cortical instability, lesser trochanter incontinuity

Kyle Classification (1994, J Bone Joint Surg (Am), 76: 924)

In 1994, Kyle introduced a classification system in JBJS journal (Am volume) that was recently adopted in the United States Hennepin national medical center. The classification system defines the femoral subtrochanteric fracture into two types according to the treatment methods.

Type I: High femoral subtrochanteric fracture. This type was further divided into three subtypes: simple, multifragmentary, and piriform fossa integrity, according to whether the piriform fossa is intact. High femoral subtrochanteric fracture with intact piriform fossa can be safely fixed by the second-generation intramedullary nail, regardless of comminution or not. Subtrochanteric fractures extending piriform fossa should be treated by sliding hip screw.

Type II: Low femoral subtrochanteric fracture, with intact lesser trochanter. This type was further divided into two subtypes: simple and multifragmentary. Low femoral subtrochanteric fracture can be treated by the first-generation intramedullary nail.

Elabdien Classification (1984, Arch Orthop Trauma Surg, 103: 241)

According to the direction of tension bone trabecular of proximal femur and the origin of the femoral marrow cavity, Elabdien et al. proposed a new location of subtrochanteric anatomical area. He put forward a new classification of femoral subtrochanteric fractures, which was divided into three types: transverse, oblique, and multifragmentary.

Zickle Classification (1976, J Bone Joint Surg (Am), 58: 866)
Zickle proposes a new classification system based on the length of oblique fracture.

Type A: The short oblique fractures, from the upper lesser trochanter to the lower lateral femoral shaft.
Type B: The long oblique fractures, from the upper lesser trochanter to the lower lateral femoral shaft.
Type C: Transverse fracture of sub-lesser trochanter near isthmus.

Watson Classification (1964, J Trauma, 4: 457)
Watson first put forward the independent classification of femoral subtrochanteric fractures, which was based on the number of fracture fragments, and the length from the incisura above the femoral neck to the origin of fracture and to the fracture line. The author set up the reference code, accordingly. But this classification didn't get popularized.

Kinast Classification (1989)
Arbeitsgemeinschaft für Osteosynthesefragen/Association for the Study of Internal Fixation has established a complete set of classification system for long-bone fractures. But for the complex subtrochanteric femoral fractures, they did not give a clear classification. In 1989, Kinast et al. reported the use of the "indirect reduction" technique and AO 95° condylar blade plate for treating multifragmentary subtrochanteric fractures, and clinical efficacy rate achieved 100%. Kinast et al. also put forward a definitive classification of femoral subtrochanteric fractures. This classification divides subtrochanteric fractures into three types, A, B, and C. According to complexity increase of the fracture, each of the three types are subdivided into three groups and each group is divided into three subgroups. Type C got the worst clinical outcomes.

8.1.5 Chapter 3 Classification of Distal Femur Fractures

Charles Neer suggested the classification of distal femur fractures for the first time in 1976. By far, there are nearly ten kinds of classifications that could be found. According to the last 5 years' literature reports, AO classification, Seinsheimer classification, and Neer's classification are the mostly commonly used classification systems.

8.1.5.1 AO Classification (2007, Journal of Orthopaedic Trauma, 21 supplement. Muller's classification of long bone fracture, originally published in the 80s)

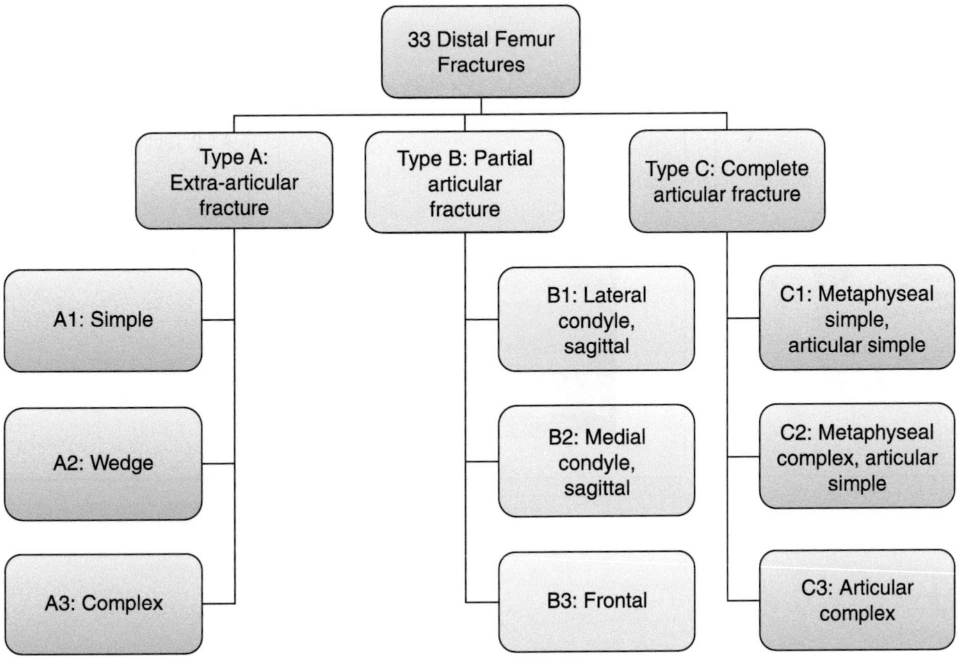

Type A: Extra-articular fracture:
- Type A1: Simple:
  - Type A1.1: Apophyseal avulsion.
  - Type A1.2: Oblique or spiral.
  - Type A1.3: Transverse.
- Type A2: Wedge:
  - Type A2.1: Intact.
  - Type A2.2: Lateral fragmented.
  - Type A2.3: Medial fragmented.
- Type A3: Complex:
  - Type A3.1: With an intermediate split fragment.
  - Type A3.2: Irregular, limited to the metaphysis.
  - Type A3.3: Irregular, extending into the diaphysis.

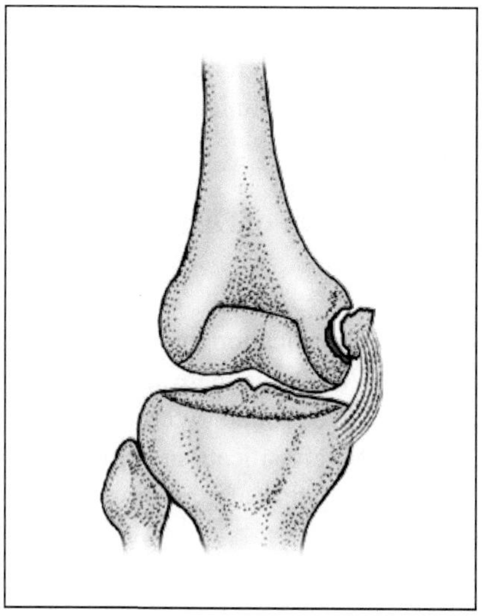

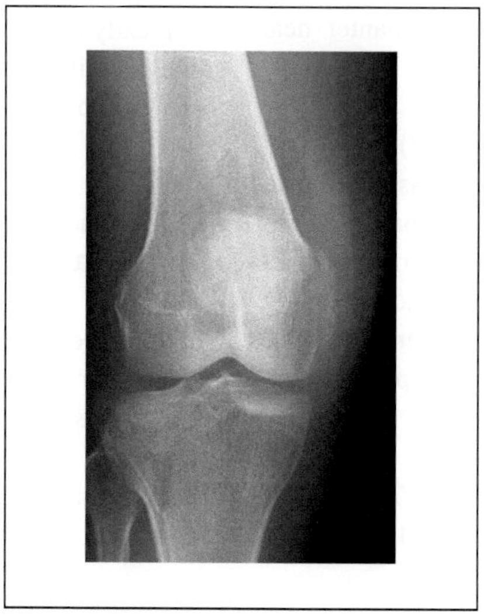

AO/OTA Classification of femoral fracture
33-A: Femur, distal, extra-articular fractures.
A1: Simple
A1.1: Apophyseal avulsion

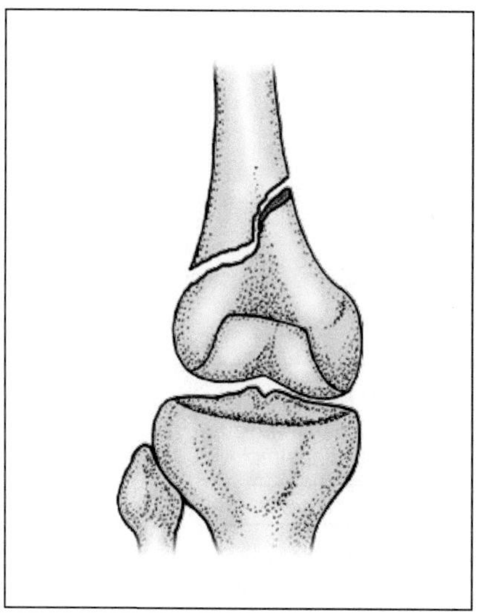

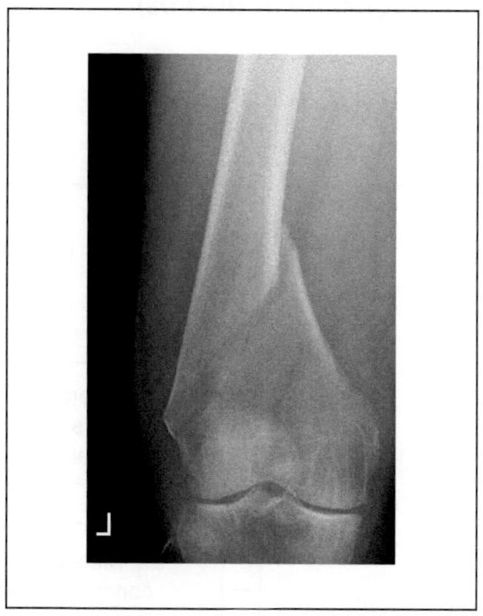

AO/OTA Classification of femoral fracture
33-A: Femur, distal, extra-articular fractures.
A1: Simple
A1.2: Oblique or spiral

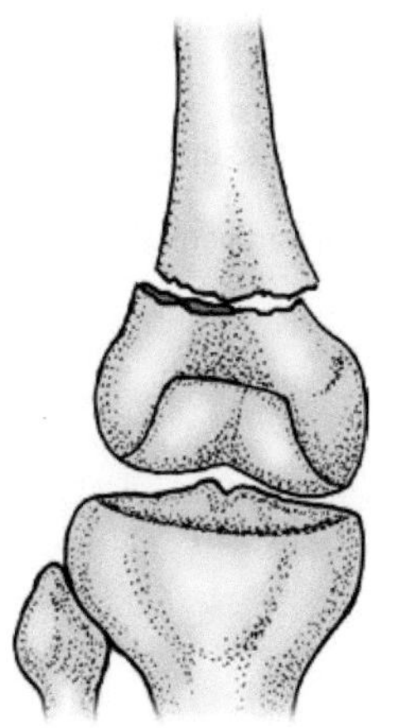

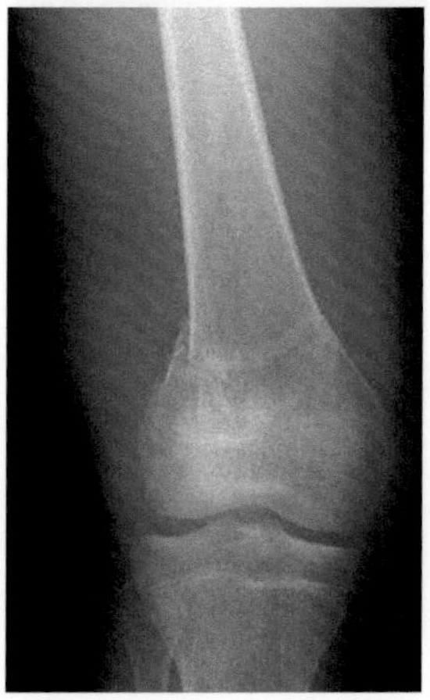

AO/OTA Classification of femoral fracture
33-A: Femur, distal, extra-articular fractures.
A1: Simple:
A1.3: Transverse

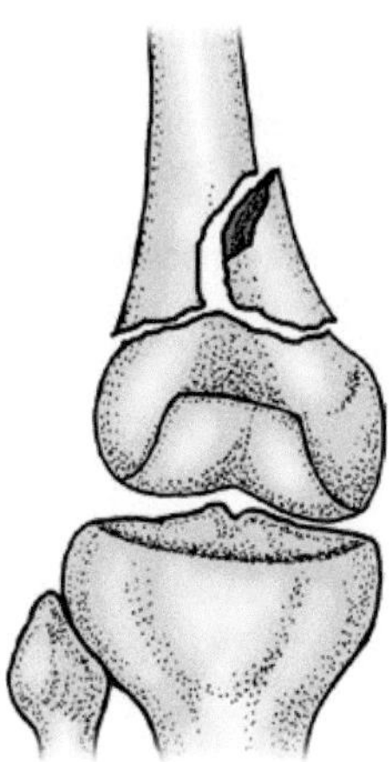

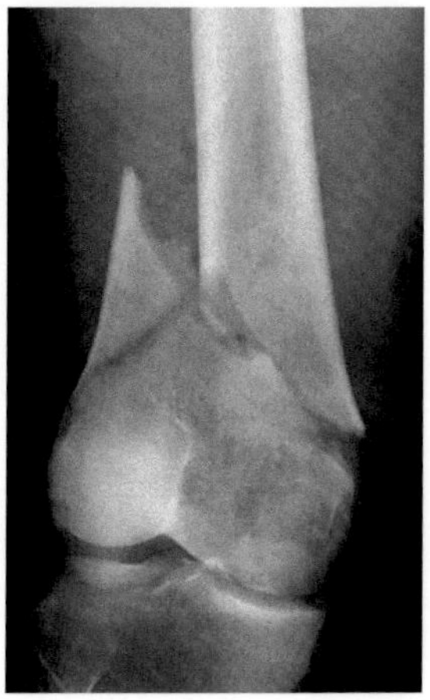

AO/OTA Classification of femoral fracture
33-A: Femur, distal, extra-articular fractures.
A2: Wedge
A2.1: Intact

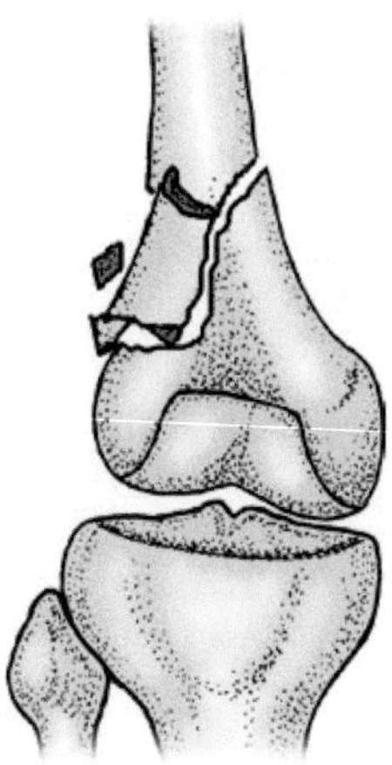

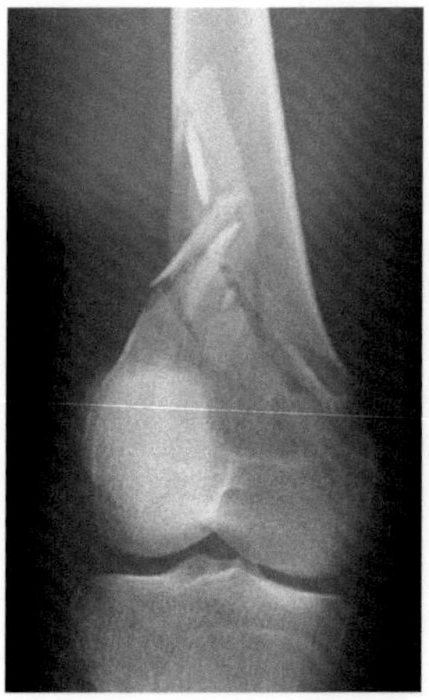

AO/OTA Classification of femoral fracture
33-A: Femur, distal, extra-articular fractures.
A2: Wedge
A2.2: Lateral fragmented

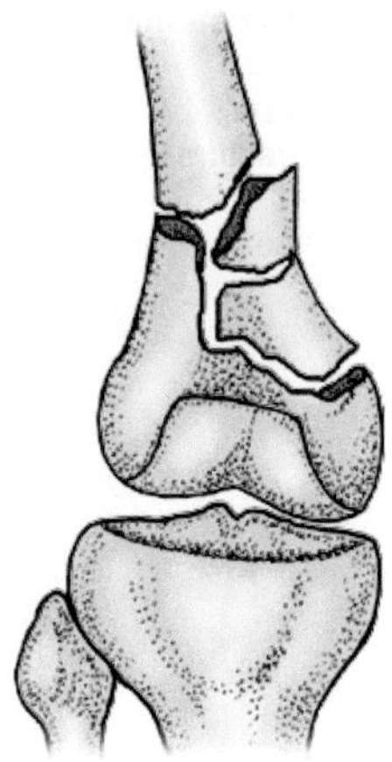

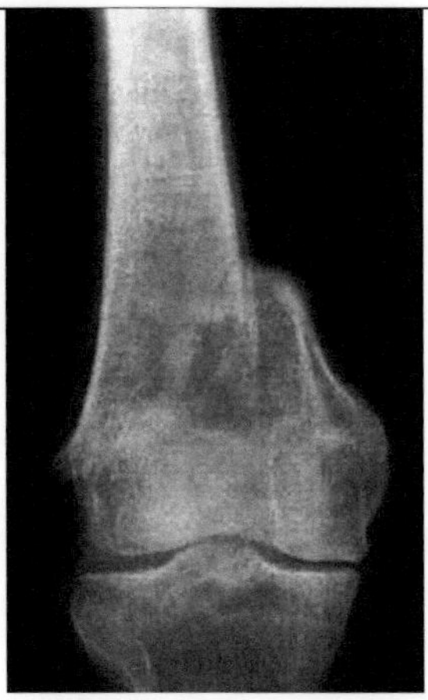

AO/OTA Classification of femoral fracture
33-A: Femur, distal, extra-articular fractures.
A2: Wedge
A2.3: Medial fragmented

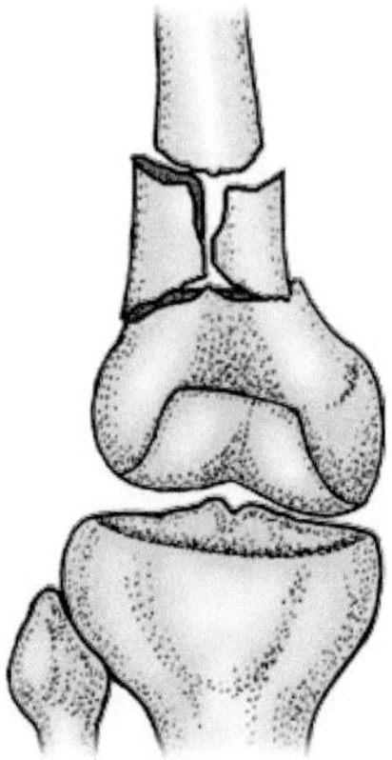

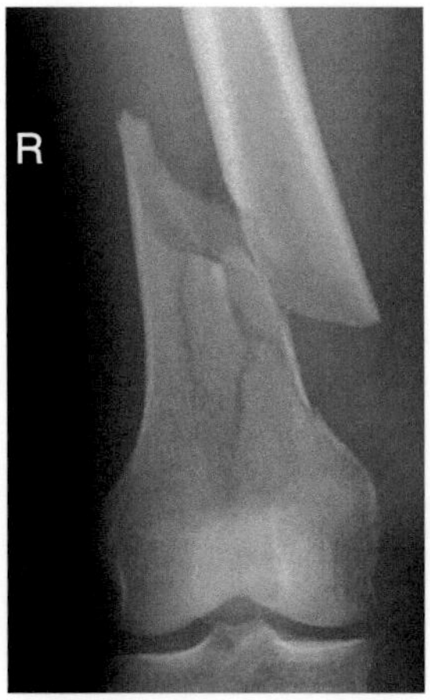

AO/OTA Classification of femoral fracture
33-A: Femur, distal, extra-articular fractures.
A3: Complex
A3.1: With an intermediate split fragment

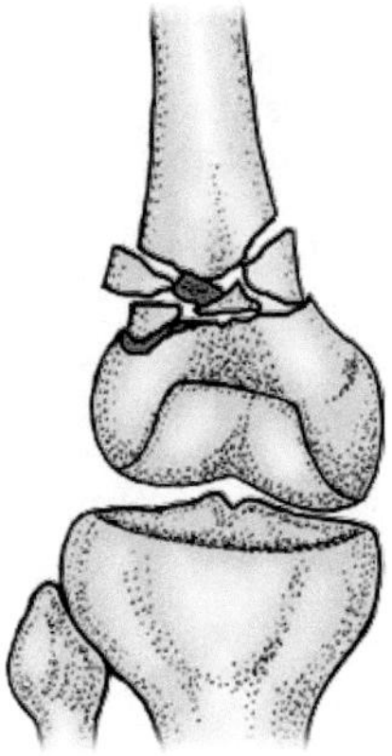

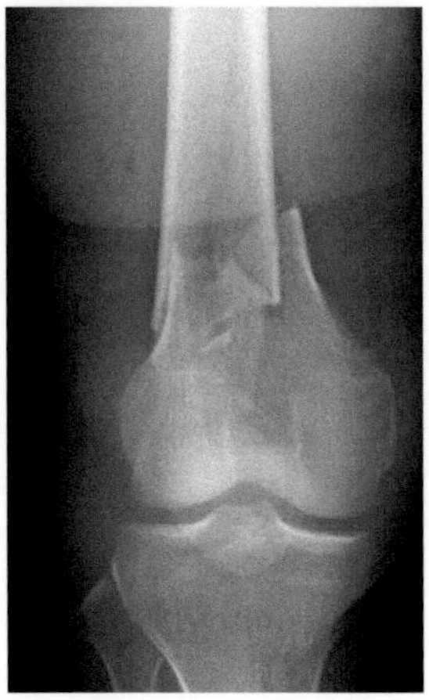

AO/OTA Classification of femoral fracture
33-A: Femur, distal, extra-articular fractures.
A3: Complex
A3.2: Irregular, limited to the metaphysis

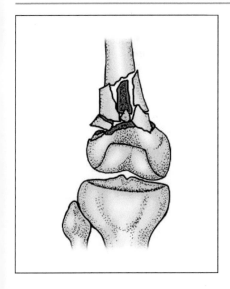

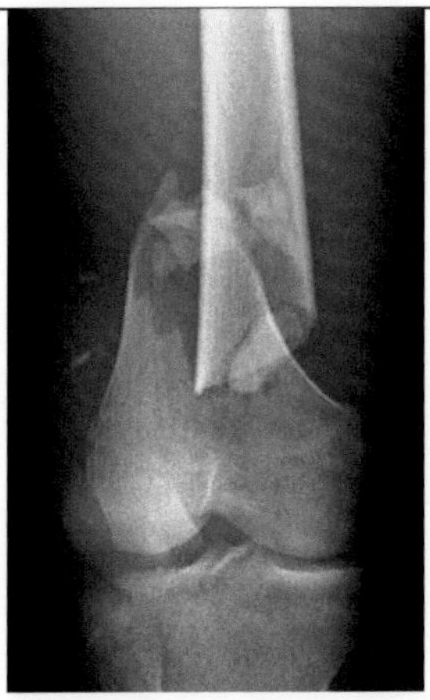

AO/OTA Classification of femoral fracture
33-A: Femur, distal, extra-articular fractures.
A3: Complex
A3.3: Irregular, extending into the diaphysis

Type B: Femur, distal, partial articular fractures:
- Type B1: Lateral condyle, sagittal fractures.
  - Type B1.1: Simple, through the notch.
  - Type B1.2: Simple, through the load-bearing surface.
  - Type B1.3: Complex, through the load-bearing surface.
- Type B2: Medial condyle, sagittal fractures:
  - Type B2.1: Simple, through the notch.
  - Type B2.2: Simple, through the load-bearing surface.
  - Type B2.3: Complex, through the load-bearing surface.
- Type B3: Frontal fractures:
  - Type B3.1: Anterior and lateral flake fracture.
  - Type B3.2: Unicondylar posterior.
  - Type B3.3: Bicondylar posterior.

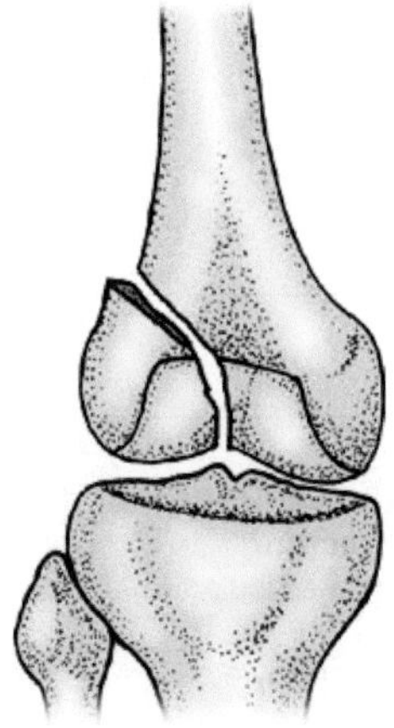

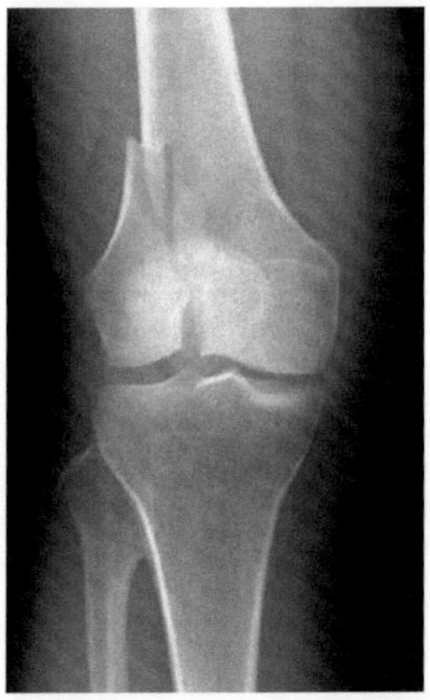

AO/OTA classification of femoral fractures
33-B: Femur distal, partial articular fractures.
B1: Lateral condyle, sagittal
B1.1: Simple, through the notch

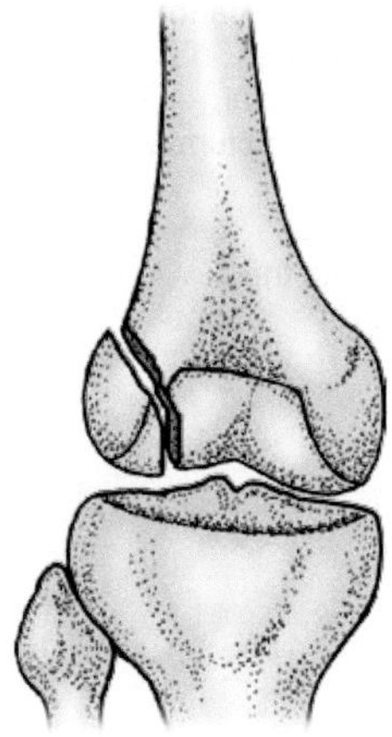

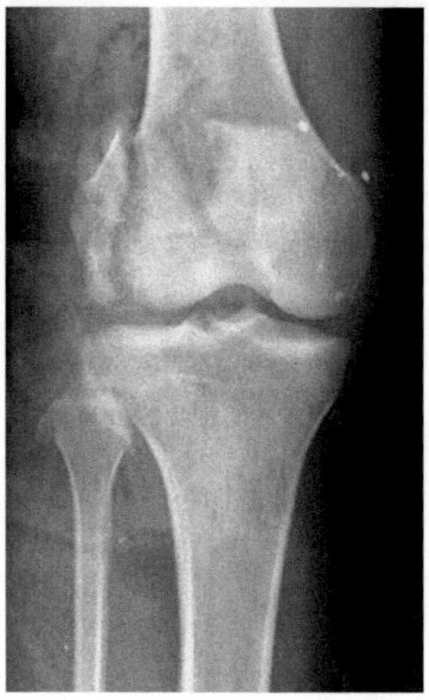

AO/OTA classification of femoral fractures
33-B: Femur distal,
partial articular fractures.
B1: Lateral condyle,
sagittal
B1.2: Simple,
through the load-bearing
surface

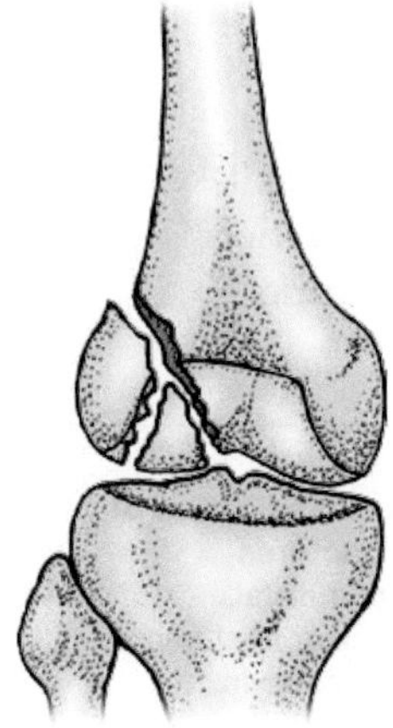

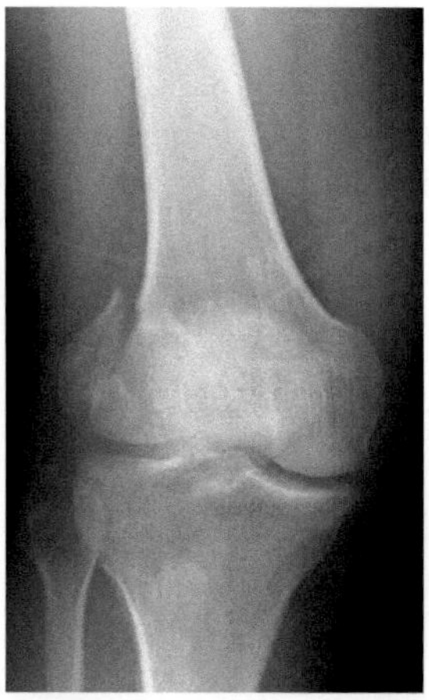

AO/OTA classification of femoral fractures
33-B: Femur distal,
partial articular fractures.
B1: Lateral condyle,
sagittal
B1.3: Complex, through
the load-bearing surface

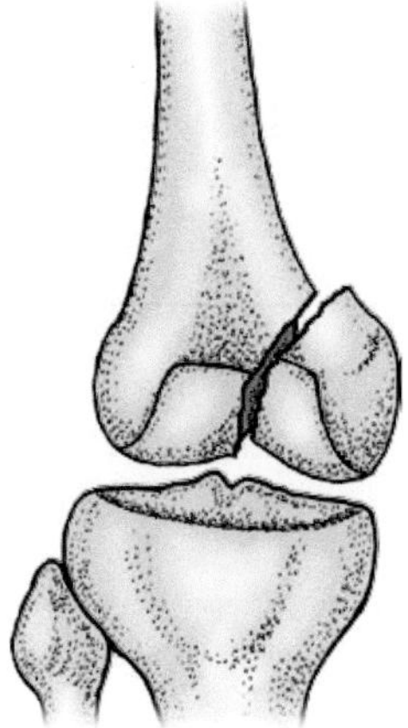

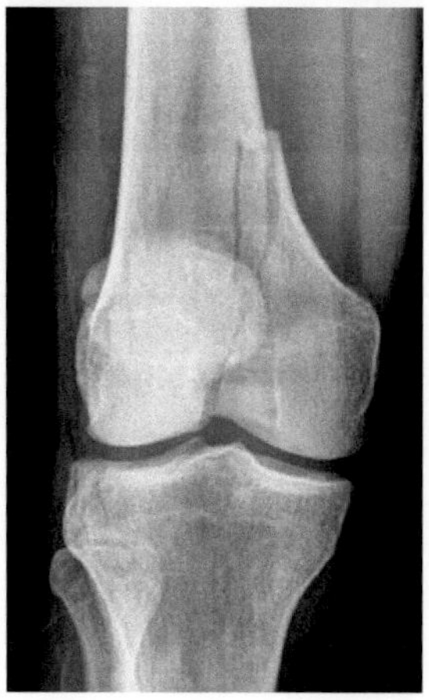

AO/OTA classification of femoral fracture
33-B: Partial-articular
fractures.
B2: Medial condyle,
sagittal
B2.1: Simple, through the
notch

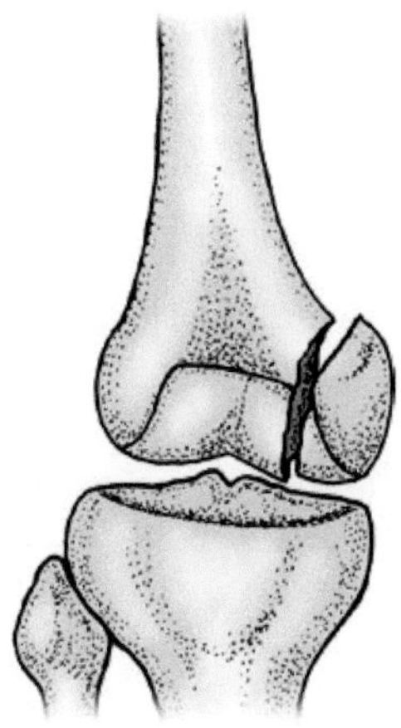

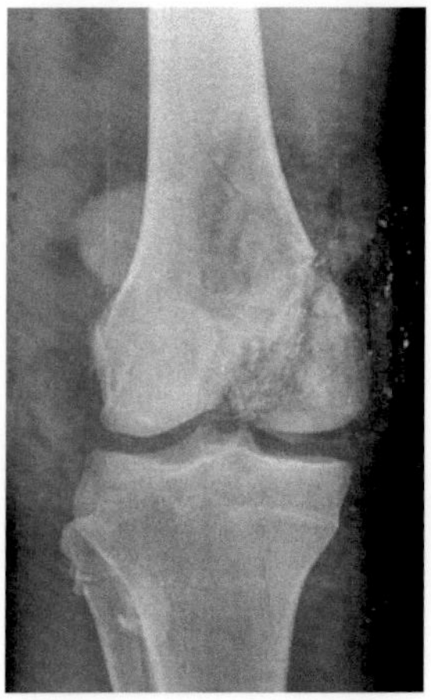

AO/OTA classification of femoral fracture
33-B: Partial-articular fractures.
B2: Medial condyle, sagittal
B2.2: Simple, through the load-bearing surface

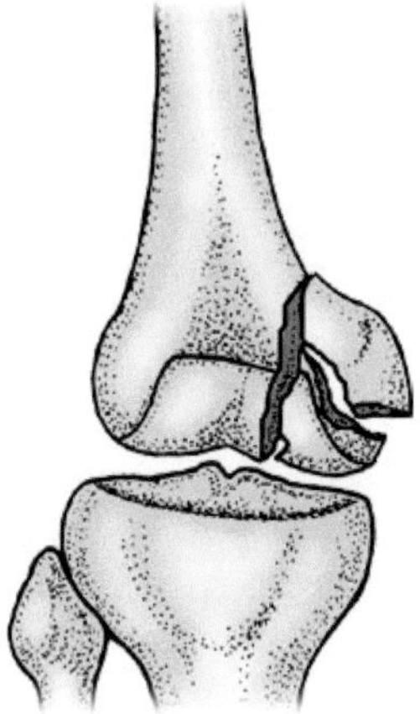

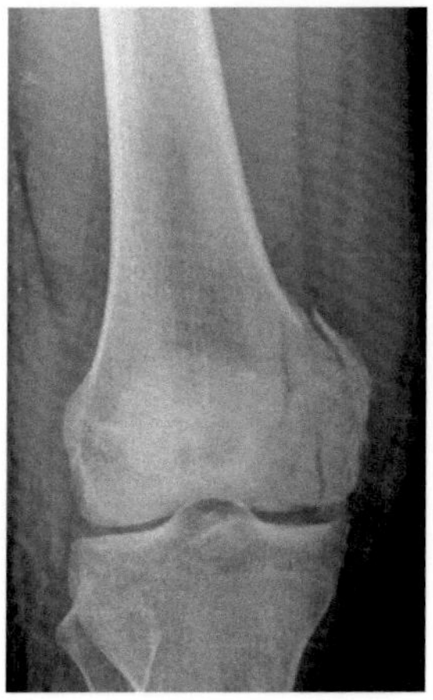

AO/OTA classification of femoral fracture
33-B: Partial-articular fractures.
B2: Medial condyle, sagittal
B2.3: Complex, through the load-bearing surface

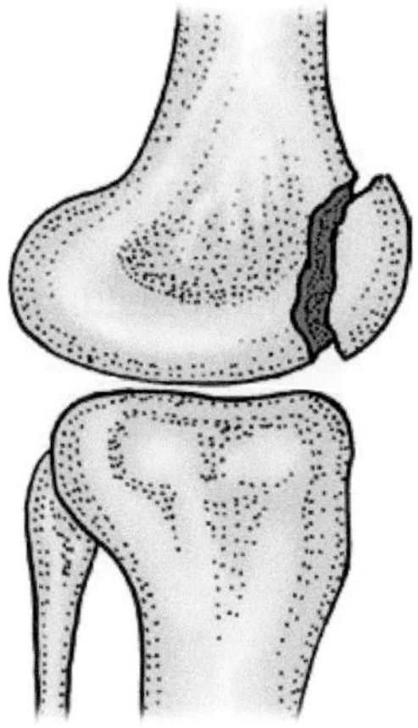

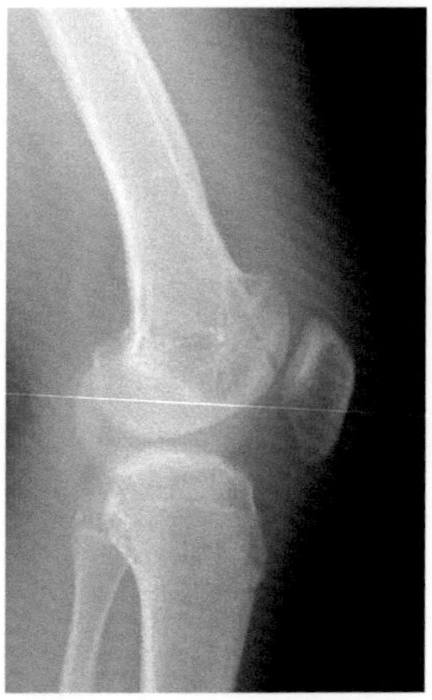

AO/OTA classification of femoral fracture
33-B: Partial-articular fractures.
B3: Frontal
B3.1: Anterior and lateral flake fracture

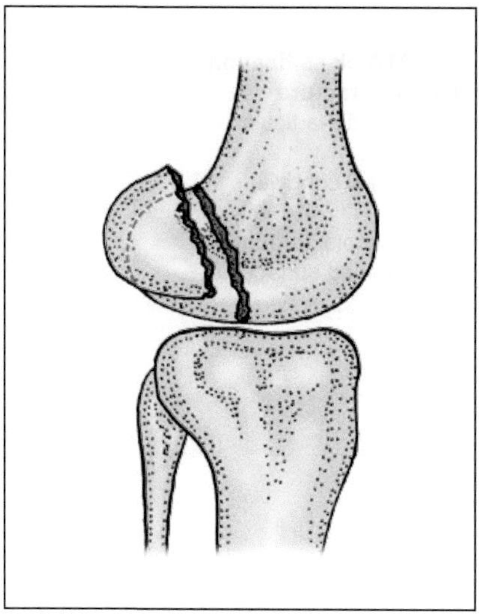

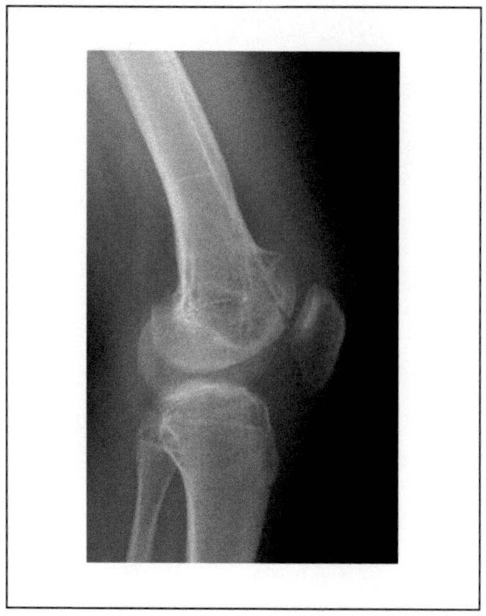

AO/OTA classification of femoral fracture
33-B: Partial-articular fractures.
B3: Frontal
B3.2: Unicondylar posterior

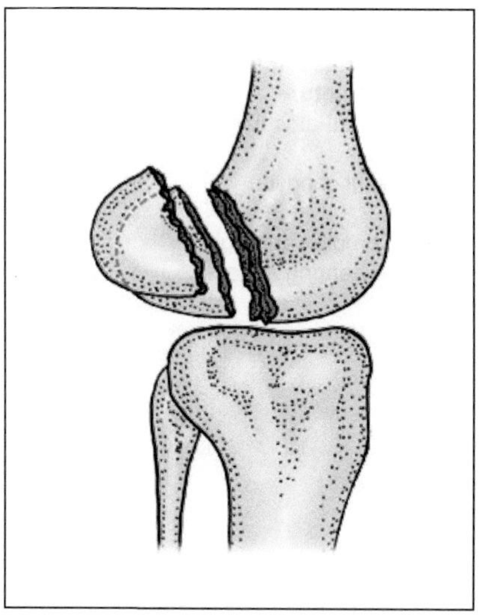

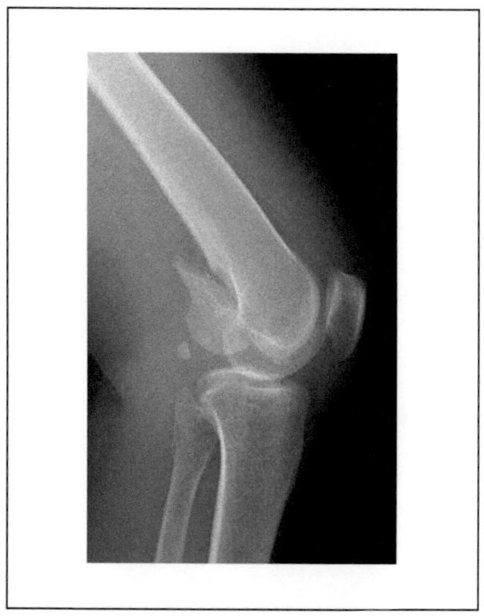

AO/OTA classification of femoral fracture
33-B: Partial-articular fractures.
B3: Frontal
B3.3: Bicondylar posterior

Type C: Complete articular fracture
- Type C1: Metaphyseal and articular simple:
  - Type C1.1: T- or Y-shaped fracture with slight displacement.
  - Type C1.2: Y-shaped fracture with marked displacement.
  - Type C1.3: T-shaped fracture.
- Type C2: Metaphyseal complex, articular simple:
  - Type C2.1: With an intact wedge fragment.
  - Type C2.2: With a fragmented wedge.
  - Type C2.3: Metaphyseal complex fracture.
- Type C3: Articular complex:
  - Type C3.1: Metaphyseal simple, articular multifragmentary.
  - Type C3.2: Metaphyseal multifragmentary, articular multifragmentary.
  - Type C3.3: Metaphysio-diaphyseal multifragmentary fracture.

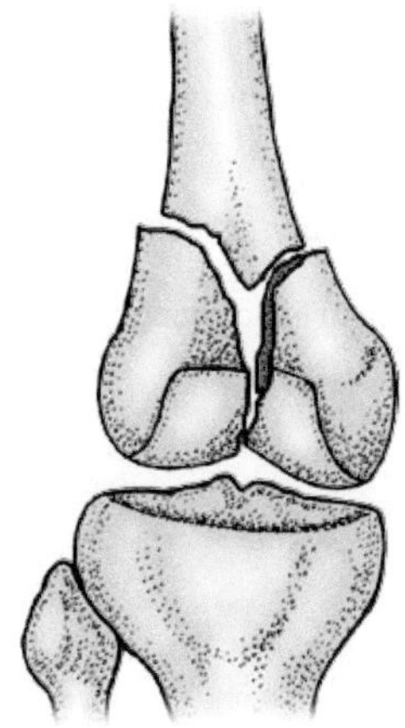

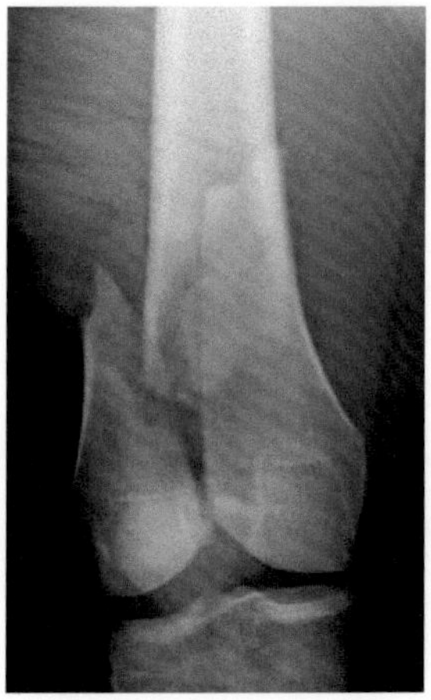

AO/OTA classification of femoral fracture
33-C: Complete articular fracture.
C1: Metaphyseal simple, articular simple
C1.1: T- or Y-shaped fracture with slight displacement

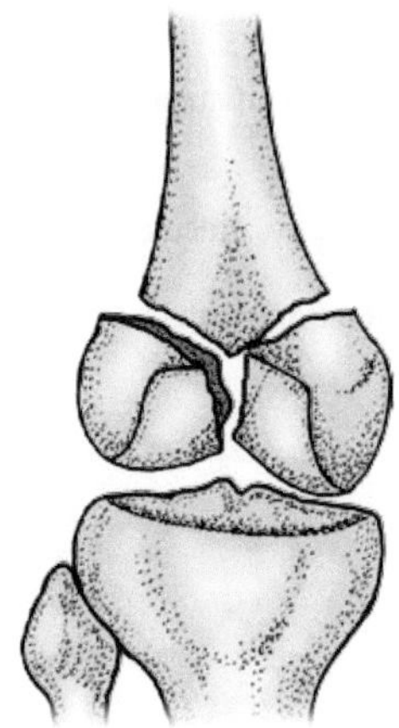

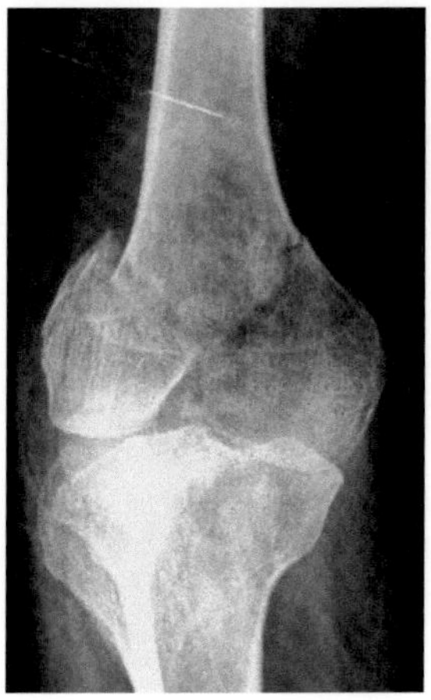

AO/OTA classification of femoral fracture
33-C: Complete articular fracture.
C1: Metaphyseal simple, articular simple
C1.2: Y-shaped fracture with marked displacement

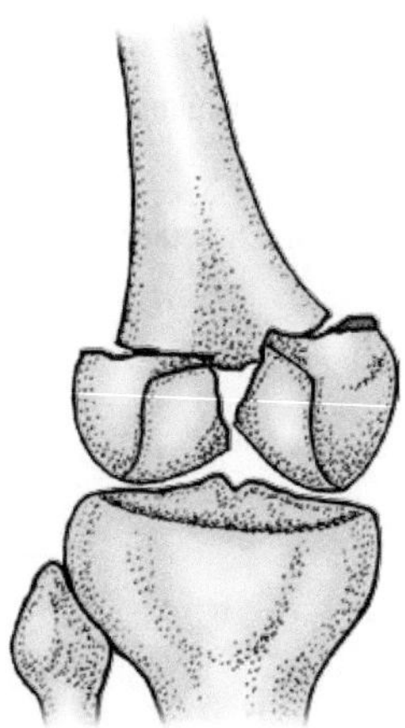

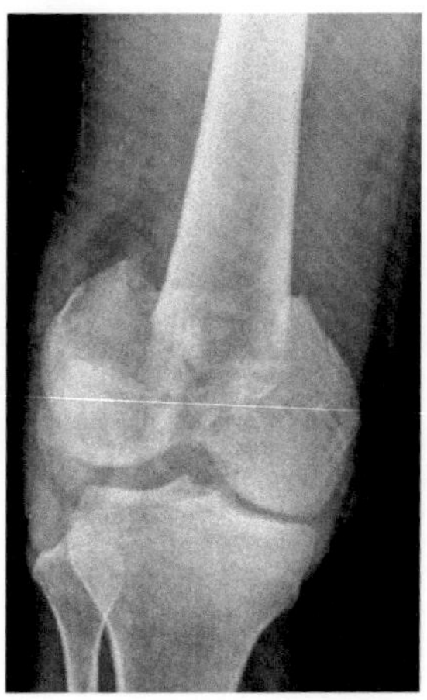

AO/OTA classification of femoral fracture
33-C: Complete articular fracture.
C1: Metaphyseal simple, articular simple
C1.3: T-shaped fracture

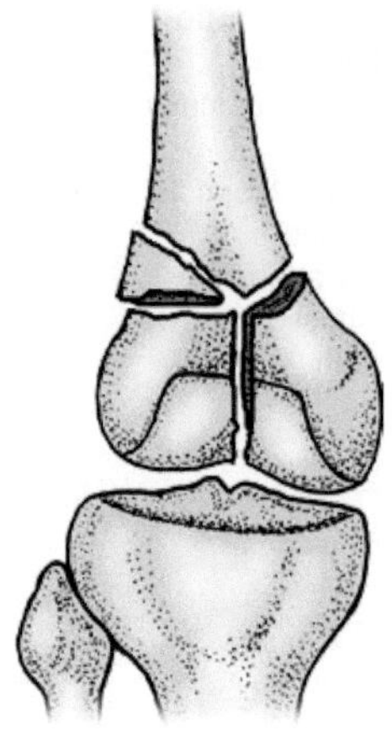

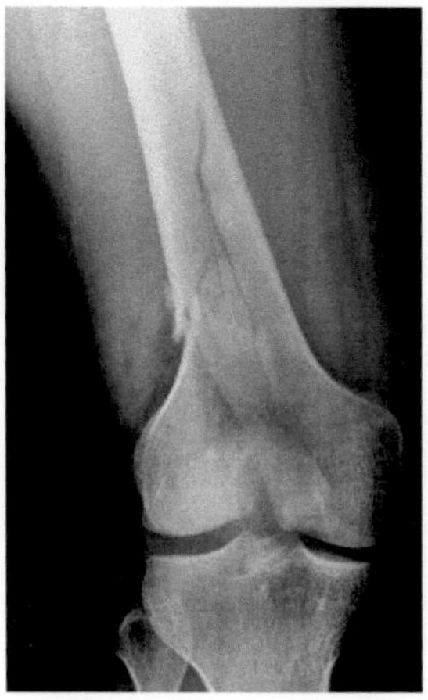

AO/OTA classification of femoral fracture
33-C: Complete articular fracture.
C2: Metaphyseal multifragmentary, articular simple
C2.1: With an intact wedge fragment

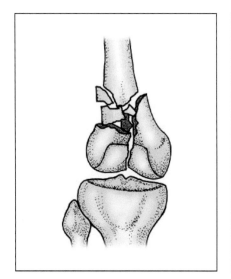

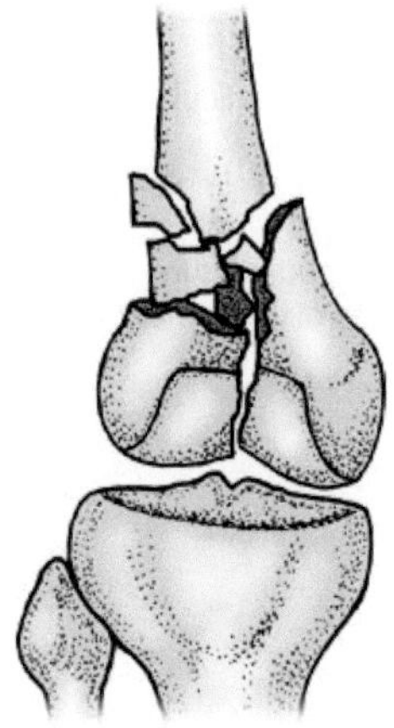

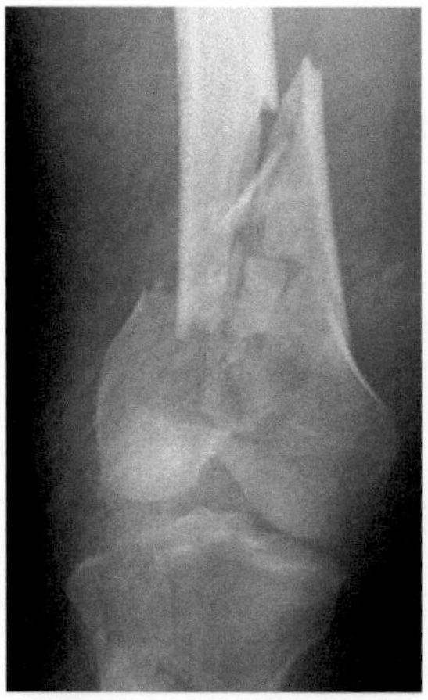

AO/OTA classification of femoral fracture
33-C: Complete articular fracture.
C2: Metaphyseal multifragmentary, articular simple
C2.2: With a fragmented wedge

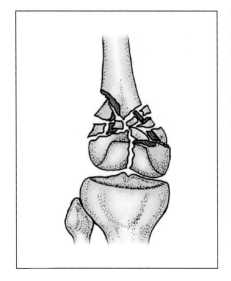

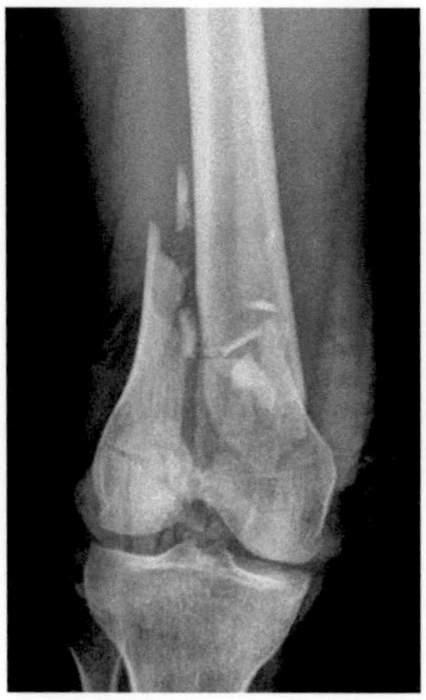

AO/OTA classification of femoral fracture
33-C: Complete articular fractures.
C2: Metaphyseal multifragmentary, articular simple
C2.3: Metaphyseal complex

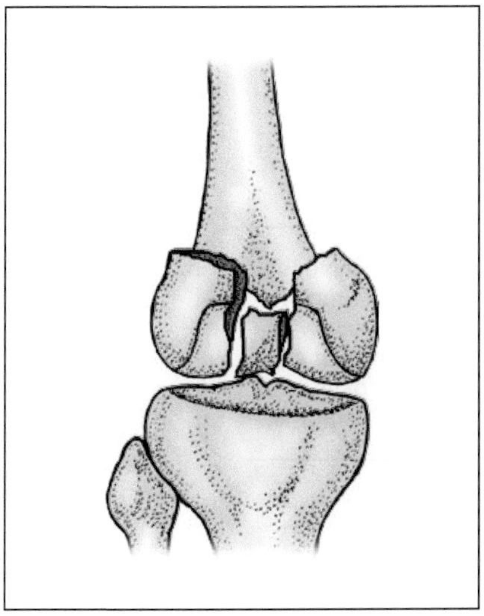

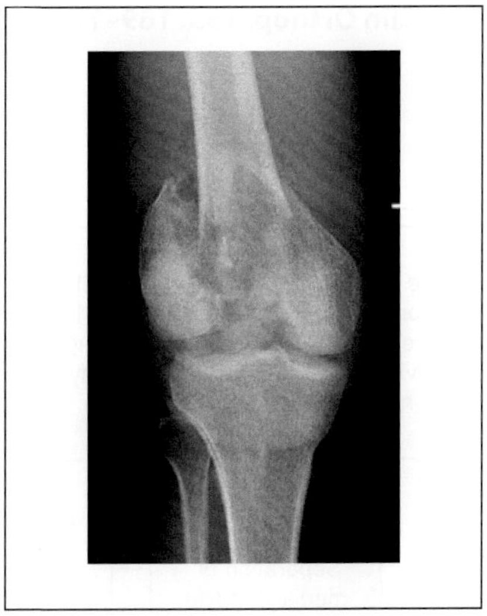

AO/OTA classification of femoral fracture
33-C: Complete articular fractures.
C3: Articular multifragmentary
C3.1: Metaphyseal simple, articular multifragmentary

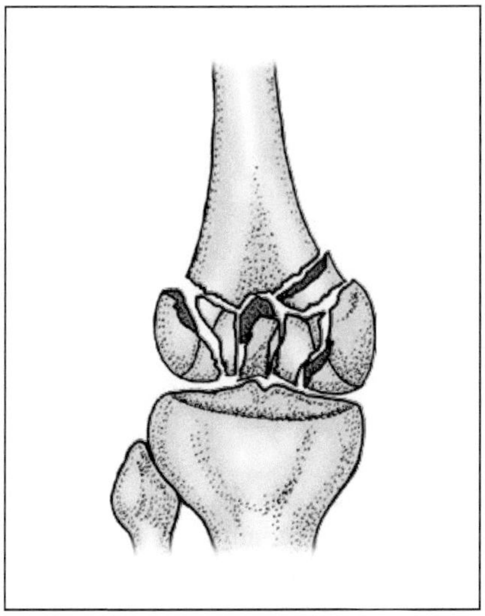

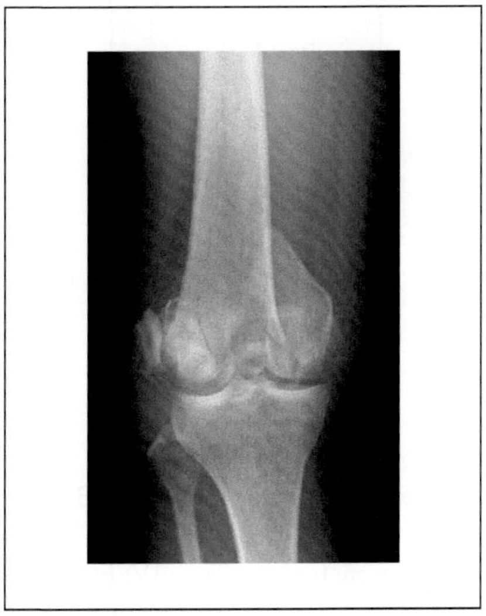

AO/OTA classification of femoral fracture
33-C: Complete articular fractures.
C3: Articular multifragmentary
C3.2: Metaphyseal multifragmentary, articular multifragmentary

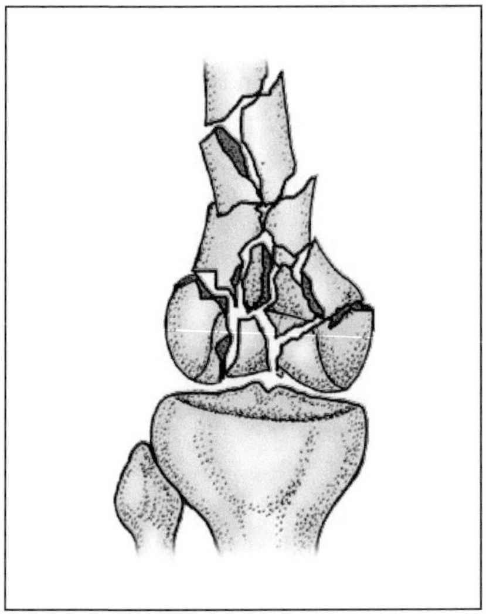

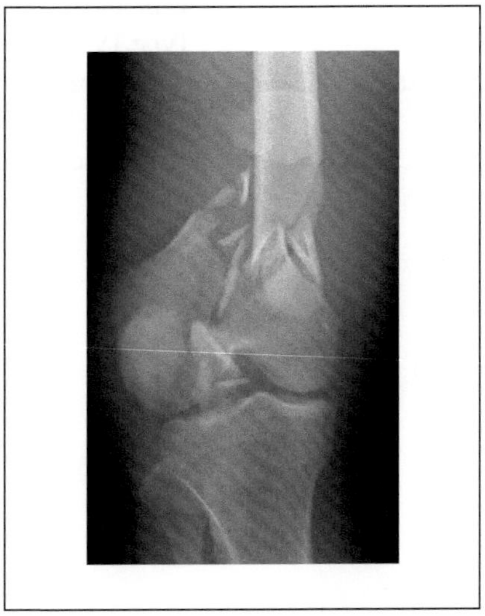

AO/OTA classification of femoral fracture
33-C: Complete articular fractures.
C3: Articular multifragmentary
C3.3: Metaphysiodiaphyseal multifragmentary

8.1.5.2 Seinsheimer Classification (1980, Clin Orthop, 153: 169–179)

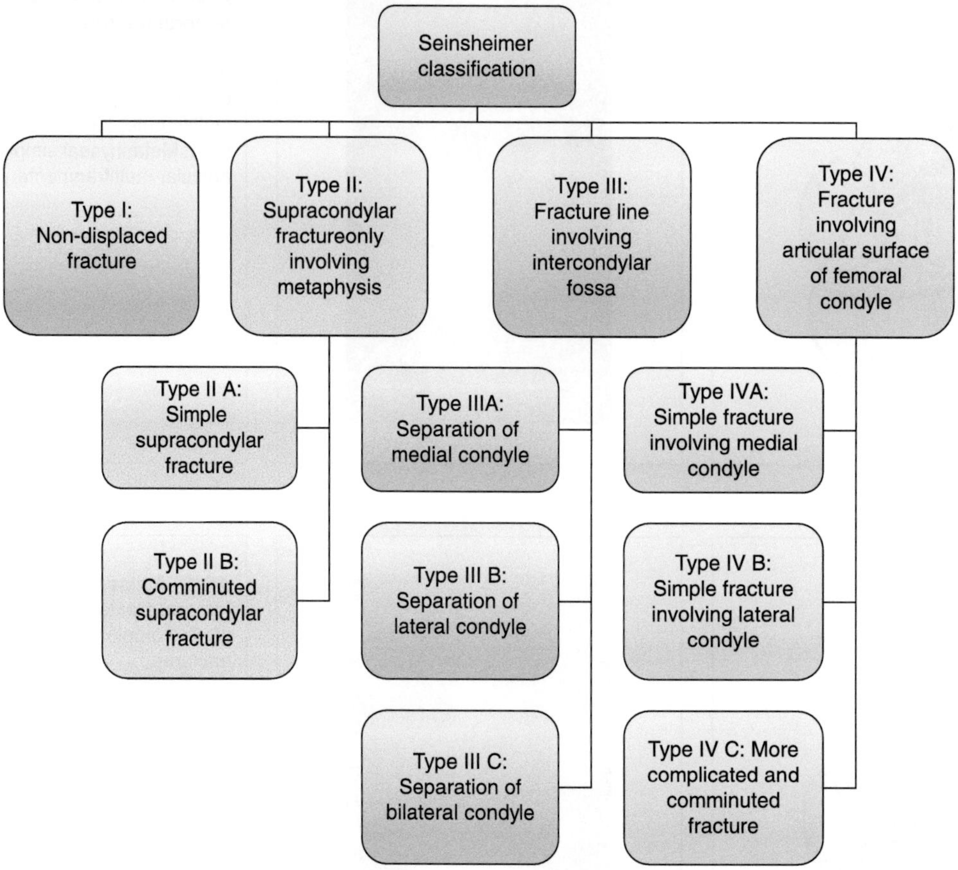

Type I: Non-displaced fractures with any fragment less than 2 mm displacement.

Type II: Simple supracondylar fracture involving metaphysis, extra-articular fracture, fracture not involving intercondyle.

Type IIA: Simple supracondylar fracture.

Type IIB: Comminuted supracondylar fracture.

Type III: Fracture involving intercondylar fossa, in which one or both condyles are separate fragments.

Type IIIA: Separation of medial condyle.

Type IIIB: Separation of lateral condyle.

Type IIIC: Separation of bilateral condyles.

Type IV: Fracture involving articular surface of femoral condyle articular surface.

Type IVA: Simple fracture involving medial condyle.

Type IVB: Simple fracture involving lateral condyle.

Type IVC: More complicated and comminuted fracture. The fracture may involve single condyle, intercondylar fossa, bilateral condyle, or three parts, which always are accompanied with metaphyseal comminution.

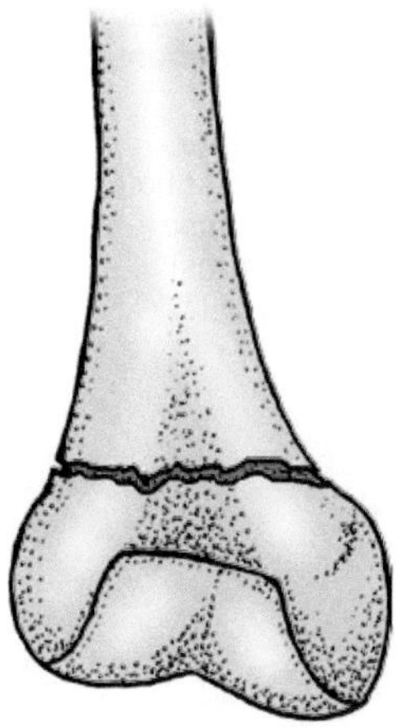

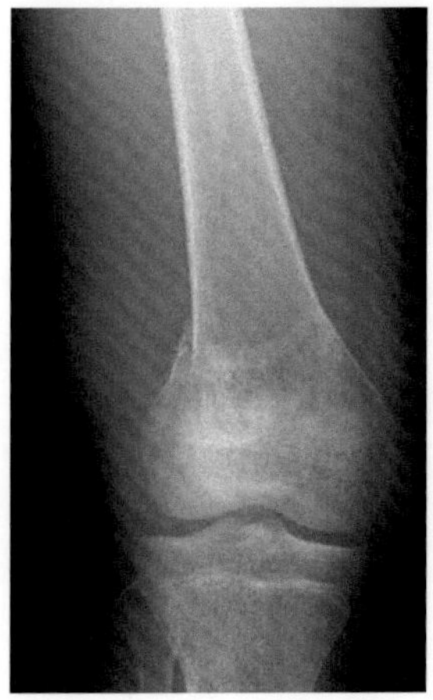

Seinsheimer classification of distal femoral fracture.
Type I : Non-displaced fractures with any fragment less than 2mm displacement.

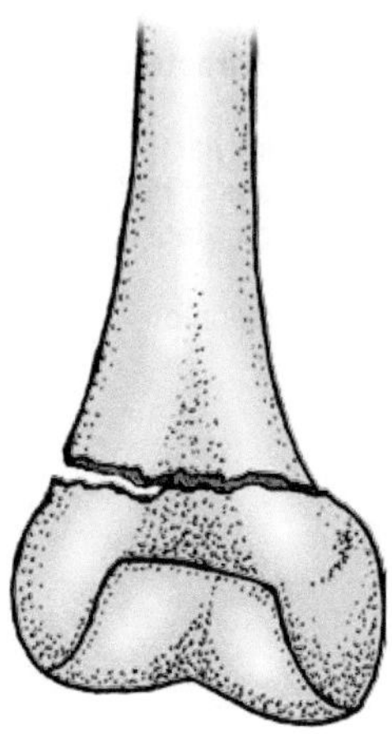

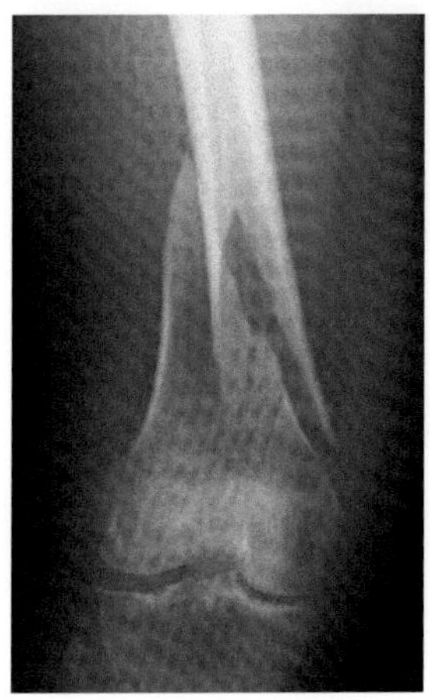

Seinsheimer classification of distal femoral fracture.
Type II: Simple supracondylar fracture involving metaphysis, extra-articular fracture, fracture not involving intercondyle.
IIA: Simple supracondylar fracture

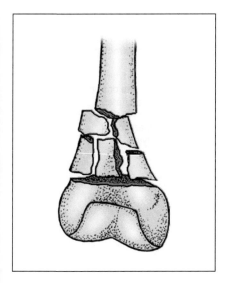

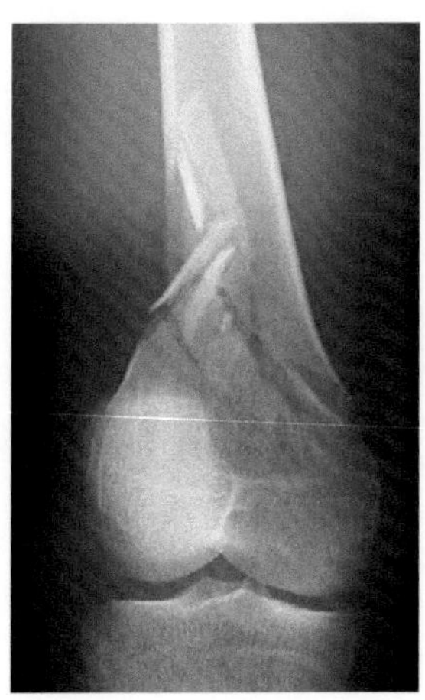

Seinsheimer classification of distal femoral fracture.
Type II: Simple supracondylar fracture involving metaphysis, extra-articular fracture, fracture not involving intercondyle.
Type IIB: Comminuted supracondylar fracture

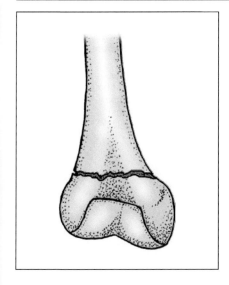

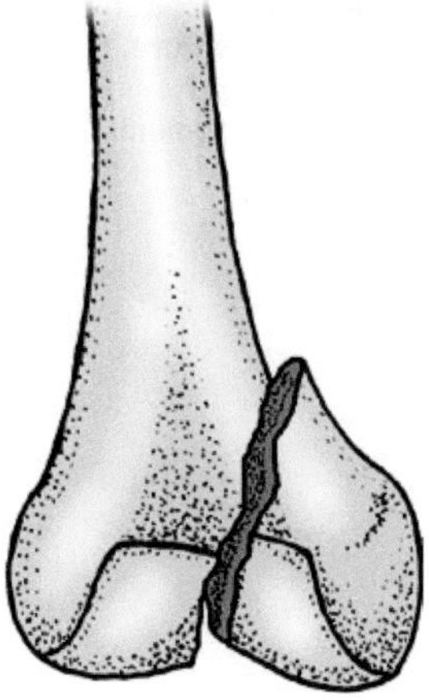

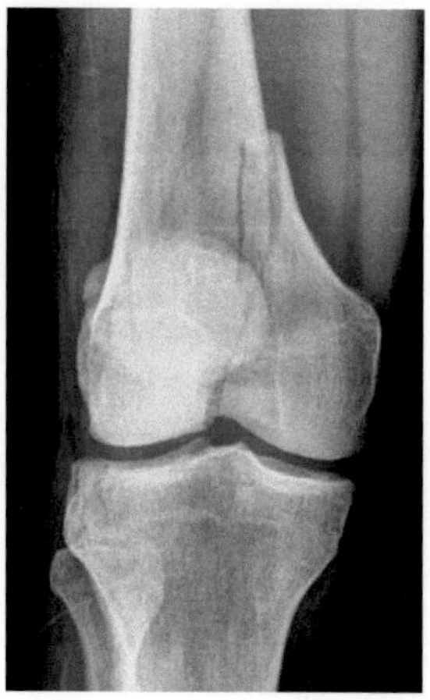

Seinsheimer classification of distal femoral fracture.
Type III Fracture involving intercondylar fossa, in which one or both condyles are separated fragments. Type IIIA: Separation of medial condyle

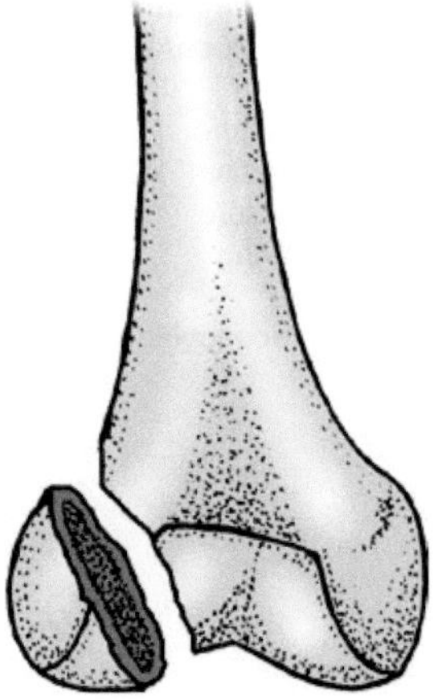

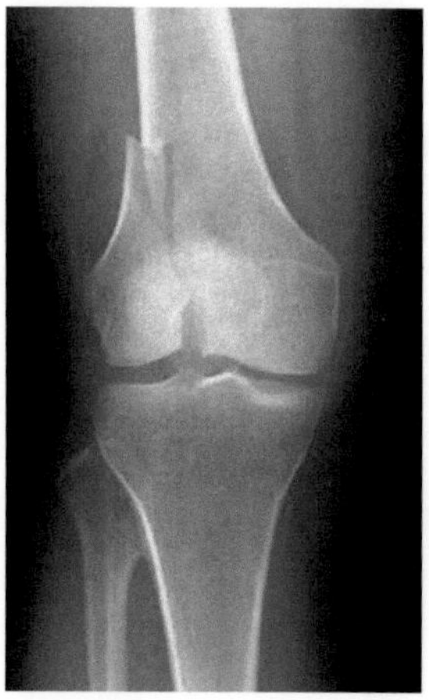

Seinsheimer classification of distal femoral fracture.
Type III Fracture involving intercondylar fossa, in which one or both condyles are separated fragments.
Type IIIB: Separation of lateral condyle

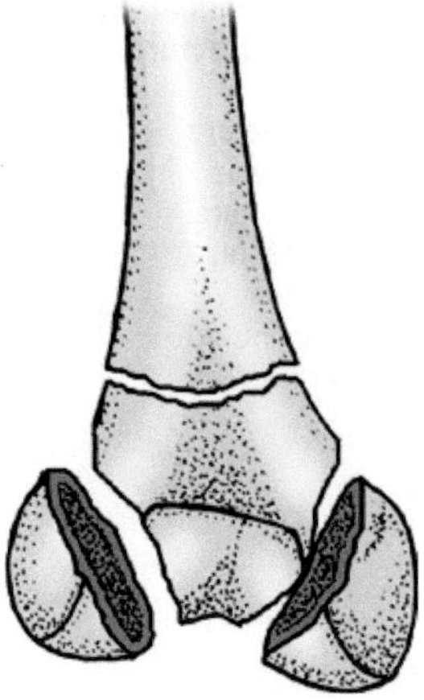

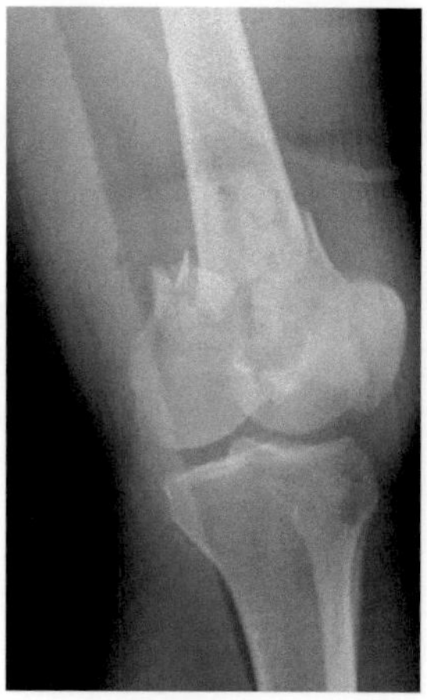

Seinsheimer classification of distal femoral fracture.
Type III Fracture involving intercondylar fossa, in which one or both condyles are separated fragments.
Type IIIC: Separation of bilateral condyles

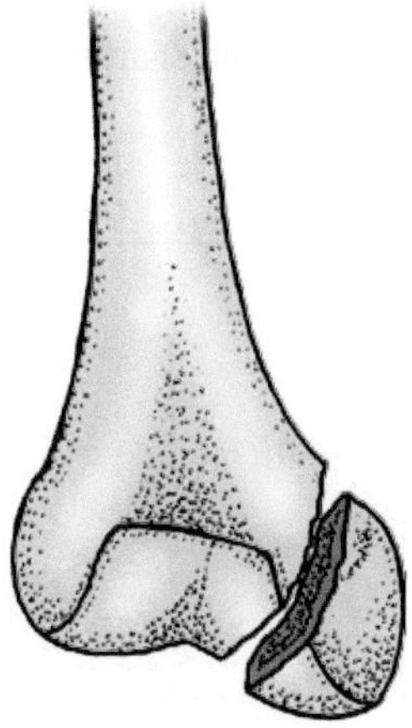

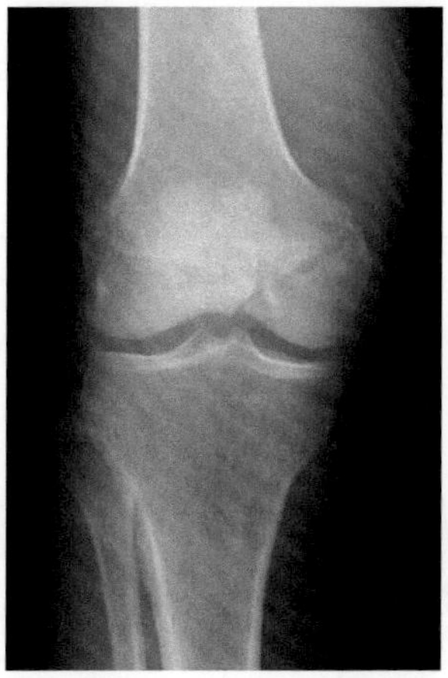

The Seinsheimer classification of distal femur fracture
Type IV: Fracture involving articular surface of femoral condyle articular surface.
Type IVA: Simple fracture involving medial condyle

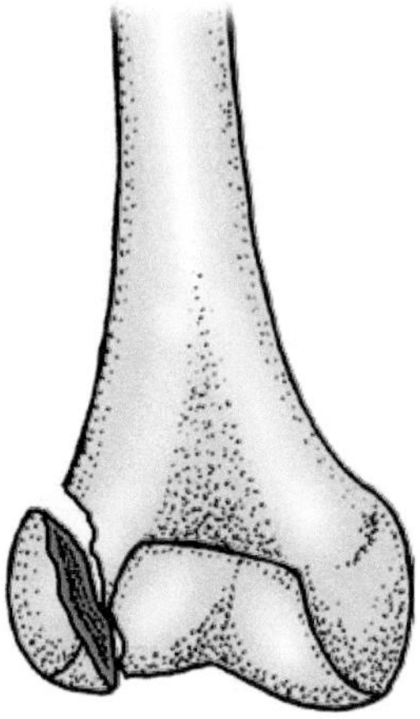

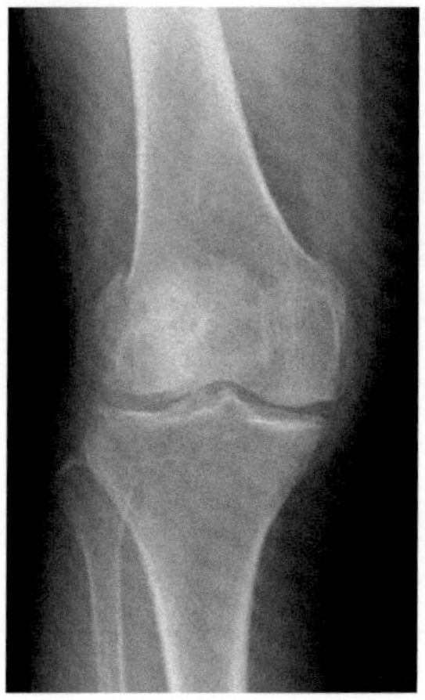

The Seinsheimer classification of distal femur fracture
Type IV: Fracture involving articular surface of femoral condyle articular surface.
Type IVB: Simple fracture involving lateral condyle

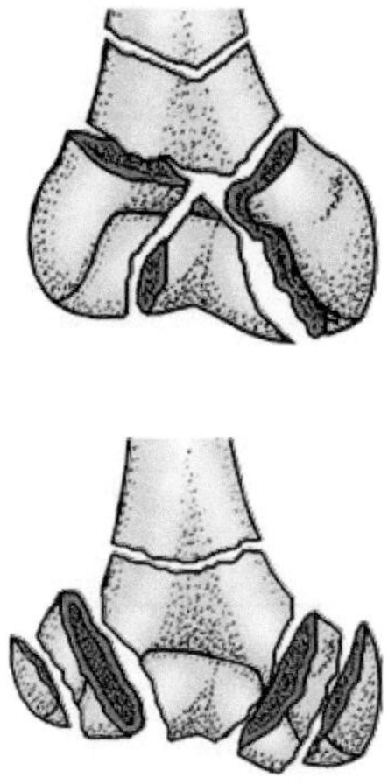

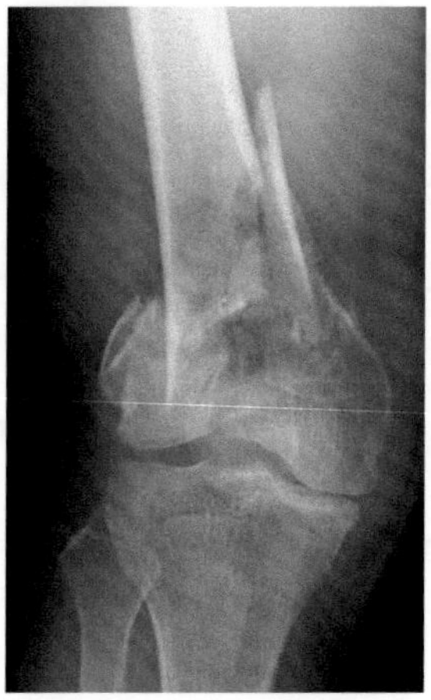

The Seinsheimer classification of distal femur fracture
Type IV: fracture involving articular surface of femoral condyle articular surface.
Type IVC More complex and comminuted fractures, including fracture involving single condyle and fossa intercondylar double condyle or both three parts are affected, often associated with metaphyseal comminution

8.1.5.3 Neer's Classification (1967, J Bone Joint Surg (Am), 49: 591–613)

Type I: Minimal displacement.
Type II: Displacement of the condyles:
  Type IIA: Medial condyle displacement.
  Type IIB: Lateral condyle displacement.
Type III: Concomitant supracondylar and shaft fractures.

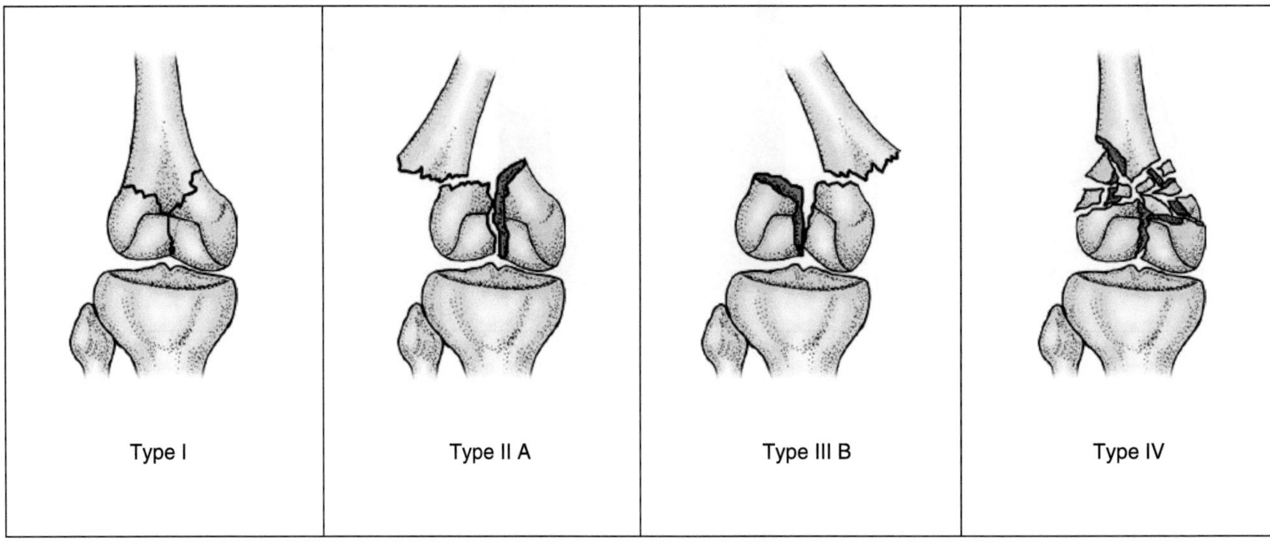

8.1.5.4 Hohl Classification (1991, Philadelphia: JB Lippincottco)

Type I: Non-displacement.
Type II: Impacted fracture.
Type III: Displacement.
Type IV: Comminuted fracture.

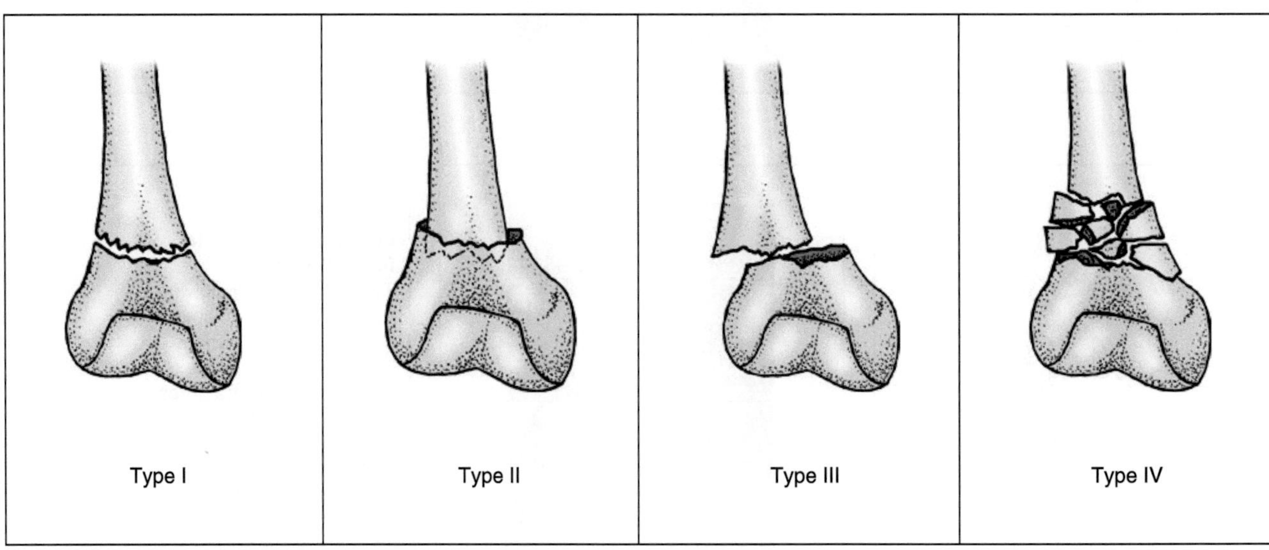

8.1.6 Section 4 Femoral Periprosthetic Fracture Classification

Khan MA and O'Driscoll M firstly proposed the classification of femoral periprosthetic fractures in 1977 (J Bone Joint Surg Br. 1977. 59 (1): 36–41). So far more than a dozen kinds of femoral periprosthetic fracture classification after hip arthroplasty can be found. Vancouver classification, AAOS classification, and Johansson classification were the most commonly used classification systems, based on the literature reports of the nearly last 5 years.

8.1.6.1 Vancouver Classification (1995, Instr Course Lect, 44: 293–304)

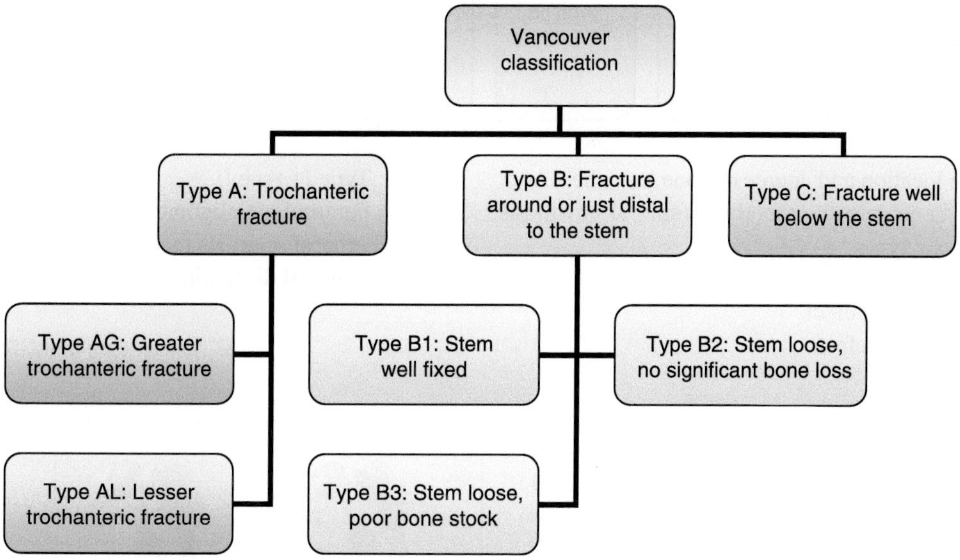

Type A: Trochanteric fracture:
  Type AG: Greater trochanteric fracture.
  Type AL: Lesser trochanteric fracture.
Type B: Fracture around or just distal to the stem:
  Type B1: Stem well fixed.
  Type B2: Stem loose, no significant bone loss.
  Type B3: Stem loose, poor bone stock.
Type C: Fracture below the stem.

Vancouver classification was made referring not only to the fracture site, but also to the stability of the original prosthesis and patients' bone quality. This classification plays an important role in comprehensively guiding intraoperative and postoperative treatment selection and formulation and is the currently most widely used method and easy to accept.

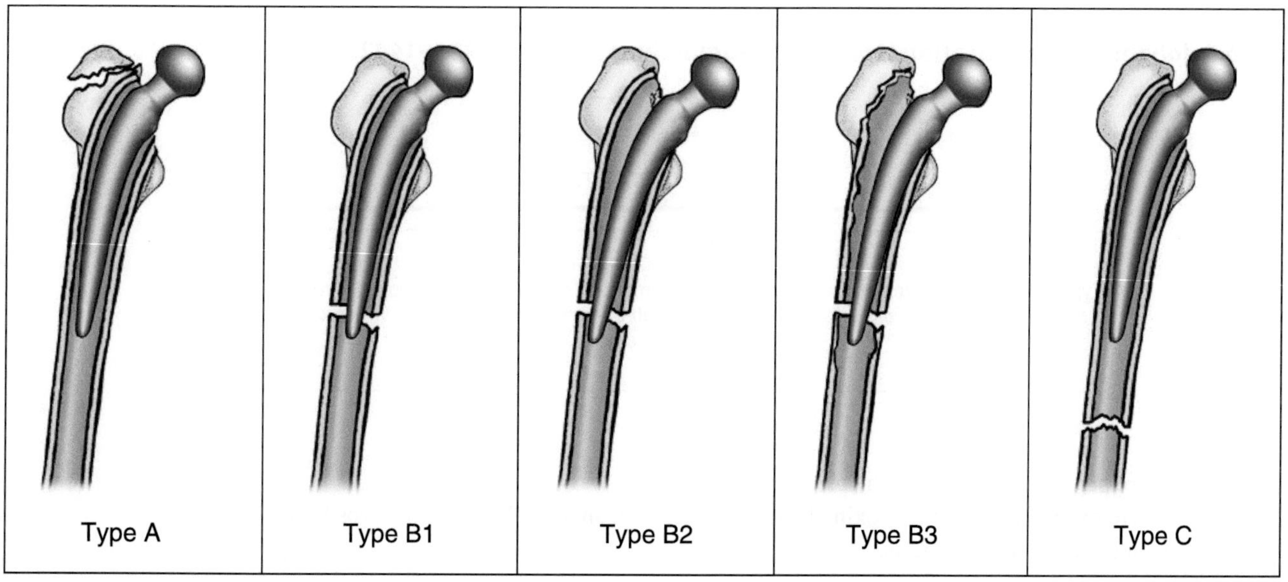

8.1.6.2 AAOS Classification (1993, Clin Orthop, 296: 133–139)

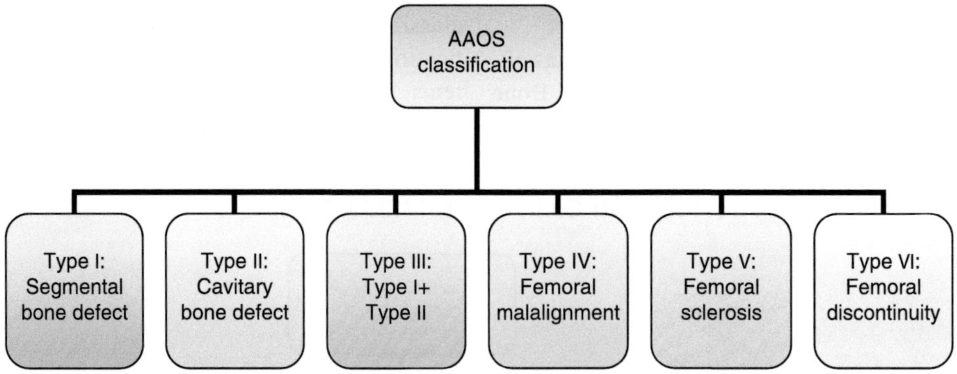

According to the location and degree of bone loss, the AAOS classification of bone defects around the femoral prosthesis was divided into six types.

Type I: Segmental bone defect.
Type II: Cavitary bone defect.
Type III: Type I+ type II.
Type IV: Femoral malalignment (angle or rotation).
Type V: Femoral sclerosis (acute stenosis or occlusion).
Type VI: Femoral discontinuity.

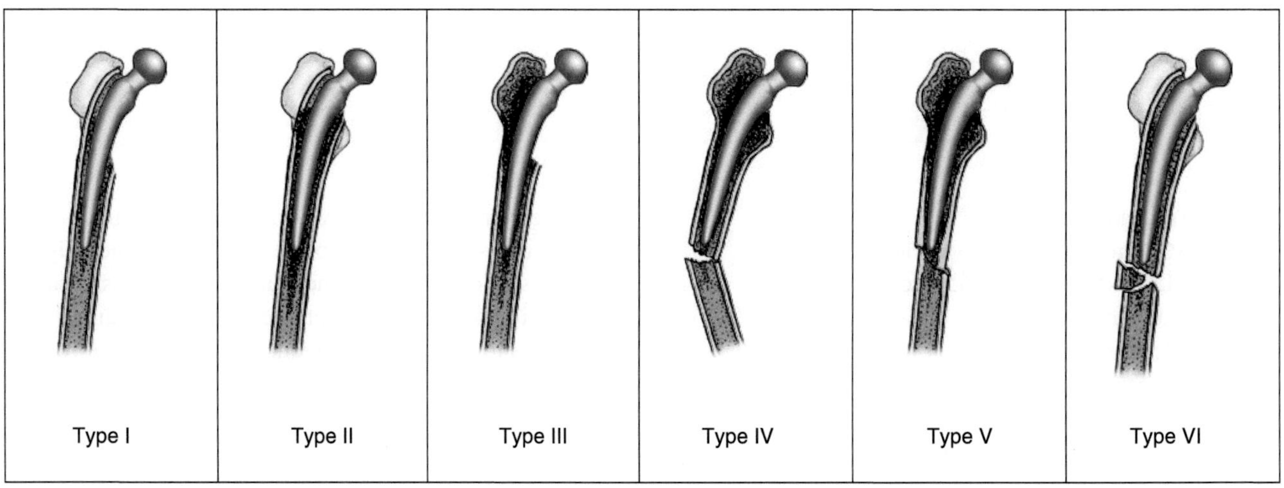

8.1.6.3 Johansson Classification (1981, J Bone Joint Surg (Am), 63: 1435–1442)

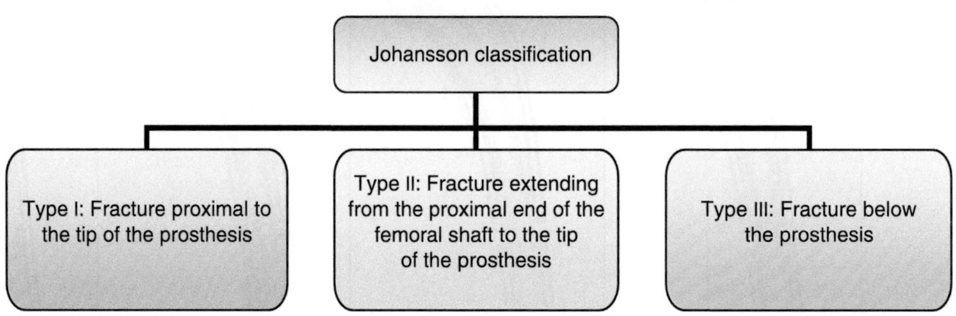

Type I: Fracture proximal to the tip of the prosthesis.
Type II: Fracture extending from the proximal end of the femoral shaft to the tip of the prosthesis.
Type III: Fracture below the prosthesis.

The Johansson classification is concise, detailing the relationship between location of the prosthesis and the fracture. This classification is one of the commonly used classification systems, to a certain extent identifying the guidance of prosthetic stability on clinical treatment selection, but not taking some factors such as bone quality of the femoral shaft into account.

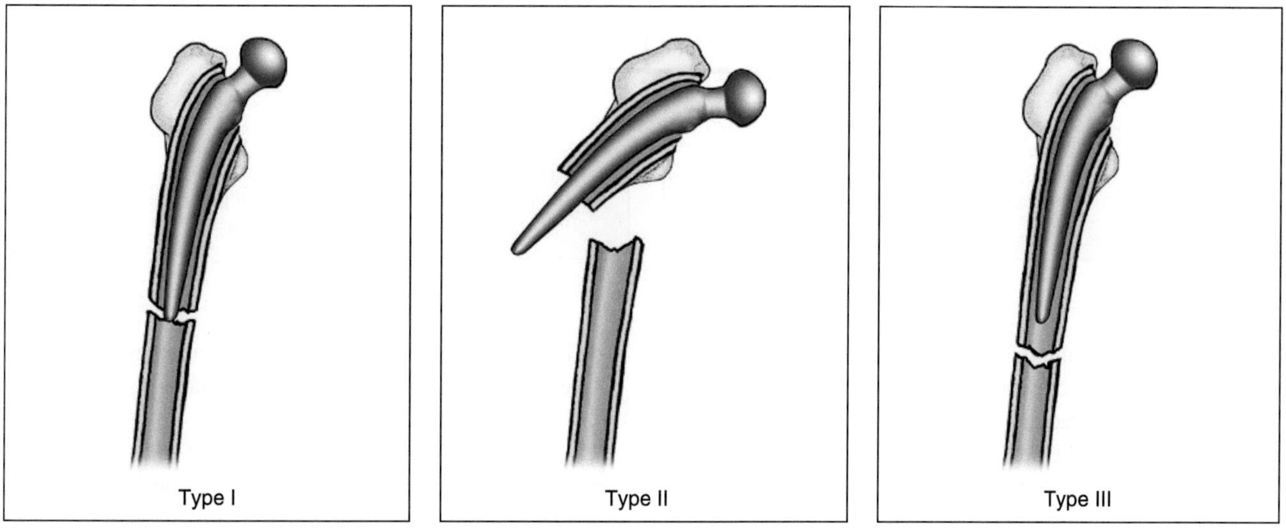

8.1.6.4 Bethea Classification (1982, Clin Orthop, 170: 95–106)

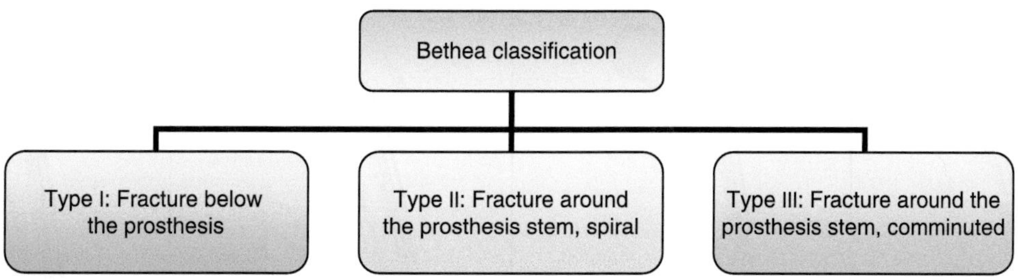

Type I: Fracture below the prosthesis.
Type II: Fracture around the prosthesis stem, spiral.
Type III: Fracture around the prosthesis stem, comminuted.

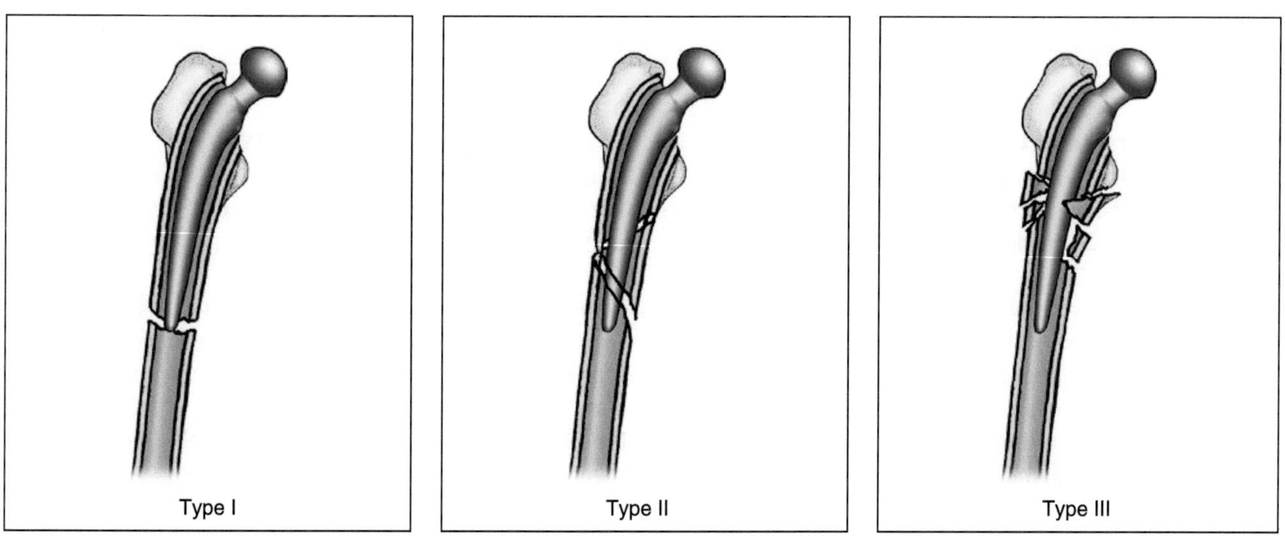

8.1.6.5 Cooke-Newman Classification (Bethea modified classification, 1988, J Bone Joint Surg (Br), 70: 386–389)

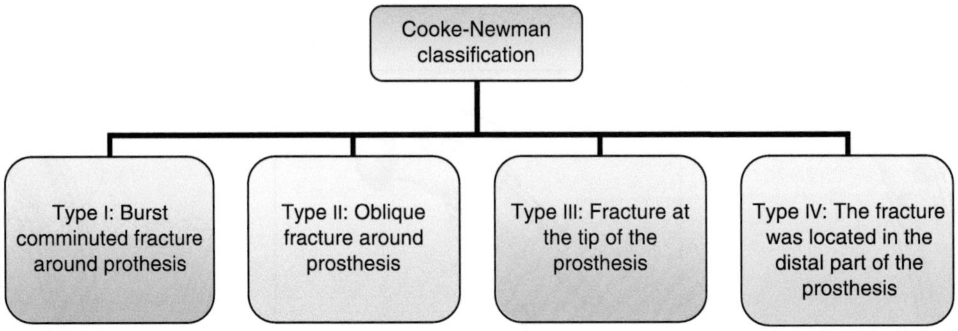

Type I: Burst comminuted fracture around prosthesis, both prosthesis and fracture are unstable.

Type II: Oblique fracture around prosthesis, the fractures were stable, but the prosthesis was unstable.

Type III: Fracture at the tip of the prosthesis, the fracture is unstable, but the prosthesis is stable.

Type IV: Fractures entirely distal to the prosthesis, the fracture is unstable, but the prosthesis is stable.

Cooke-Newman classification refers to the most important factor affecting the stability of the femoral prosthesis, which better guides the selection of treatment options.

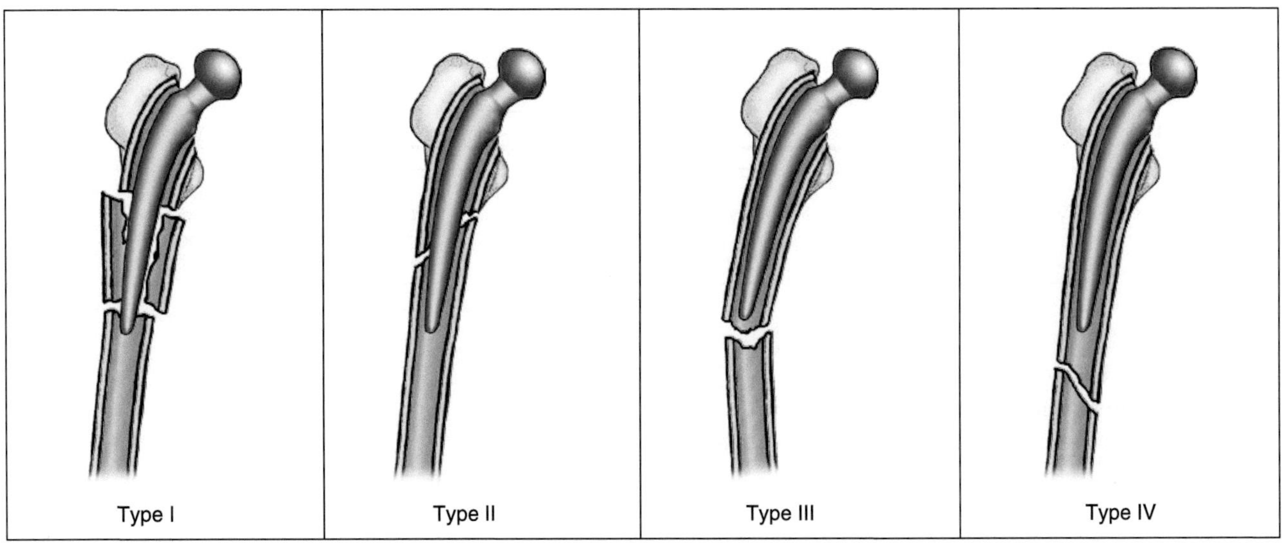

8.1.6.6 Towers-Beals Classification (1999, Orthop Clin North Am, 30: 235–247)

According to fracture location, fracture, and prosthesis stability, the fracture is divided into four types.

Type I: Fractures involving the proximal femur, often accompanied by avulsion fracture of greater or lesser trochanter.

Type II: Fractures involving the femoral shaft but not extending to the prosthetic tip, stable.

Type III: Fractures extending to the prosthetic tip.

Type IV: Distal femoral fractures, not involving the prosthesis.

8.1.6.7 Mark Classification (in 1999)

Mark et al. proposed a classification for femoral periprosthetic fractures based on the choice of treatment options in 1999.

Type I: Stable fractures and reliable prosthesis fixation.

Type II: Unstable fractures and reliable prosthesis fixation.

Type III: Fracture and prosthesis are unstable, but the femoral bone mass was normal.

Type IV: Fracture and prosthesis are unstable, accompanied by femoral bone defect and bone loss.

Mark classification refers to the stability of the prosthesis and fracture and the quality of the femoral shaft, with good guidance for the choice of treatment options, and helps to predict postoperative outcomes.

8.1.6.8 Whittaker Classification (in 1974)

Whittaker et al. divided femoral periprosthetic fractures into three types in 1974.

Type I: Intertrochanteric fracture.
Type II: Oblique or spiral fracture around the prosthesis stem.
Type III: Complex and severe fractures, with separation of distal fracture fragments.

Whittaker classification is the earliest classification for femoral periprosthetic fractures in literature, which is simply based on the fracture site, briefly and clearly.

8.1.6.9 Other Classifications

These include Schwartz classification, Jensen classification, Kavanag classification, Mont-Maar classification, Xiangjin Lin classification, and Yujie Liu classification.

Classifications of Patellar Fracture

9

Yingze Zhang and Yanbin Zhu

9.1 AO/OTA Classification (2007, Journal of Orthopaedic Trauma)

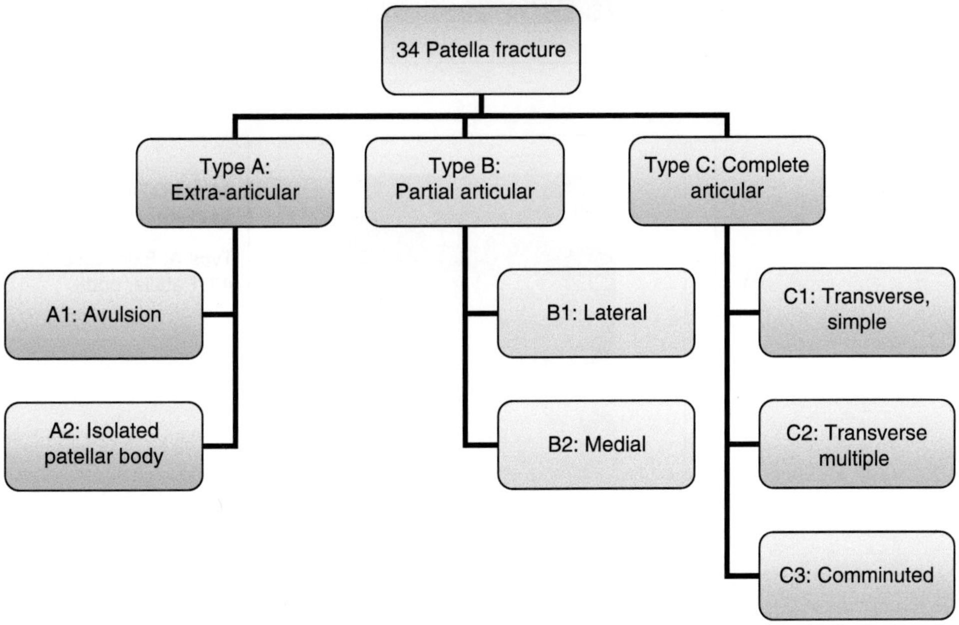

Type A: Extra-articular fracture
- A1: Avulsion
- A2: Patella body

Type B: Partial-articular vertical fracture
- B1: Lateral fracture
  - B1.1: Lateral simple fracture
  - B1.2: Lateral comminuted fracture
- B2: Medial fracture
  - B2.1: Medial simple fracture
  - B2.2: Medial comminuted fracture

Type C: Complete articular, transverse fracture
- C1: Transverse, simple fracture
  - C1.1: Transverse, middle
  - C1.2: Transverse, proximal
  - C1.3: Transverse, distal
- C2: Comminuted (with three fragments)
  - C2.1: Transverse, middle
  - C2.2: Transverse, proximal
  - C2.3: Transverse, distal
- C3: Complex comminuted (with >3 fragments)
  - C3.1: with 4 fragments
  - C3.2: with >4 fragments

Y. Zhang (✉) • Y. Zhu
Department of Orthopedics,
The Third Hospital of Hebei Medical University,
Shijiazhuang, China
e-mail: yzzhangdr@126.com, yzling_liu@163.com

Y. Zhang (ed.), *Clinical Classification in Orthopaedics Trauma*, https://doi.org/10.1007/978-981-10-6044-1_9

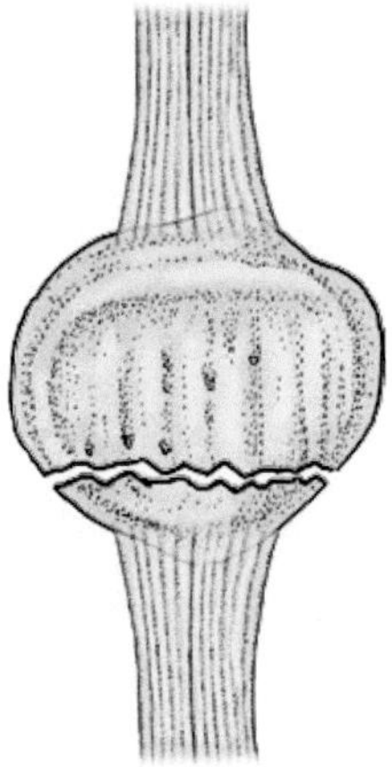

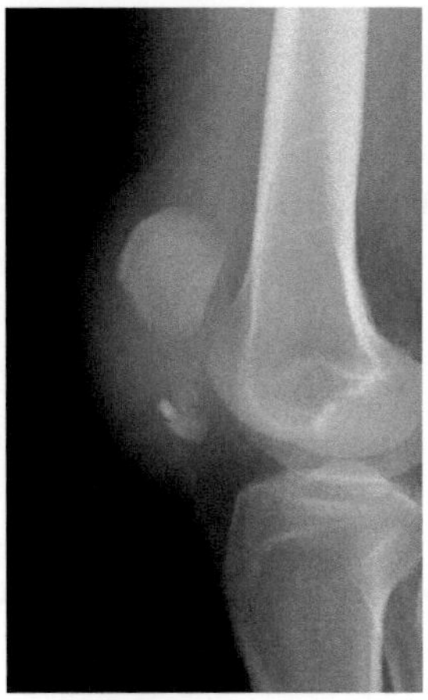

34 AO/OTA classification of patellar fracture

Type A: Extra-articular.
A1: Avulsion

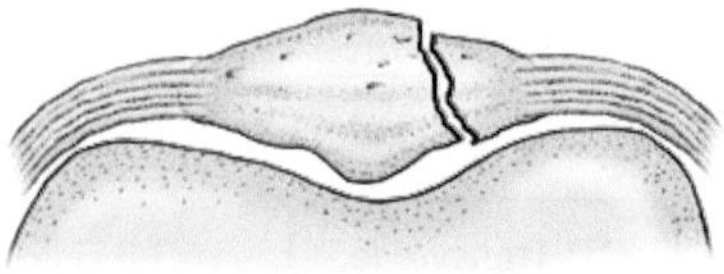

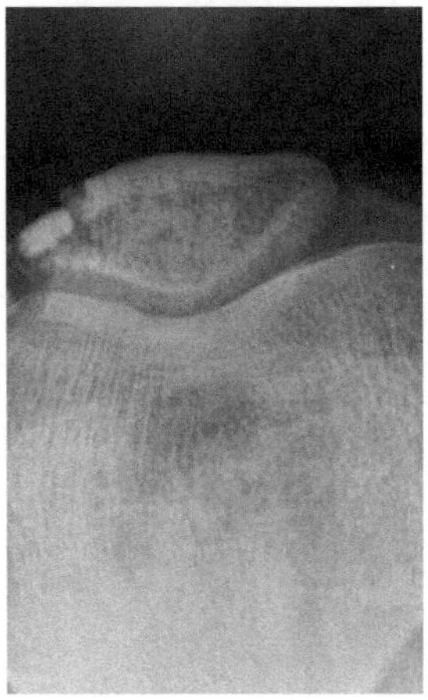

34 AO/OTA classification of patellar fracture

Type A: Extra-articular.
A2: Patellar body

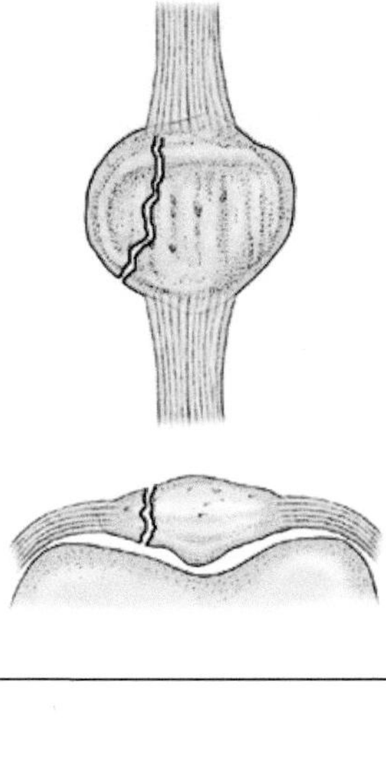

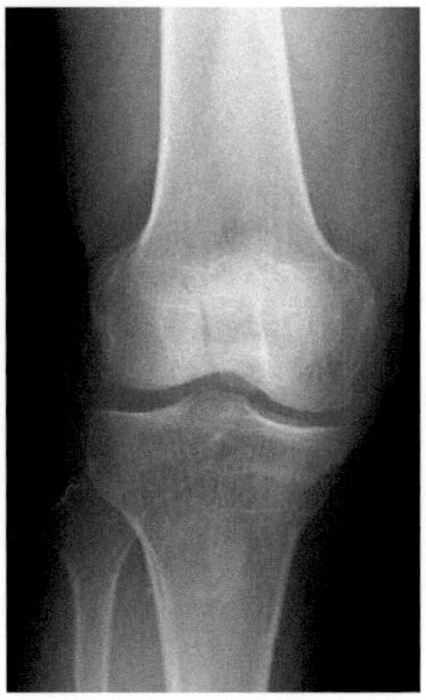

34 AO/OTA classification of patellar fracture

Type B: Partial articular vertical fracture.
B1: Lateral
B1.1: Lateral, simple

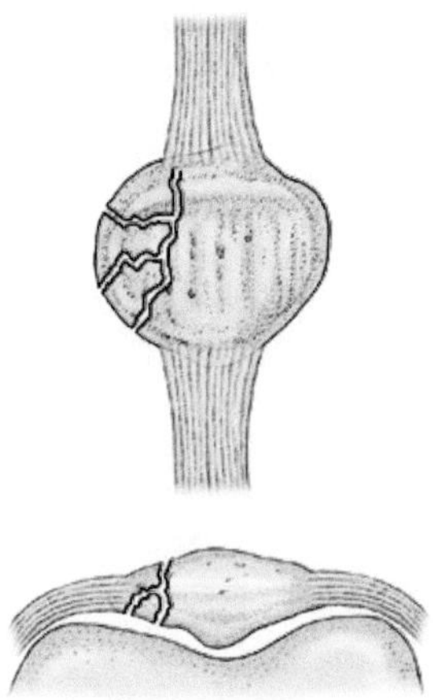

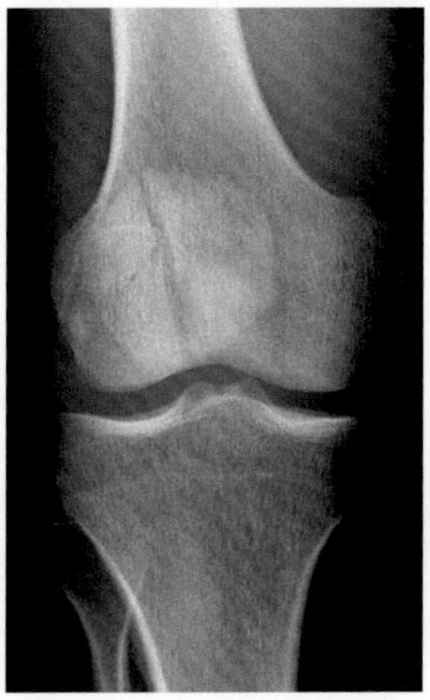

34 AO/OTA classification of patellar fracture

Type B: Partial articular vertical fracture.
B1: Lateral
B1.2: Lateral, comminuted

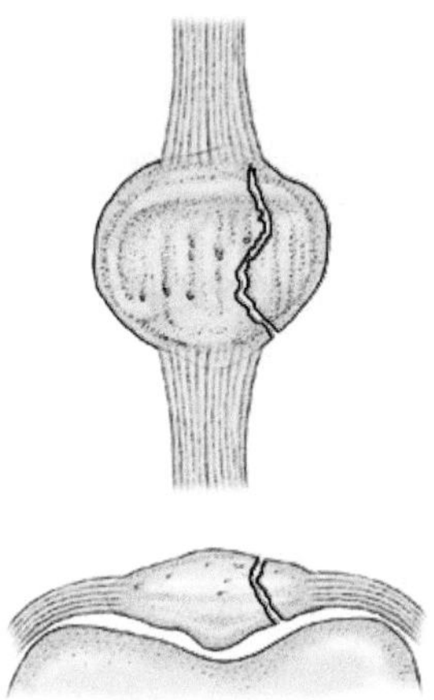

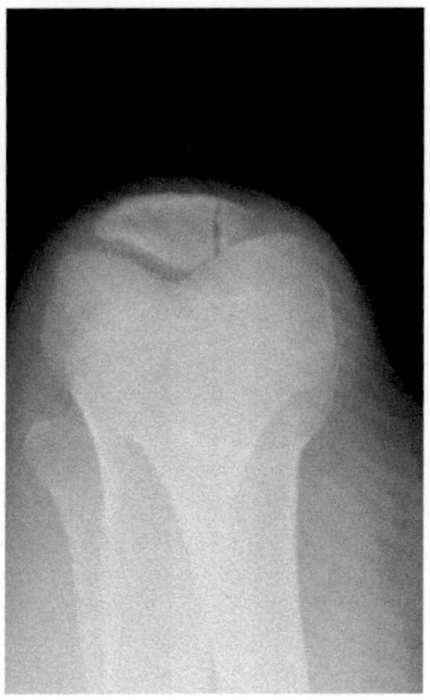

34 AO/OTA classification of patellar fracture

Type B: Partial articular. vertical fracture.
B2: Medial
B2.1: Medial, simple

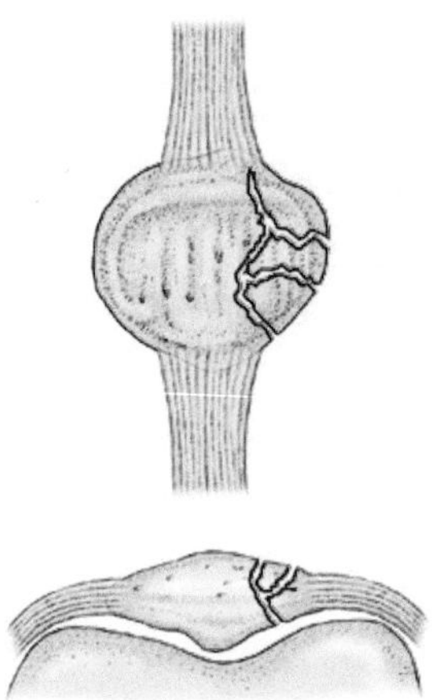

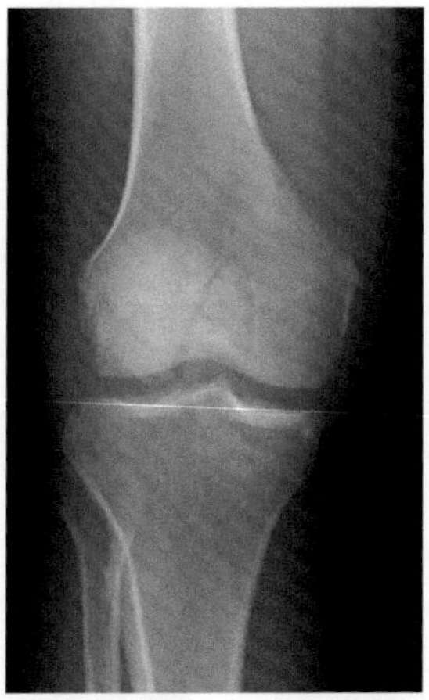

34 AO/OTA classification of patellar fracture

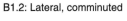

Type B: Partial articular. vertical fracture.
B2: Medial
B2.2: Medial, comminuted

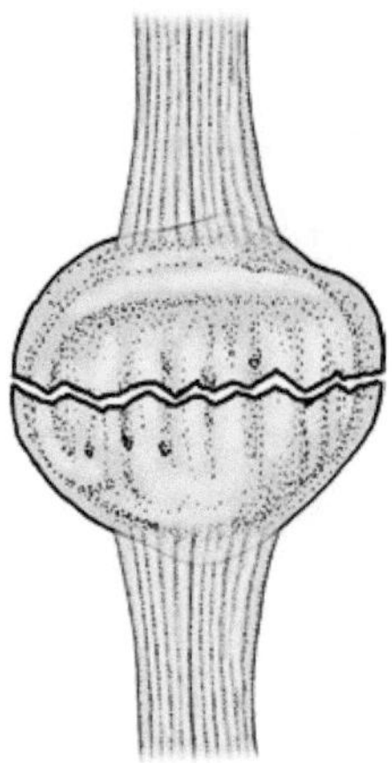

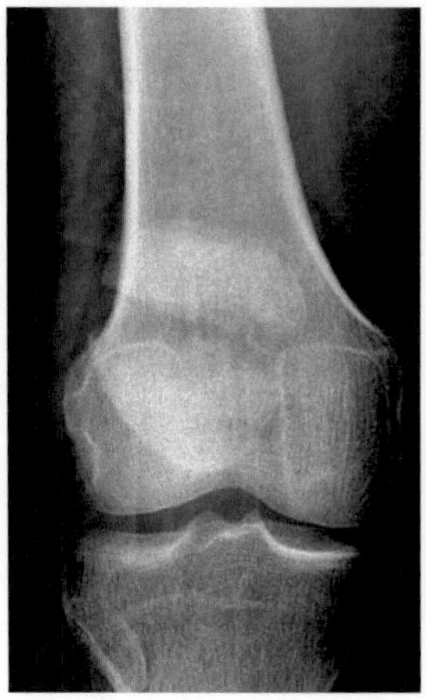

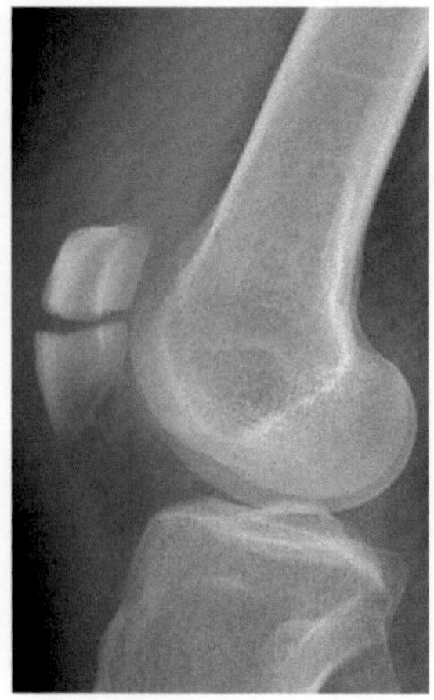

34 AO/OTA classification of patellar fracture

Type C: Complete articular, transverse.
C1: Simple
C1.1: Middle

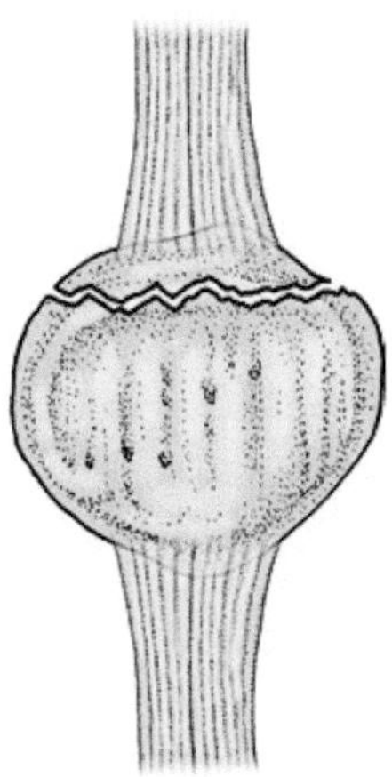

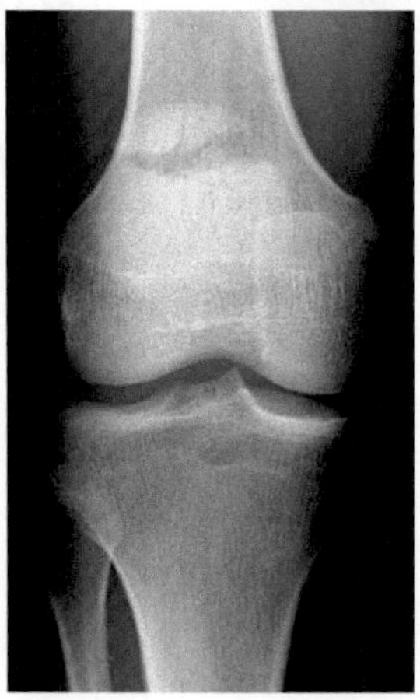

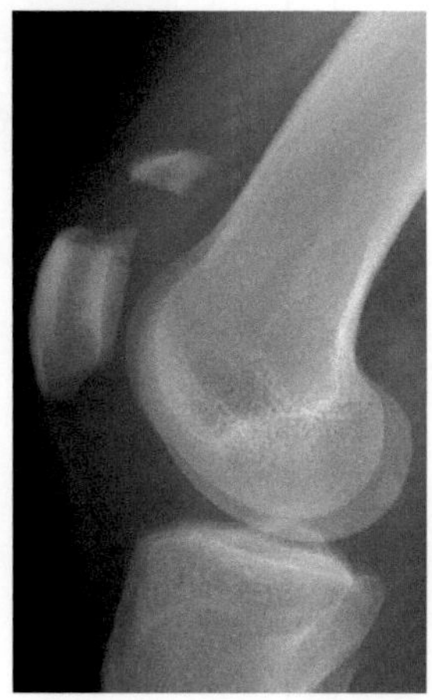

34 AO/OTA classification of patellar fracture

Type C: Complete articular, transverse.
C1: Simple
C1.2: Proximal

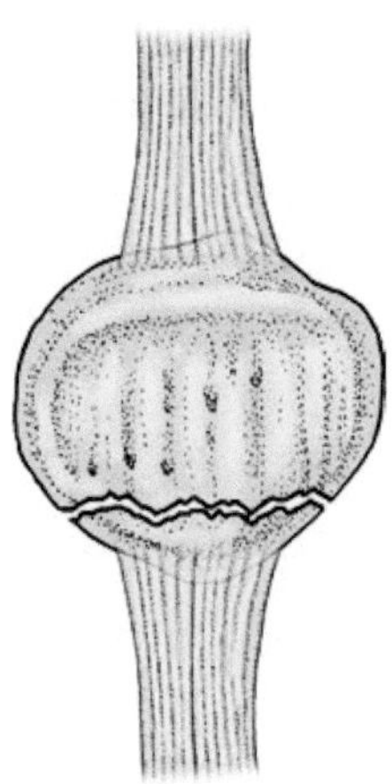

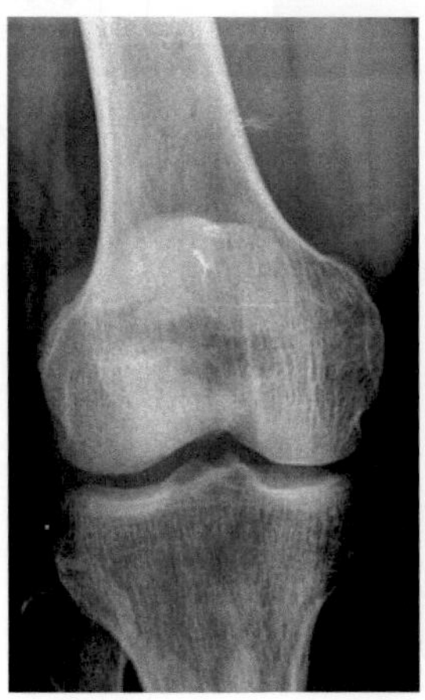

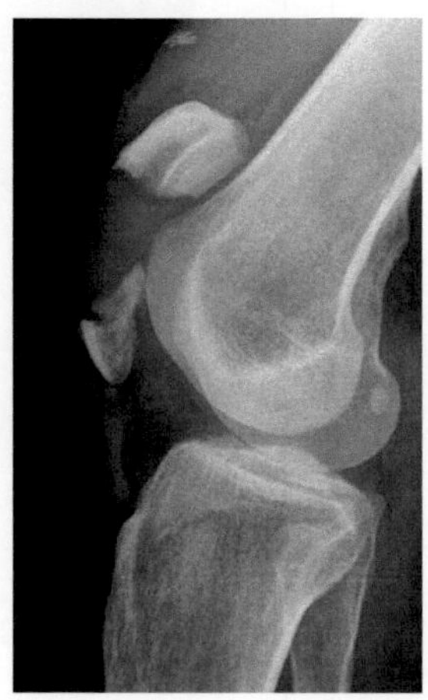

34 AO/OTA classification of patellar fracture

Type C: Complete articular, transverse.
C1: Simple
C1.3: Distal

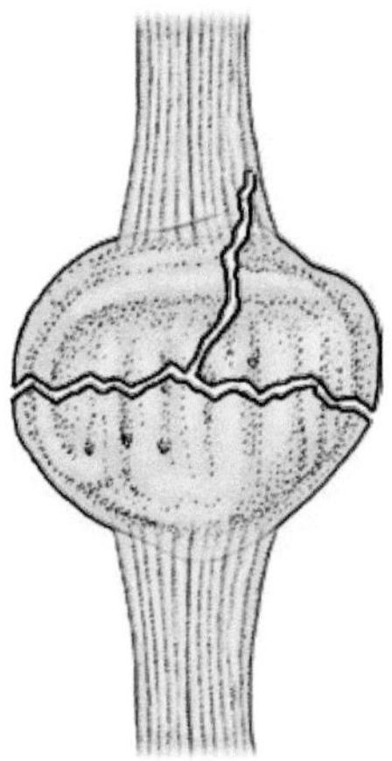

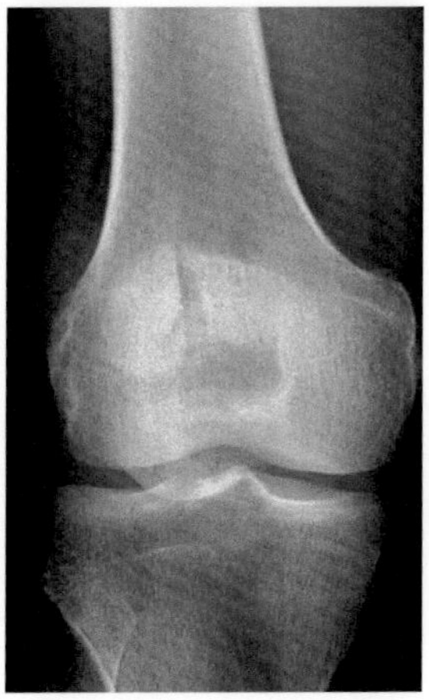

34 AO/OTA classification of patellar fracture

Type C: Complete articular, transverse.
C2: Comminuted (with 3 fragments)
C2.1: Middle

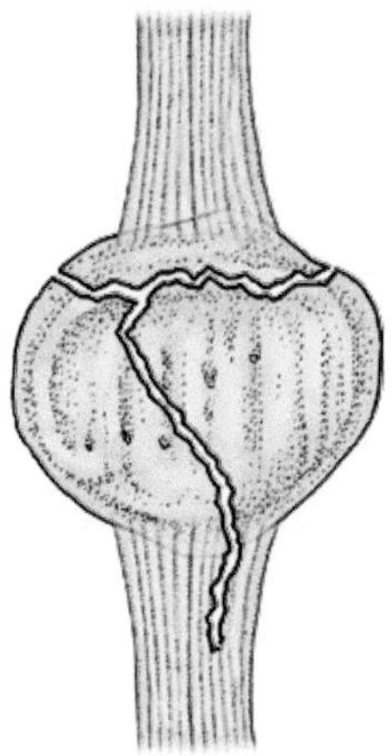

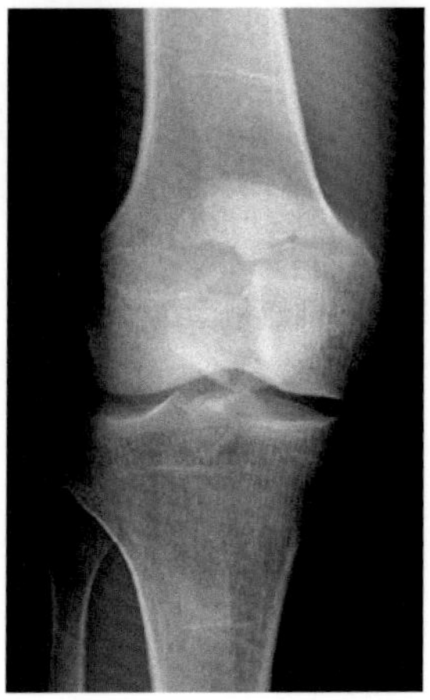

34 AO/OTA classification of patellar fracture

Type C: Complete articular, transverse.
C2: Comminuted (with 3 fragments)
C2.2: Proximal

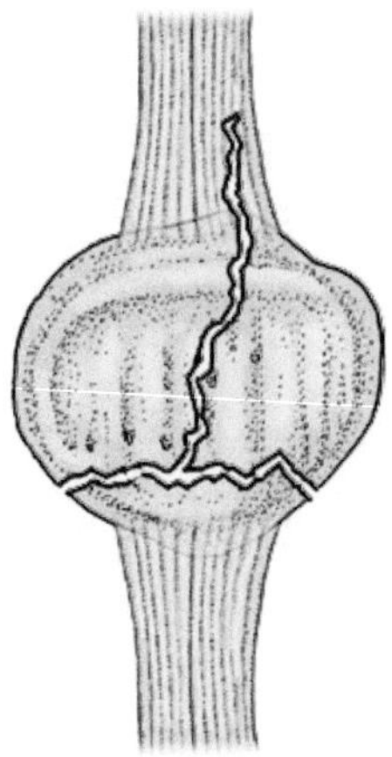

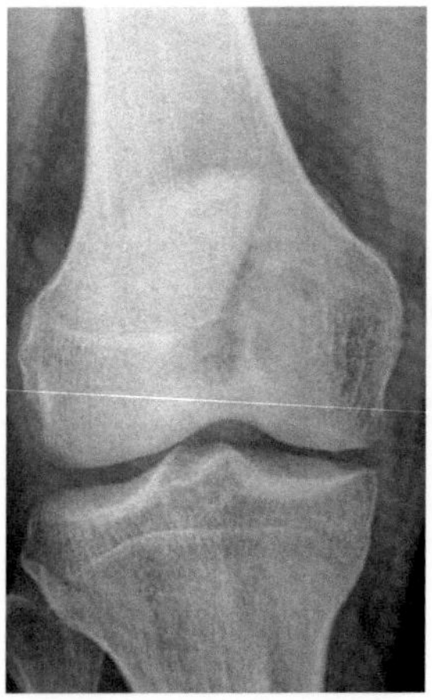

34 AO/OTA classification of patellar fracture

Type C: Complete articular, transverse.
C2: Comminuted (with 3 fragments)
C2.3: Distal

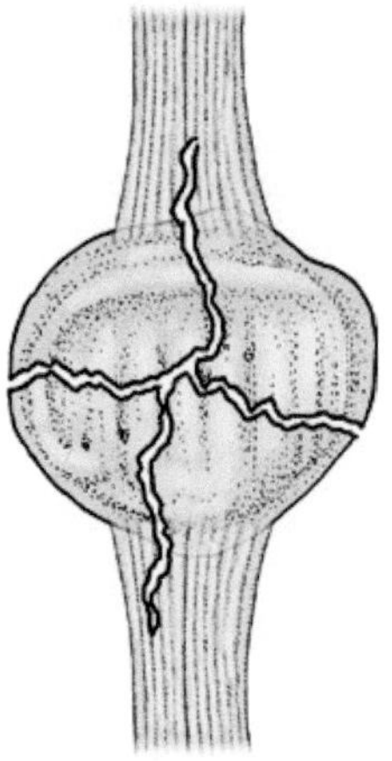

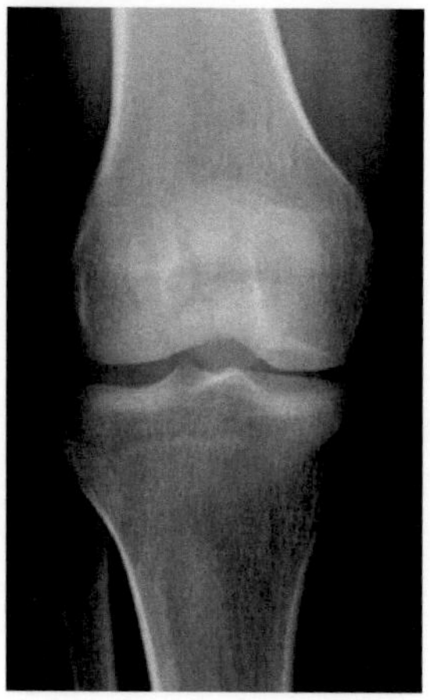

34 AO/OTA classification of patellar fracture

Type C: Complete articular, transverse.
C3: Transverse, comminuted (with > 3 fragments)
C3.1: with 4 fragments

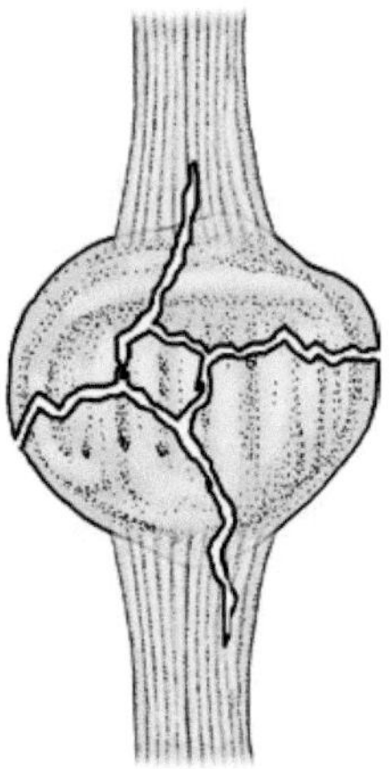

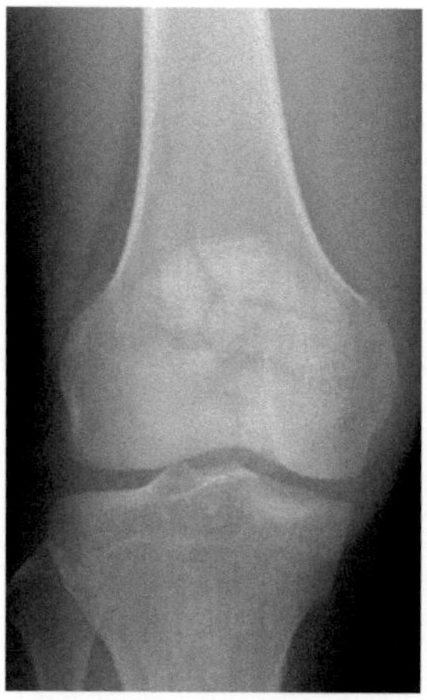

34 AO/OTA classification of patellar fracture

Type C: Complete articular, transverse.
C3: Transverse, comminuted (with > 3 fragments)
C3.2: With > 4 fragments

9.2 Regazzoni Classification

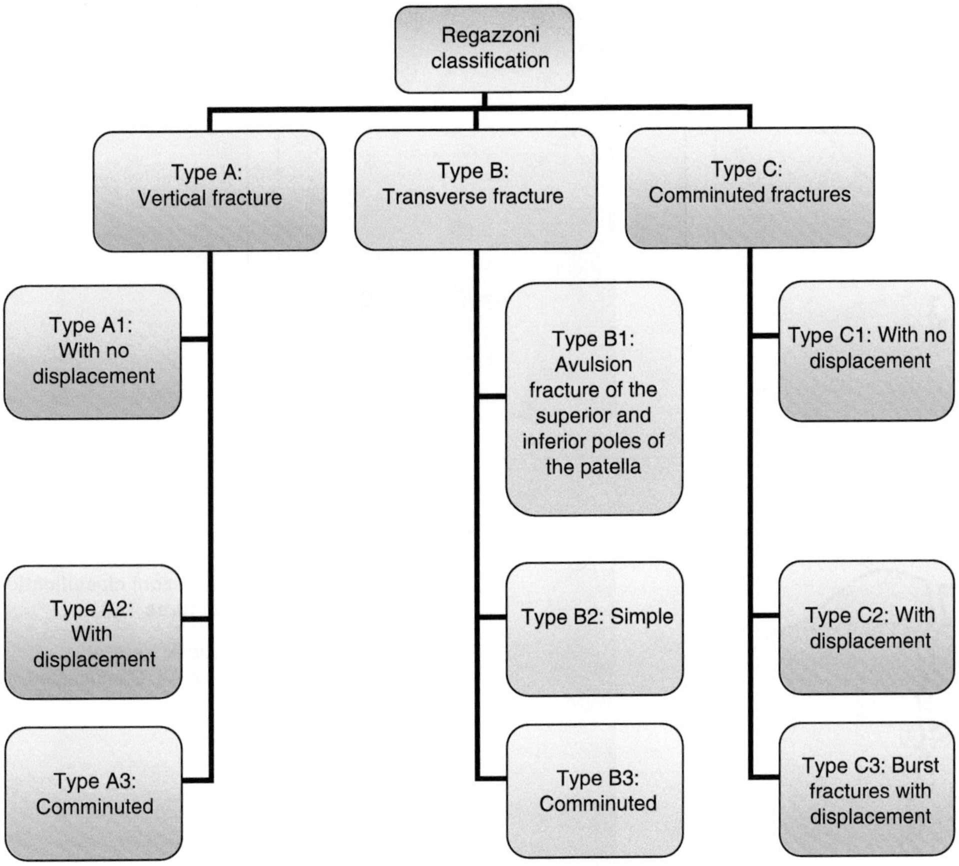

Type A: vertical fracture
- Type A1: with no displacement
- Type A2: with displacement
- Type A3: comminuted

Type B: transverse fracture
- Type B1: avulsion fracture of the superior and inferior poles of the patella (<5 mm in diameter of the superior pole, <15 mm in diameter of the inferior pole)
- Type B2: simple and B3 comminuted

Type C: comminuted fractures
- Type C1: with no displacement
- Type C2: with displacement of less than 2 mm
- Type C3: burst fractures with displacement of more than 2 mm

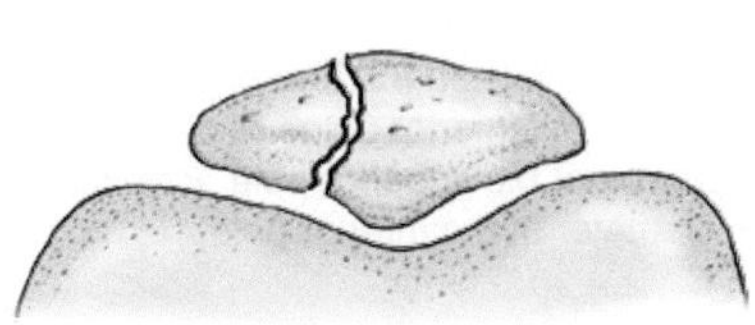

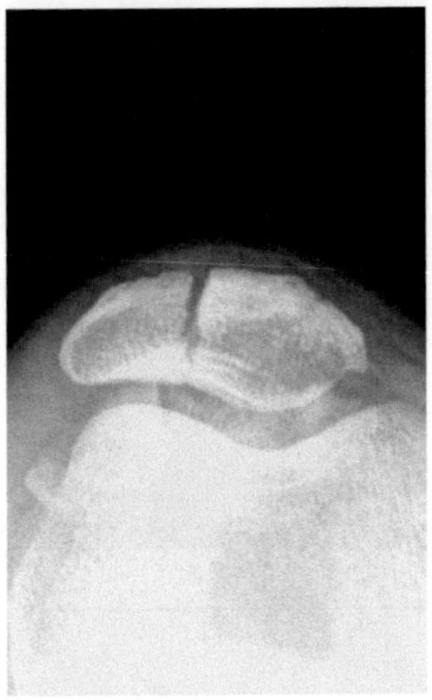

Regazzoni classification of patellar fractures

Type A: Vertical.
Type A1: with displacement

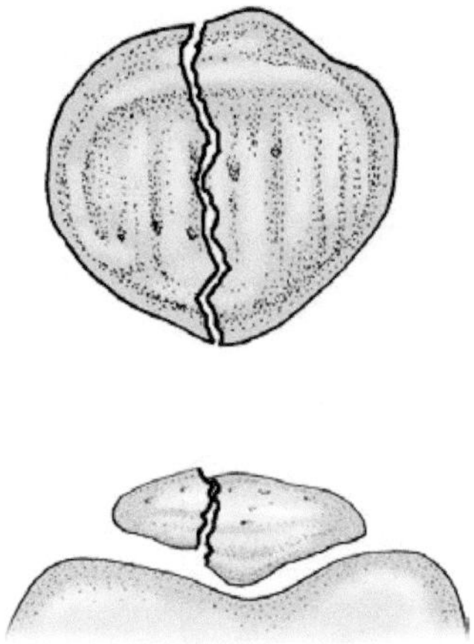

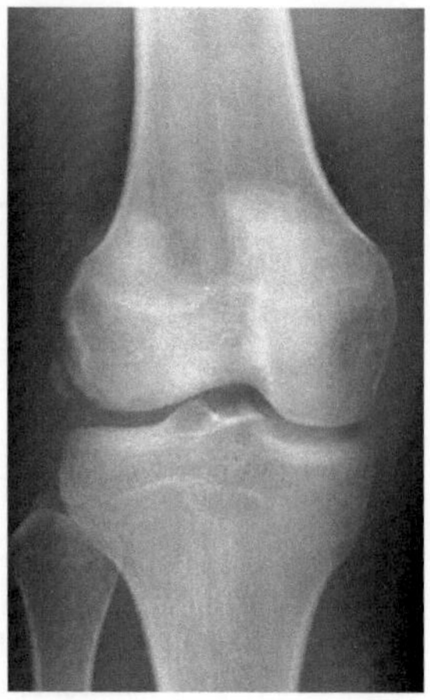

Regazzoni classification of patellar fractures

Type A: Vertical.
Type A2: with displacement

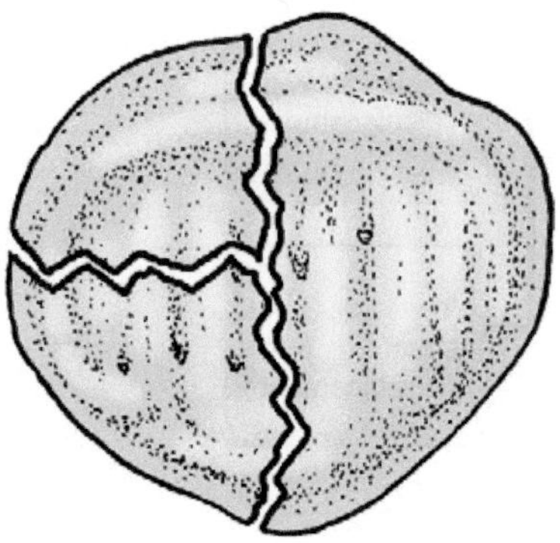

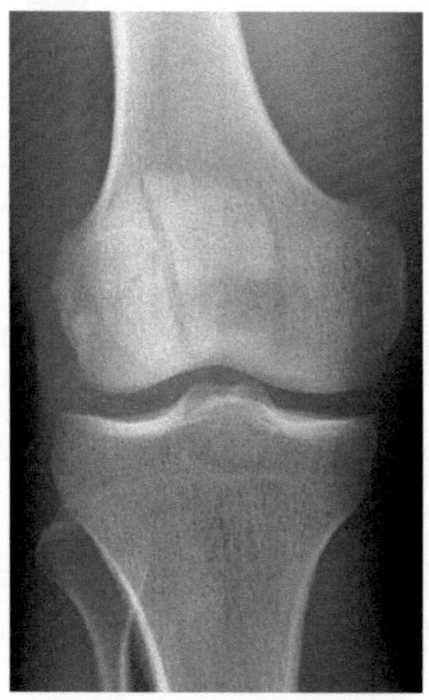

Regazzoni classification of patellar fractures

Type A: Vertical.
Type A3: Comminuted

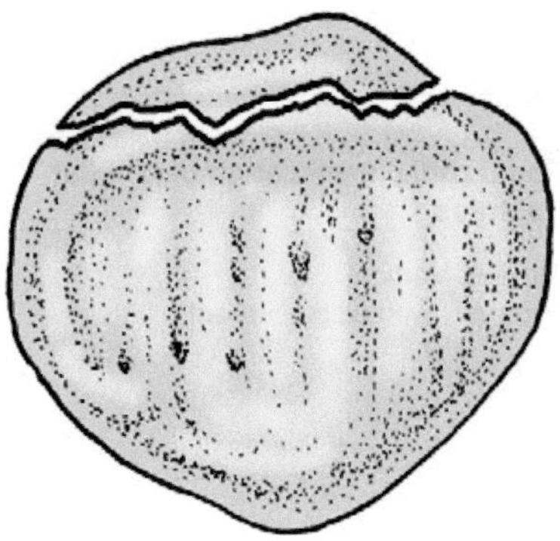

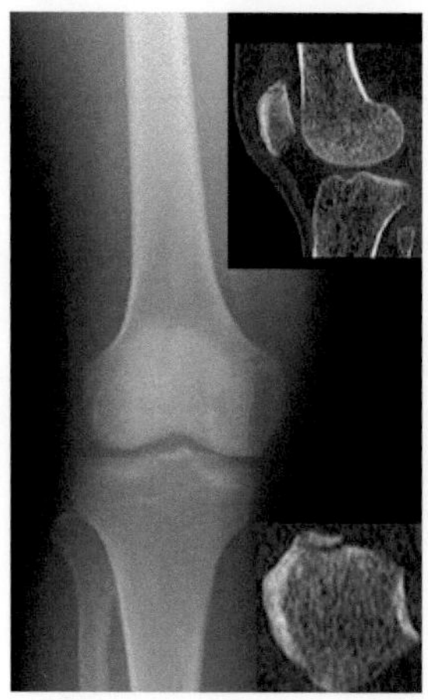

Regazzoni classification of patellar fractures

Type B: Transverse.
Type B1: Avulsion fracture of the superior and inferior poles (< 5 mm in diameter of the superior pole. < 15 mm in diameter of the inferior pole)

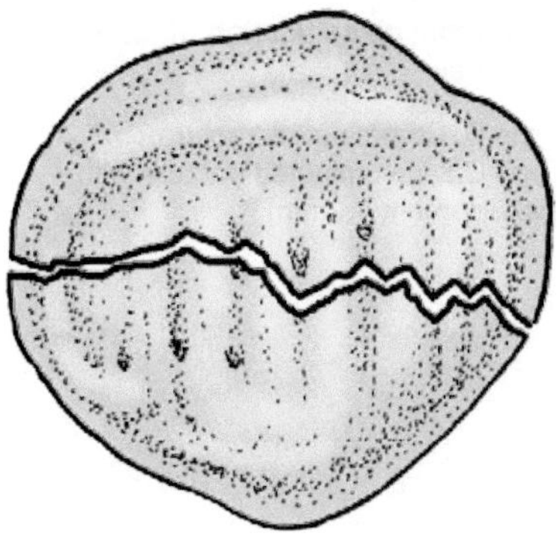

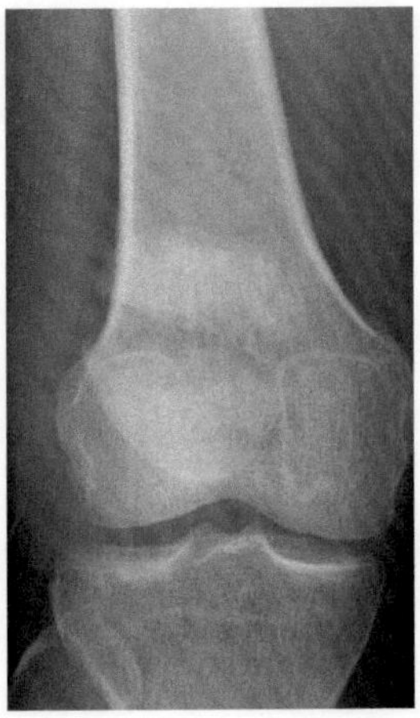

Regazzoni classification of patellar fractures

Type B: Transverse fracture.
Type B2: Simple transverse fracture

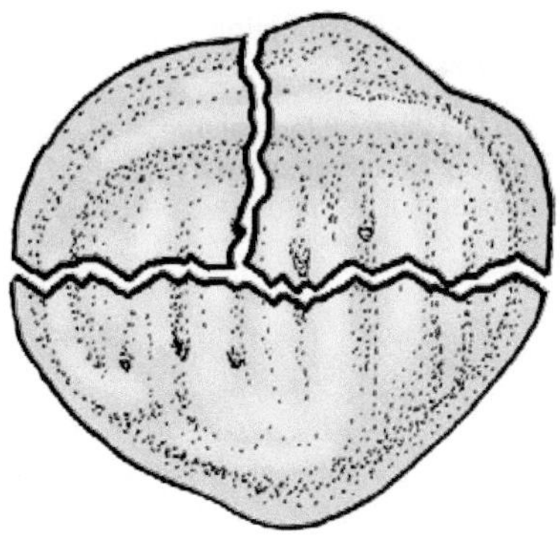

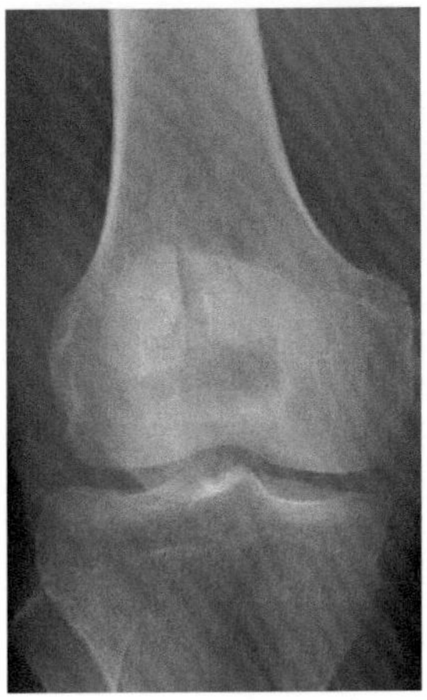

Regazzoni classification of patellar fractures

Type B: Transverse fracture.
Type B3: Comminuted transverse fracture

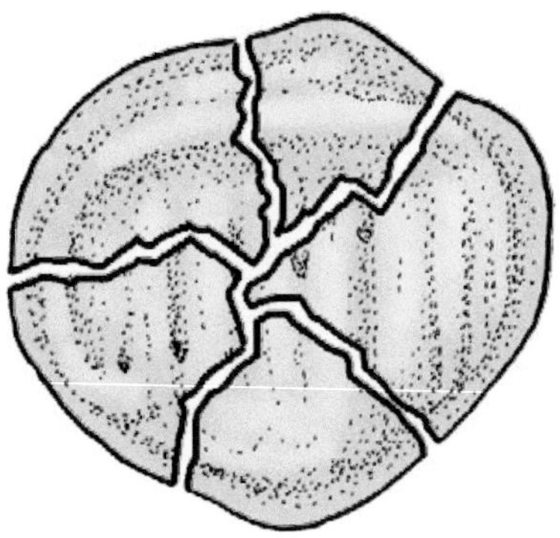

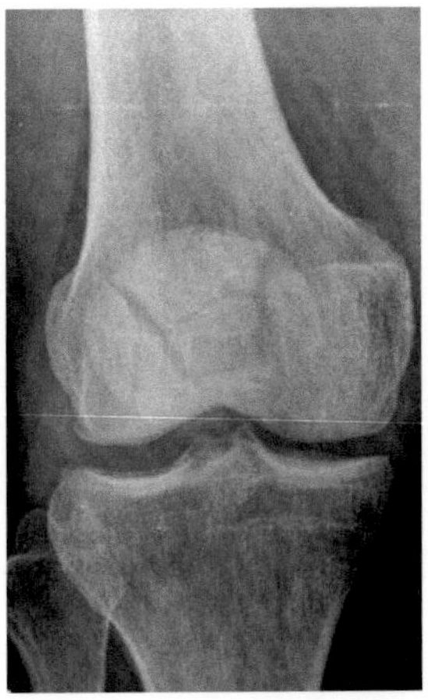

Regazzoni classification of patellar fractures

Type C: Comminuted fracture.
Type C1: Comminuted fracture with no displacement

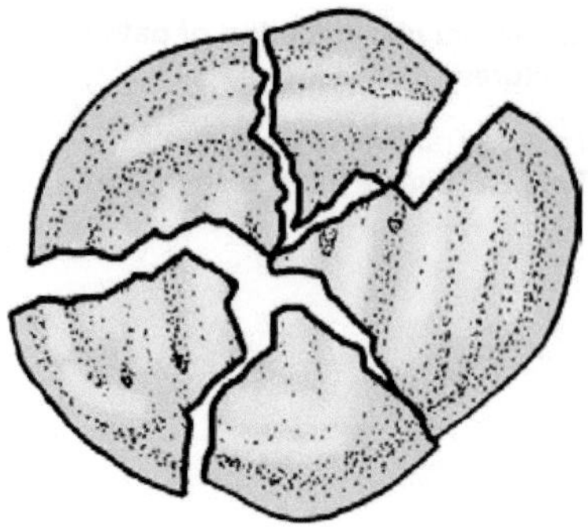

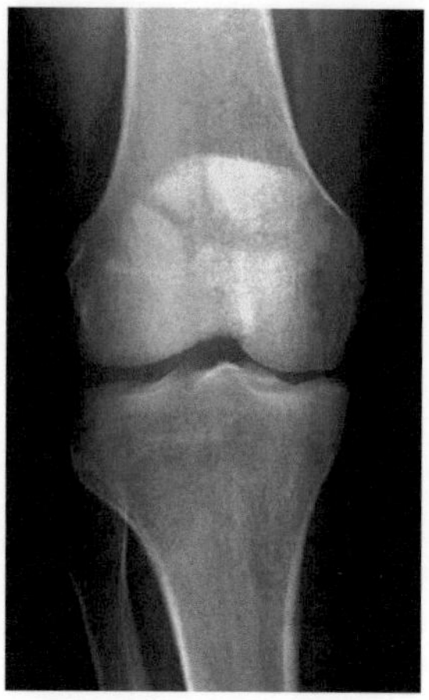

Regazzoni classification of patellar fractures

Type C: Comminuted fracture.
Type C2: Comminuted fracture with displacement (<2mm)

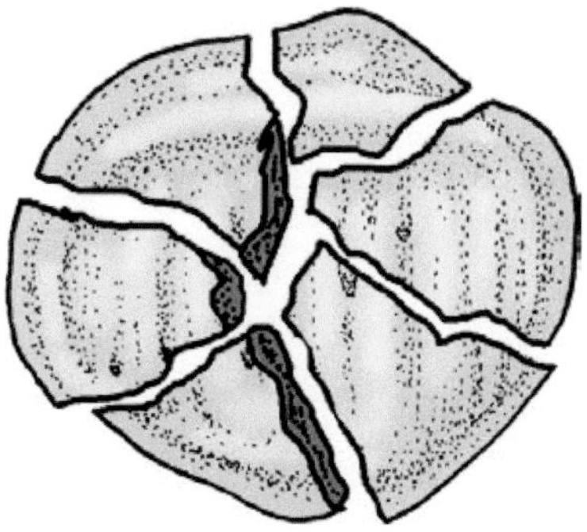

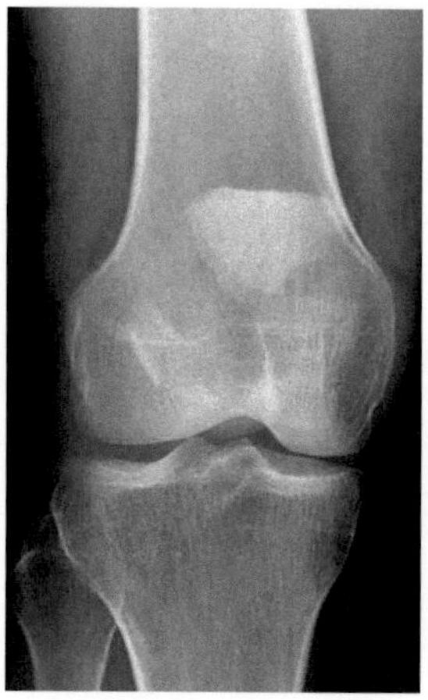

Regazzoni classification of patellar fractures

Type C: Comminuted fracture.
Type C3: Burst fracture with displacement (≥2mm)

9.3 Sanders Classification

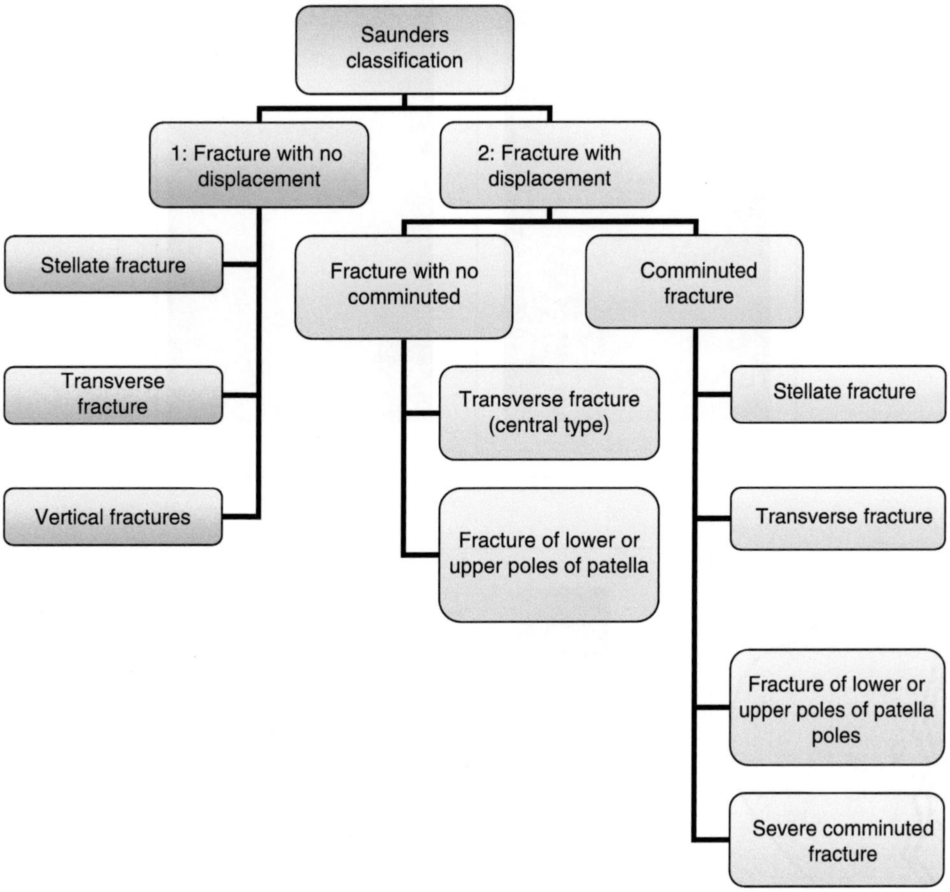

Type 1: Sanders classified patella fractures with no displacement into three types:
- Type 1.1: Stellate fracture
- Type 1.2: Transverse fracture
- Type 1.3: Vertical fractures

Type 2: Fracture with displacement:
- Type 2.1: Fracture with no comminution
  - Type 2.1.1: Transverse fracture (central type)
  - Type 2.1.2: Fracture of the patella poles (superior and inferior)
- Type 2.2: Comminuted fracture:
  - Type 2.2.1: Stellate fracture
  - Type 2.2.2: Transverse fracture
  - Type 2.2.3: Fracture of the patella poles
  - Type 2.2.4: Severe comminuted fracture

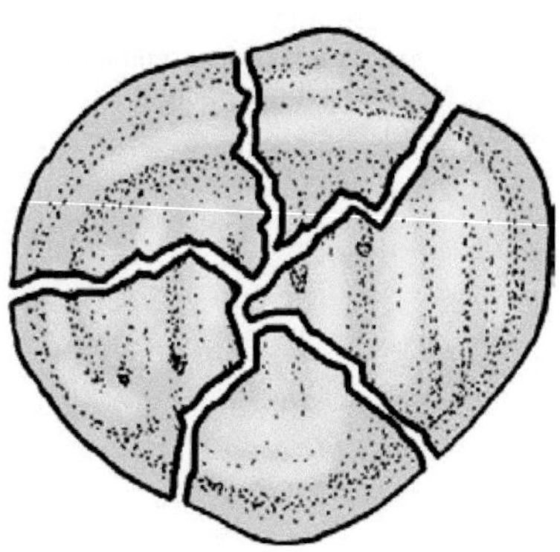

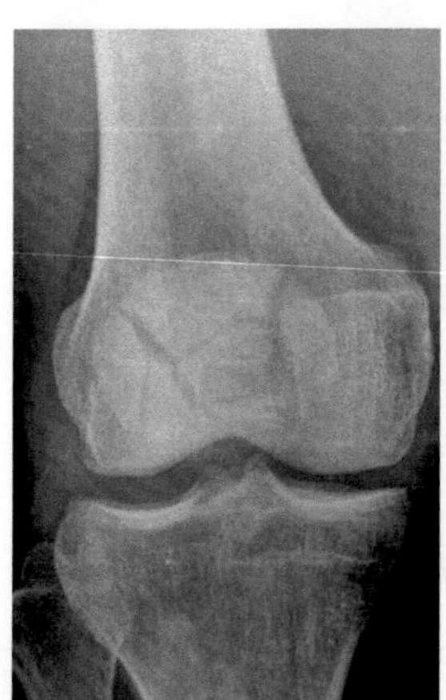

Saunders classification of patella fractures

Type 1: Fracture with no displacement.
Type 1.1: Stellate fracture

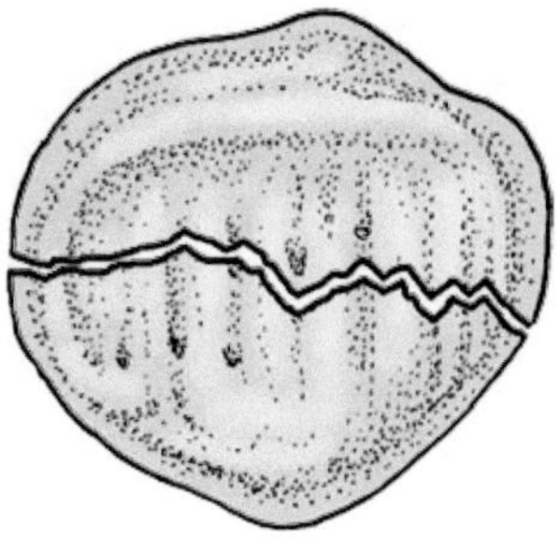

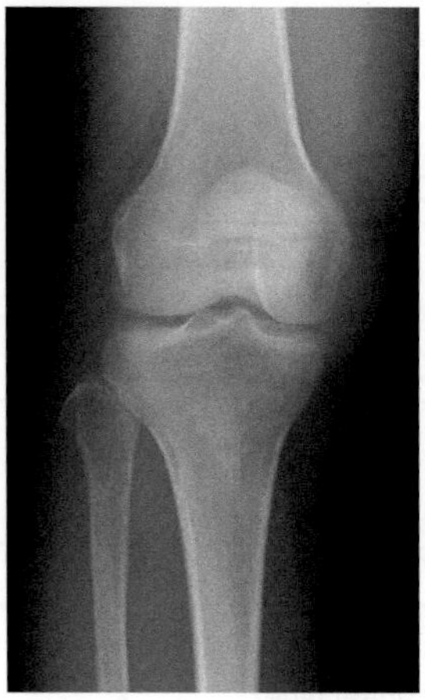

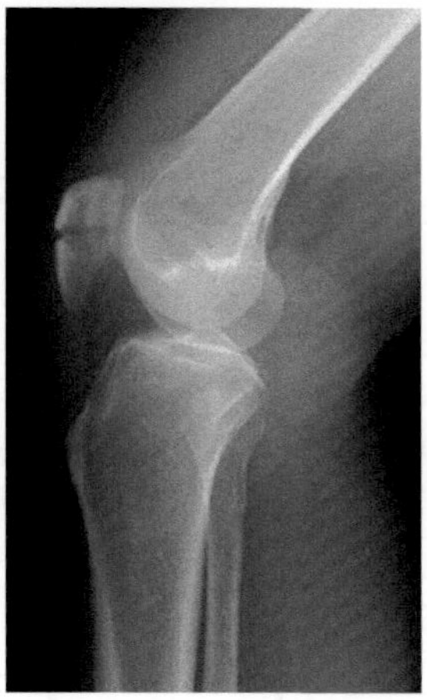

Saunders classification of patella fractures

Type 1: Fracture with no displacement.
Type 1.2: Transverse fracture

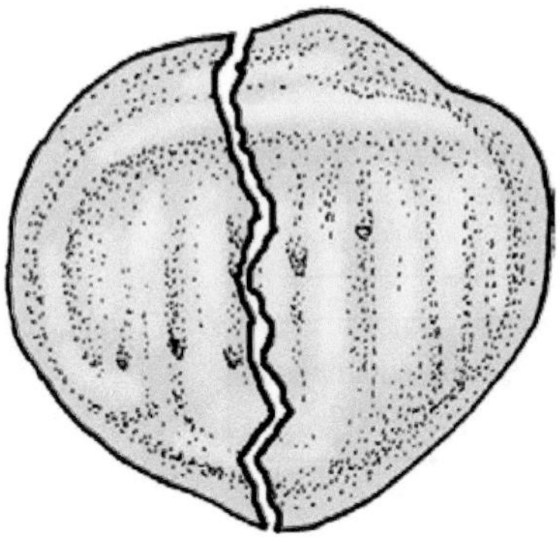

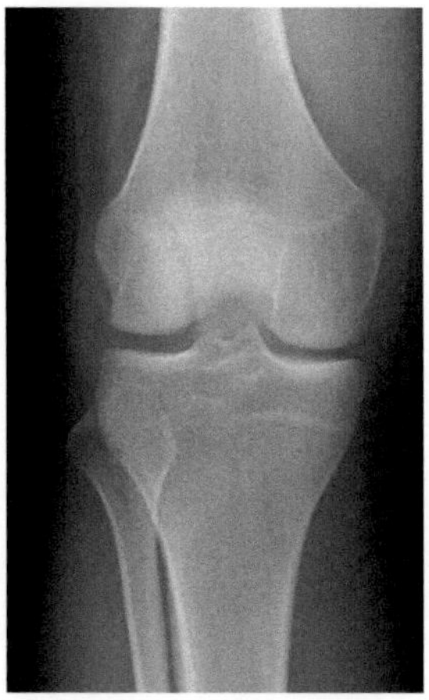

Saunders classification of patella fractures

Type 1: Fracture with no displacement.
Type 1.3: Vertical fractures

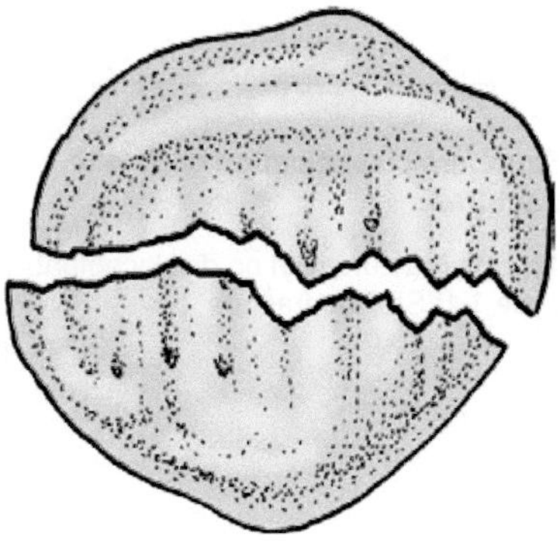

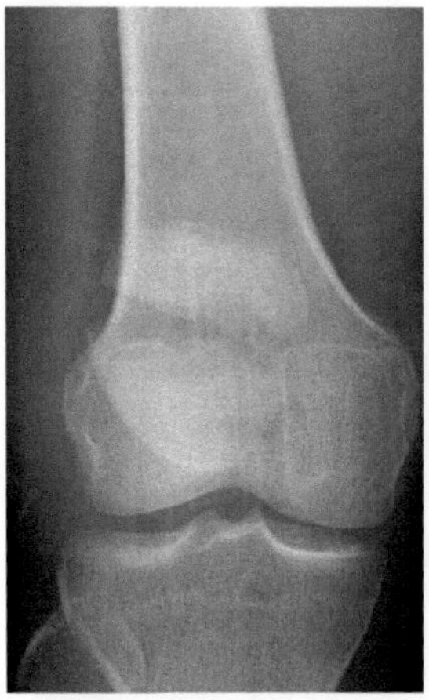

Saunders classification of patella fractures

Type 2: Fracture with displacement.
Type 2.1: Fracture with no comminution
Type 2.1.1: Transverse fracture (central type)

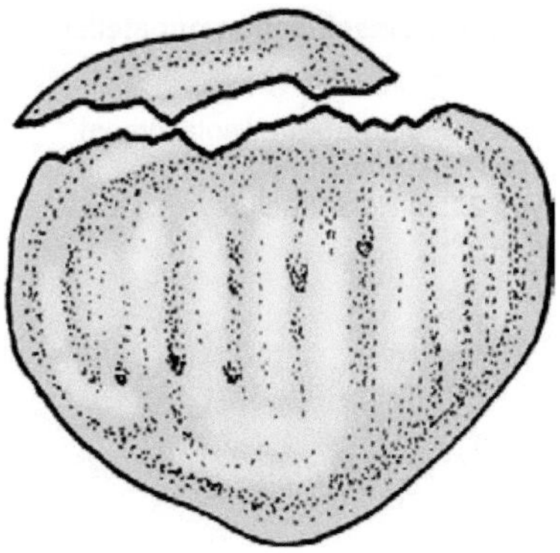

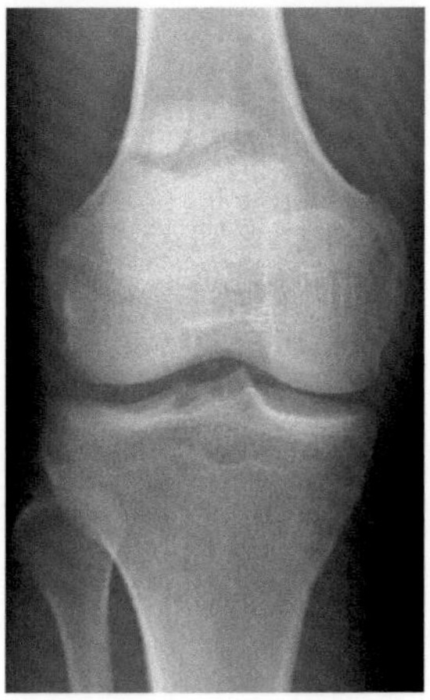

Saunders classification of patellar fractures

Type 2: Fracture with displacement.
Type 2.1: Non-comminution
Type 2.1.2: Polar(upper or inferior)

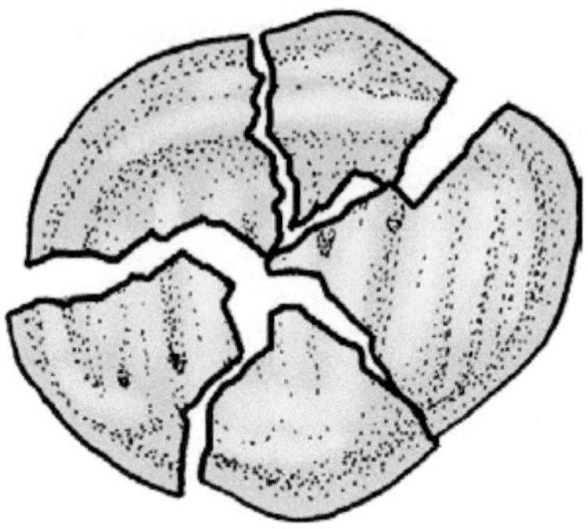

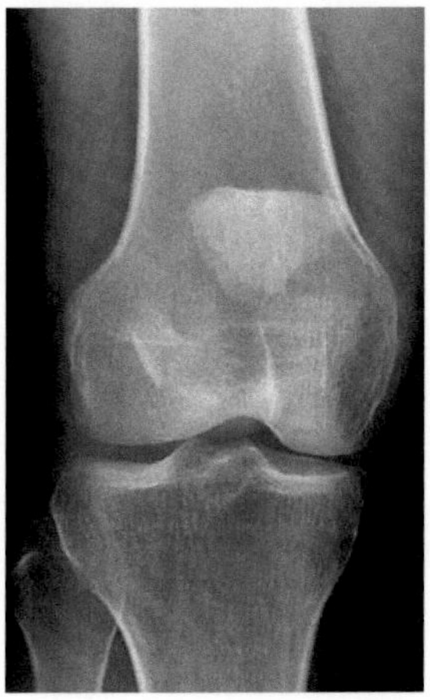

Saunders classification of patellar Fracture

Type 2: Fracture with displacement.
Type 2.2: Comminuted
Type 2.2.1: Stellate fracture

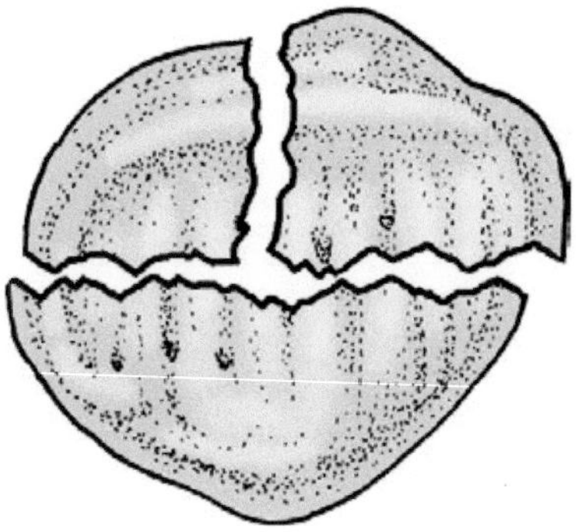

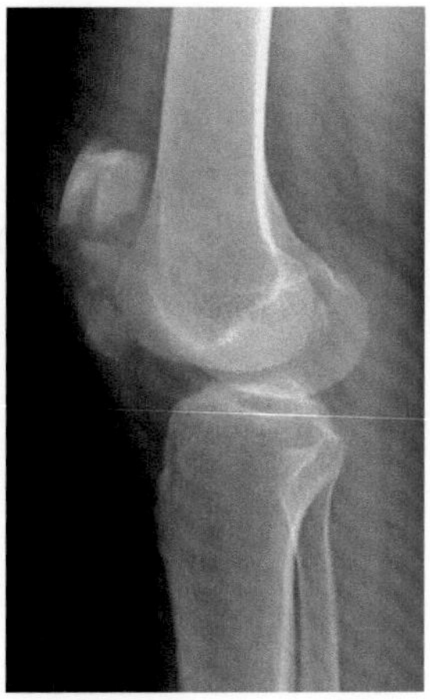

Saunders classification of patellar fractures

Type 2: Fracture with displacement.
Type 2.2: Comminuted
Type 2.2.2: Transverse

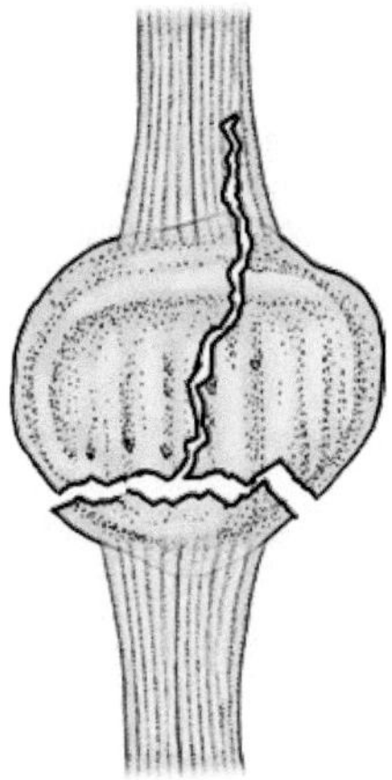

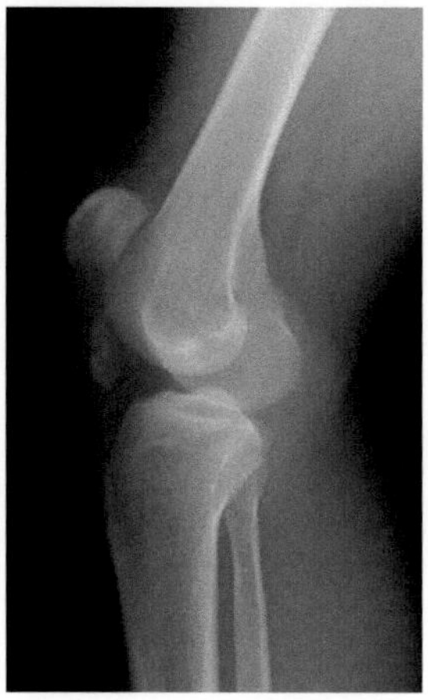

Saunders classification of patellar fractures

Type 2: Fracture with displacement.
Type 2.2: Comminuted
Type 2.2.3: Polar fracture

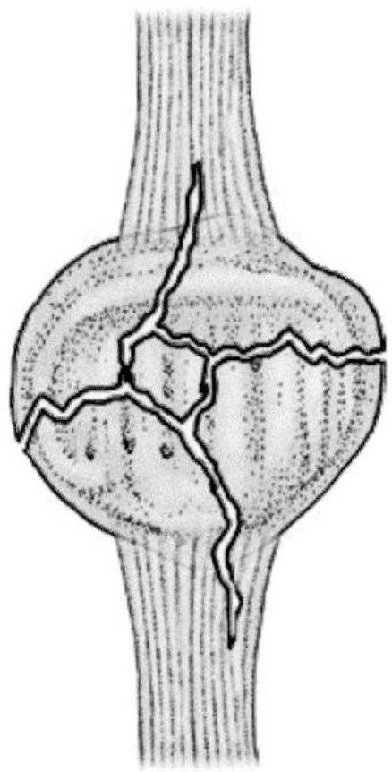

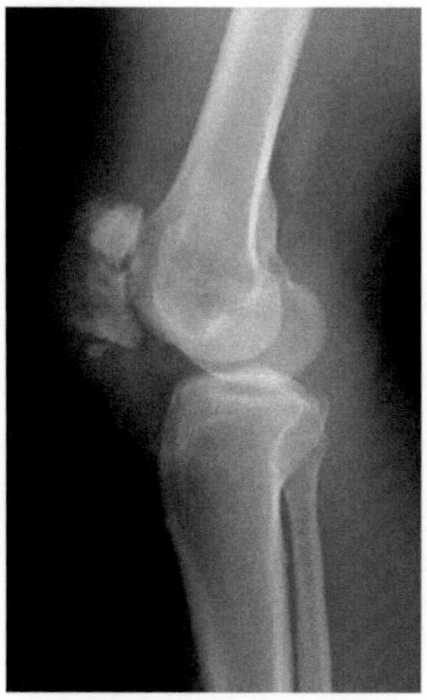

Saunders classification of patellar Fracture

Type 2: Fracture with displacement.
Type 2.2: Comminuted
Type 2.2.4: Severely comminuted

9.4 Rockwood Classification (1996, Fracture in Adult. 4th Ed. Philadelphia: JB Lippincott-Raven Publishers)

Type I: Non-displacement
Type II: Transverse
Type III: Bottom or inferior pole
Type IV: Non-displaced comminuted
Type V: Displaced comminuted
Type VI: Vertical
Type VII: Osteochondral

Classification of Tibial and Fibular Fractures

10

Yingze Zhang and Juan Wang

10.1 Proximal Tibial and Fibular Fractures

Proximal tibial fractures were first described by Sir Astley Cooper in 1825. Since the early attempt at classifying tibial plateau fractures by Muller in 1990, there have been ~10 classification systems of proximal tibial and fibular fractures proposed by researchers; among them, the Schatzker classification is the most commonly cited system, followed by the AO/OTA classification according to our 5-year literature review.

10.1.1 Schatzker Classification (1979, Clin Orthop, 138:94–104)

Type I: Split fracture of the lateral tibial plateau. The wedge fragment is not depressed.

Type II: Split and depression of the lateral tibial plateau.

Type III: Pure depression of the lateral tibial plateau.

Type IV: Medial tibial plateau fracture, often involving the tibial spine.

Type V: Split fracture involving both tibial plateau regions.

Type VI: Fracture through the metaphysis of the tibia.

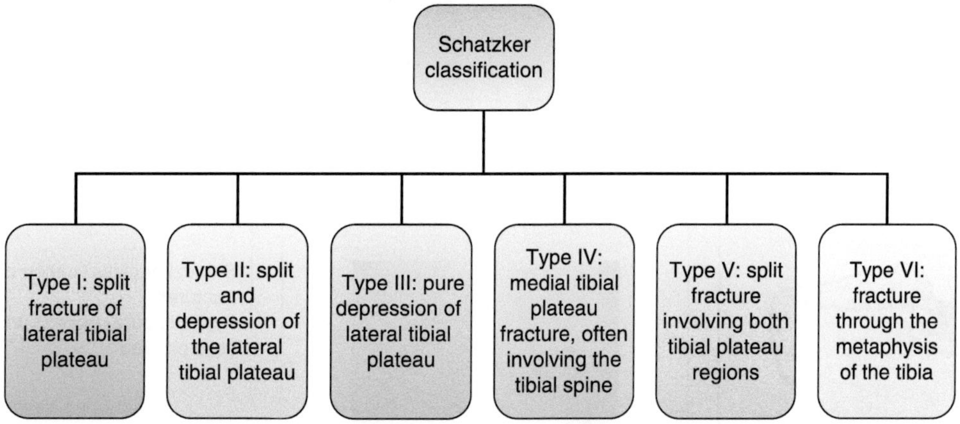

Y. Zhang (✉) • J. Wang
Department of Orthopedics,
The Third Hospital of Hebei Medical University,
Shijiazhuang, China
e-mail: yzzhangdr@126.com, yzling_liu@163.com

Y. Zhang (ed.), *Clinical Classification in Orthopaedics Trauma*, https://doi.org/10.1007/978-981-10-6044-1_10

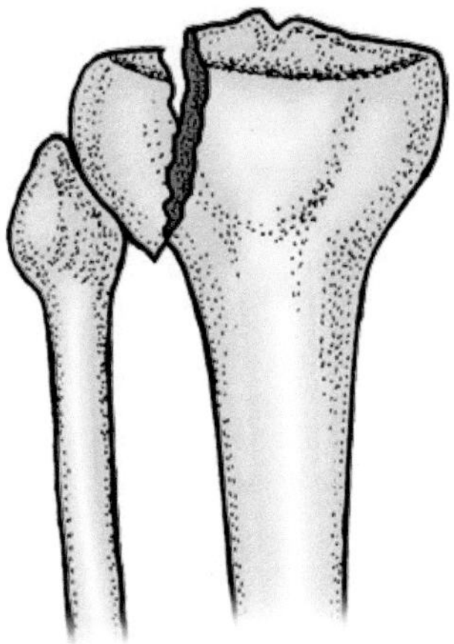

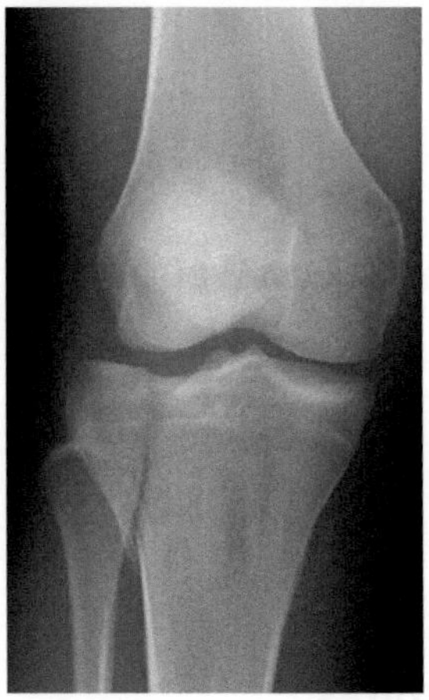

Schatzker classification of tibial plateau fractures
Type I : split fracture of the lateral tibial plateau. The wedge fragment is not depressed

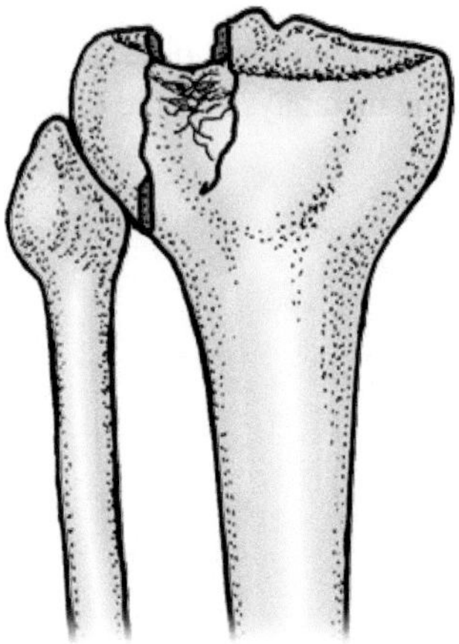

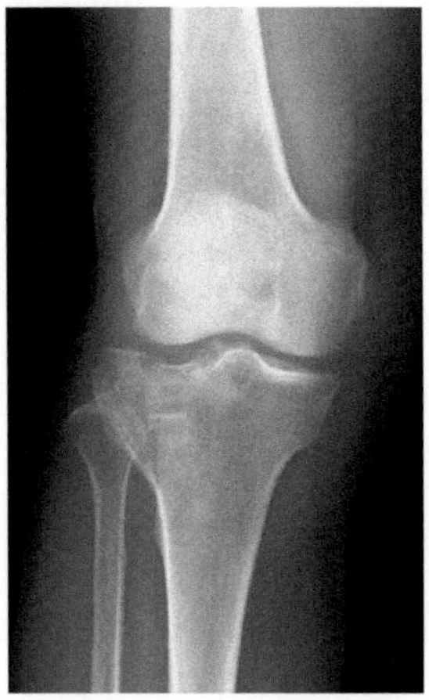

Schatzker classification of tibial plateau fractures
Type II : split and depression of the lateral tibial plateau

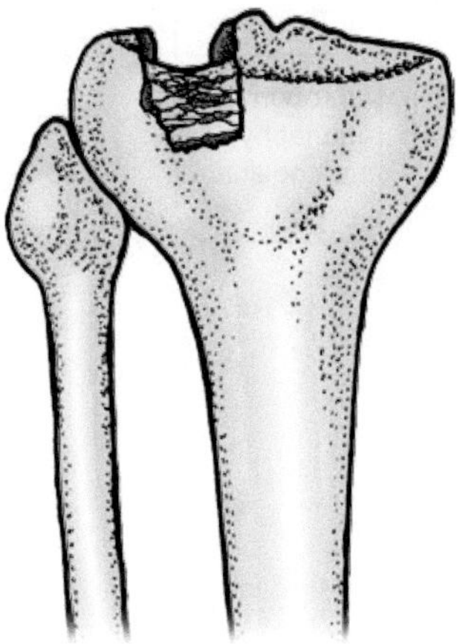

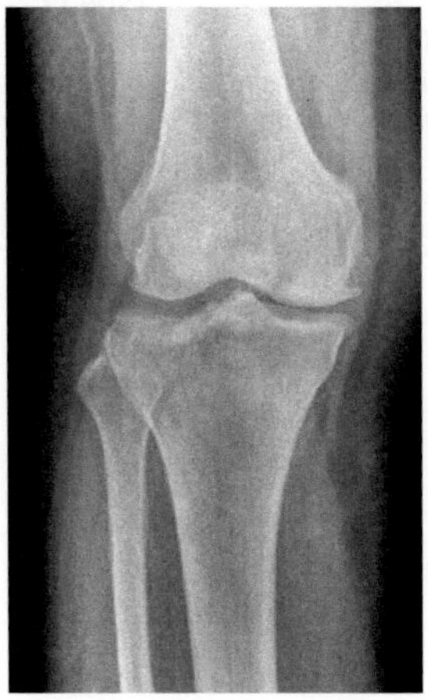

Schatzker classification of tibial plateau fractures
Type III : pure depression of the lateral tibial plateau

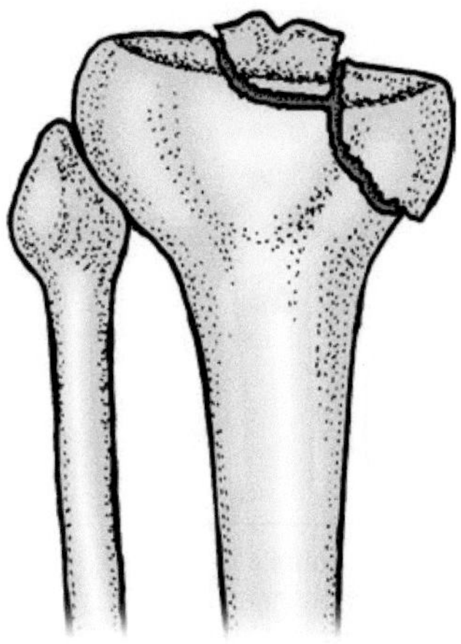

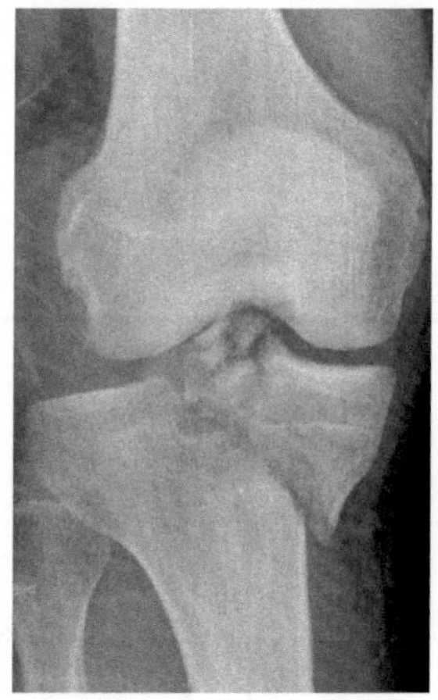

Schatzker classification of tibial plateau fractures
Type IV: medial tibial plateau fracture, often involving the tibial spines

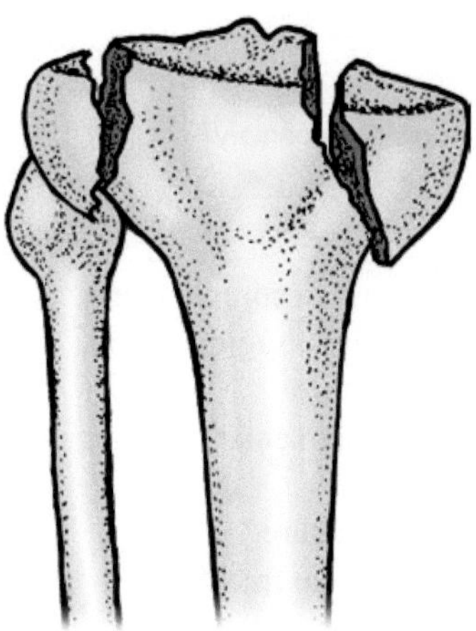

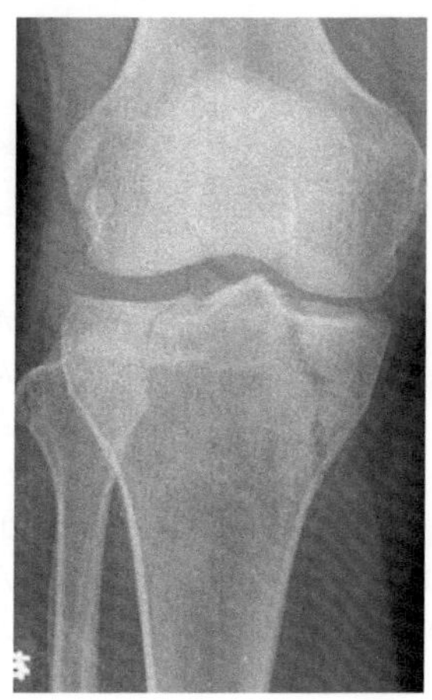

Schatzker classification of tibial plateau fractures
Type V: split fracture involving both tibial plateau regions

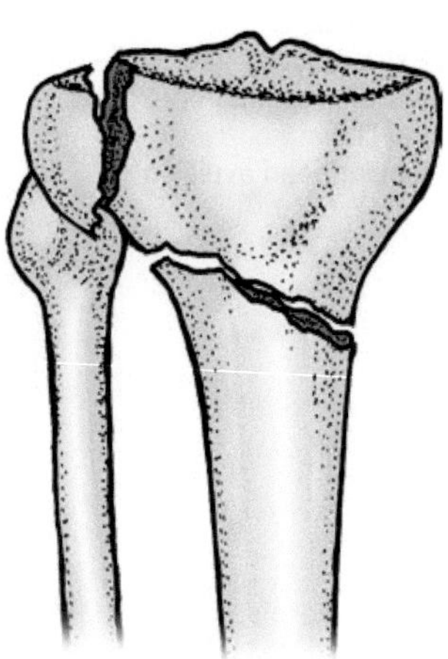

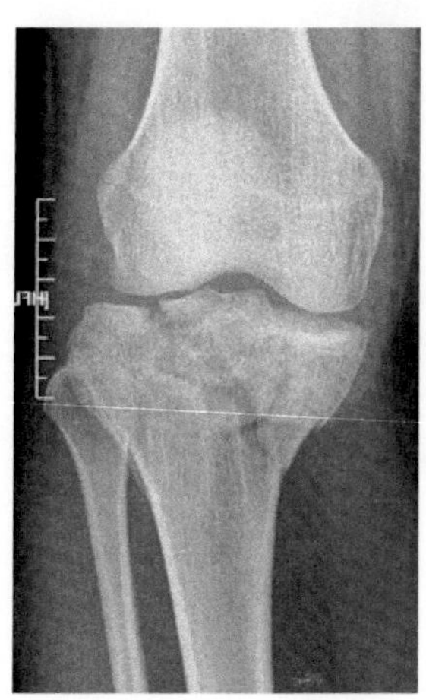

Schatzker classification of tibial plateau fractures
Type VI: fracture through the metaphysis of the tibia

10.1.2 AO/OTA Classification (2007, Journal of Orthopaedic Trauma. 21 supplement; firstly proposed in 1980s, revised in 2007)

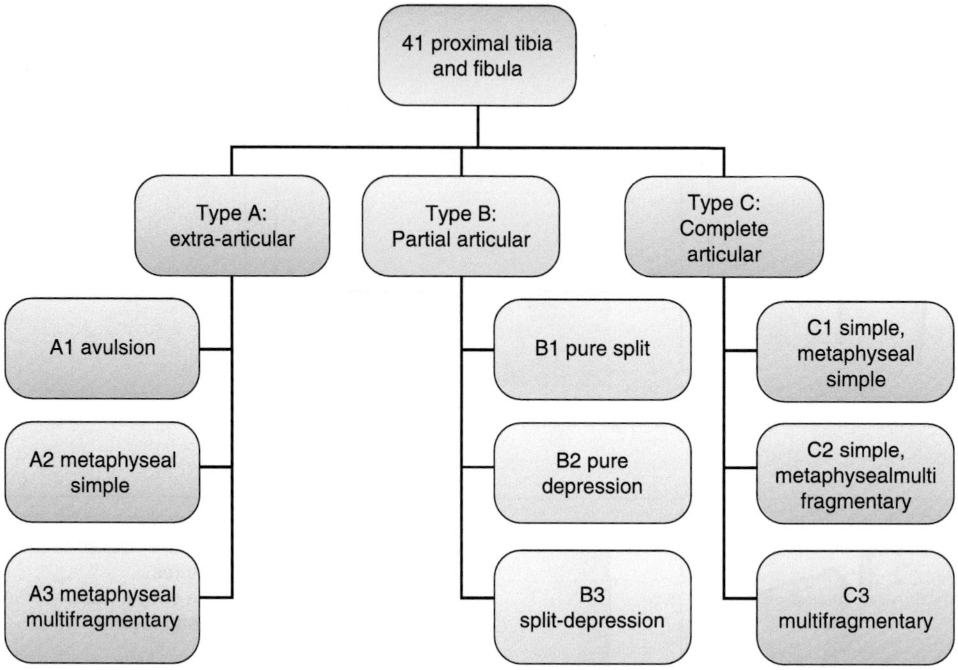

Type A: Extra-articular fracture:
- Type A1: Avulsion fracture of proximal tibia and fibula. This type is subdivided into:
  - Type A1.1: Fibular head avulsion.
  - Type A1.2: Tibial tubercle avulsion.
  - Type A1.3: Cruciate ligament insertion avulsion.
- Type A2: Metaphyseal simple fracture of proximal tibia, subdivided into:
  - Type A2.1: Oblique fracture in coronal plane.
  - Type A2.2: Oblique fracture in sagittal plane.
  - Type A2.3: Transverse fracture.
- Type A3: Metaphyseal multifragmentary fracture of proximal tibia, subdivided into:
  - Type A3.1: Intact wedge fracture.
  - Type A3.2: Fragmented wedge fracture.
  - Type A3.3: Comminuted fracture.

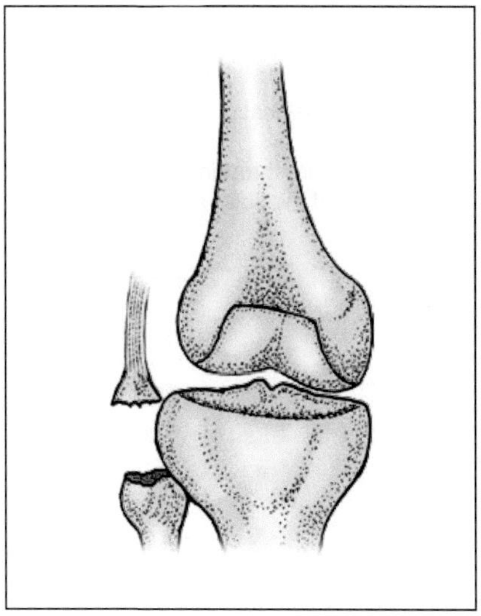

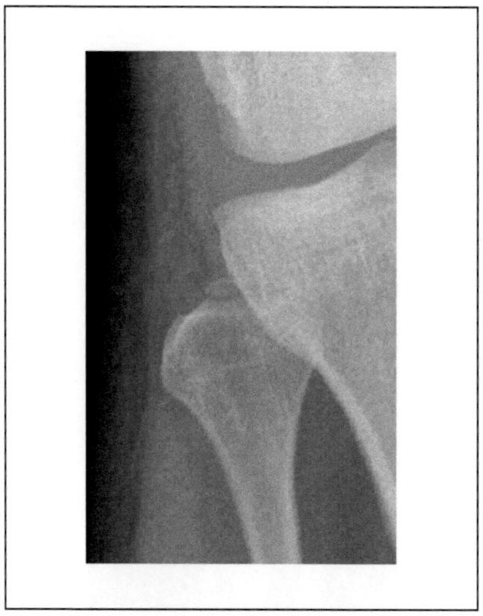

AO/OTA classification of proximal tibia and fibula
41-A Extra-articular fracture
A1 Avulsion fracture of proximal tibia and fibula:
A1.1 Fibular head avulsion

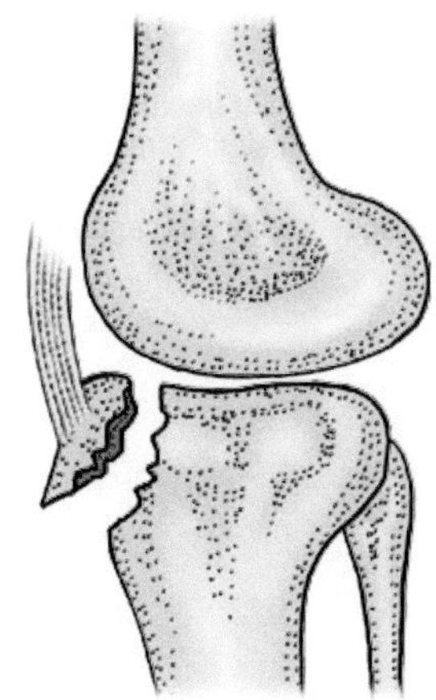

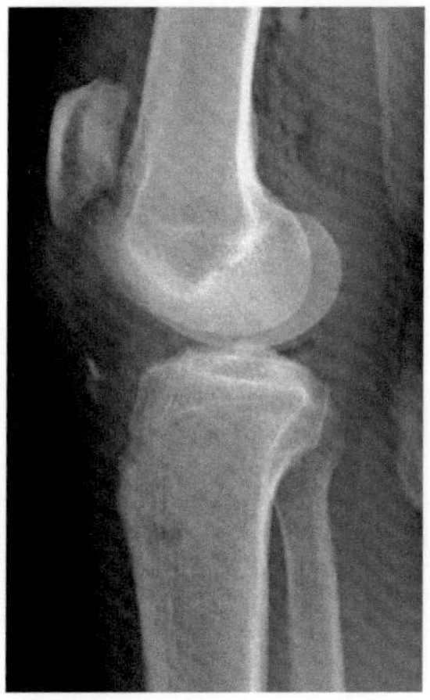

AO/OTA classification of proximal tibia and fibula
41-A Extra-articular fracture
A1 Avulsion fracture of proximal tibia and fibula:
A1.2 Tibial tubercle avulsion

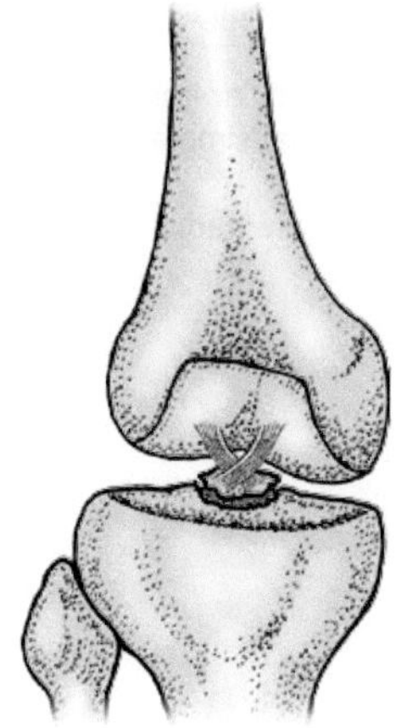

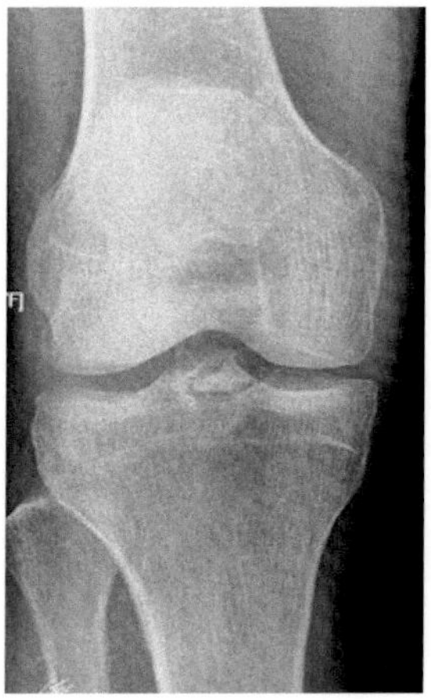

AO/OTA classification of proximal tibia and fibula
41-A Extra-articular fracture
A1 Avulsion fracture of proximal tibia and fibula:
A1.3 Cruciate ligament insertion avulsion

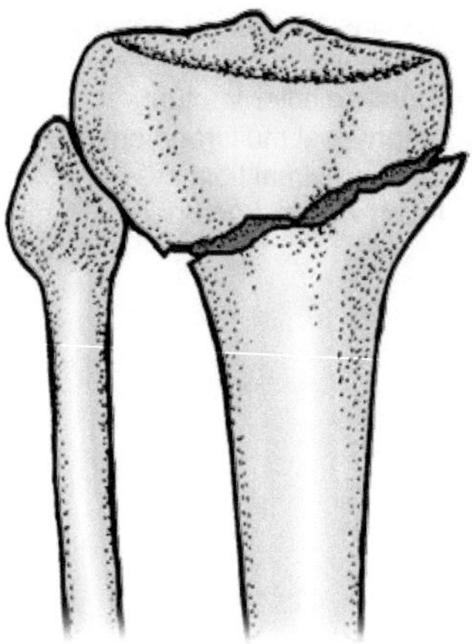

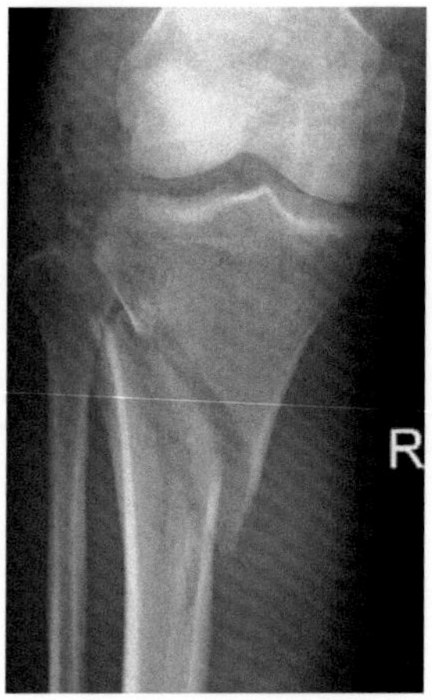

AO/OTA classification of proximal tibia and fibula
41-A Extra-articular fracture
A2 Metaphyseal simple fracture of proximal tibia:
A2.1 Oblique fracture in coronal plane

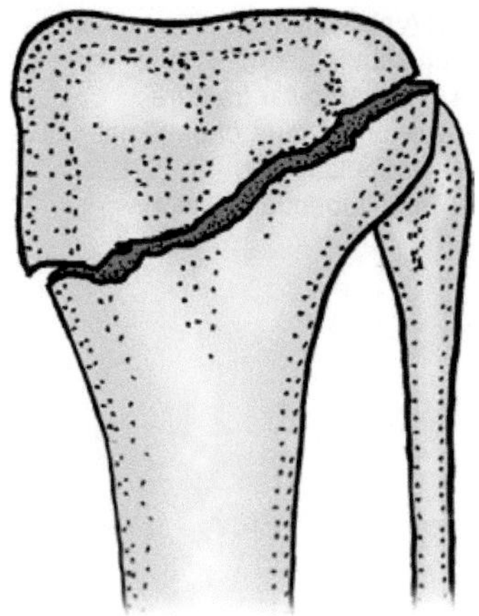

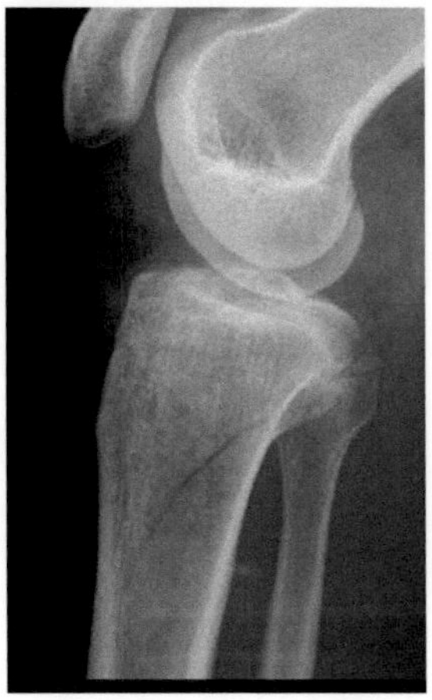

AO/OTA classification of proximal tibia and fibula
41-A Extra-articular fracture
A2 Metaphyseal simple fracture of proximal tibia:
A2.2 Oblique fracture in sagittal plane

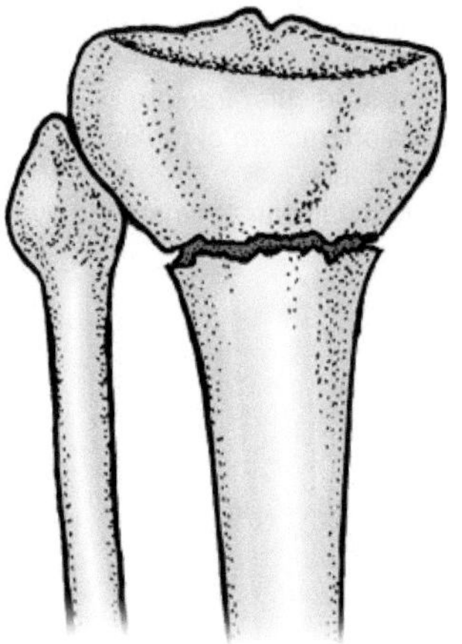

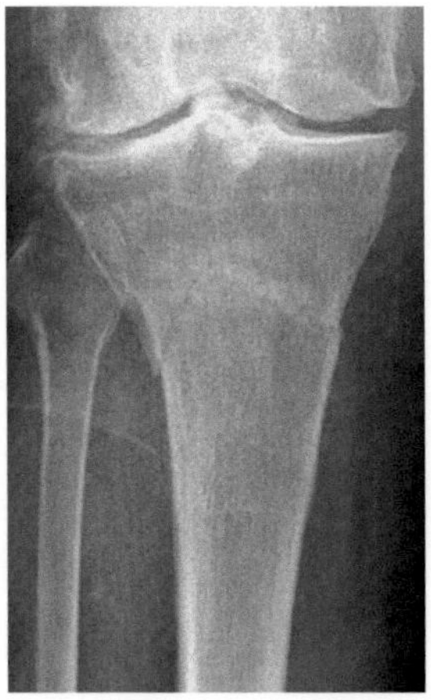

AO/OTA classification of proximal tibia and fibula
41-A Extra-articular fracture
A2 Metaphyseal simple fracture of proximal tibia:
A2.3 Transverse fracture

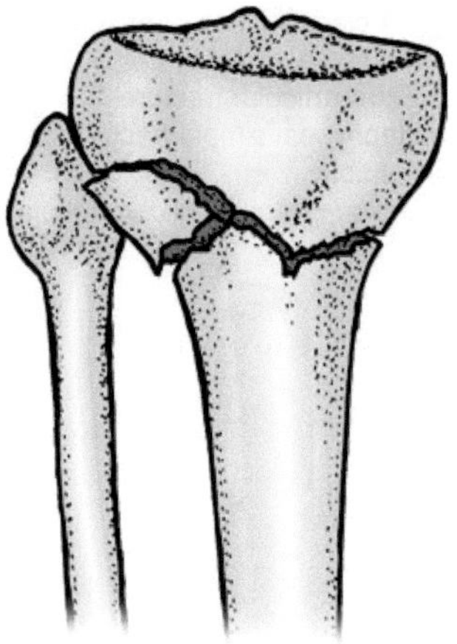

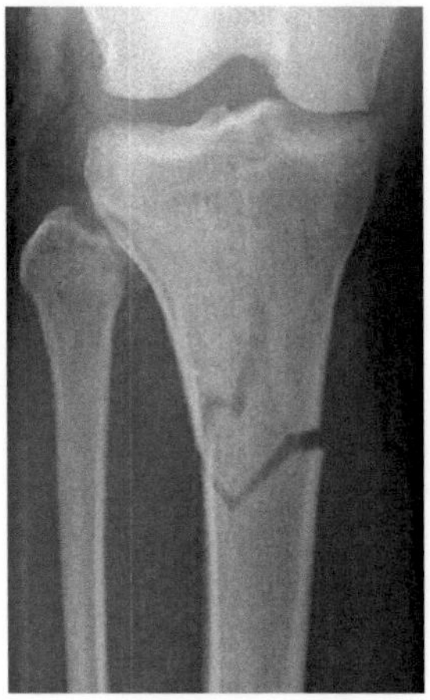

AO/OTA classification of proximal tibia and fibula
41-A Extra-articular fracture
A3 Metaphyseal multifragmentary fracture of proximal tibia:
A3.1 Intact wedge fracture

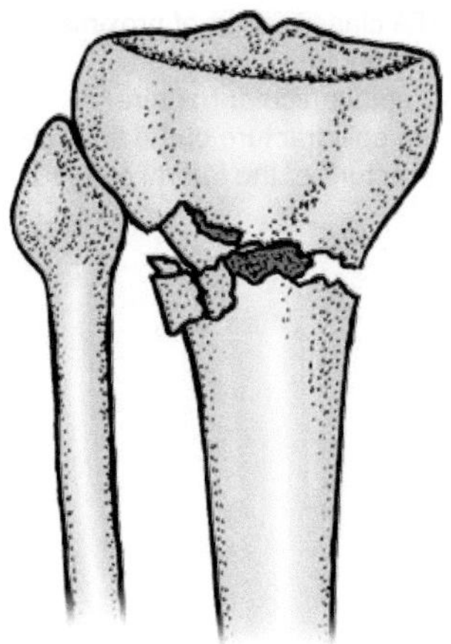

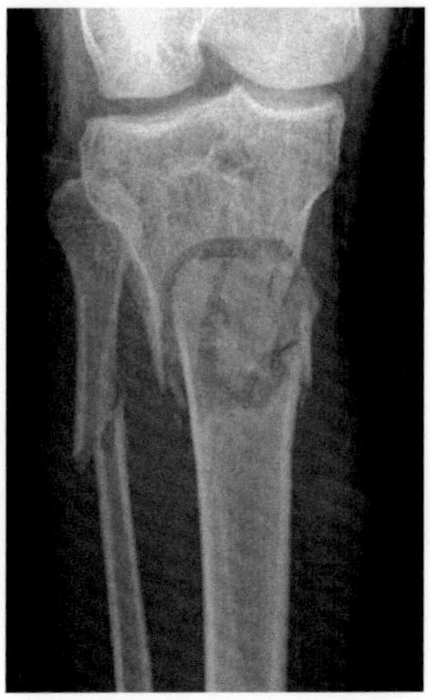

AO/OTA classification of proximal tibia and fibula
41-A Extra-articular fracture
A3 Metaphyseal multifragmentary fracture of proximal tibia:
A3.2 Fragmented wedge fracture

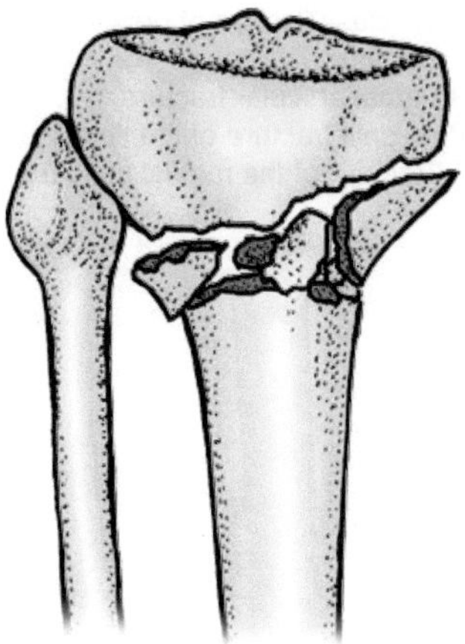

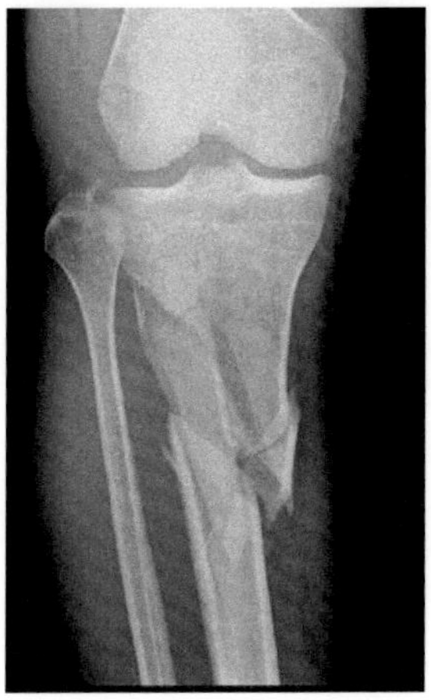

AO/OTA classification of proximal tibia and fibula
41-A Extra-articular fracture
A3 Metaphyseal multifragmentary fracture of proximal tibia:
A3.3 Complex fracture

Type B: Partial articular fracture:
- Type B1: Pure split fracture of the tibial plateau, subdivided into:
  - Type B1.1: Fracture of the lateral plateau.
  - Type B1.2: Fracture of the medial plateau.
  - Type B1.3: Oblique fracture of one of the plateaus, involving tibial spines.
- Type B2: Pure depression fracture of the tibial plateau, subdivided into:
  - Type B2.1: Total depression of the lateral plateau.
  - Type B2.2: Limited depression of the lateral plateau.
  - Type B2.3: Depression of the medial plateau.
- Type B3: Split-depression fracture of the tibial plateau, subdivided into:
  - Type B3.1: Fracture of the lateral plateau.
  - Type B3.2: Fracture of the medial plateau.
  - Type B3.3: Fracture of one of the plateaus, involving tibial spines.

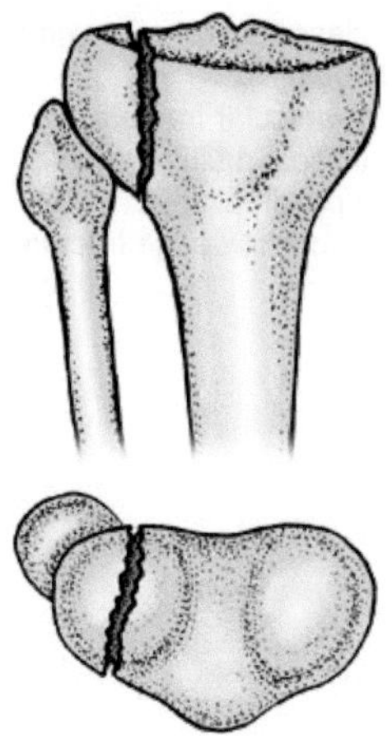

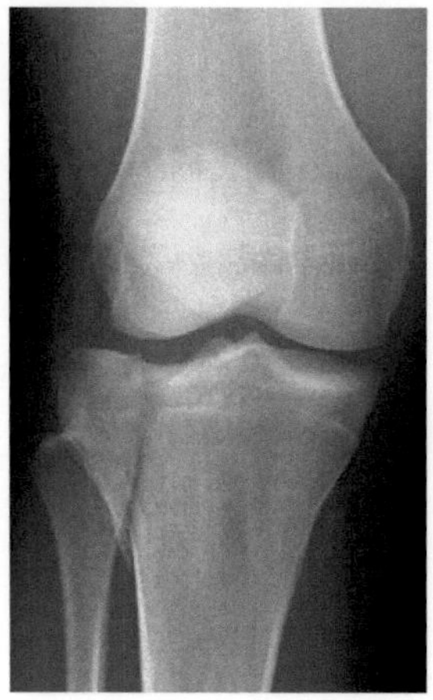

AO/OTA classification of proximal tibia and fibula
41-B Partial articular fracture
B1 Pure split fracture of the tibial plateau:
B1.1 Fracture of the lateral plateau

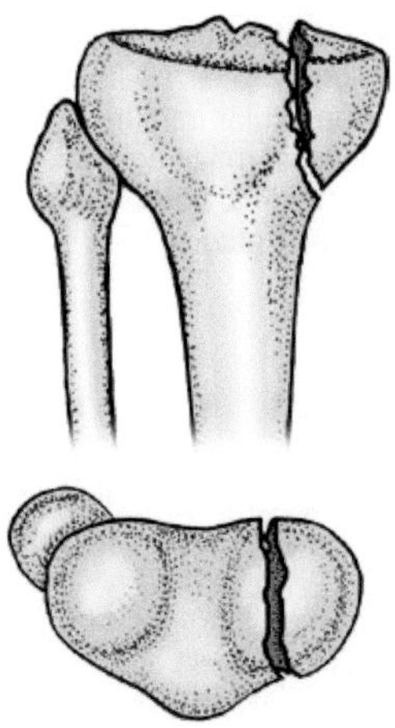

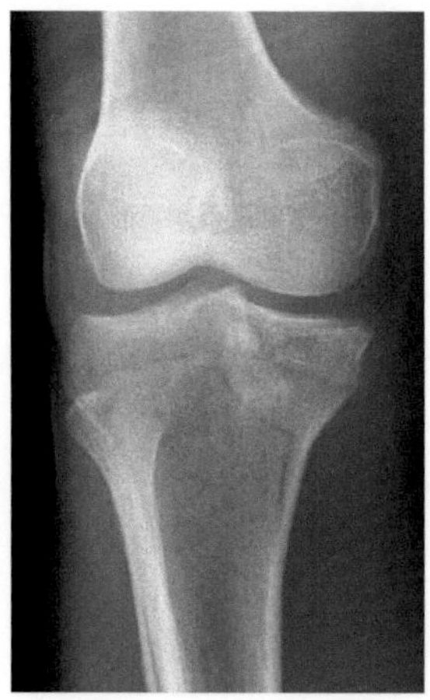

AO/OTA classification of proximal tibia and fibula
41-B Partial articular fracture
B1 Pure split fracture of the tibial plateau:
B1.2 Fracture of the medial plateau

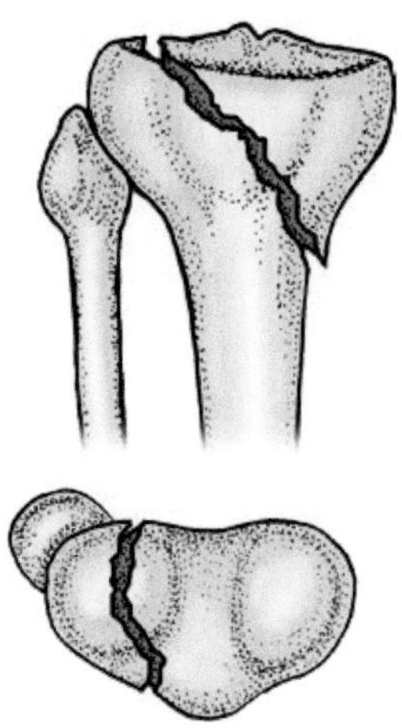

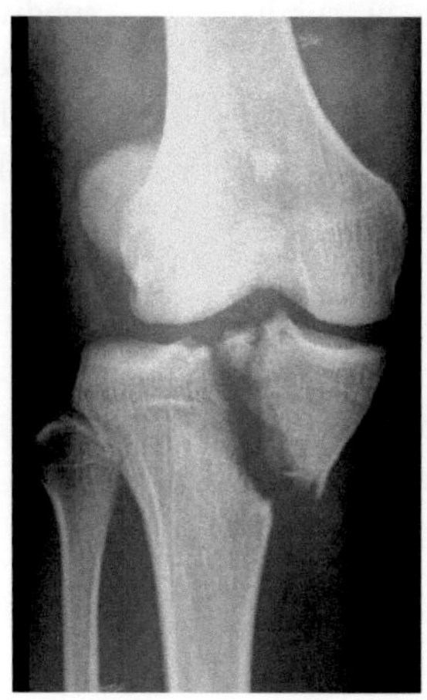

AO/OTA classification of proximal tibia and fibula
41-B Partial articular fracture
B1 Pure split fracture of the tibial plateau:
B1.3 Oblique fracture of one of the plateaus, involving tibial spines

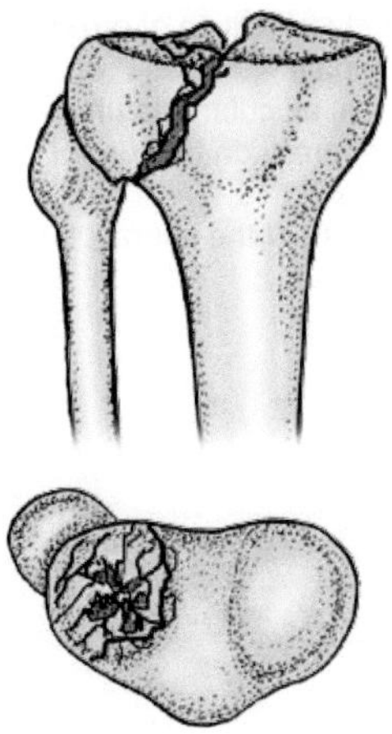

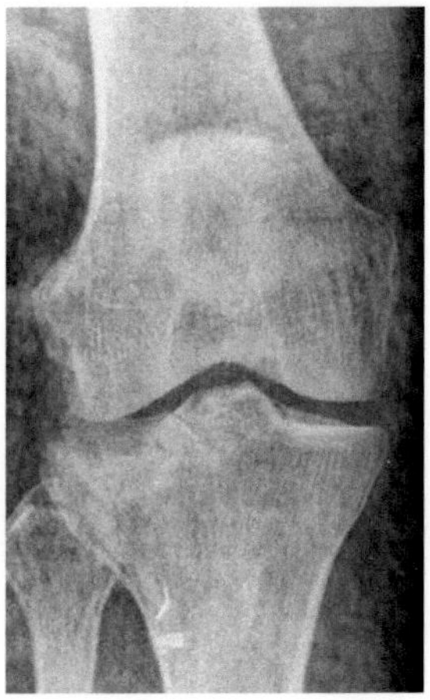

AO/OTA classification of proximal tibia and fibula
41-B Partial articular fracture
B2 Pure depression fracture of the tibial plateau:
B2.1 Total depression of the lateral plateau

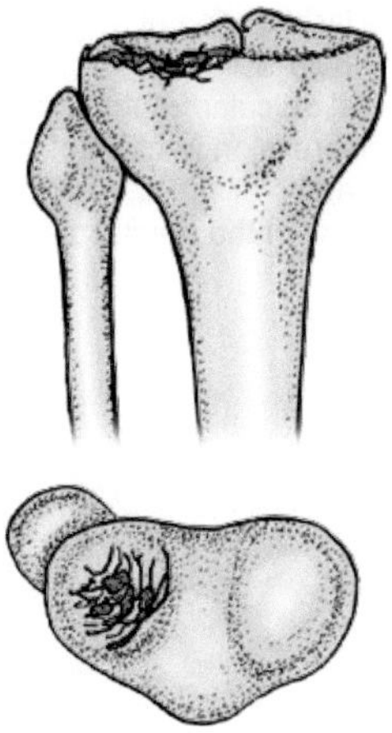

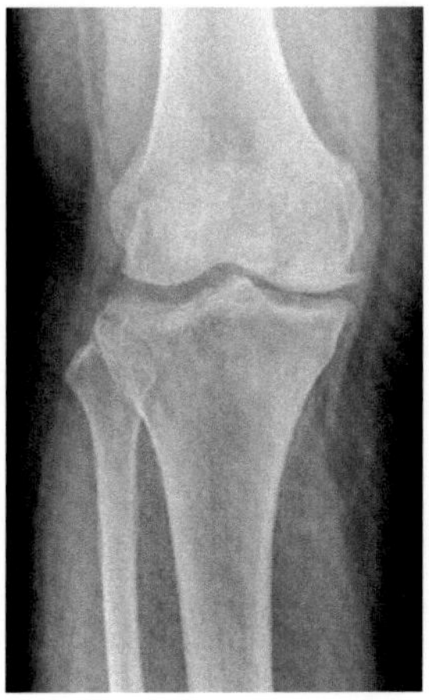

AO/OTA classification of proximal tibia and fibula
41-B Partial articular fracture
B2 Pure depression fracture of the tibial plateau:
B2.2 Limited depression of the lateral plateau

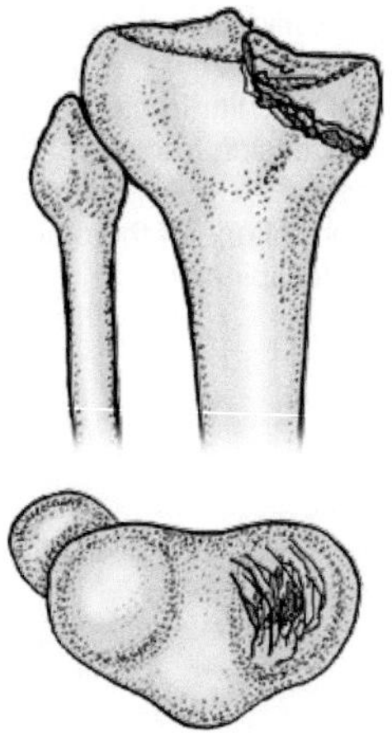

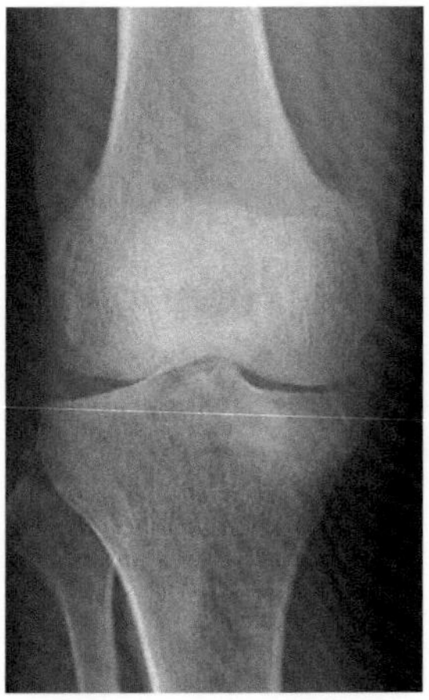

AO/OTA classification of proximal tibia and fibula
41-B Partial articular fracture
B2 Pure depression fracture of the tibial plateau:
B2.3 Depression of the medial plateau

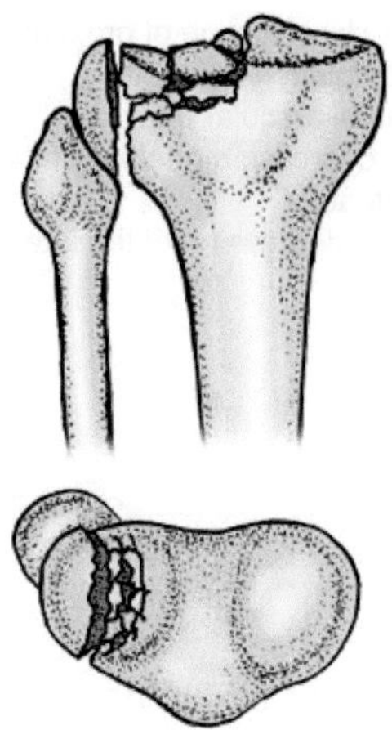

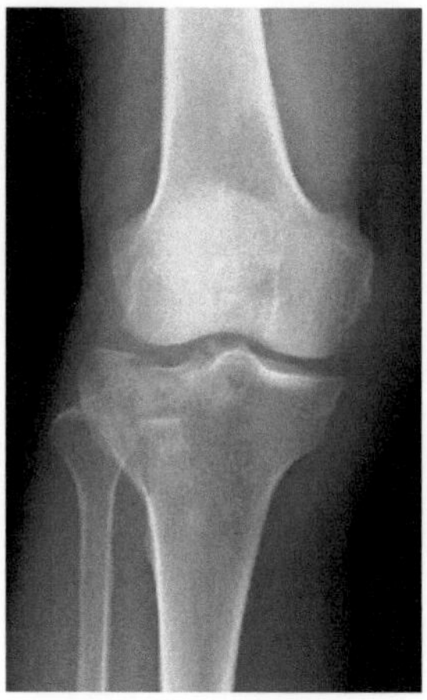

AO/OTA classification of proximal tibia and fibula
41-B Partial articular fracture
B3 Split-depression fracture of the tibial plateau:
B3.1 Fracture of the lateral plateau

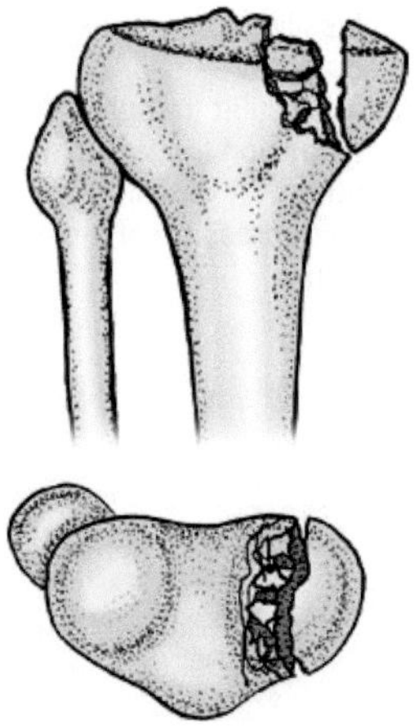

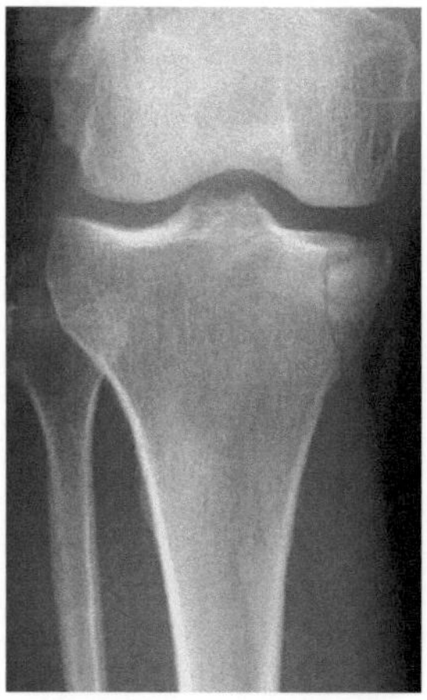

AO/OTA classification of proximal tibia and fibula
41-B Partial articular fracture
B3 Split-depression fracture of the tibial plateau:
B3.2 Fracture of the medial plateau

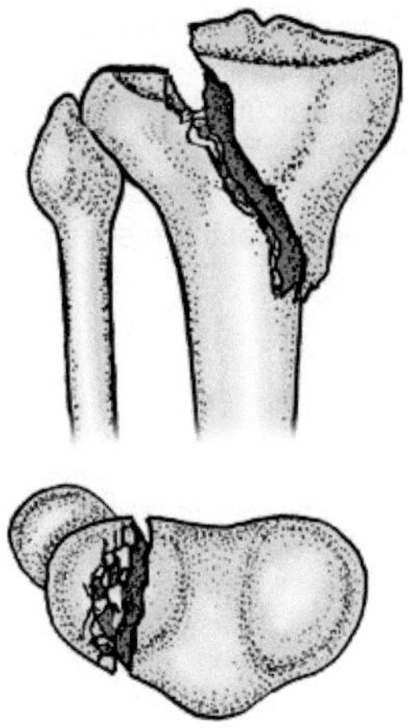

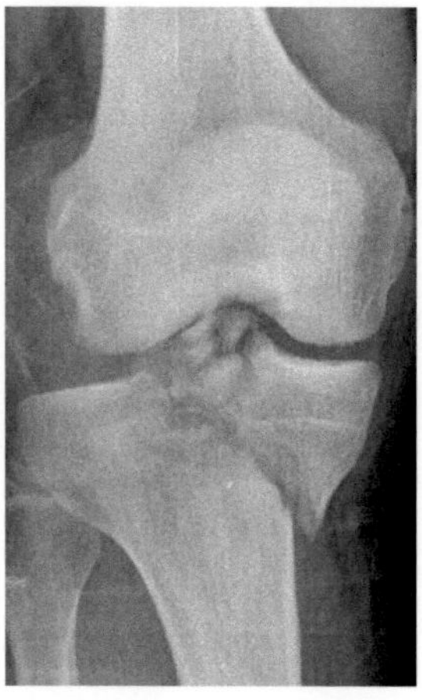

AO/OTA classification of proximal tibia and fibula
41-B Partial articular fracture
B3 Split-depression fracture of the tibial plateau:
B3.3 Fracture of one of the plateaus, involving tibial spines

Type C: Complete articular fracture:
- Type C1: Simple articular and metaphyseal fracture, subdivided into:
  - Type C1.1: Non- or slight displacement.
  - Type C1.2: Displaced fracture of one condyle.
  - Type C1.3: Displaced fracture of both condyles.
- Type C2: Articular simple, metaphyseal multifragmentary fracture, subdivided into:
  - Type C2.1: Intact wedge metaphyseal fragment.
  - Type C2.2: Fragmented wedge metaphysis.
  - Type C2.3: Complex metaphyseal fracture.
- Type C3: Multifragmentary articular fracture, subdivided into complex fractures of:
  - Type C3.1: The lateral plateau.
  - Type C3.2: The medial plateau.
  - Type C3.3: Both plateaus.

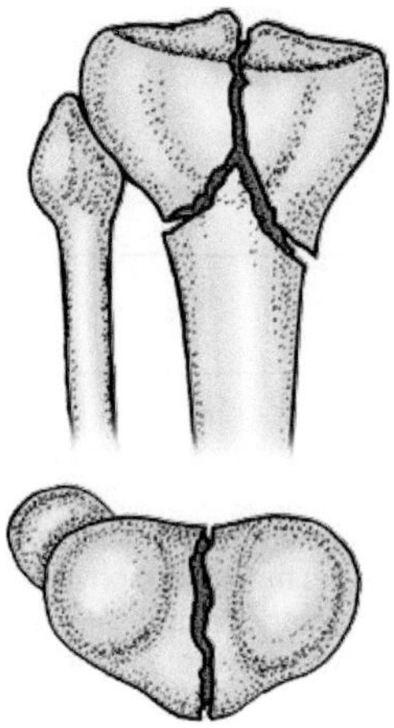

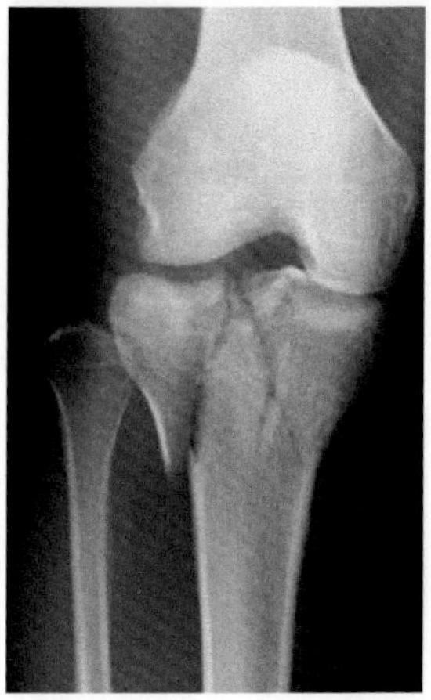

AO/OTA classification of proximal tibia and fibula
41-C Complete articular fracture
C1 Simple articular and metaphyseal fracture:
C1.1 Non- or slight displacement

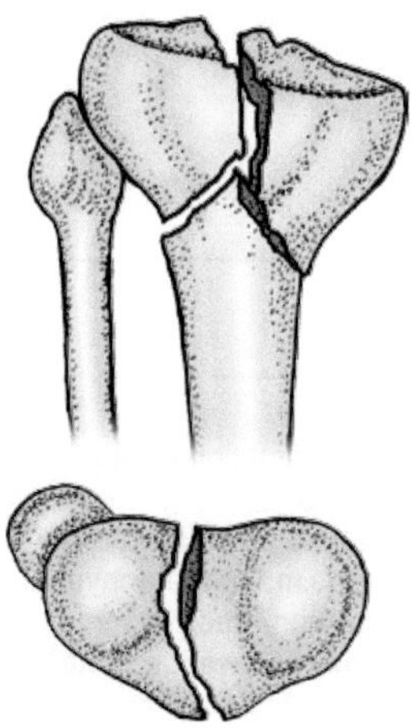

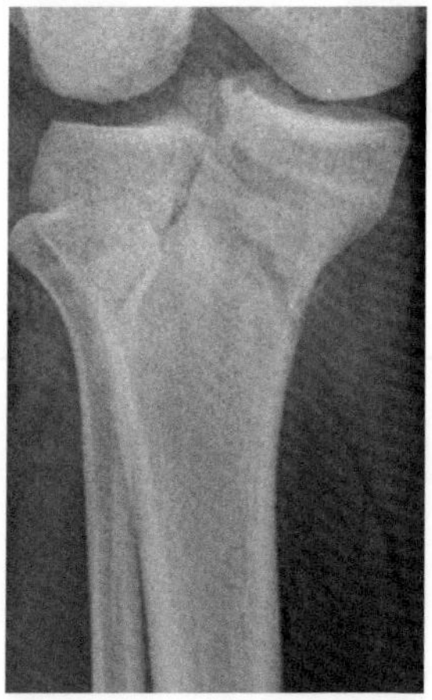

AO/OTA classification of proximal tibia and fibula
41-C Complete articular fracture
C1 Simple articular and metaphyseal fracture:
C1.2 Displaced fracture of one condyle

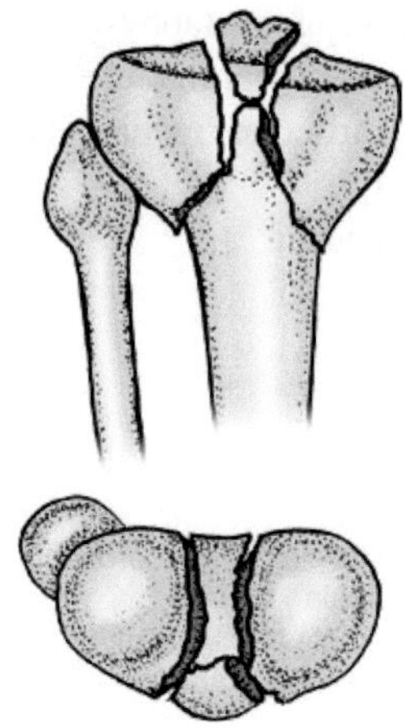

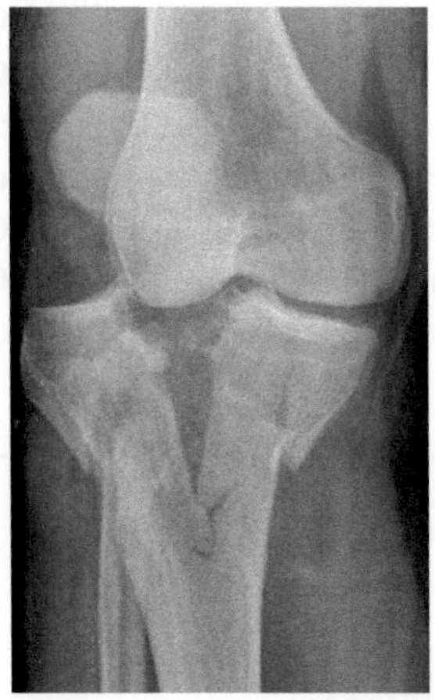

AO/OTA classification of proximal tibia and fibula
41-C Complete articular fracture
C1 Simple articular and metaphyseal fracture:
C1.3 Displaced fracture of both condyles

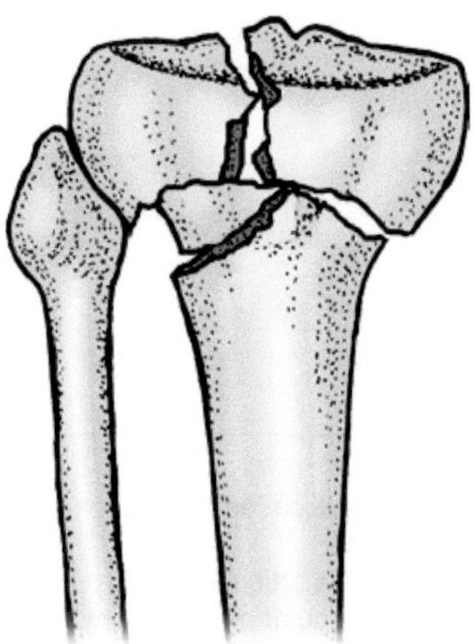

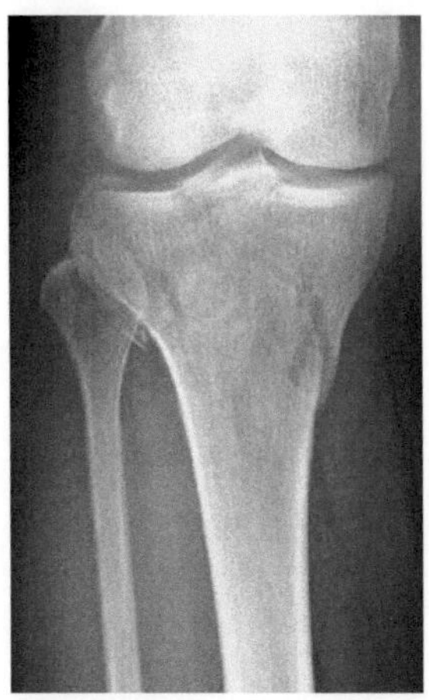

AO/OTA classification of proximal tibia and fibula
41-C Complete articular fracture
C2 Articular simple, metaphyseal multifragmentary fracture:
C2.1 Intact wedge metaphyseal fragment

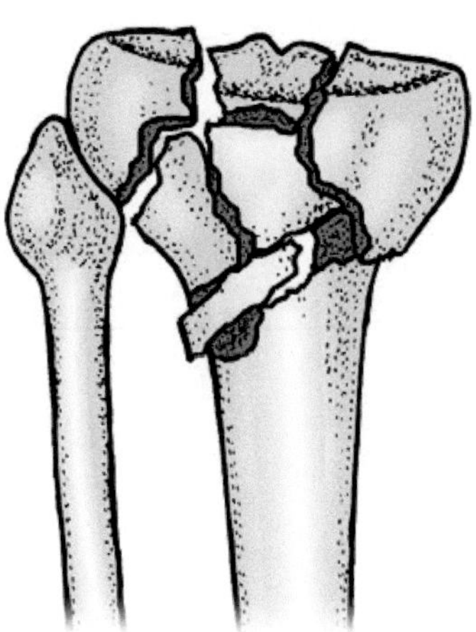

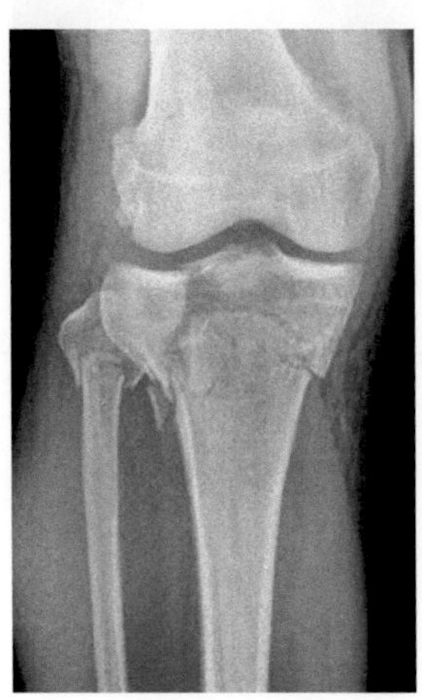

AO/OTA classification of proximal tibia and fibula
41-C Complete articular fracture
C2 Articular simple, metaphyseal multifragmentary fracture:
C2.2 Fragmented wedge metaphysis

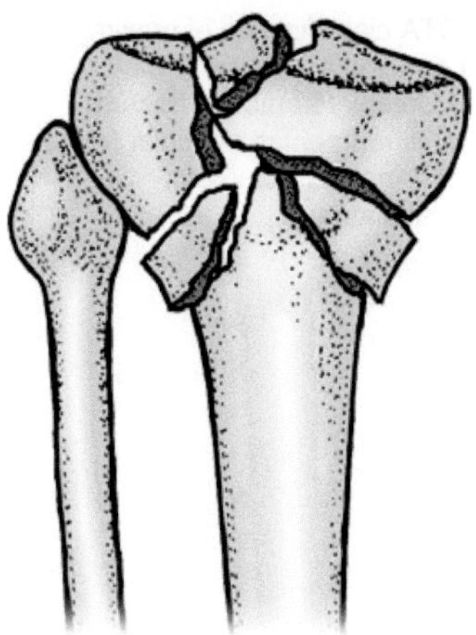

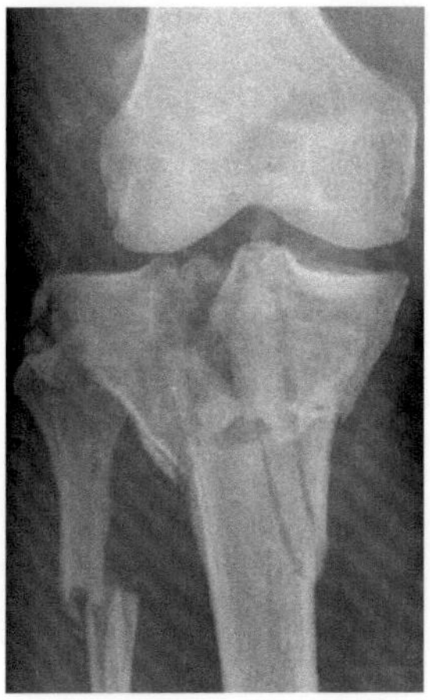

AO/OTA classification of proximal tibia and fibula
41-C Complete articular fracture
C2 Articular simple, metaphyseal multifragmentary fracture:
C2.3 Complex metaphyseal fracture

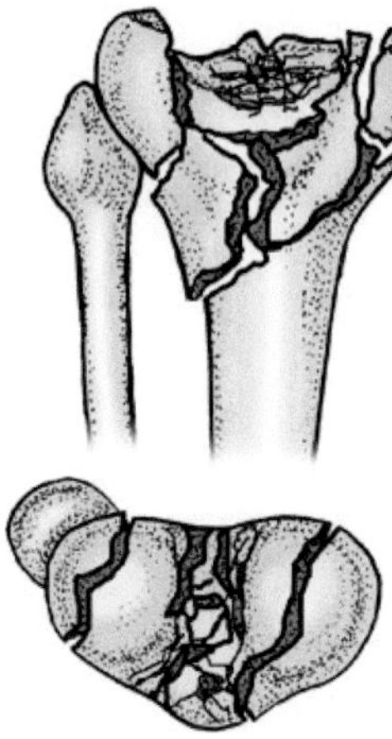

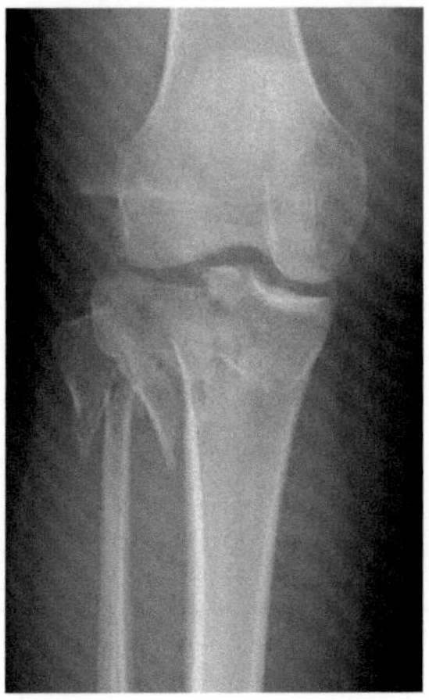

AO/OTA classification of proximal tibia and fibula
41-C Complete articular fracture
C3 Multifragmentary articular fracture:
C3.1 Complex fractures of the lateral plateau

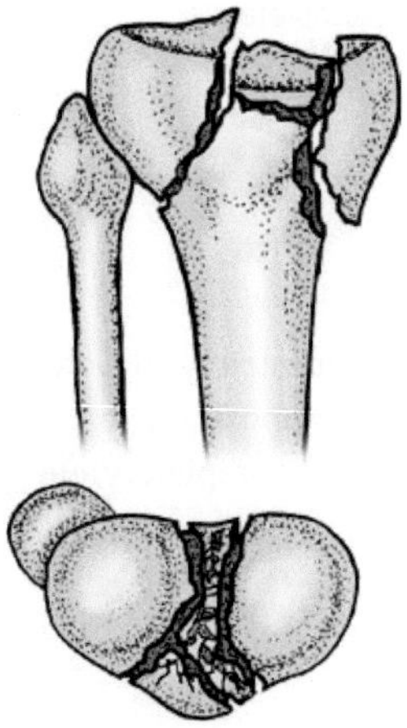

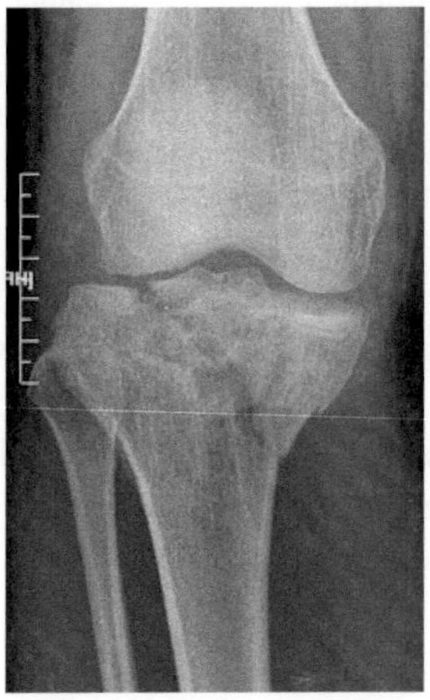

AO/OTA classification of proximal tibia and fibula
41-C Complete articular fracture
C3 Multifragmentary articular fracture:
C3.2 Complex fractures of the medial plateau

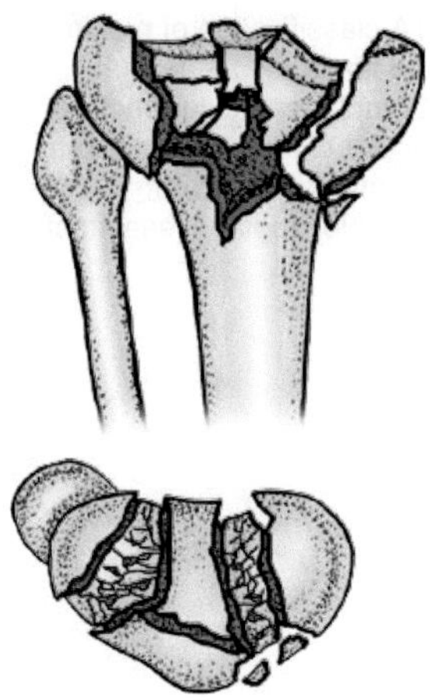

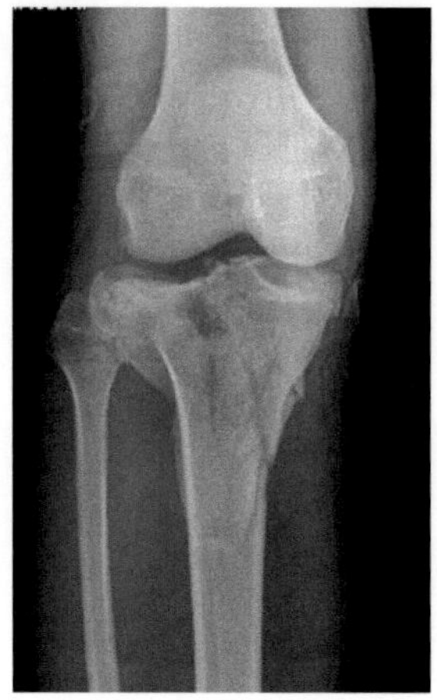

AO/OTA classification of proximal tibia and fibula
41-C Complete articular fracture
C3 Multifragmentary articular fracture:
C3.3 Complex fractures of bilateral plateaus

10.1.3 Meyers Classification (1959, J Bone Joint Surg (Am), 41:209–222)

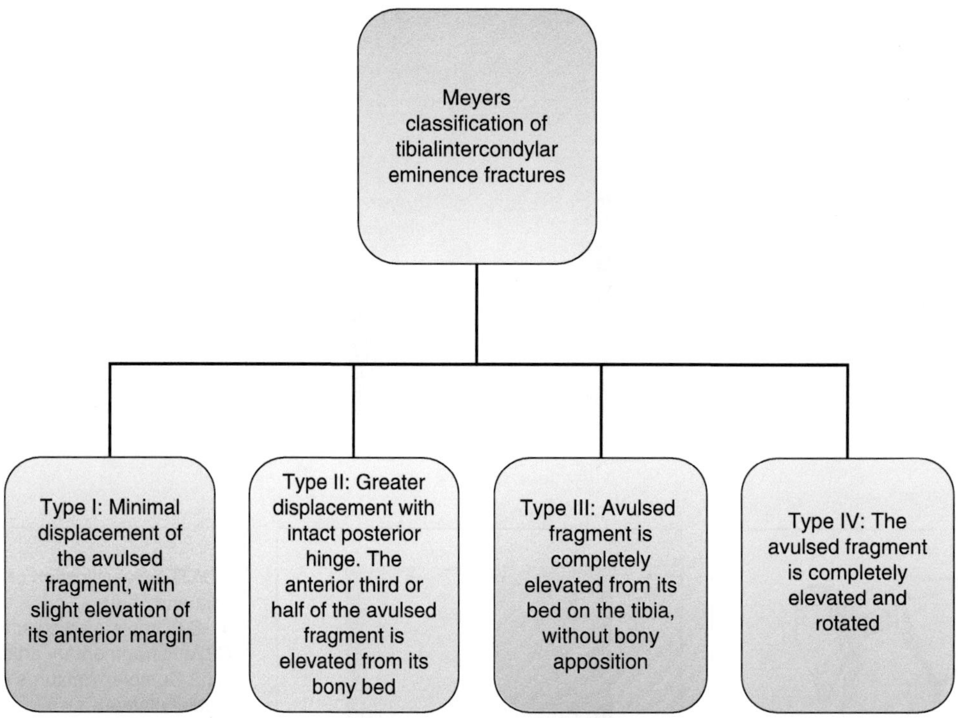

Type I: Minimal displacement of the avulsed fragment, with slight elevation of its anterior margin.

Type II: Greater displacement with intact posterior hinge. The anterior third or half of the avulsed fragment is elevated from its bony bed, producing a beaklike deformity on the lateral radiograph.

Type III: Avulsed fragment is completely elevated from its bed on the tibia, without bony apposition.

Type IV: The avulsed fragment is completely elevated and rotated.

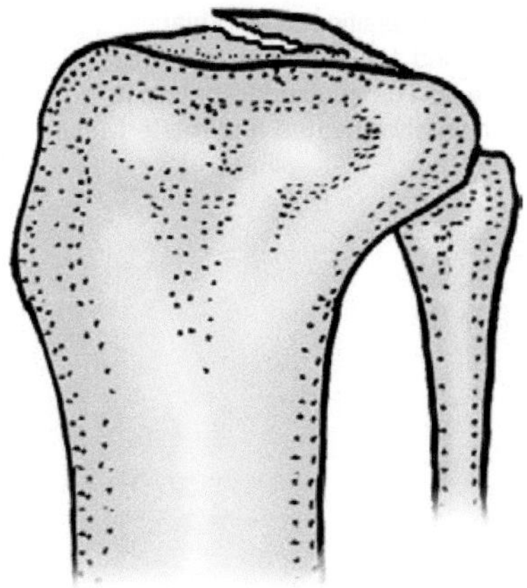

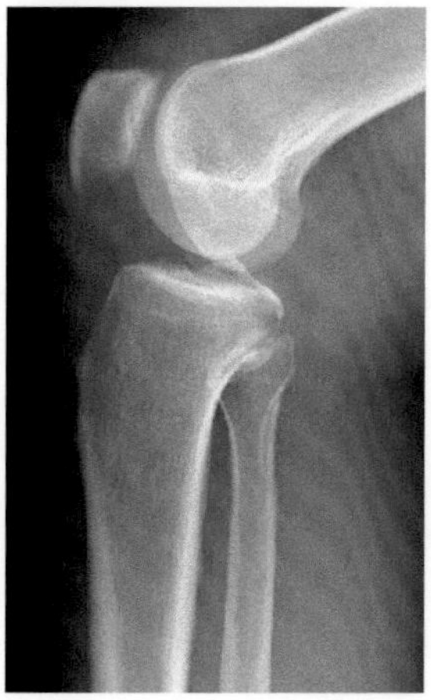

Meyers classification of tibial intercondylar eminence fractures
Type I : Minimal displacement of the avulsed fragment, with slight elevation of its anterior margin

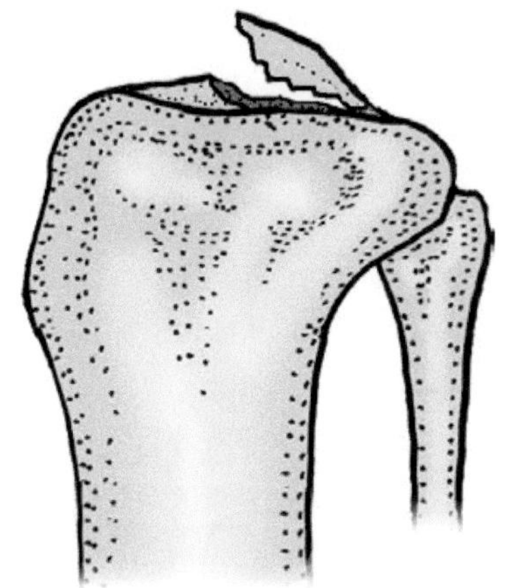

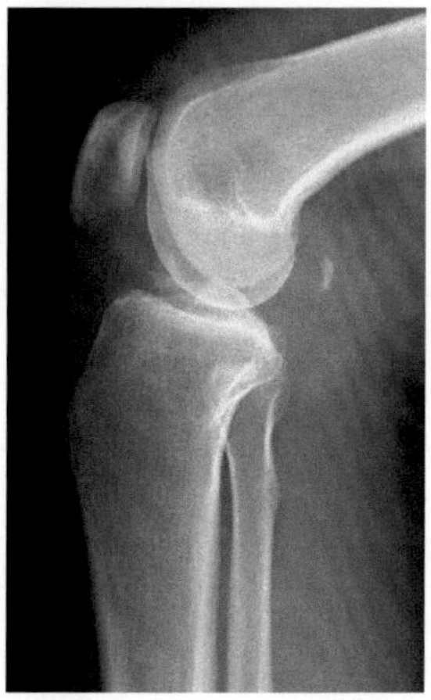

Meyers classification of tibial intercondylar eminence fractures
Type II: Greater displacement with intact posterior hinge. The anterior third or half of the avulsed fragment is elevated from its bony bed, producing a beaklike deformity on the lateral radiograph

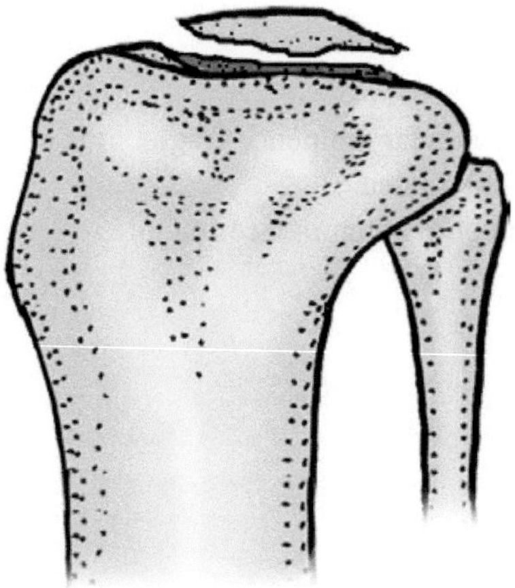

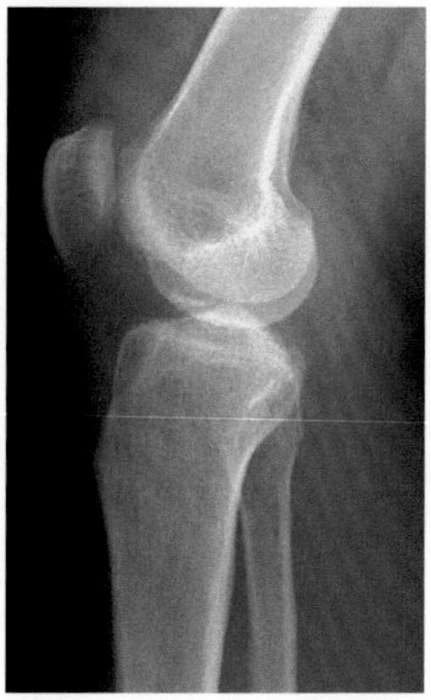

Meyers classification of tibial intercondylar eminence fractures
Type III: Avulsed fragment is completely elevated from its bed on the tibia, without bony apposition

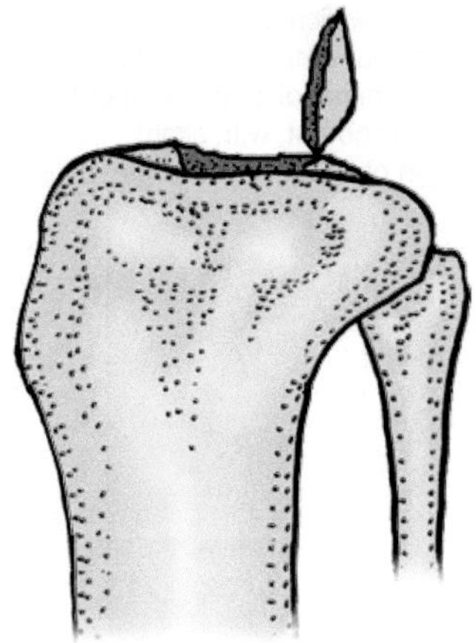

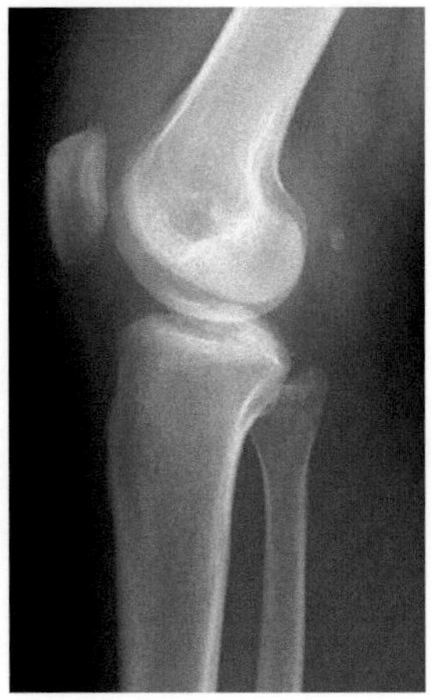

Meyers classification of tibial intercondylar eminence fractures
Type IV: The avulsed fragment is completely elevated and rotated

10.1.4 Meyers-Mckeever-Zaricznyj Classification (1977, J Bone Joint Surg (Am), 59:1111–1114)

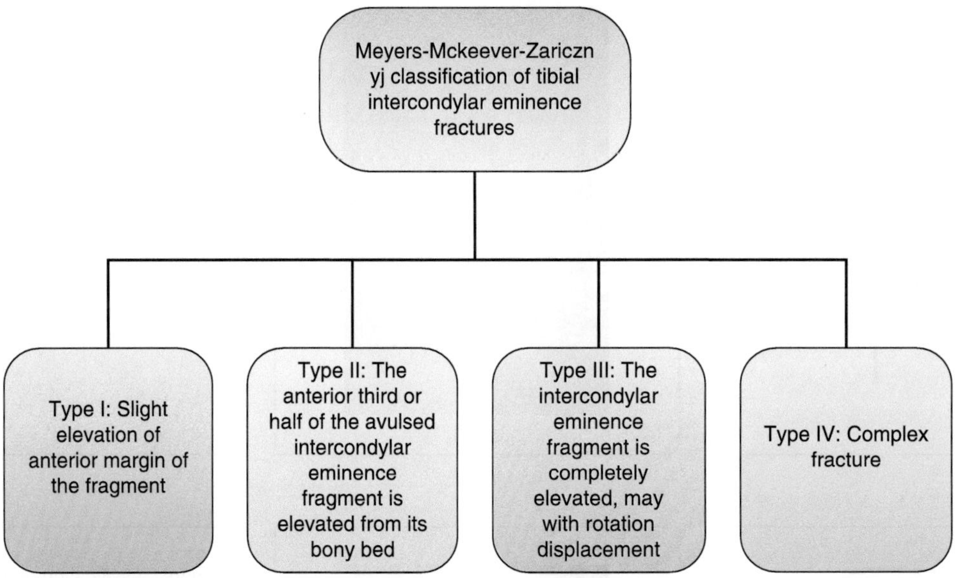

Type I: Slight elevation of anterior margin of the intercondylar eminence fragment.

Type II: The anterior third or half of the avulsed intercondylar eminence fragment is elevated from its bony bed, producing a beaklike deformity on the lateral radiograph.

Type III:

Type IIIa: The intercondylar eminence fragment is completely elevated from its bed on the tibia, without bony apposition.

Type IIIb: The intercondylar eminence fragment is completely elevated and rotated.

Type IV: Complex intercondylar eminence fracture.

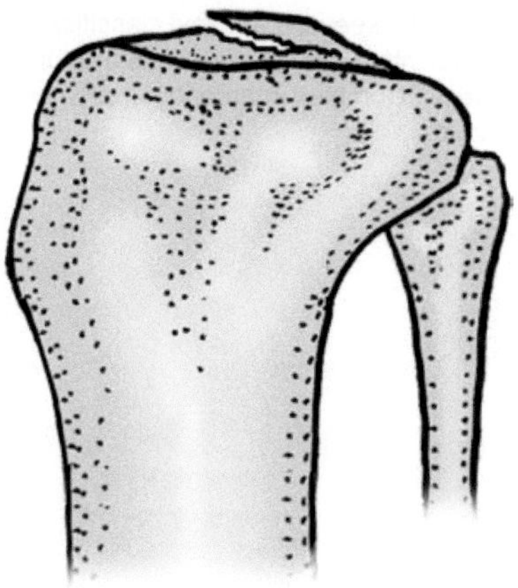

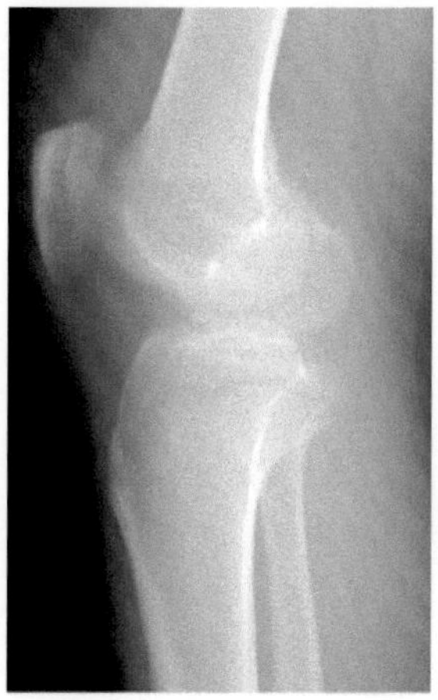

Meyers-Mckeever-Zaricznyj classification of tibial intercondylar eminence fractures
Type I : Slight elevation of anterior margin of the intercondylar eminence fragment

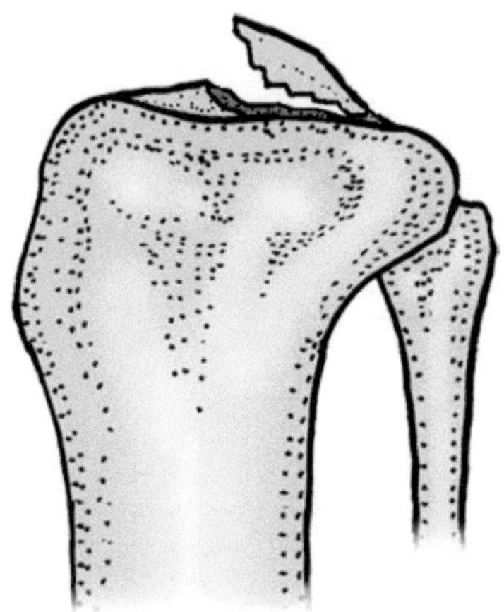

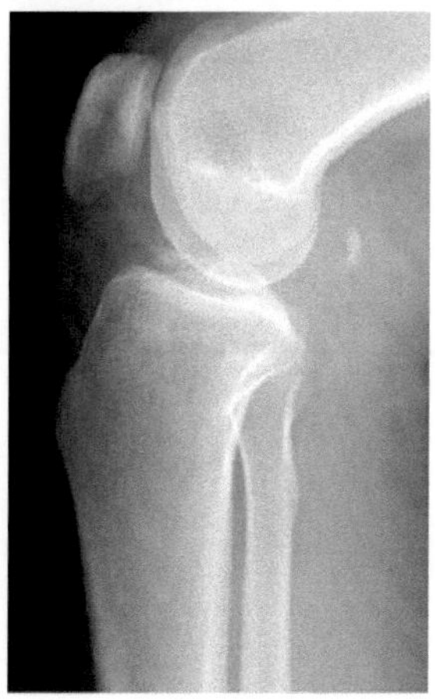

Meyers-Mckeever-Zaricznyj classification of tibial intercondylar eminence fractures
Type II: The anterior third or half of the avulsed intercondylar eminence fragment is elevated from its bony bed, producing a beaklike deformity on the lateral radiograph

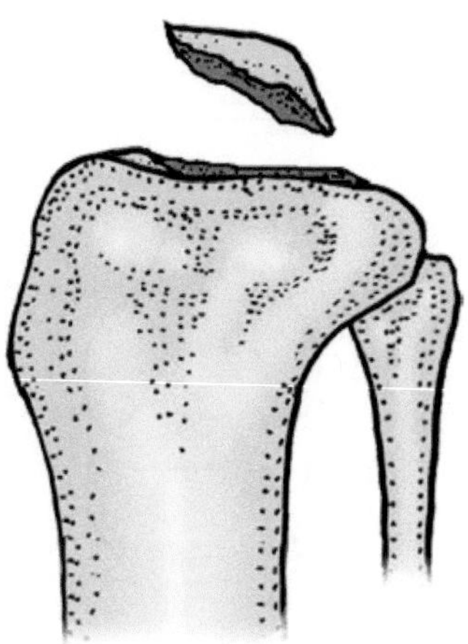

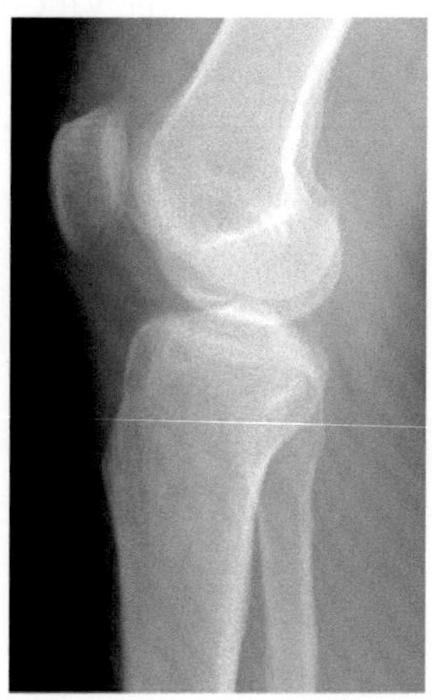

Meyers-Mckeever-Zaricznyj classification of tibial intercondylar eminence fractures
Type III: IIIa The intercondylar eminence fragment is completely elevated from its bed on the tibia, without bony apposition; IIIb The intercondylar eminence fragment is completely elevated and rotated

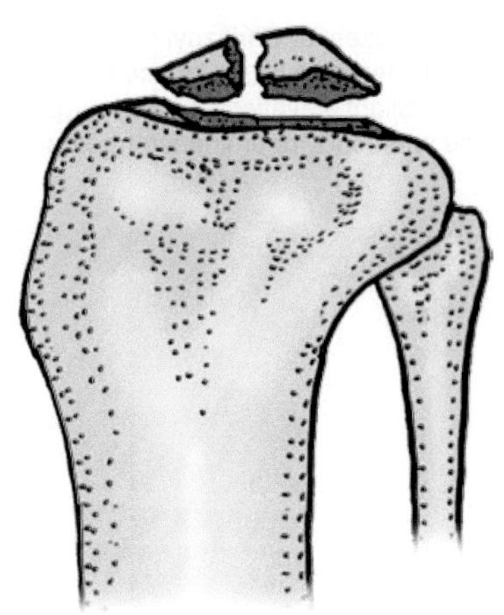

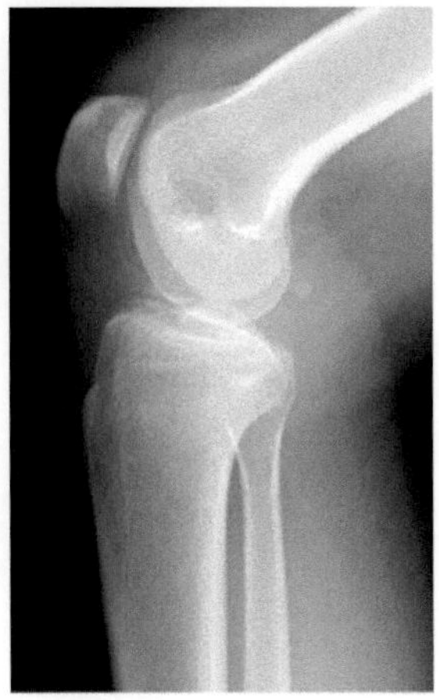

Meyers-Mckeever-Zaricznyj classification of tibial intercondylar eminence fractures
Type IV : Complex intercondylar eminence fracture

10.1.5 Hohl Classification (1967, J Bone Joint Surg (Am), 49:1455–1467)

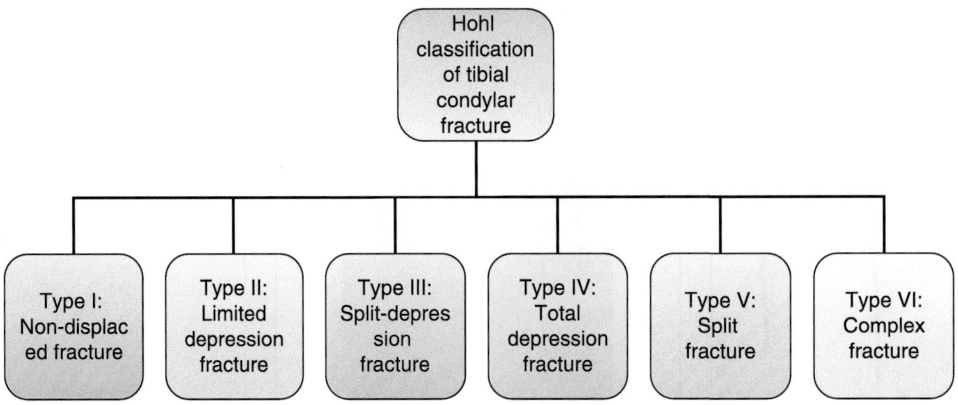

Hohl classification categorized the tibial intercondylar eminence fractures into six types:

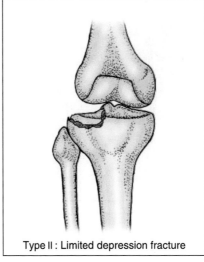

Type I: Non-displaced fracture
Type II: Limited depression fracture
Type III: Split-depression fracture
Type IV: Total depression fracture
Type V: Split fracture
Type VI: Complex fracture

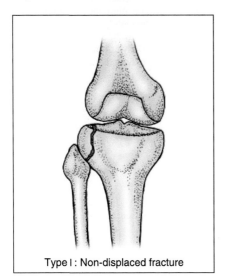

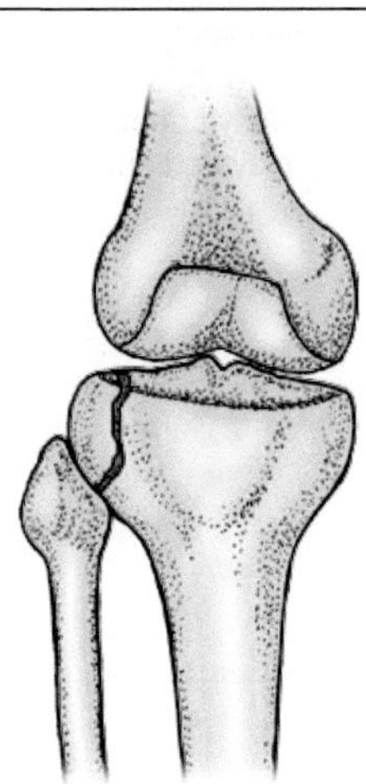

Type I : Non-displaced fracture

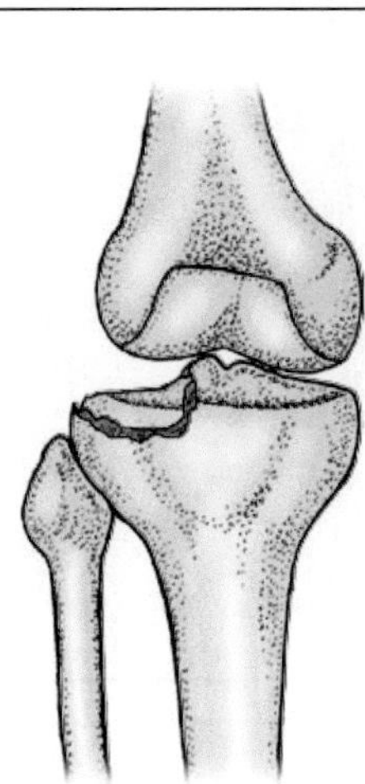

Type II : Limited depression fracture

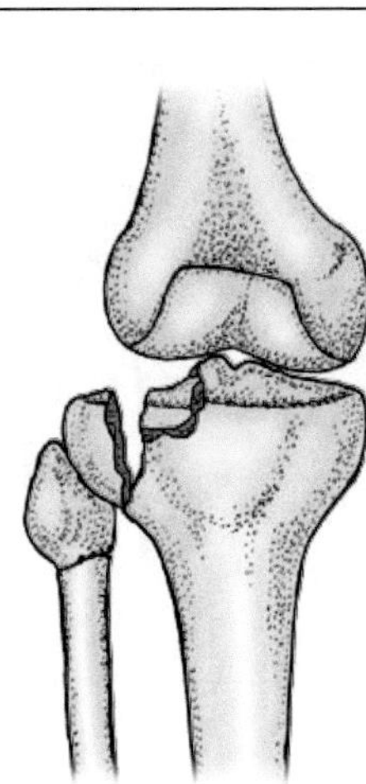

Type III : Split-depression fracture

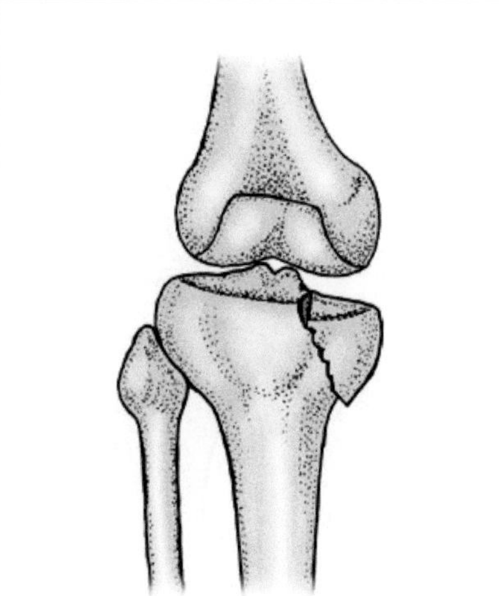

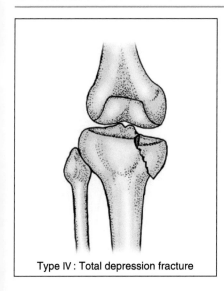

Type IV : Total depression fracture

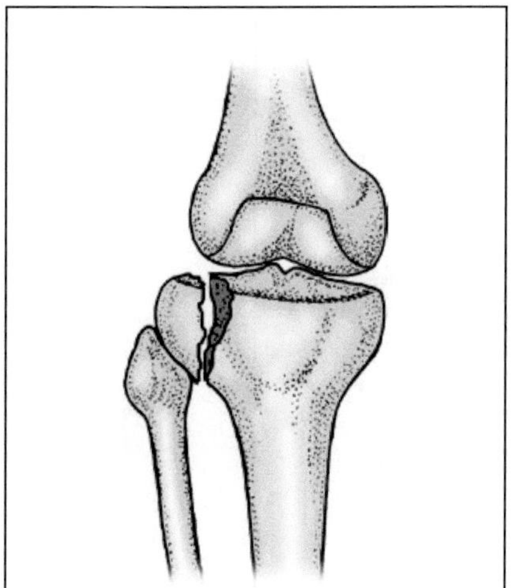

Type V : Split fracture

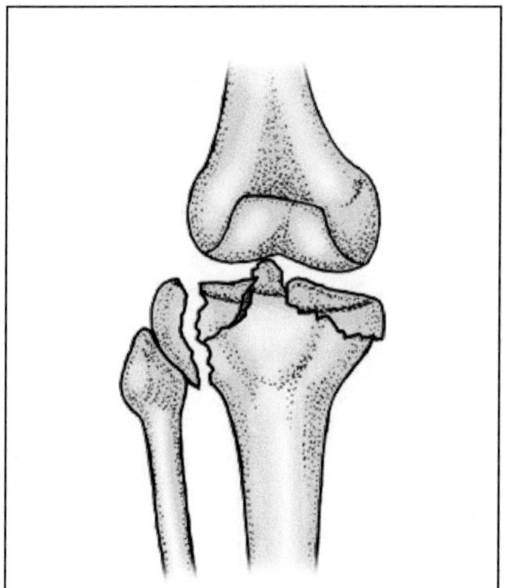

Type VI : Complex fracture

10.1.6 Modified Hohl Classification (1991, Fractures in Adults. 3rd. Philadelphia: J B Lippincott)

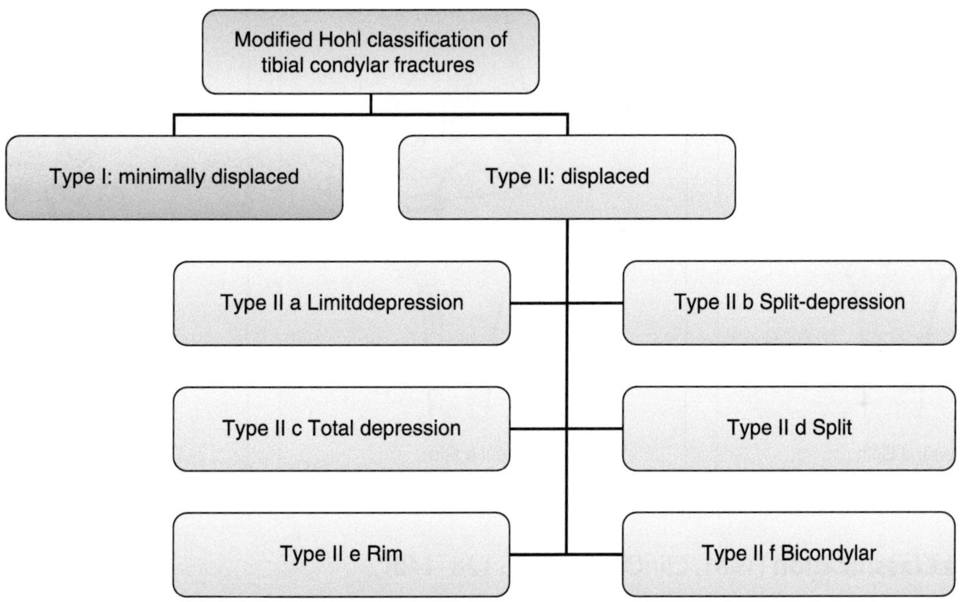

Hohl modified his classification with combination of the Moore classification and categorized tibial condylar fractures into the following types:

Type I: Minimally displaced fracture, with plateau depression or displacement no more than 4 mm.

Type II: Displaced fracture. This type is subdivided into:

- Type IIa: Limited depression.
- Type IIb: Split depression.
- Type IIc: Total depression.
- Type IId: Split.
- Type IIe: Rim (including rim avulsion subtype and rim depression subtype).
- Type IIf: Bicondylar fracture.

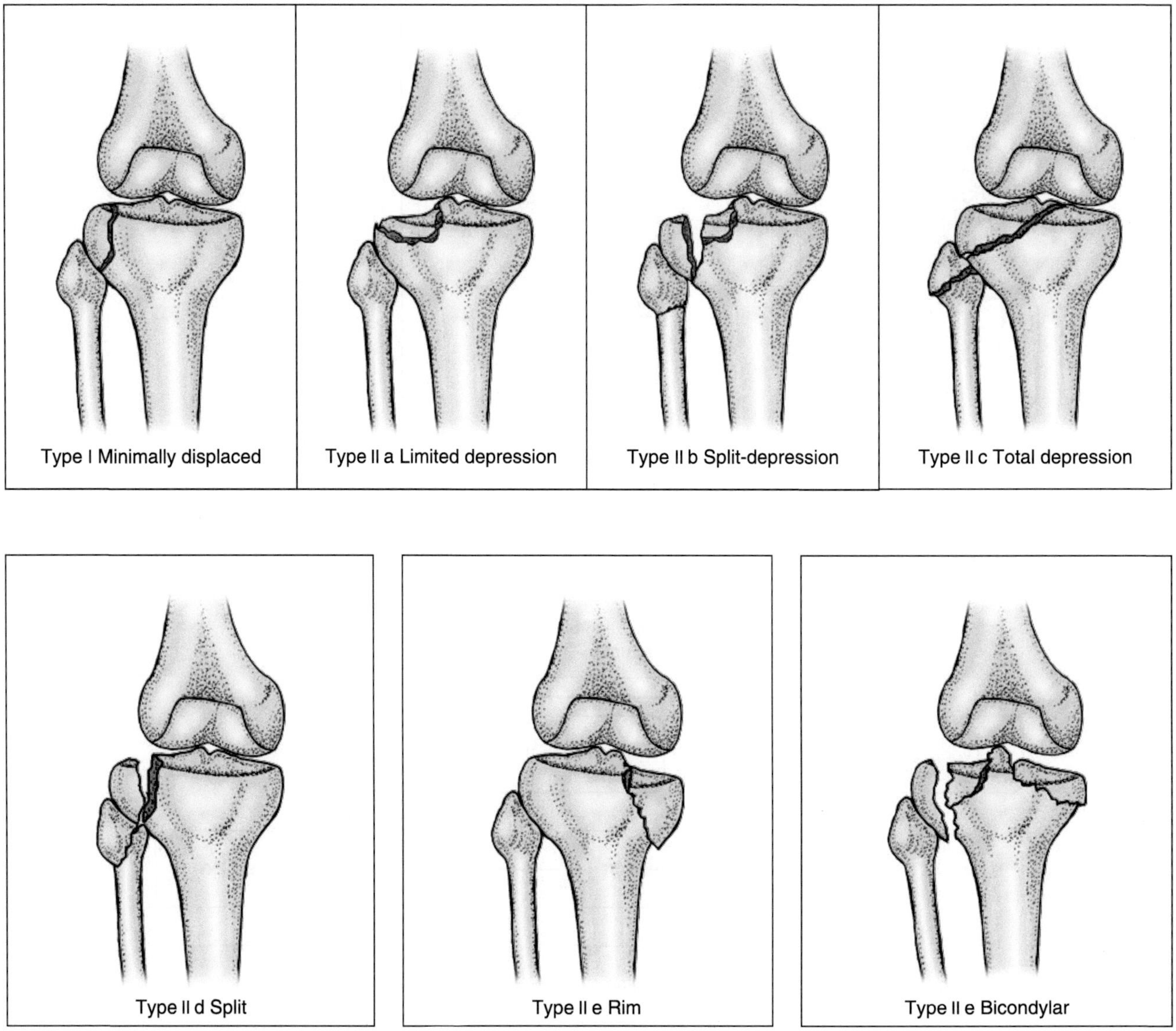

10.1.7 Moore Classification (1981, ClinOrthop, 156:128–140)

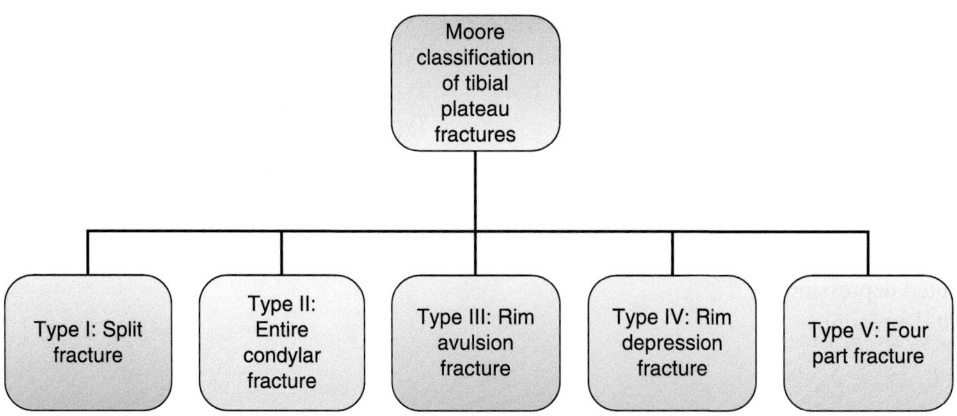

This classification system includes five groups:

Type I: Split fracture.
Type II: Entire condylar fracture.
Type III: Rim avulsion fracture.
Type IV: Rim depression fracture.
Type V: Four-part fracture.

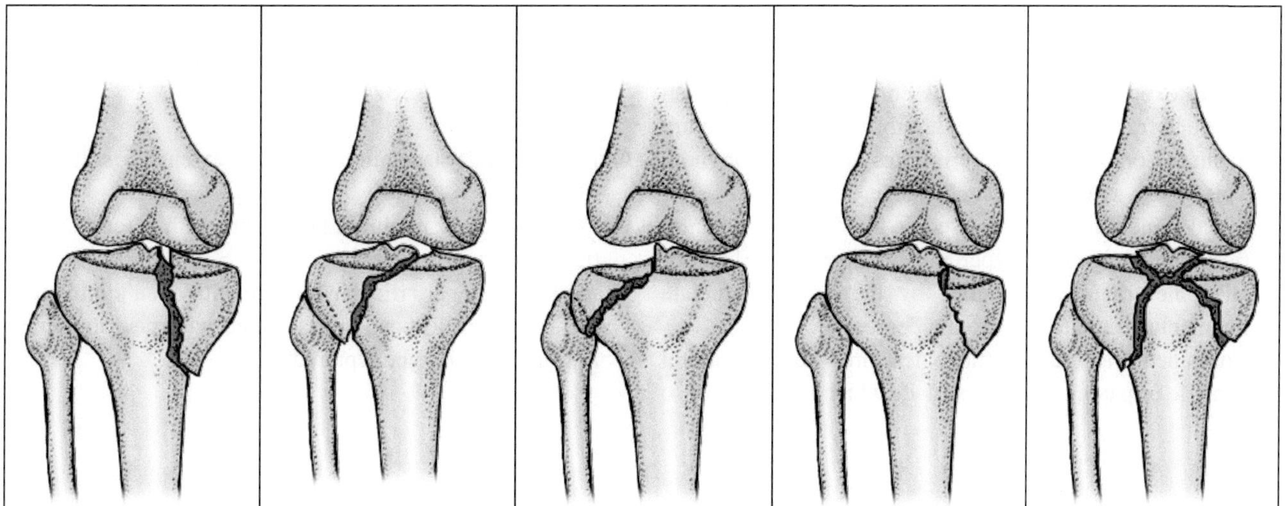

Type I: Split fracture | Type II: Entire condylar fracture | Type III: Rim avulsion fracture | Type IV: Rim depression fracture | Type V: Four part fracture

10.1.8 **Khan Classification** (2000, Clin Orthop Relat Res, 375:231)

Khan et al. devised a comprehensive classification of the tibial plateau fracture, using contemporary classifications as a database. They grouped these fractures alphanumerically as lateral (L), medial (M), posterior (P), anterior (A), rim (R), bicondylar (B), and subcondylar (S), and proposed subtypes.

10.1.9 **Modified Schatzker Classification by Honkonen-Jarvinen** (1992, J Bone Joint Surg (Br), 74:840–847)

Honkonen and Jarvinen have modified Schatzker classification to take residual angulation into account. They divided type VI fractures into two types: VIA medially tilted and VIB laterally tilted.

10.1.10 **Luo CF Classification** (2008)

A group of Chinese surgeons have proposed a three-column classification of tibial plateau fractures based on the findings of CT. On transverse CT imaging at the level of the tip of the fibula head, the midpoint of the two tibial spines was defined as the focal point (point O). The most anterior part of the tibial tuberosity, medial-posterior ridge of the tibial plateau, and most anterior point of the fibular head were defined as points A, B, and C, respectively. The tibial plateau was separated by lines OA, OB, and OC into three columns: anterolateral, anteromedial, and posterior. They suggested to use this new system as a helpful tool for surgical planning.

10.1.11 **Arthroscopic Classification** (2001)

The arthroscopic classification of tibial plateau fractures proposed by Hou XK et al. included the following types:

1. Linear crack: The crack of tibial plateau cartilage may extend to the subchondral bone. The probe can't be inserted into the slit.
2. Peripheral fracture: The fracture line usually is located beneath the meniscus, which is only visualized after elevating the meniscus by probe. This type of fracture is non-displaced and thus difficult to be discovered on X-ray film.
3. Fissure: This type mostly is split fracture on X-ray, with broad fracture line that is deep into cancellous bone. The edge of the cartilage fissure is ragged and uneven, occasionally having small cartilage fragments. It is easy to insert the probe into the split.

4. Depression: The cartilage fragment is depressed along with the bone fragment, forming a pit involving the weight-bearing area. Sometimes the probe is not able to reach its bottom. The cartilage fragment is one-piece or slightly cracked.
5. Split depression: The characteristics of split pattern and depression pattern are coexisting.
6. Complex fracture: The tibial plateau fracture is comminuted, exposing the cancellous bone. The gap between the bone fragments is filled with fibrin clot. Concomitant meniscus or other structure injuries are quite common. This type is a management challenge.
7. Tibial spine fracture: Arthroscopic findings include anterior cruciate ligament hyperemia and loosening. The tibial spine fragment is pulled by the anterior cruciate ligament and rotated to varying degrees.
8. Combined fracture: Cartilage fractures at the femoral condyle or patella articular surface which is reciprocal to the tibial plateau fracture site are observed arthroscopically in minority cases, due to complicated injury mechanism. The lesions are shallow and indiscoverable on plain X-rays.

10.1.12 Collins-Temple Classification of Open Knee Injuries (1988, Clin Orthop, 243:384–387)

Grade I: Single laceration, without extensive soft-tissue injury.

Grade II: Single or multiple laceration, with extensive soft-tissue injury or defect.

Grade III: Open periarticular fracture with open joint injury.

Grade IV: Open dislocation associated with neuromuscular injuries needed to be repaired.

10.2 Tibial and Fibular Shaft Fractures

Our review of the literature for the last 5 years regarding fractures of the tibial and fibular shafts revealed that the AO/OTA classification system had been the most commonly used classification, followed by the anatomic classification among the ~10 classification systems that we searched

10.2.1 AO/OTA Classification System (2007, Journal of Orthopaedic Trauma. 21 supplement; the AO classification of long bone fractures was initially proposed by Muller in 1980s and modified in 2007)

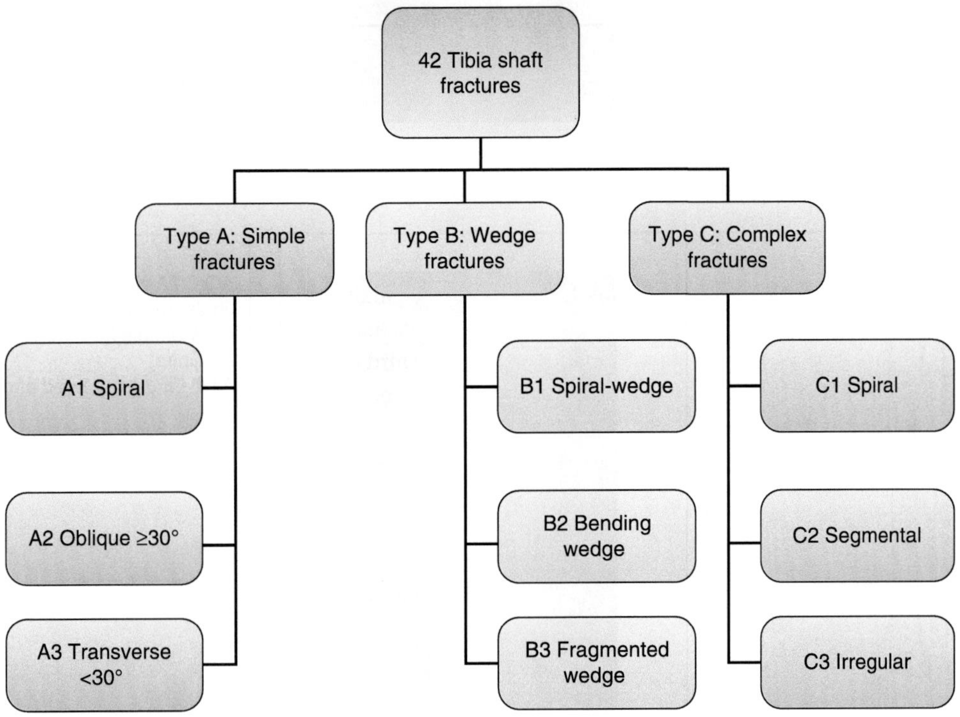

Type A: Simple fracture:
- Type A1: Spiral:
  - Type A1.1: Intact fibula.
  - Type A1.2: Fibula fractured at different level.
  - Type A1.3: Fibula fractured at same level.
- Type A2: Oblique (≥30°):
  - Type A2.1: Intact fibula.
  - Type A2.2: Fibula fractured at different level.
  - Type A2.3: Fibula fractured at same level.
- Type A3: Transverse (<30°):
  - Type A3.1: Intact fibula.
  - Type A3.2: Fibula fractured at different level.
  - Type A3.3: Fibula fractured at same level.

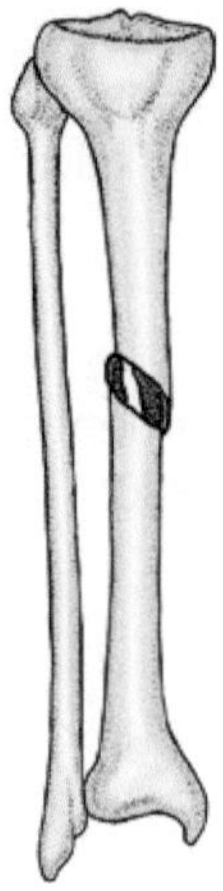

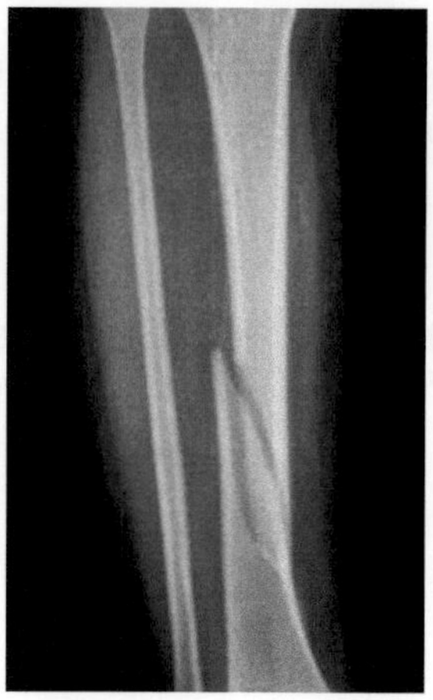

AO/OTA classification of tibia and fibula fractures
42- A Simple fracture
A1 Spiral
A1.1 Intact fibula

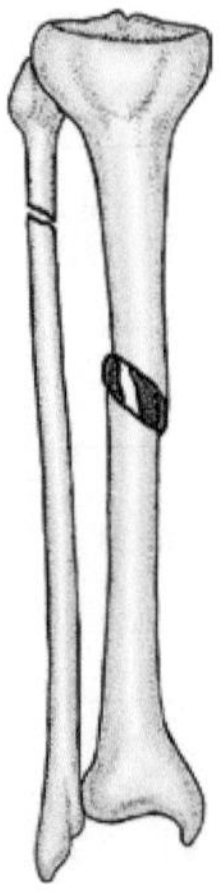

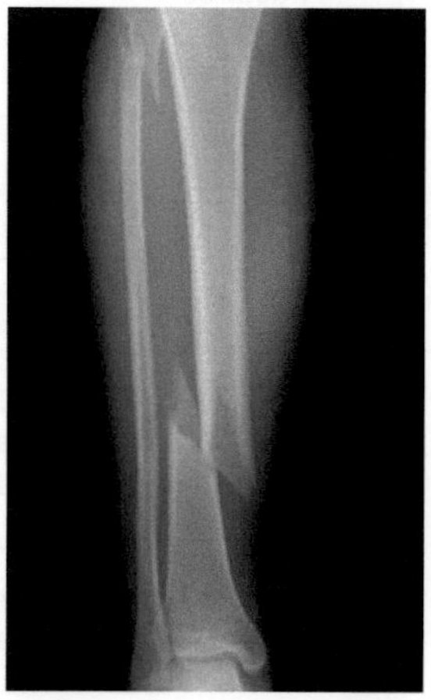

AO/OTA classification of tibia and fibula fractures
42-A Simple fracture
A1 Spiral
A1.2 Fibula fractured at different level

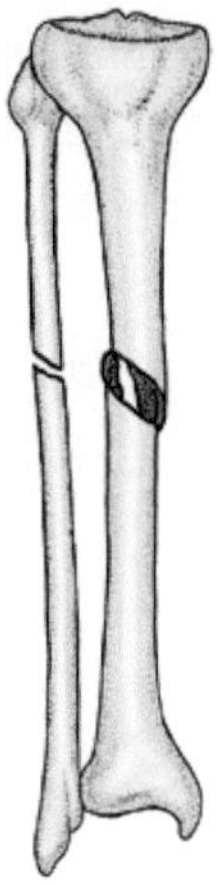

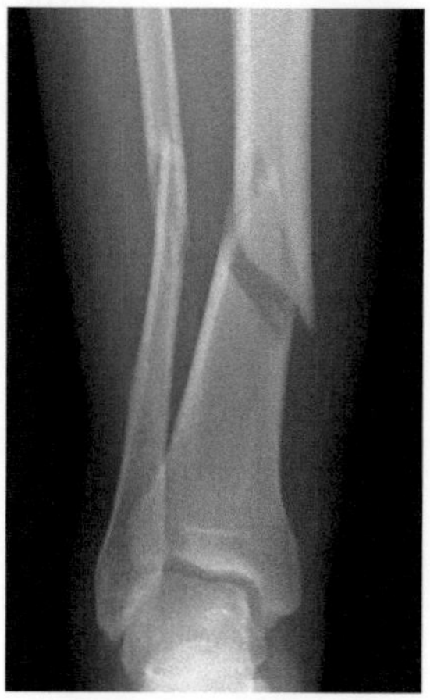

AO/OTA classification of tibia and fibula fractures
42-A Simple fracture
A1 Spiral
A1.3 Fibula fractured at same level

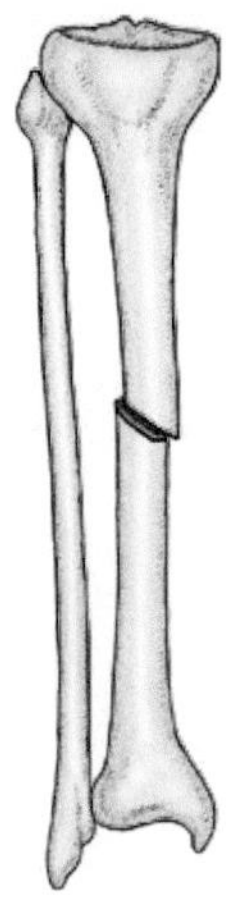

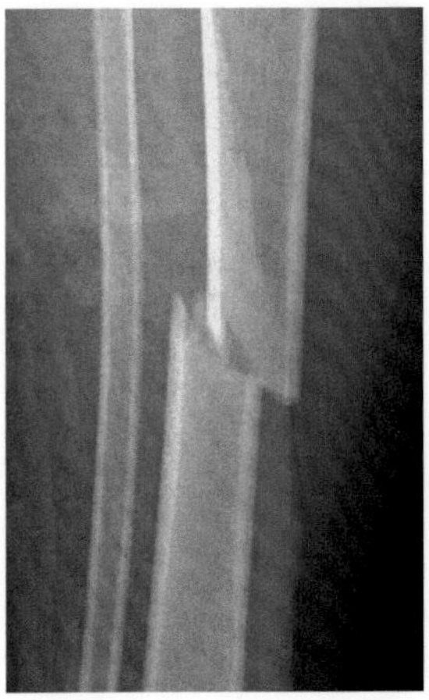

AO/OTA classification of tibia and fibula fractures
42-A Simple fracture
A2 Oblique (≥30°)
A2.1 Intact fibula

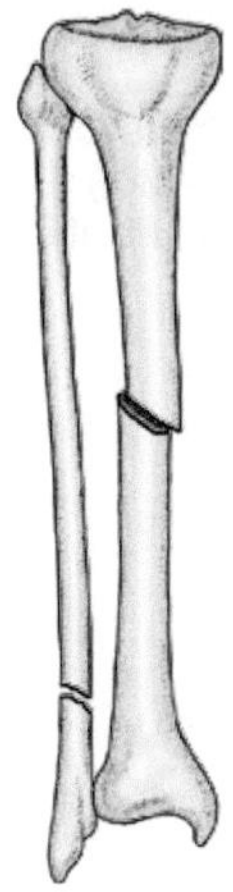

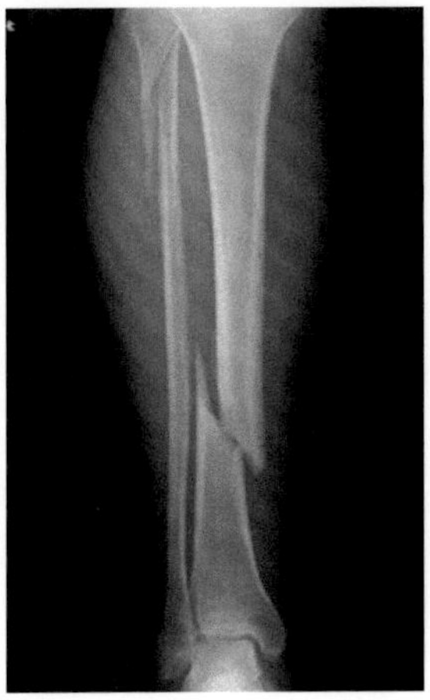

AO/OTA classification of tibia and fibula fractures
42-A Simple fracture
A2 Oblique (≥30°)
A2.2 Fibula fractured at different level

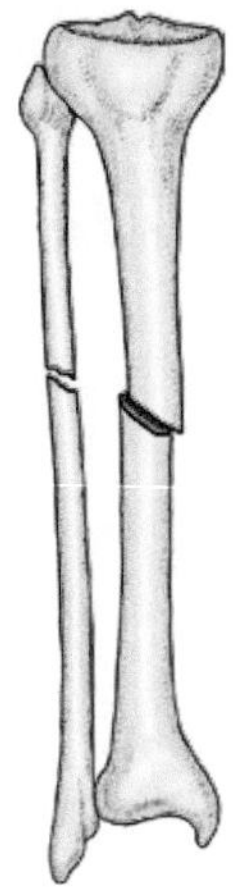

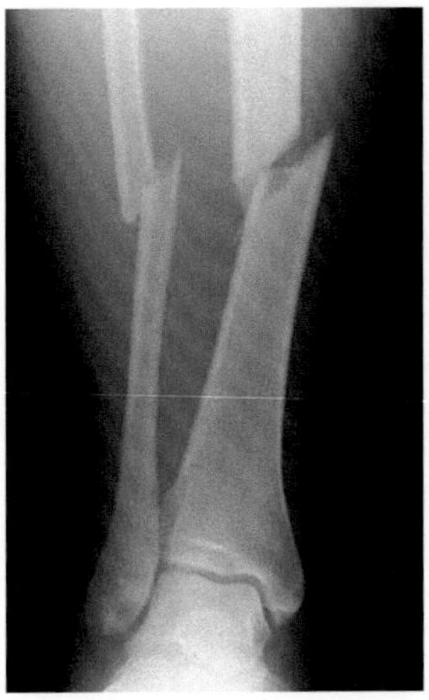

AO/OTA classification of tibia and fibula fractures
42-A Simple fracture
A2 Oblique (≥30°)
A2.3 Fibula fractured at same level

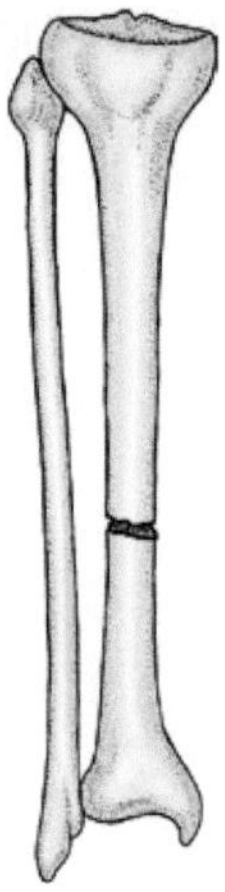

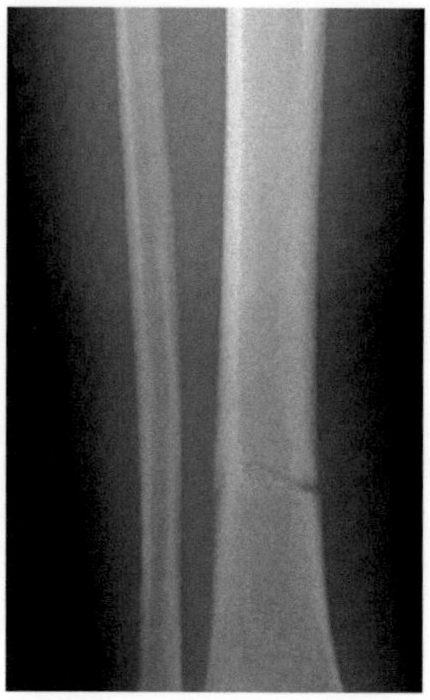

AO/OTA classification of tibia and fibula fractures
42-A Simple fracture
A3 Transverse (<30°)
A3.1 Intact fibula

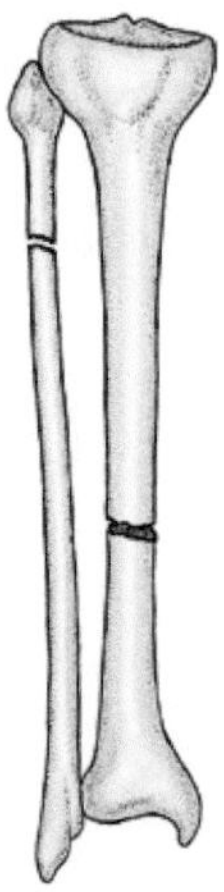

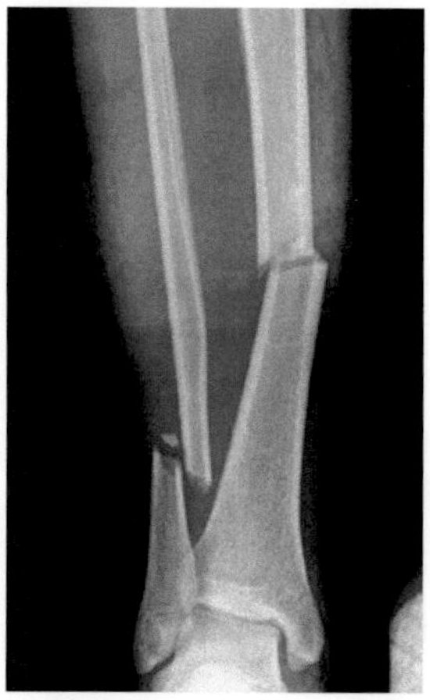

AO/OTA classification of tibia and fibula fractures
42-A Simple fracture
A3 Transverse (<30°)
A3.2 Fibula fractured at different level

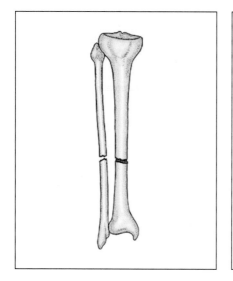

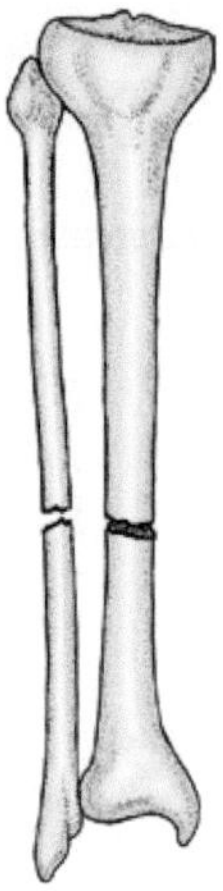

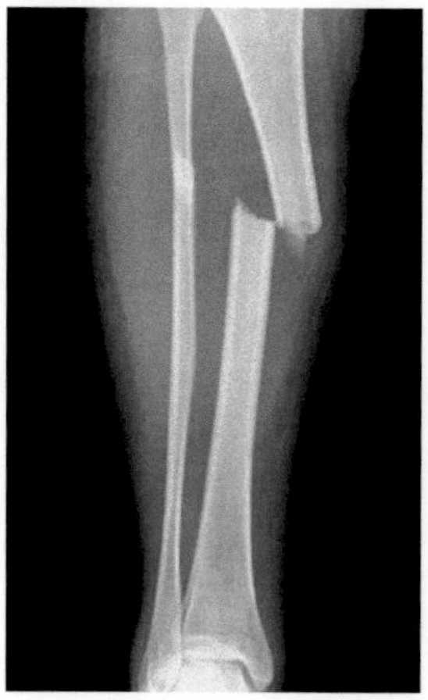

AO/OTA classification of tibia and fibula fractures
42-A Simple fracture
A3 Transverse (<30°)
A3.3 Fibula Fractured at same level

Type B: Wedge fracture:
- Type B1: Spiral wedge:
  - Type B1.1: Intact fibula.
  - Type B1.2: Fibula fractured at different level.
  - Type B1.3: Fibula fractured at same level.
- Type B2: Bending wedge:
  - Type B2.1: Intact fibula.
  - Type B2.2: Fibula fractured at different level.
  - Type B2.3: Fibula fractured at same level.
- Type B3: Fragmented wedge:
  - Type B3.1: Intact fibula.
  - Type B3.2: Fibula fractured at different level.
  - Type B3.3: Fibula fractured at same level.

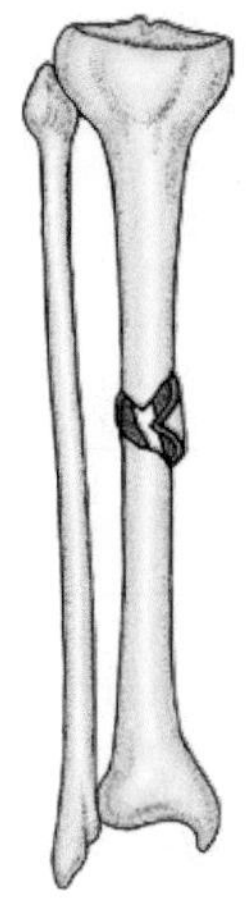

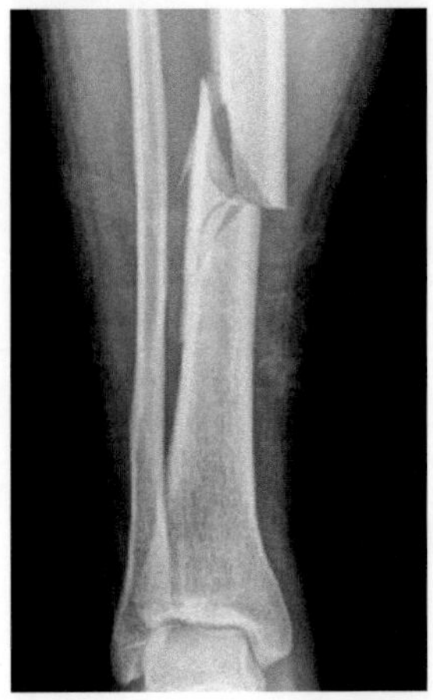

AO/OTA classification of tibia and fibula fractures
42-B Wedge fracture
B1 Spiral wedge
B1.1 Intact fibula

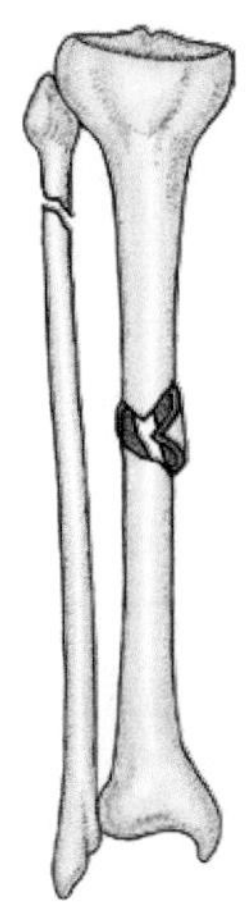

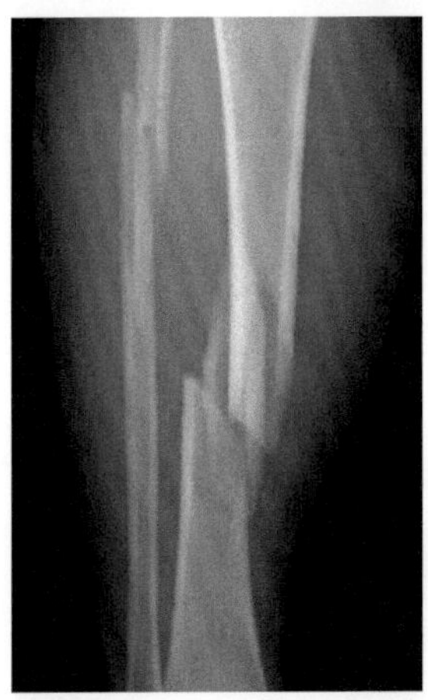

AO/OTA classification of tibia and fibula fractures
42-B Wedge fracture
B1 Spiral wedge
B1.2 Fibula fractured at different levels

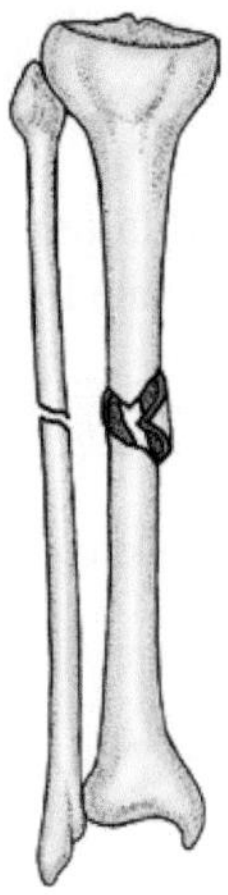

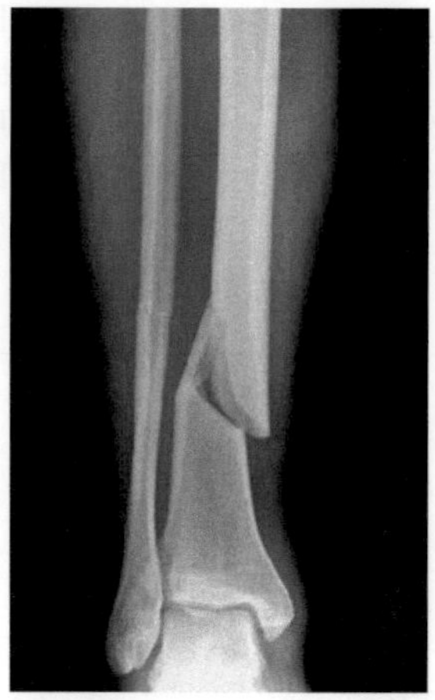

AO/OTA classification of tibia and fibula fractures
42-B Wedge fracture
B1 Spiral wedge
B1.3 Fibula fractured at same level

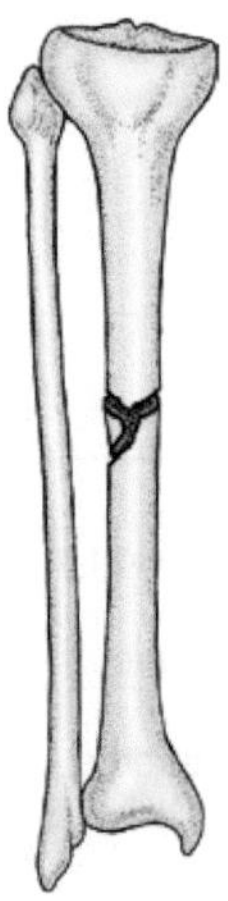

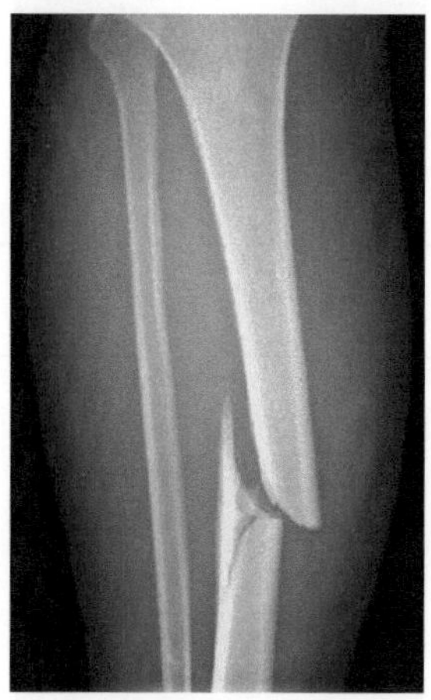

AO/OTA classification of tibia and fibula fractures
42-B Wedge fracture
B2 Bending wedge
B2.1 Intact fibula

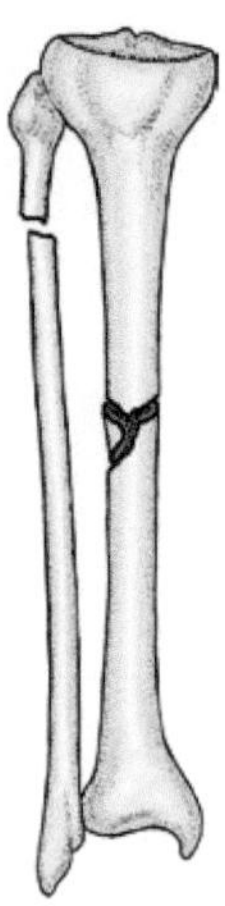

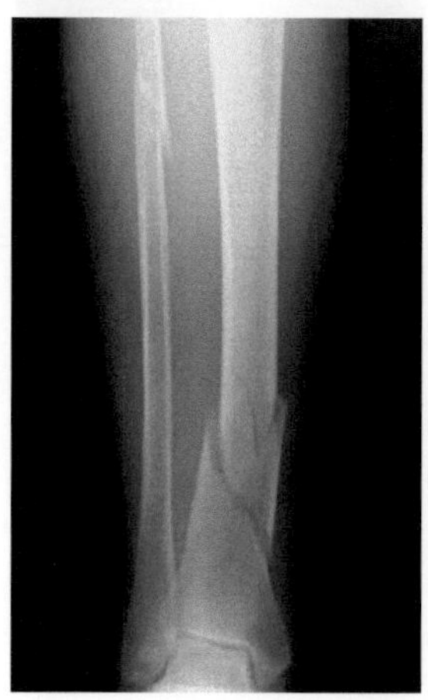

AO/OTA classification of tibia and fibula fractures
42-B Wedge fracture
B2 Bending wedge
B2.2 Fibula fractured at different levels

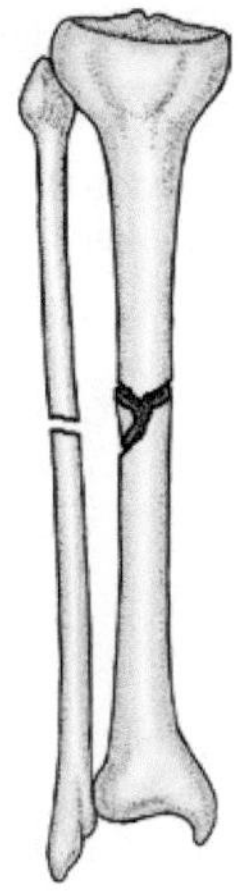

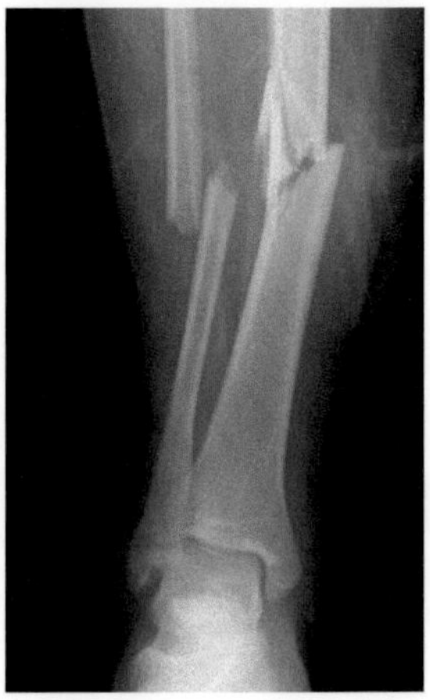

AO/OTA classification of tibia and fibula fractures
42-B Wedge fracture
B2 Bending wedge
B2.3 Fibula fractured at same level

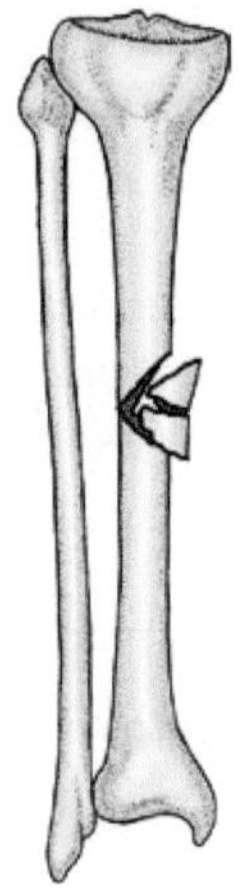

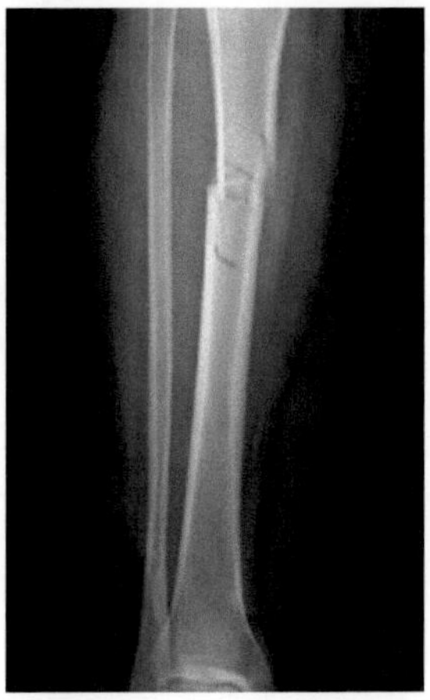

AO/OTA classification of tibia and fibula fractures
42-B Wedge fracture
B3 Fragmented wedge B3.1 intact fibula

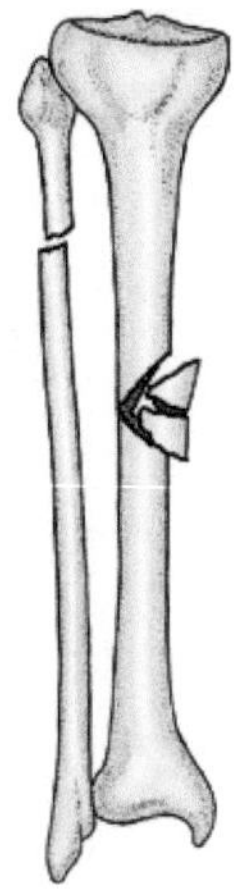

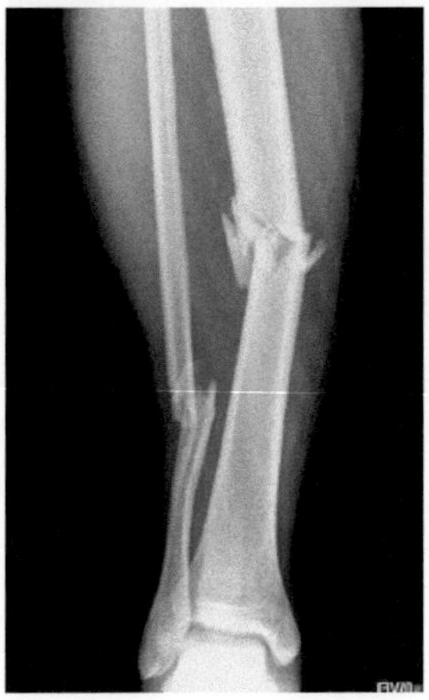

AO/OTA classification of tibia and fibula fractures
42-B Wedge fracture
B3 Fragmented wedge B3.2 fibula fractured at different levels

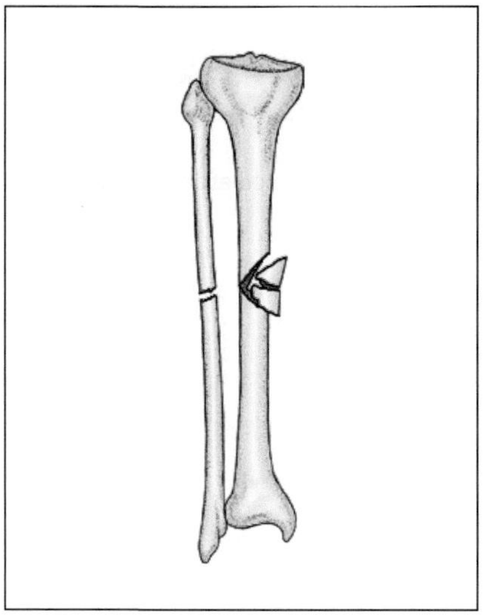

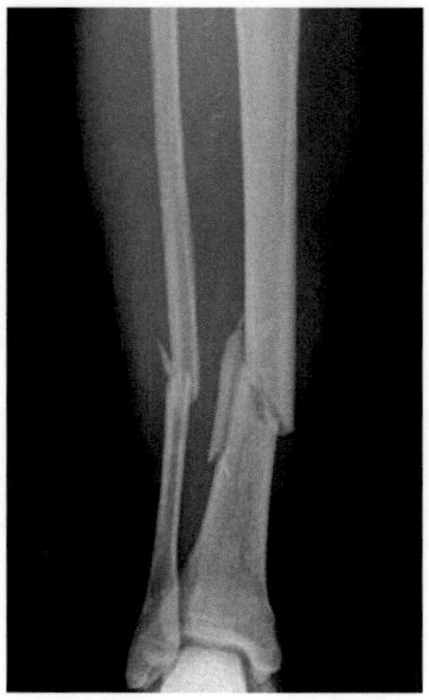

AO/OTA classification of tibia and fibula fractures
42-B Wedge fracture
B3 Fragmented wedge B3.3 fibula fractured at same level

Type C: Complex fracture, having multi fragmentary intermediate zone between intact proximal and distal segments:

- Type C1: Spiral fracture:
  - Type C1.1: With two intermediate fragments.
  - Type C1.2: With three intermediate fragments.
  - Type C1.3: With more than three intermediate fragments.
- Type C2: Segmental fracture:
  - Type C2.1: With an intermediate segmental fragment.
  - Type C2.2: With an intermediate segmental fragment and additional wedge fragment(s).
  - Type C2.3: With 2 or more intermediate segmental fragments.
- Type C3: Irregular fracture:
  - Type C3.1: With two or three intermediate fragments.
  - Type C3.2: Limited shattering (<4 cm).
  - Type C3.3: Extensive shattering (≥4 cm).

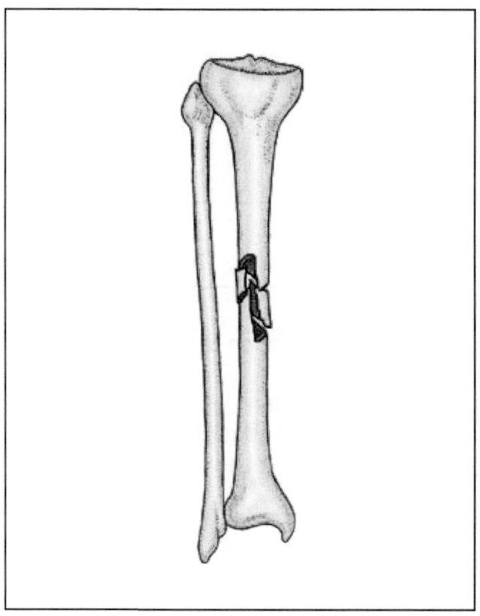

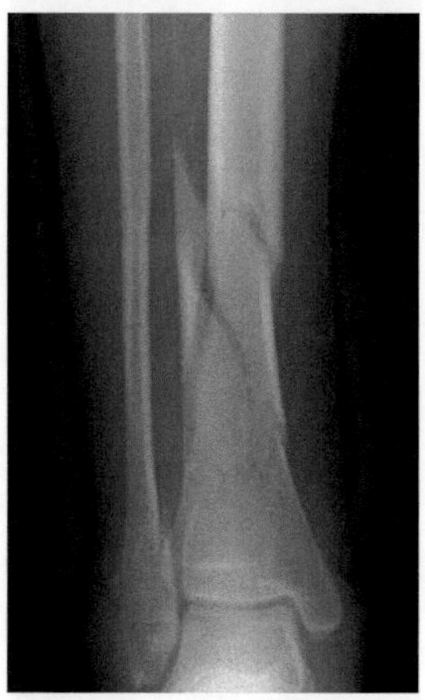

AO/OTA classification of tibia and fibula fractures
42-C Complex fracture
C1 Spiral fracture
C1.1 With 2 intermediate fragments

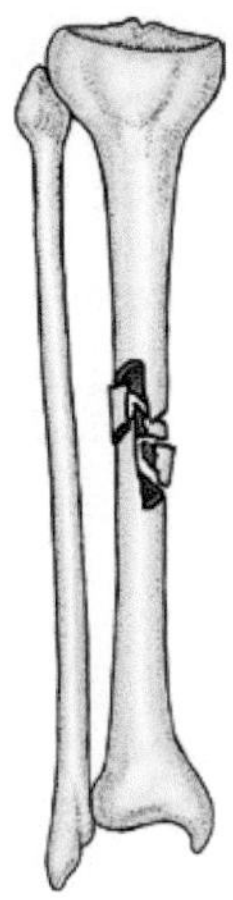

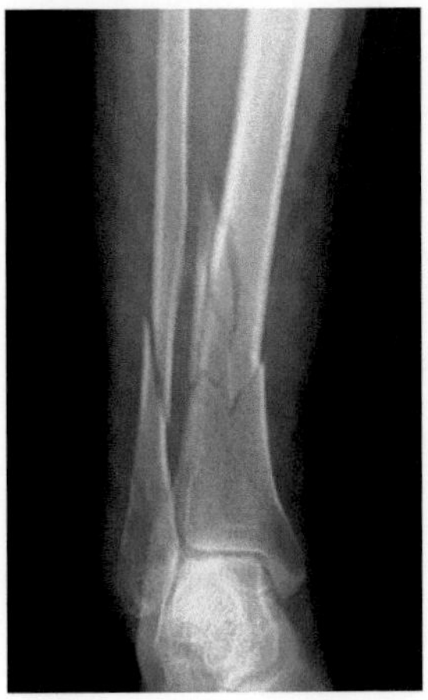

AO/OTA classification of tibia and fibula fractures
42-C Complex fracture
C1 Spiral fracture
C1.2 With 3 intermediate fragments

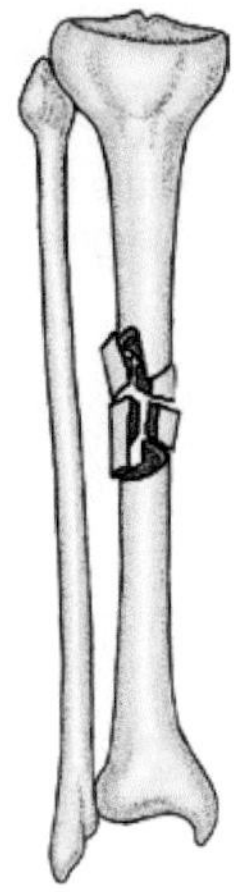

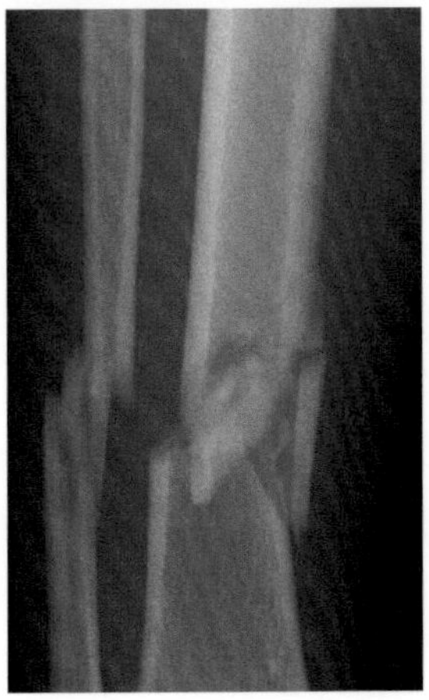

AO/OTA classification of tibia and fibula fractures
42-C Complex fracture
C1 Spiral fracture
C1.3 With more than 3 intermediate fragments

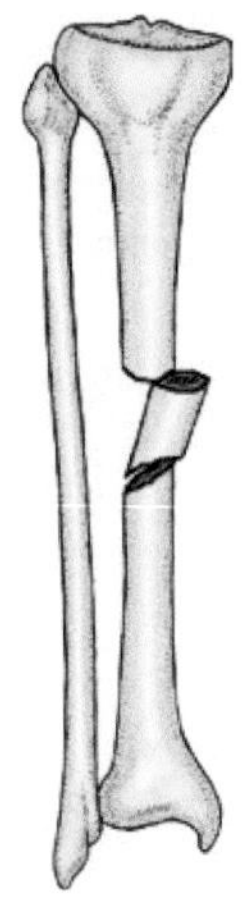

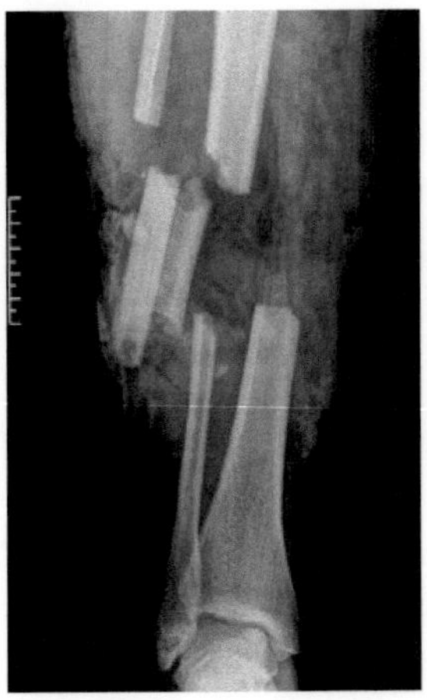

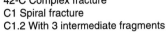

AO/OTA classification of tibia and fibula fractures
42-C Complex fracture
C2 Segmental fracture C2.1 with an intermediate segmental fragment

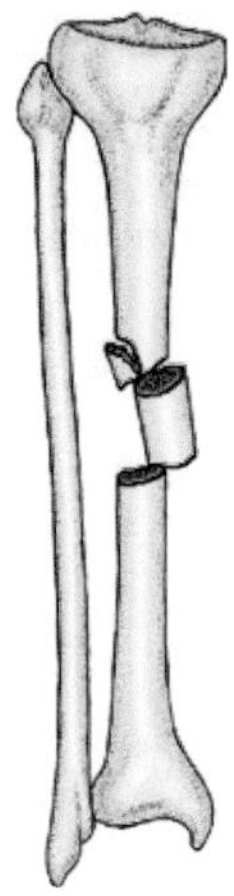

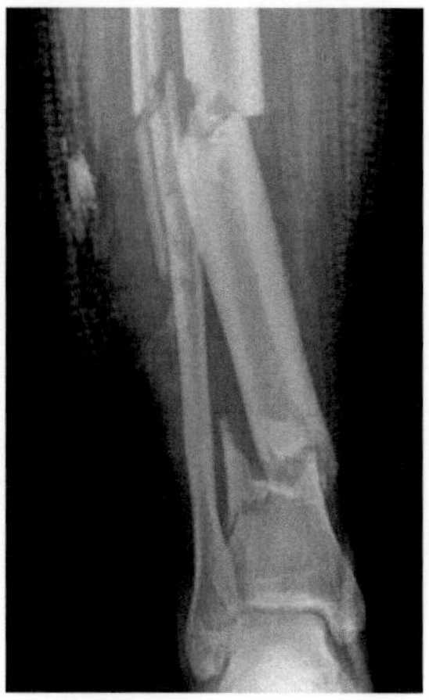

AO/OTA classification of tibia and fibula fractures
42-C Complex fracture
C2 Segmental fracture C2.2 with an intermediate segmental fragment and additional wedge fragment(s)

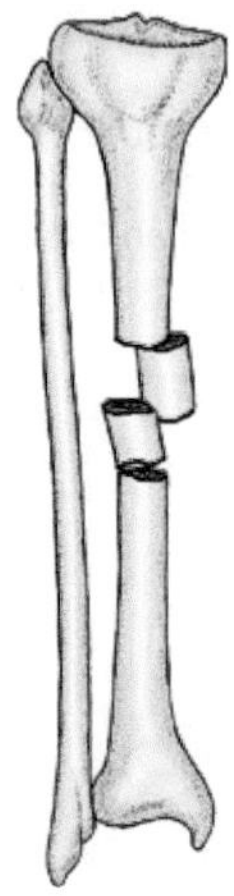

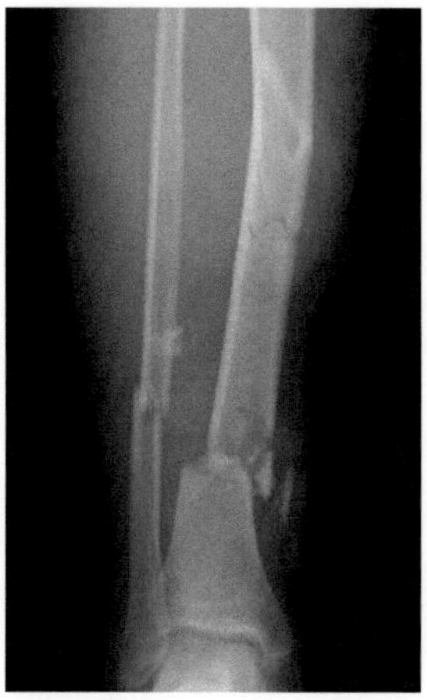

AO/OTA classification of tibia and fibula fractures
42-C Complex fracture
C2 Segmental fracture C2.3 with 2 or more intermediate segmental fragments

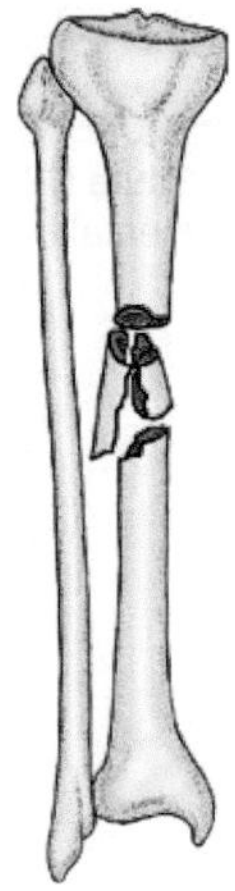

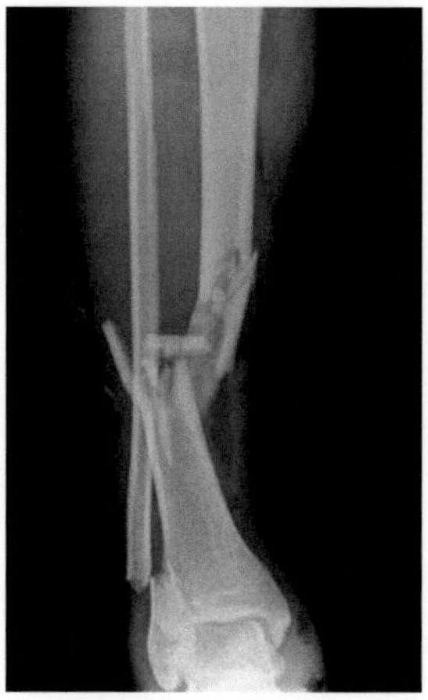

AO/OTA classification of tibia and fibula fractures
42-C Complex fracture
C3 Irregular fracture C3.1 with 2 or 3 intermediate fragments

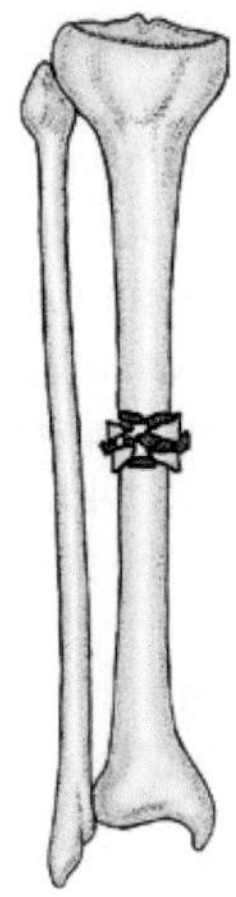

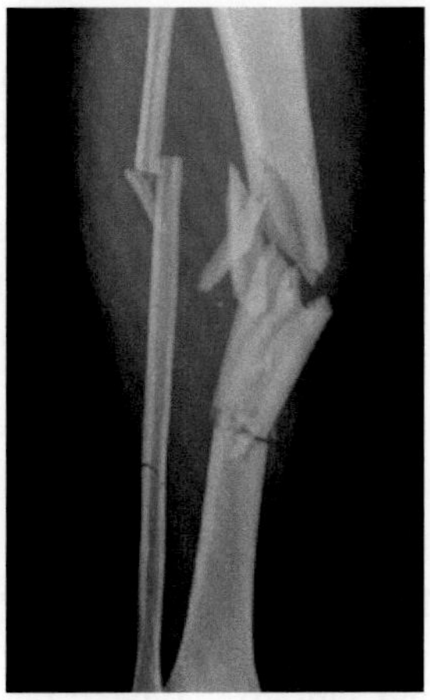

AO/OTA classification of tibia and fibula fractures
42-C Complex fracture
C3 Irregular fracture C3.2 limited shattering(<4cm)

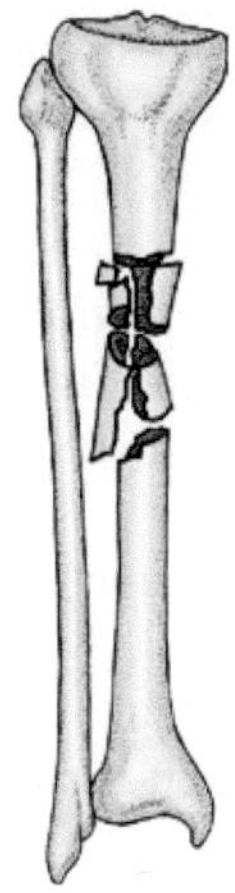

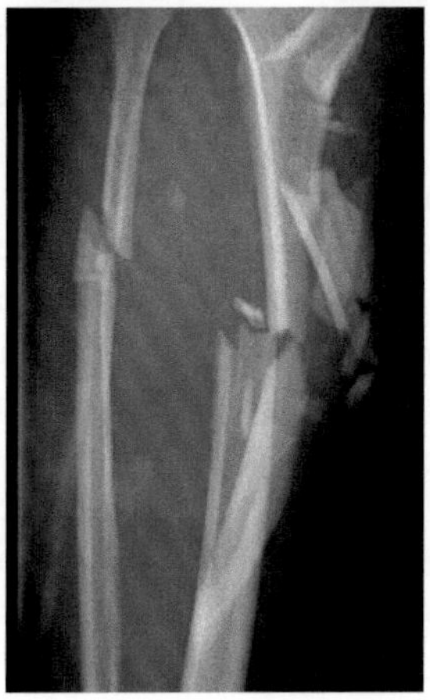

AO/OTA classification of tibia and fibula fractures
42-C Complex fracture
C3 Irregular fracture C3.3 extensive shattering(≥4cm)

10.2.2 **Modified Ellis Classification** (1998, Skeletal Trauma. 2nd ed. WB Saunders: Harcount Publishers Limited)

Characteristics	Displacement (%)	Comminution	Wound	Energy	Fracture pattern
Mild	0–50	No or minimal	Open grade I (Gustilo), closed grade 0 (Tscherne)	Low	Spiral
Moderate	50–100	Minimal, butterfly segment	Open grade II, closed grade I	Moderate	Transverse or oblique
Major	100	Two or more free segments	Open grades III–V, closed grades II–III	High, crushing	Transverse or fragmented

10.2.3 Anatomic Classification

This classification divides these fractures into four types: transverse, oblique, spiral, and complex.

10.2.4 Classification by Fracture Pattern

This classification divides these fractures into four types: transverse, oblique, spiral, and complex.

10.2.5 Classification by Soft-Tissue Integrity

This classification includes two types (open and closed) based on the integrity of the soft-tissue envelope.

10.2.6 Classification of Open Tibial Fractures

10.2.6.1 Gustilo-Anderson Classification (1976, JBJS, 58-A:453–458)

Type I: Fractures of this type have a clean wound of <1 cm with minimal or no contamination. The wound results from a perforation from the inside out by one of the fracture ends, with minor soft-tissue damage and no contusion. Type I fractures are simple fractures, including spiral or short oblique fractures; these are rarely complex fractures.

Type II: An open fracture with a laceration greater than 1 cm without extensive soft-tissue damages, flaps, or avulsions. This type is associated with mild-to-moderate contusion, moderate complex fracture, and moderate contamination.

Type III: Either an open segmental fracture, an open fracture with extensive soft-tissue damages, or a traumatic amputation, which is highly contaminated. These fractures usually result from high-energy trauma.

Type IIIA: Open fractures with adequate soft-tissue coverage of a fractured bone despite extensive soft-tissue lacerations or flaps

Type IIIB: Open fractures with extensive soft-tissue loss, with periosteal stripping and bone exposure. These injuries are usually associated with massive contamination and will often need further soft-tissue coverage procedures (i.e., free or rotational flap creations)

Type IIIC: Open fractures associated with arterial injuries requiring repair, independent of the fracture type.

10.2.6.2 Wang YC Classification

Type 1: Open fracture with skin breakage from the inside out.

Type 2: Open fracture with skin breakage from the outside in.

Type 3: Latent open fracture.

10.2.6.3 Zhu BT Classification

This classification divides open tibial fractures into three types according to the wound dimension, soft-tissue damage severity, and extent of contamination:

Type I: The wound resulting from a perforation from the inside out by one of the fracture ends is less than 3 cm, with minor soft-tissue contusion and no apparent contamination.

Type II: The wound is 3–15 cm, apparently contaminated, with moderate soft-tissue damage.

Type III: The wound is larger than 15 cm, severely contaminated, associated with smashed soft-tissue damages and neuromuscular injuries.

10.3 Distal Tibial and Fibular Fracture

As early as 1816, Dupuytren used cadaver experiments to produce ankle fractures. Subsequently, French authors have referred to low and high Dupuytren fractures. NielLauge-Hansen, a Danish physician who studied ankle fractures during the 1940s and 1950s, ultimately created the most detailed and comprehensive classification system of ankle injuries.

The Danis classification was first described by Danis in 1949 and was later modified and popularized by Weber in 1972.

To date, there have been ~10 classification systems for distal tibial and fibular fractures. Based on our review of literature over the last 5 years, the most commonly used system was the AO/OTA classification, followed by the Lauge-Hansen classification and Danis-Weber classification.

10.3.1 **AO/OTA Classification** (2007, Journal of Orthopaedic Trauma. 21 supplement; the AO classification of long bone fractures was initially proposed by Muller in 1980s and revised in 2007)

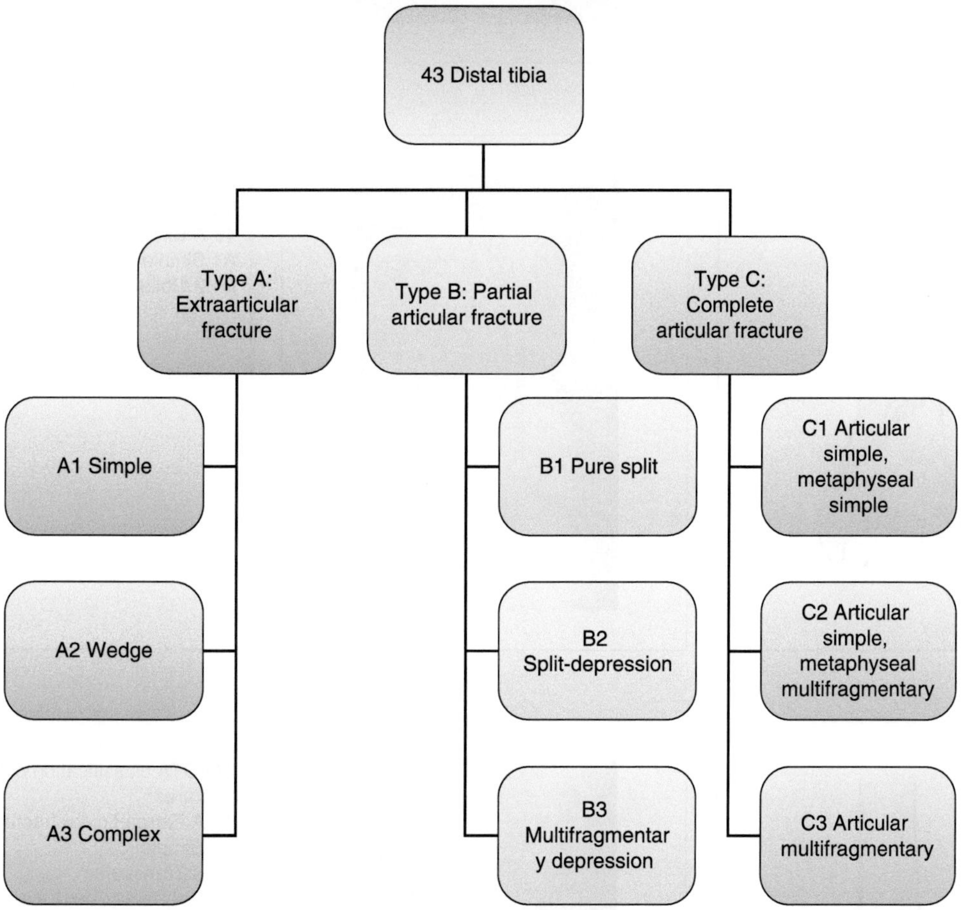

Type A: Extra-articular fracture:
- Type A1: Simple:
  - Type A1.1: Spiral.
  - Type A1.2: Oblique.
  - Type A1.3: Transverse.
- Type A2: Wedge:
  - Type A2.1: Posterolateral impaction.
  - Type A2.2: Anteromedial wedge.
  - Type A2.3: Extending into diaphysis.
- Type A3: Complex:
  - Type A3.1: With three intermediate fragments.
  - Type A3.2: More than three intermediate fragments.
  - Type A3.3: Extending into diaphysis.

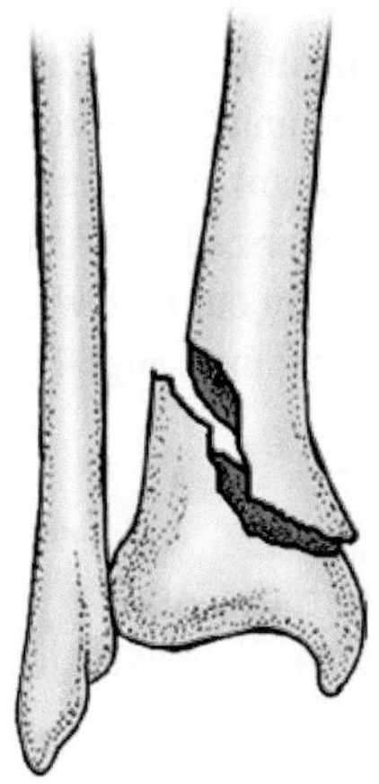

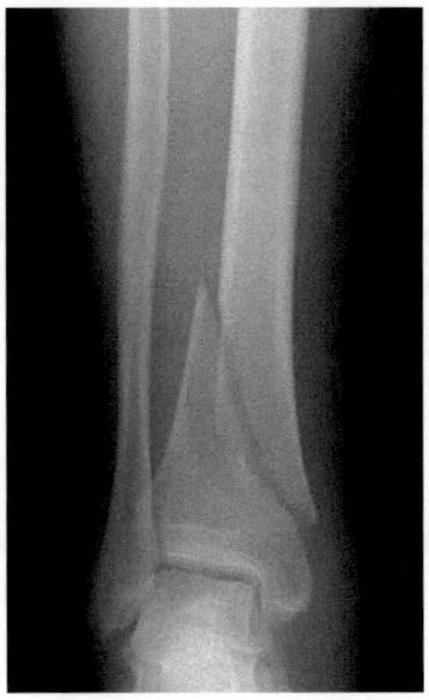

AO/OTA classification of tibia and fibula fractures
43-A Extraarticular fracture
A1 Simple
A1.1 Spiral

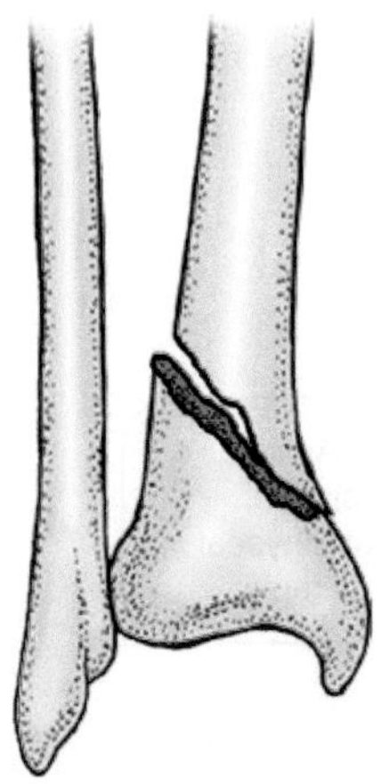

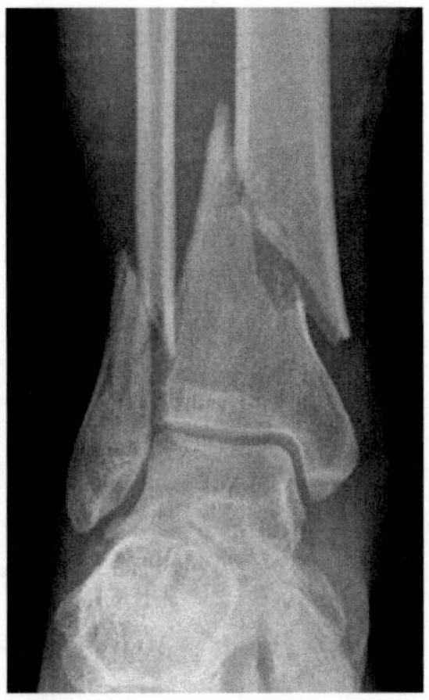

AO/OTA classification of tibia and fibula fractures
43-A Extraarticular fracture
A1 Simple
A1.2 Oblique

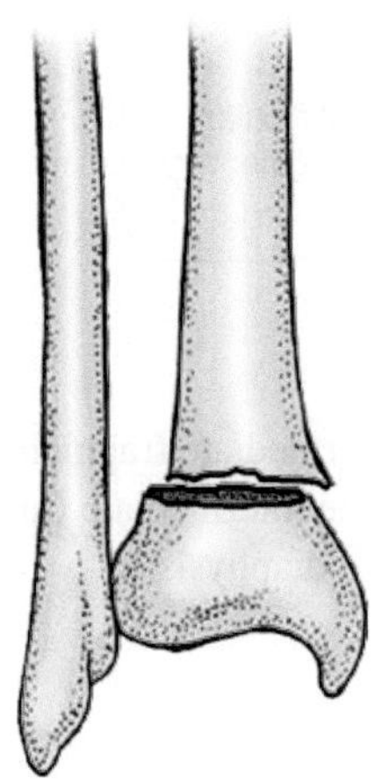

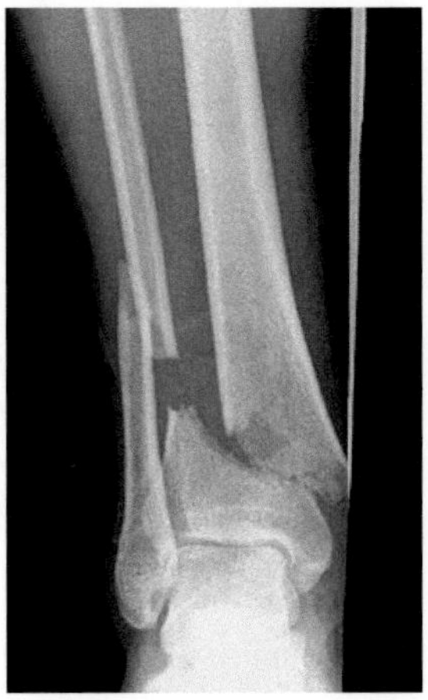

AO/OTA classification of tibia and fibula fractures
43-A Extraarticular fracture
A1 Simple
A1.3 Transverse

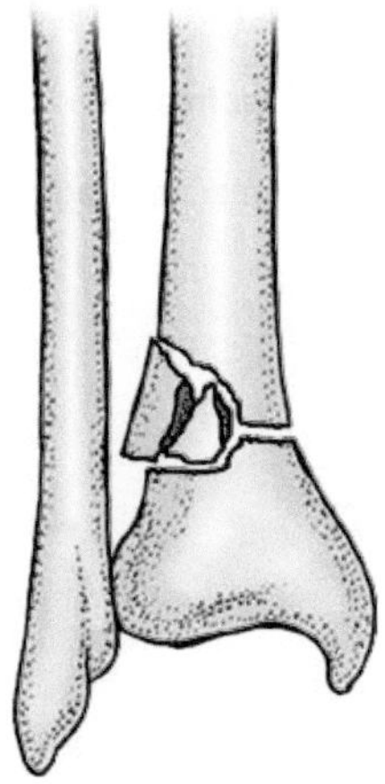

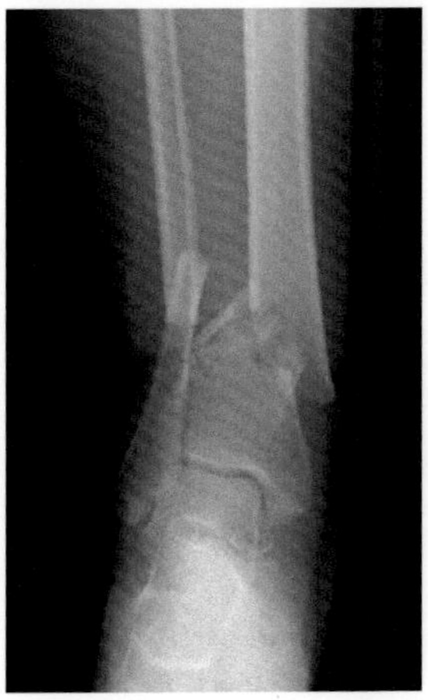

AO/OTA classification of tibia and fibula fractures
43-A Extraarticular fracture
A2 Wedge
A2.1 Posterolateral impaction

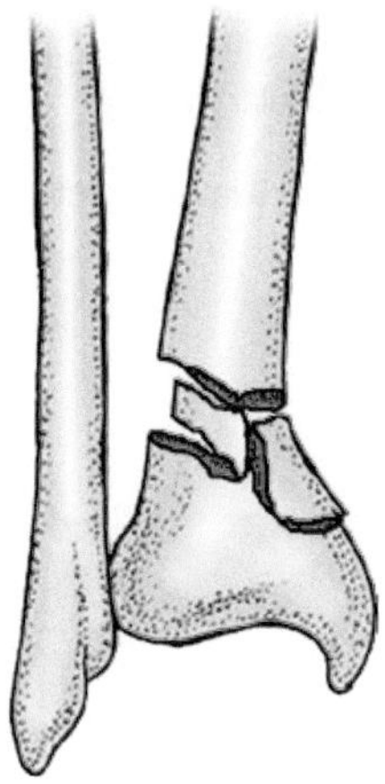

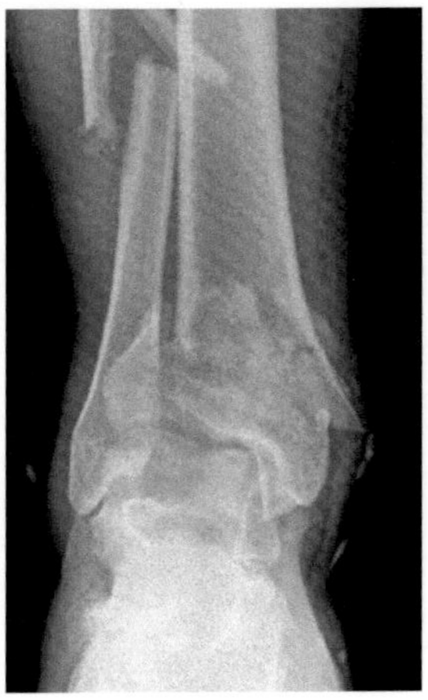

AO/OTA classification of tibia and fibula fractures
43-A Extraarticular fracture
A2 Wedge
A2.2 Anteromedial wedge

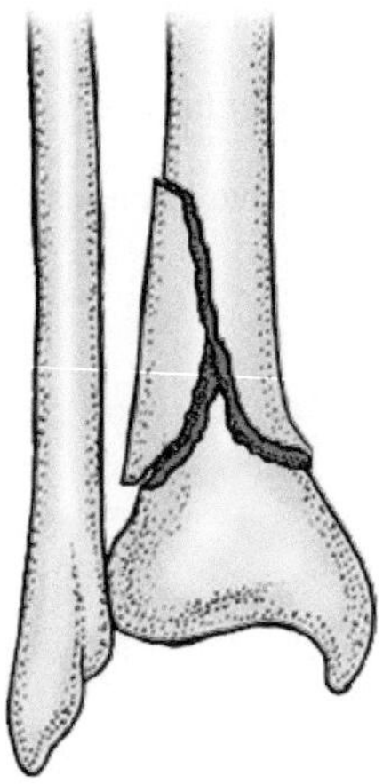

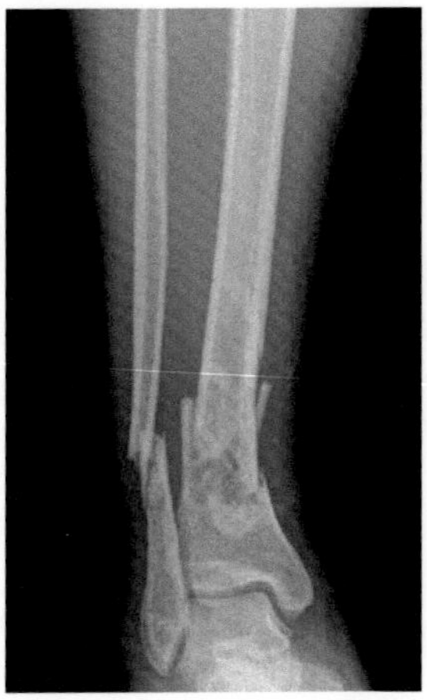

AO/OTA classification of tibia and fibula fractures
43-A Extraarticular fracture
A2 Wedge
A2.3 Extending into diaphysis

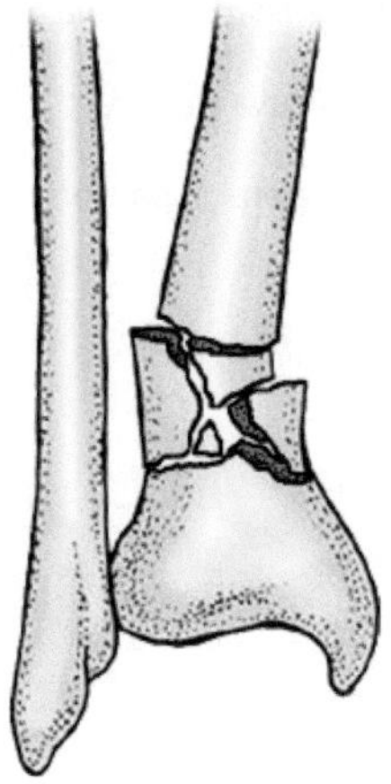

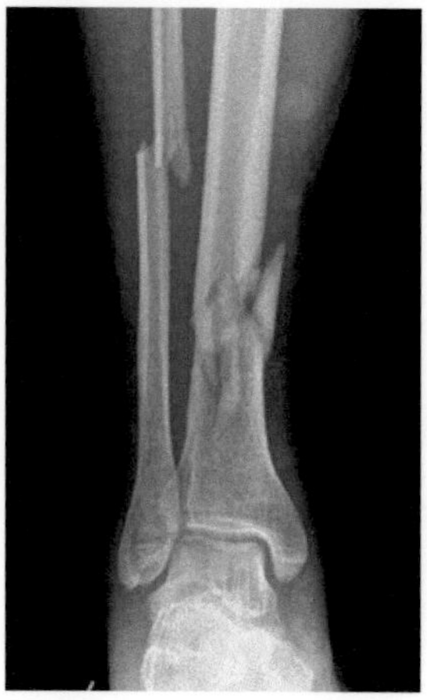

AO/OTA classification of tibia and fibula fractures
43-A Extraarticular fracture
A3 Complex
A3.1 With 3 intermediate fragments

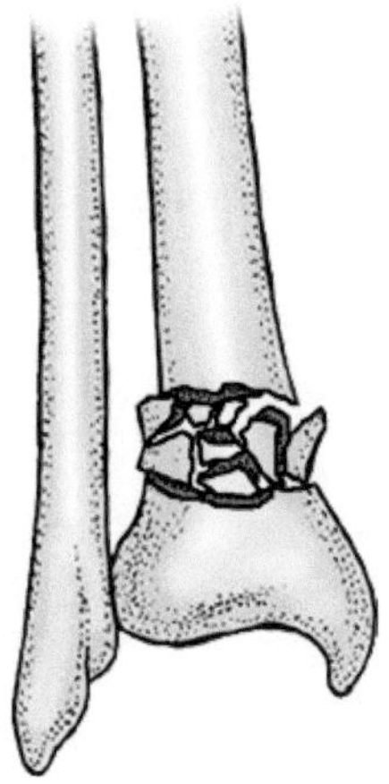

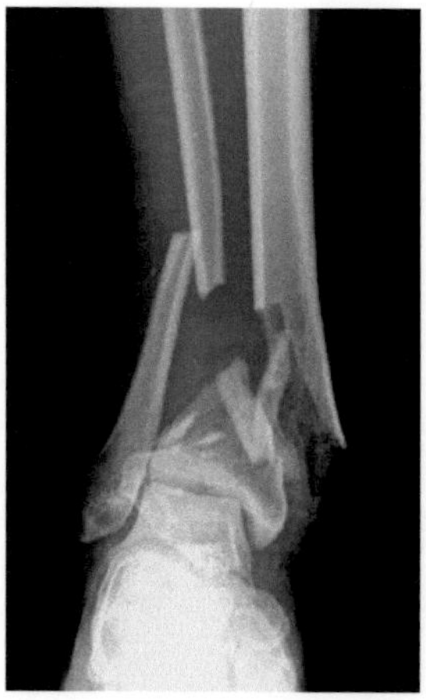

AO/OTA classification of tibia and fibula fractures
43-A Extraarticular fracture
A3 Complex
A3.2 More than 3 intermediate fragments

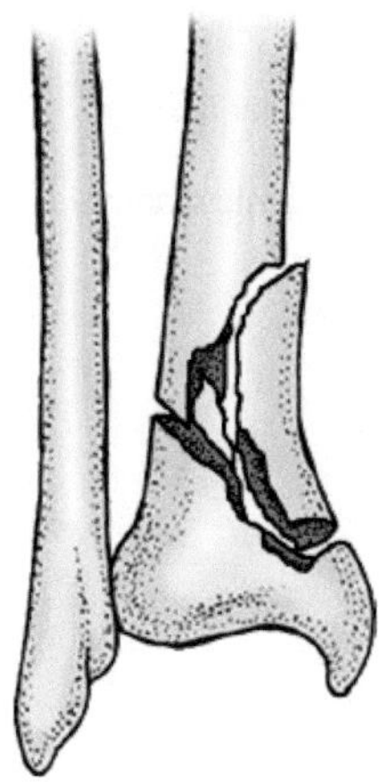

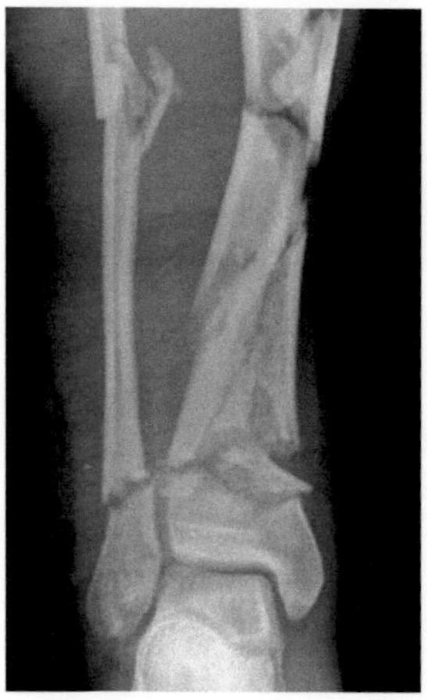

AO/OTA classification of tibia and fibula fractures
43-A Extraarticular fracture
A3 Complex
A3.3 Extending into diaphysis

Type B: Partial articular fracture:

- Type B1: Pure split:
  - Type B1.1: Frontal.
  - Type B1.2: Sagittal.
  - Type B1.3: Metaphyseal multifragmentary.
- Type B2: Split depression:
  - Type B2.1: Frontal.
  - Type B2.2: Sagittal.
  - Type B2.3: Of the central fragment.
- Type B3: Multifragmentary depression:
  - Type B3.1: Frontal.
  - Type B3.2: Sagittal.
  - Type B3.3: Metaphyseal multifragmentary.

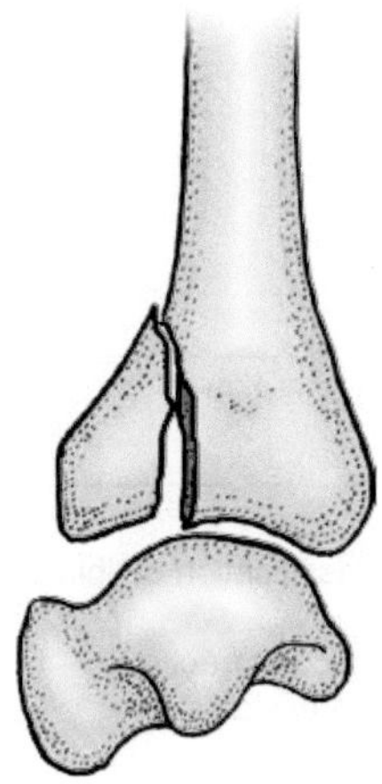

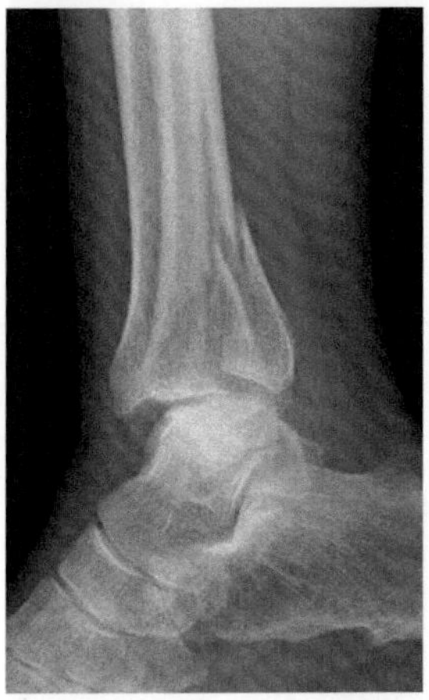

AO/OTA classification of tibia and fibula fractures
B Partial articular fracture
B1 Pure split
B1.1 Frontal

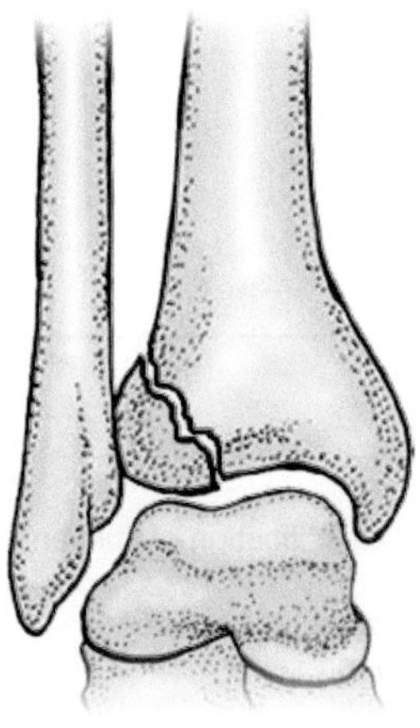

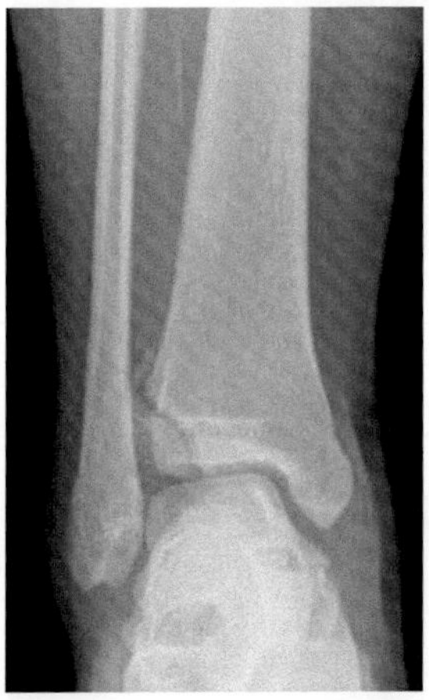

AO/OTA classification of tibia and fibula fractures
B Partial articular fracture
B1 Pure split
B1.2 Sagittal

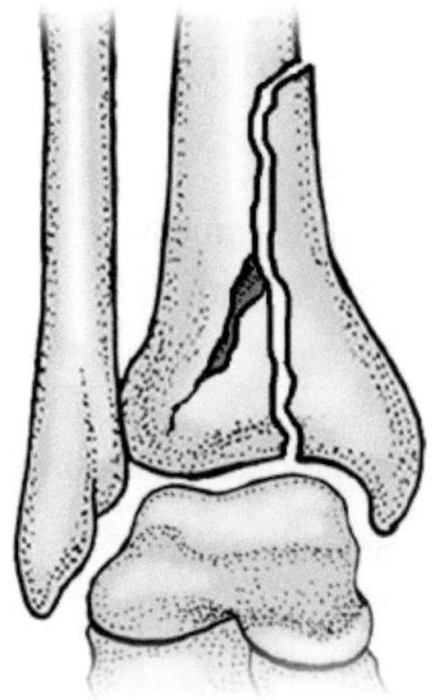

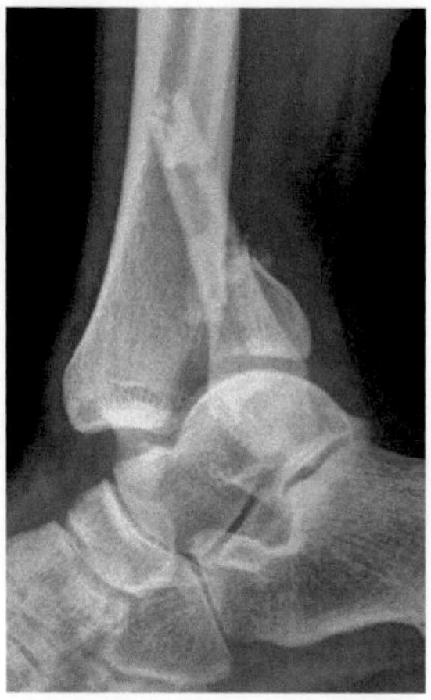

AO/OTA classification of tibia and fibula fractures
B Partial articular fracture
B1 Pure split
B1.3 Metaphyseal multifragmentary

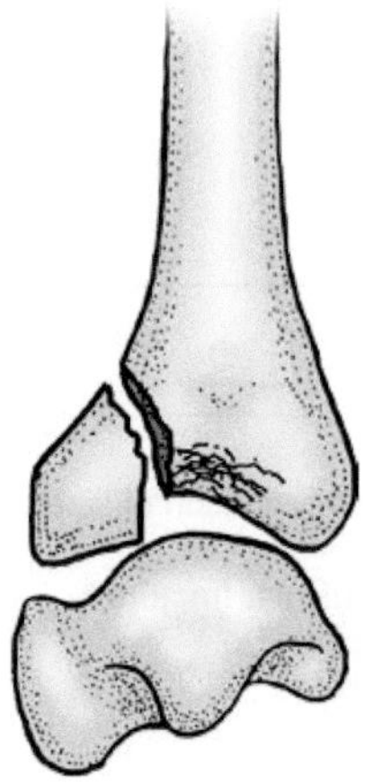

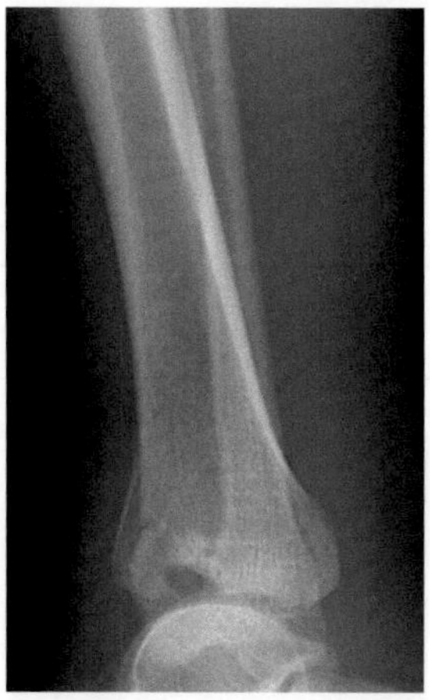

AO/OTA classification of tibia and fibula fractures
B Partial articular fracture
B2 Split-depression
B2.1 Frontal

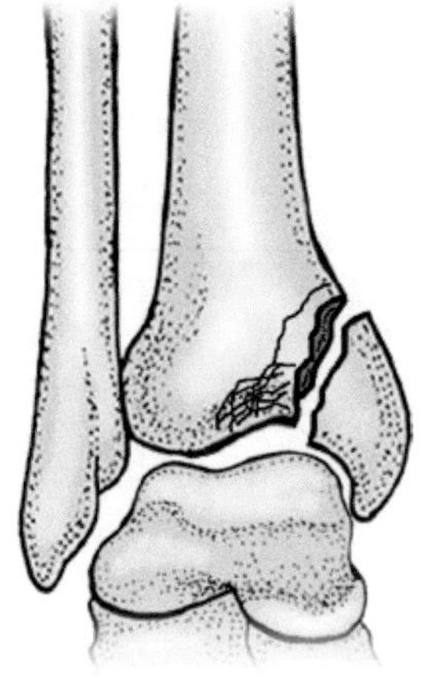

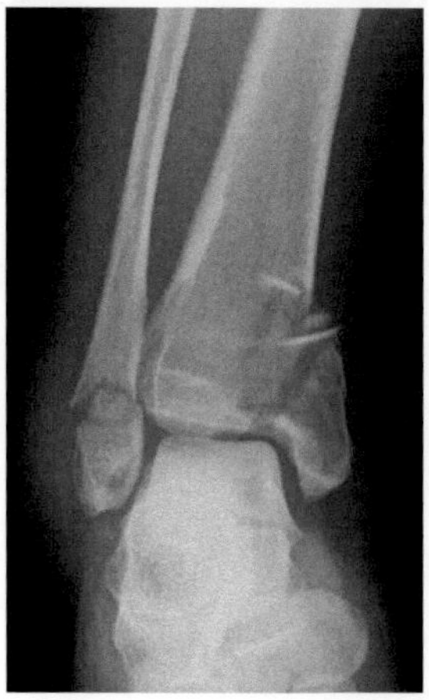

AO/OTA classification of tibia and fibula fractures
B Partial articular fracture
B2 Split-depression
B2.2 Sagittal

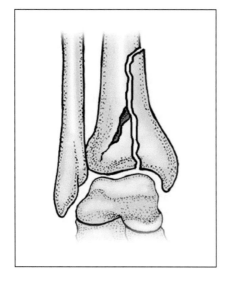

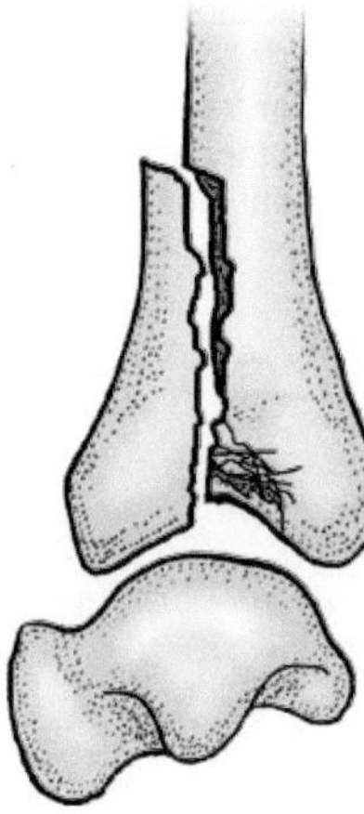

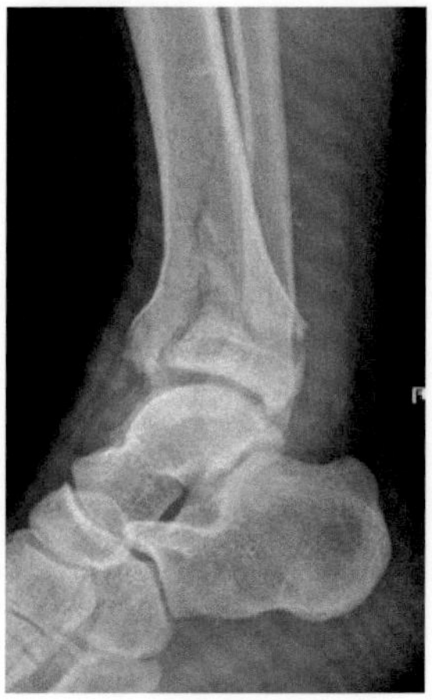

AO/OTA classification of tibia and fibula fractures
B Partial articular fracture
B2 Split-depression
B2.3 Of the central fragment

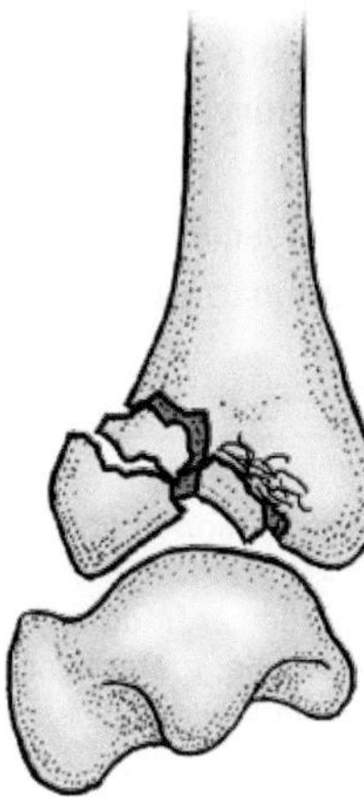

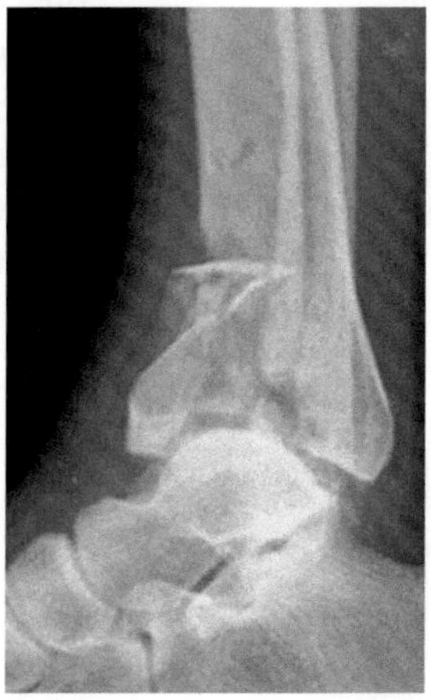

AO/OTA classification of tibia and fibula fractures
B Partial articular fracture
B3 Multifragmentary depression
B3.1 Frontal

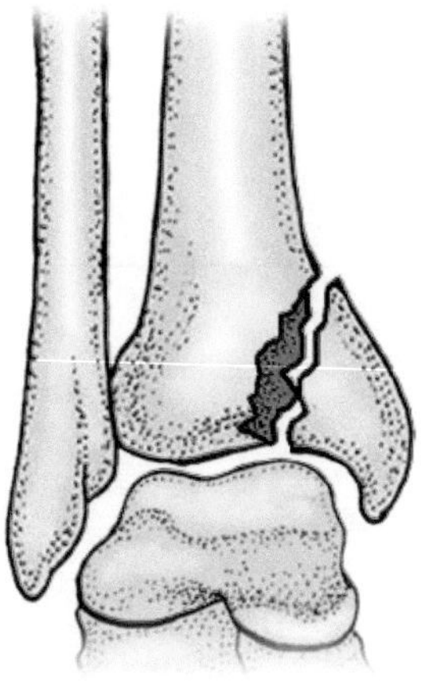

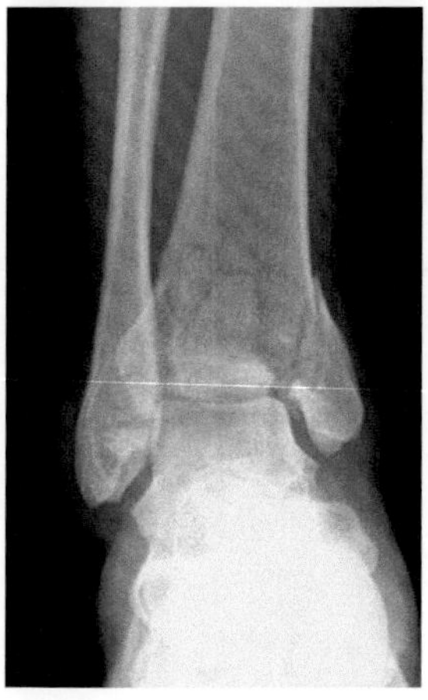

AO/OTA classification of tibia and fibula fractures
B Partial articular fracture
B3 Multifragmentary depression
B3.2 Sagittal

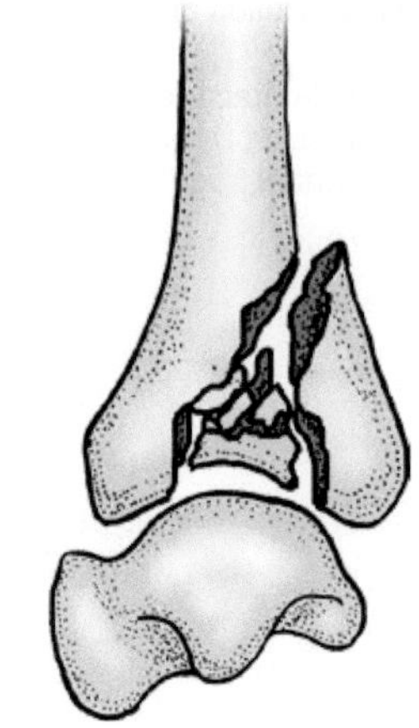

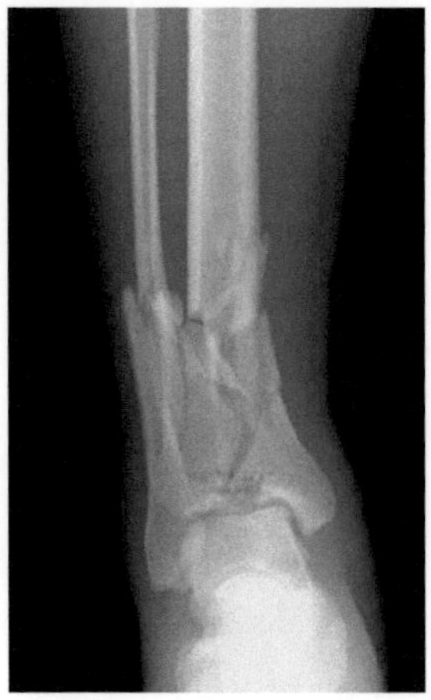

AO/OTA classification of tibia and fibula fractures
B Partial articular fracture
B3 Multifragmentary depression
B3.3 Metaphyseal multifragmentary

Type C: Complete articular fracture:

- Type C1: Articular simple, metaphyseal simple:
  - Type C1.1: Without impaction.
  - Type C1.2: With epiphyseal depression.
  - Type C1.3: Extending into diaphysis.
- Type C2: Articular simple, metaphyseal multifragmentary:
  - Type C2.1: With asymmetric impaction.
  - Type C2.2: Without asymmetric impaction.
  - Type C2.3: Extending into diaphysis.
- Type C3: Articular multifragmentary:
  - Type C3.1: Epiphyseal.
  - Type C3.2: Epiphysio-metaphyseal.
  - Type C3.3: Epiphysio-metaphysio-diaphyseal.

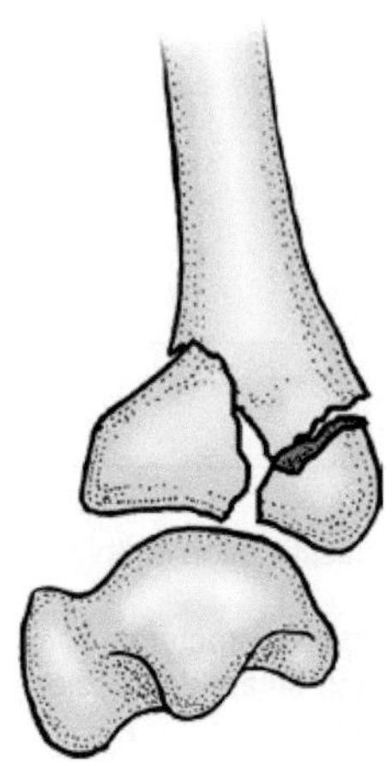

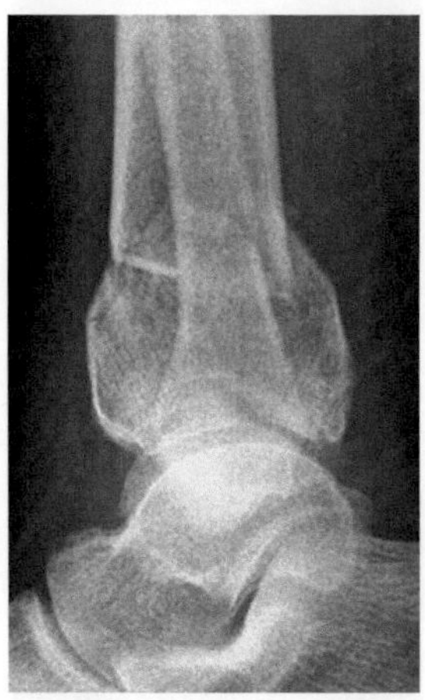

AO/OTA classification of tibia and fibula fractures
C Complete articular fracture
C1 Articular simple, metaphyseal simple
C1.1 Without impaction

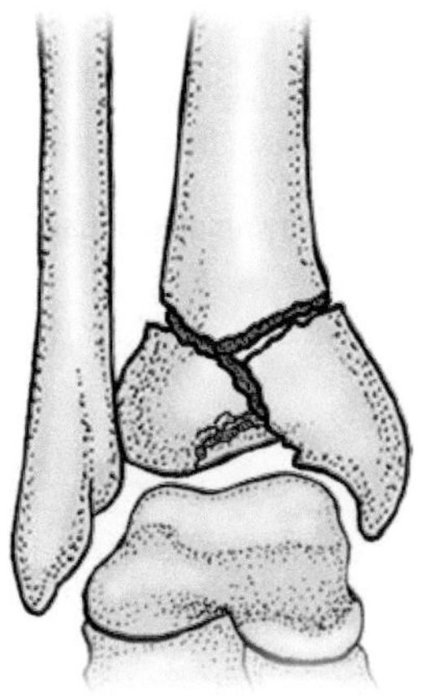

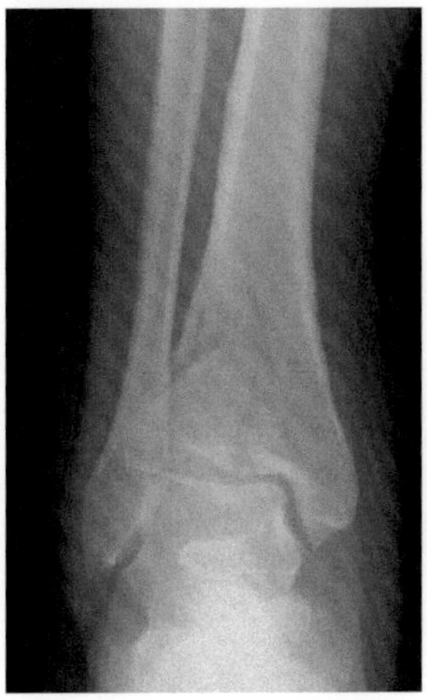

AO/OTA classification of tibia and fibula fractures
C Complete articular fracture
C1 Articular simple, metaphyseal simple
C1.2 With epiphyseal depression

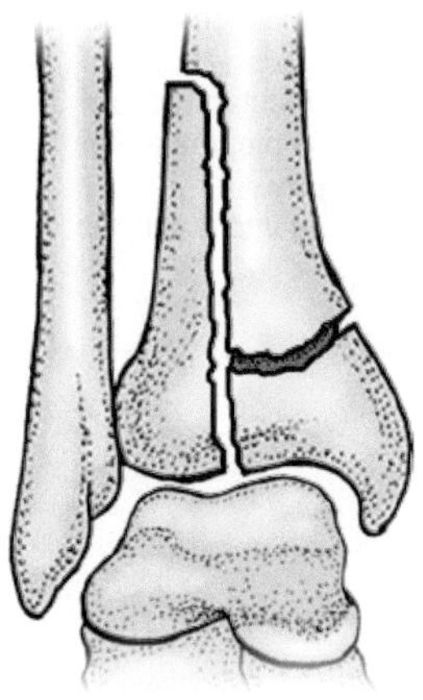

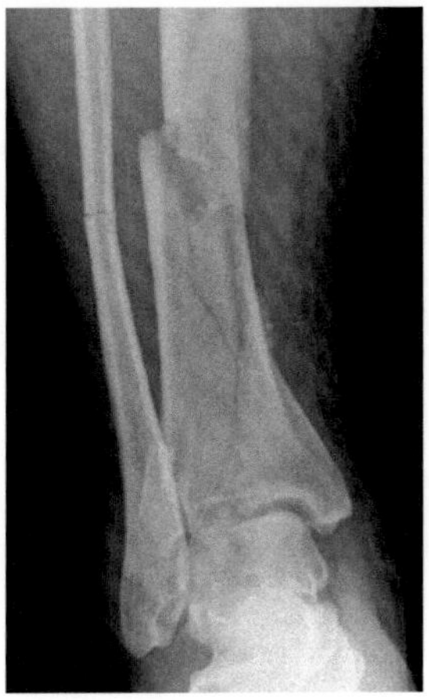

AO/OTA classification of tibia and fibula fractures
C Complete articular fracture
C1 Articular simple, metaphyseal simple
C1.3 Extending into diaphysis

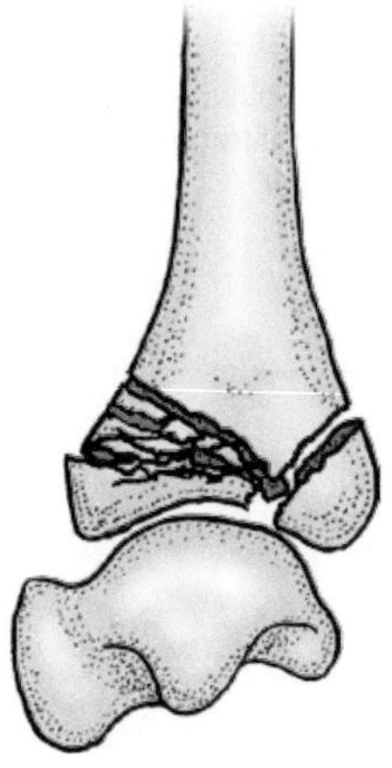

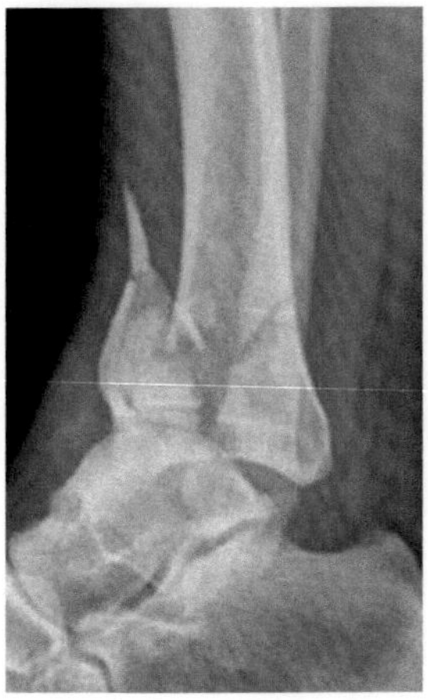

AO/OTA classification of tibia and fibula fractures
C Complete articular fracture
C2 Articular simple, metaphyseal multifragmentary
C2.1 With asymmetric impaction

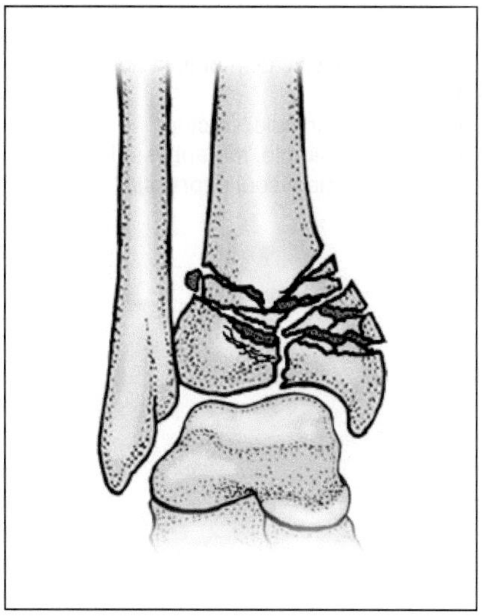

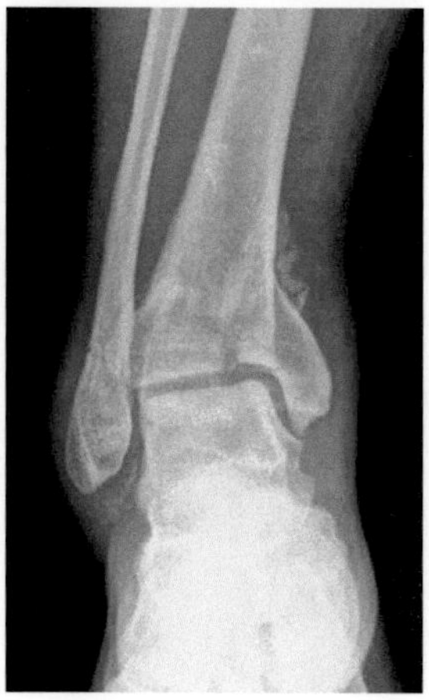

AO/OTA classification of tibia and fibula fractures
C Complete articular fracture
C2 Articular simple, metaphyseal multifragmentary
C2.2 Without asymmetric impaction

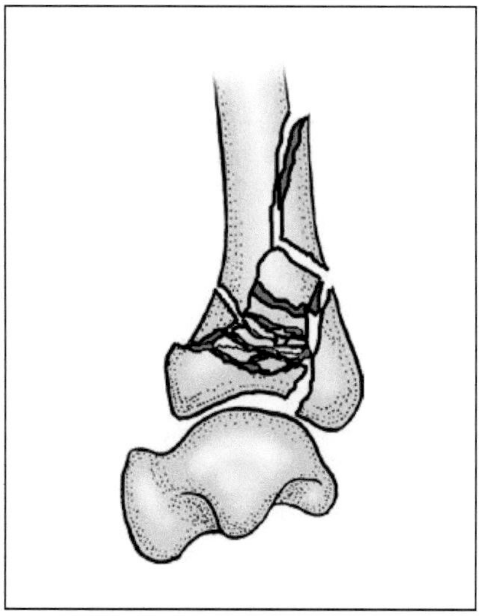

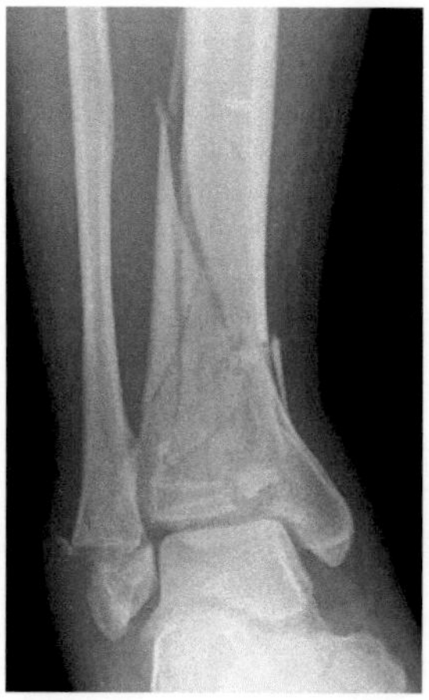

AO/OTA classification of tibia and fibula fractures
C Complete articular fracture
C2 Articular simple, metaphyseal multifragmentary
C2.3 Extending into diaphysis

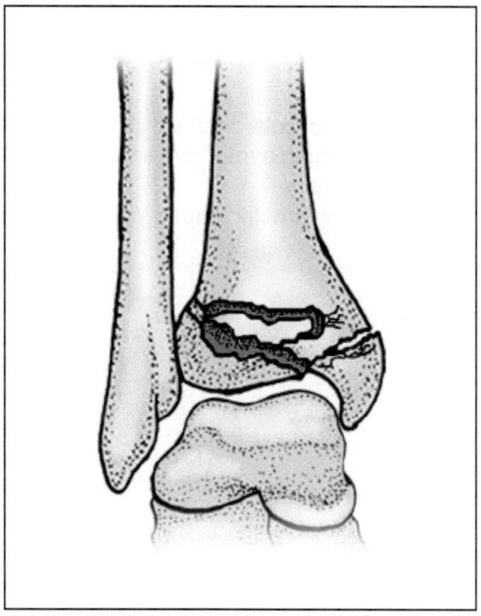

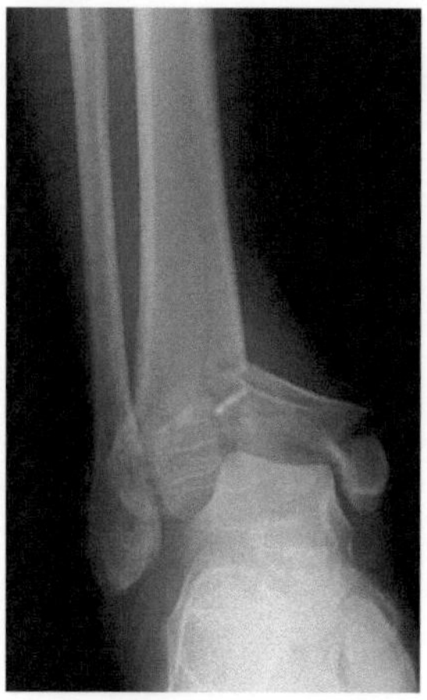

AO/OTA classification of tibia and fibula fractures
C Complete articular fracture
C3 Articular multifragmentary
C3.1 Epiphyseal

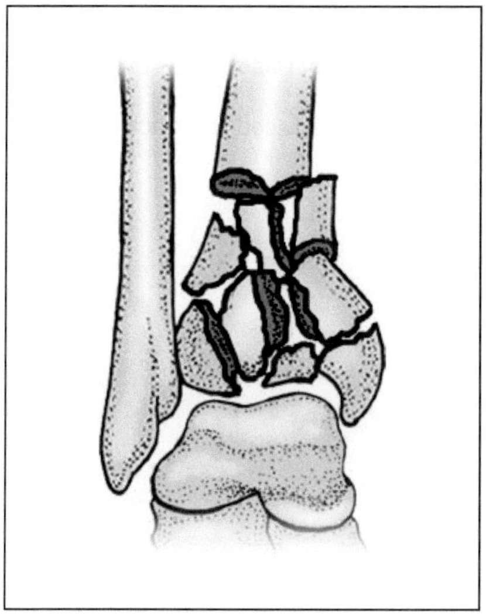

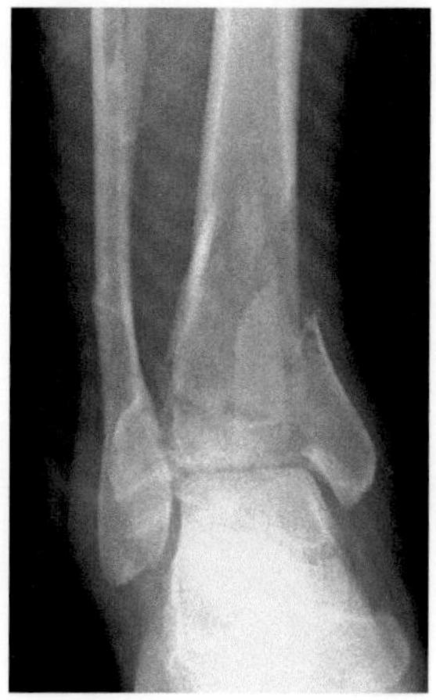

AO/OTA classification of tibia and fibula fractures
C Complete articular fracture
C3 Articular multifragmentary
C3.2 Epiphysio-metaphyseal

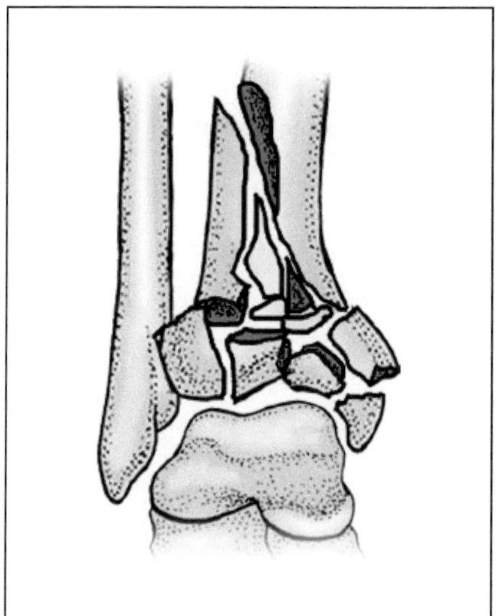

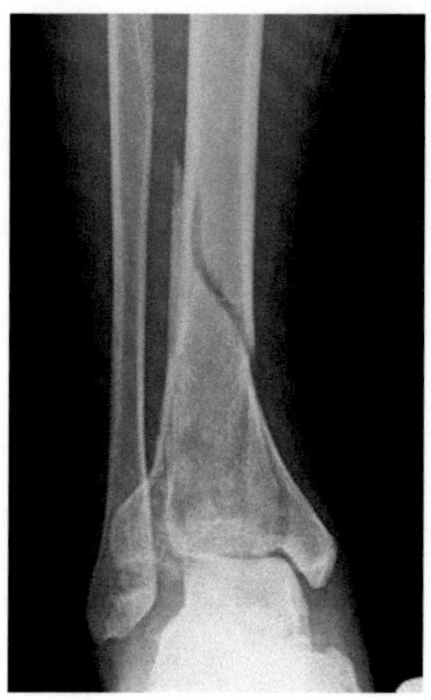

AO/OTA classification of tibia and fibula fractures
C Complete articular fracture
C3 Articular multifragmentary
C3.3 Epiphysio-metaphysio-diaphyseal

10.3.2 Ruedi-Allgower Classification of Pilon Fracture (1979, Clin Orthop Relat Res, 138:105–110)

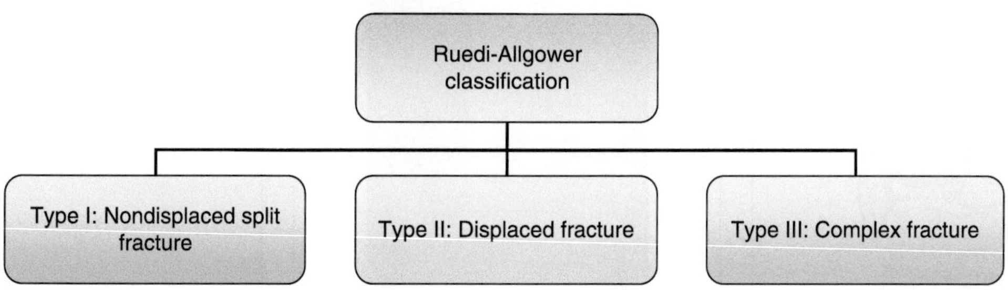

Type I: Non-displaced split fractures, which can be treated conservatively.

Type II: Displaced fractures with no comminution or impaction, moderately compromising the smoothness of the articular surface.

Type III: Complex fractures with a high degree of comminution and displacement, severely compromising the smoothness of the articular surface.

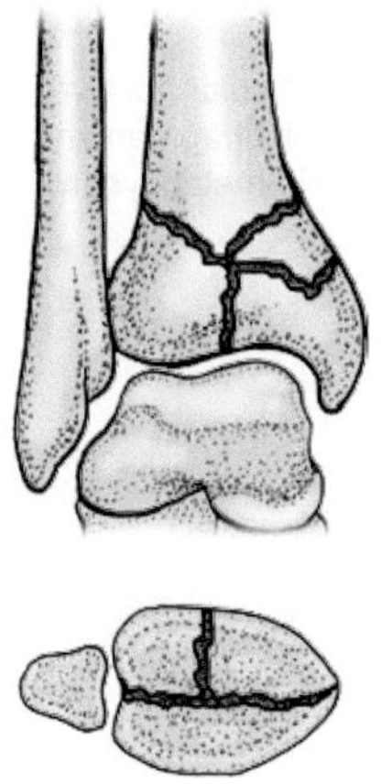

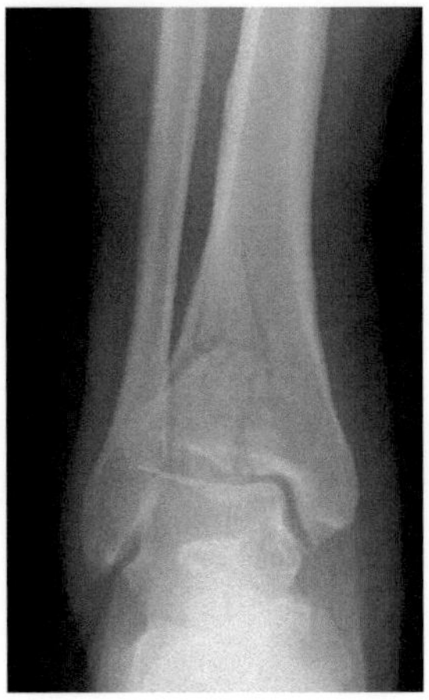

Ruedi-Allgower classification of Pilon. fracture
Type I: Nondisplaced split fracture

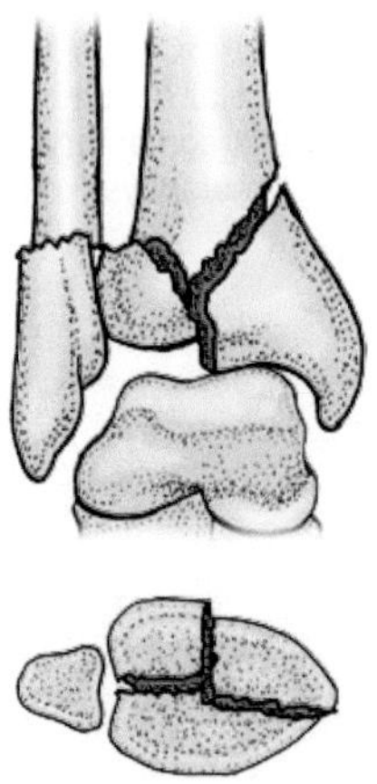

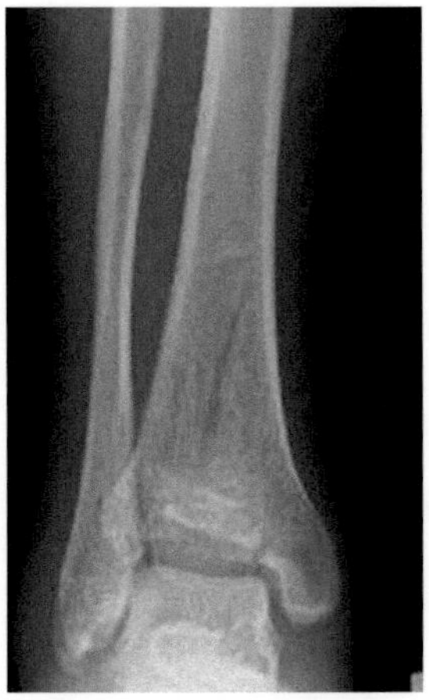

Ruedi-Allgower classification of Pilon fracture
Type II: Displaced fracture

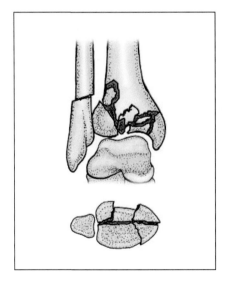

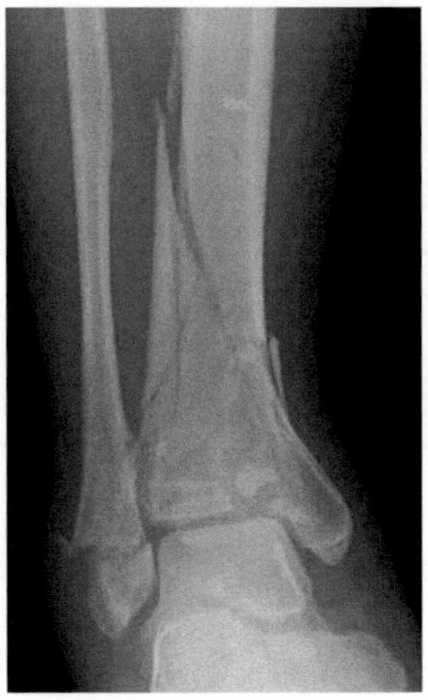

Ruedi-Allgower classification of Pilon fracture
Type III: Complex fracture

10.3.3 Classifications of Ankle Fractures

10.3.3.1 **Lauge-Hansen Classification** (1950, Arch Surg, 60:957–985)

Ankle injuries are divided into five types based on the position of the foot at the time of the traumatic event (supination or pronation) and the direction of the deforming forces on the talus (abduction, adduction, or external rotation): supination-adduction (SA), supination-external rotation (SER), pronation-abduction (PA), pronation-external rotation (PER), and pronation-dorsal flexion. Each type is subdivided into different stages according to the severity of the injury.

Supination-Adduction (SA)

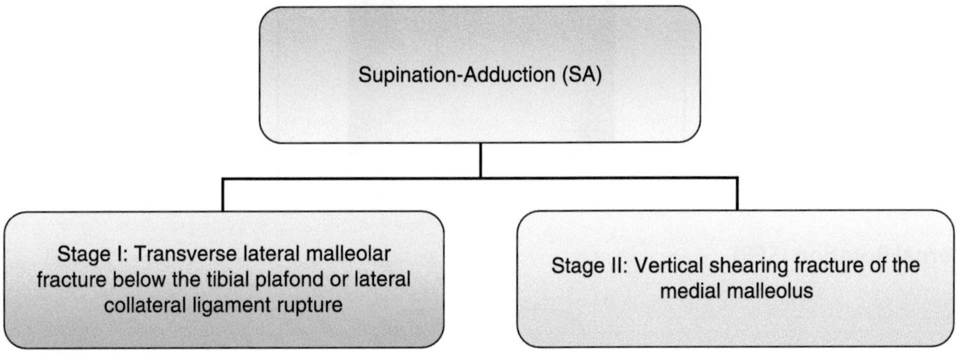

Stage I: Transverse lateral malleolar fracture below the tibial plafond or lateral collateral ligament rupture.
Stage II: Vertical shearing fracture of the medial malleolus.

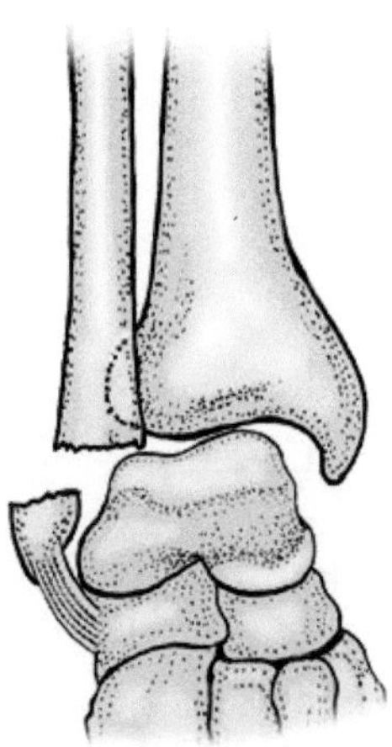

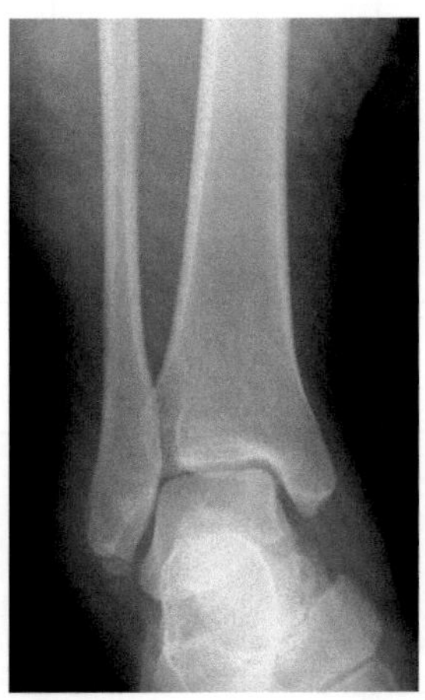

Lauge-Hansen classification of ankle fractures
Supination-Adduction (SA)
Stage I: Transverse lateral malleolar fracture below the tibial plafond or lateral collateral ligament rupture

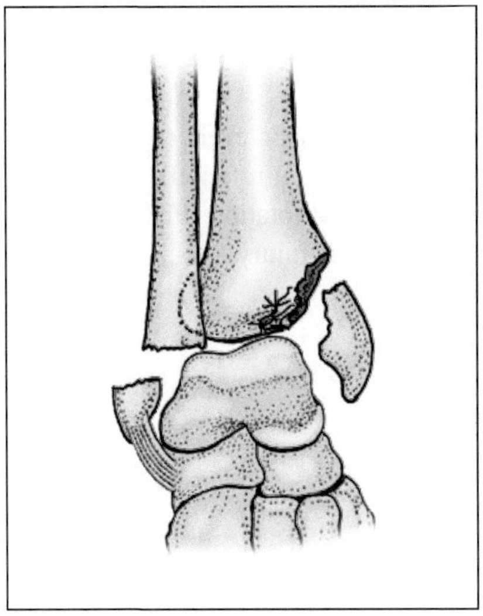

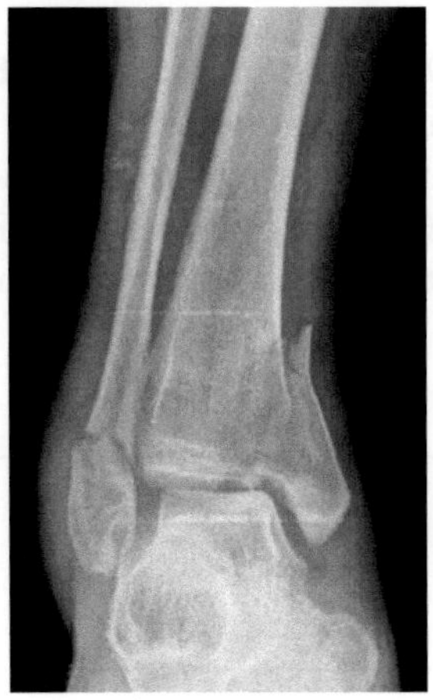

Lauge-Hansen classification of ankle fractures
Supination-Adduction (SA)
Stage II: Vertical shearing fracture of the medial malleolus

Supination-External Rotation (SER)

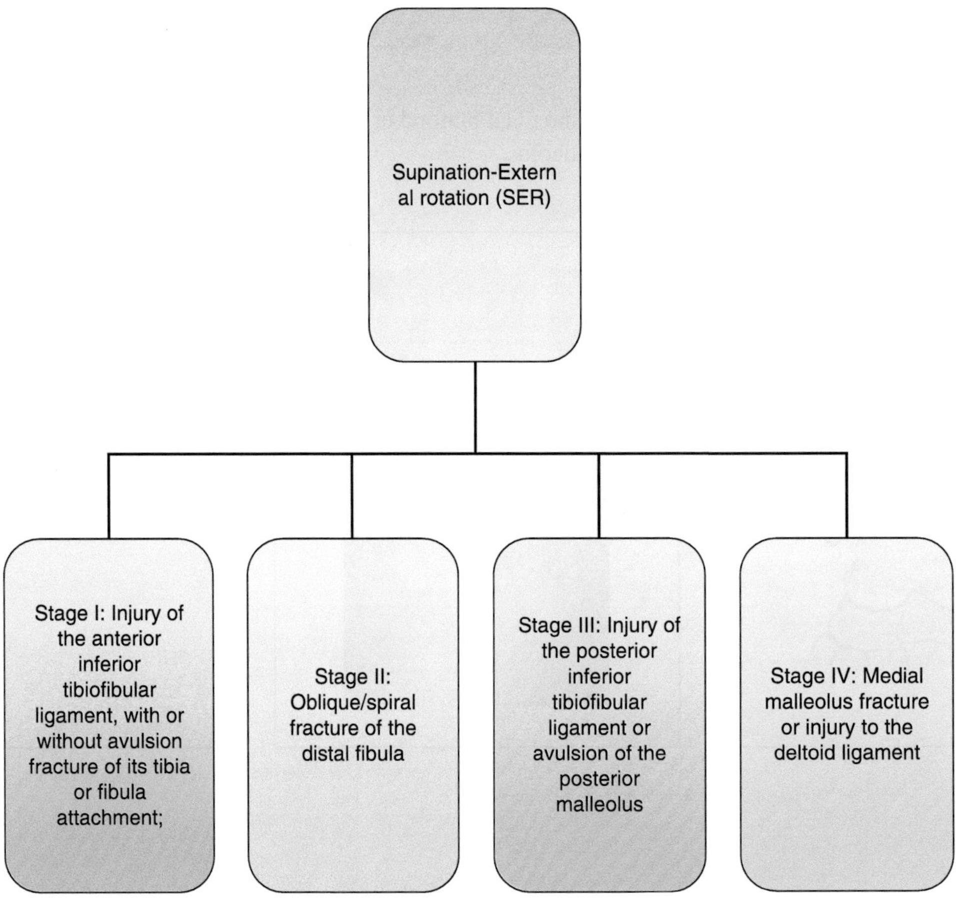

Stage I: Injury of the anterior inferior tibiofibular ligament, with or without avulsion fracture of its tibia or fibula attachment.

Stage II: Oblique/spiral fracture of the distal fibula, with fracture line extending from anteroinferior to posterosuperior.

Stage III: Injury of the posterior inferior tibiofibular ligament or avulsion of the posterior malleolus.

Stage IV: Medial malleolus fracture or injury to the deltoid ligament.

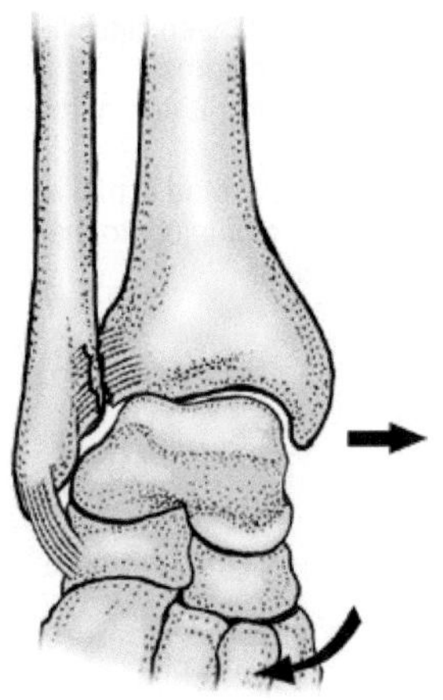

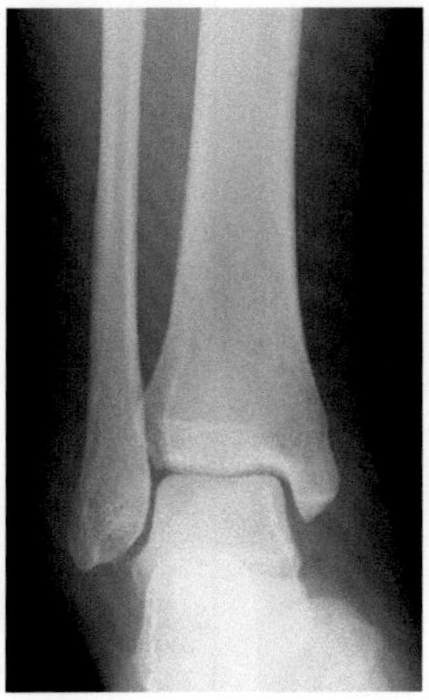

Lauge-Hansen classification of ankle fractures
Supination-External rotation (SER)
Stage I: Injury of the anterior inferior tibiofibular ligament, with or without avulsion fracture of its tibia or fibula attachment

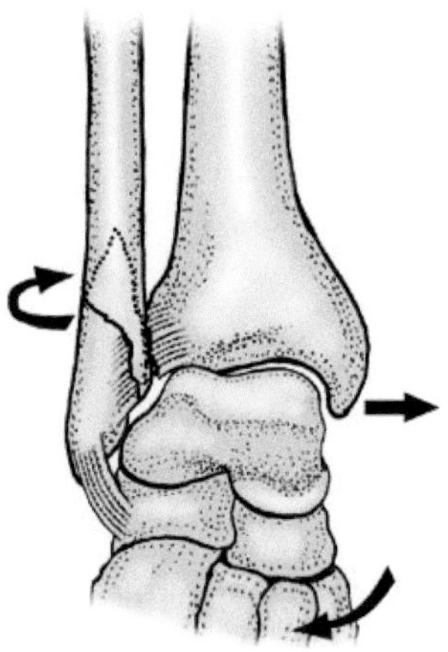

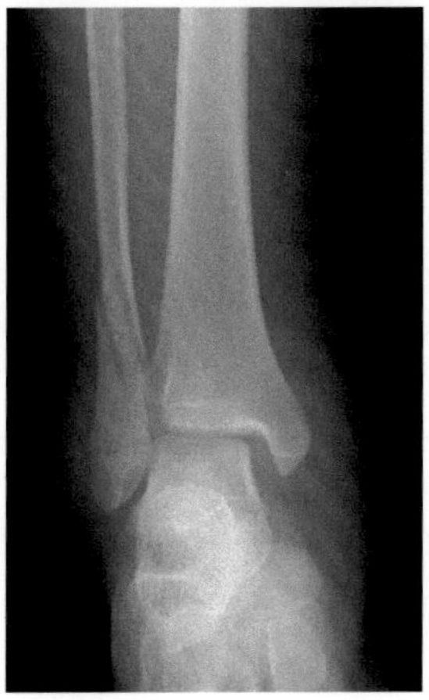

Lauge-Hansen classification of ankle fractures
Supination-External rotation (SER)
Stage I: Oblique/spiral fracture of the distal fibula, with fracture line extending from anteroinferior to posterosuperior fibula

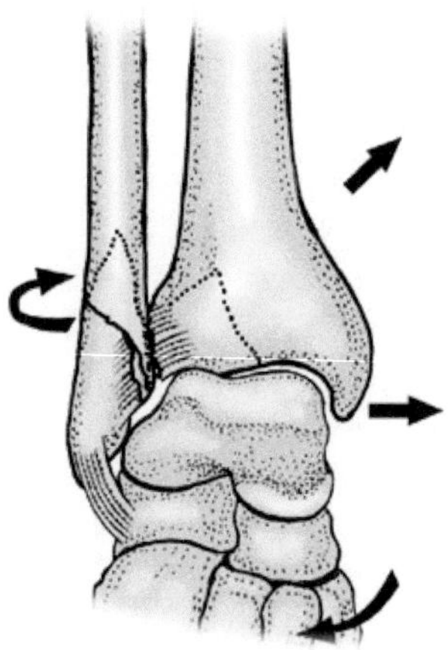

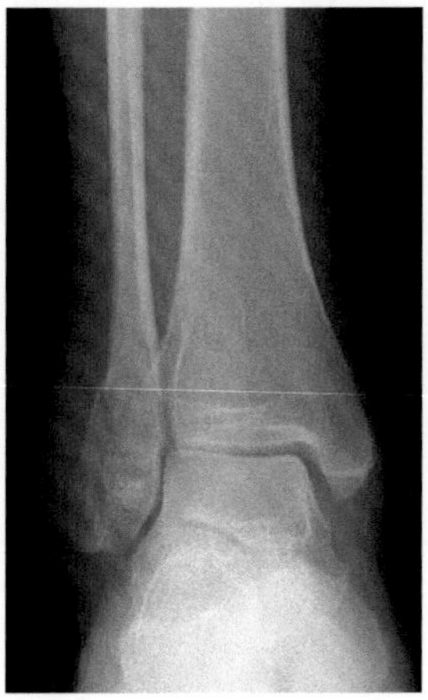

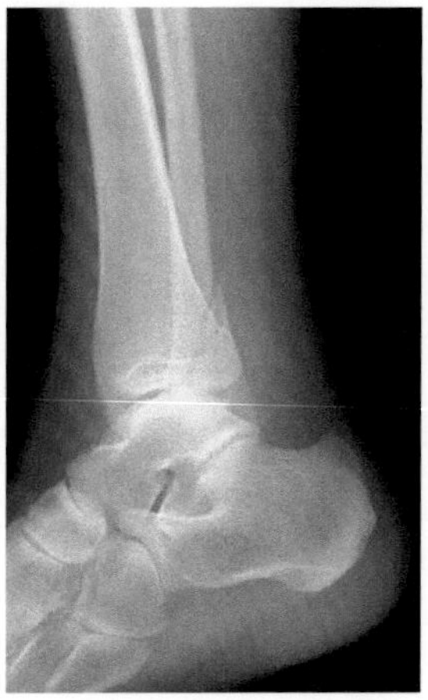

Lauge-Hansen classification of ankle fractures
Supination-External rotation (SER)
Stage III: Injury of the posterior inferior tibiofibular ligament or avulsion of the posterior malleolus

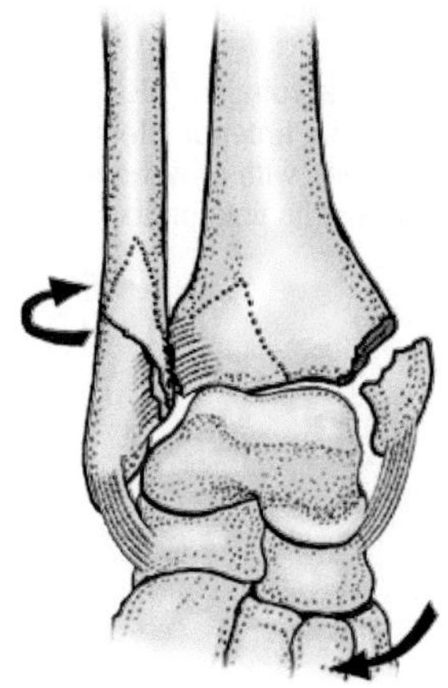	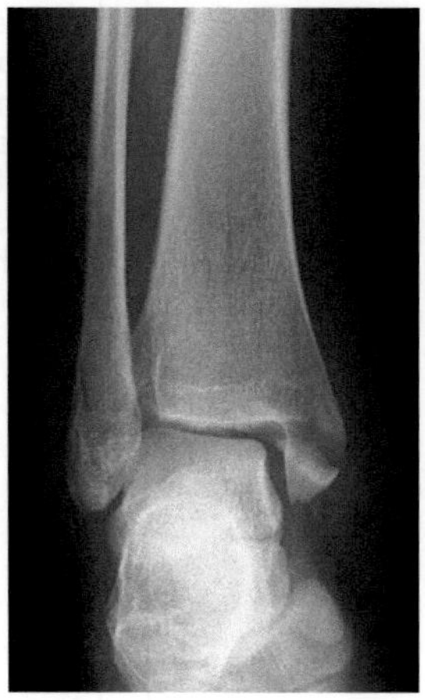	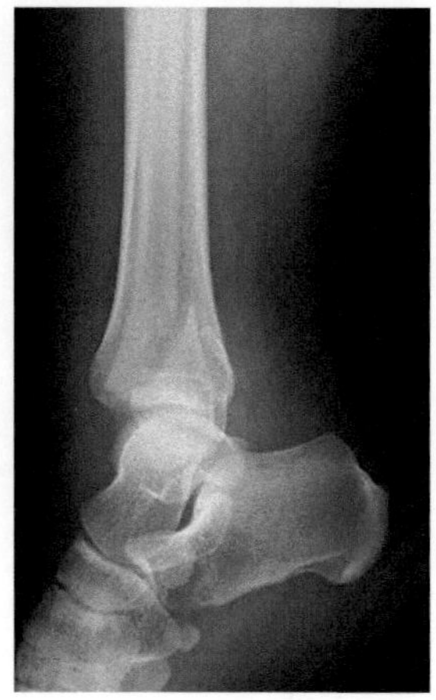	Lauge-Hansen classification of ankle fractures Supination-External rotation (SER) Stage IV: Medial malleolus fracture or injury to the deltoid ligament

Pronation-Abduction (PA)

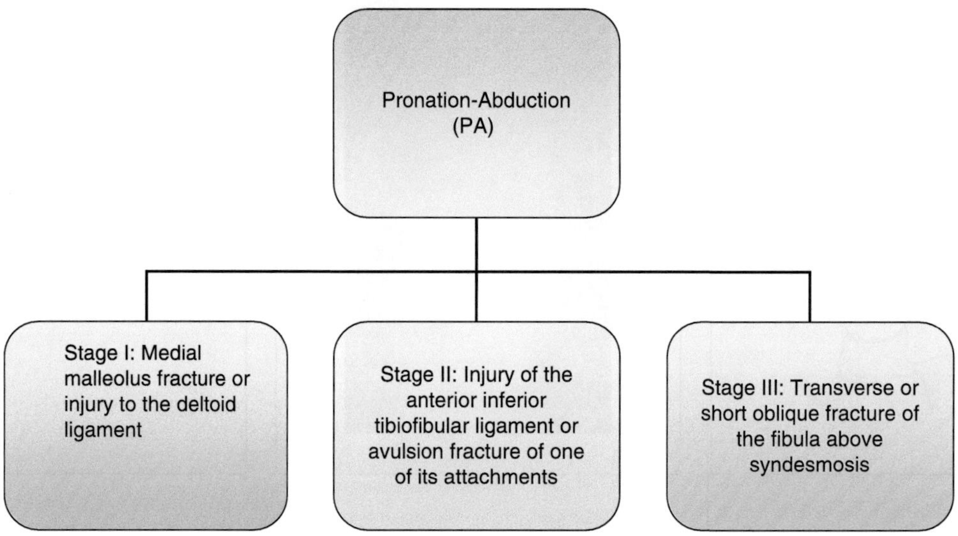

Stage I: Medial malleolus fracture or injury to the deltoid ligament.

Stage II: Injury of the anterior inferior tibiofibular ligament or avulsion fracture of one of its attachments.

Stage III: Transverse or short oblique fracture of the fibula above syndesmosis.

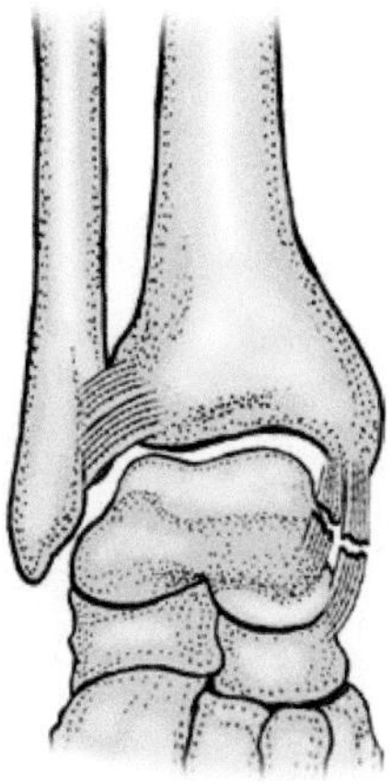

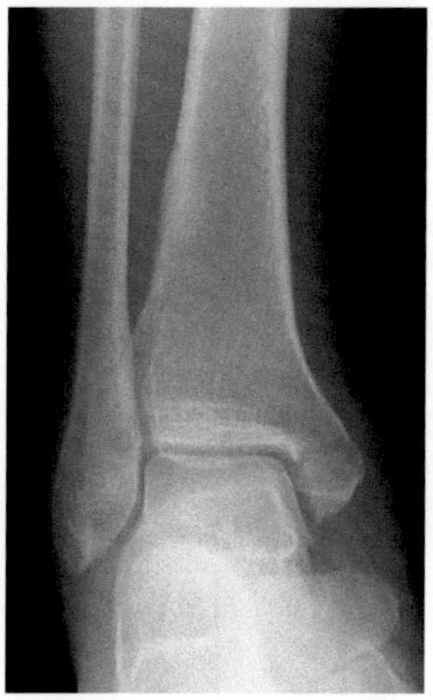

Lauge-Hansen classification of ankle fractures
Pronation-Abduction (PA)
Stage I: Medial malleolus fracture or injury to the deltoid ligament

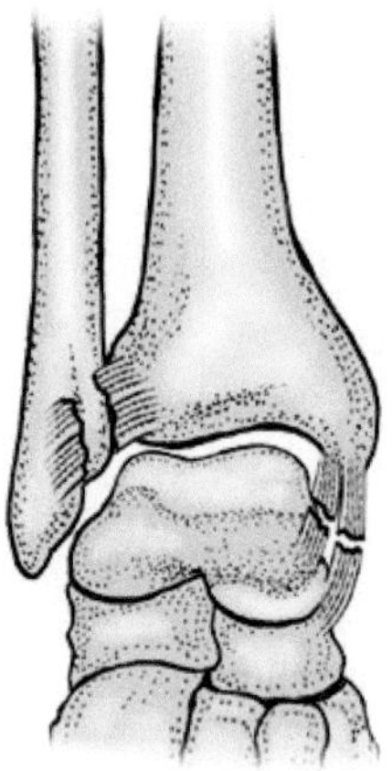

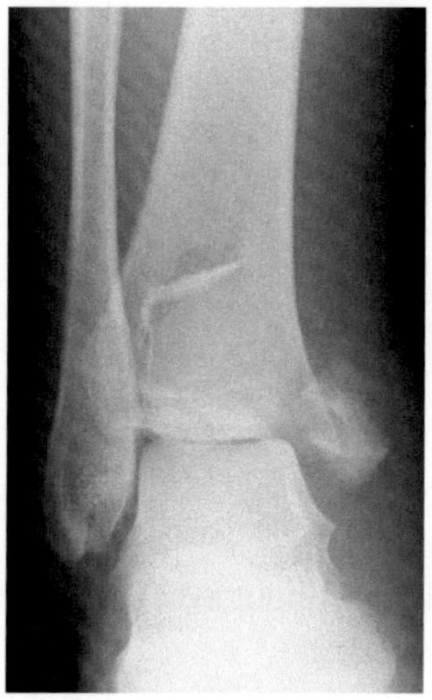

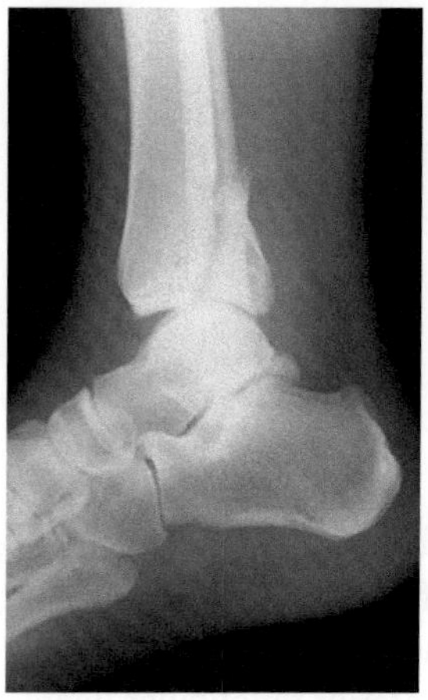

Lauge-Hansen classification of ankle fractures
Pronation-Abduction (PA)
Stage II: Injury of the anterior inferior tibiofibular ligament or avulsion fracture of one of its attachments

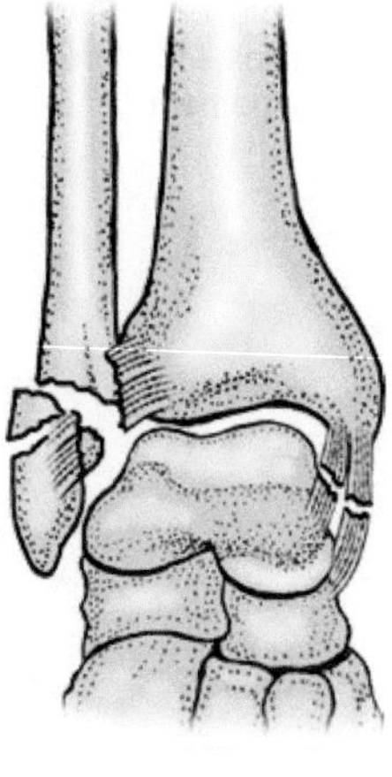

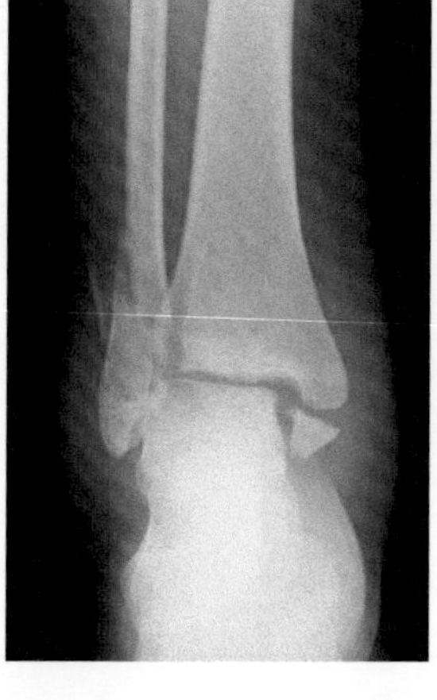

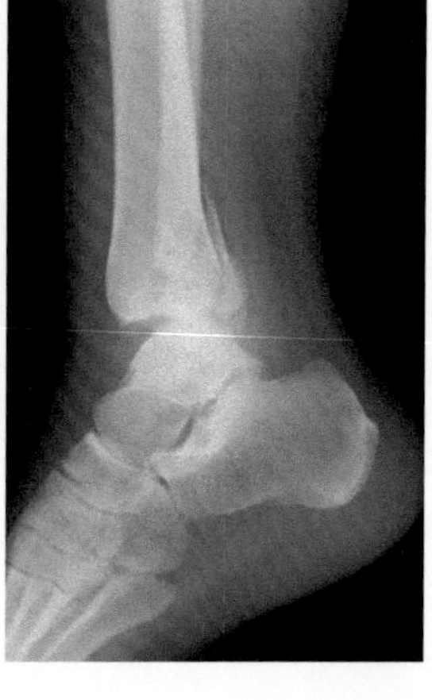

Lauge-Hansen classification of ankle fractures
Pronation-Abduction (PA)
Stage III: Transverse or short oblique fracture of the fibula above syndesmosis

Pronation-External Rotation (PER)

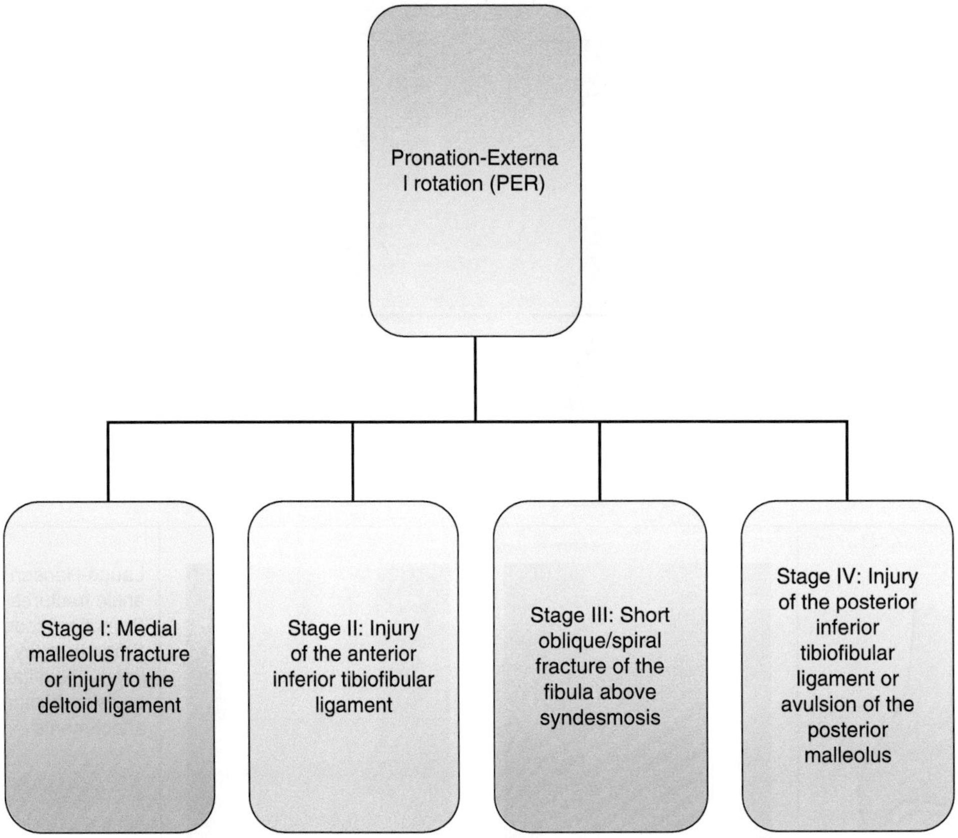

Stage I: Medial malleolus fracture or injury to the deltoid ligament.
Stage II: Injury of the anterior inferior tibiofibular ligament, with or without avulsion of one of its attachments.
Stage III: Short oblique/spiral fracture of the fibula above syndesmosis.
Stage IV: Injury of the posterior inferior tibiofibular ligament or avulsion of the posterior malleolus.

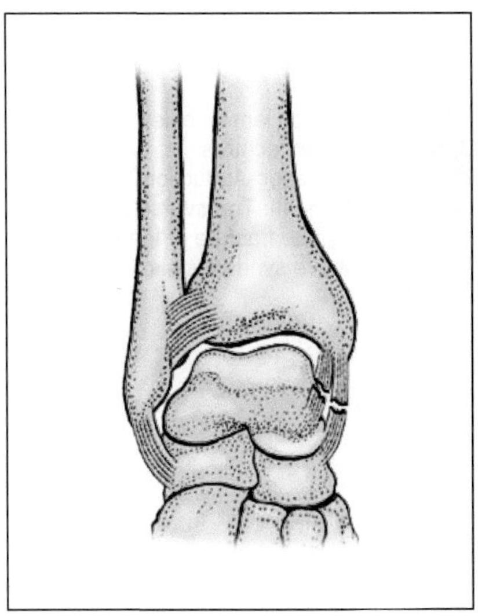

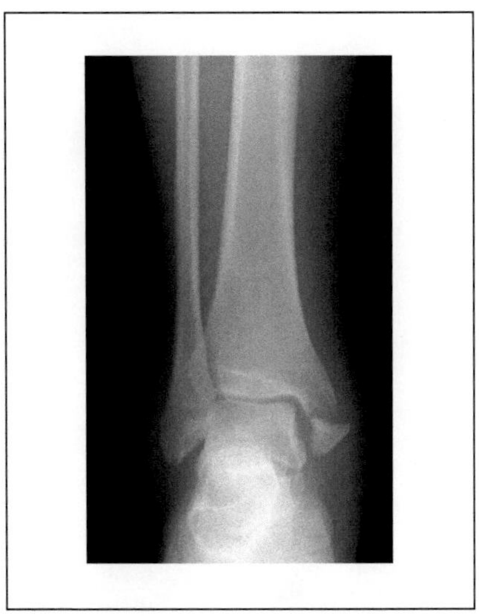

Lauge-Hansen classification of ankle fractures
Pronation-External rotation (PER):
Stage I: Medial malleolus fracture or injury to the deltoid ligament

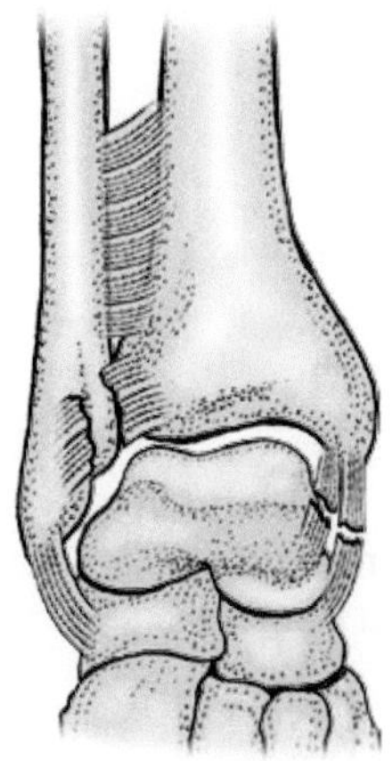

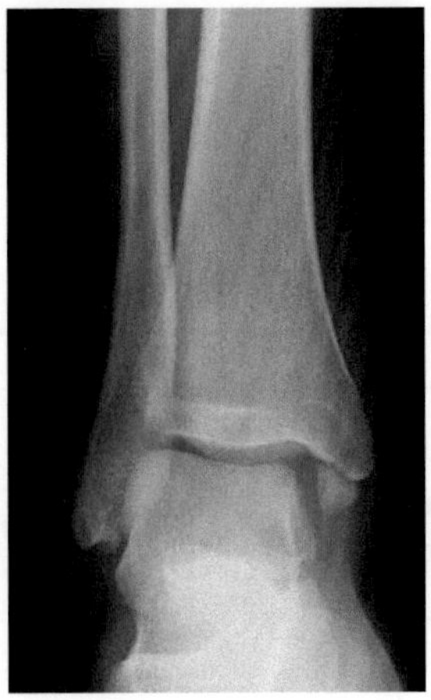

Lauge-Hansen classification of ankle fractures
Pronation-External rotation (PER):
Stage II: Injury of the anterior inferior tibiofibular ligament, with or without avulsion of one of its attachments

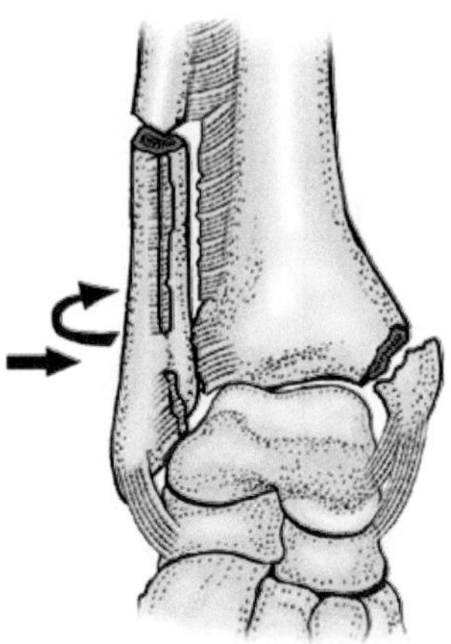

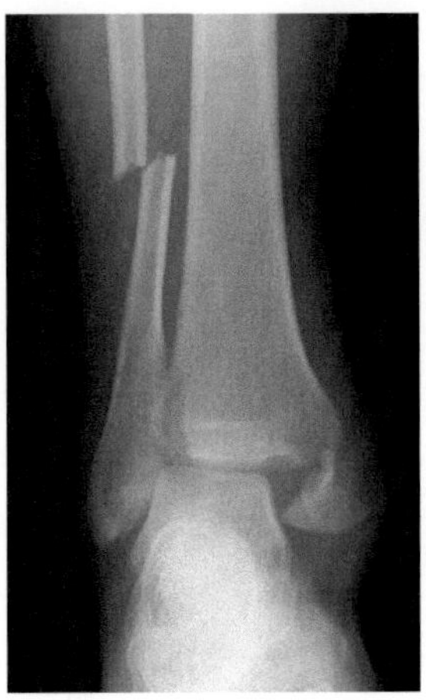

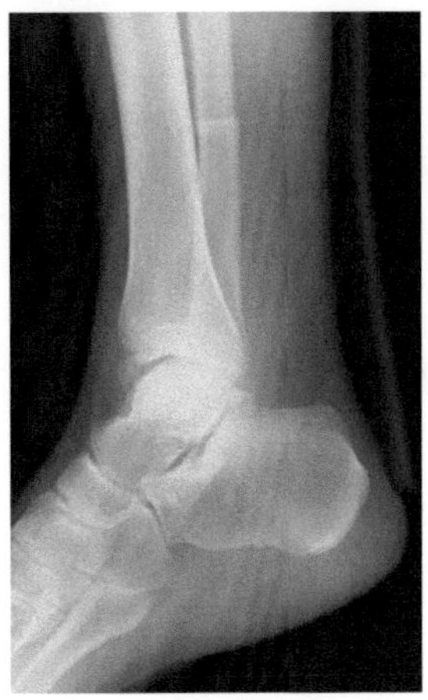

Lauge-Hansen classification of ankle fractures
Pronation-External rotation (PER)
Stage III: Short oblique/spiral fracture of the fibula above syndesmosis

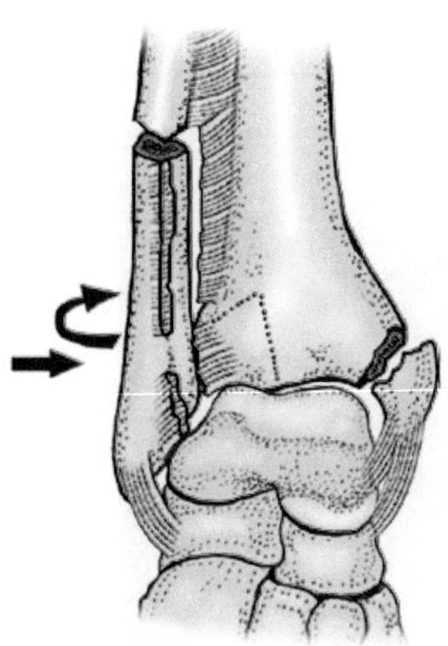

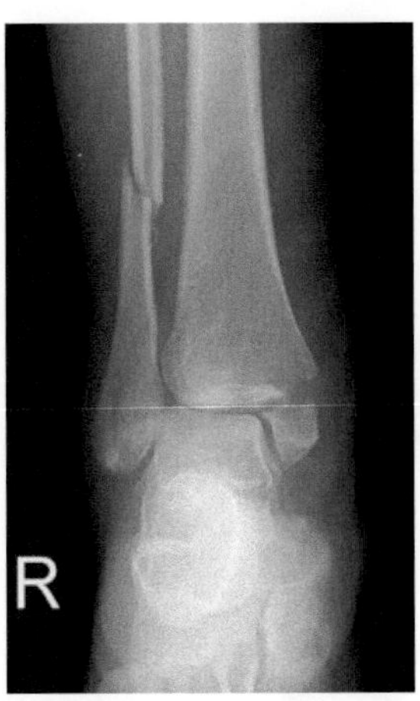

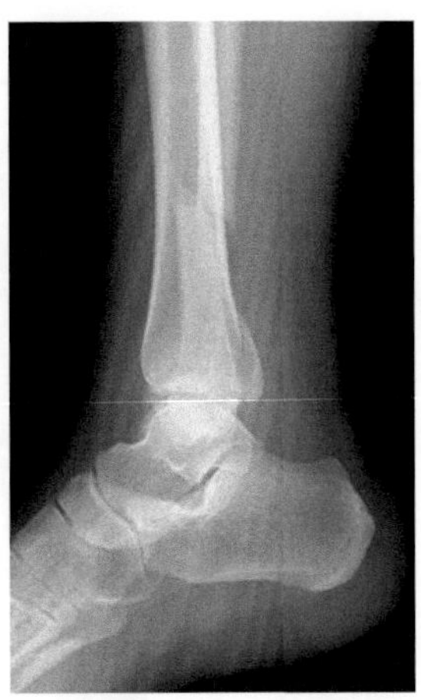

Lauge-Hansen classification of ankle fractures
Pronation-External rotation (PER)
Stage IV: Injury of the posterior inferior tibiofibular ligament or avulsion of the posterior malleolus

Pronation-Dorsal A? 旋前-背屈损伤(PDA)

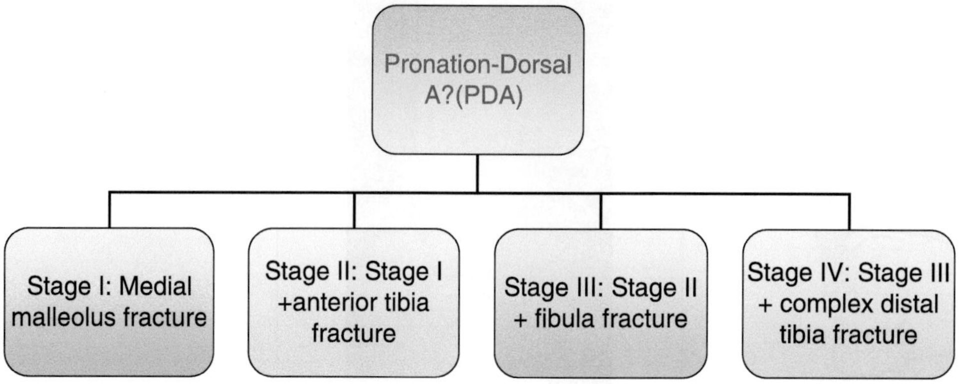

Stage I: Oblique medial malleolus fracture.
Stage II: Stage I+ anterior tibia fracture.
Stage III: Stage II+ fibula fracture.
Stage IV: Stage III + complex distal tibia fracture involving articular surface.

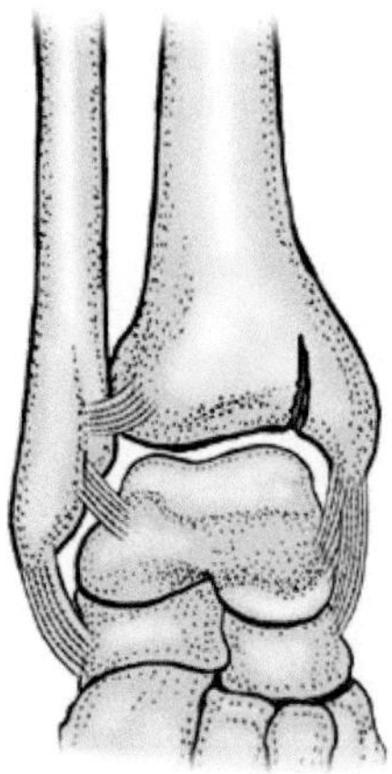
Pronation-Dorsal A?(PDA): Stage I

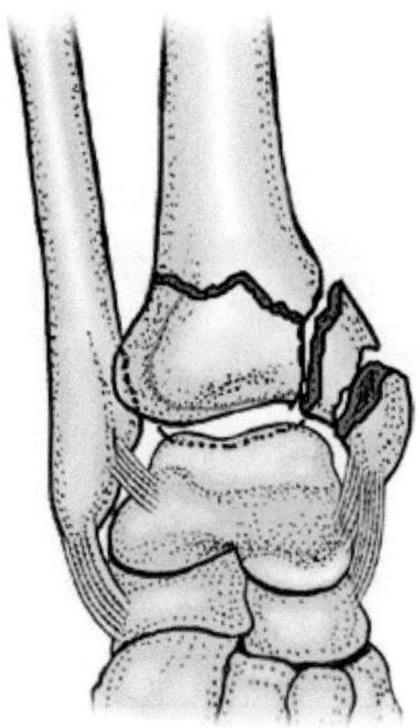
Pronation-Dorsal A?(PDA): Stage II

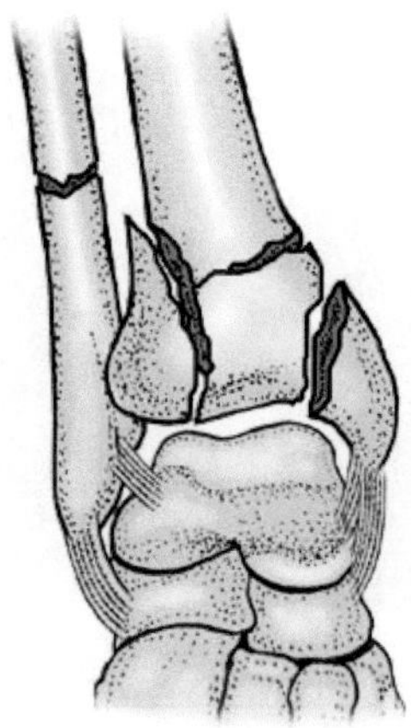
Pronation-Dorsal A?(PDA): Stage III

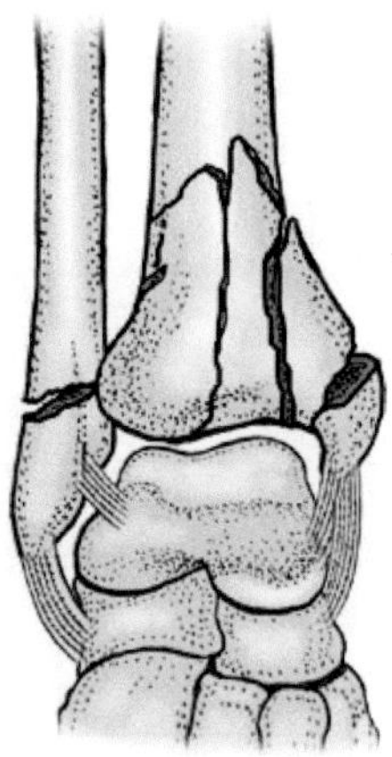
Pronation-Dorsal A?(PDA): Stage IV

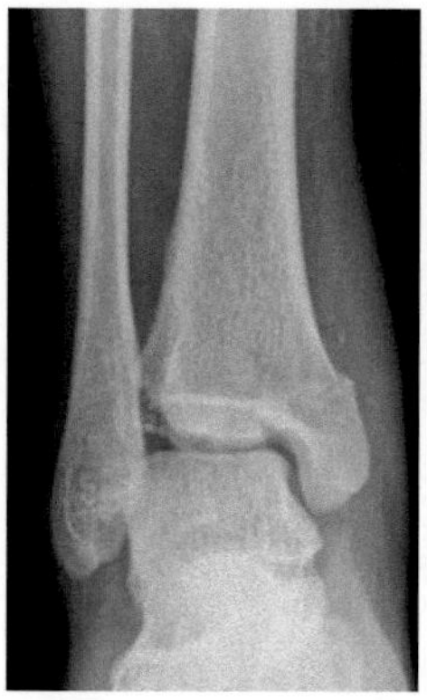
Stage I: Oblique medial malleolus fracture

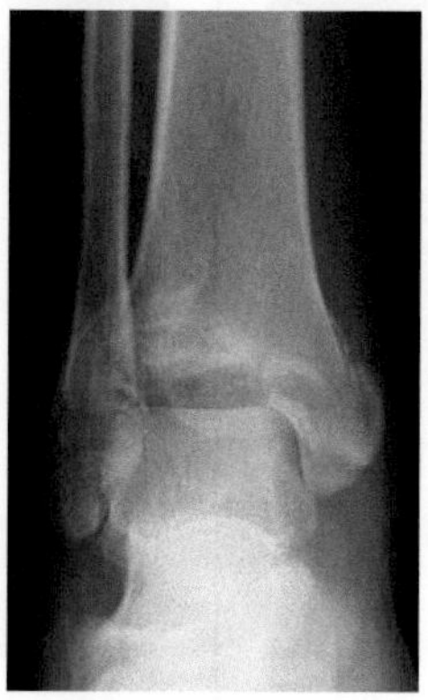
Stage III: Stage II(Stage I + anterior tibia fracture) + fibula fracture

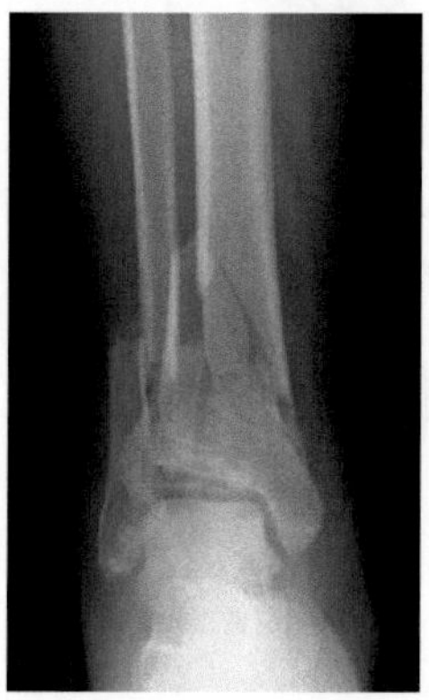
Stage IV: Stage III + complex distal tibia fracture involving articular surface

10.3.3.2 **Denis-Weber Classification** (1966, Die Verletjungen des boerenspurnggelenkes, in aktuelleproblome in der chirurgie. Bern: Verlag Hans Huber)

The Denis-Weber classification of ankle fractures is a very useful system initially proposed by Robert Denis in 1949 and subsequently modified by Weber in 1972, which is consulted by the AO classification system as well. This classification is based on the relationship of the fibular fracture to the syndesmosis. High fibular fractures usually indicate more severe syndesmosis injuries, larger displacements, and increased necessity for open surgery and internal fixation.

Type

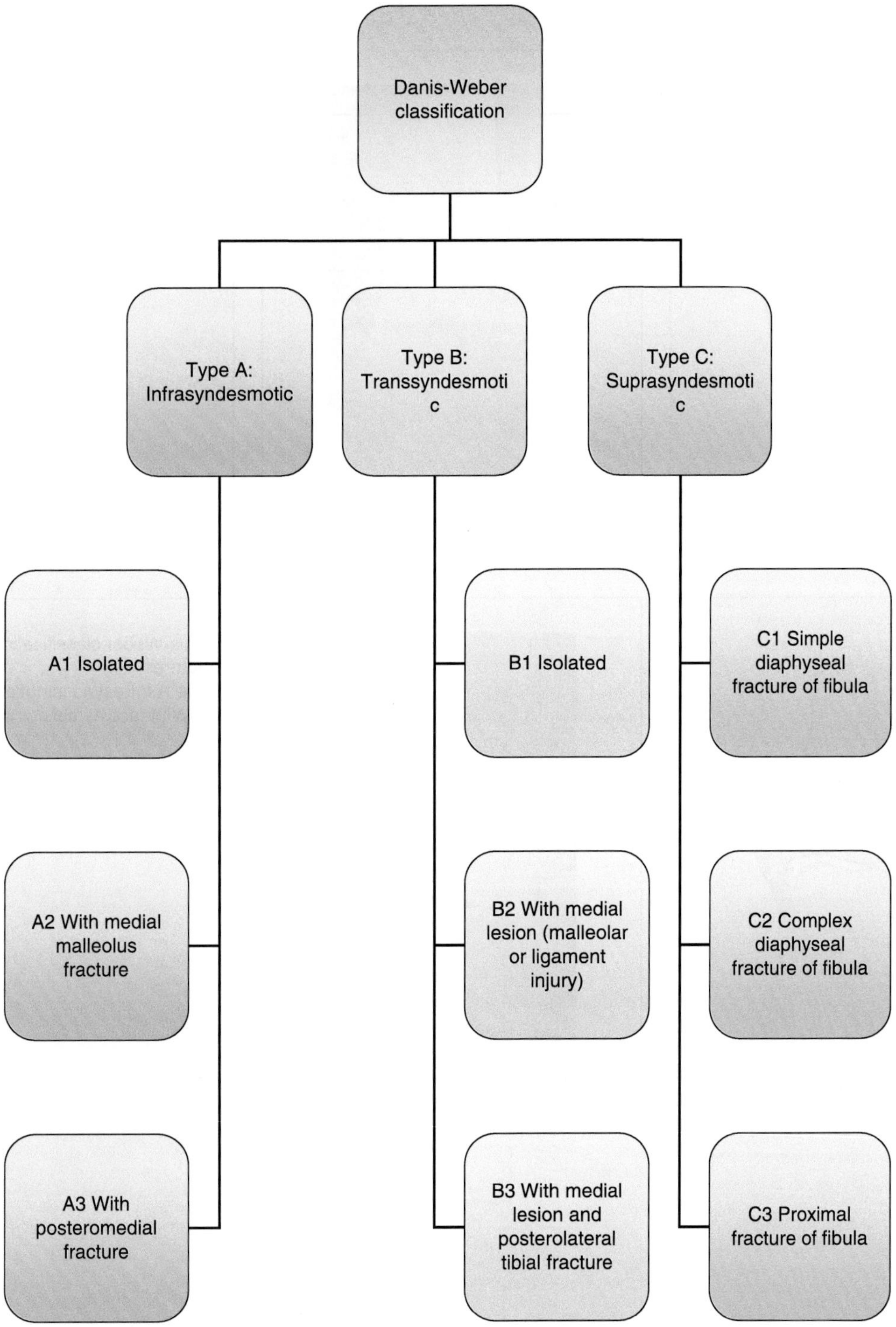

Type A: Infrasyndesmotic (fracture of fibula below the syndesmosis):
- Type A1: Isolated.
- Type A2: With medial malleolus fracture.
- Type A3: With posteromedial fracture.

Type B: Transsyndesmotic (fracture of fibula at syndesmosis level):
- Type B1: Isolated.
- Type B2: With medial lesion (malleolar or ligament injury).
- Type B3: With medial lesion and posterolateral tibial fracture.

Type C: Suprasyndesmotic (fracture of fibula above syndesmosis):
- Type C1: Simple diaphyseal fracture of fibula.
- Type C2: Complex diaphyseal fracture of fibula.
- Type C3: Proximal fracture of fibula.

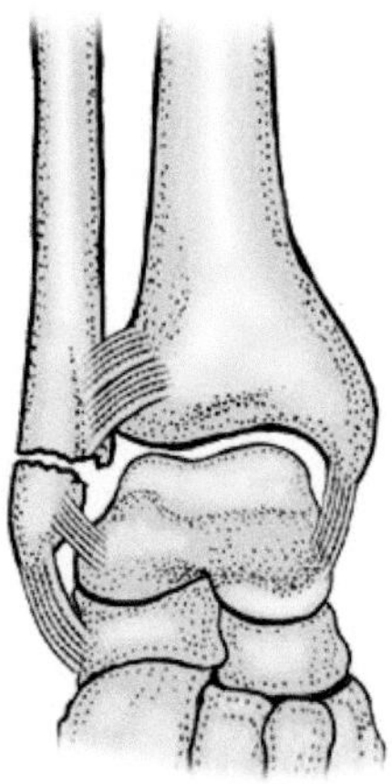
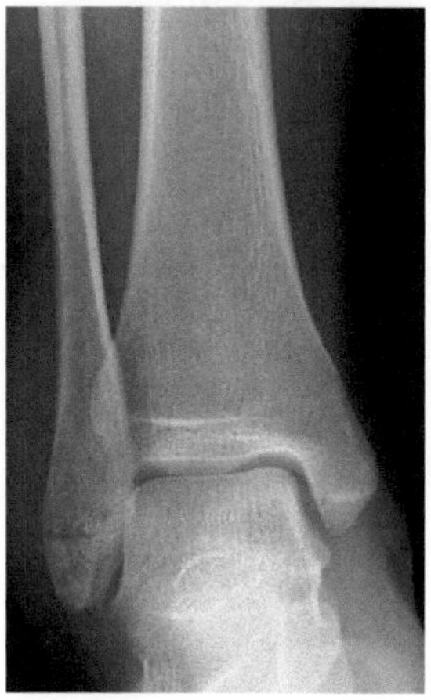

Denis-Weber classification of ankle fractures
Type A Infrasyndesmotic
A1 Isolated

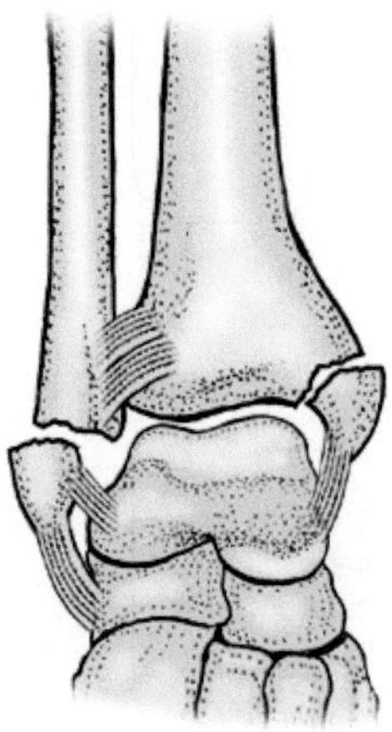
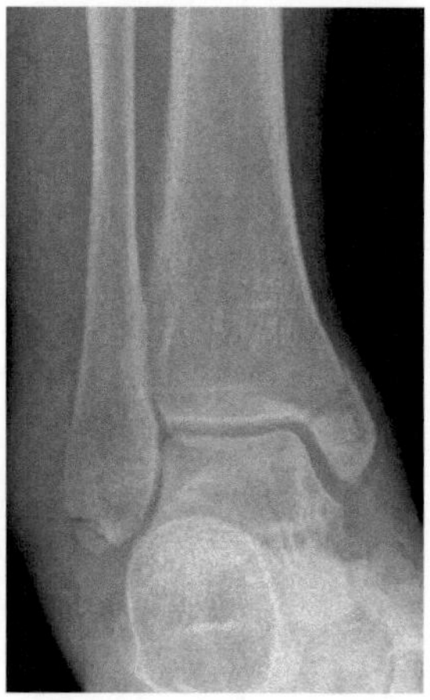

Denis-Weber classification of ankle fractures
Type A Infrasyndesmotic
A2 With medial malleolus fracture

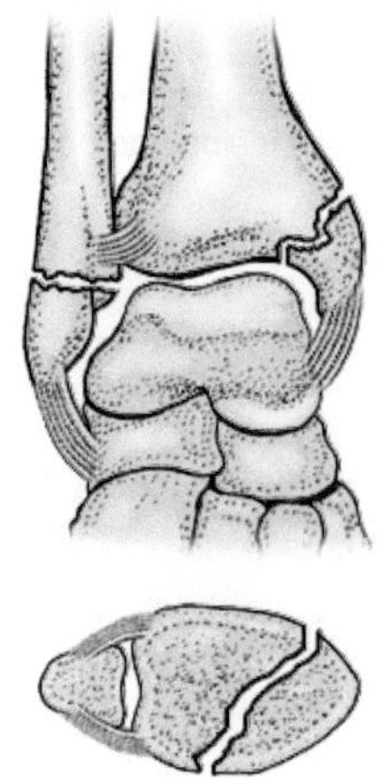

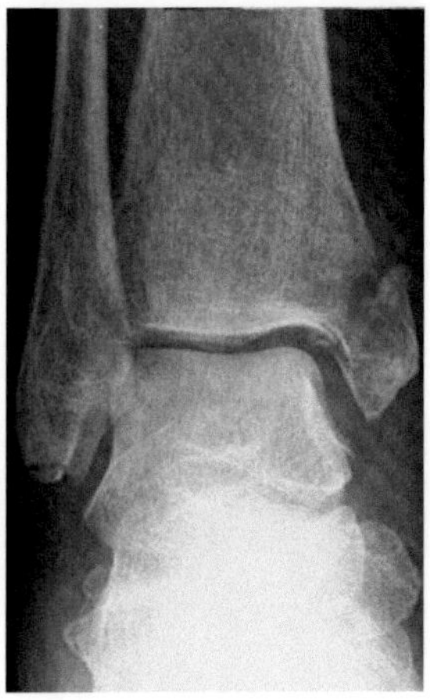

Denis-Weber classification of ankle fractures
Type A Infrasyndesmotic
A3 With posteromedial fracture

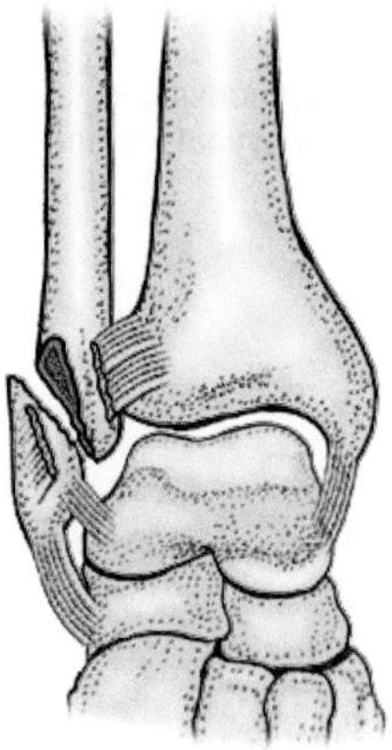

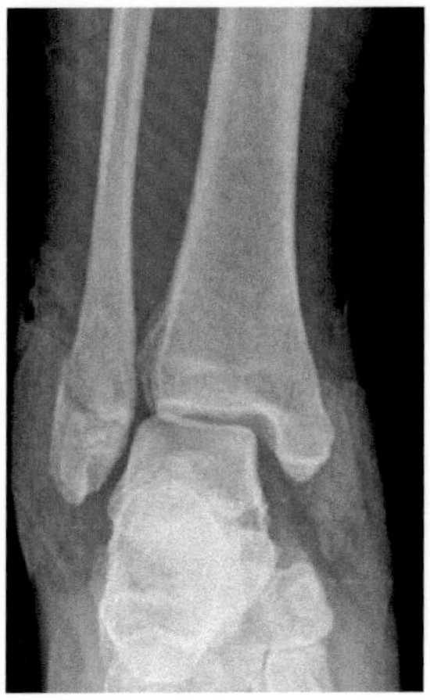

Denis-Weber classification of ankle fractures
Type B Transsyndesmotic
B1 Isolated

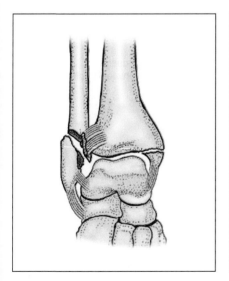

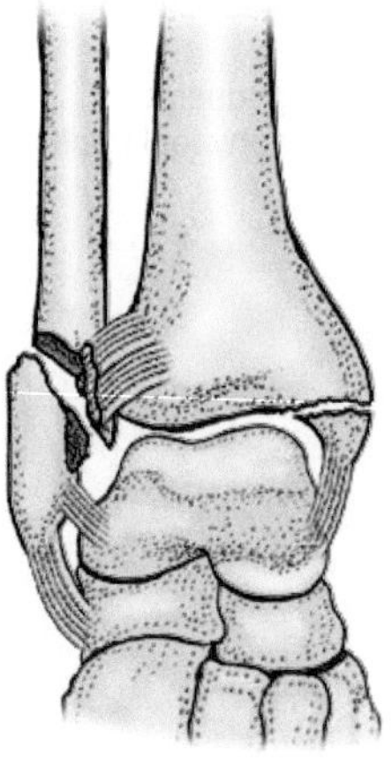

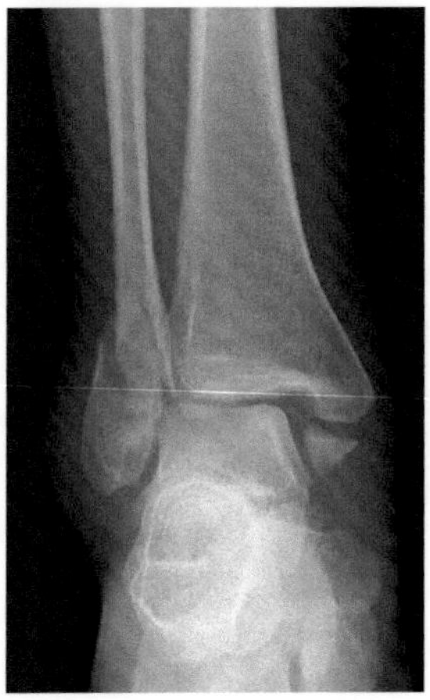

Denis-Weber classification of ankle fractures
Type B Transsyndesmotic
B2 With medial lesion (malleolar or ligament injury)

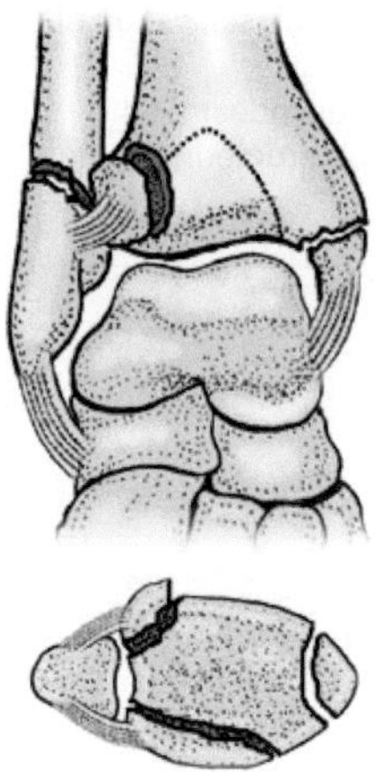

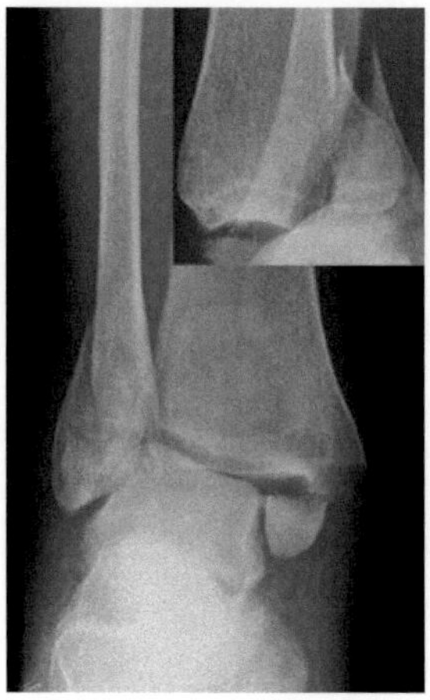

Denis-Weber classification of ankle fractures
Type B Transsyndesmotic
B3 With medial lesion and posterolateral tibial fracture

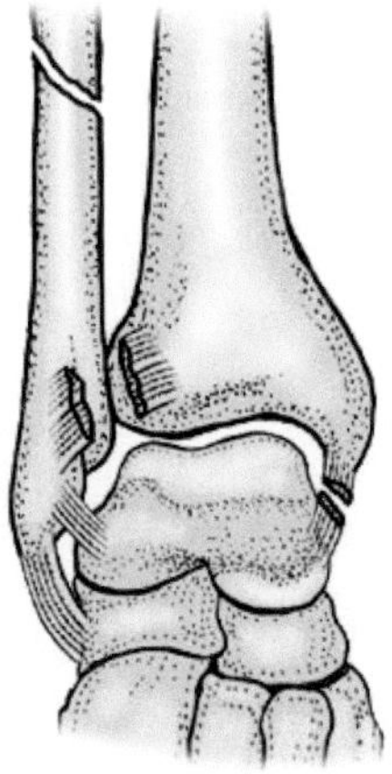

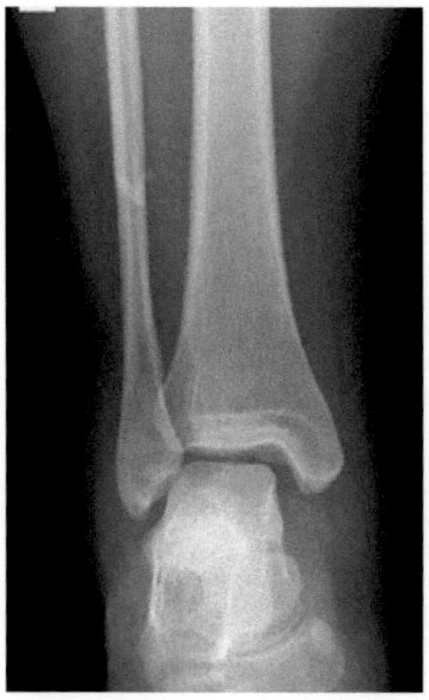

Denis-Weber classification of ankle fractures
Type C Suprasyndesmotic
C1 Simple diaphyseal fracture of fibula

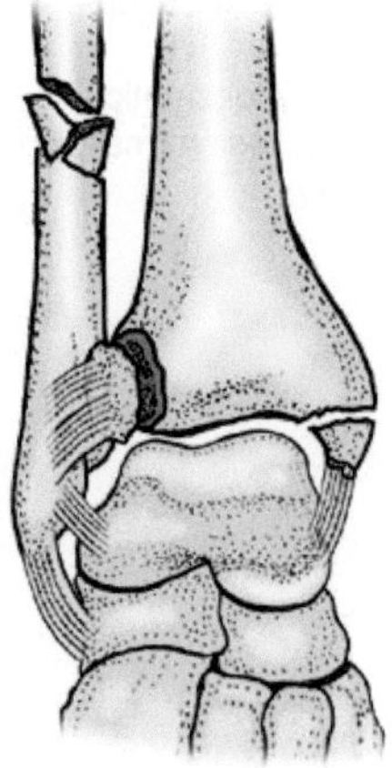

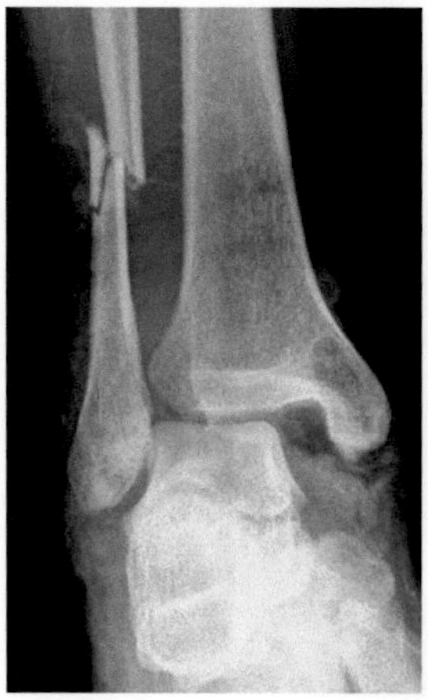

Denis-Weber classification of ankle fractures
Type C Suprasyndesmotic
C2 Complex diaphyseal fracture of fibula

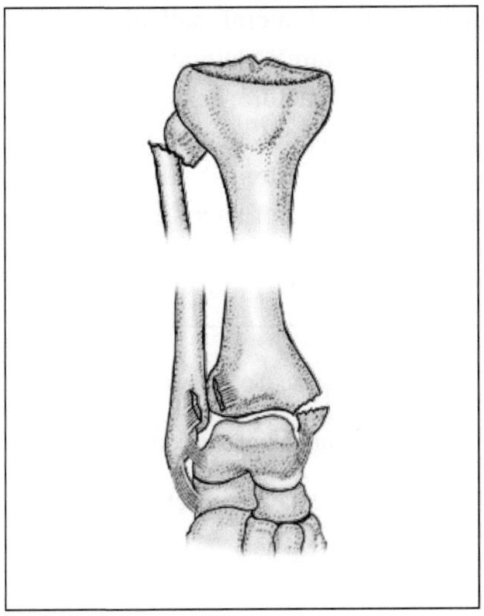

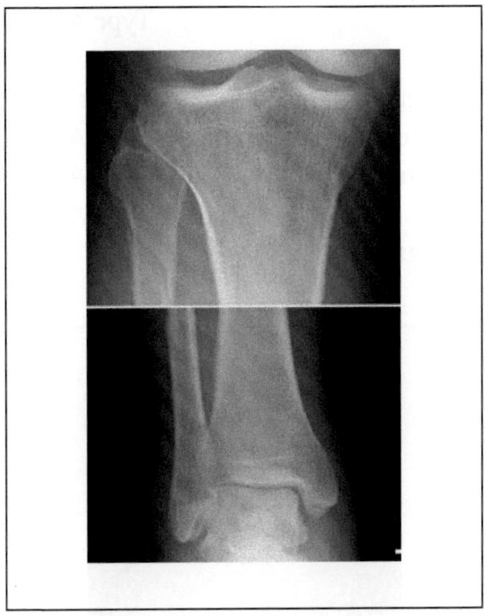

Denis-Weber classification of ankle fractures
Type C Suprasyndesmotic
C3 Proximal fracture of fibula

10.3.3.3 **AO/OTA Classification** (2007 revised version, Journal of Orthopaedic Trauma, 21 supplement; the AO classification of long bone fracture was firstly proposed by Muller in 1980s)

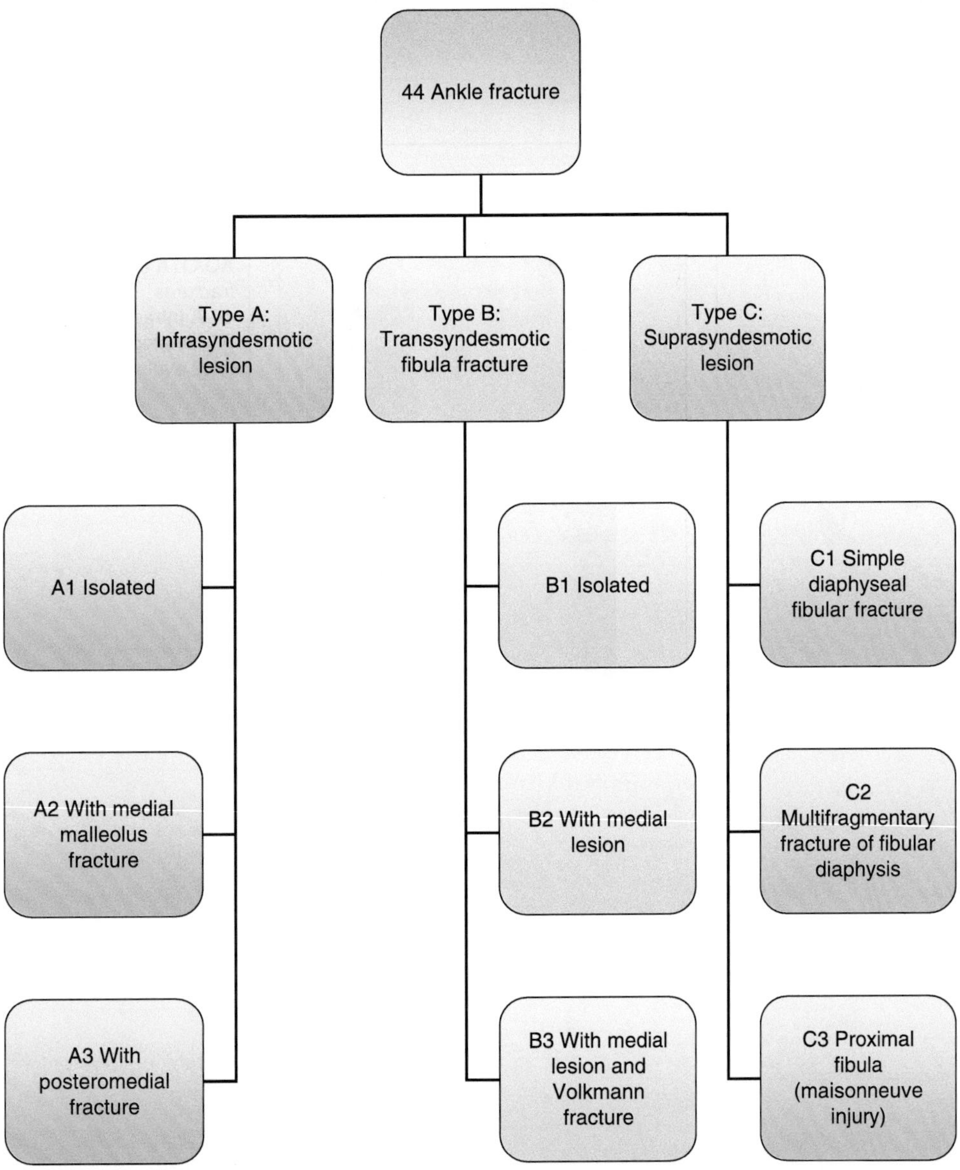

Type A: Infrasyndesmotic lesion:
- Type A1: Isolated:
  - Type A1.1: Rupture of lateral collateral ligament.
  - Type A1.2: Avulsion of tip of lateral malleolus.
  - Type A1.3: Transverse fracture of lateral malleolus.
- Type A2: With medial malleolus fracture:
  - Type A2.1: Rupture of lateral collateral ligament.
  - Type A2.2: Avulsion of tip of lateral malleolus.
  - Type A2.3: Transverse fracture of lateral malleolus.
- Type A3: With posteromedial fracture:
  - Type A3.1: Rupture of lateral collateral ligament.
  - Type A3.2: Avulsion of tip of lateral malleolus.
  - Type A3.3: Transverse fracture of lateral malleolus.

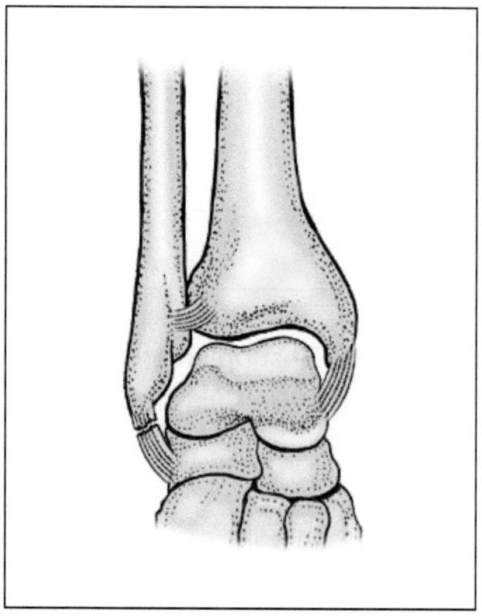

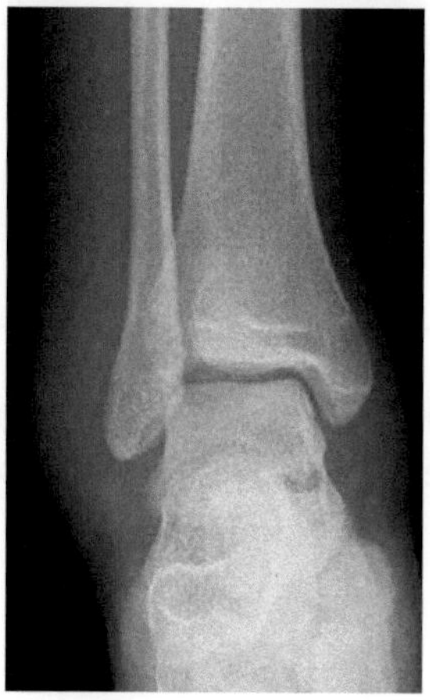

AO/OTA classification of tibia and fibula fractures
44-A Infrasyndesmotic lesion
A1 Isolated
A1.1 rupture of lateral collateral ligament

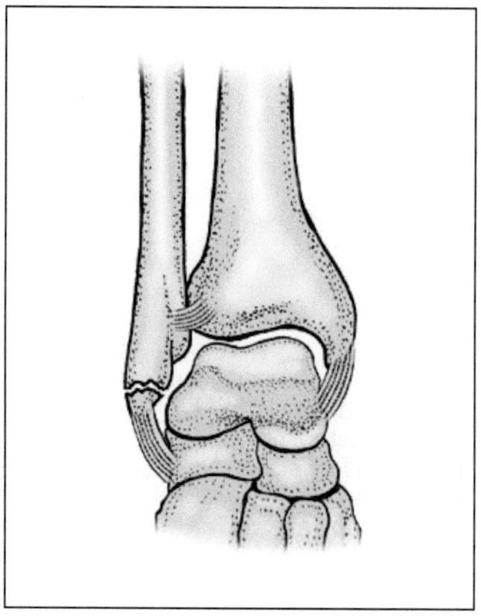

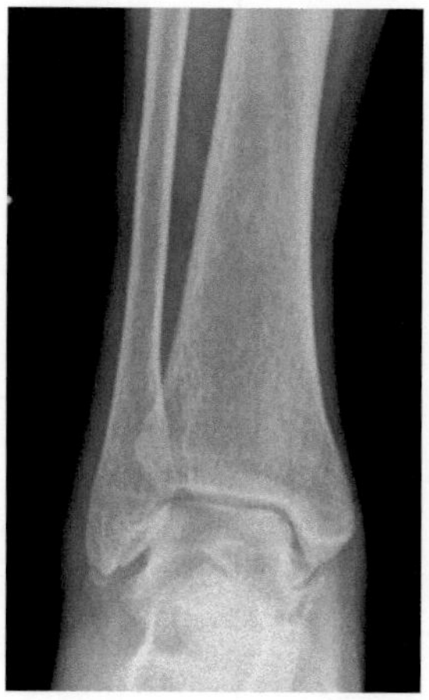

AO/OTA classification of tibia and fibula fractures
44-A Infrasyndesmotic lesion
A1 Isolated
A1.2 avulsion of tip of lateral malleolus

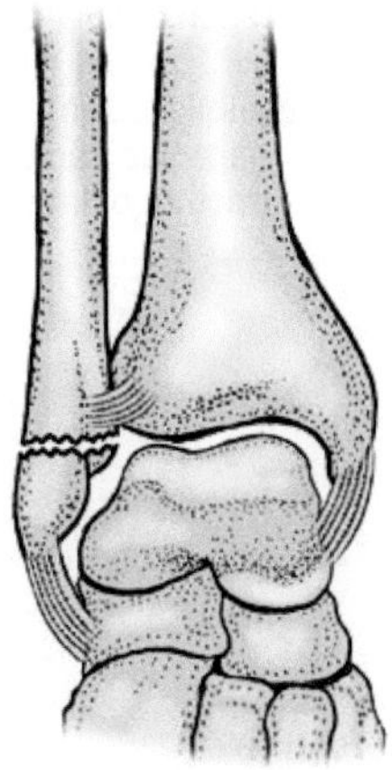

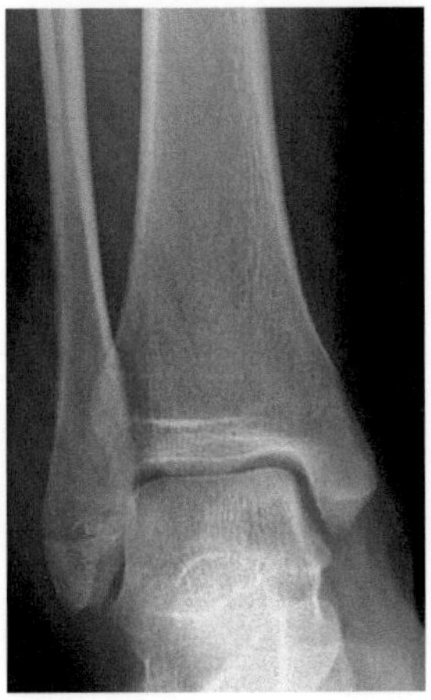

AO/OTA classification of tibia and fibula fractures
44-A Infrasyndesmotic lesion
A1 Isolated
A1.3 transverse fracture of lateral malleolus

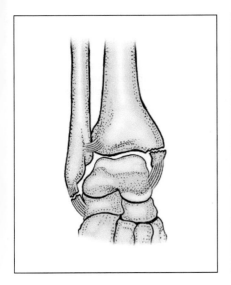

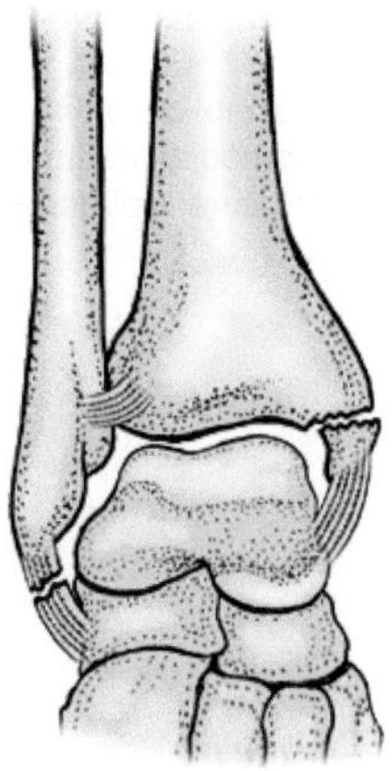

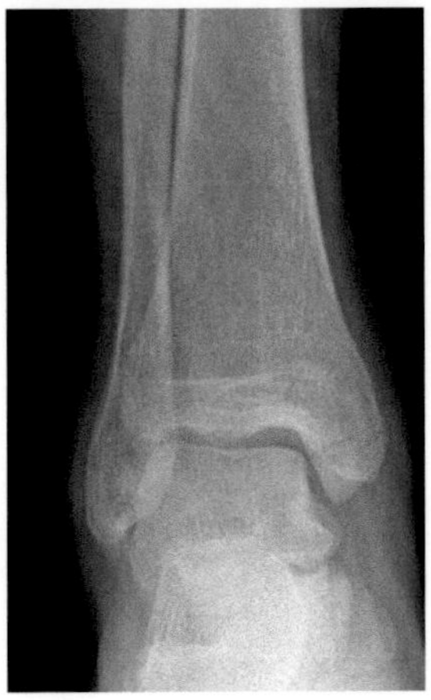

AO/OTA classification of tibia and fibula fractures
44-A Infrasyndesmotic lesion
A2 With medial malleolus fracture
A2.1 rupture of lateral collateral ligament

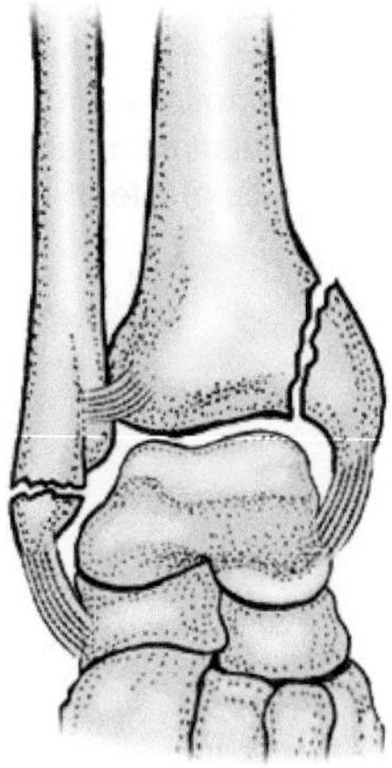

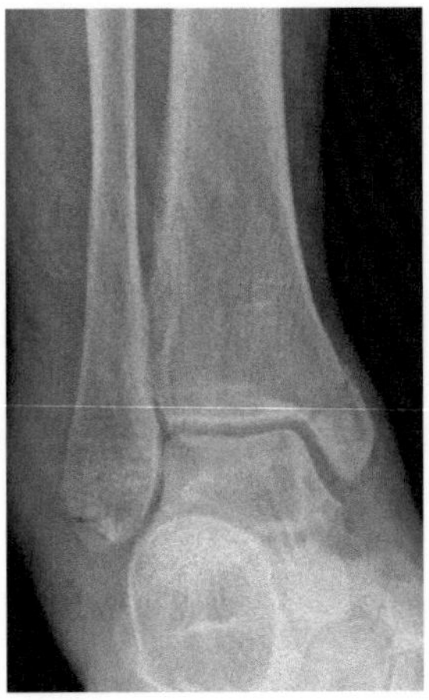

AO/OTA classification of tibia and fibula fractures
44-A Infrasyndesmotic lesion
A2 With medial malleolus fracture
A2.2 avulsion of tip of lateral malleolus

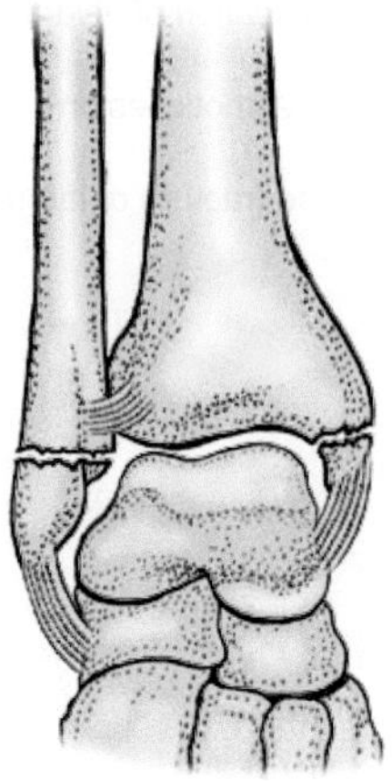

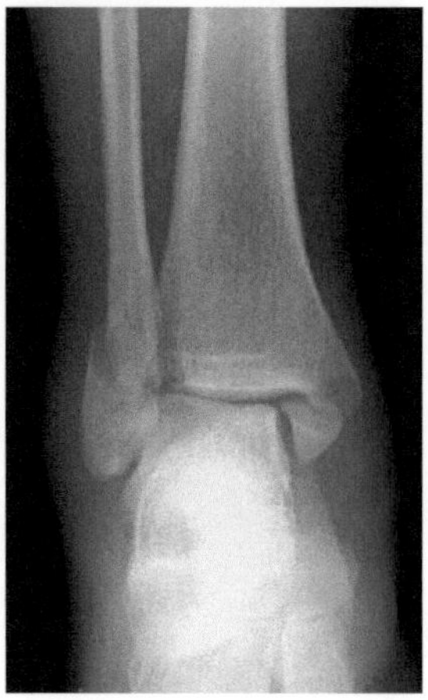

AO/OTA classification of tibia and fibula fractures
44-A Infrasyndesmotic lesion
A2 With medial malleolus fracture
A2.3 transverse fracture of lateral malleolus

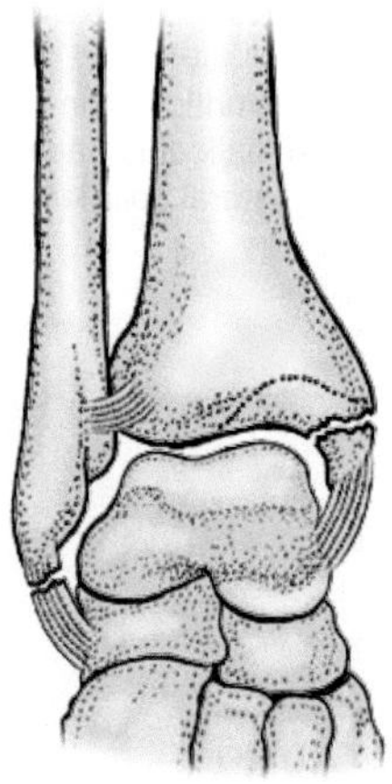

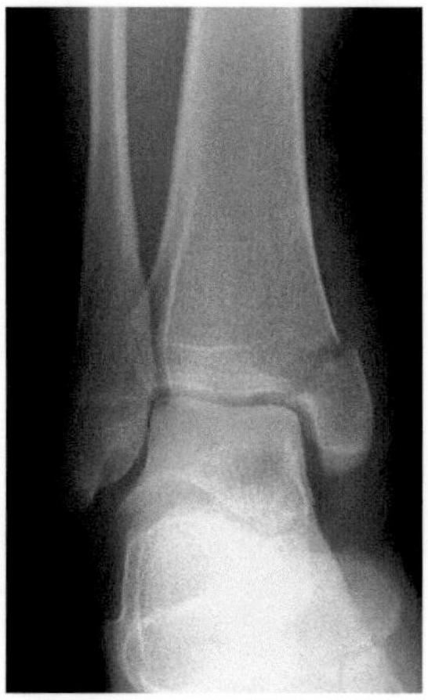

AO/OTA classification of tibia and fibula fractures
44-A Infrasyndesmotic lesion
A3 With posteromedial fracture
A3.1 rupture of lateral collateral ligament

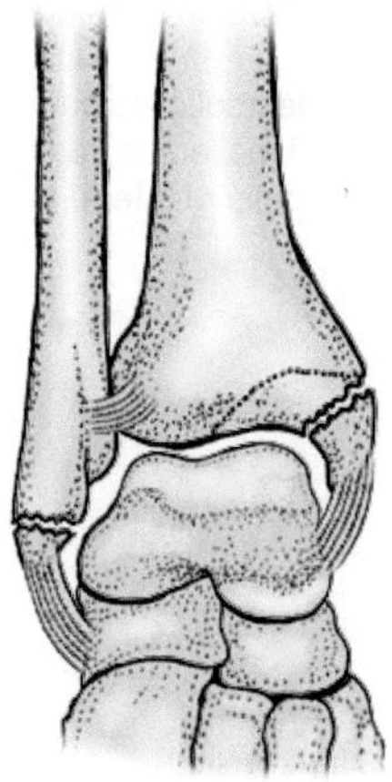

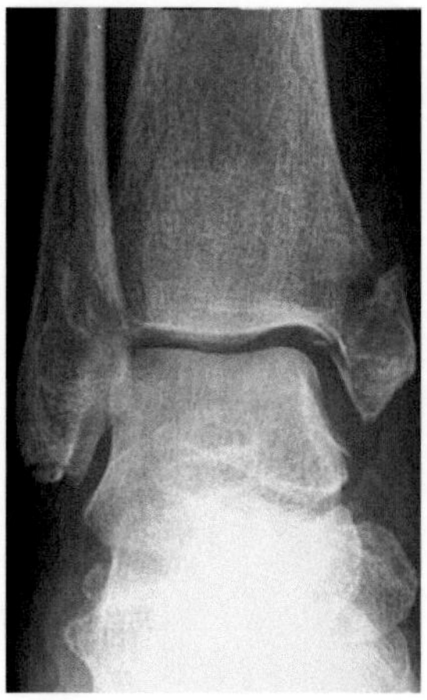

AO/OTA classification of tibia and fibula fractures
44-A Infrasyndesmotic lesion
A3 With posteromedial fracture
A3.2 avulsion of tip of lateral malleolus

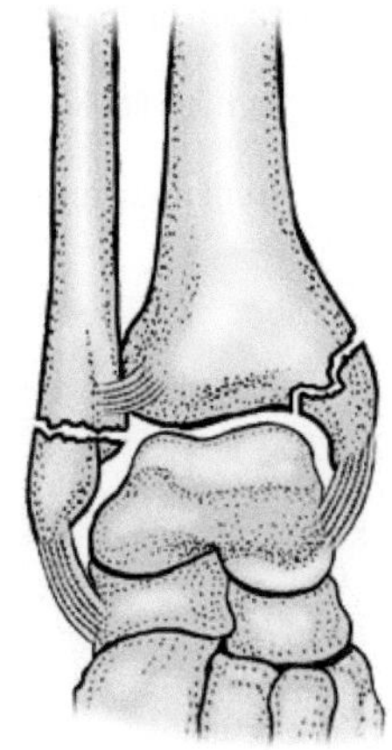

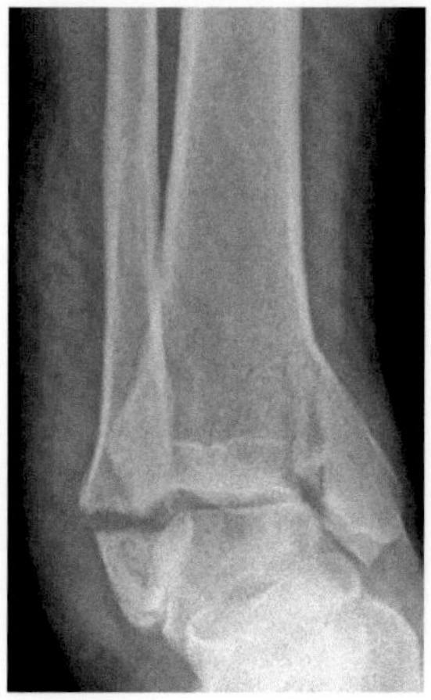

AO/OTA classification of tibia and fibula fractures
44-A Infrasyndesmotic lesion
A3 With posteromedial fracture
A3.3 transverse fracture of lateral malleolus

Type B: Transsyndesmotic fibula fracture:
- Type B1: Isolated:
  - Type B1.1: Simple.
  - Type B1.2: Simple with rupture of anterior syndesmosis.
  - Type B1.3: Multifragmentary.
- Type B2: With medial lesion:
  - Type B2.1: Simple with rupture of medial collateral and anterior syndesmosis.
  - Type B2.2: Simple with fracture of medial malleolus and rupture of anterior syndesmosis.
  - Type B2.3: Multifragmentary with medial lesion.
- Type B3: With medial lesion and Volkmann (fracture of posterolateral rim):
  - Type B3.1: Simple with medial collateral ligament rupture.
  - Type B3.2: Simple with fracture of medial malleolus.
  - Type B3.3: Multifragmentary with fracture of medial malleolus.

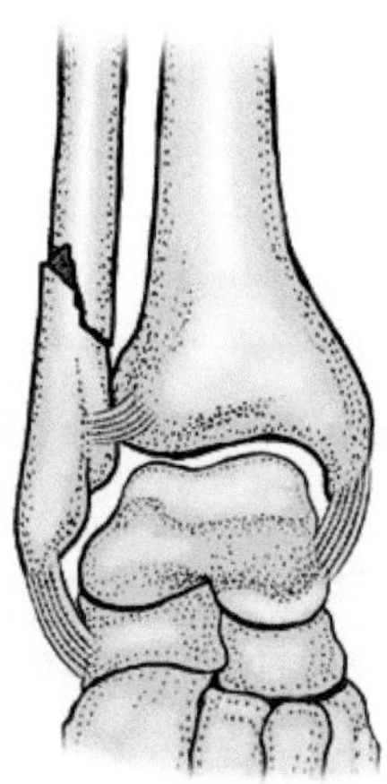

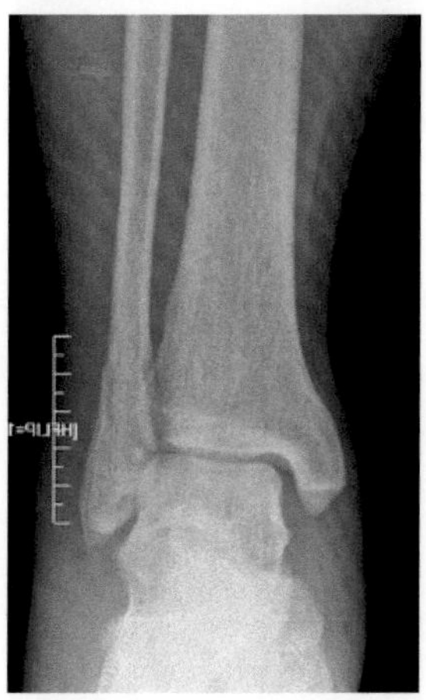

AO/OTA classification of tibia and fibula fractures
44-B Transsyndesmotic fibula fracture
B1 Isolated
B1.1 simple

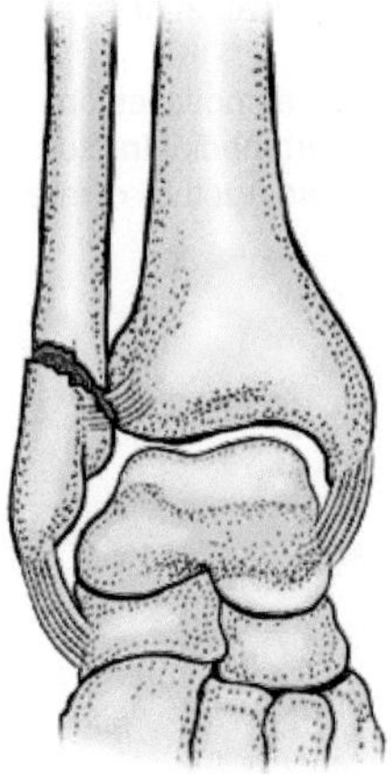

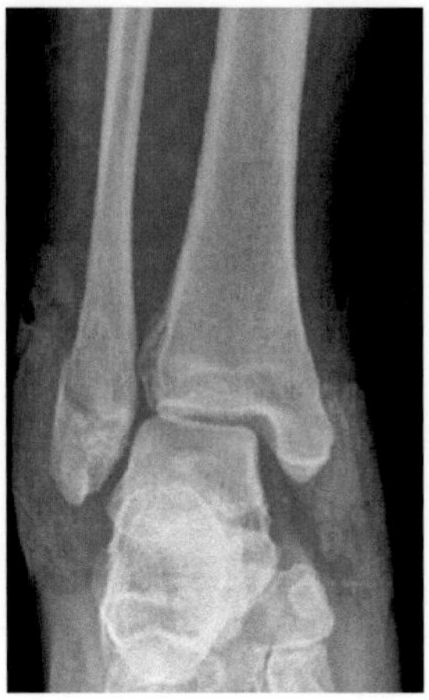

AO/OTA classification of tibia and fibula fractures
44-B Transsyndesmotic fibula fracture
B1 Isolated
B1.2 simple with rupture of anterior syndesmosis

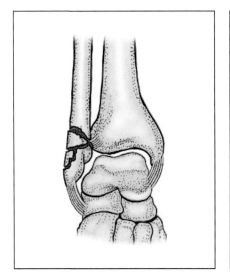

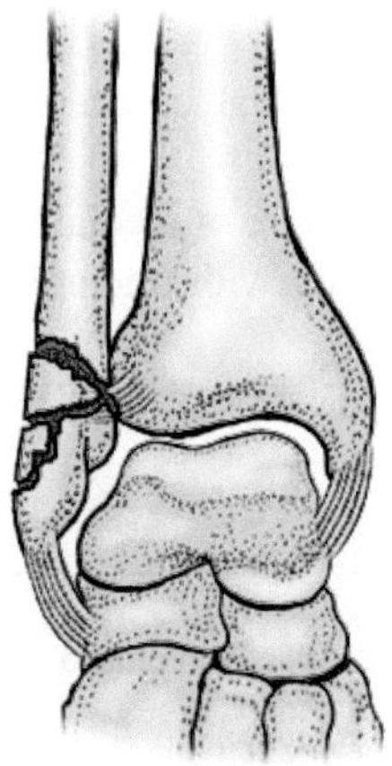

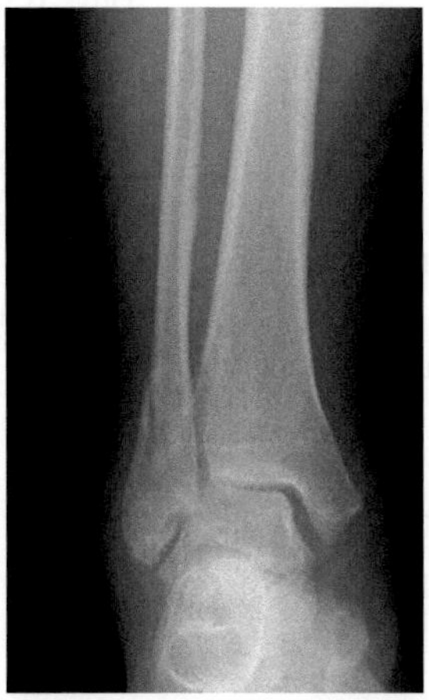

AO/OTA classification of tibia and fibula fractures
44-B Transsyndesmotic fibula fracture
B1 Isolated
B1.3 multifragmentary

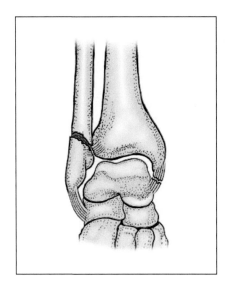

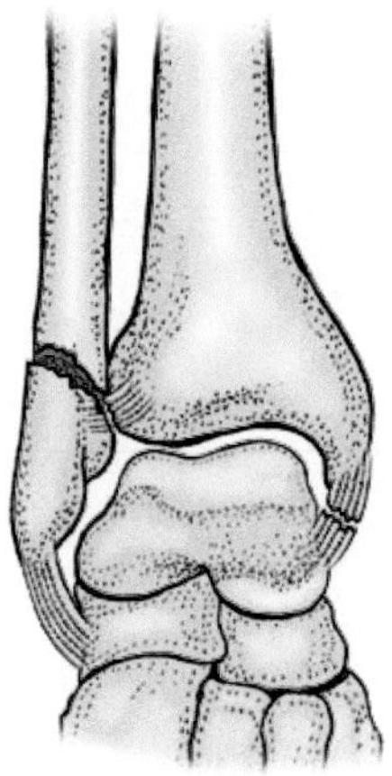

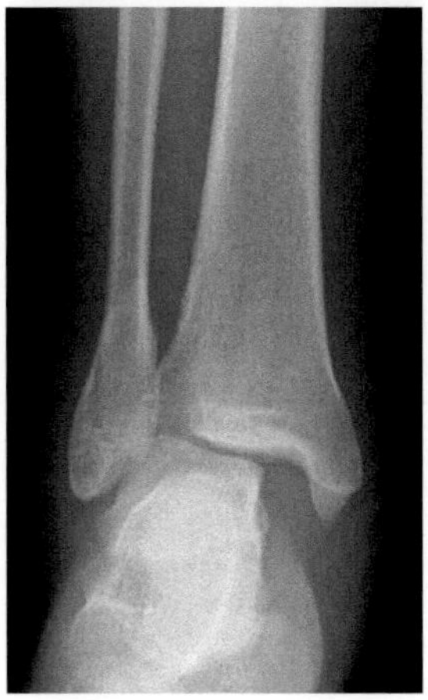

AO/OTA classification of tibia and fibula fractures
44-B Transsyndesmotic fibula fracture
B2 With medial lesion
B2.1 simple with rupture of medial collateral and anterior syndesmosis

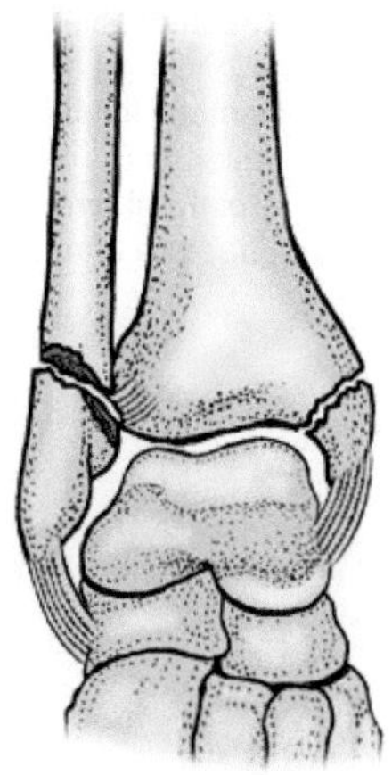

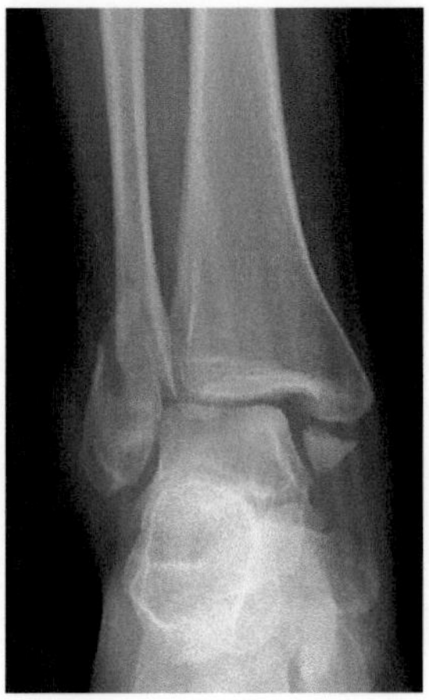

AO/OTA classification of tibia and fibula fractures
44-B Transsyndesmotic fibula fracture
B2 With medial lesion
B2.2 simple with fracture of medial malleolus and rupture of anterior syndesmosis

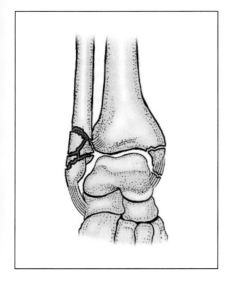

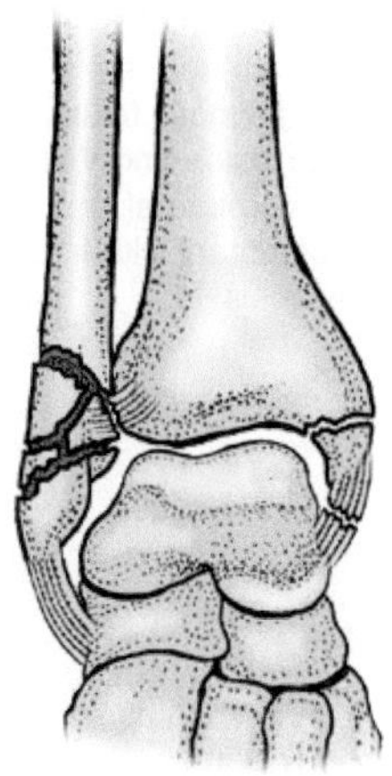

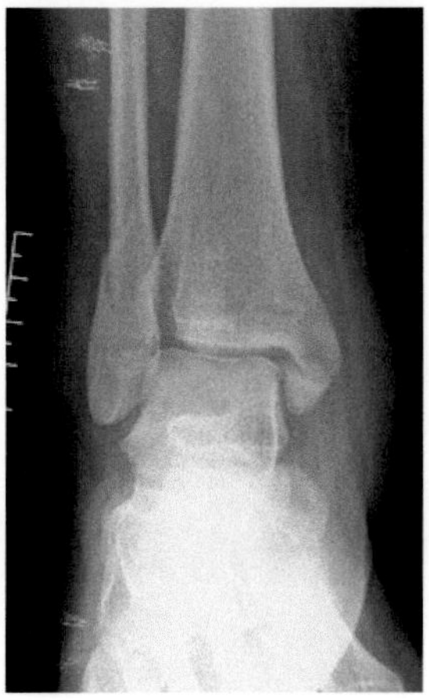

AO/OTA classification of tibia and fibula fractures
44-B Transsyndesmotic fibula fracture
B2 With medial lesion B2.3 multifragmentary with medial lesion

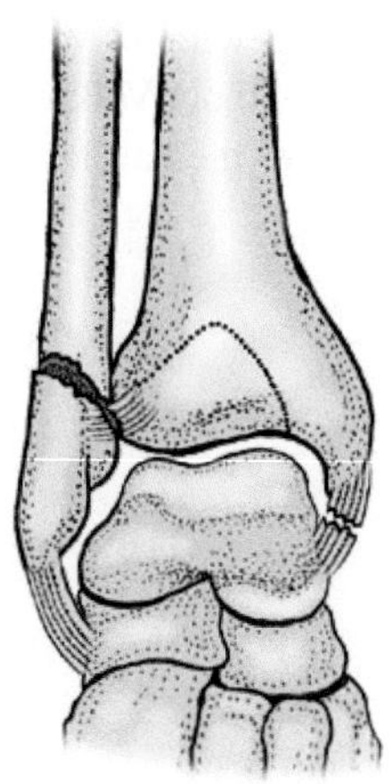

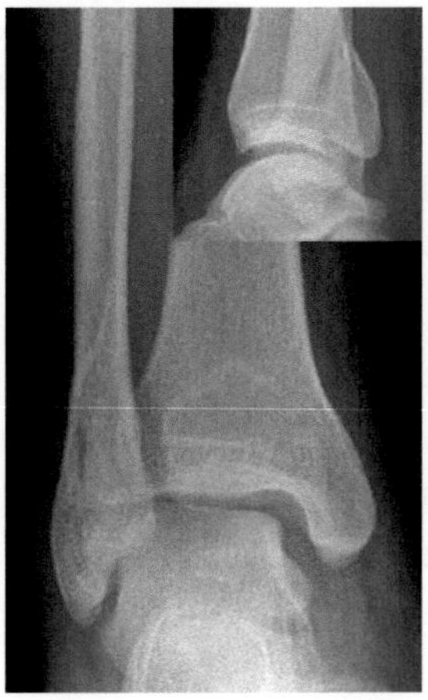

AO/OTA classification of tibia and fibula fractures
44-B Transsyndesmotic fibula fracture
B3 With medial lesion and Volkmann (fracture of posterolateral rim)
B3.1 simple with medial collateral ligament rupture

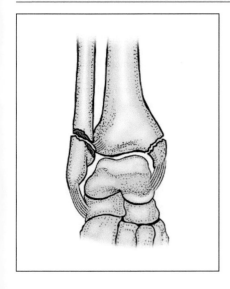

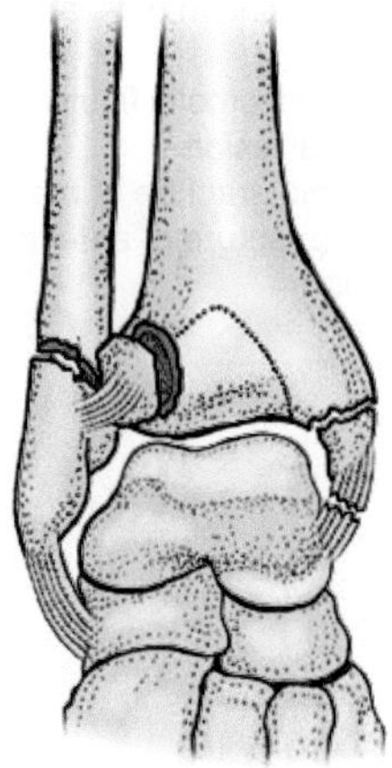

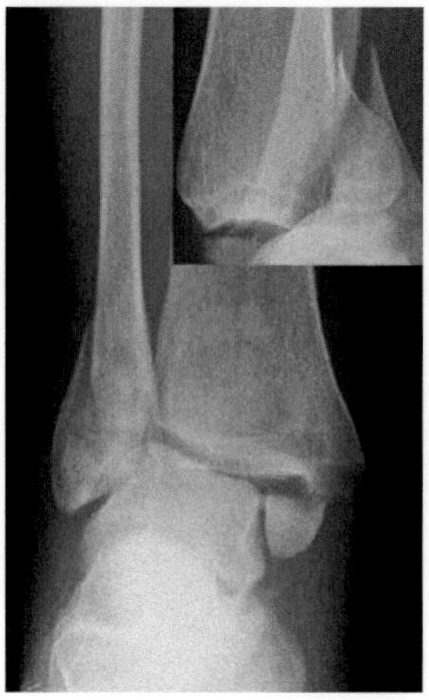

AO/OTA classification of tibia and fibula fractures
44-B Transsyndesmotic fibula fracture
B3 With medial lesion and Volkmann (fracture of posterolateral rim)
B3.2 simple with fracture of medial malleolus

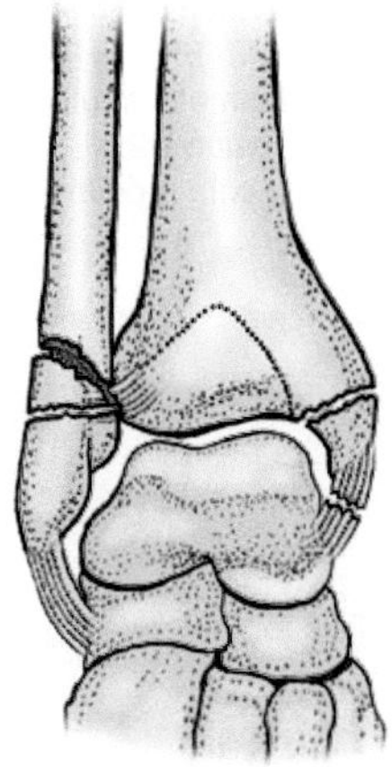

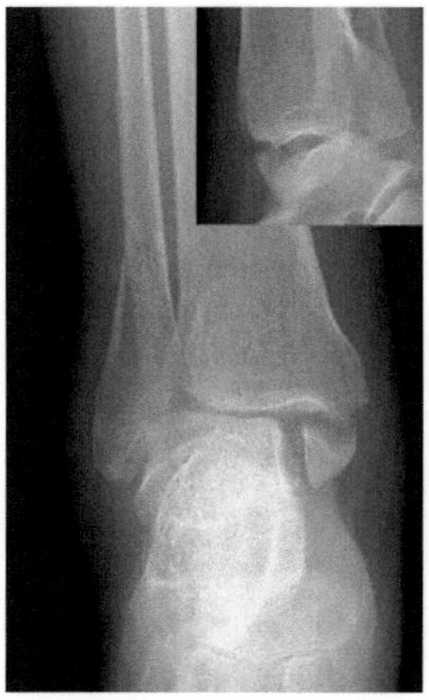

AO/OTA classification of tibia and fibula fractures
44-B Transsyndesmotic fibula fracture
B3 With medial lesion and Volkmann (fracture of posterolateral rim)
B3.3 multifragmentary with fracture of medial malleolus

Type C: Suprasyndesmotic lesion:

- Type C1: Simple diaphyseal fibular fracture:
  - Type C1.1: With rupture of medial collateral ligament.
  - Type C1.2: With fracture of medial malleolus.
  - Type C1.3: With fracture of medial malleolus and a Volkmann (Dupuytren).
- Type C2: Multifragmentary fracture of fibular diaphysis:
  - Type C2.1: With rupture of medial collateral ligament.
  - Type C2.2: With fracture of medial malleolus.
  - Type C2.3: With fracture of medial malleolus and a Volkmann (Dupuytren).
- Type C3: Proximal fibula (Maisonneuve injury):
  - Type C3.1: Without shortening, without Volkmann.
  - Type C3.2: With shortening, without Volkmann.
  - Type C3.3: Dislocation with medial lesion and a Volkmann.

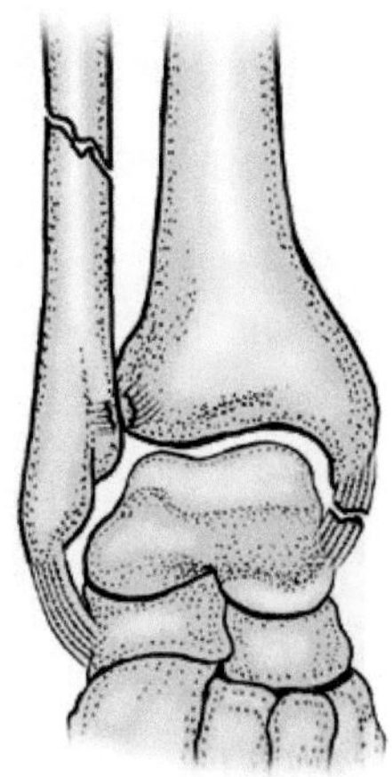
44-C1.1

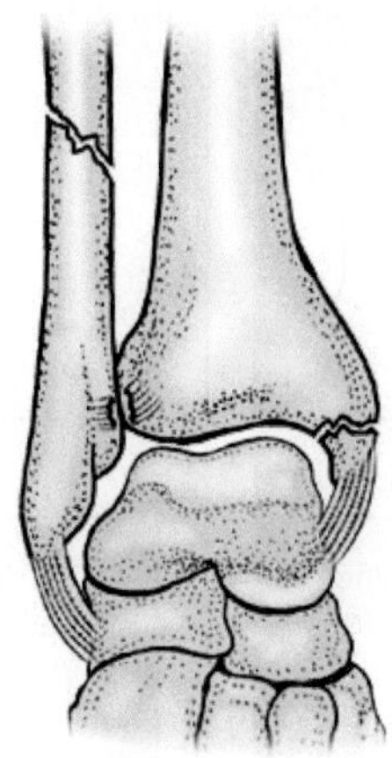
44-C1.2

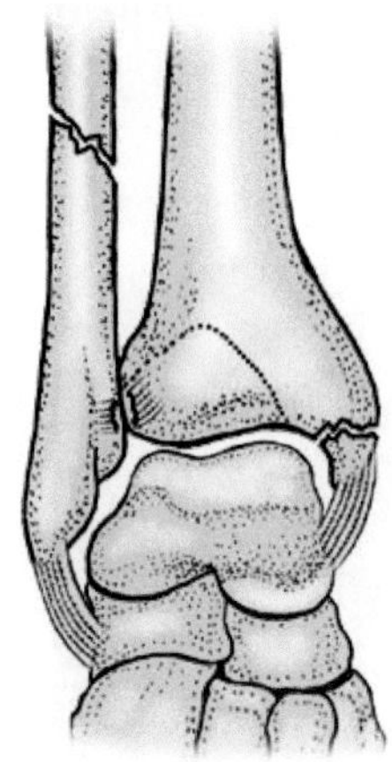
44-C1.3

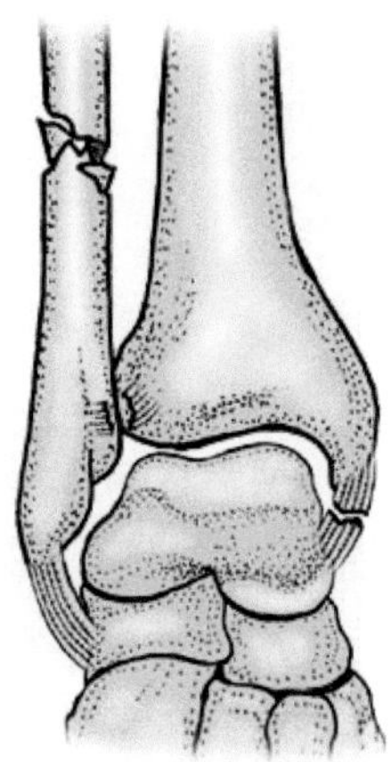
44-C2.1

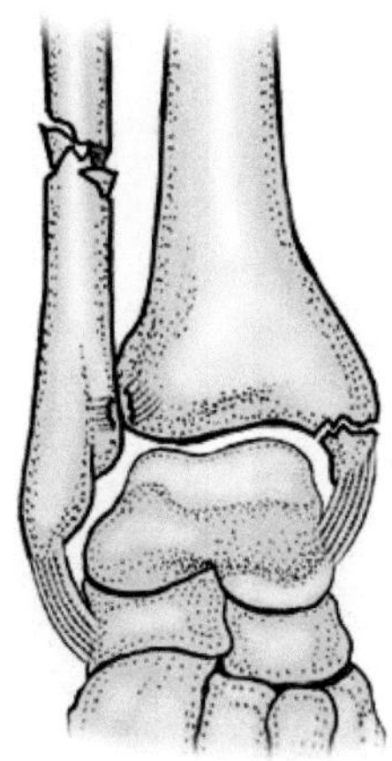
44-C2.2

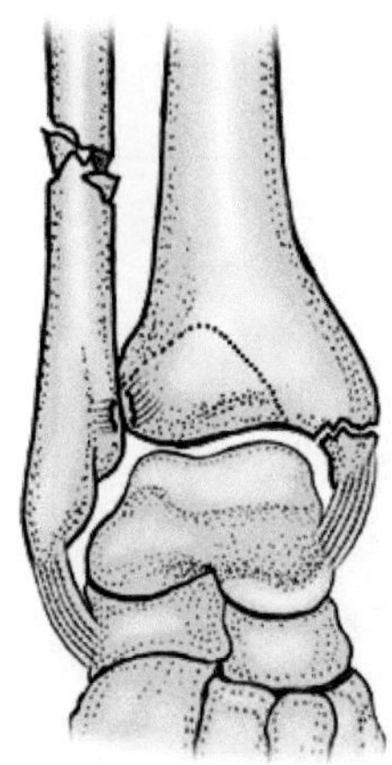
44-C2.3

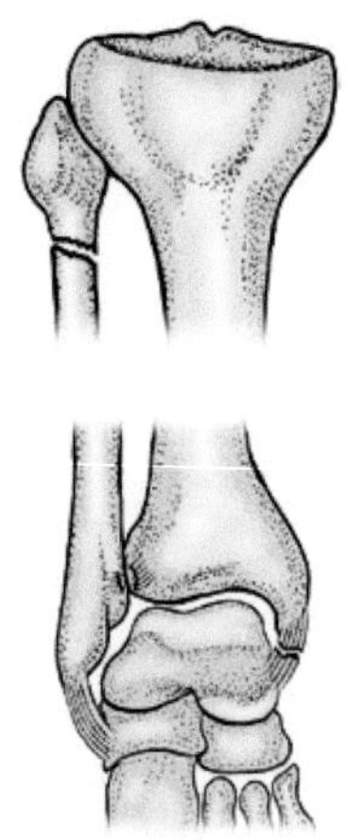
44-C3.1

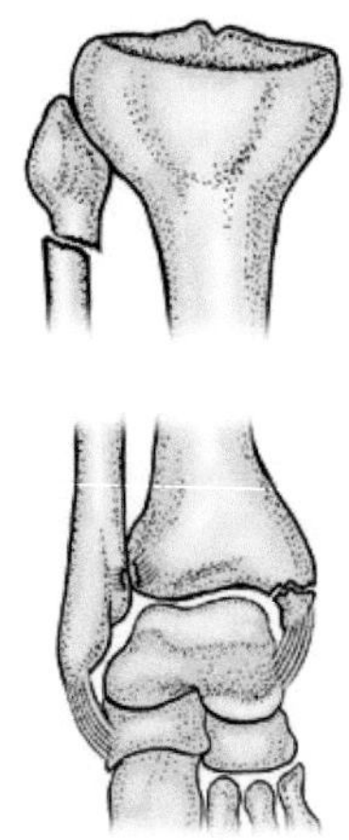
44-C3.2

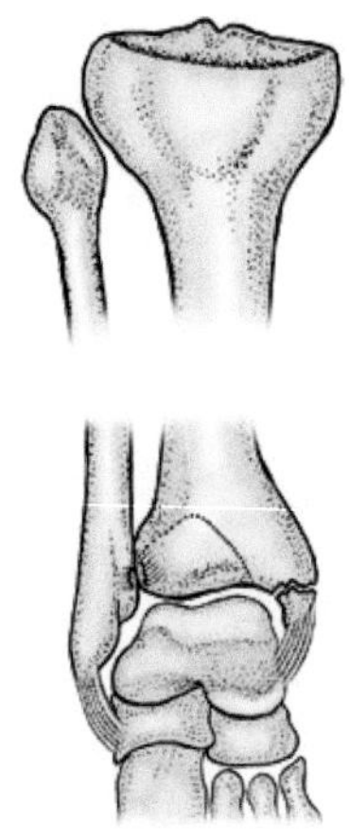
44-C3.3

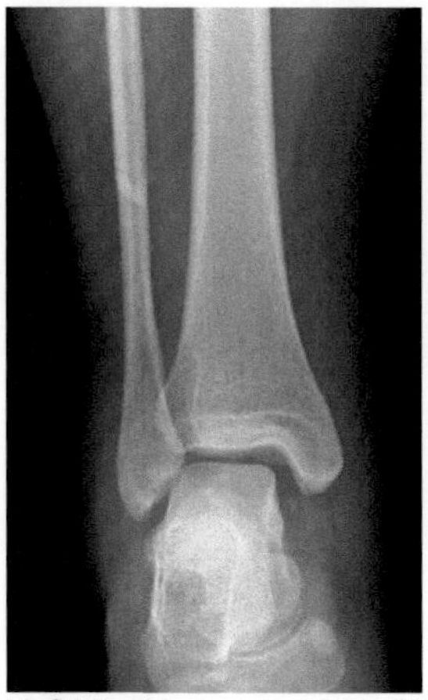
44-C1.1 with rupture of medial collateral ligament

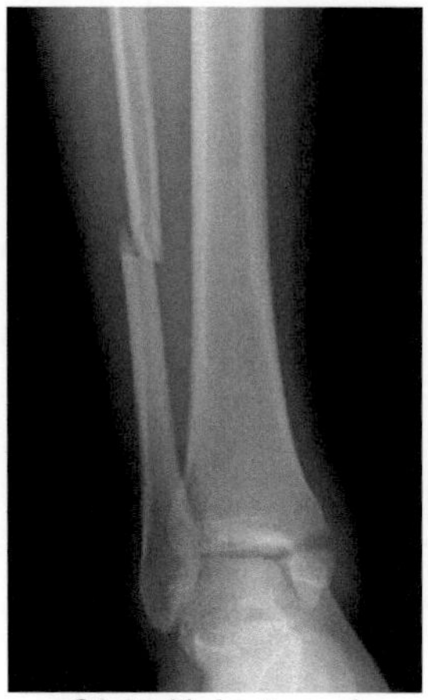
C1.2 with fracture of medial malleolus

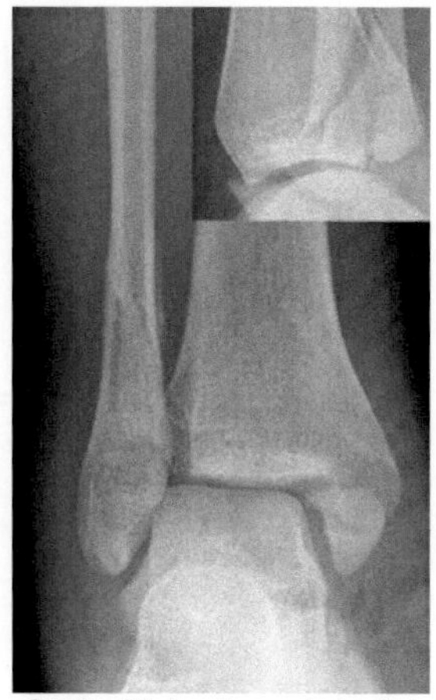
C1.3 with fracture of medial malleolus and a Volkmann

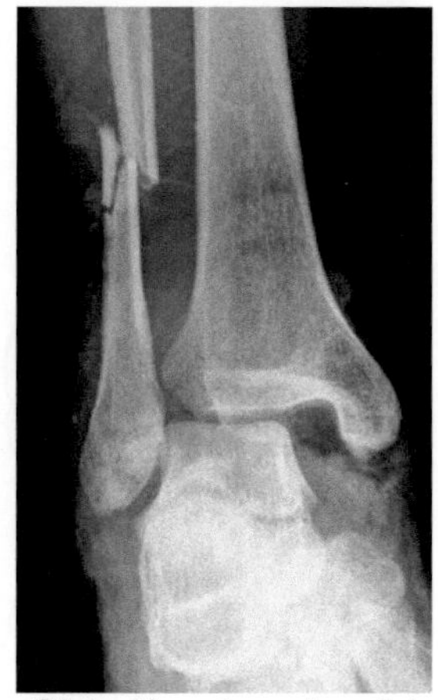
C2.1 with rupture of medial collateral ligament

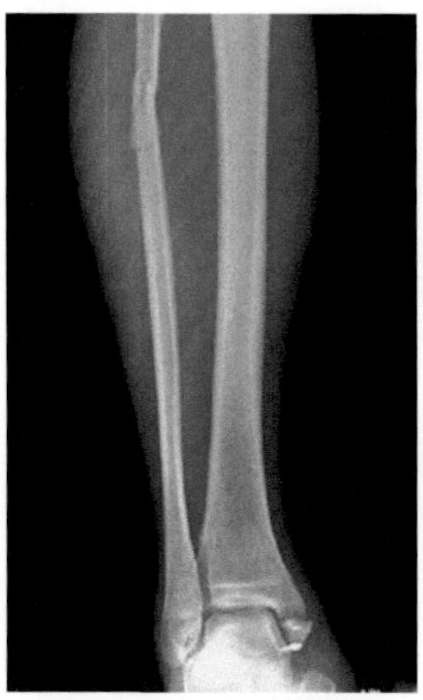
C2.2 with fracture of medial malleolus

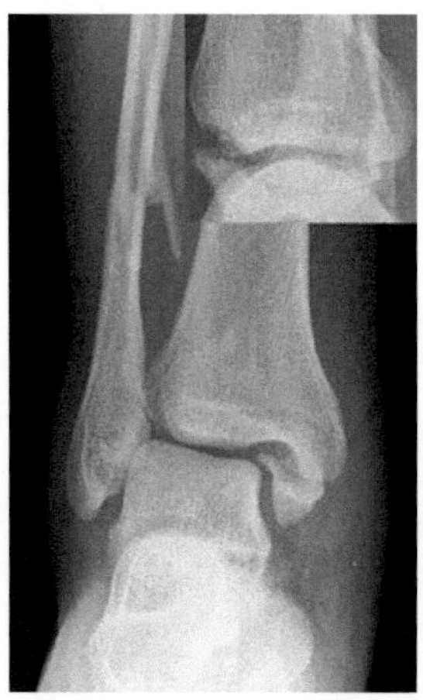
C2.3 with fracture of medial malleolus and a Volkmann

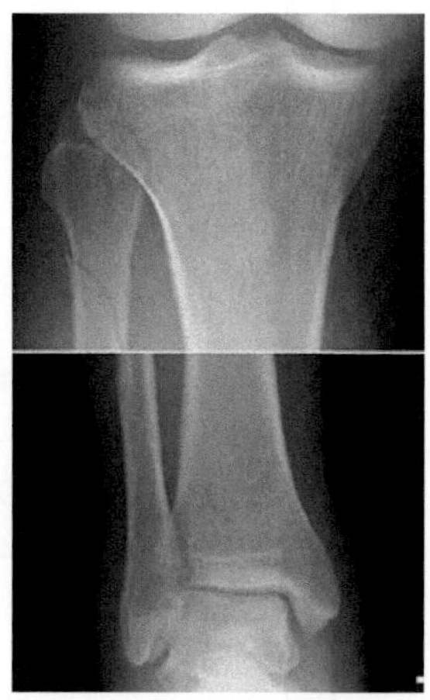
C3.1 without shortening, without Volkmann

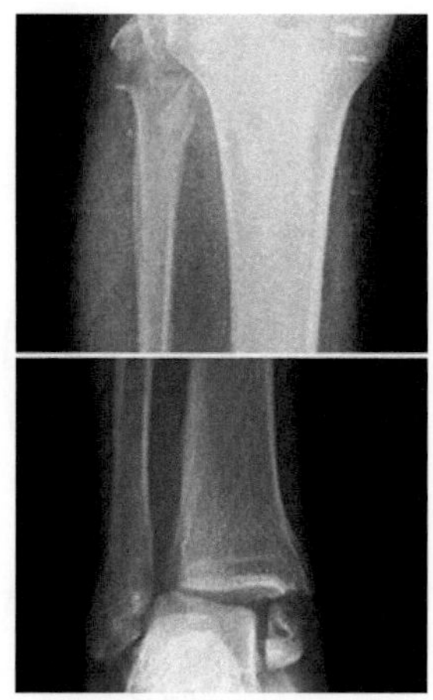
C3.2 with shortening, without Volkmann

10.3.3.4 **Ashurst-Bromer Classification** (1922, Arch Surg, 4:51–129; Ashurst-Bromer-Rockwood and greens fractures in adult, fourth edition 1996, s p 2201)

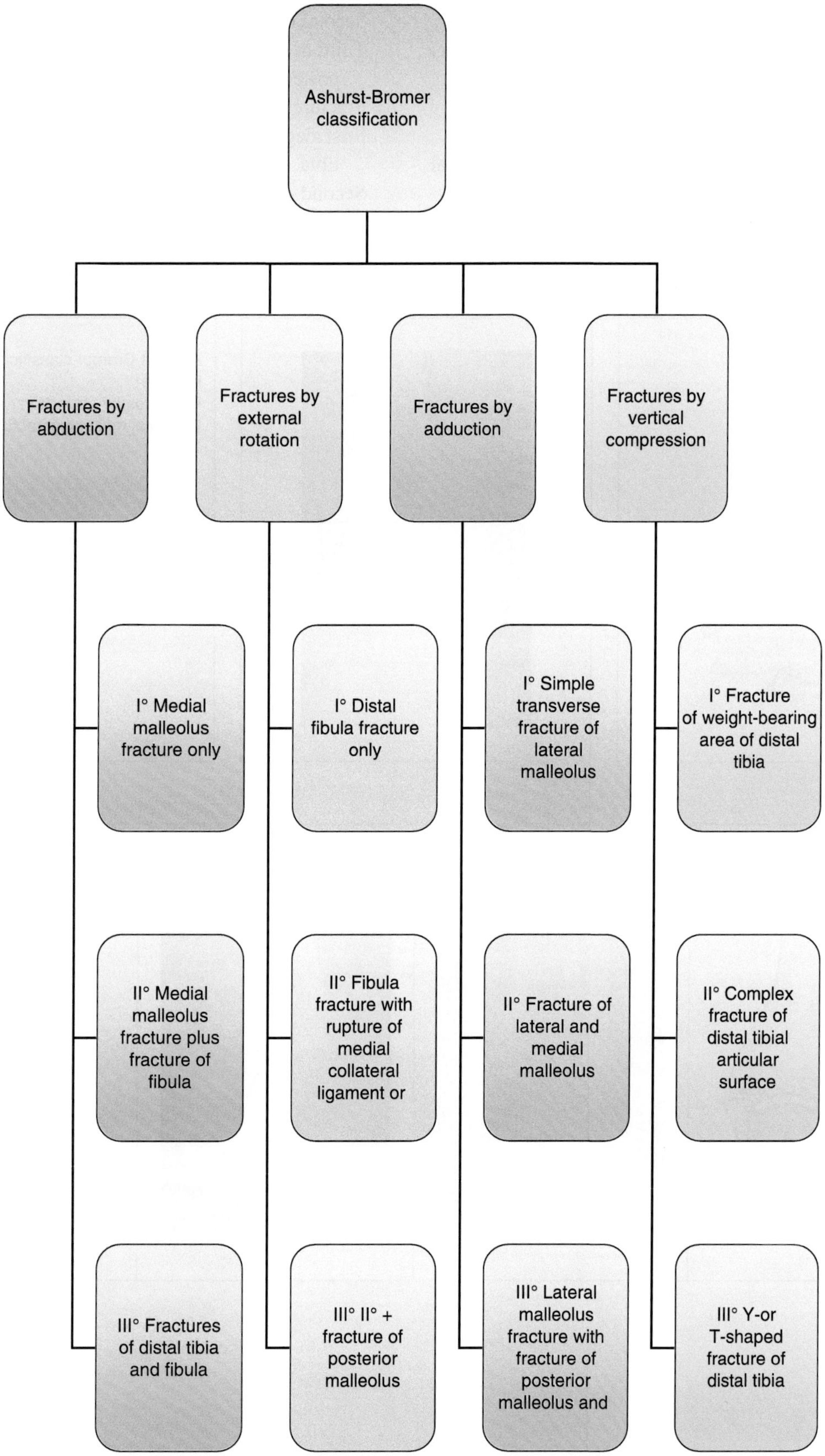

(a) Fractures by abduction:
First degree: Medial malleolus fracture only.
Second degree: Medial malleolus fracture plus fracture of fibula.
Third degree: Fractures of distal tibia (supramalleolar) and fibula.

(b) Fractures by external rotation:
First degree: Distal fibula fracture only.
Second degree: Fibula fracture with rupture of medial collateral ligament or fracture of medial malleolus.
Third degree: Second degree plus fracture of posterior malleolus.

(c) Fractures by adduction:
First degree: Simple transverse fracture of lateral malleolus.
Second degree: Fracture of lateral and medial malleolus.
Third degree: Lateral malleolus fracture with fracture of posterior malleolus and distal tibia.

(d) Fractures by vertical compression:
First degree: Fracture of weight-bearing area of distal tibia.
Second degree: Complex fracture of distal tibial articular surface.
Third degree: Y- or T-shaped fracture of distal tibia.

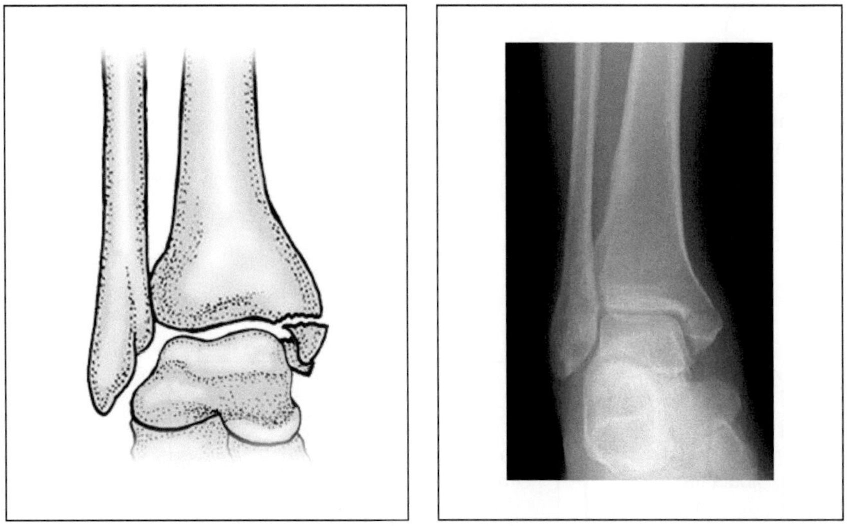

Ashurst-Bromer classification of ankle fracture
Fractures by abduction
I° Medial malleolus fracture only

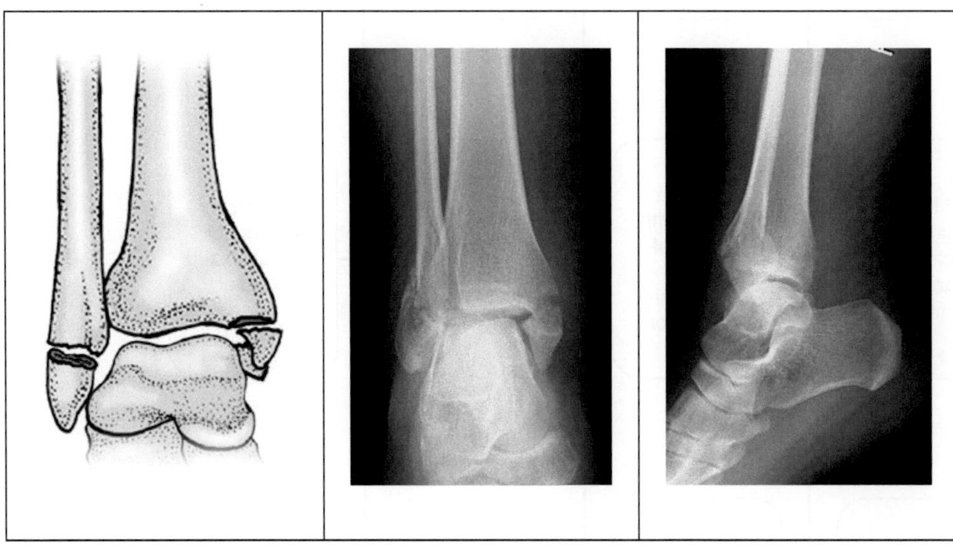

Ashurst-Bromer classification of ankle Fractures by abduction
II° Medial malleolus fracture plus fracture of fibula

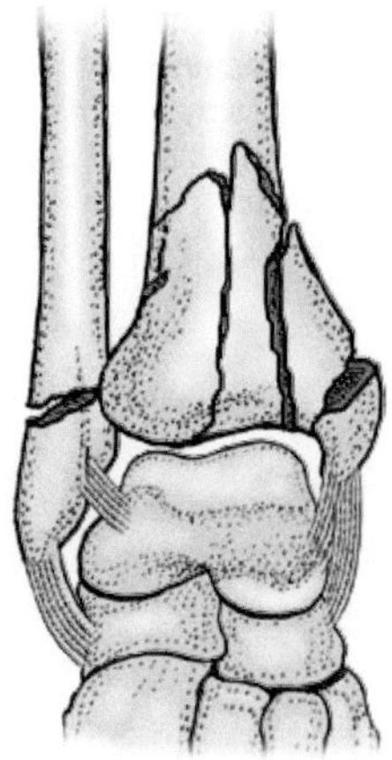

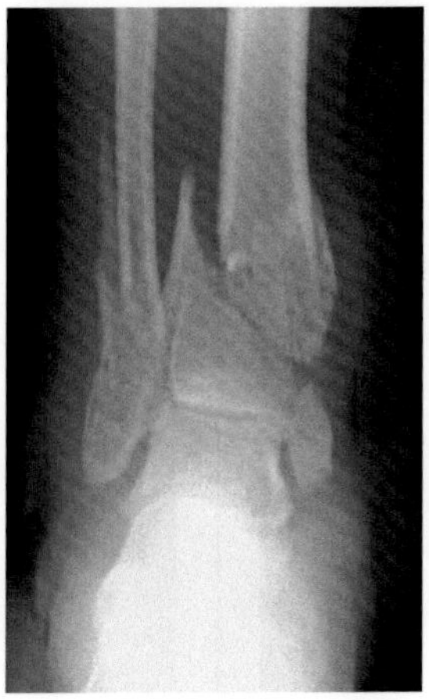

Ashurst-Bromer classification of ankle
Fractures by abduction
III° Fractures of distal tibia and fibula

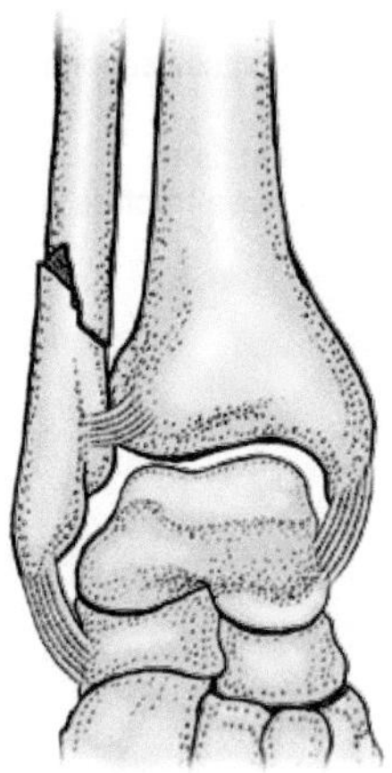

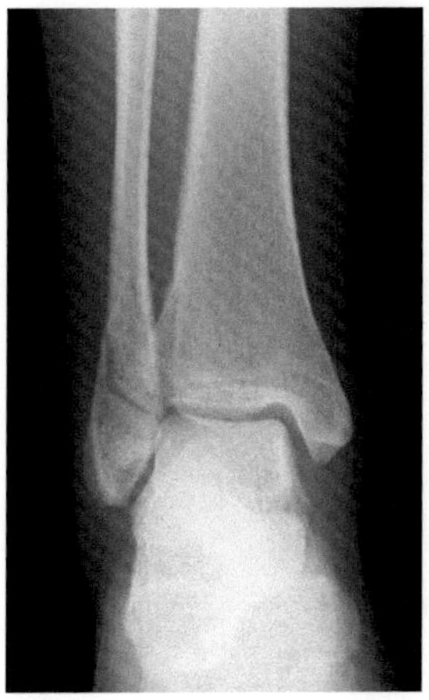

Ashurst-Bromer classification of ankle fracture
Fractures by external rotation
I° Distal fibula fracture only

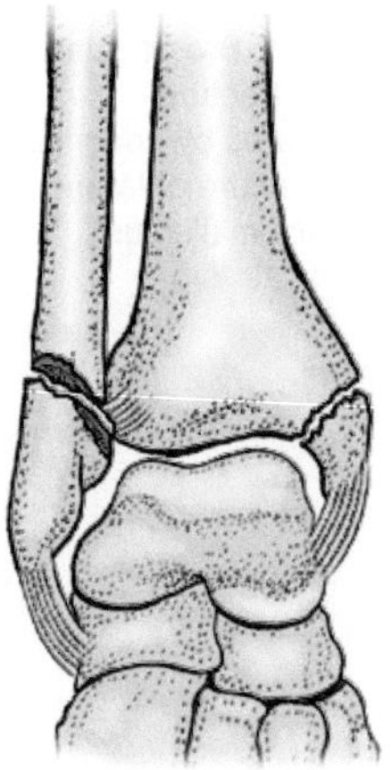

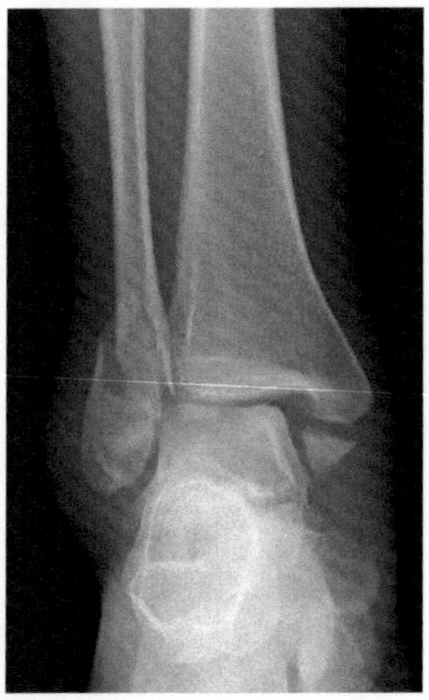

Ashurst-Bromer classification of ankle fracture
Fractures by external rotation
II° Fibula fracture with rupture of medial collateral ligament or fracture of medial malleolus

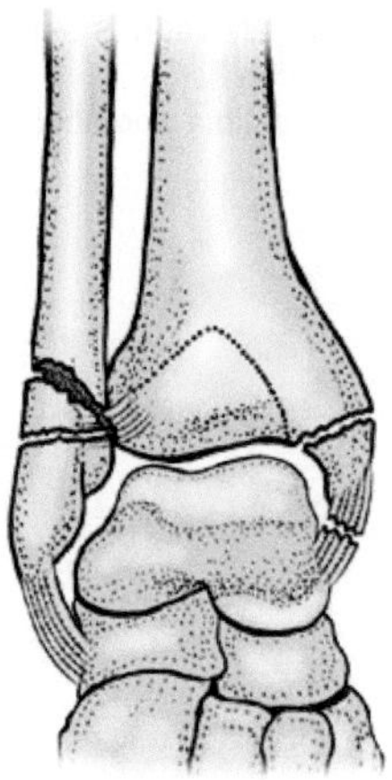
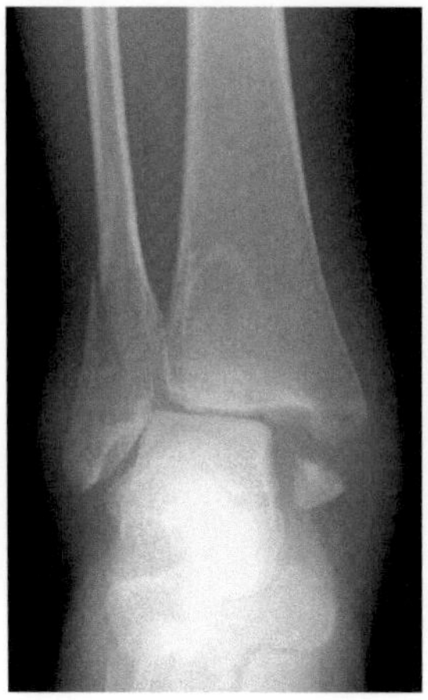
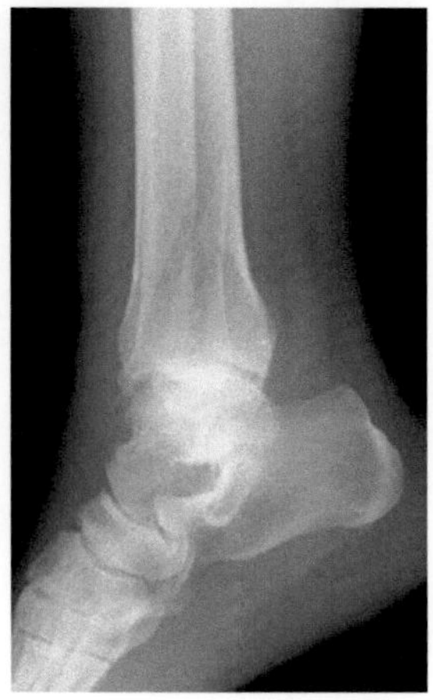

Ashurst-Bromer classification of ankle fracture
Fractures by external rotation
III° II° + fracture of posterior malleolus

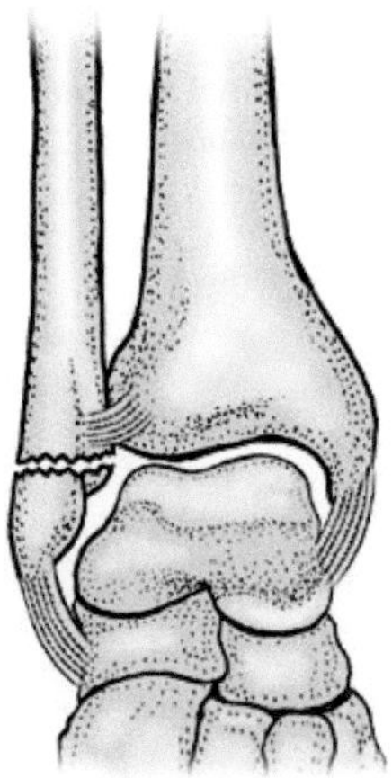
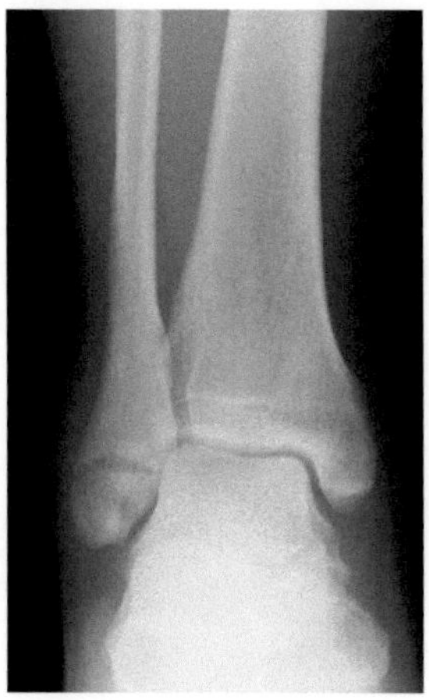

Ashurst-Bromer classification of ankle fracture
Fractures by adduction
I° Simple transverse fracture of lateral malleolus

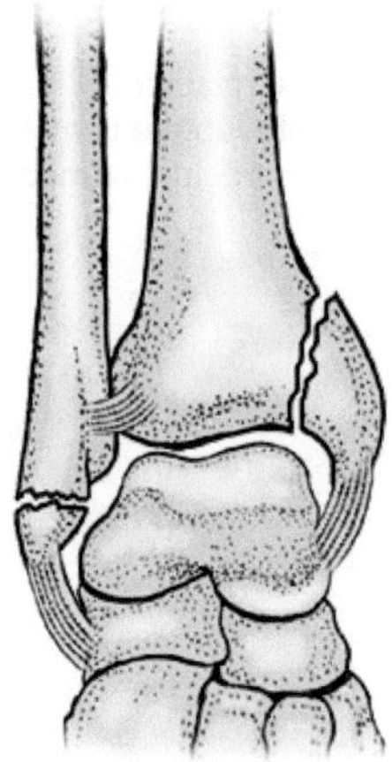
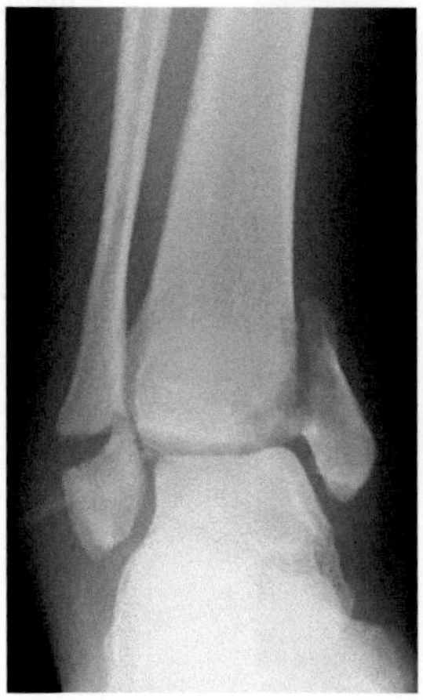
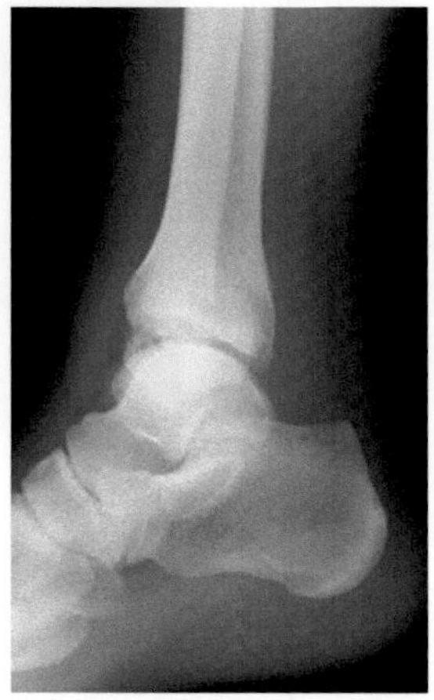

Ashurst-Bromer classification of ankle fracture
Fractures by adduction
II° Fracture of lateral and medial malleolus

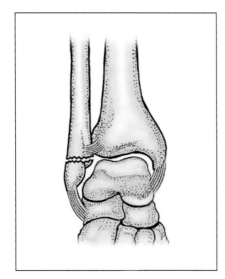

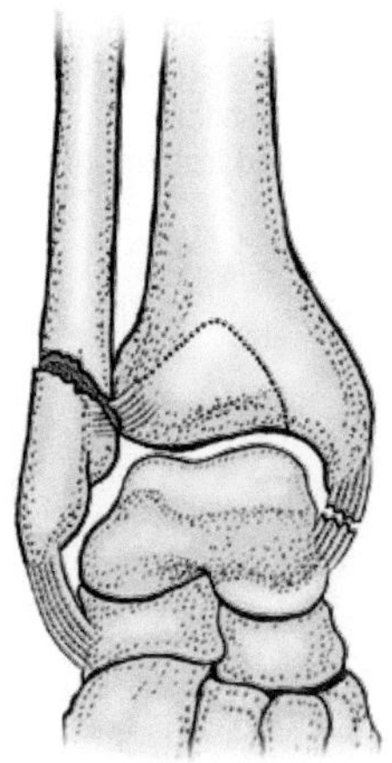

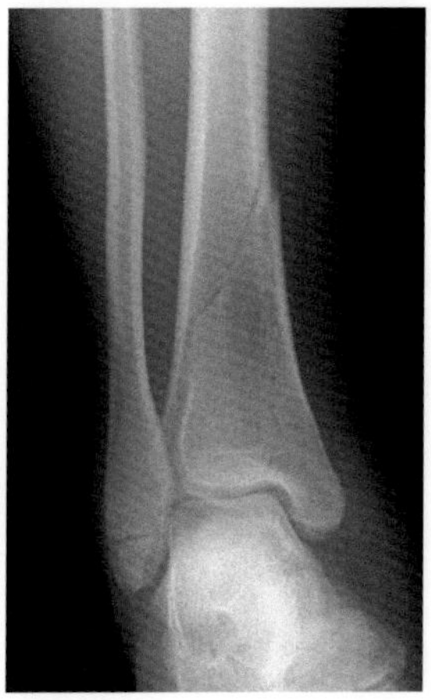

Ashurst-Bromer classification of ankle fracture
Fractures by adduction
III° Lateral malleolus fracture with fracture of posterior malleolus and distal tibia

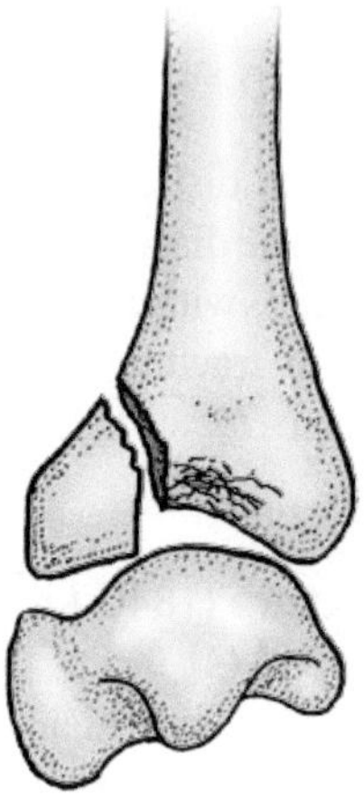

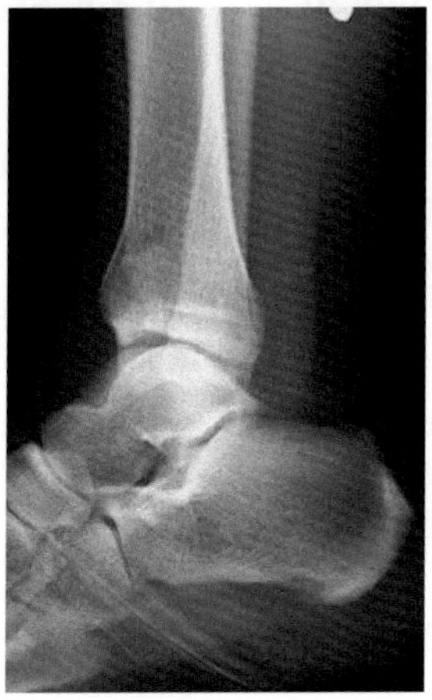

Ashurst-Bromer classification of ankle fracture
Fractures by vertical compression
I° Fracture of weight-bearing area of distal tibia

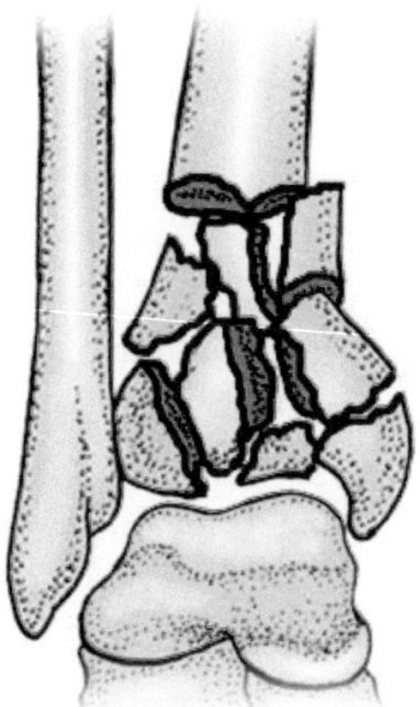

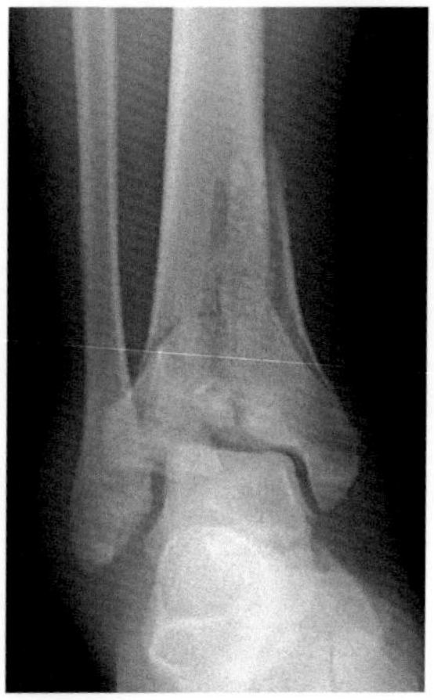

Ashurst-Bromer classification of ankle fracture
Fractures by vertical compression
II° Complex fracture of distal tibial articular surface

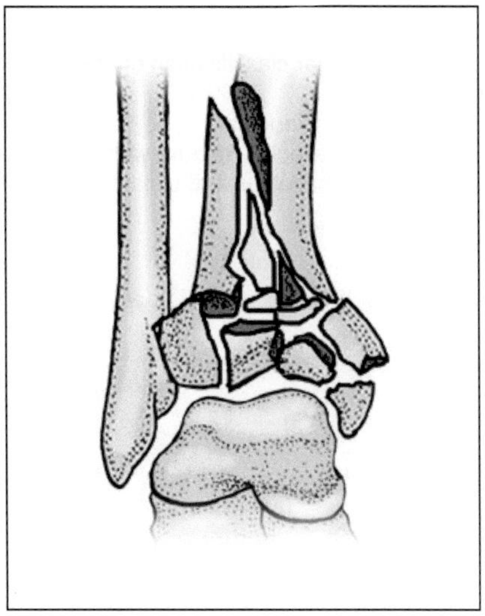

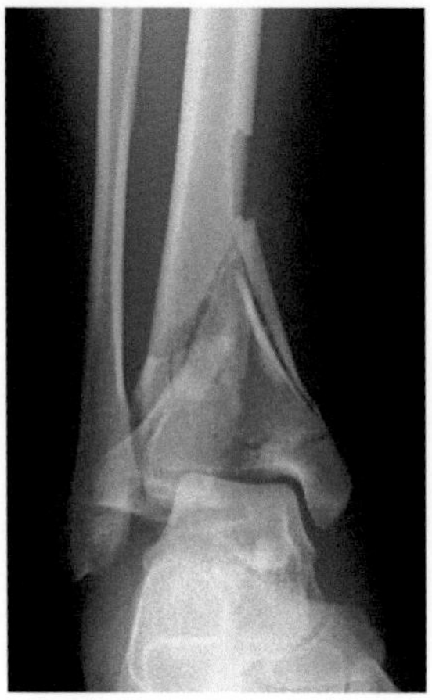

Ashurst-Bromer classification of ankle fracture
Fractures by adduction
III° Y- or T-shaped fracture of distal tibia

10.3.3.5 Clinical Classification by Wang Q (2000)

This classification is simple and practical, but lacks the evaluation of the mechanism and degree of injury.

Type I: Single fracture: Subtype a: medial malleolus fracture; b: lateral malleolus fracture; c: posterior malleolus fracture; d: syndesmosis separation.

Type II: Double fracture: ab: fracture of medial and lateral malleolus; ac: fracture of medial and posterior malleolus; cd: posterior malleolus fracture and syndesmosis separation; bc: fracture of lateral and posterior malleolus; ad: medial malleolus fracture and syndesmosis separation; bd: lateral malleolus fracture and syndesmosis separation.

Type III: Triple fracture: abc: trimalleolar fracture; abd: fracture of medial and lateral malleolus with syndesmosis separation; acd: fracture of medial and posterior malleolus and syndesmosis separation; bcd: fracture of lateral and posterior malleolus and syndesmosis separation.

Type IV: Depression fracture of anterior rim of distal tibia.

Type V: Injuries of collateral ligament: a: medial, b: lateral, ab: medial and lateral.

Type VI: Physeal injuries in children.

10.3.4 Fracture Types Named After People

10.3.4.1 Pilon Fracture

Pilon fracture is the fracture of the distal one-third of the tibia involving the tibiotalar joint. The distal articular surface of the tibia is severely comminuted, with bone defects and cancellous bone compression. This fracture is often associated with lower fibular fractures (~75 to 85%) and severe soft-tissue contusions.

10.3.4.2 Maisonneuve Fracture (1840, Arch Gen Med. 7:165–187, 433–474)

Maisonneuve fractures refer to proximal fibular fractures caused by external rotation, often combined with medial malleolus fracture, triangular ligament tear, anterior talofibular ligament rupture, interosseous ligament injury, tibiofibular ligament tear, posterior malleolus fracture, and other injuries.

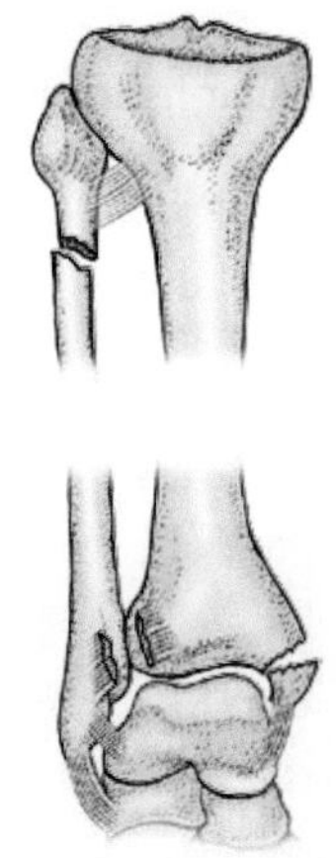

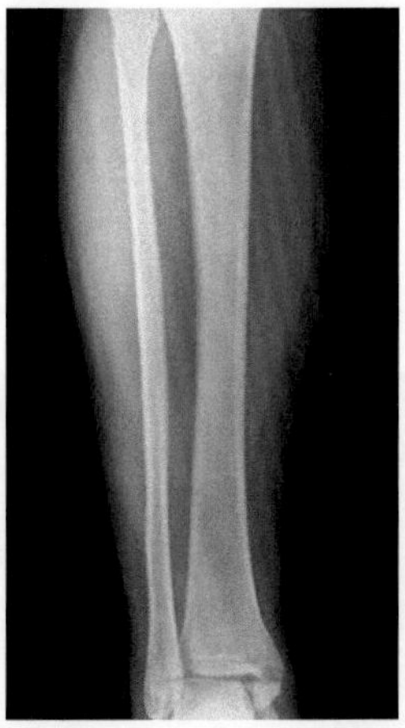

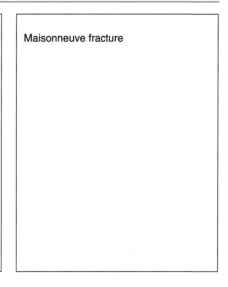

Maisonneuve fracture

10.3.4.3 Lefort-Wagstaffe Fracture (1886, Bull Gen Ther, 110:193–199)

This fracture refers to the vertical avulsion fracture of the fibular attachment of the tibiofibular ligament.

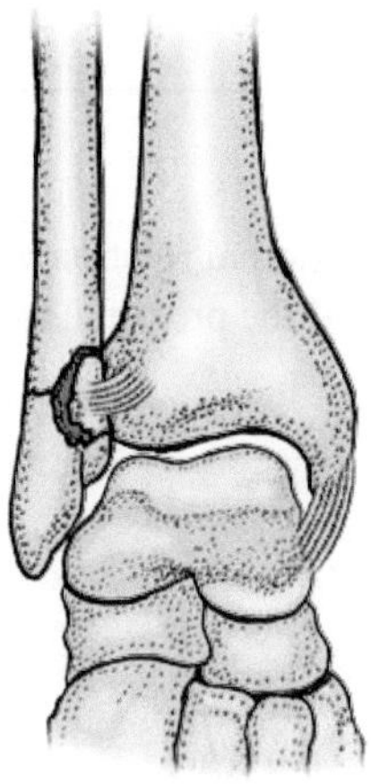

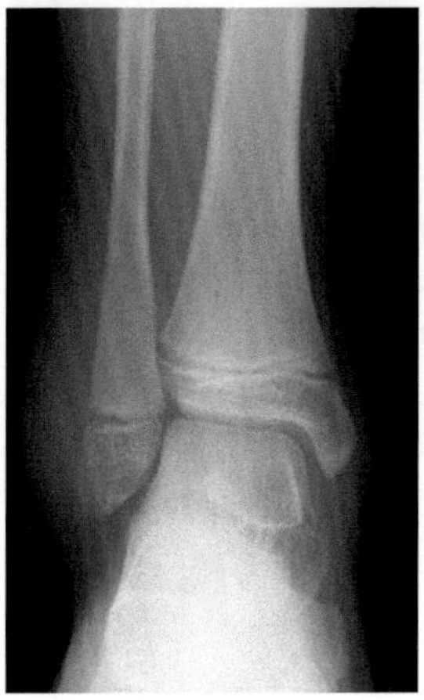

Lefort-Wagstaffe fracture

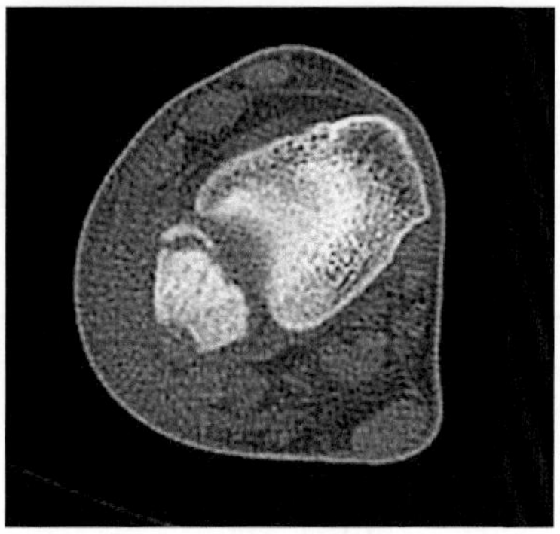

10.3.4.4 **Tillaux-Chaput Fracture** (1907, Les Fractures Mallolaires du Cou-de-pied et les Accidents du Travail. Paris, MassonCie)

Type A: Avulsion fracture of the anterolateral rim of tibia caused by traction of the anterior tibiofibular ligament.
Type B: Type A with medial lesion.

Accompanied by medial damage

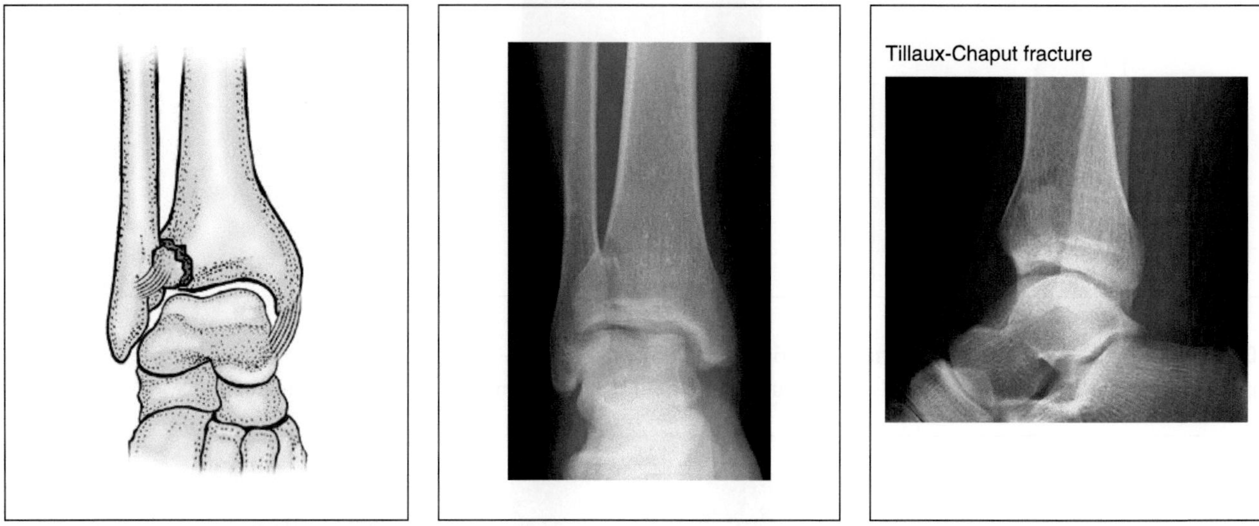

10.3.4.5 **Bosworth Fracture (1947)**

Bosworth fracture is an ankle fracture dislocation that is difficult to reduce, related to extreme external rotation and plantar flexion of the ankle. The distal fibula is fractured, with an associated fixed posterior dislocation of the proximal fibular fragment which becomes trapped behind the posterior tibia.

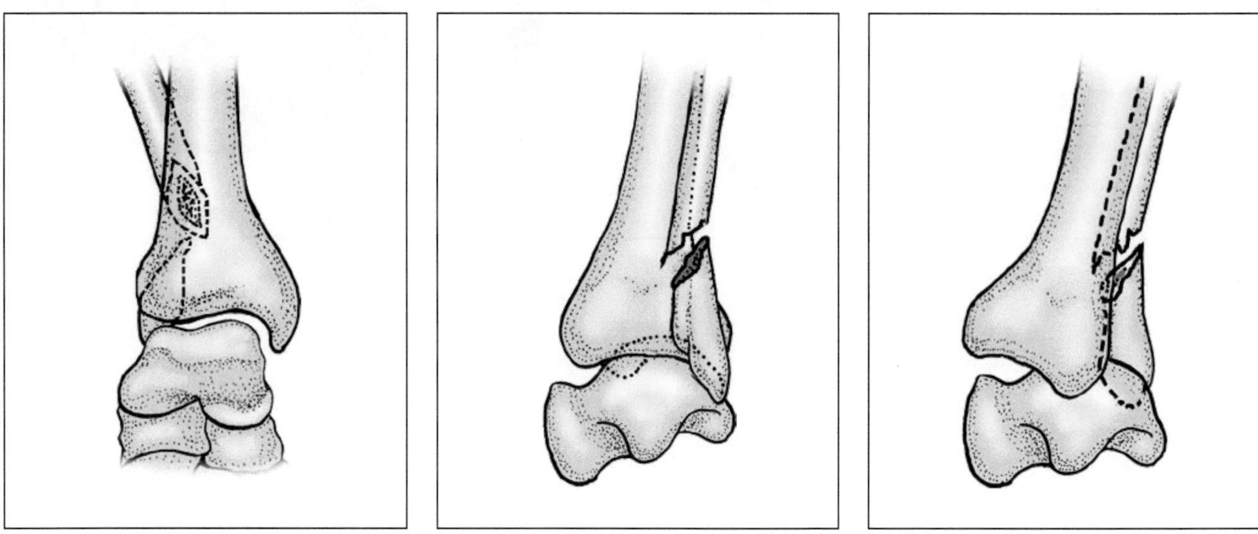

10.3.4.6 **Dupuytren Fracture** (1819, Annu Med Chir Hop Hosp Civils Paris, 1:1)

This fracture refers to a fracture of the middle or distal third of the fibula accompanied by avulsion fracture of the medial malleolus, rupture of the inferior tibiofibular ligament, and disruption of the syndesmosis, which is caused by an extreme abduction of the ankle.

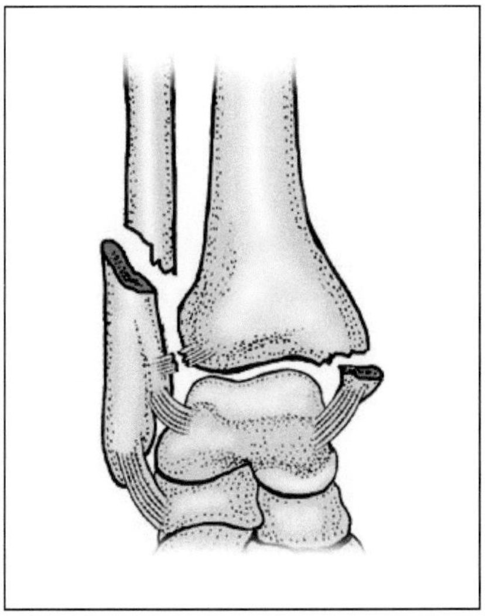

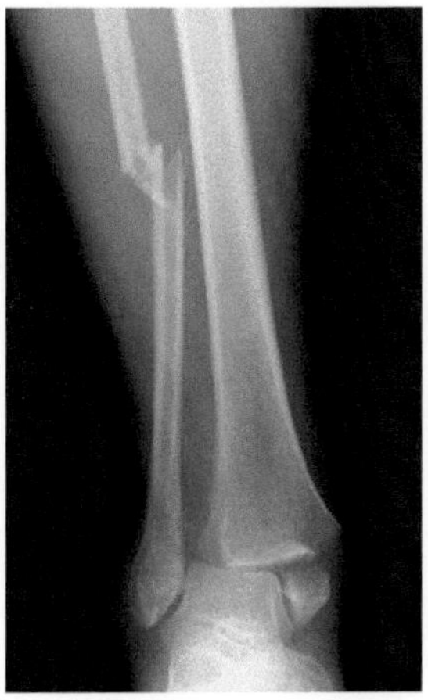

Dupuytren fracture

10.3.4.7 **Gosselin Fracture**

The Gosselin fracture is a V-shaped fracture of the distal tibia, which extends into the ankle joint and fractures the tibial plafond into anterior and posterior fragments. This fracture was named after the French author Leon Athanese Gosselin (1815–1887) who firstly described it.

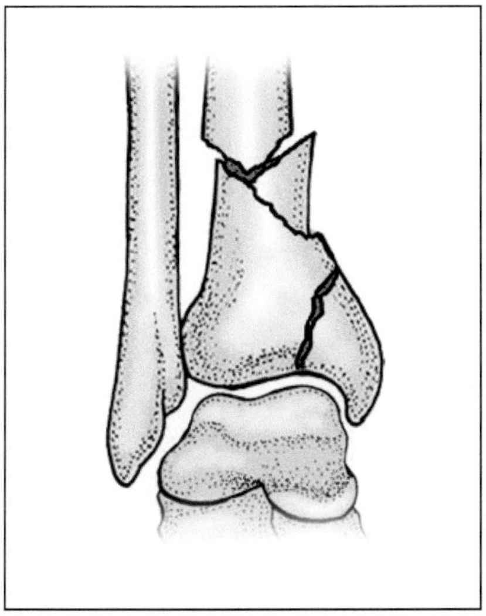

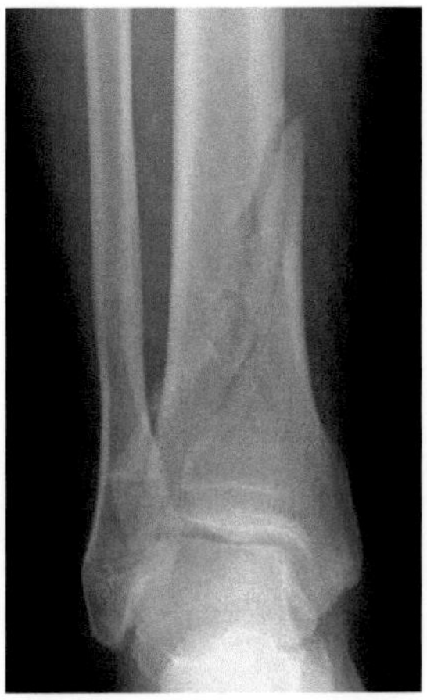

Gosselin fracture

Classification of Foot Fractures

11

Yingze Zhang and Haotian Wu

11.1 Section 1 Classification of Talar Fractures

There are many classifications of talar fractures; the most commonly used classifications are the anatomic classification and the Hawkins classification of talar neck fractures.

11.1.1 Anatomy Classification

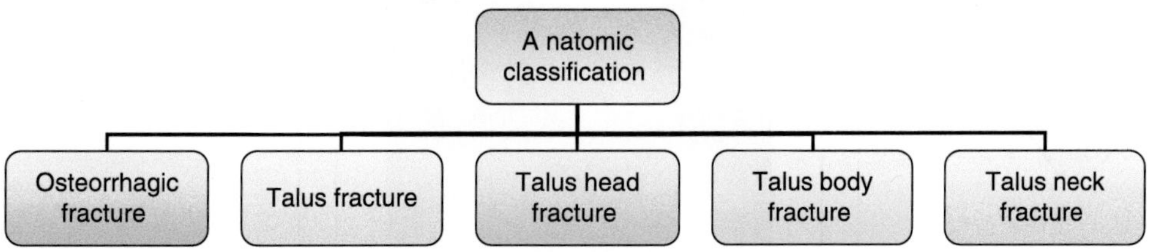

Lateral process fracture of the talus
Posterior process fracture of the talus
Talus head fracture
Talus body fracture

Talus neck fracture

Y. Zhang (✉) • H. Wu
Department of Orthopedics,
The Third Hospital of Hebei Medical University,
Shijiazhuang, China
e-mail: yzzhangdr@126.com, yzling_liu@163.com

Y. Zhang (ed.), *Clinical Classification in Orthopaedics Trauma*, https://doi.org/10.1007/978-981-10-6044-1_11

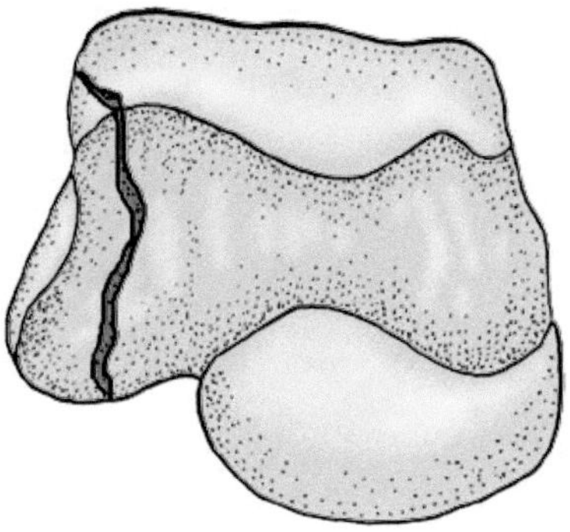

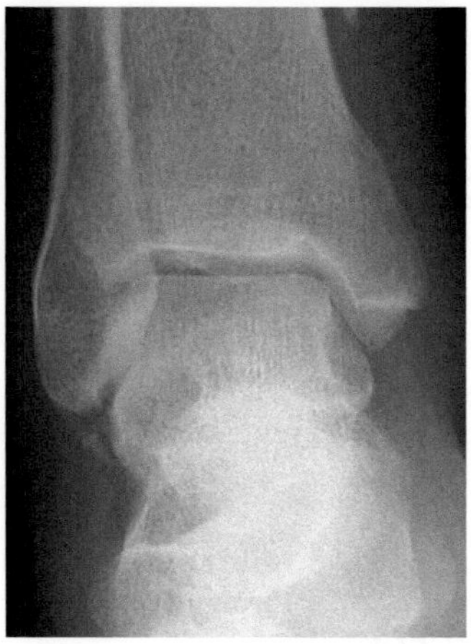

Anatomy classification
Lateral process fracture of the talus

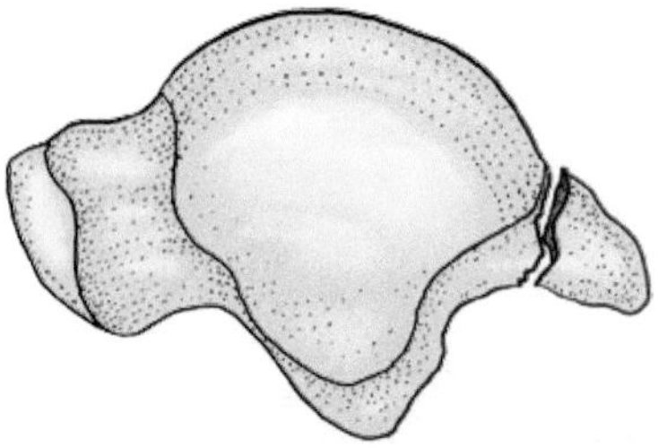

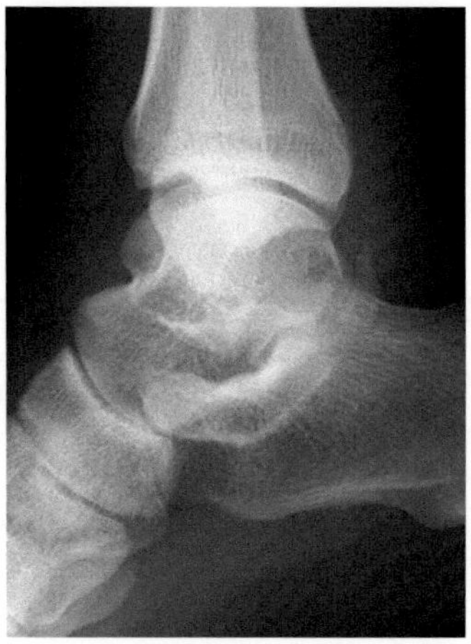

Anatomy classification
Posterior process fracture of the talus

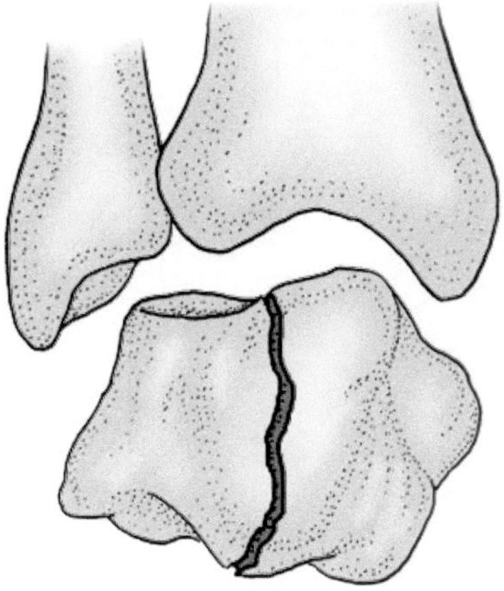

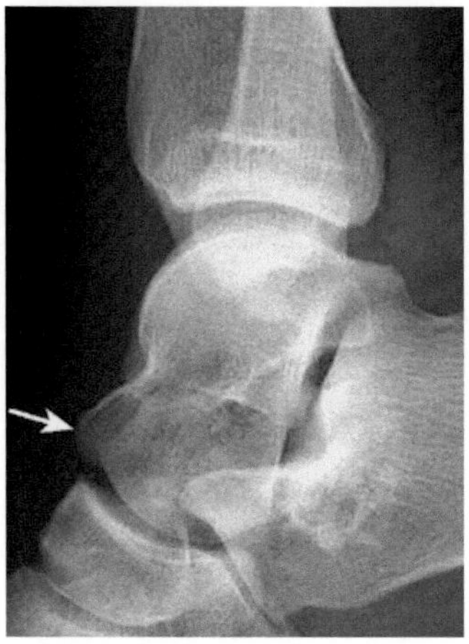

Anatomy classification
Talus head fracture

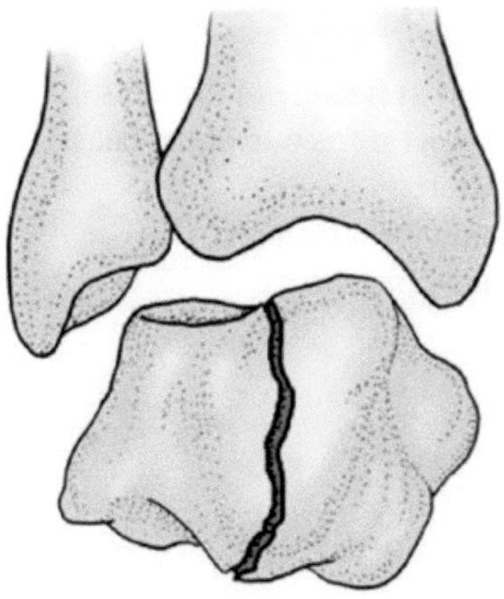

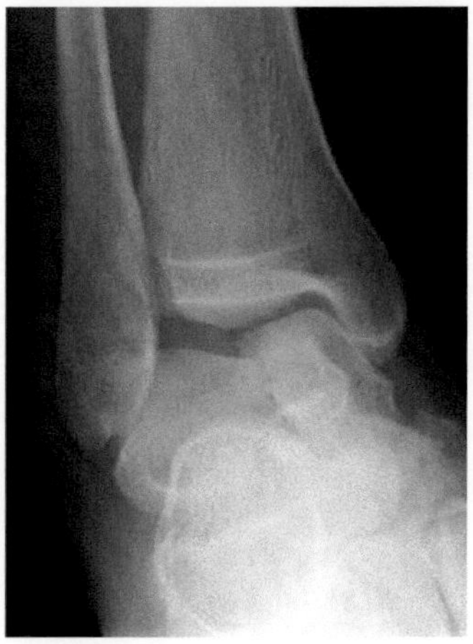

Anatomy classification
Talus body fracture

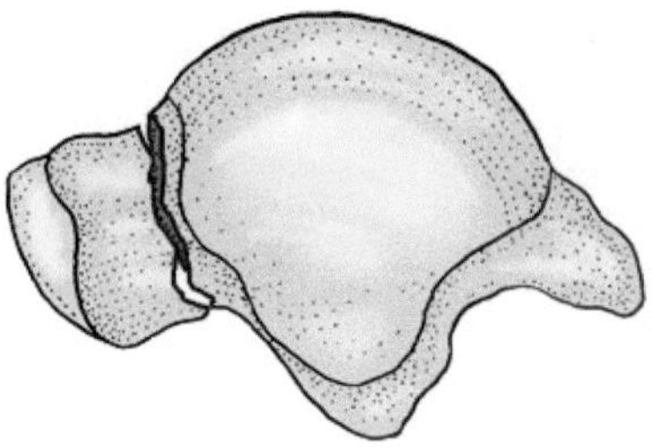

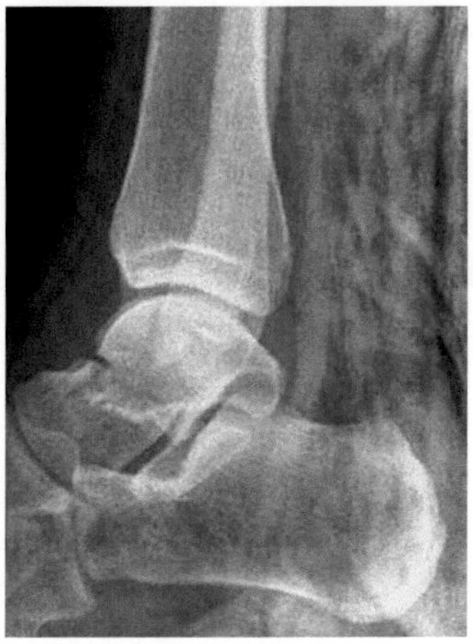

Anatomy classification
Talus body fracture

11.1.2 AO/OTA Classification of Talus Fractures (2007, Journal of Orthopaedic Trauma. 21 supplement)

81: Talus fractures:
- Type A: Talus head or talus process or avulsion fracture:
  - A1: Avulsion fracture:
    - A1.1: Avulsion fracture of talus anterior process.
    - A1.2: Avulsion fracture of other sites.
  - A2: Talus process fractures:
    - A2.1: Lateral process fracture of the talus.
    - A2.2: Posterior process fracture of the talus.
  - A3: Talus head fracture:
    - A3.1: Non-comminuted fracture.
    - A3.2: Comminuted fracture.

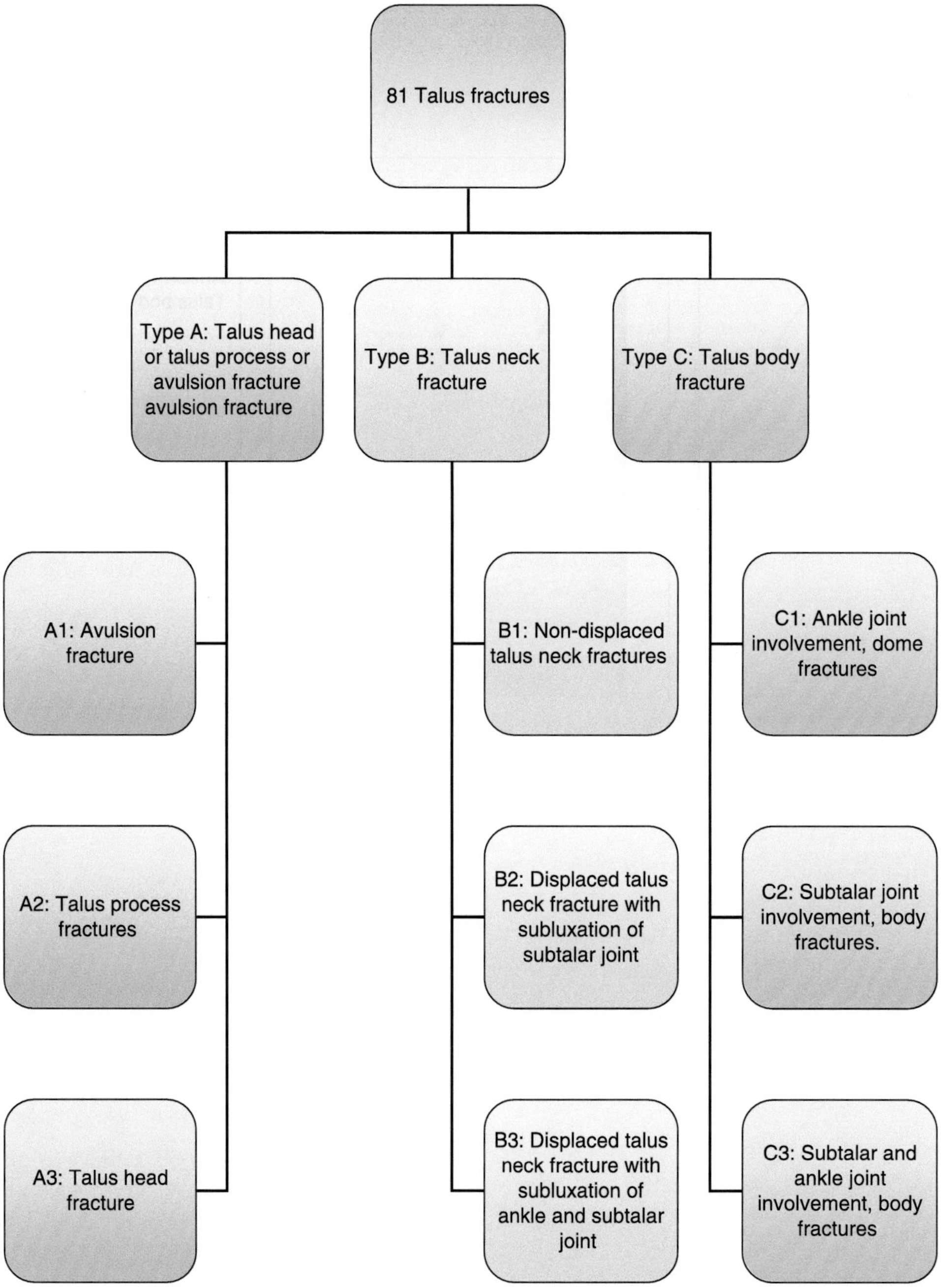

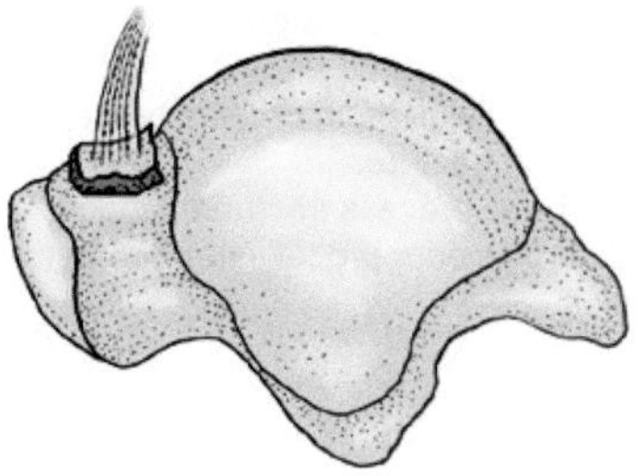

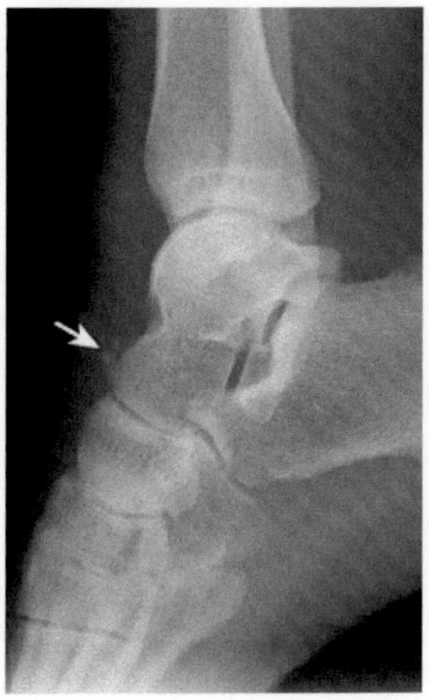

AO/OTA classification
81 Talus fractures
Type A: Talus head or talus process or avulsion fracture.
A1: Avulsion fracture.
A1.1: Avulsion fracture of talus anterior process

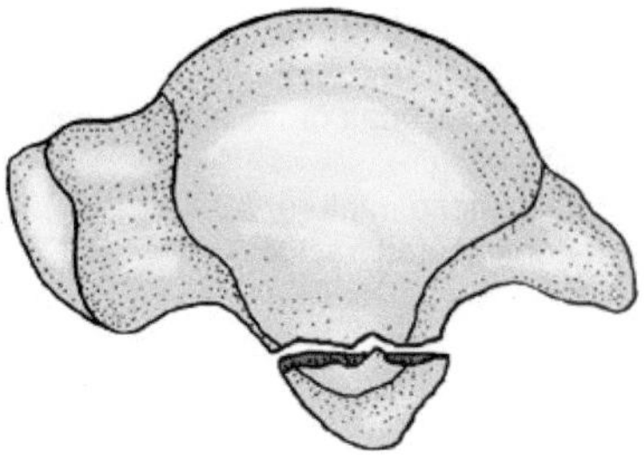

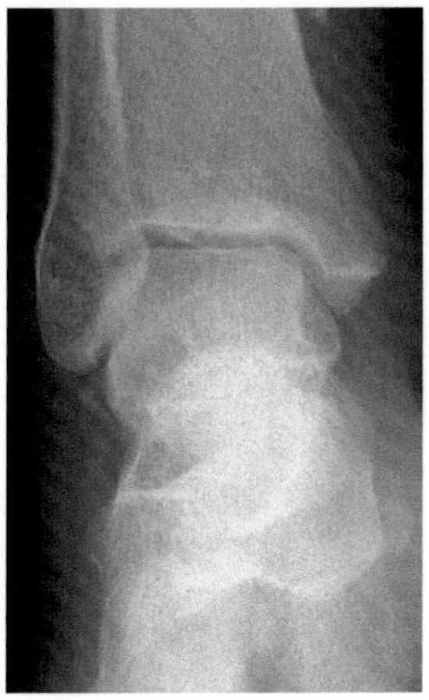

AO/OTA classification
81 Talus fractures
Type A: Talus head or talus process or avulsion fracture.
A1: Avulsion fracture.
A1.2: Avulsion fracture of other sites

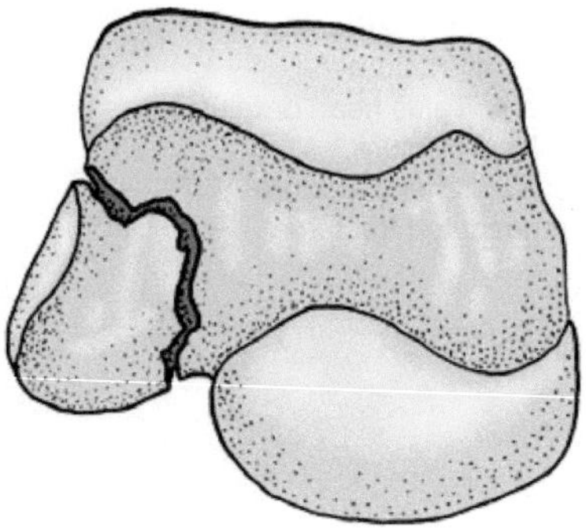

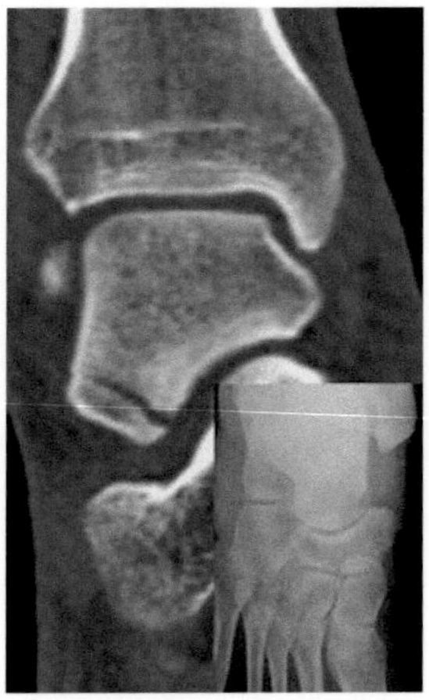

AO/OTA classification
81 Talus fractures
Type A: Talus head or talus process or avulsion fracture.
A2: Talus process fractures.
A2.1: Lateral process fracture of the talus

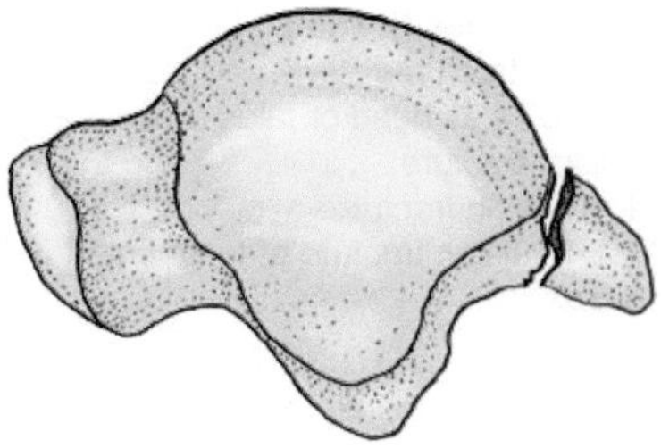

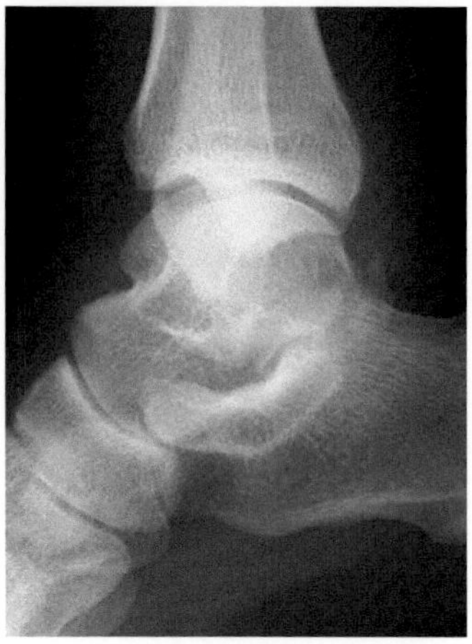

AO/OTA classification
81 Talus fractures
Type A: Talus head or talus process or avulsion fracture.
A2: Talus process fractures.
A2.2: Posterior process fracture of the talus

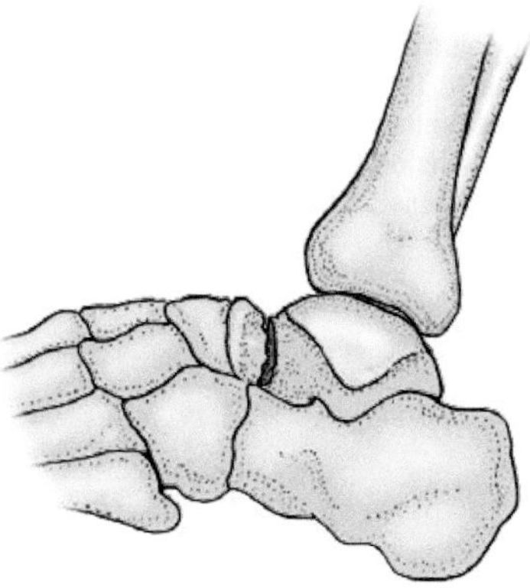

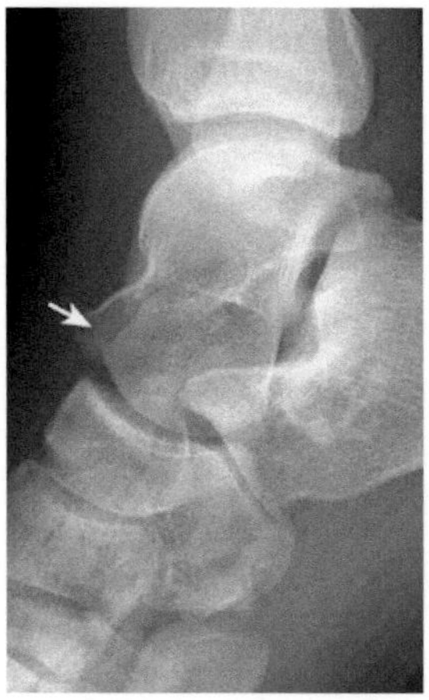

AO/OTA classification
81 Talus fracture
Type A: Talus head or talus process or avulsion fracture.
A3: Talus head fracture. A3.1: Non-comminuted fracture

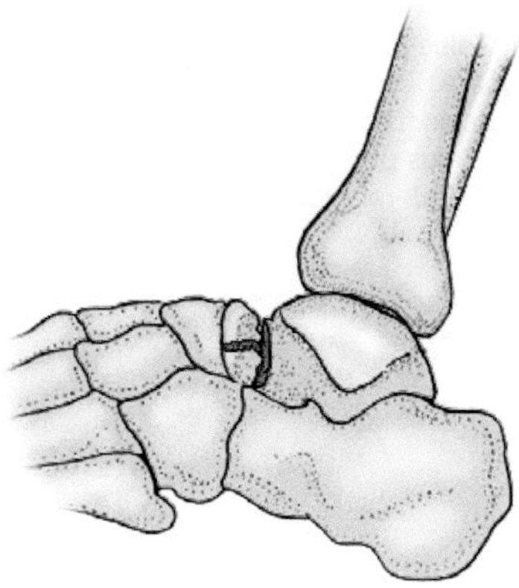

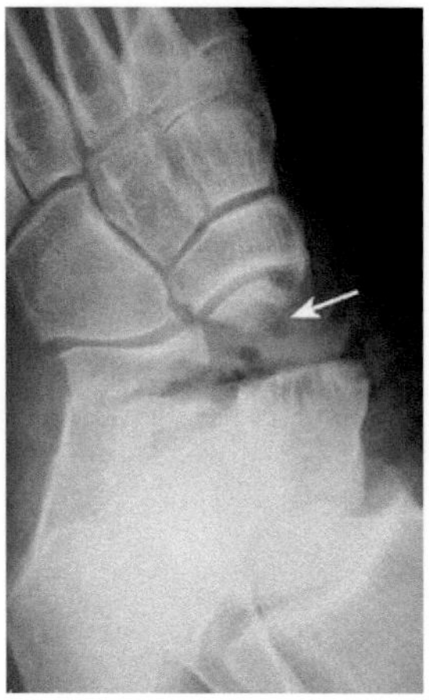

AO/OTA classification
81 Talus fracture
Type A: Talus head or talus process or avulsion fracture.
A3: Talus head fracture A3.2: Comminuted fracture

Type B: Talus neck fracture
 Type B1: Non-displaced talus neck fractures
 Type B2: Displaced talus neck fracture with subluxation of subtalar joint
  Type B2.1: Non-comminuted fracture
  Type B2.2: Comminuted fracture
  Type B2.3: Involves talus head
 Type B3: Displaced talus neck fracture with subluxation of ankle and subtalar joint
  Type B3.1: Non-comminuted fracture
  Type B3.2: Comminuted fracture
  Type B3.3: Involves talus head

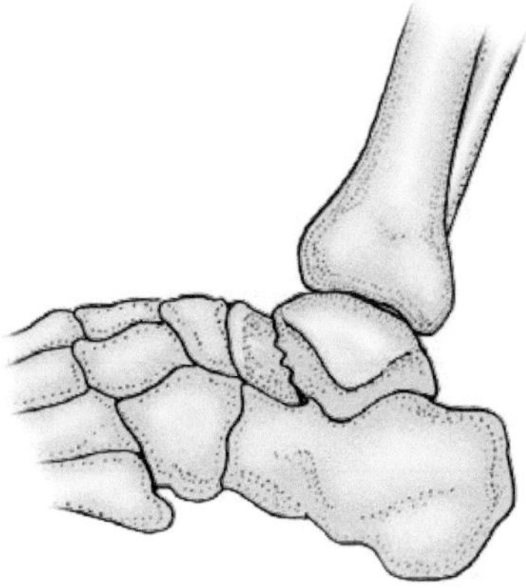

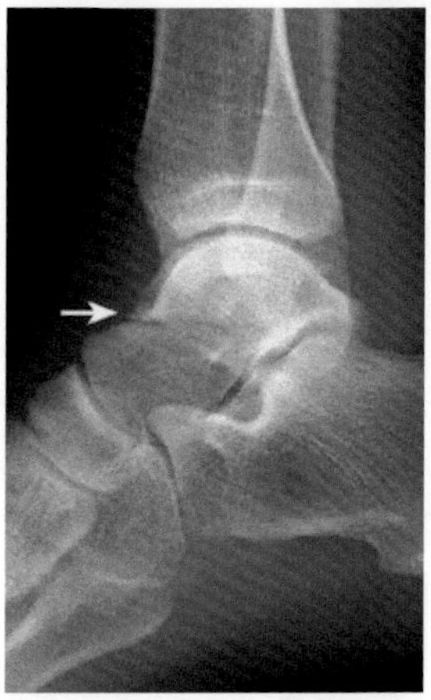

AO/OTA classification
81 Talus fractures
Type B: Talus neck fracture.
B1: Nondisplaced talus neck fractures

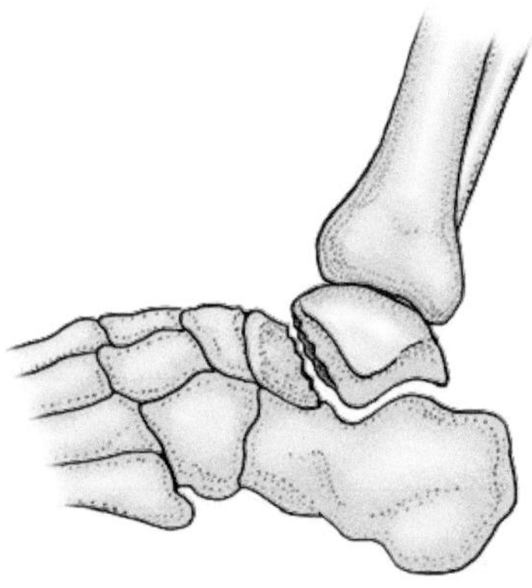

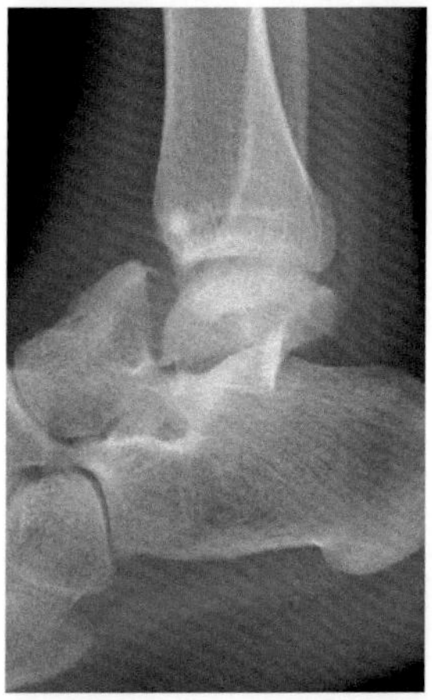

AO/OTA classification
81 Talus fractures
Type B: Talus neck fracture.
B2: Displaced talus neck fracture with subluxation of subtalar joint.
B2.1: Non-comminuted fracture

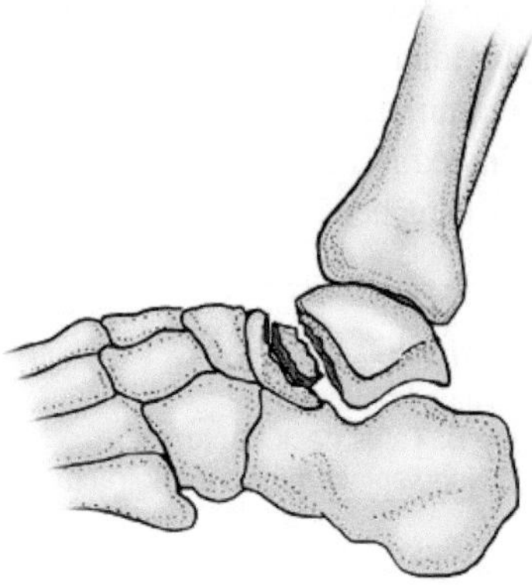

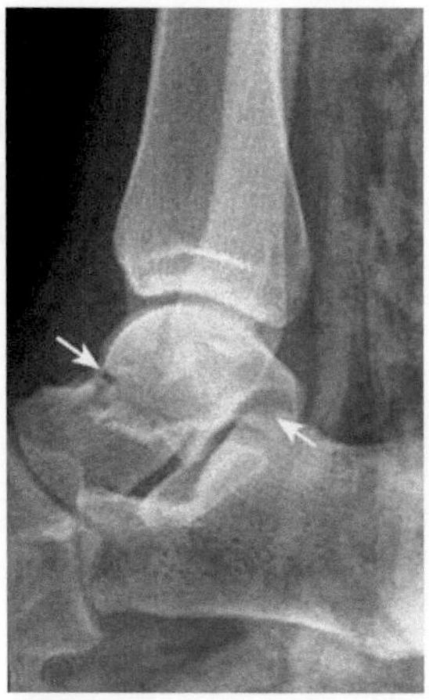

AO/OTA classification
81 Talus fractures
Type B: Talus neck fracture.
B2: Displaced talus neck fracture with subluxation of subtalar joint.
B2.2: Comminuted fracture

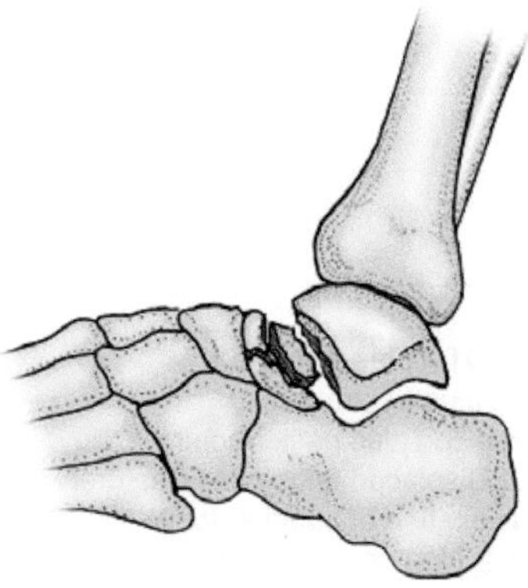

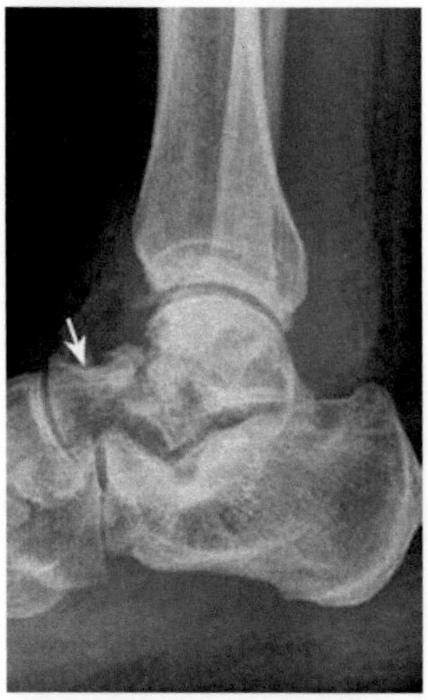

81 Talus fractures
Type B Talus neck fracture.
B2 Displaced talus neck fracture with subluxation of subtalar joint.
B2.3 Involves talus head

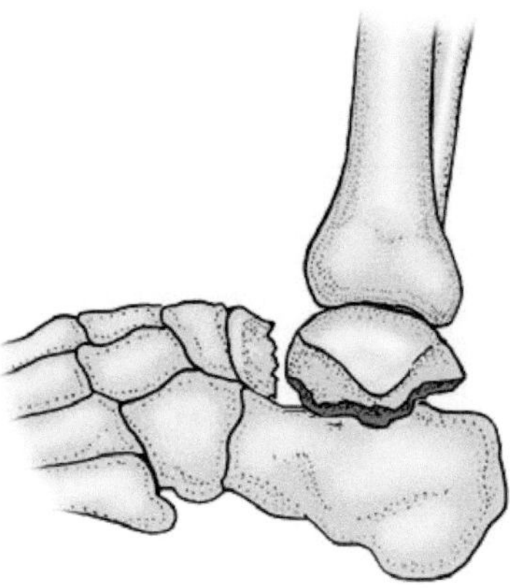

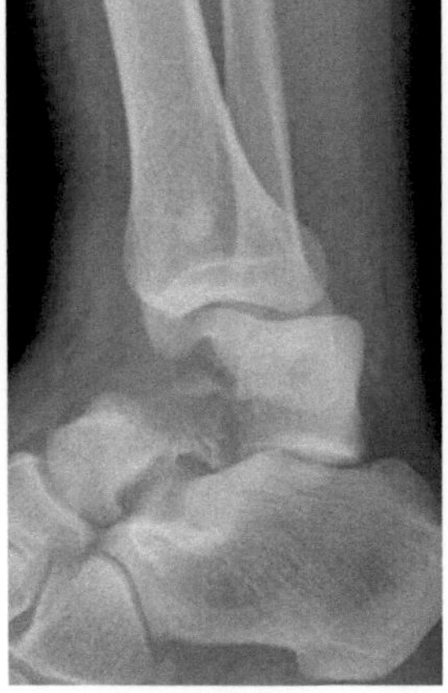

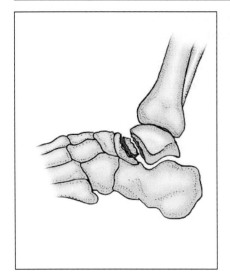

AO/OTA classification
81 Talus fractures
Type B: Talus neck fracture.
B3: Displaced talus neck fracture with subluxation of ankle and subtalar joint.
B3.1: Non-comminuted fracture

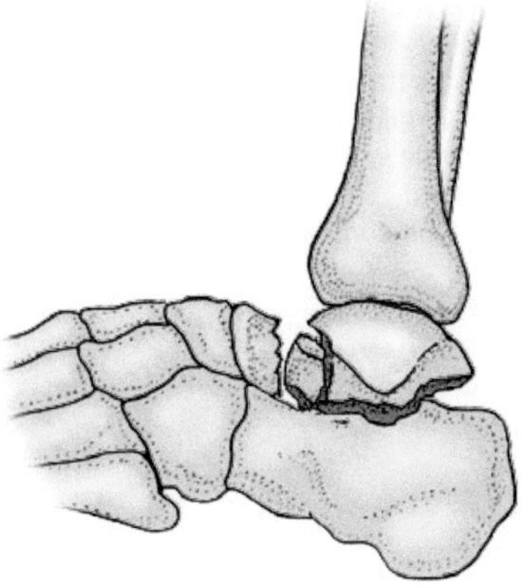

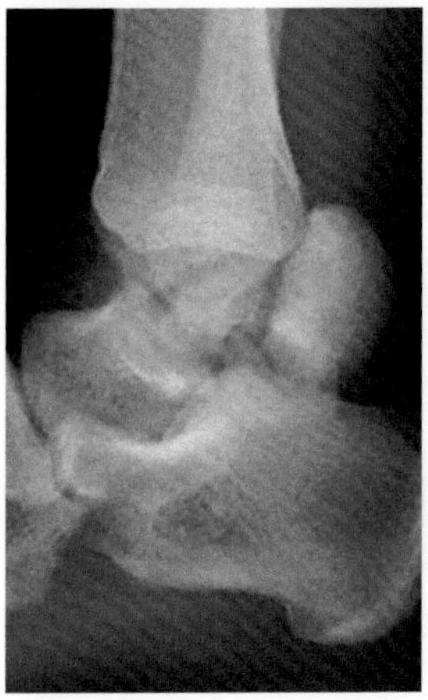

AO/OTA classification
81 Talus fractures
Type B: Talus neck fracture.
B3: Displaced talus neck fracture with subluxation of ankle and subtalar joint.
B3.2; Comminuted fracture

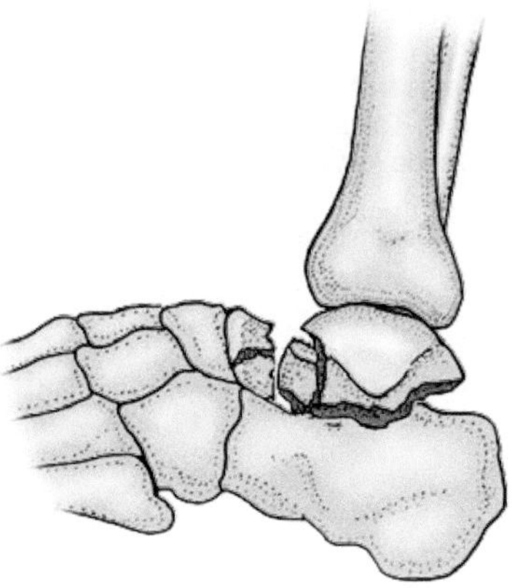

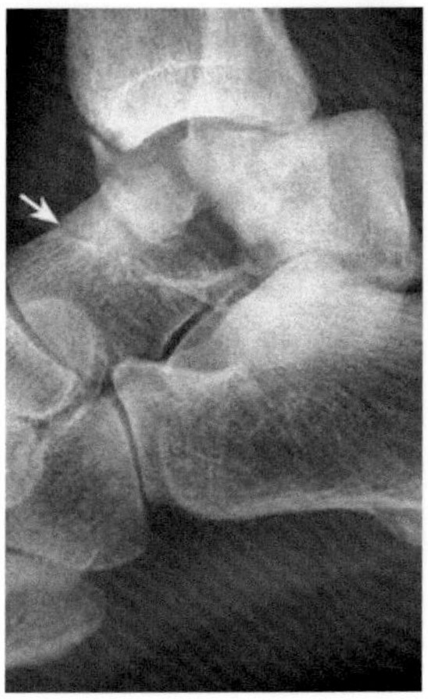

AO/OTA classification
81 Talus fractures
Type B: Talus neck fracture.
B3: Displaced talus neck fracture with subluxation of ankle and subtalar joint.
B3.3: Involves talus head

Type C: Talus body fracture:
- Type C1: Ankle joint involvement, dome fractures:
  - Type C1.1: Non-comminuted fracture.
  - Type C1.2: Comminuted fracture.
- Type C2: Subtalar joint involvement, body fractures:
  - Type C2.1: Non-comminuted fracture.
  - Type C2.2: Comminuted fracture.
- Type C3: Subtalar and ankle joint involvement, body fractures:
  - Type C3.1: Noncomminuted fracture.
  - Type C3.2: Comminuted fracture.

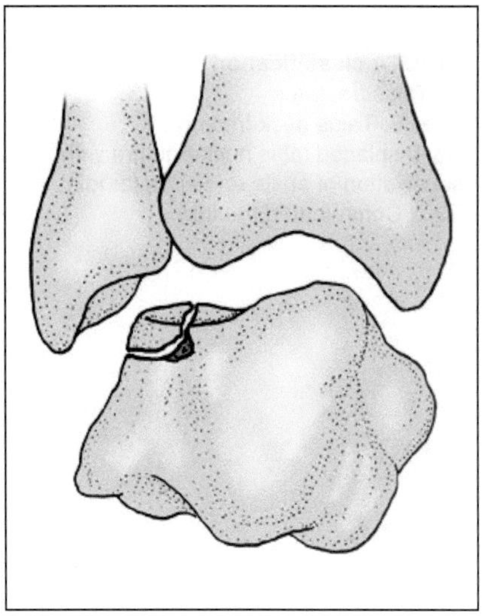

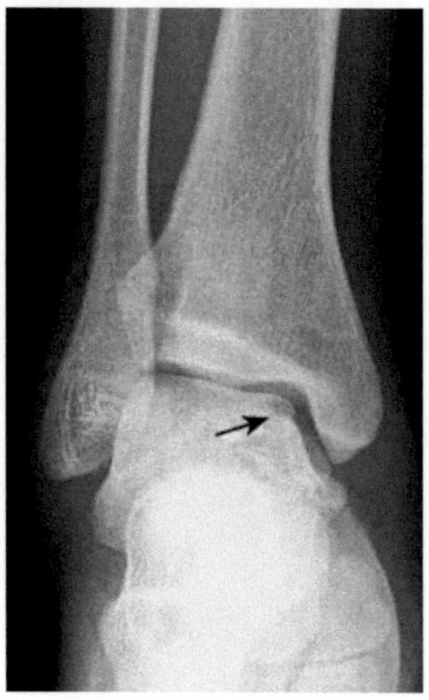

AO/OTA classification

81 Talus fractures
Type C: talus body fracture.
C1: Ankle joint involvement, dome fractures.
C1.1 Non-comminuted fracture

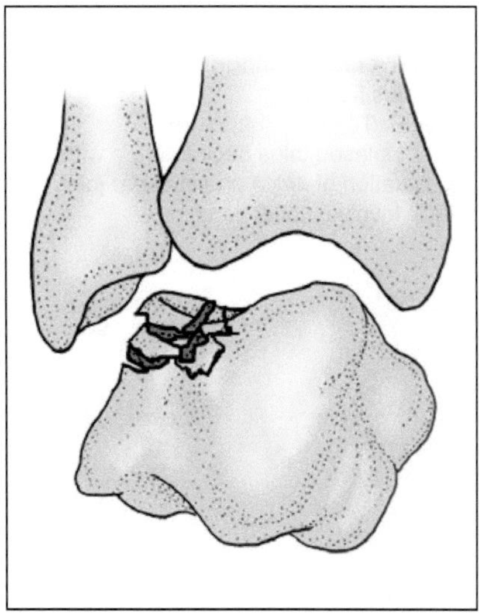

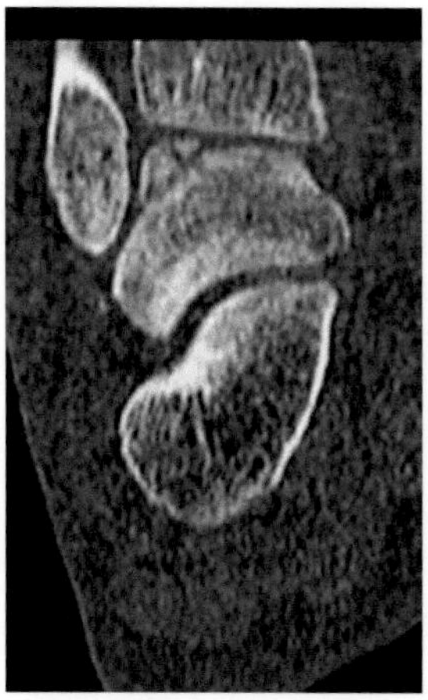

AO/OTA classification

81 Talus fractures
Type C: Talus body fracture.
C1: Ankle joint involvement, dome fractures.
C1.2: Comminuted fracture

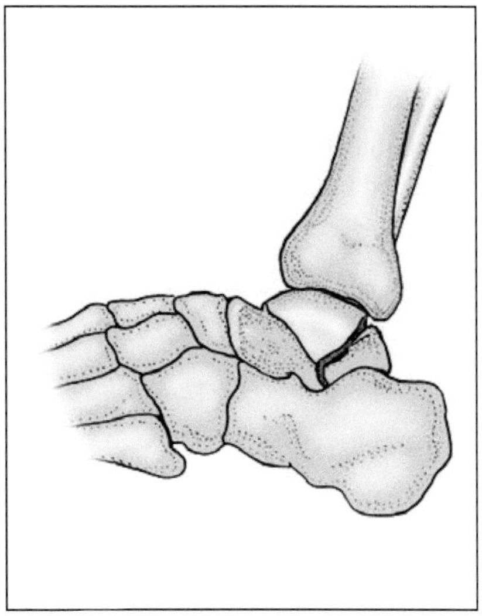

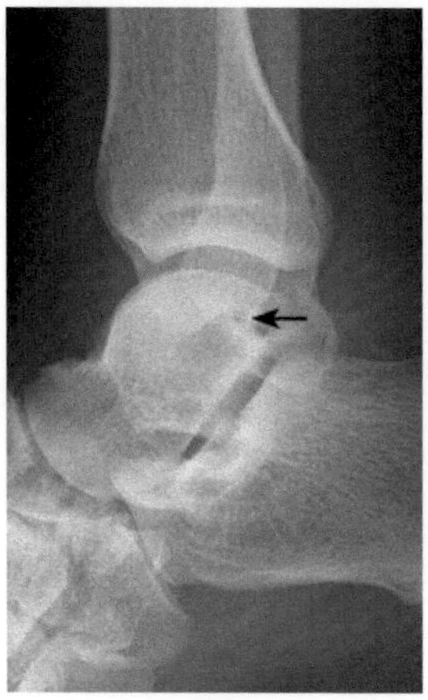

AO/OTA classification

81 Talus fractures
Type C: talus body fracture.
C2: Subtalar joint involvement, body fractures.
C2.1: Non-comminuted fracture

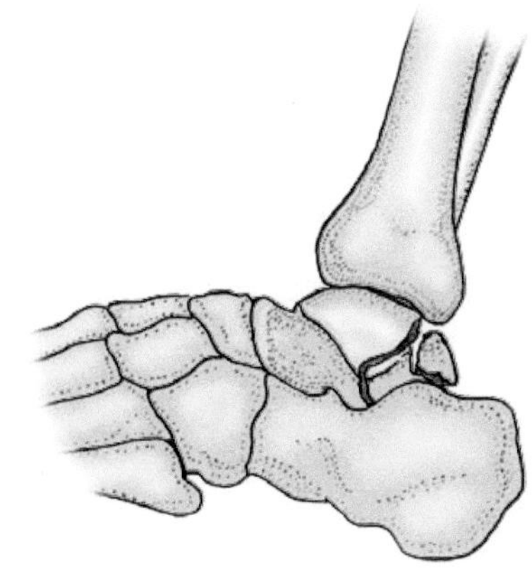

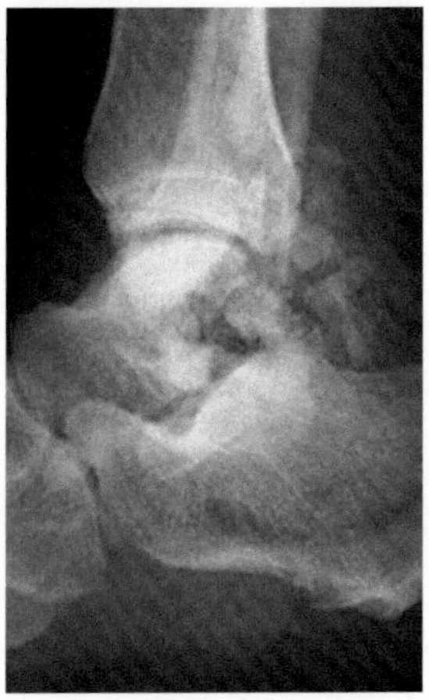

AO/OTA classification

81 Talus fractures
Type C: Talus body fracture.
C2: Subtalar joint involvement, body fractures.
C2.2: Comminuted fracture

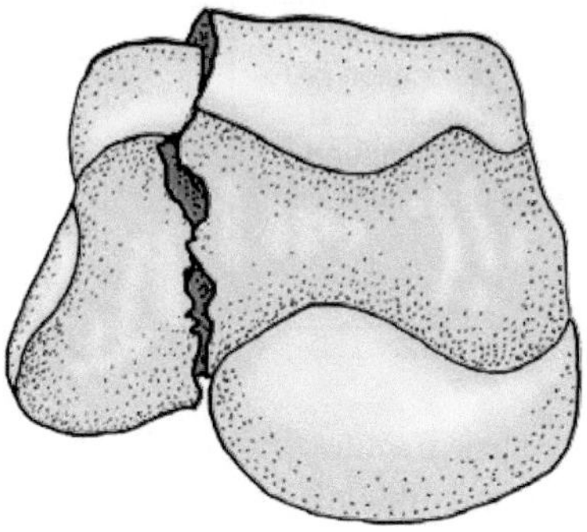

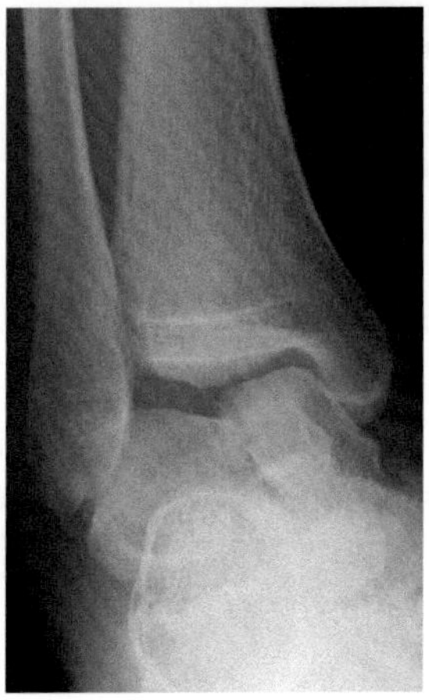

AO/OTA classification

81 Talus fractures
Type C: Talus body fracture.
C3: Subtalar and ankle joint involvement, body fractures.
C3.1: Non-comminuted fracture

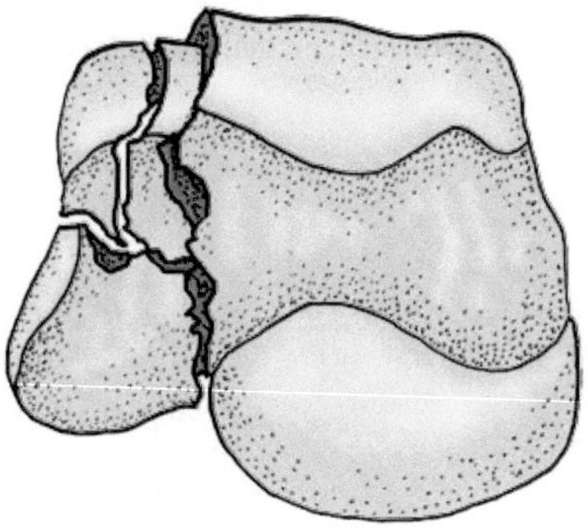

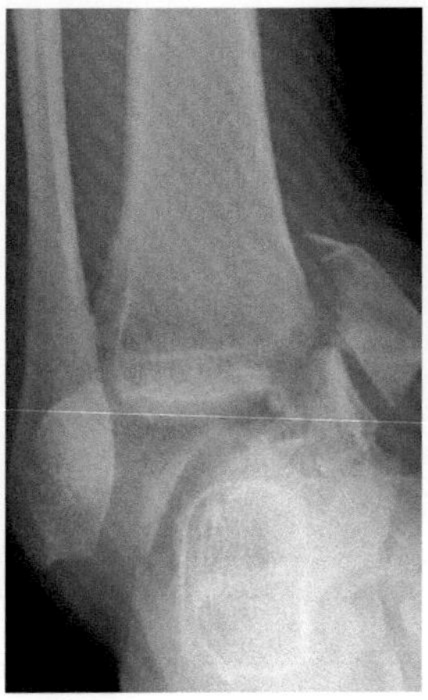

AO/OTA classification

81 Talus fractures
Type C: talus body fracture.
C3: Subtalar and ankle joint involvement, body fractures.
C3.2: Comminuted fracture

11.1.3 Hawkins Classification of Talus Neck Fractures (1970, J Bone Joint Surg [Am], 52:991–1002)

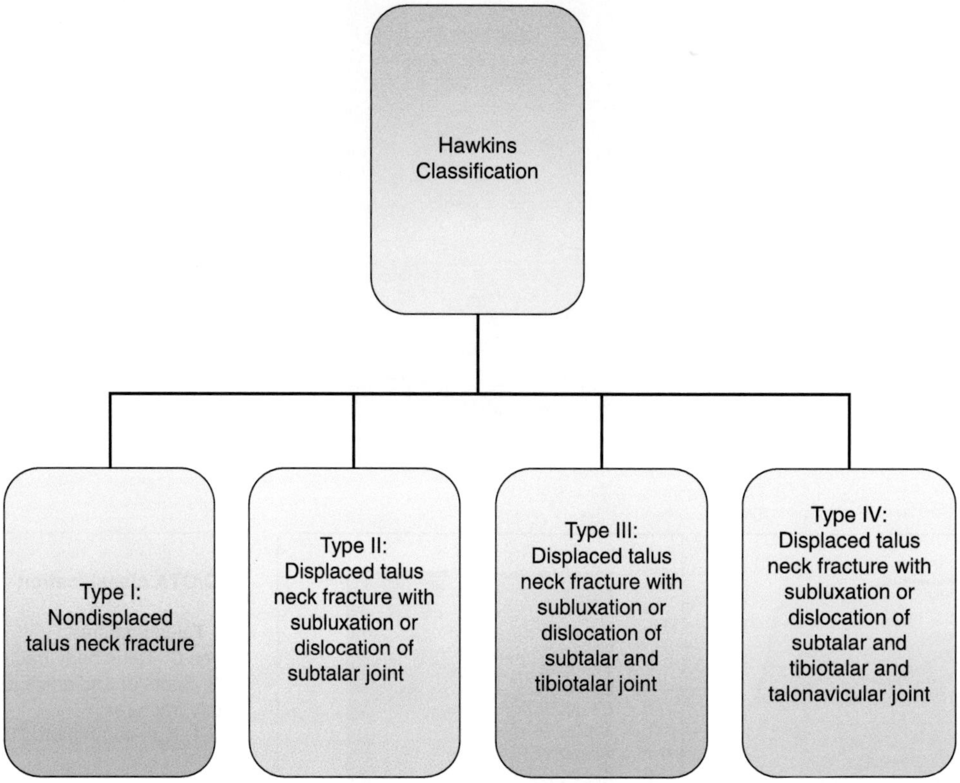

Type I: Nondisplaced talus neck fracture.

Type II: Displaced talus neck fracture with subluxation or dislocation of subtalar joint.

Type III: Displaced talus neck fracture with subluxation or dislocation of subtalar and tibiotalar joint.

Type IV: Displaced talus neck fracture with subluxation or dislocation of subtalar and tibiotalar and talonavicular joint (1978, J Bone Jiont Surg [Am], 60:143-156).

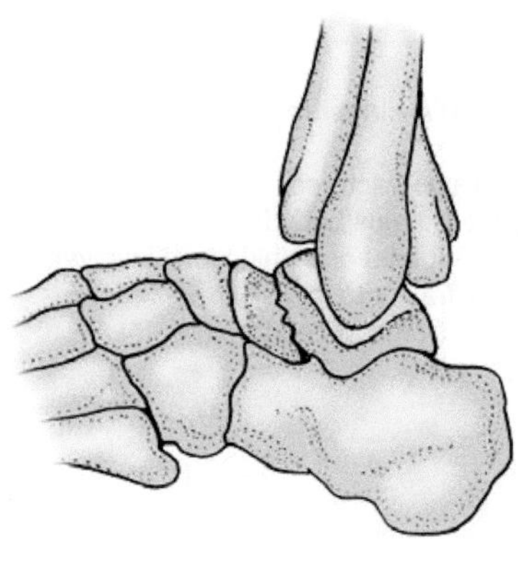

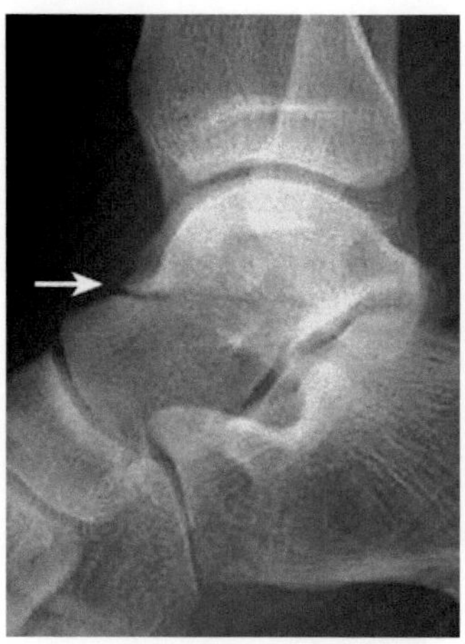

Hawkins classification of talus neck fractures

Type I: Nondisplaced talus neck fracture

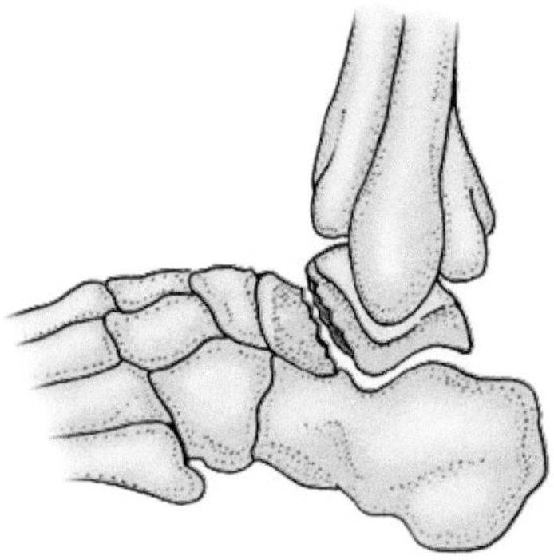

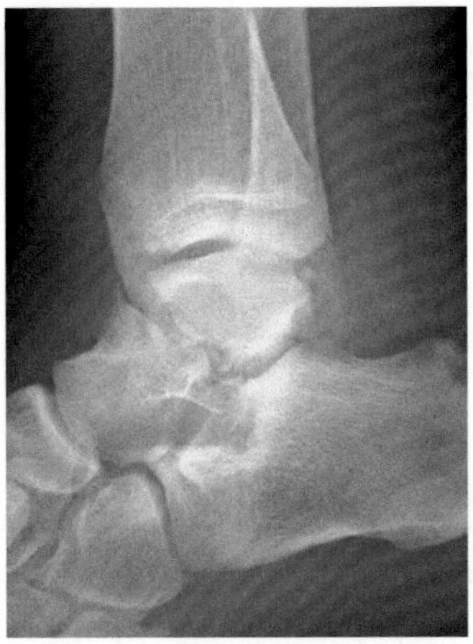

Hawkins classification of talus neck fractures

Type II: Displaced talus neck fracture with subluxation or dislocation of subtalar joint

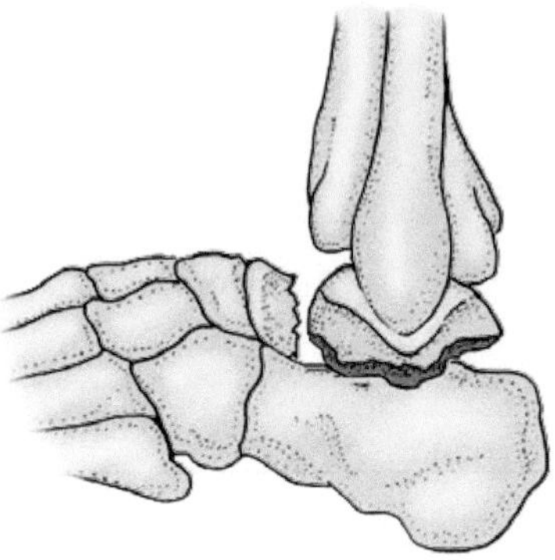

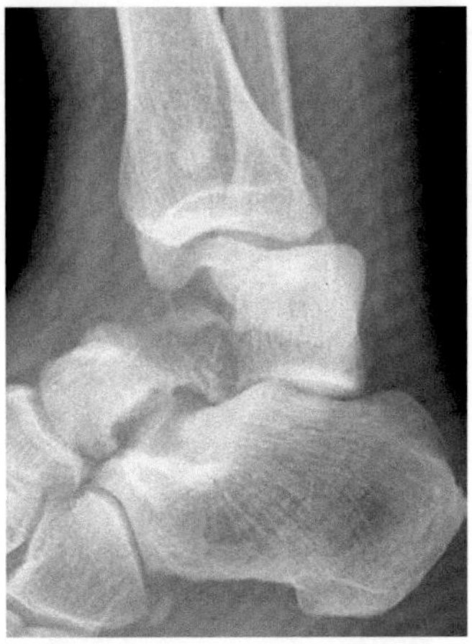

Hawkins classification of talus neck fractures

Type III: Displaced talus neck fracture with subluxation or dislocation of subtalar and tibiotalar joint

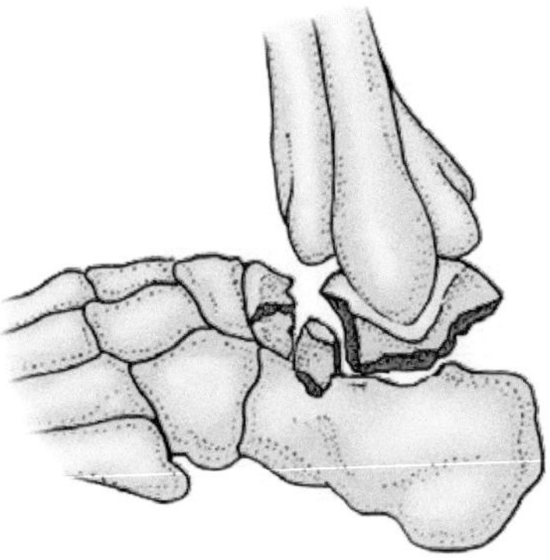

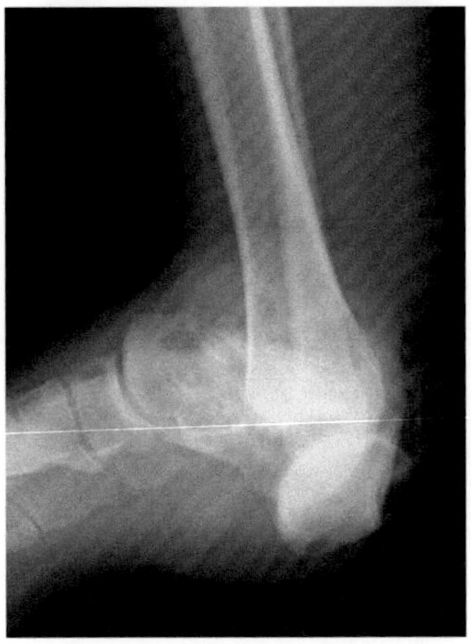

Hawkins classification of talus neck fractures

Type IV: Displaced talus neck fracture with subluxation or dislocation of subtalar and tibiotalar and talonavicular joint

11.1.4 The Classification of Talus Body Fractures

11.1.4.1 Sneppen Classification (1997, Acta Orthop Scand, 48:317–324)

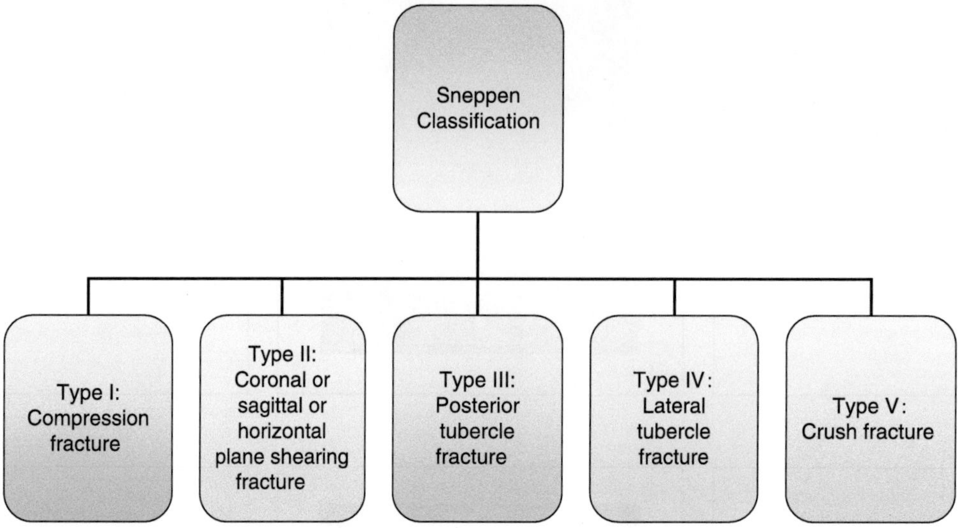

Type I: Compression fracture.
Type II: Coronal or sagittal or horizontal plane shearing fracture.
Type III: Posterior tubercle fracture.
Type IV: Lateral tubcrcle fracture.
Type V: Crush fracture.

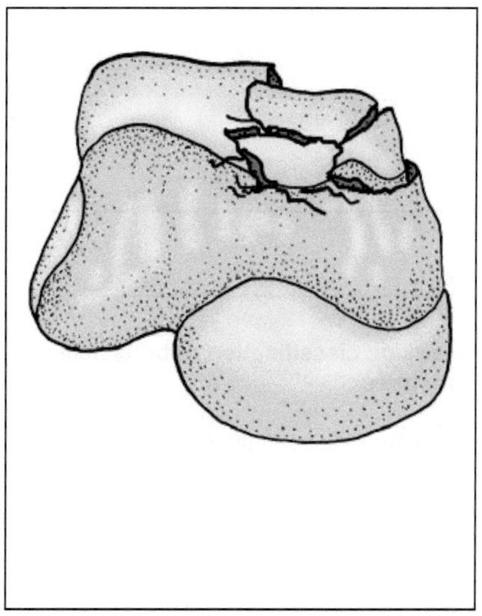

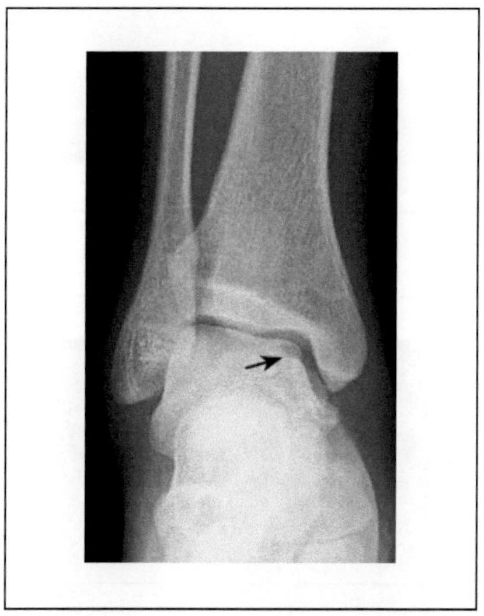

Sneppen classification of talus body fracture

Type I: Compression fracture

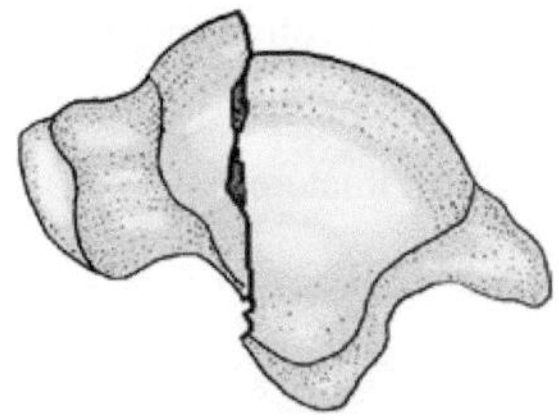

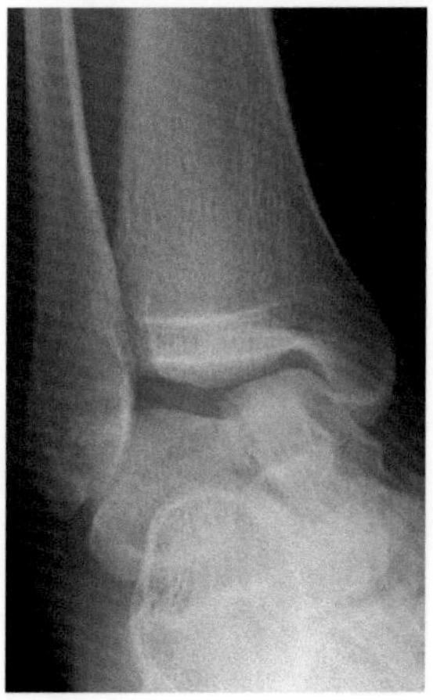

Sneppen classification of talus body fracture

Type II: Coronal or sagittal or horizontal plane shearing fracture

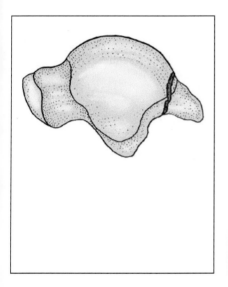

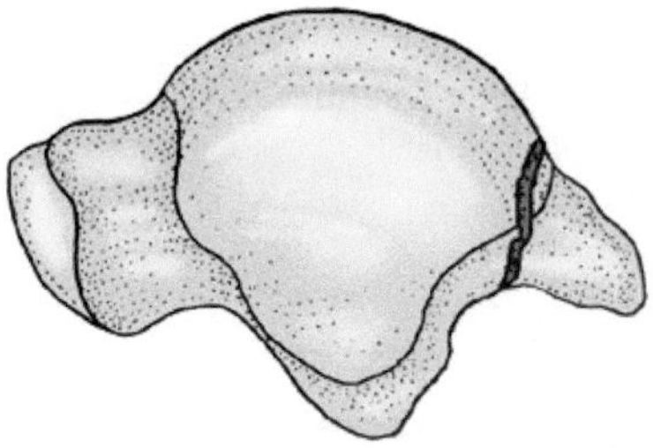

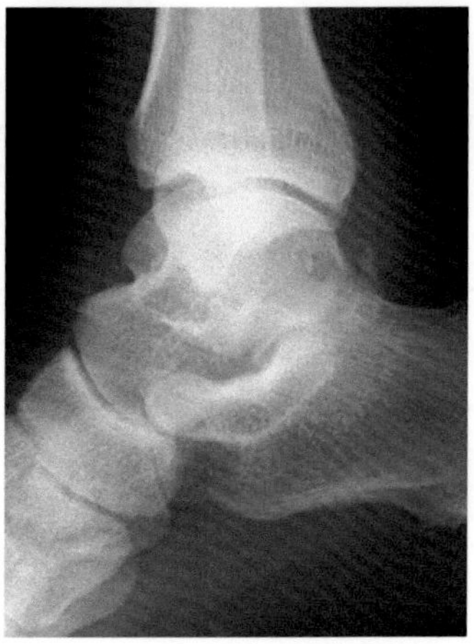

Sneppen classification of talus body fracture

Type III: Posterior tubercle fracture

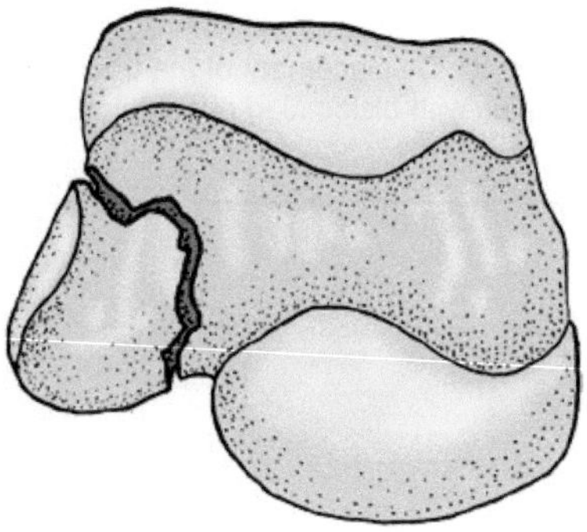

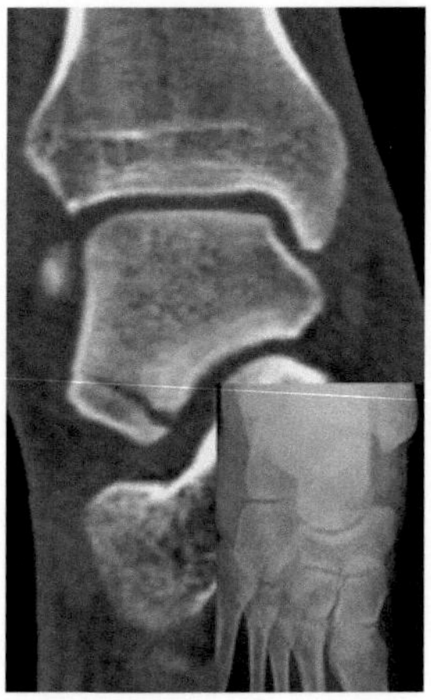

Sneppen classification of talus body fracture

Type IV: Lateral tubercle fracture

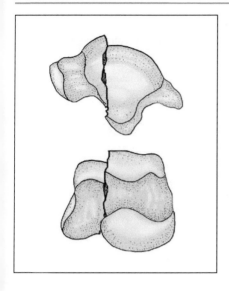

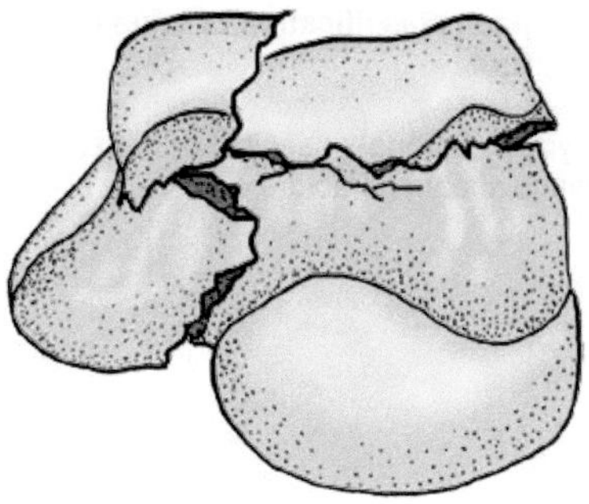

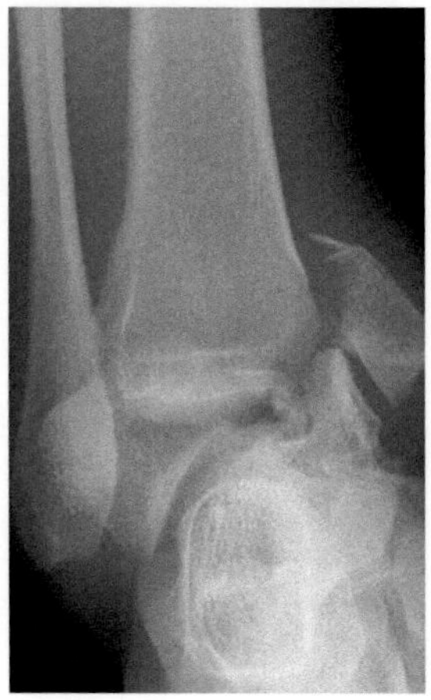

Sneppen classification of talus body fracture

Type V: Crush fracture

11.1.4.2 Boyd-Knight Classification (1942)

Type I: Coronal or sagittal plane shearing fracture
- Type IA: Non-displaced talus fracture.
- Type IB: Displacement of the trochlea of talus.
- Type IC: Displacement of the trochlea of talus with dislocation of subtalar joint.
- Type ID: Talus body dislocated from the subtalar and trochlear joint.

Type II: Horizontal plane shearing fracture:
- Type IIA: Non-displaced.
- Type IIB: Displaced.

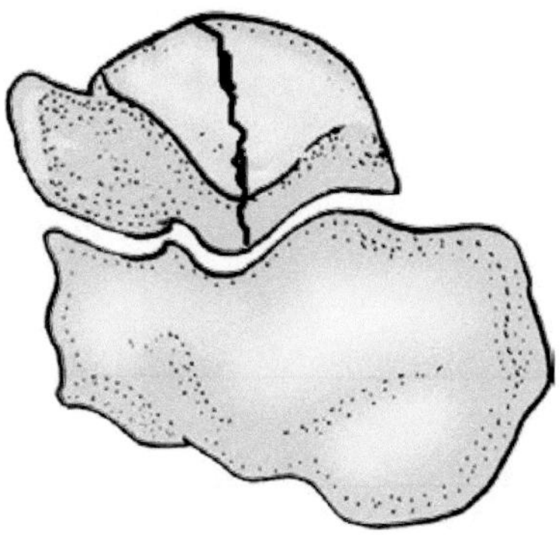

Type I: Coronal or sagittal plane shearing fracture
Type IA: Nondisplced talus fracture

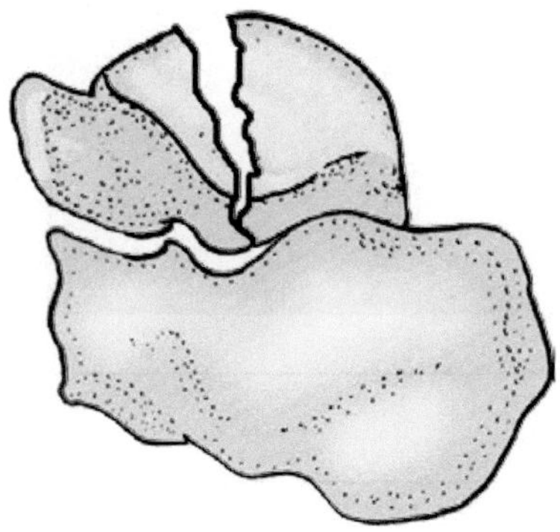

Type IB: Displacement of the trochlea of talus

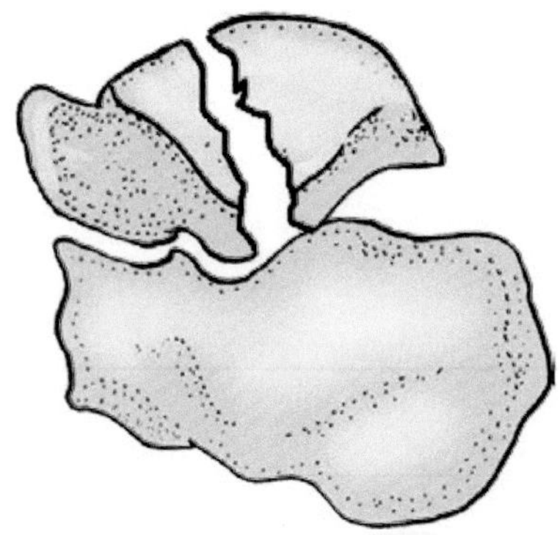

Type IC: Displacement of the trochlea of talus with dislocation of subtalar joint

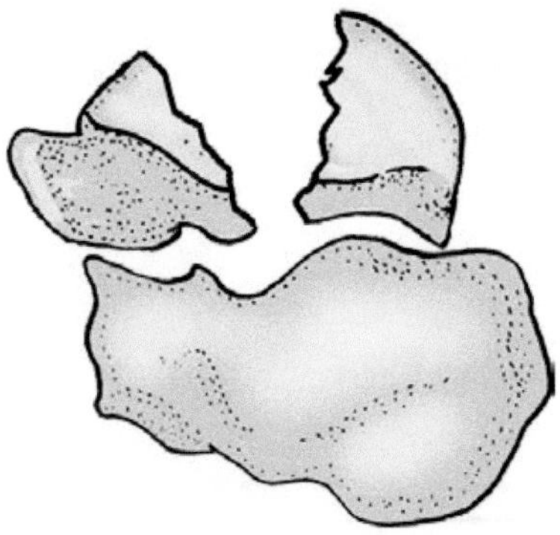

Type 1D: Talus body dislocated from the subtalar and trochlear joint

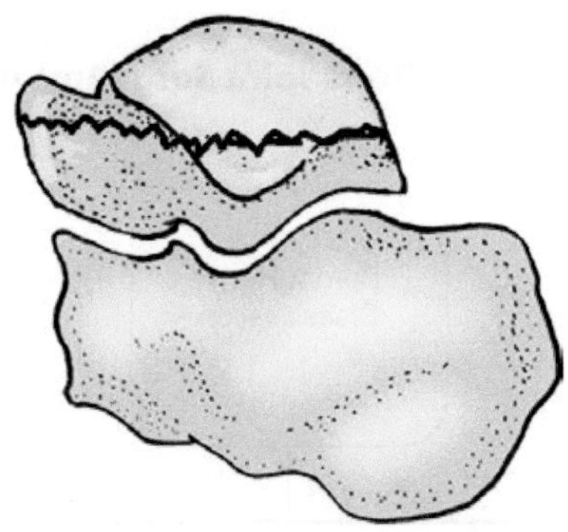

Type II: Horizontal plane shearing fracture
Type IIA: Nondisplaced

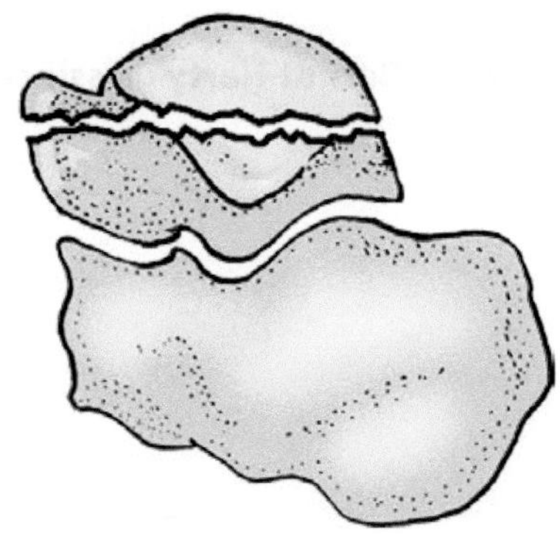

Type IIB: Displaced

11.1.5 Delee Classification of Talus Fractures (1986, Surgery of the foot. 5th ed. St. Louis: C V Mosby, 656)

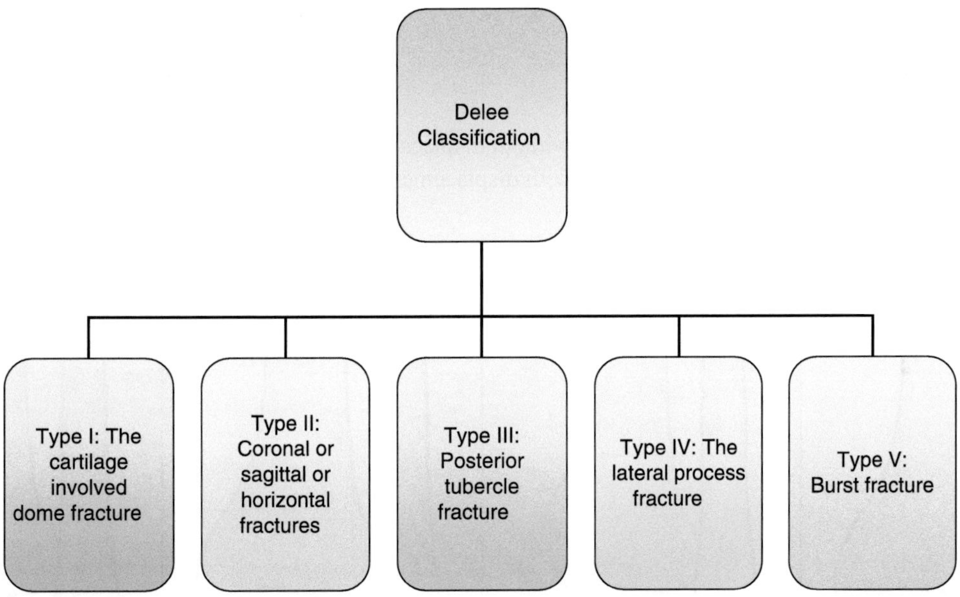

Type I: The cartilage involved dome fracture.
Type II: Coronal or sagittal or horizontal fractures.
Type III: Posterior tubercle fracture.
Type IV: The lateral process fracture.
Type V: Burst fracture.

11.1.6 The Classification of Talus Osteochondral Fracture

11.1.6.1 Berndt-Harty Classification (1959, J Bone Joint Surg [Am], 41:988–1020)

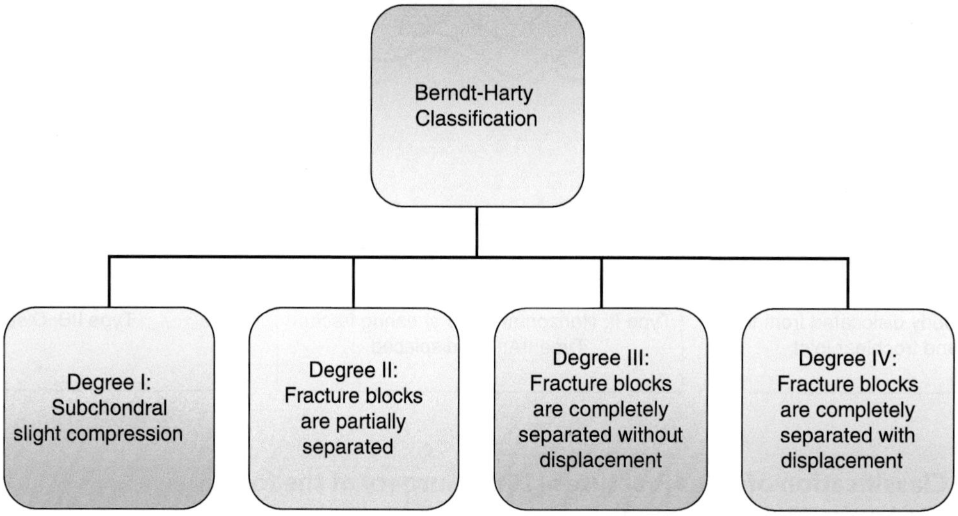

Fractures are divided into four degrees according to the X-ray.

Degree I: Subchondral slight compression.
Degree II: Fracture blocks are partially separated.
Degree III: Fracture blocks are completely separated without displacement.
Degree IV: Fracture blocks are completely separated with displacement.

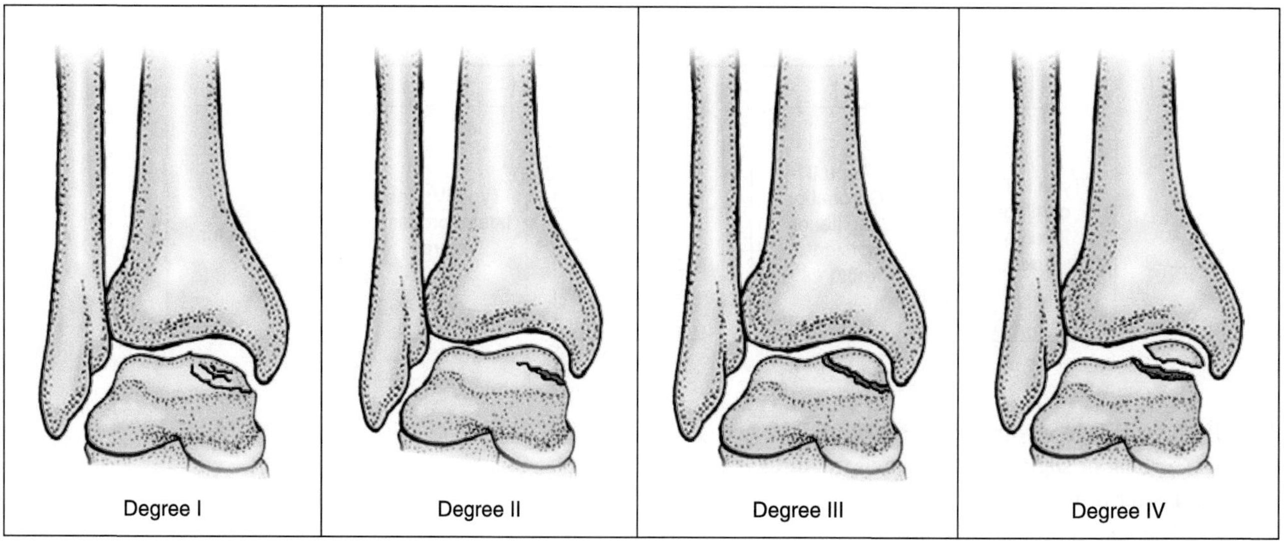

11.1.6.2 Hepple's MRI Classification (1999)

Type I: Simple cartilage injury.

Type IIa: Cartilage injury, accompanied with subchondral fractures and marrow edema.

Type IIb: Cartilage injury, accompanied with subchondral fractures.

Type III: Fracture without displacement.

Type IV: Fracture with displacement.

Type V: Subchondral bone cyst formation.

11.1.6.3 Ferkel-Sgaglione CT Classification (1990)

Type I: Cystic lesions in the dome of the talus, the dome is intact.

Type IIa: Cystic lesions connect to the surface of the talus dome.

Type IIb: Articular surface cleft, the surface fracture block without displacement.

Type III: Non-displaced fracture with translucent zone.

Type III: Displaced fracture.

Type V: Subchondral bone cyst formation.

11.1.6.4 Pritsch's Ankle Arthroscopy Classification of Talar Cartilage Fracture (1986, J Bone Joint Surg [Am], 68:862–865)

Degree I: Articular cartilage is complete, hard, and shiny.

Degree II: Articular cartilage is complete but soft.

Degree III: Articular cartilage wear.

11.2 Section 2 Classification of Calcaneal Fractures

In literature, there are >10 classifications of calcaneal fractures. According to the reports over the last 5 years, the most commonly used classifications are the Sanders classification and Essex-Lopresti classification.

11.2.1 Sanders Classification (1993, Orthop Relat Res, 290:87–95)

Classification principle: Based on the findings of coronal and axial CT, calcaneal fractures are divided into four types according to the posterior facet. At the widest undersurface of the posterior facet of the talus, the articular surface is divided into three equal columns by two lines that are then extended across the calcaneal posterior facet; with the addition of a third line just medial to the medial edge of the posterior facet, the posterior facet of the calcaneus could be arbitrarily divided into three potential fragments: medial, central, and lateral. These fragments plus the sustentaculum tali resulted in a total of four potential articular pieces.

Type I: All non-displaced fractures regardless of the number of fracture lines.
Type II: Two-part fractures of the posterior facet, displacement ≥2 mm.
  Type IIa: Fracture line lateral.
  Type IIb: Fracture line medial.
  Type IIc: Fracture line sustentaculum tali.
Type III: Three-part fractures with a centrally depressed fragment; subtypes IIIAB, IIIAC, and IIIBC.
Type IV: Four-part articular fractures; highly comminuted.

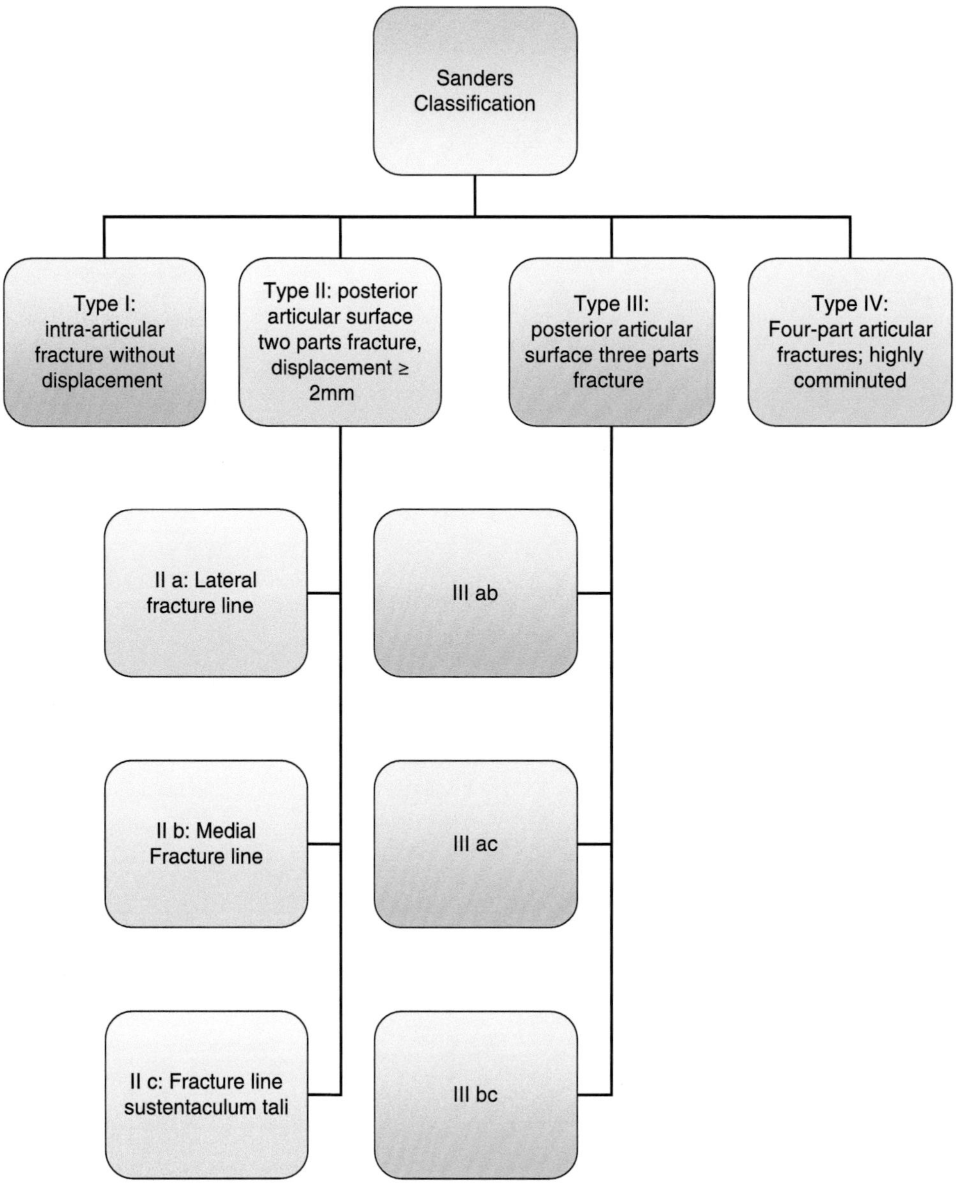

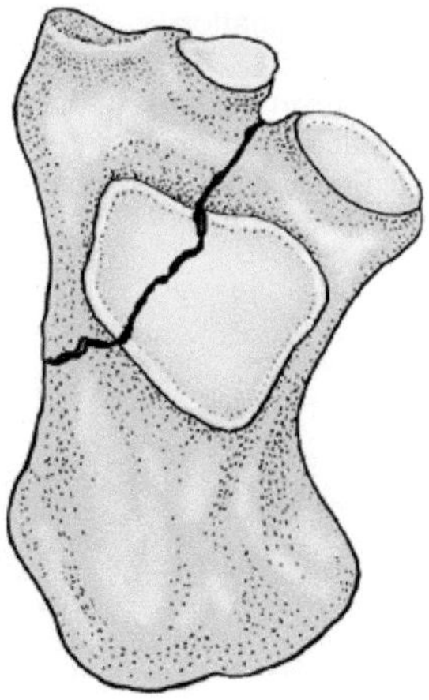

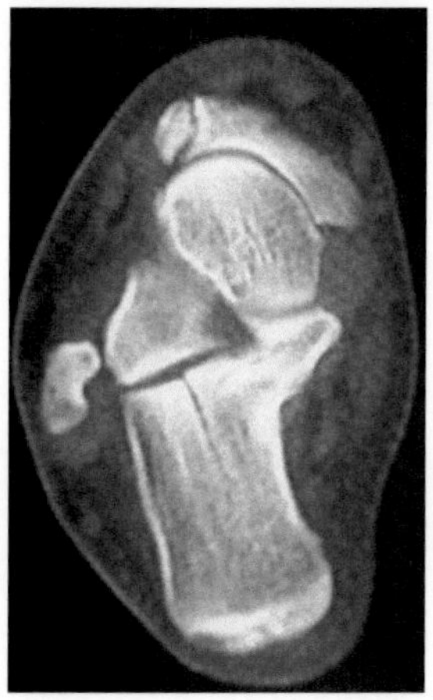

Sanders classification

Type I: All non-displaced fractures regardless of the number of fracture lines

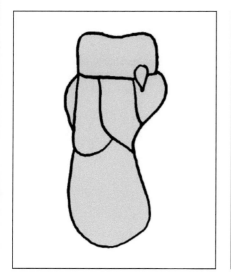

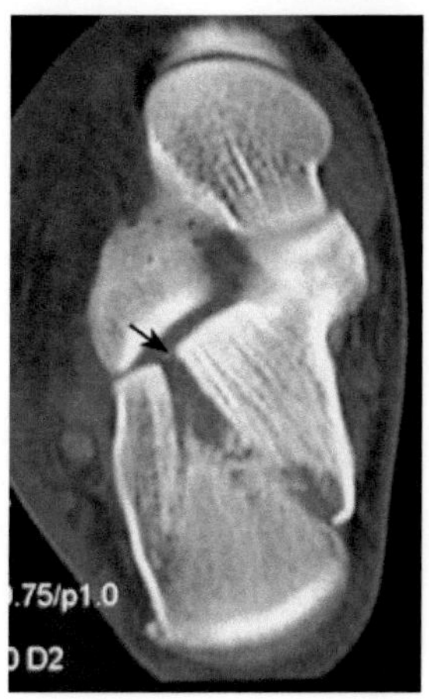

Sanders classification

Type II: Two-part fractures of the posterior facet, displacement≥2mm.
II a: Lateral fracture line

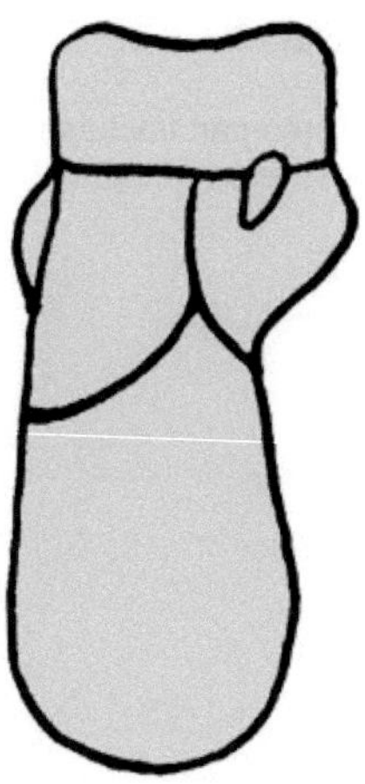

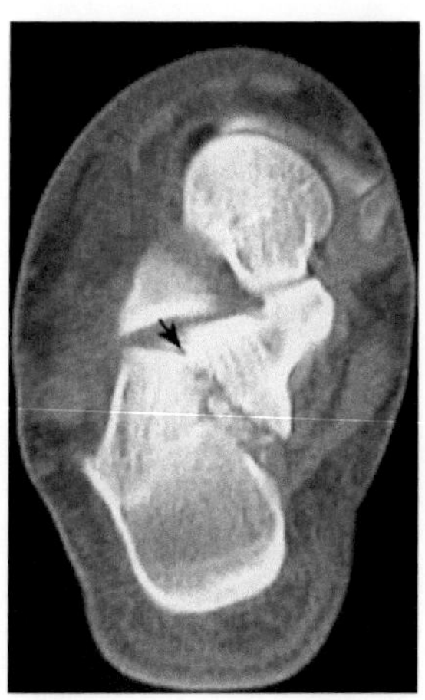

Sanders classification

Type II: Two-part fractures of the posterior facet, displacement≥2mm.
II b: Medial Fracture line

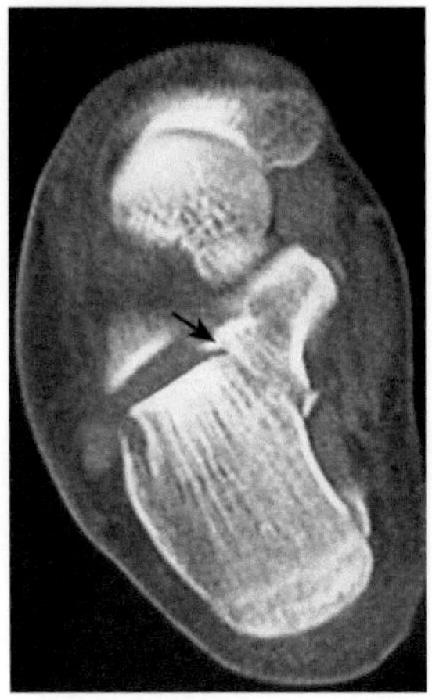

Sanders classification

Type II: Two-part fractures of the posterior facet, displacement≥2mm.
Type II c: Fracture line sustentaculum tali

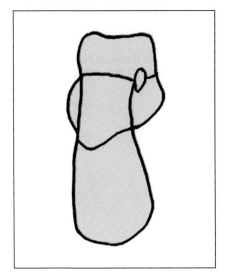

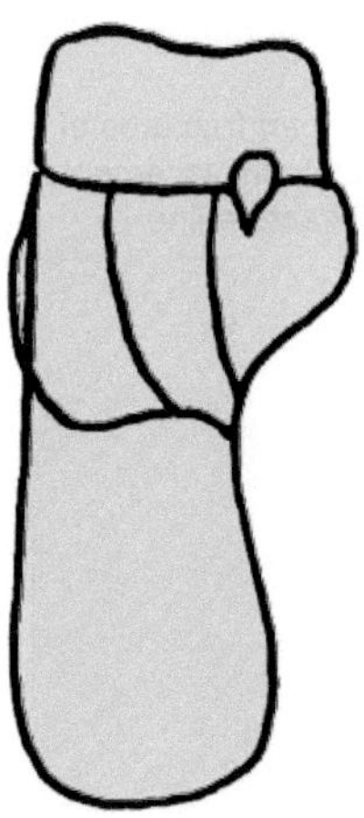

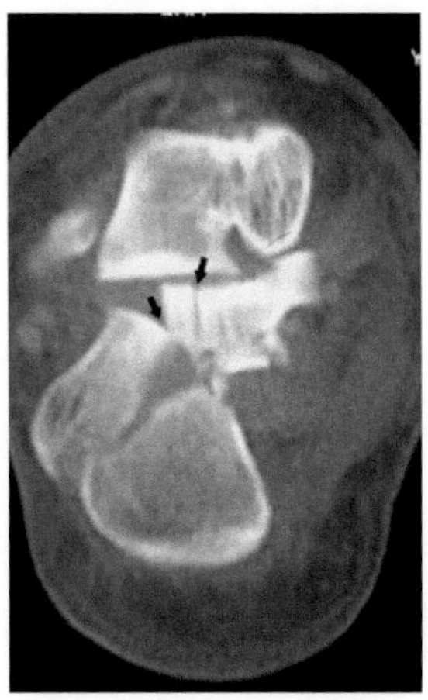

Sanders classification

Type III: Three-part fractures with a centrally depressed fragment
III ab

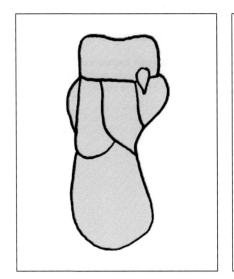

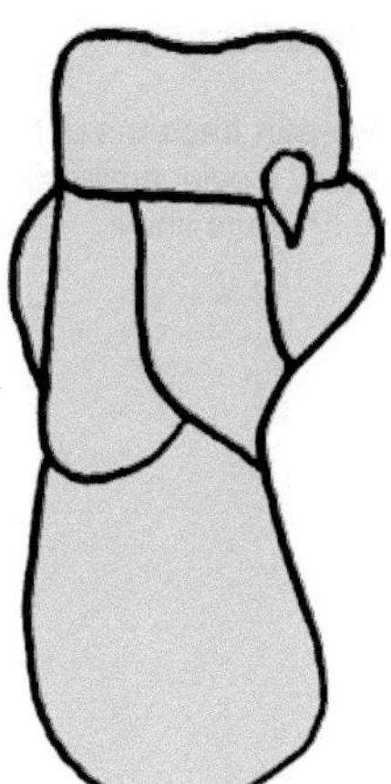

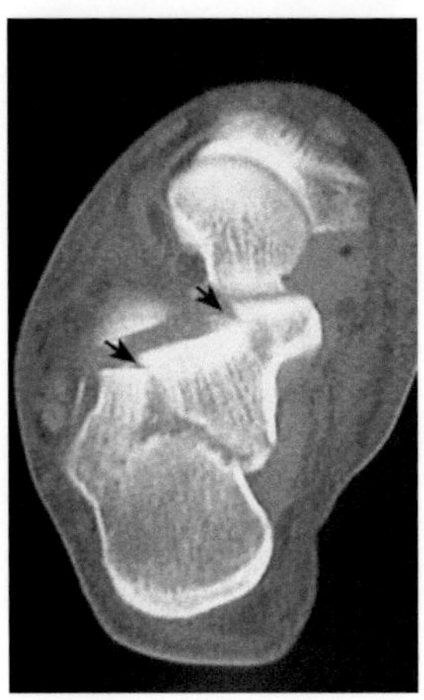

Sanders classification

Type III: Three-part fractures with a centrally depressed fragment
III ac

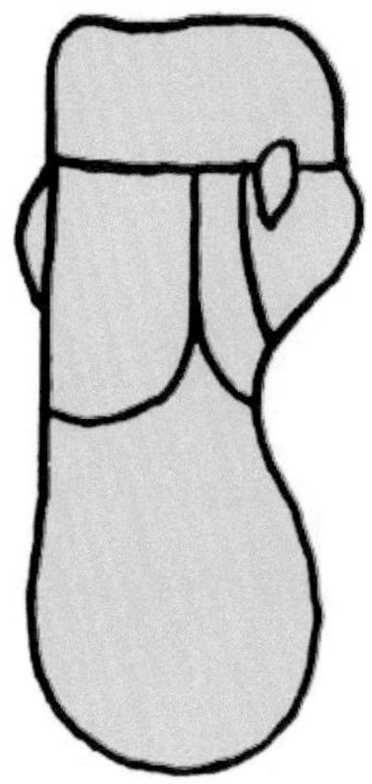

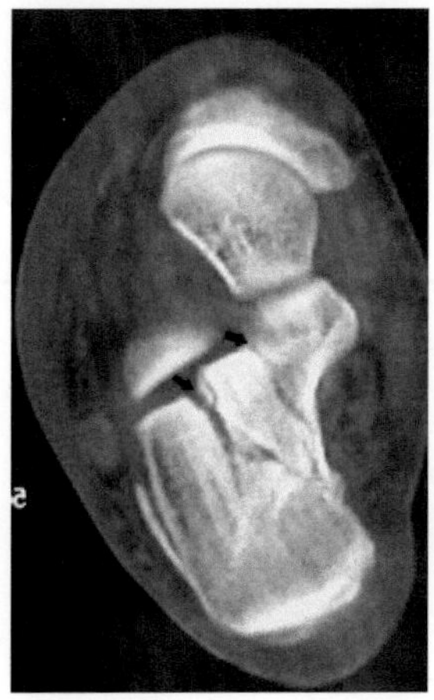

Sanders classification

Type III: Three-part fractures with a centrally depressed fragment
II b c

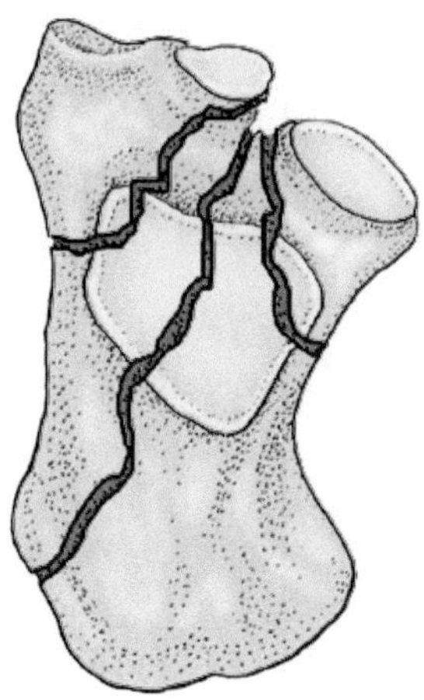

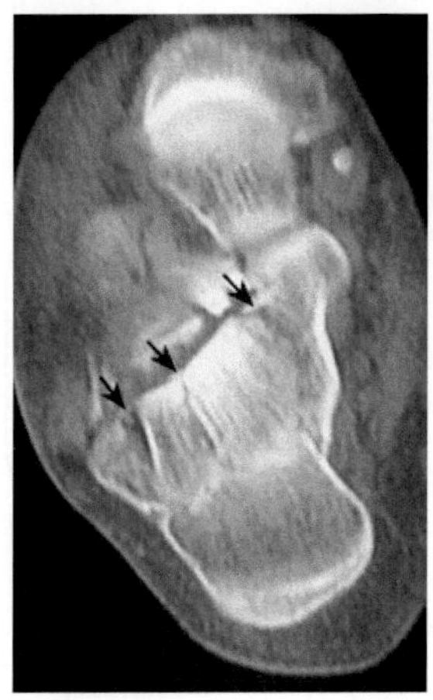

Sanders classification

Type III: Four-part articular fractures; highly comminuted

11.2.2 Essex-Lopresti Classification (1952, Br J Surg, 39:395–419)

Type I: Subtalar joint intact:
- Type I.A: Calcaneal tuberosity fracture:
  - Type I.A1: Beaklike fracture.
  - Type I.A2: Medial wall avulsion fracture.
  - Type I.A3: Vertical fracture.
  - Type I.A4: Horizontal fracture.
- Type I.B: Calcaneocuboid joint involved calcaneal fractures:
  - Type I.B1: Parrot nose type;
  - Type I.B2: Other types;

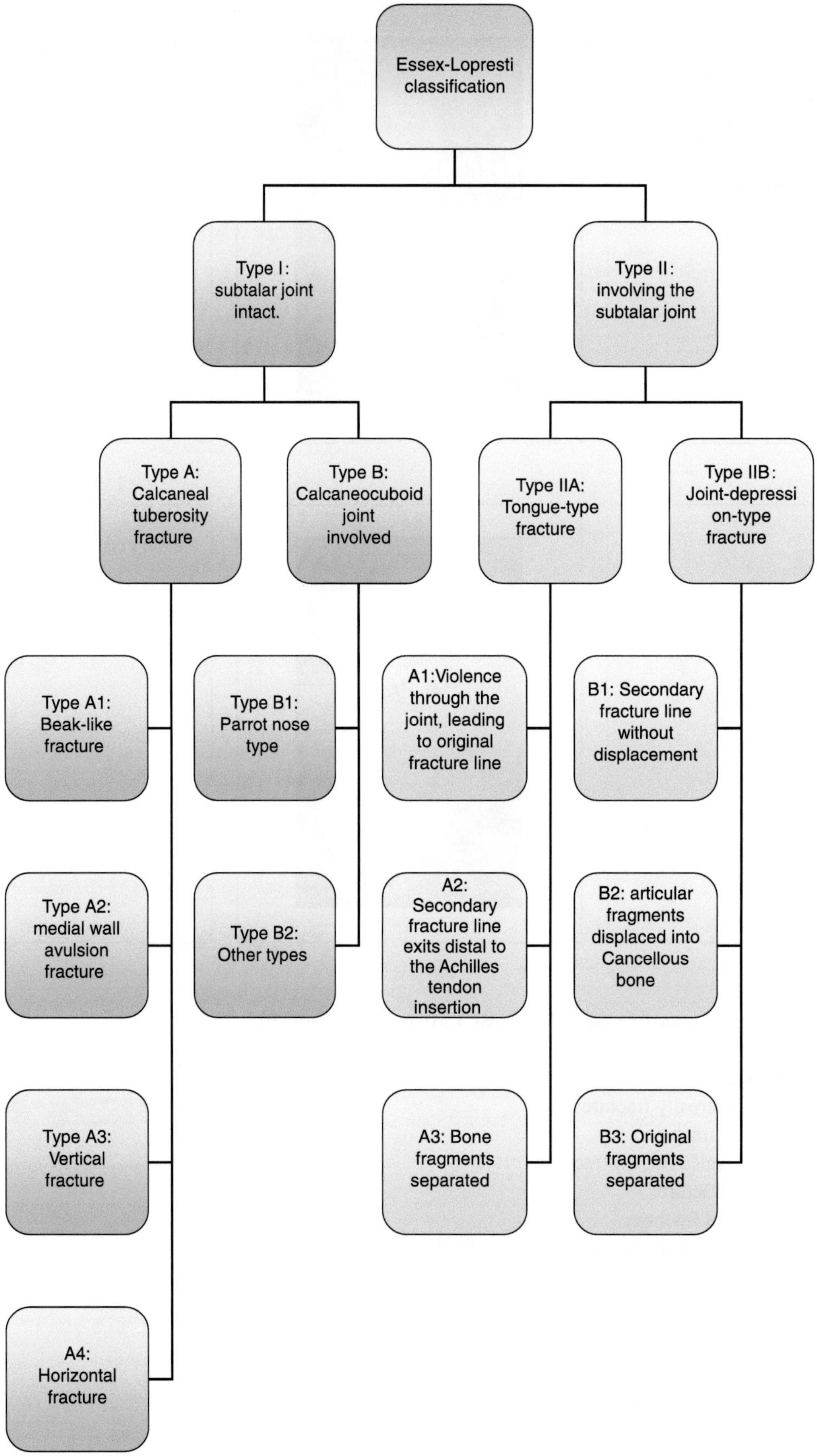
Essex-Lopresti classification
Type I: subtalar joint intact.
Type II: involving the subtalar joint
Type A: Calcaneal tuberosity fracture
Type B: Calcaneocuboid joint involved
Type IIA: Tongue-type fracture
Type IIB: Joint-depression-type fracture
Type A1: Beak-like fracture
Type B1: Parrot nose type
A1:Violence through the joint, leading to original fracture line
B1: Secondary fracture line without displacement
Type A2: medial wall avulsion fracture
Type B2: Other types
A2: Secondary fracture line exits distal to the Achilles tendon insertion
B2: articular fragments displaced into Cancellous bone
Type A3: Vertical fracture
A3: Bone fragments separated
B3: Original fragments separated
A4: Horizontal fracture

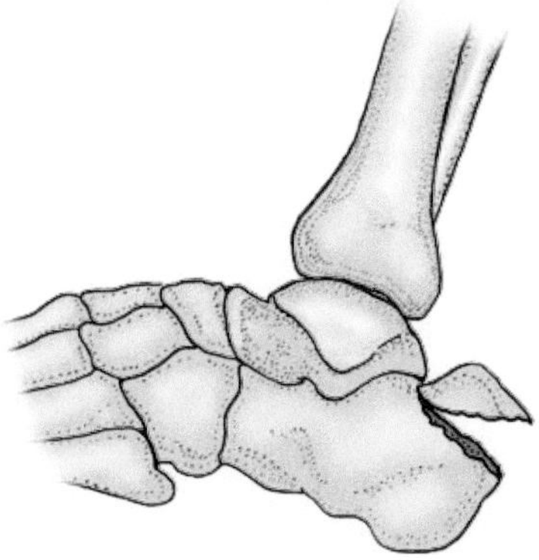

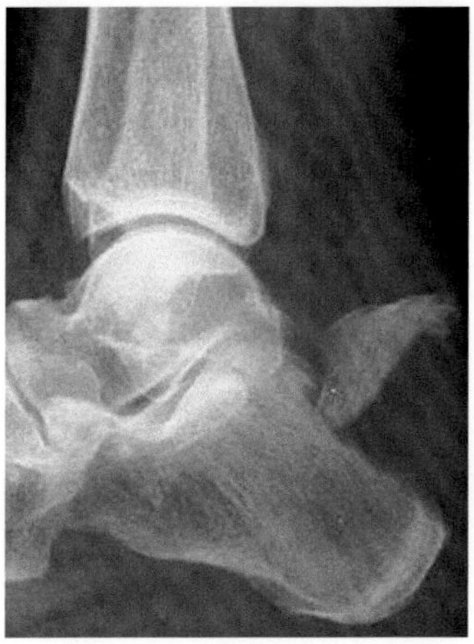

Essex-Lopresti classification

Type I: subtalar joint intact.
Type A: Calcaneal tuberosity fracture.
A1: Beak-like fracture

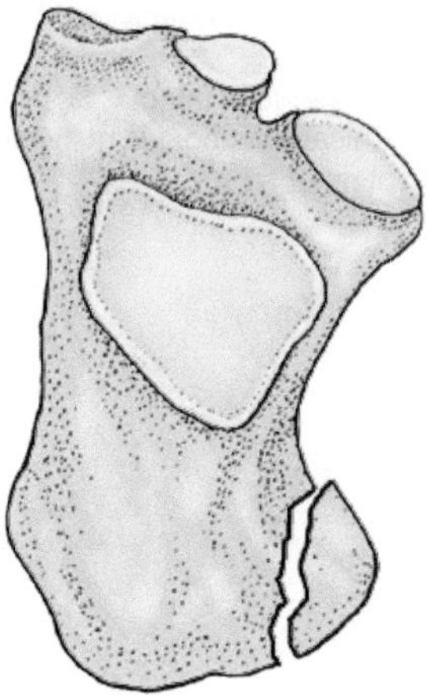

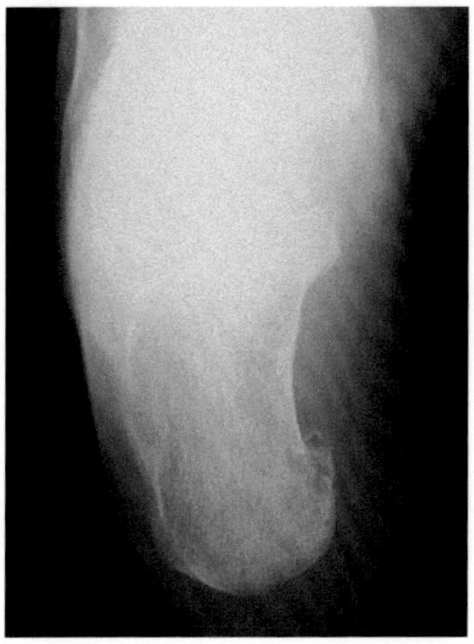

Essex-Lopresti classification

Type I: subtalar joint intact.
Type A: Calcaneal tuberosity fracture.
A2: medial wall avulsion fracture

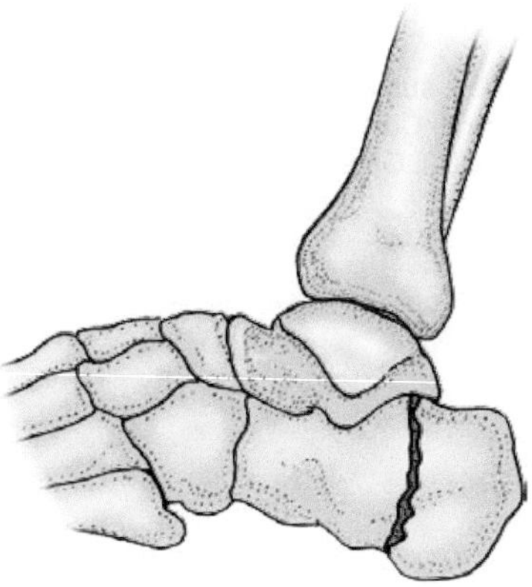

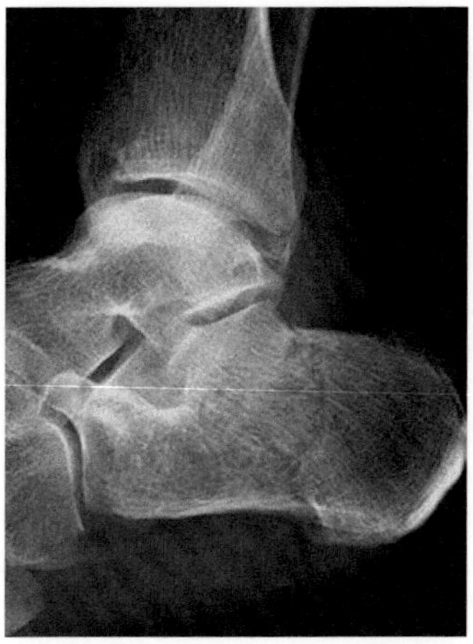

Essex-Lopresti classification

Type I: subtalar joint intact.
Type A: Calcaneal tuberosity fracture
A3: Vertical fracture

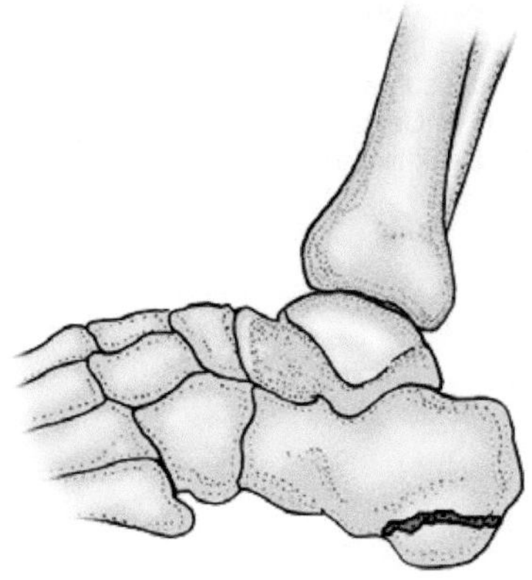

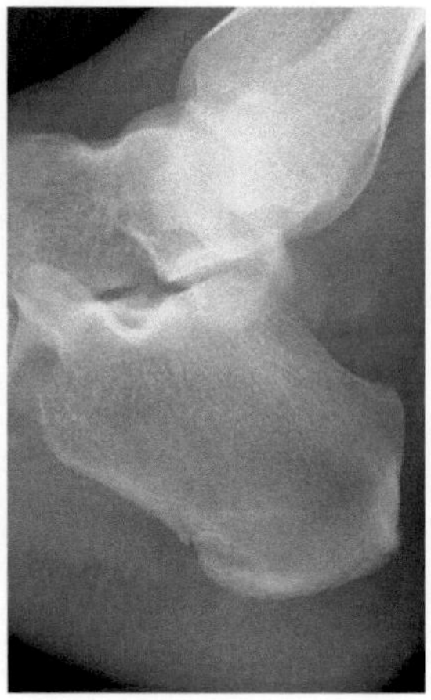

Essex-Lopresti classification

Type I: subtalar joint intact.
Type A: Calcaneal tuberosity fracture
A4 Horizontal

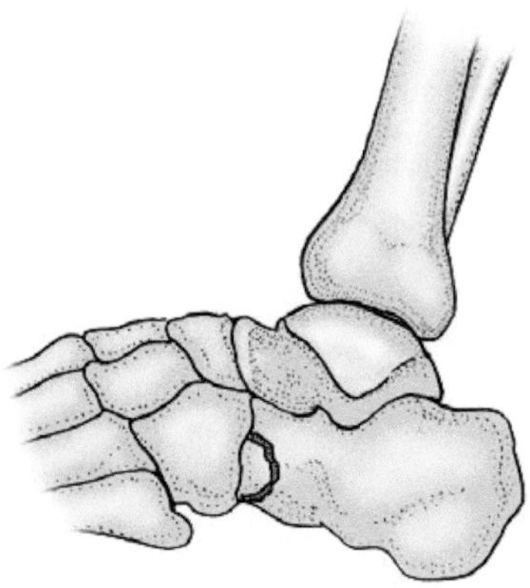

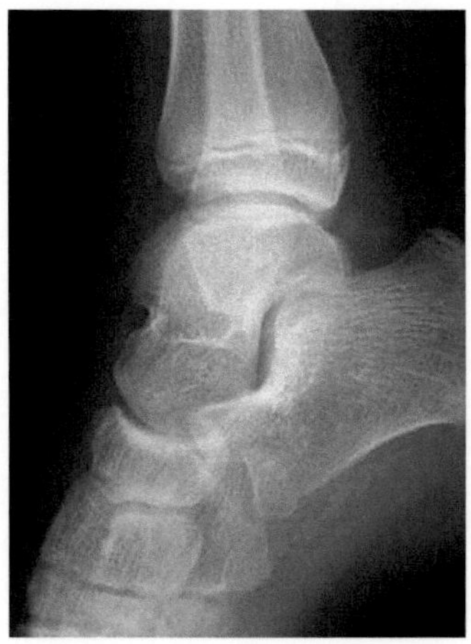

Essex-Lopresti classification

Type I: subtalar joint intact.
Type B: Calcaneocuboid joint involved.
B1: Parrot nose type

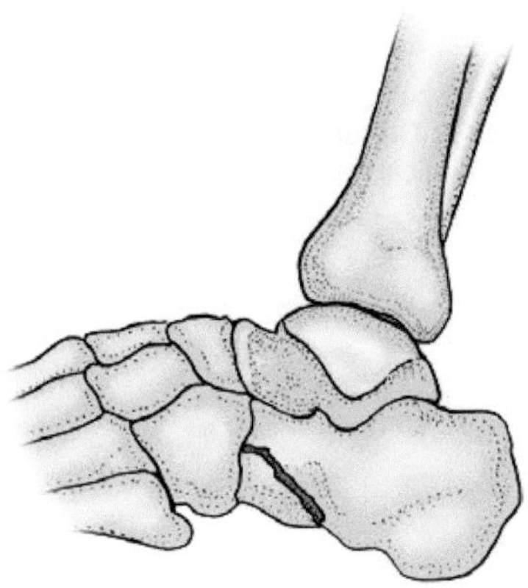

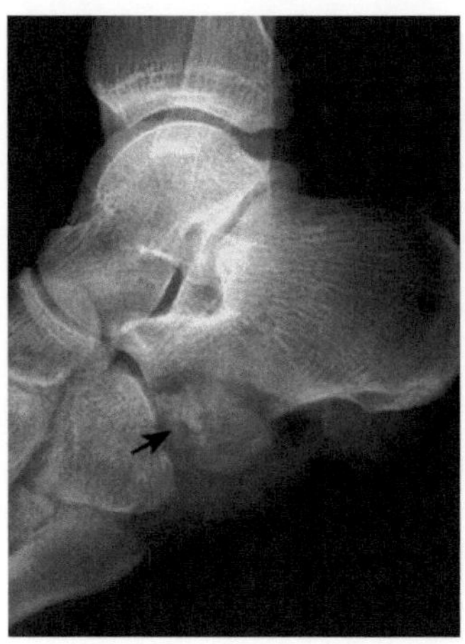

Essex-Lopresti classification

Type I: subtalar joint intact
Type B: Calcaneocuboid joint involved.
Type B2: Other types

Type II: Fractures involving the subtalar joint.

Type IIA: Tongue-type fracture.

Type IIA1: Secondary fracture line exits distal to the Achilles tendon insertion, and the tongue fragment consists of superior part of calcaneal body and lateral part of posterior facet. In the tongue-type fracture, the force runs through the subtalar joint, and thus produces the primary fracture line.

Type IIA2: Secondary fracture line exits distal to the Achilles tendon insertion, and the tongue fragment consists of superior part of calcaneal body and lateral part of posterior facet. In the tongue-type fracture, the secondary fracture line runs to the posterior rim of calcaneal tuberosity, with no displacement.

Type IIA3: Secondary fracture line exits distal to the Achilles tendon insertion; the tongue fragment consists of superior part of calcaneal body and lateral part of posterior facet. In the tongue-type fracture, the anterior portion of the fragment falls into the cancellous bone of the calcaneus body, the rear upturned, displaced.

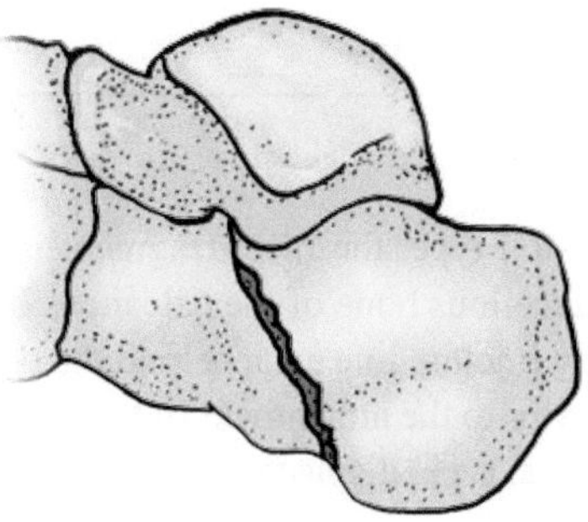

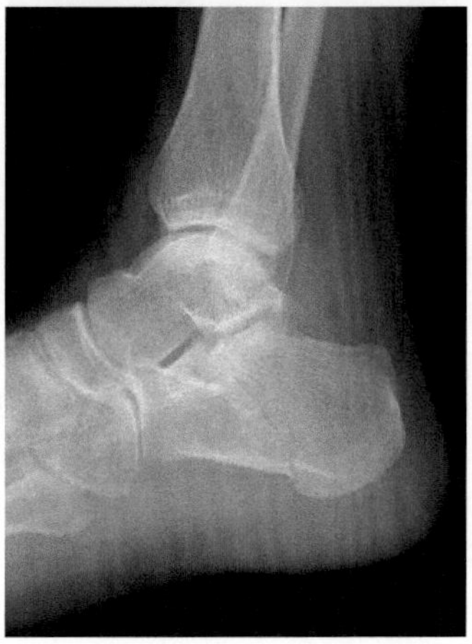

Essex-Lopresti classification

Type II: Fractures involving the subtalar joint

Type II A: Tongue-type fracture.

Type II A1: Secondary fracture line exits distal to the Achilles tendon insertion, the tongue fragment consists of superior part of calcaneal body and lateral part of posterior facet. The tongue-type fracture, the force runs through the subtalar joint, thus produces the primary fracture line

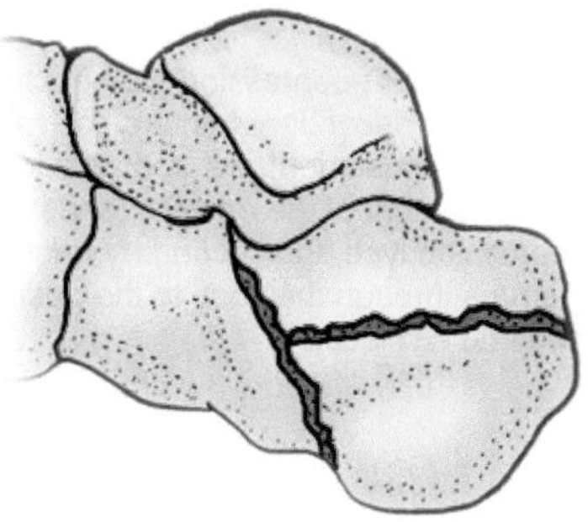

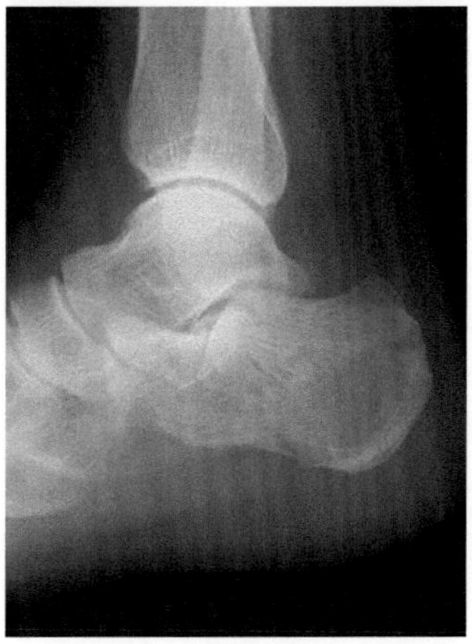

Essex-Lopresti classification

Type II: Fractures involving the subtalar joint

Type II A: Tongue-type fracture.

Type II A2: Secondary fracture line exits distal to the Achilles tendon insertion, the tongue fragment consists of superior part of calcaneal body and lateral part of posterior facet. The tongue-type fracture, the secondary fracture line runs to the posterior rim of calcaneal tuberosity, no displacement

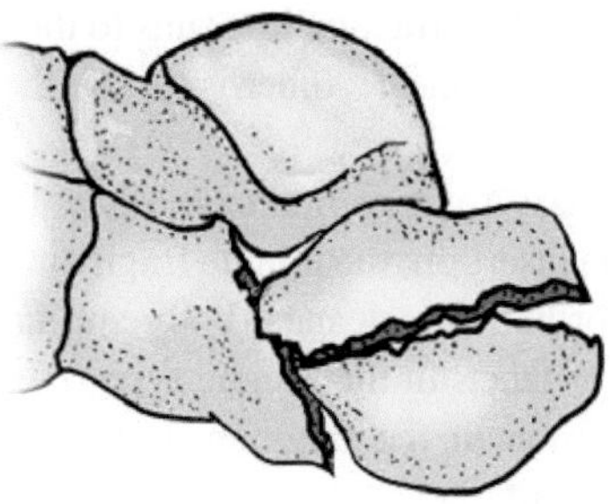

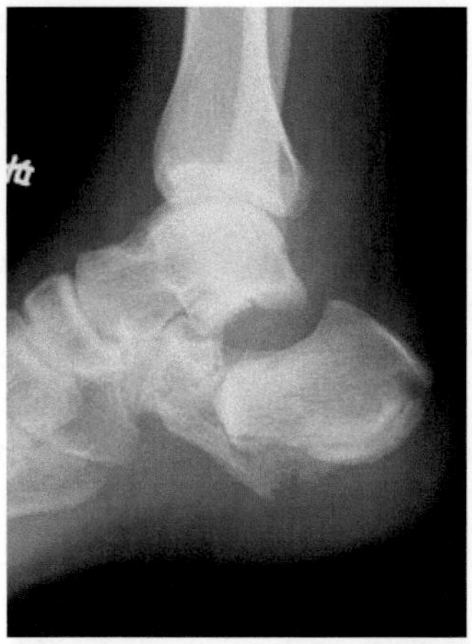

Essex-Lopresti classification

Type II: Fractures involving the subtalar joint
Type II A: Tongue-type fracture.
Type II A3: Secondary fracture line exits distal to the Achilles tendon insertion, the tongue fragment consists of superior part of calcaneal body and lateral part of posterior facet. The tongue-type fracture, the anterior portion of the fragment falls into the cancellous bone of the calcaneus body, the rear upturned, displaced

Type IIB: Joint depression-type fracture.

Type IIB1: Secondary fracture line exits behind the posterior facet and anterior to the attachment of the Achilles tendon. In depression type, the secondary fracture line runs through the body to the posterior facet, with no displacement.

Type IIB2: Secondary fracture line exits behind the posterior facet and anterior to the attachment of the Achilles tendon. In depression type, the facet fragment is displaced into the cancellous bone of the calcaneus body.

Type IIB3: Secondary fracture line exits behind the posterior facet and anterior to the attachment of the Achilles tendon. In depression type, displacement from the primary fracture line.

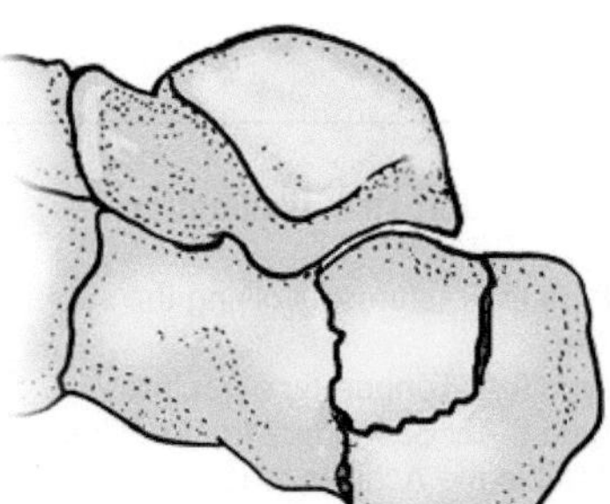

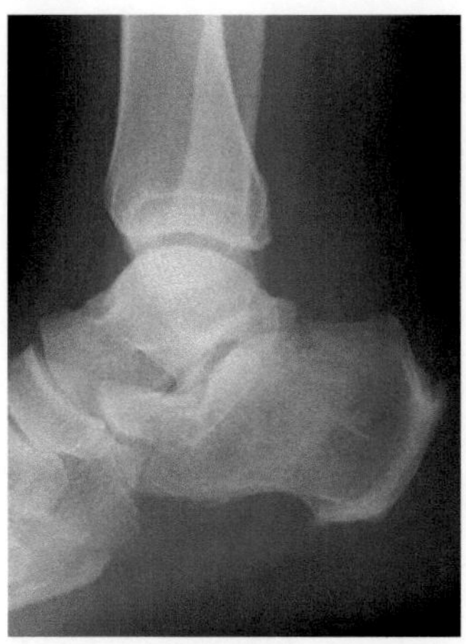

Essex-Lopresti classification of calcaneal fracture

Type II: Fractures involving the subtalar joint.
Type II B: Joint-depression-type fracture.
Type II B1: Secondary fracture line exits behind the posterior facet and anterior to the attachment of the Achilles tendon. Depression type, the secondary fracture line runs through the body to the posterior facet, no displaced

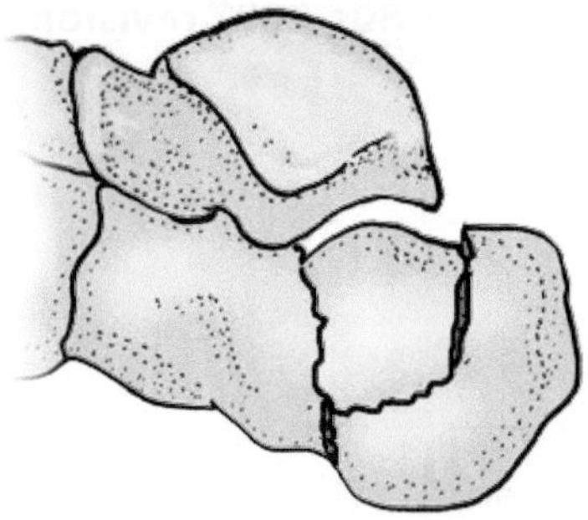

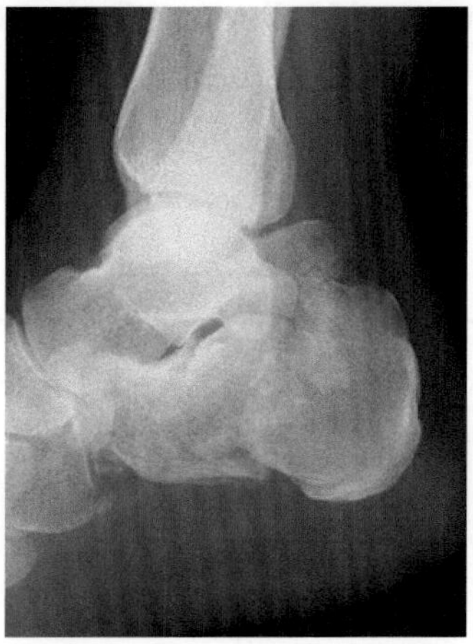

Essex-Lopresti classification of calcaneal fracture

Type II: Fractures involving the subtalar joint.
Type II B: Joint-depression-type fracture.
Type II B2: Secondary fracture line exits behind the posterior facet and anterior to the attachment of the Achilles tendon. Depression type, the facet fragment displaced into the cancellous bone of the calcaneus body

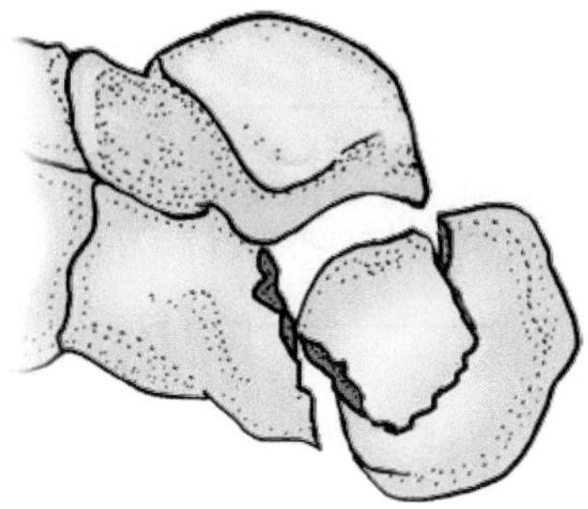

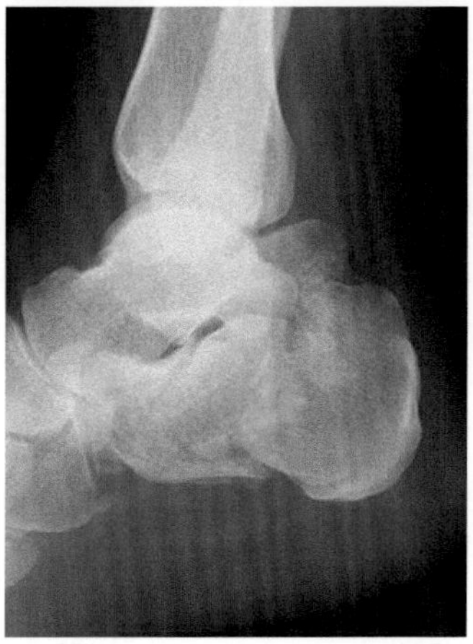

Essex-Lopresti classification of calcaneal fracture

Type II: Fractures involving the subtalar joint.
Type II B: Joint-depression-type fracture.
Type II B3: Secondary fracture line exits behind the posterior facet and anterior to the attachment of the Achilles tendon. Depression type, displaced from the primary fracture line

11.2.3 AO/OTA Classification (2007, Journal of Orthopaedic Trauma. 21 supplement; AO classification of long bone fracture of Muller was first put forward in the 80s, 2007 revision)

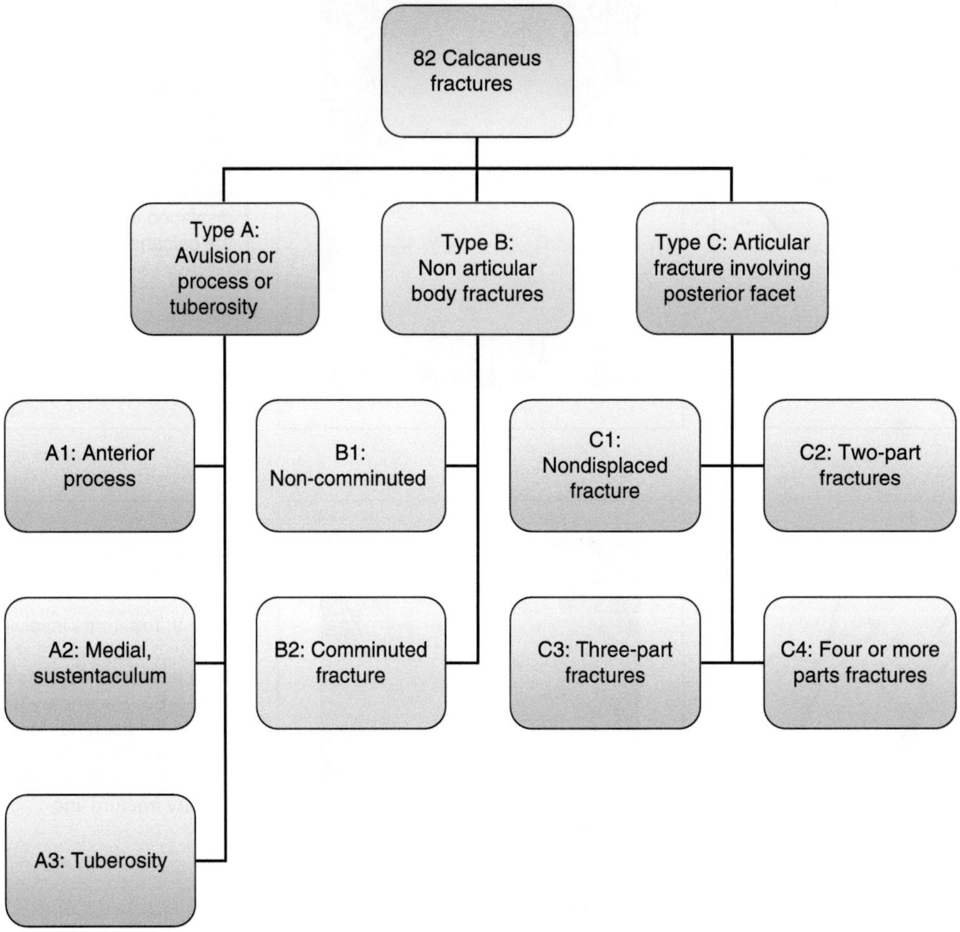

Type A: Avulsion or process or tuberosity fractures:
- Type A1: Anterior process:
  - Type A1.1: Non-comminuted fractures.
  - Type A1.2: Comminuted fractures.
- Type A2: Medial, sustentaculum tali:
  - Type A2.1: Non-comminuted fractures.
  - Type A2.2: Comminuted fractures.
- Type A3: Tuberosity:
  - Type A3.1: Non-comminuted fractures.
  - Type A3.2: Comminuted fractures.

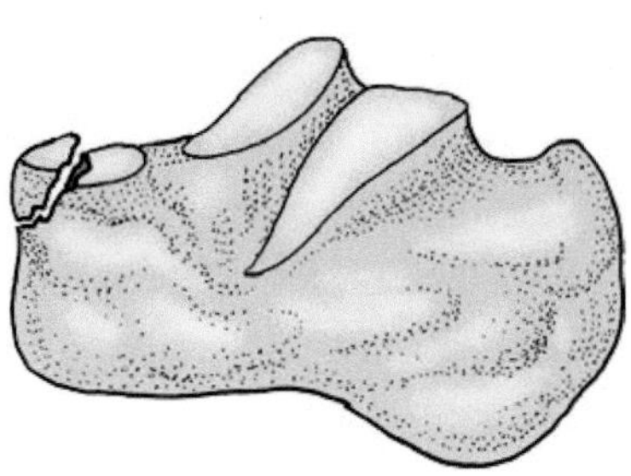

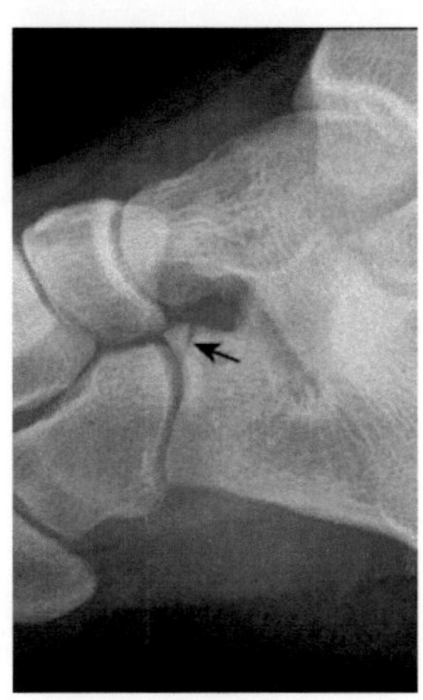

82 AO/OTA classification of calcaneal fractures

Type A: Avulsion or process or tuberosity fractures.
A1: Anterior process.
A1.1: Non-comminuted fracture

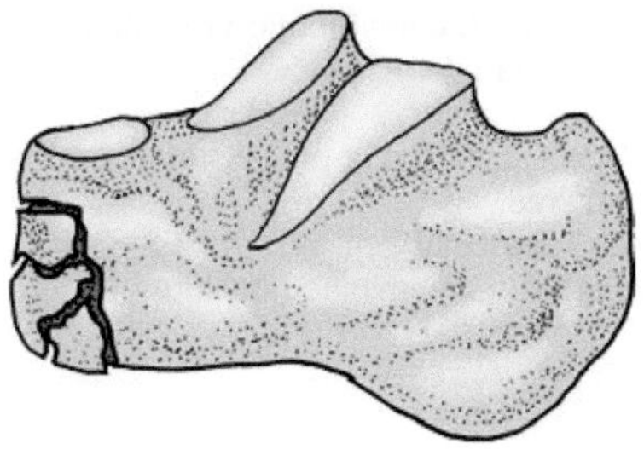

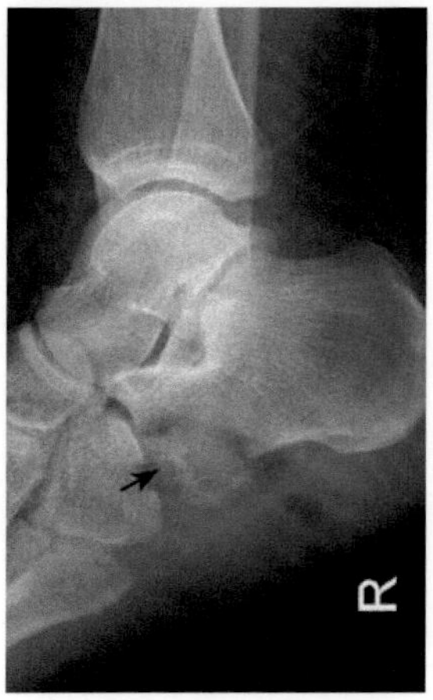

82 AO/OTA classification of calcaneal fractures

Type A: Avulsion or process or tuberosity fractures.
A1: Anterior process.
A1.1: Comminuted fractures

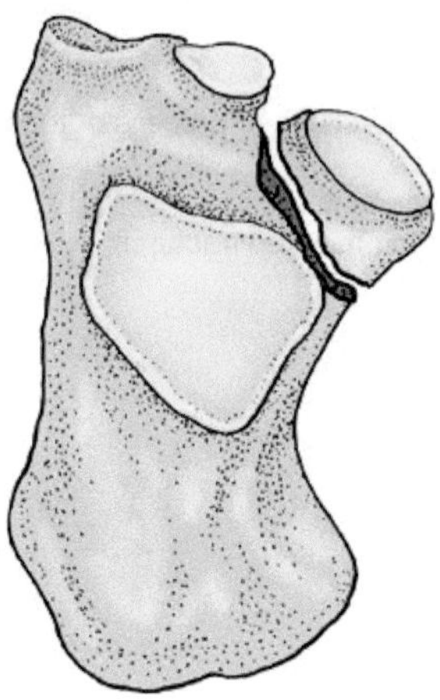

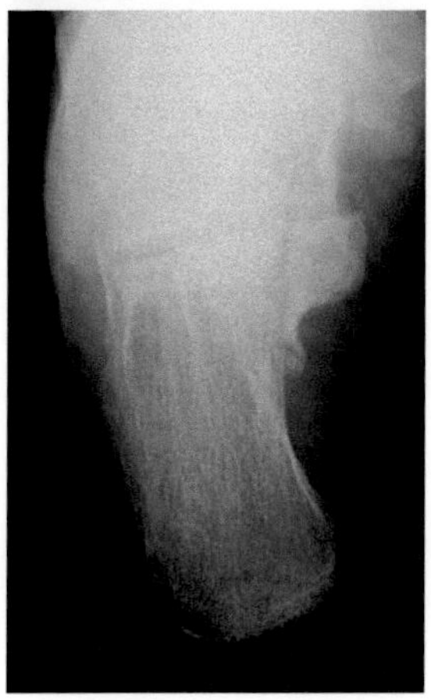

82 AO/OTA classification of calcaneal fractures

Type A: Avulsion or process or tuberosity fractures.
A2: Medial, sustentaculum tali.
A2.1: Non-comminuted fractures

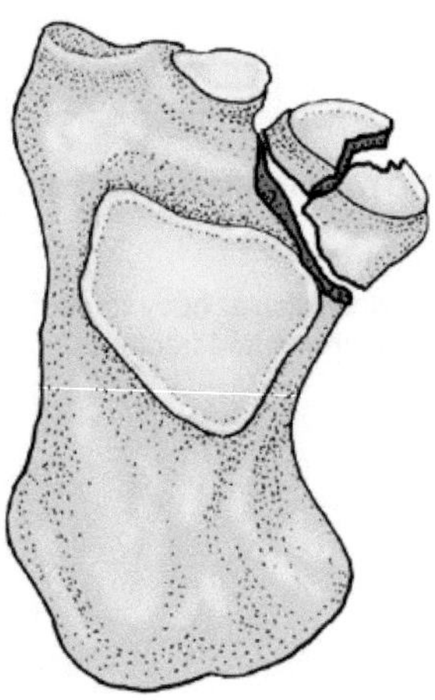

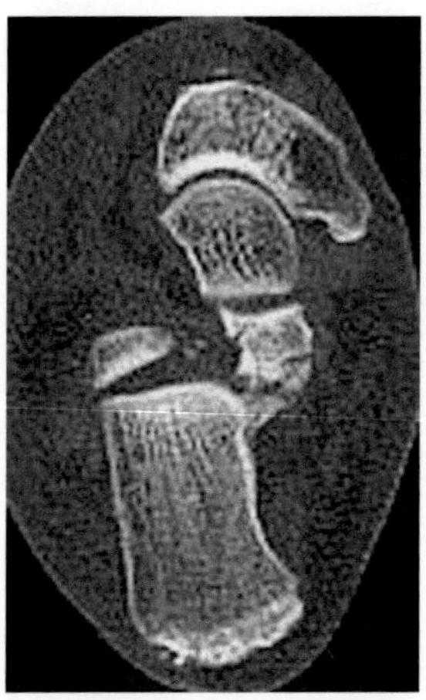

82 AO/OTA classification of calcaneal fractures

Type A: Avulsion or process or tuberosity fractures.
A2: Medial, sustentaculum tali.
A2.2: Comminuted fractures

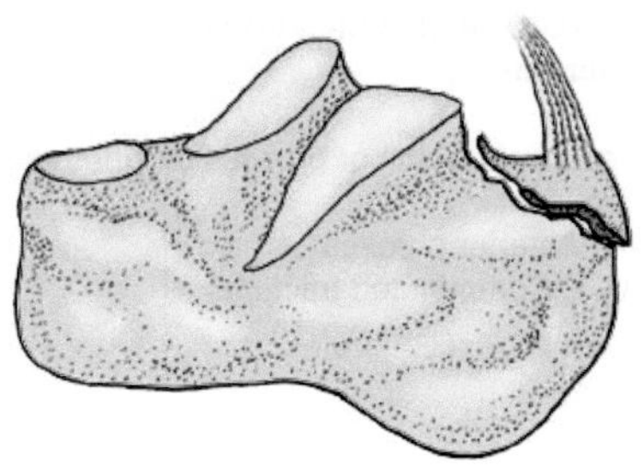

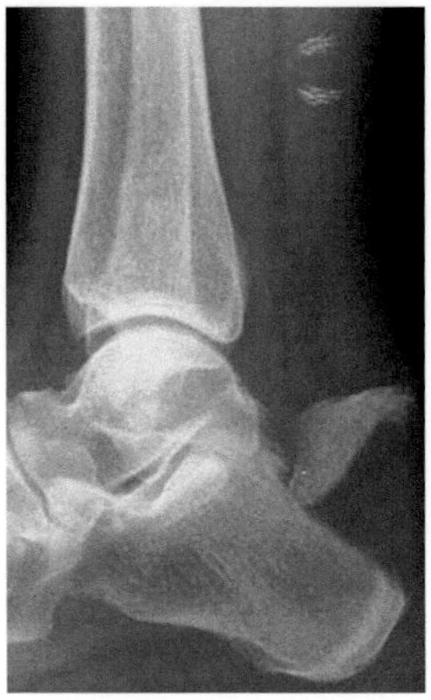

82 AO/OTA classification of calcaneal fractures

Type A: avulsion or process or tuberosity fractures.
A3: Tuberosity.
A3.1; Non-comminuted fractures

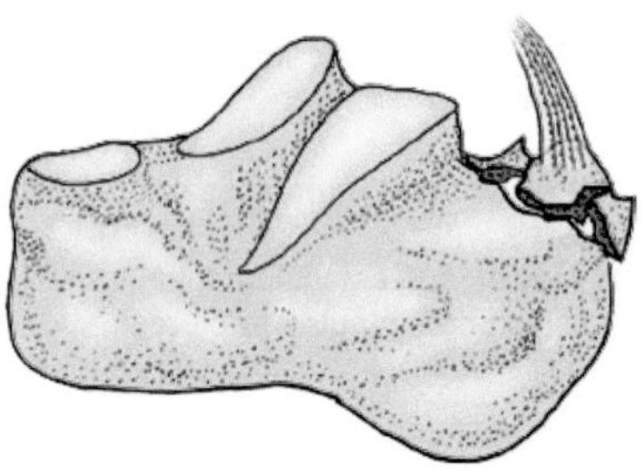

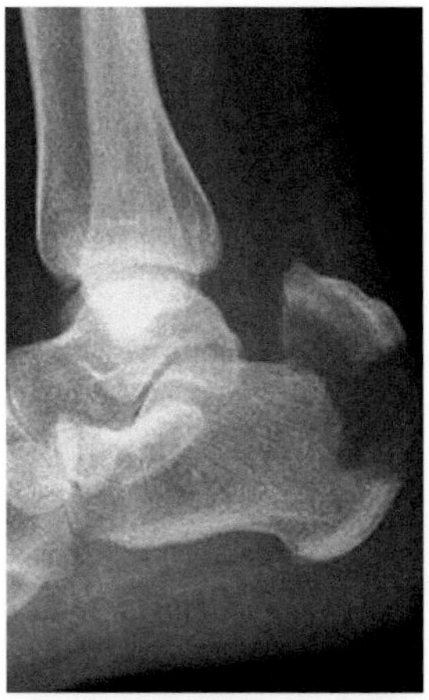

82 AO/OTA classification of calcaneal fractures

Type A: Avulsion or process or tuberosity fractures.
A3: Tuberosity.
A3.2: Comminuted fractures

Type B: Non-articular body fractures:
Type B1: Non-comminuted fractures.
Type B2: Comminuted fractures.

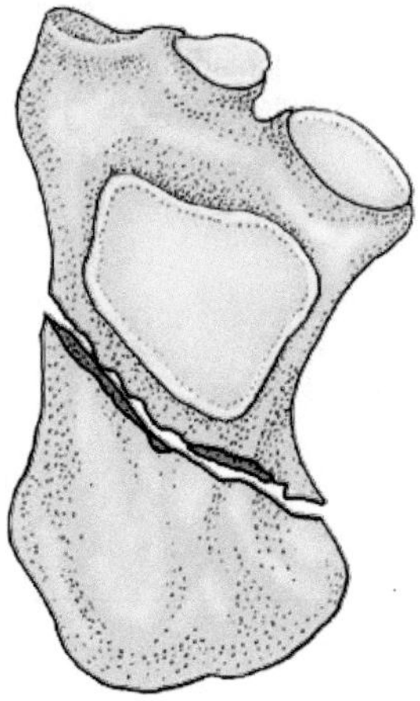

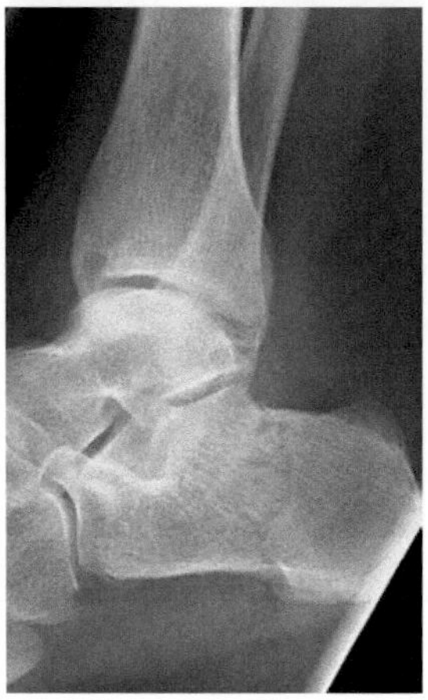

82 AO/OTA classification of calcaneal fractures

Type B: Nonarticular body fractures.
B1: Non-comminuted fractures

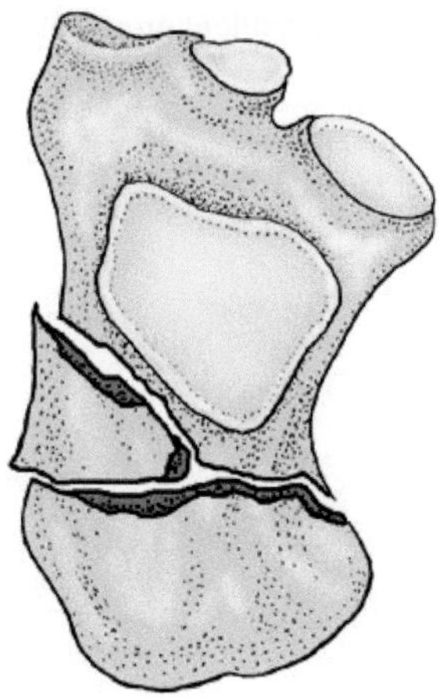

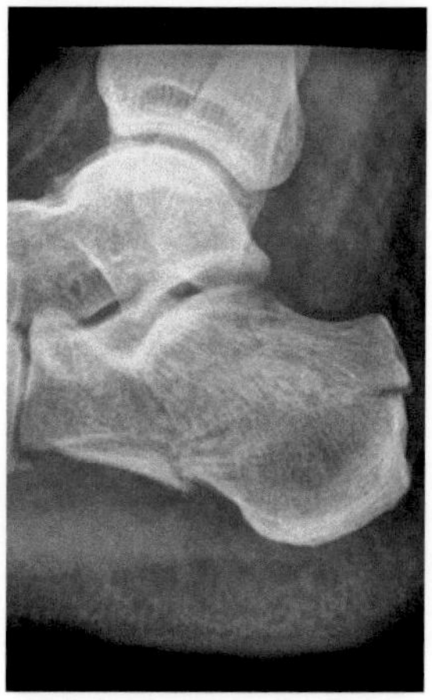

82 AO/OTA classification of calcaneal fractures

Type B: Nonarticular body fractures.
B2: Comminuted fractures

Type C: Articular fracture involving posterior facet:

- C1: Non-displaced fractures.
- C2: Two-part fractures.
- C3: Three-part fractures.
- C4: Four or more parts fractures.

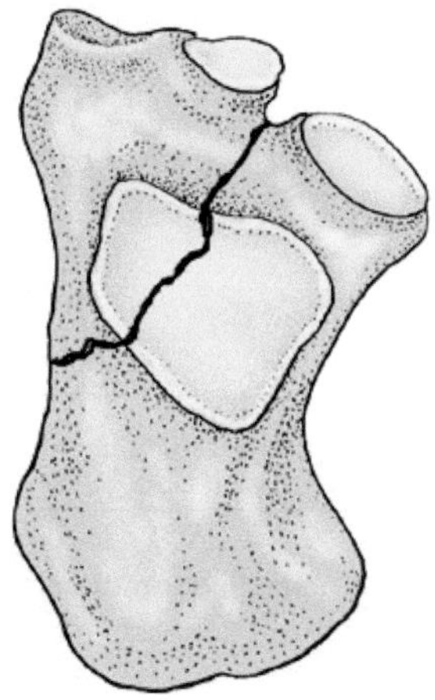

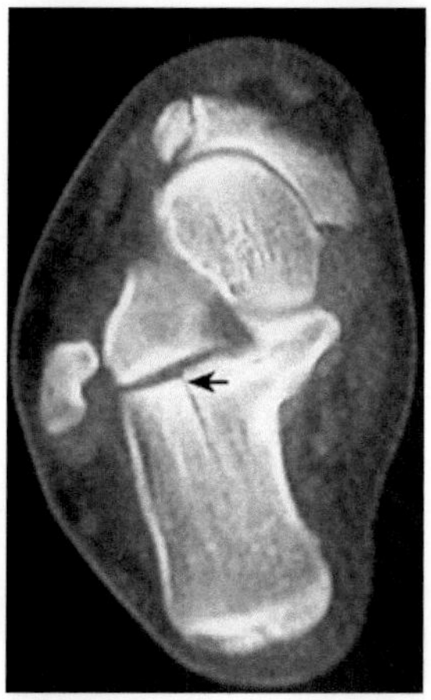

82 AO/OTA classification of calcaneal fractures

Type C: Articular fracture involving posterior facet.
C1: Nondisplaced fractures

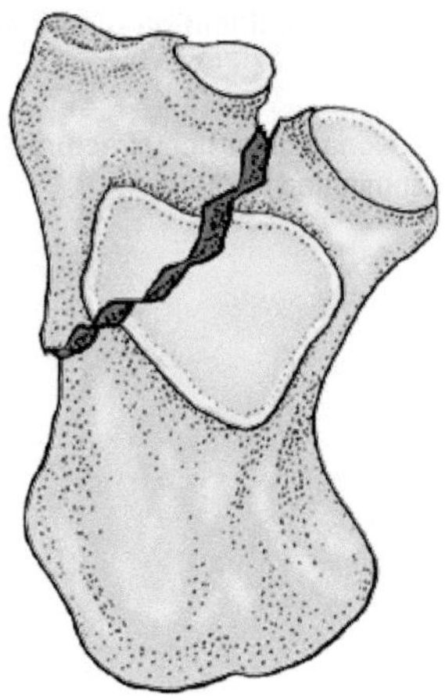

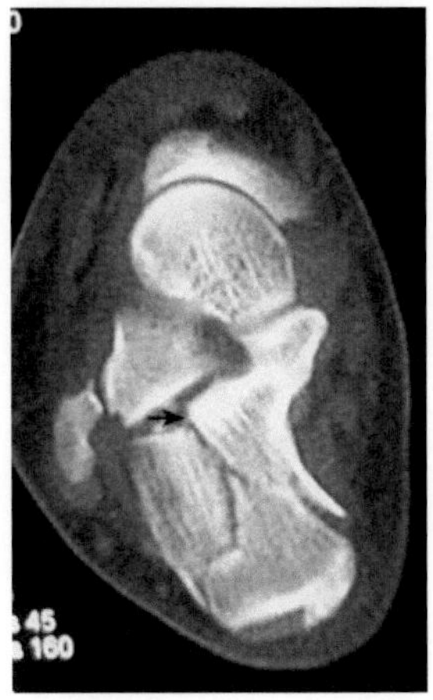

82 AO/OTA classification of calcaneal fractures

Type C: Articular fracture involving posterior facet.
C2: Two-part fractures

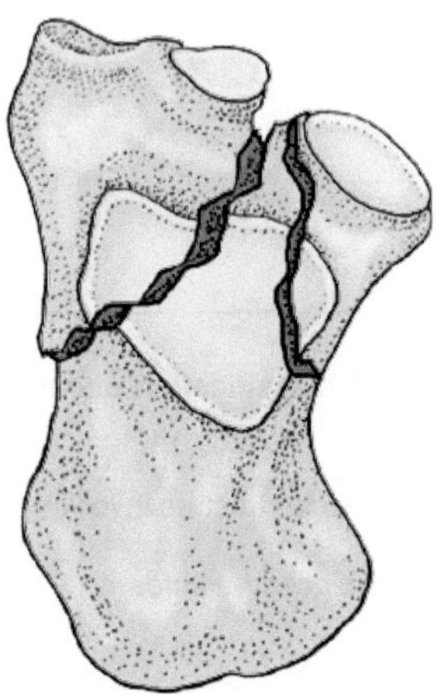

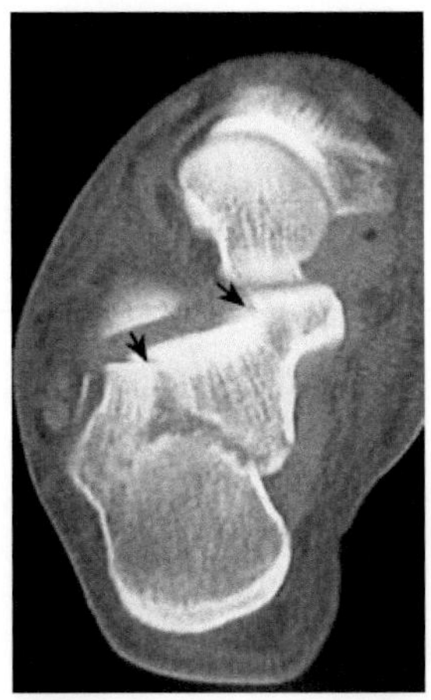

82 AO/OTA classification of calcaneal fractures

Type C: articular fracture involving posterior facet.
C3: three-part fractures

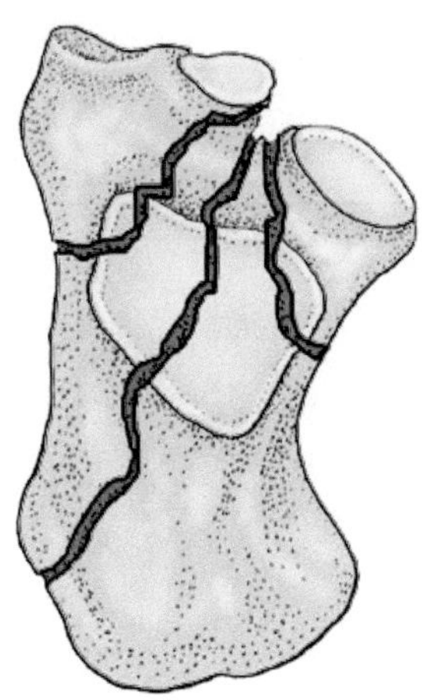

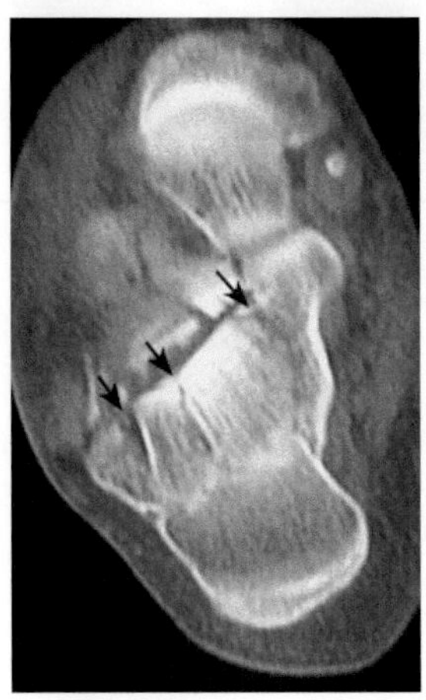

82 AO/OTA classification of calcaneal fractures

Type C: Articular fracture involving posterior facet.
C4: Four or more parts fractures

11.2.4 Intra-articular Calcaneal Fractures Classification

11.2.4.1 Soeur-Remy Classification (1975, J Bone Joint Surg [Br], 57:413–421)

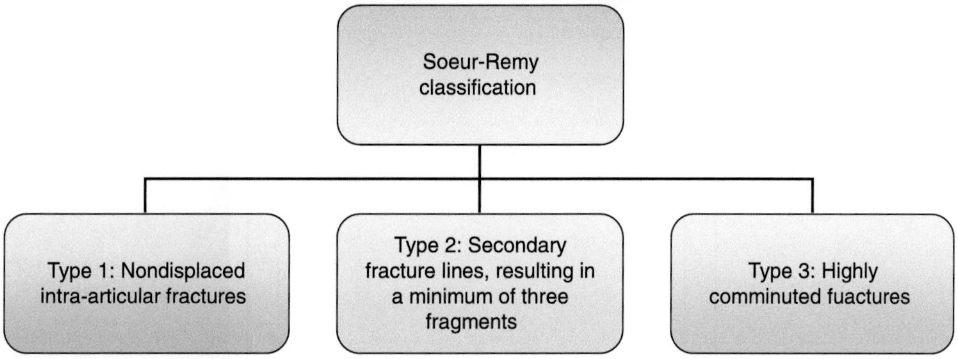

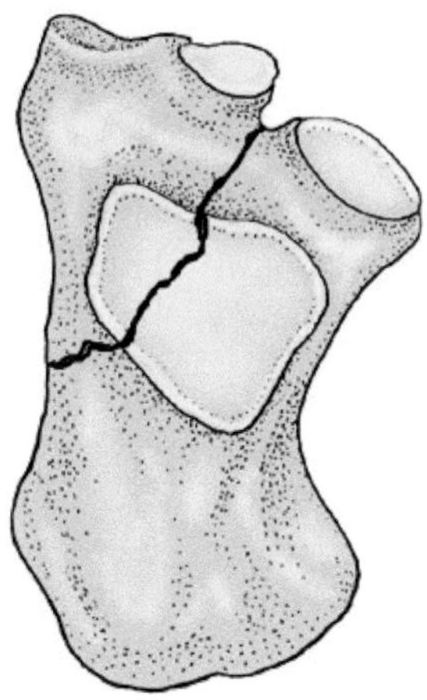

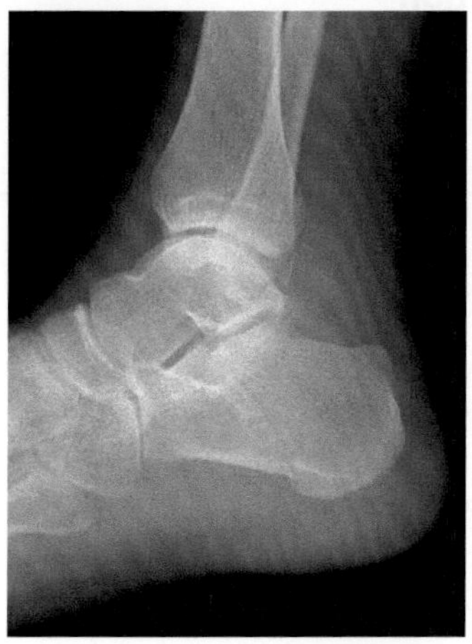

Soeur-Remy classification of calcaneal fractures

Type1: Nondisplaced intra-articular fractures

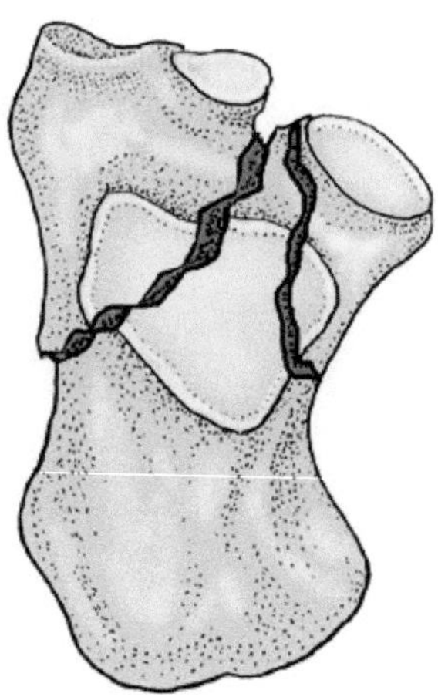

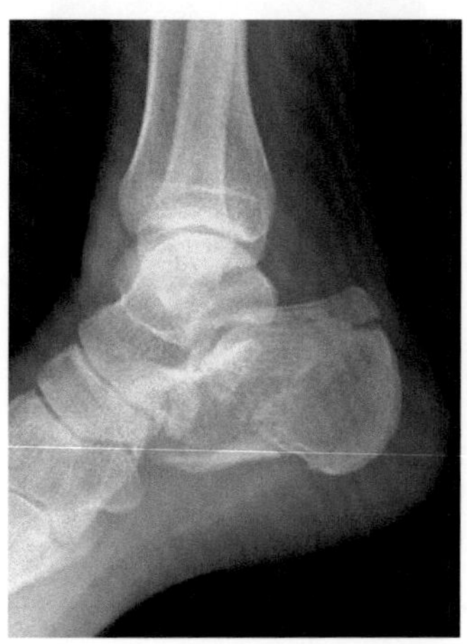

Sour-Remy classification of calcaneal fractures

Type 2: Secondary fracture lines, resulting in a minimum of three fragments

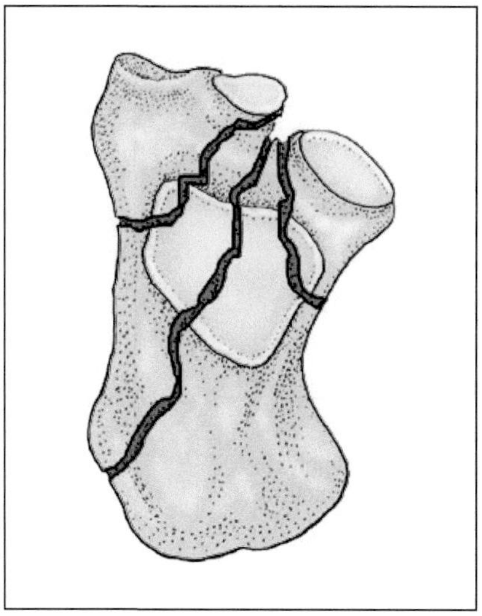

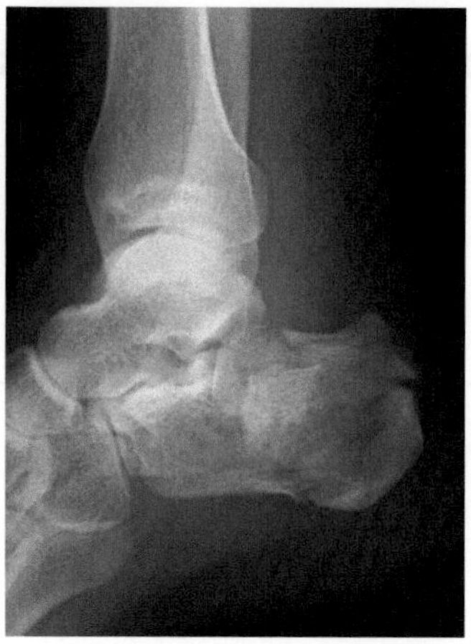

Sour-Remy classification of calcaneal fractures

Type 3: Highly comminuted fractures

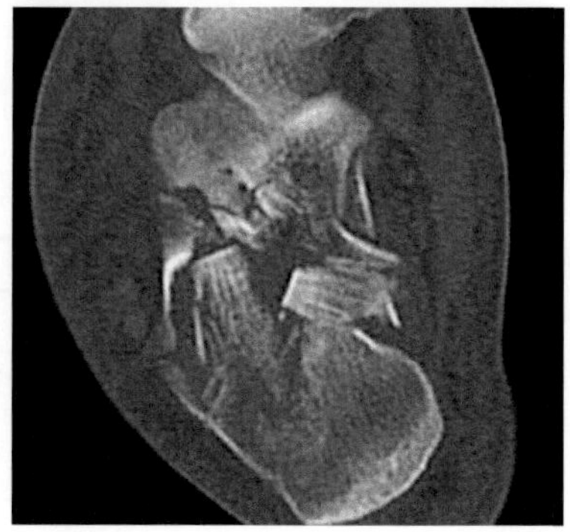

11.2.4.2 Crosby-Fitzgibbons Classification

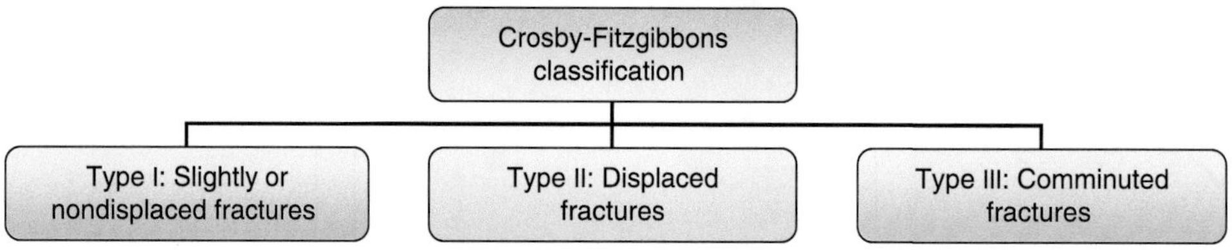

Crosby divided the fractures into three types according to CT scan:

Type I: Slightly or non-displaced posterior facet fractures.
Type II: Displaced posterior facet fractures.
Type III: Comminuted posterior facet fracture.

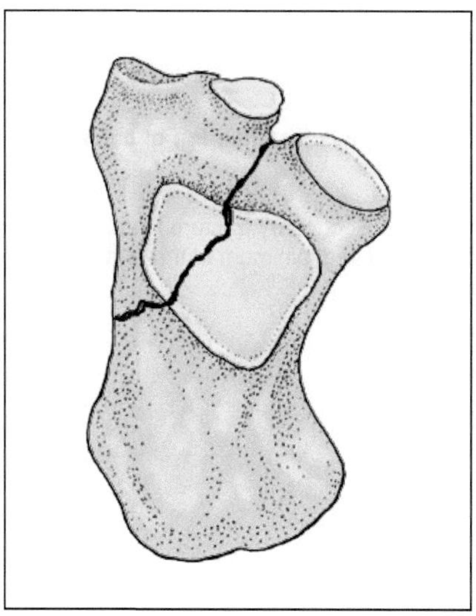

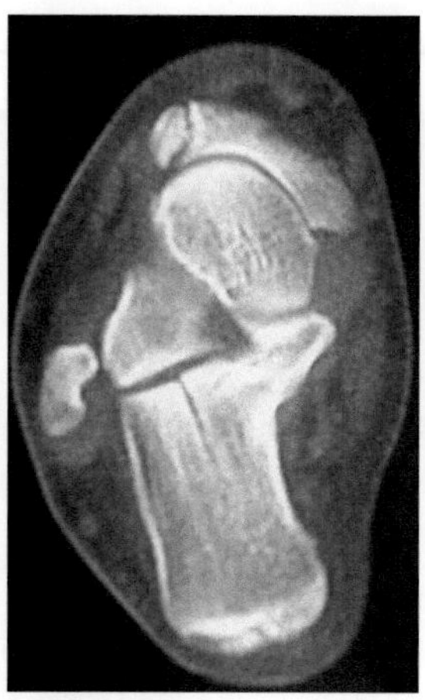

Crosby-Fitzgibbons classification of intra-articular calcaneal fractures

Type I: Slightly or nondisplaced posterior facet fractures

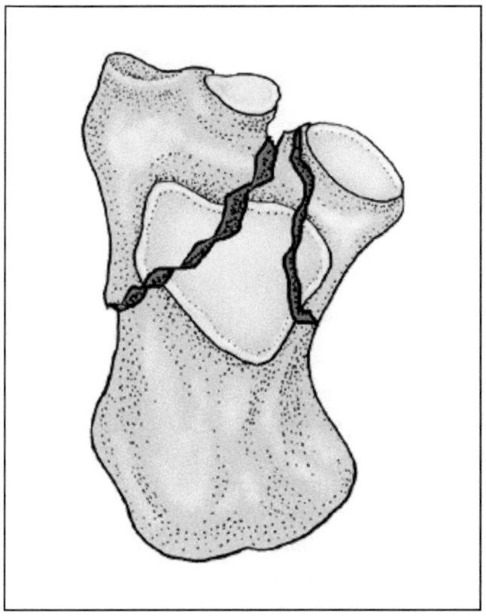

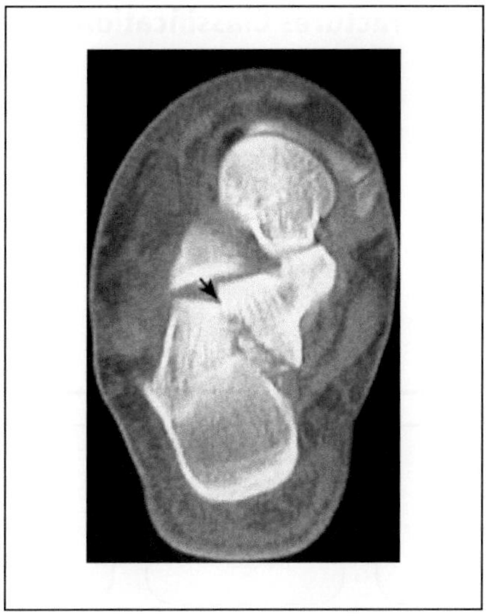

Crosby-Fitzgibbons classification of intra-articular calcaneal fractures

Type II: displaced posterior facet fractures

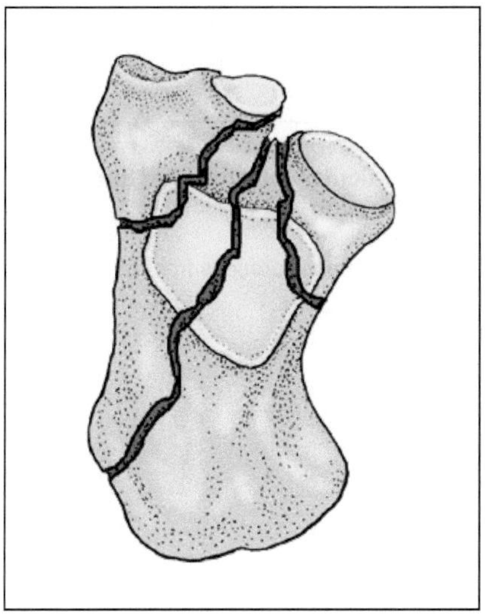

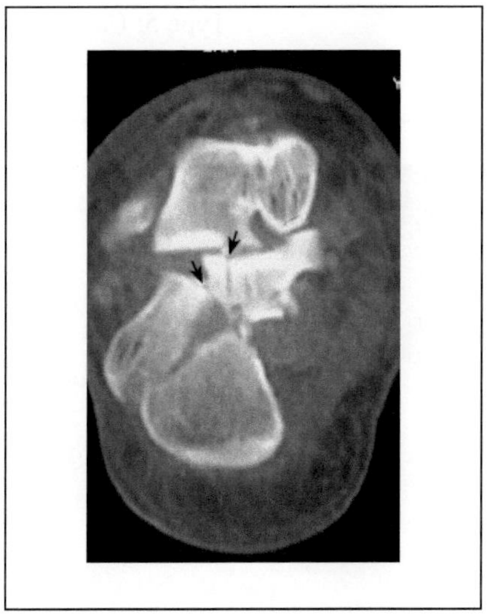

Crosby-Fitzgibbons classification of intra-articular calcaneal fractures

Type III: comminuted posterior facet fracture

11.2.4.3 Stephenson-Paley Classification (1993, J Bone Joint Surg [Am], 75:342–354)

Type A: Two parts of non-displaced shearing fractures.

Type B:
- Type B1: Tongue-type fractures.
- Type B2: Comminuted tongue-type fractures.

Type C:
- Type C1: Intra-articular depression fractures.
- Type C2: Comminuted intra-articular depression fractures.

Type D: Comprehensive intra-articular depression fractures.

11.2.4.4 Rowe Classification (1963, J Am Med Assoc, 194:920–923)

Rowe et al. combined Warrick Bremner (1953 years) and Watson Jones (1955 years) opinions, and divided calcaneal fractures into five types:

Type I:
- Type IA: Calcaneal tuberosity fractures.
- Type IB: Calcaneal sustentaculum tali fractures.
- Type IC: Calcaneal posterior tuberosity fractures.

Type II:
- Type IIA: Beak-shape fractures:
- Type IIB: Avulsion fractures of Achilles tendon insertion.

Type III: Wedge fractures, subtalar joint uninvolved.

Type IV: Fractures involving subtalar joint.

Type V: Comminuted central depression fractures.

11.2.5 Other Extra-Articular Calcaneal Fractures Classification

11.2.5.1 Anatomical Site Classification

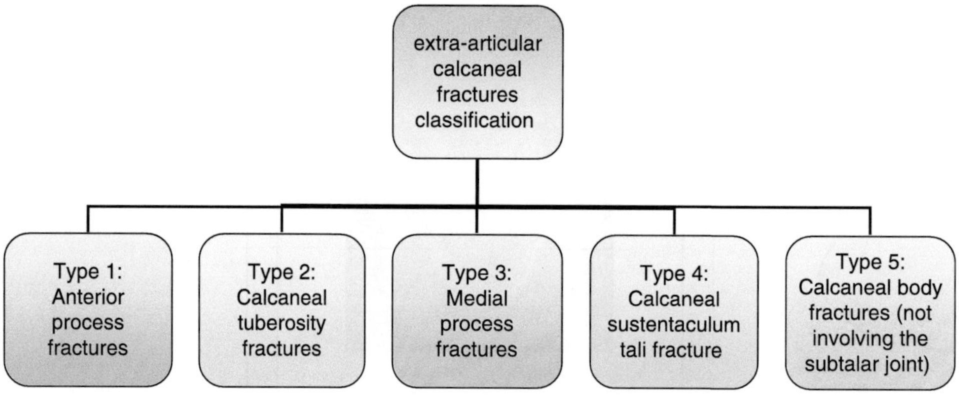

Type 1: Anterior process fractures.
Type 2: Calcaneal tuberosity fractures.
Type 3: Medial process fractures.
Type 4: Calcaneal sustentaculum tali fractures.
Type 5: Calcaneal body fractures (not involving the subtalar joint).

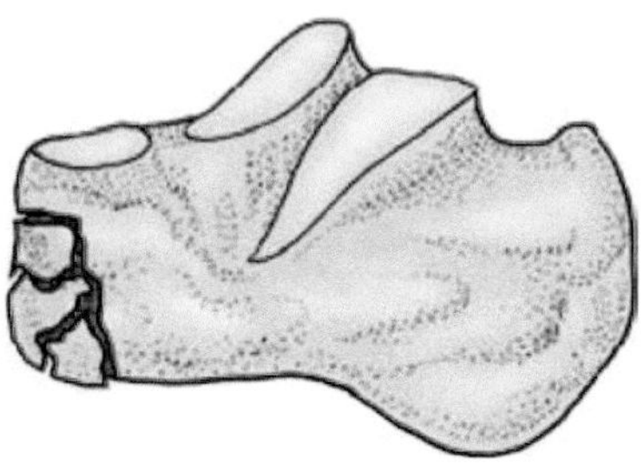

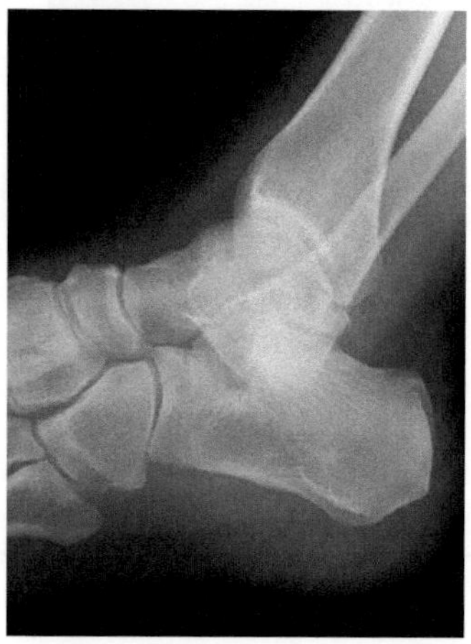

extra-articular calcaneal fractures classification

Type 1: Anterior process fractures

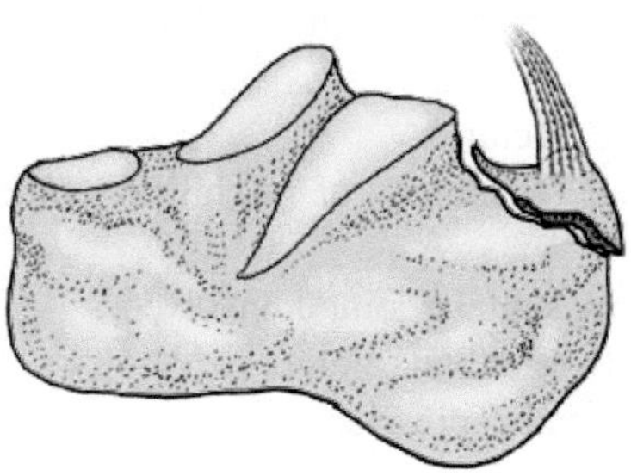

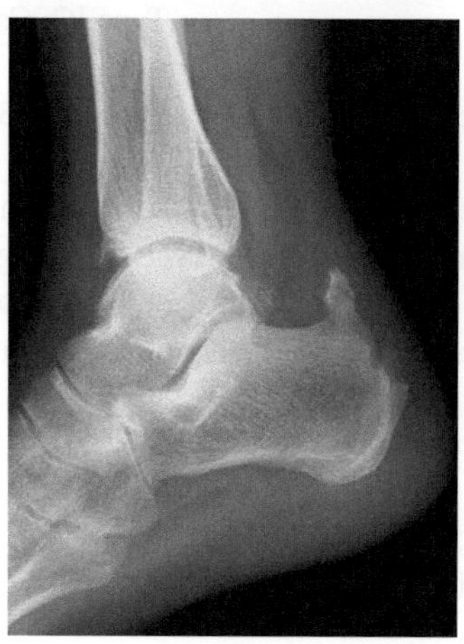

extra-articular calcaneal fractures classification

Type 2: Calcaneal tuberosity fractures

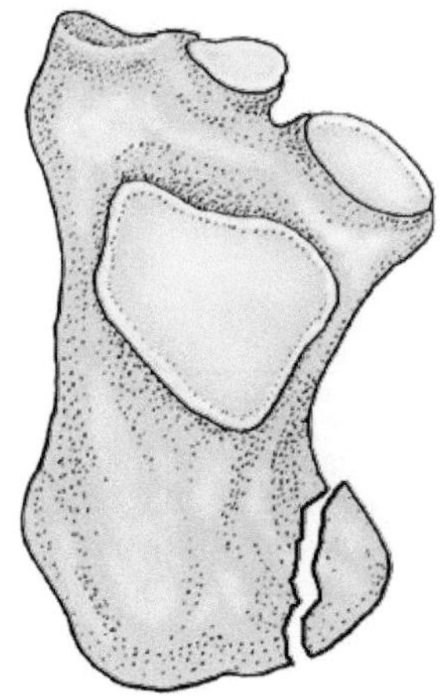

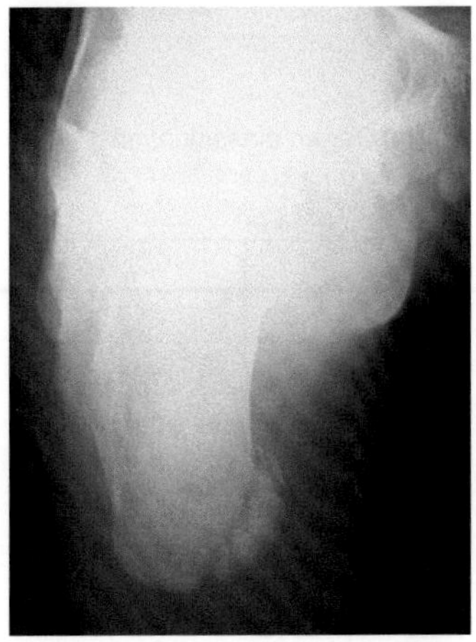

extra-articular calcaneal fractures classification

Type 3: Medial process fractures

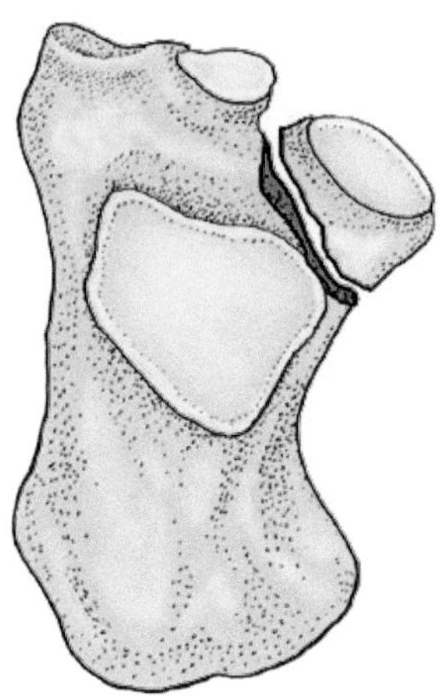

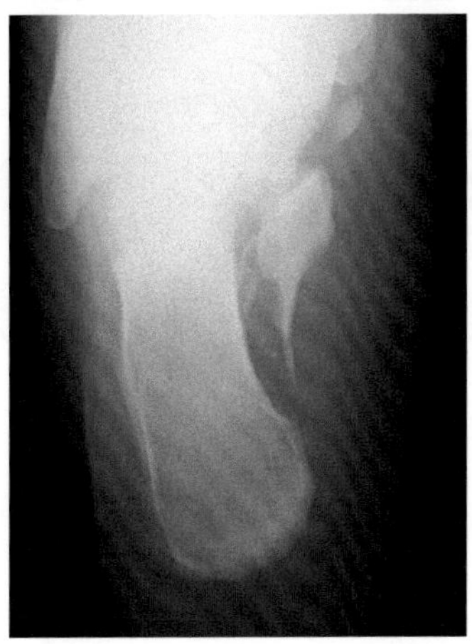

extra-articular calcaneal fractures classification

Type 4: Calcaneal sustentaculum tali fractures

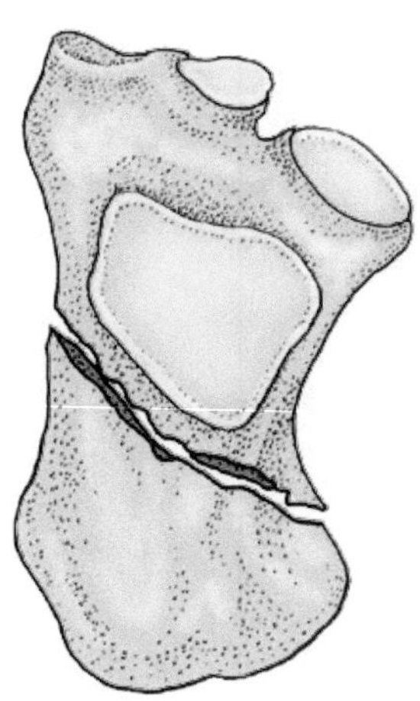

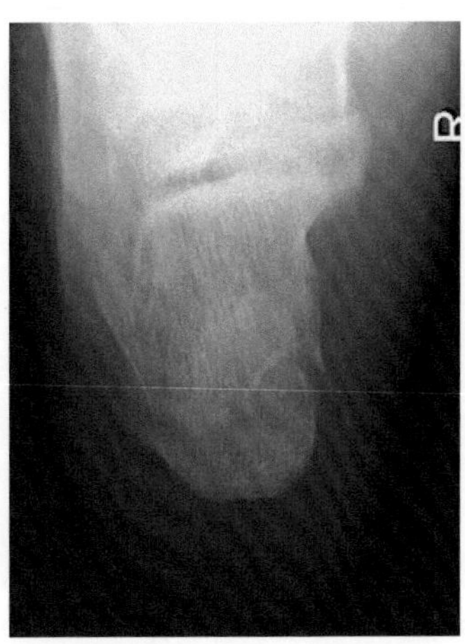

extra-articular calcaneal fractures classification

Type 5: Calcaneal body fractures (not involving the subtalar joint)

11.2.5.2 Degan Classification of Calcaneus Anterior Process Fracture

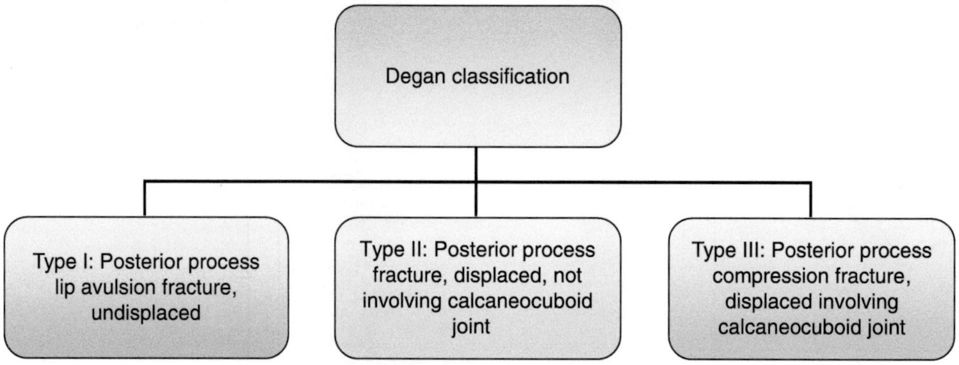

Type I: Posterior process lip avulsion fracture, non-displaced.
Type II: Posterior process avulsion fracture, displaced, not involving calcaneocuboid joint.
Type III: Posterior process compression fracture, displaced, involving calcaneocuboid joint.

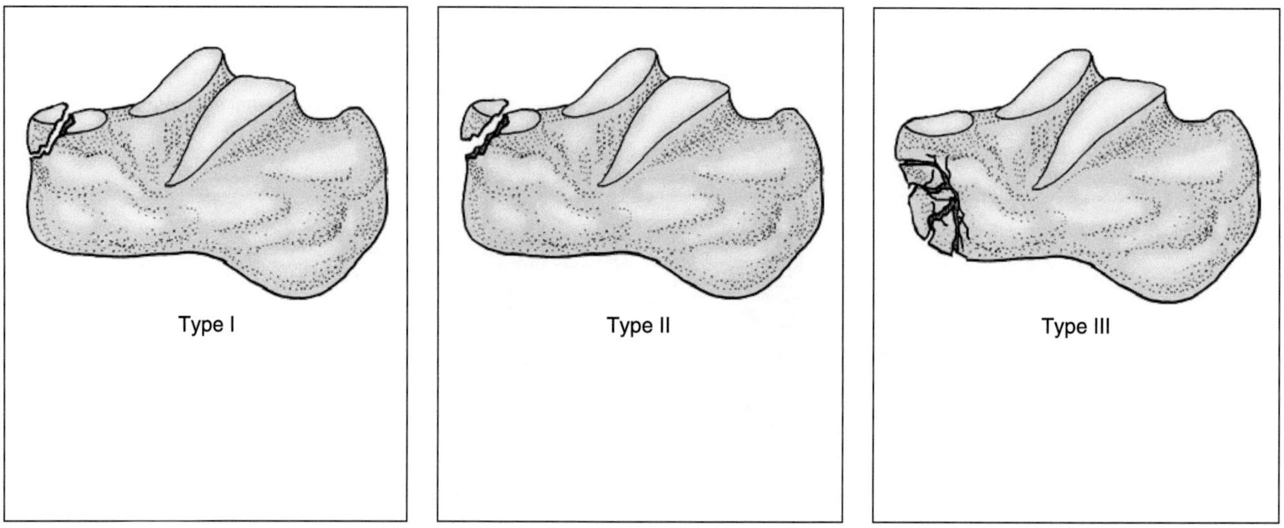

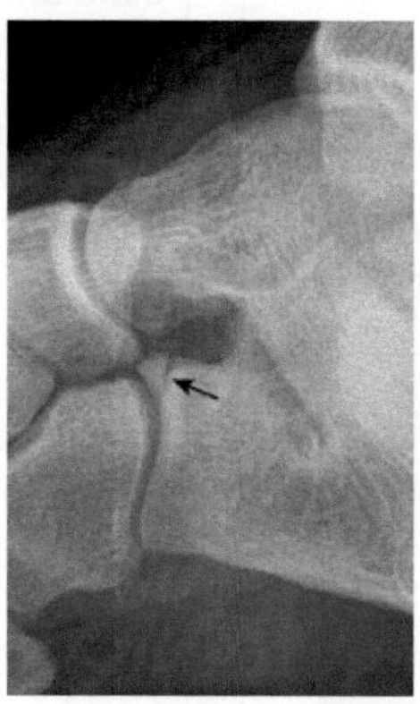

Type I: Posterior process lip avulsion fracture, undisplaced

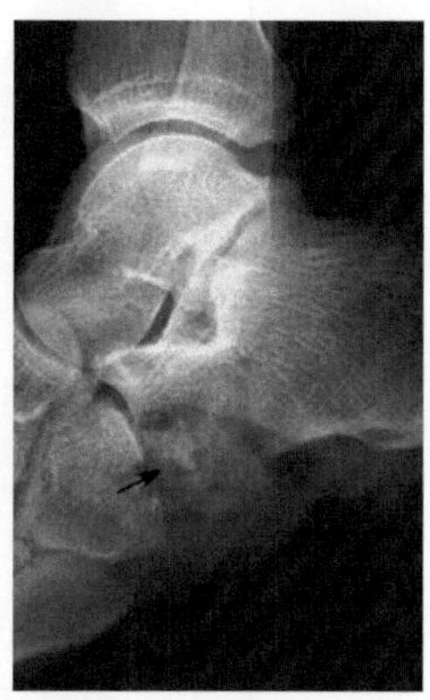

Type III: Posterior process compression fracture, displaced, involving calcaneocuboid joint

11.2.5.3 Extra-Articular Fracture Mixed Classification (2008, Arch Orthop Trauma Surg, 128:1099–1106)

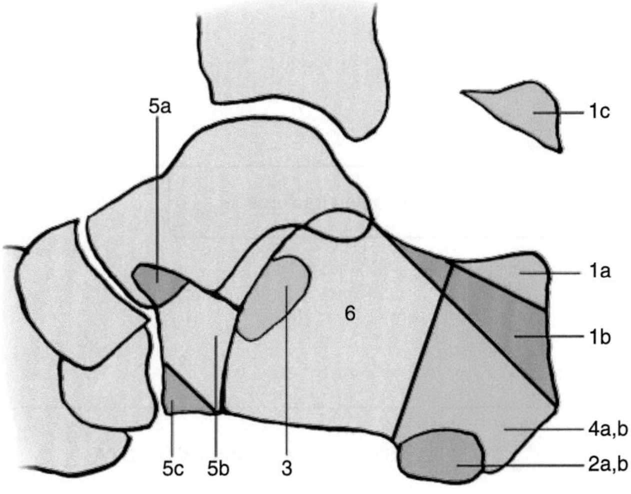

Type 1a: Beaklike fractures, non-displaced.
Type 1c: Beaklike fractures, displaced.
Type 1b: Avulsion fracture of Achilles tendon insertion.
Type 2a, 2b: Medial or lateral process fractures.
Type 3: Sustentaculum tali fractures.
Type 4a: Vertical tuberosity fractures;
Type 4b: Epiphysis avulsion fractures.
Type 5a: Anterosuperior avulsion or compression fractures.
Type 5b: Calcaneocuboid joint fractures.
Type 5c: Distal inferolateral fractures.
Type 6a: Extensor tendon avulsion fractures.
Type 6b: Plantar fascia avulsion fractures.
Type 6c: Lateral joint capsule avulsion fractures.

11.2.5.4 Yicong Wang Classification (2001, Bone and Joint Injury. 3rd ed. Peking: People's Medical Publishing House)

Type I: Anterior tuberosity fractures.
Subdivided into anterior tuberosity avulsion fractures and calcaneocuboid joint compression fractures.
Type II: Tuberosity fractures.
Subdivided into posterior calcaneal avulsion fractures and posterosuperior calcaneal beaklike fractures.
Type III: Medial or lateral process fractures.
Type IV: Sustentaculum tali fractures.
Type V: Body fractures.

11.2.6 Calcaneal Fracture of Linsenmaier Classification According to Three-Dimensional Reconstruction of CT Scan (2003, Eur Radiol, 13:2315–2322)

According to involving facet, fragment of lateral subtalar joint, and the degree of fragment displacement, calcaneal fracture was divided into six types.

Type I: Non-displaced extra-articular fractures.
Type II: Displaced extra-articular fractures.
Subdivided into heel width increasing (B), height decreasing (C,) and axial displacement of calcaneocuboid joint (D).
Type III: Non-displaced intra-articular fractures.
Type IV: Displaced intra-articular, two-part fractures of the posterior subtalar joint.
Subdivided into displaced posterior subtalar facet (A), heel width increasing (B), height decreasing (C), and axial displacement of calcaneocuboid joint (D).
Type V: Displaced intra-articular, three-part fractures of posterior subtalar joint.
Subdivided into displaced posterior subtalar facet (A), heel width increasing (B), height decreasing (C), and axial displacement of calcaneocuboid joint (D).
Type VI: Comminuted intra-articular fractures, four or more parts of the posterior subtalar joint.
Subdivided into displaced posterior subtalar facet (A), heel width increasing (B), height decreasing (C), and axial displacement of calcaneocuboid joint (D).

11.2.7 Classification of Calcaneocuboid Joint Fractures

Type I: Non-displaced facet fractures.
Type II: One fracture line in articular surface, fracture line in sagittal or transverse plane, displaced or calcaneocuboid joint subluxation.
Type III: Two fracture lines in articular surface, fracture lines in sagittal or transverse plane, displaced or calcaneocuboid joint subluxation.
Type IV: Comminuted fractures, three or more fracture lines in articular surface, displaced or calcaneocuboid joint subluxation.

11.3 Section 3 Classification of Other Tarsal Fractures

11.3.1 Classification of Navicular Fractures

11.3.1.1 AO/OTA Classification

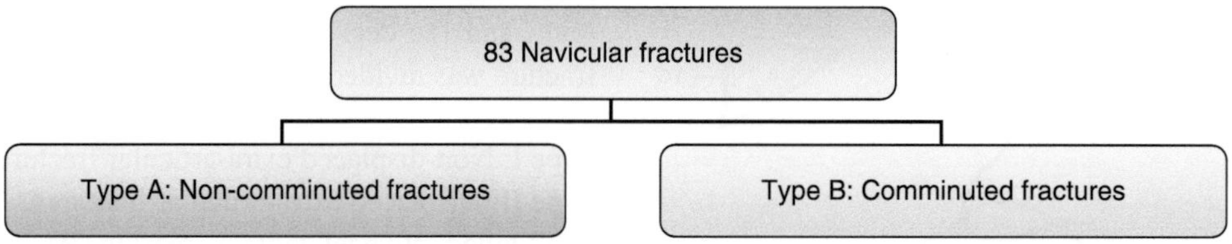

Type A: Non-comminuted fractures.
Type B: Comminuted fractures.

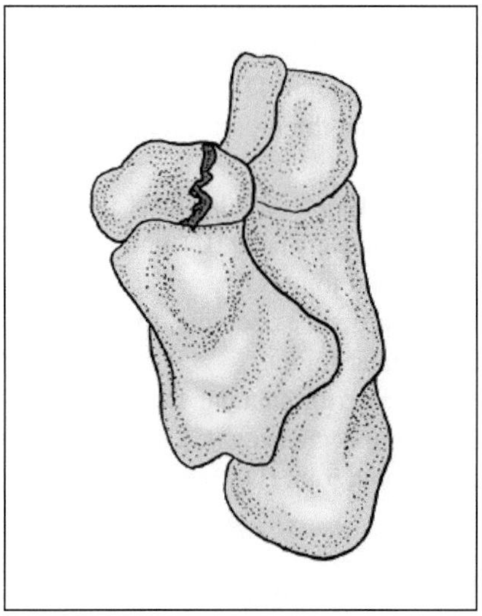

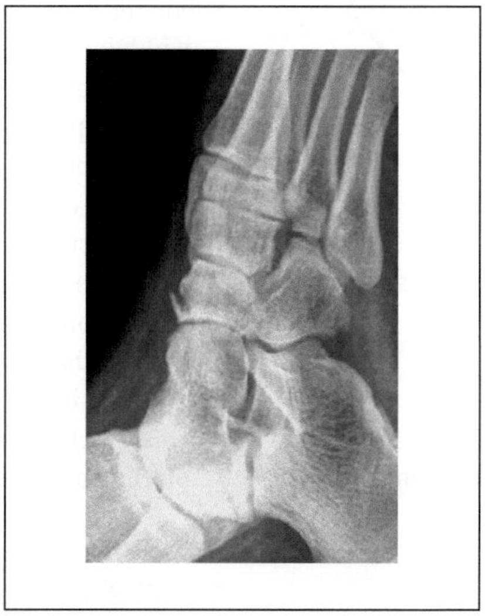

83 Navicular fractures OA/OTA classification

Type A: Non-comminuted fractures

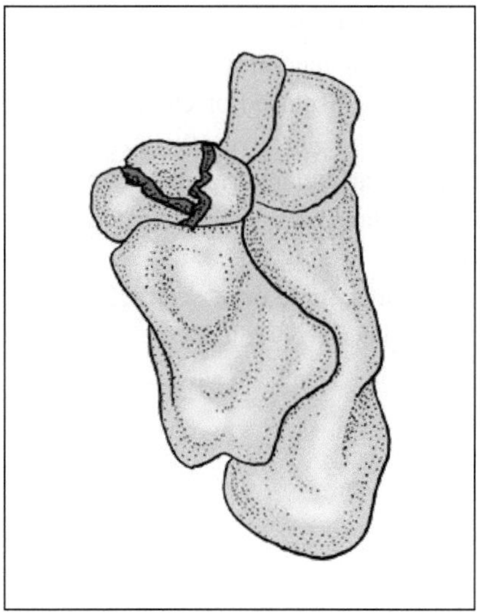

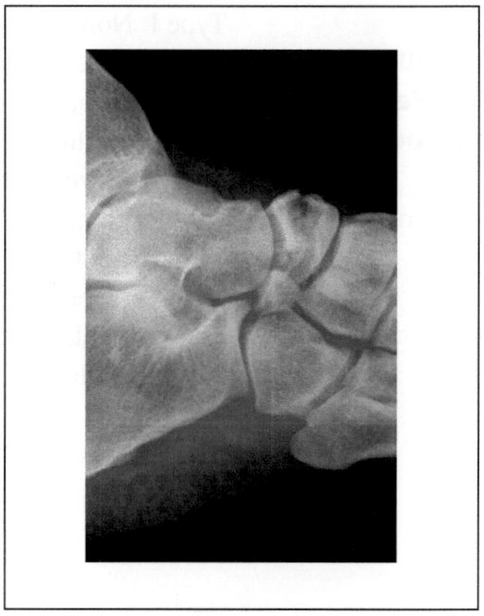

83 Navicular fractures OA/OTA classification

Type B: Comminuted fractures

11.3.1.2 Eichenholtz-Levin Classification (2006, Springer-Verlag London Limited)

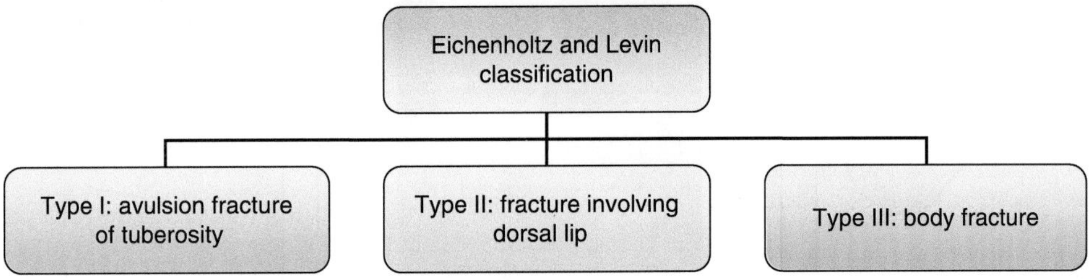

Type I: Avulsion fracture of tuberosity.
Type II: Fracture involving dorsal lip.
Type III: Body fracture.

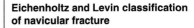

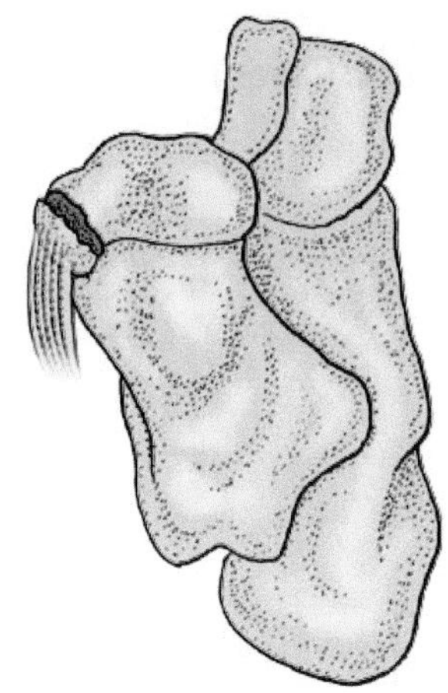

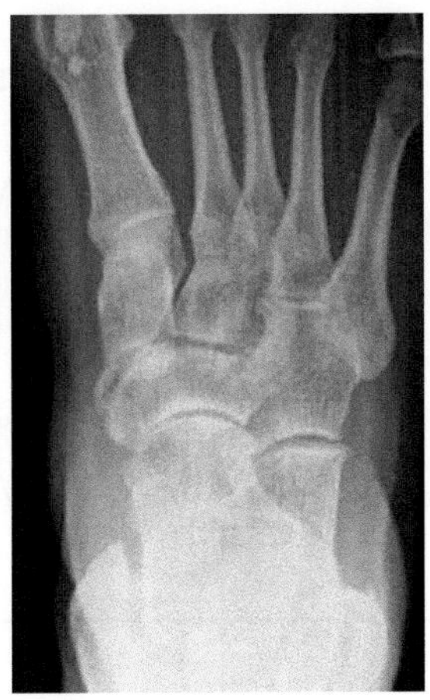

Eichenholtz and Levin classification of navicular fracture

Type I: Avulsion fracture of tuberosity

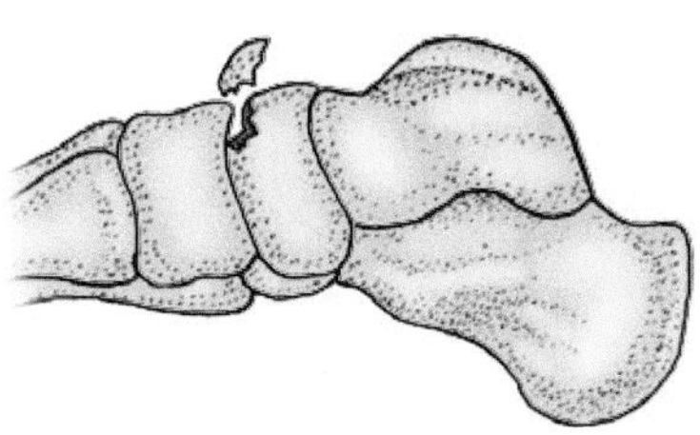

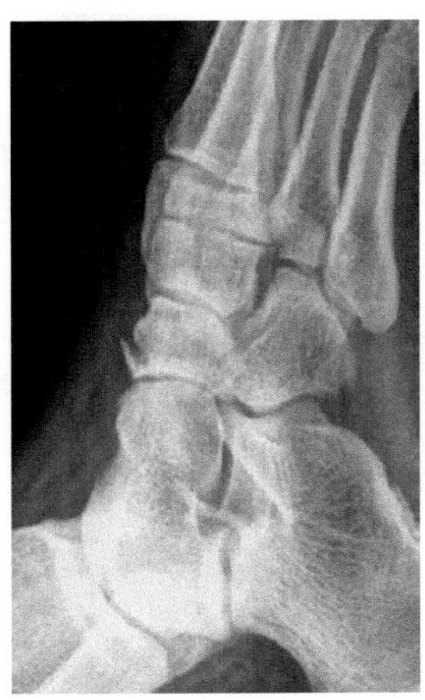

Eichenholtz and Levin classification of navicular fracture

Type II: Fracture involving dorsal lip

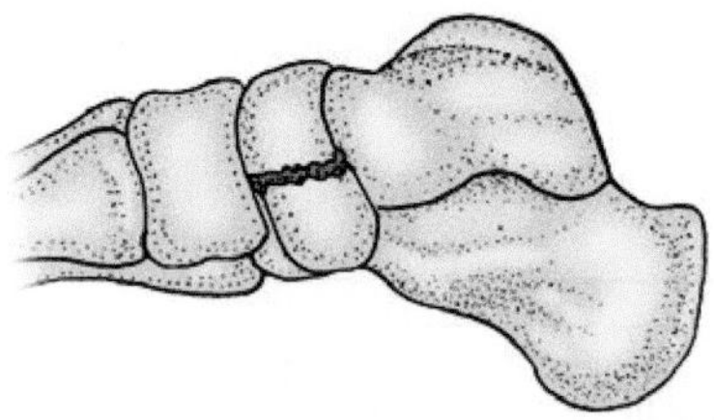

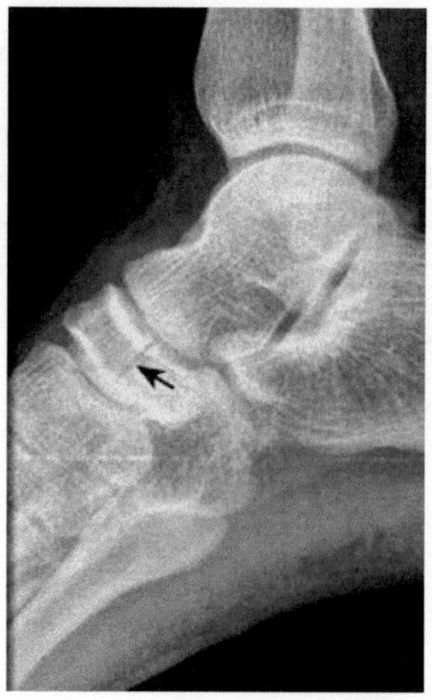

Eichenholtz and Levin classification of navicular fracture

Type III: Body fracture

11.3.1.3 Sageorzan Classification (1993, Orthopaedic Trauma Protocols. New York: Raven)

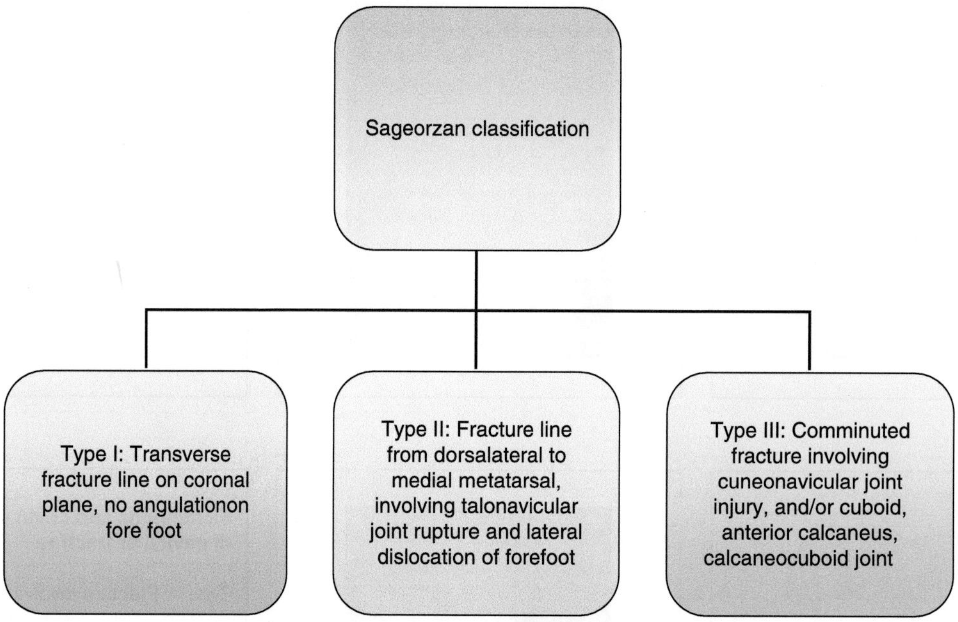

Type I: Transverse fracture line on coronal plane, no angulation of forefoot.

Type II: Fracture line from dorsolateral to medial metatarsal, involving talonavicular joint rupture and lateral dislocation of forefoot.

Type III: Comminuted fracture involving cuneonavicular joint injury, and/or cuboid, anterior calcaneus, calcaneocuboid joint fracture.

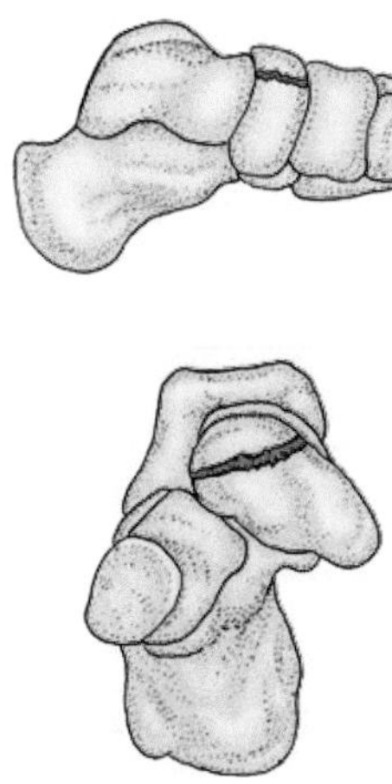

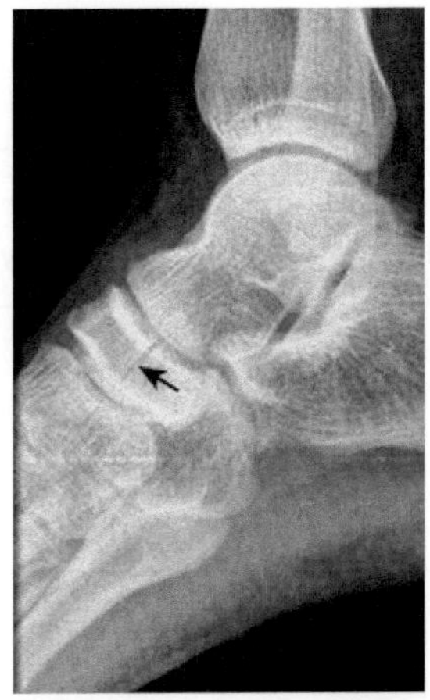

Sageorzan classification of navicular fracture

Type I: Transverse fracture line on coronal plane, no angulation of forefoot

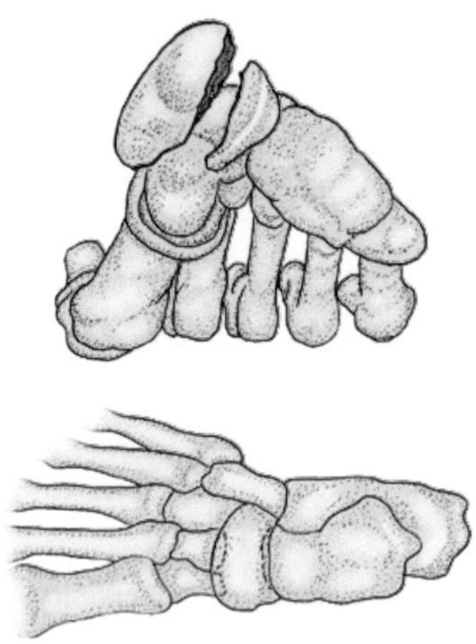

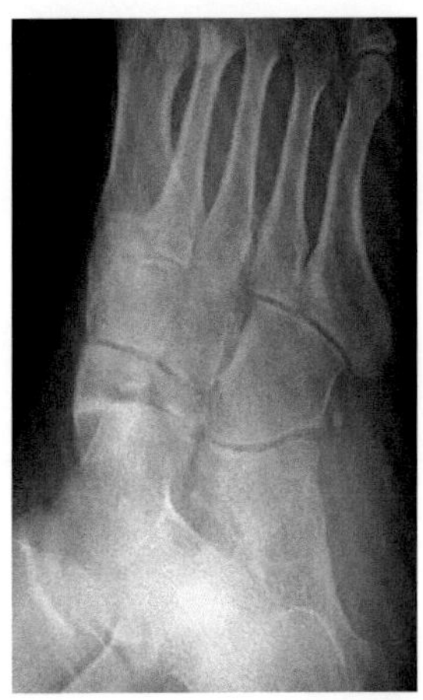

Sageorzan classification of navicular fracture

Type II: Fracture line from dorsalateral to medial metatarsal, involving talonavicular joint rupture and lateral dislocation of forefoot

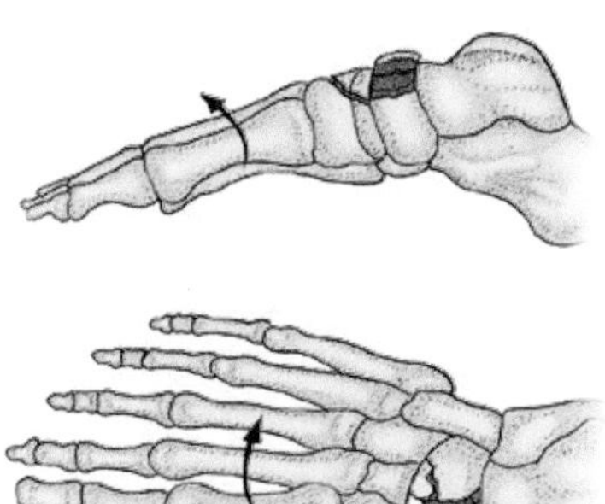

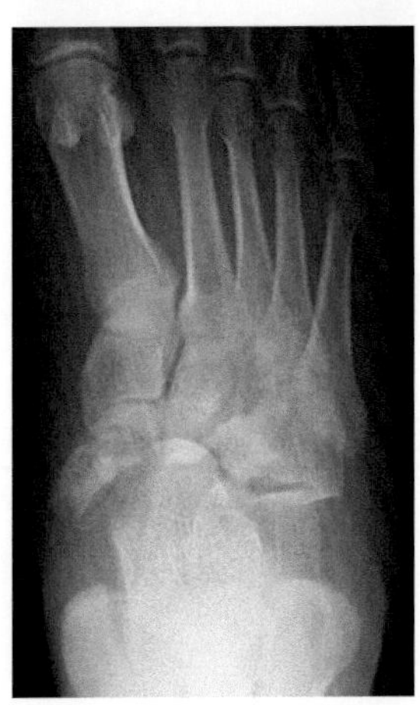

Sageorzan classification of navicular fracture

Type III: Comminuted fracture involving cuneonavicular joint injury, and/or cuboid, anterior calcaneus, calcaneocuboid joint fracture

11.3.2 AO/OTA Classification of Cuboid Fracture

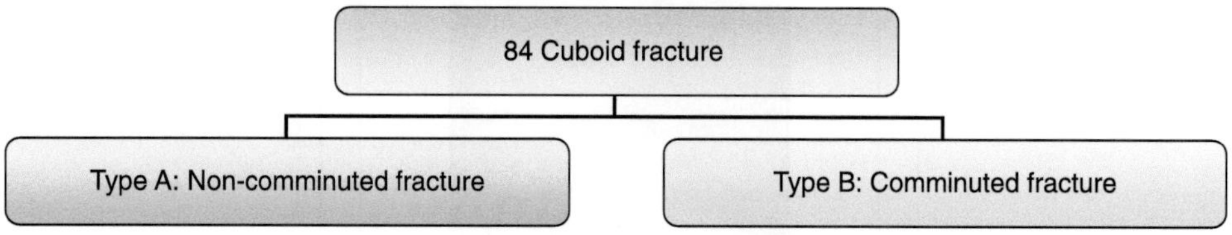

Type A: Non-comminuted fracture.
Type B: Comminuted fracture.

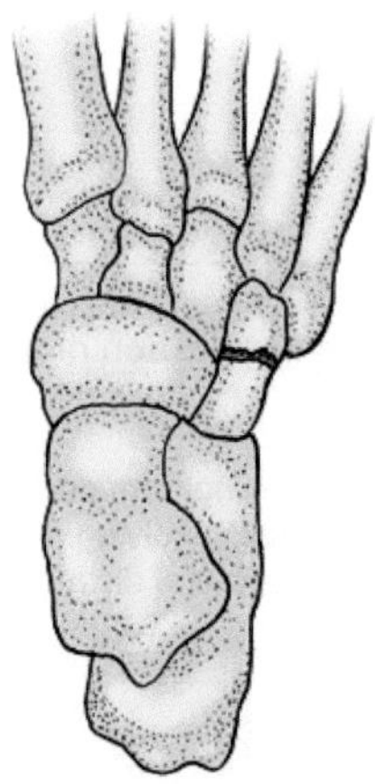

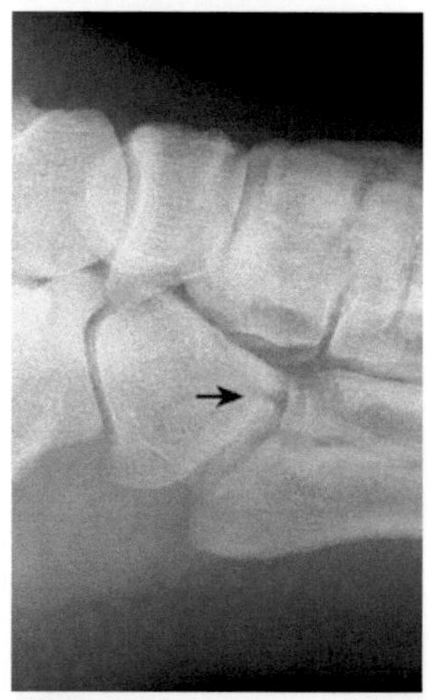

AO/OTA classification of cuboid fracture

Type A: Non-comminuted fracture

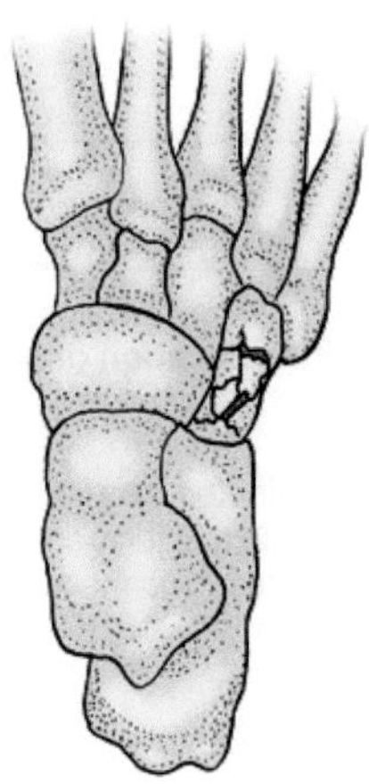

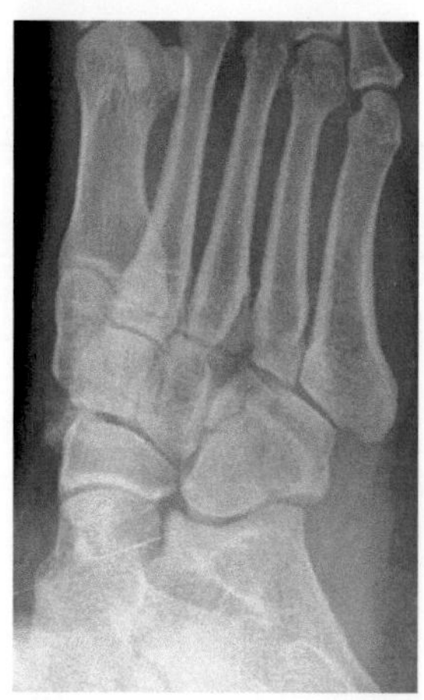

AO/OTA classification of cuboid fracture

Type B: Comminuted fracture

11.3.3 AO/OTA Classification of Cuneiform Fracture

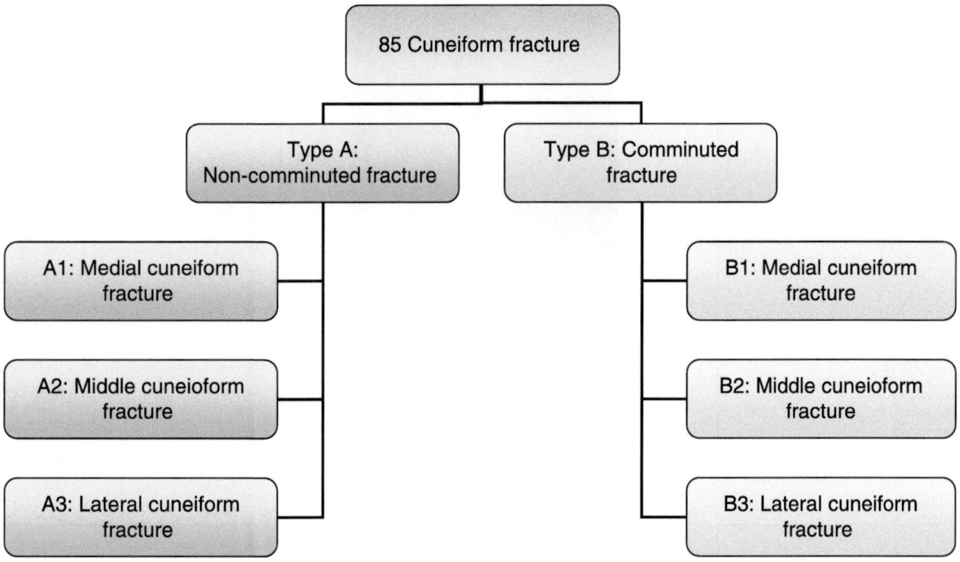

Type A: Non-comminuted fracture:
- Type A1: Medial cuneiform fracture.
- Type A2: Middle cuneiform fracture.
- Type A3 lateral cuneiform fracture.

Type B: Comminuted fracture:
- Type B1: Medial cuneiform fracture.
- Type B2: Middle cuneiform fracture.
- Type B3: Lateral cuneiform fracture.

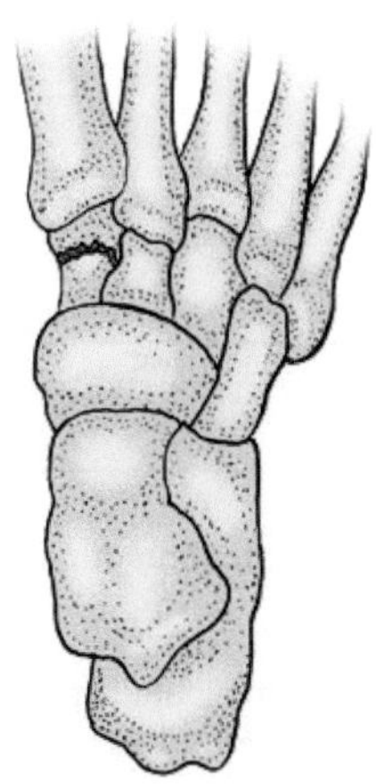

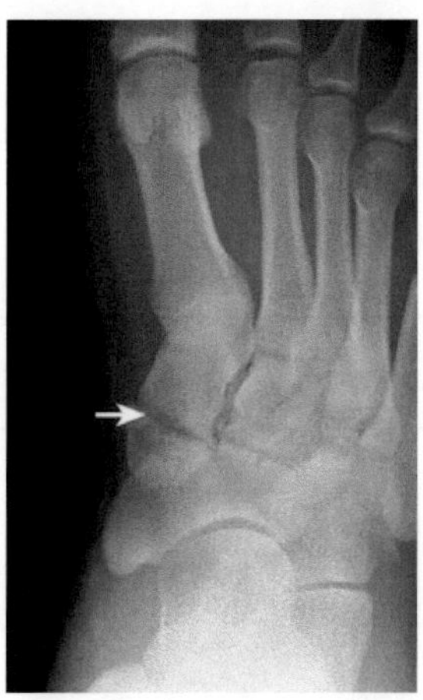

AO/OTA classification of cuneiform fracture

Type A: Non-comminuted fracture.
A1: Medial cuneiform fracture

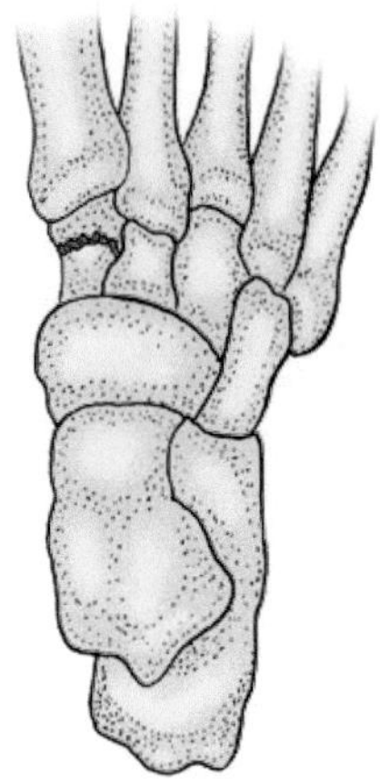

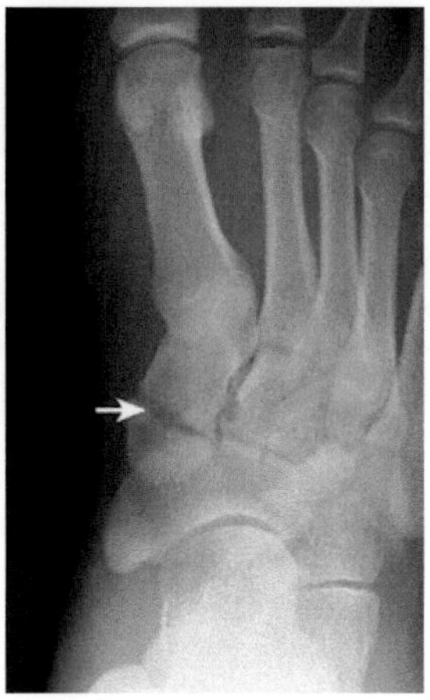

AO/OTA classification of cuneiform fracture

Type A: Non-comminuted fracture.
A1: Medial cuneiform fracture

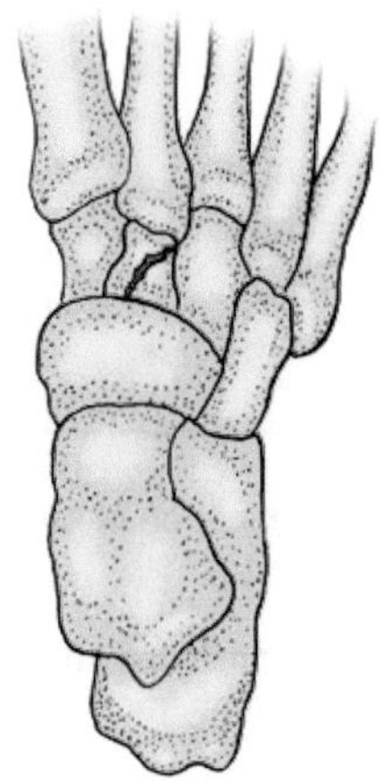

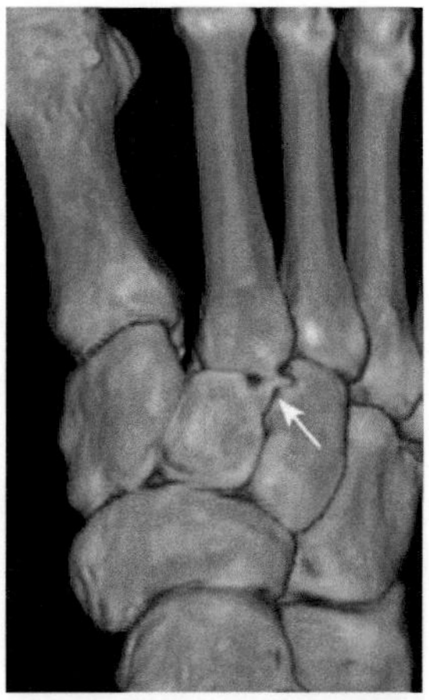

AO/OTA classification of cuneiform fracture

Type A: Non-comminuted fracture.
A2: Middle cuneioform fracture

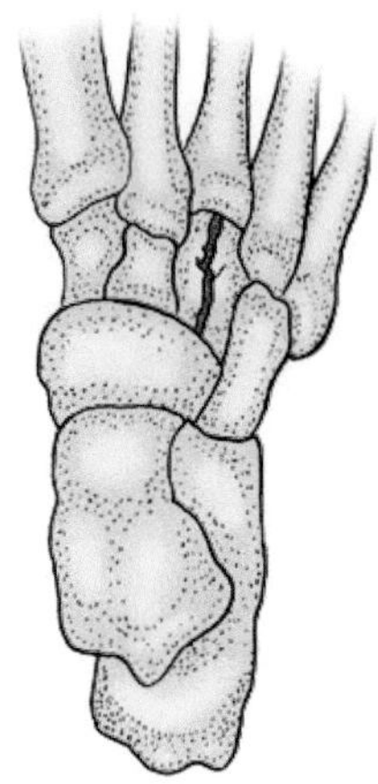

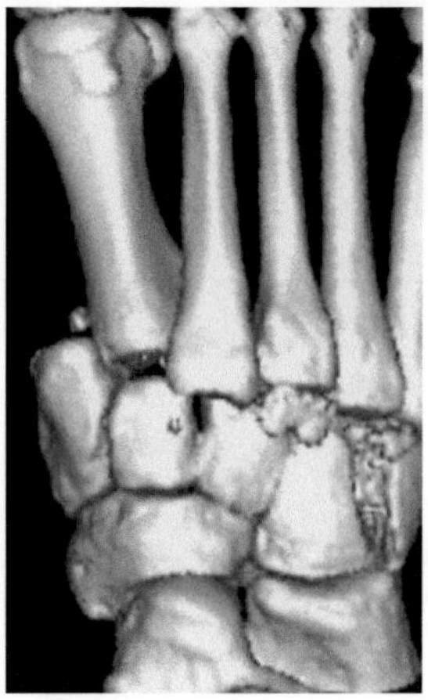

AO/OTA classification of cuneiform fracture

Type A: Non-comminuted fracture.
A3: Lateral cuneiform fracture

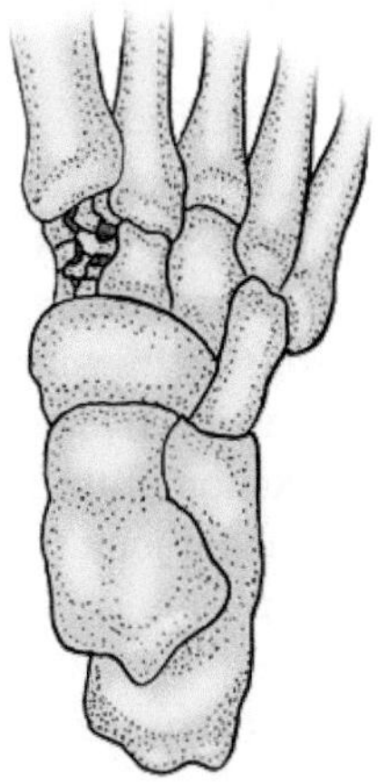

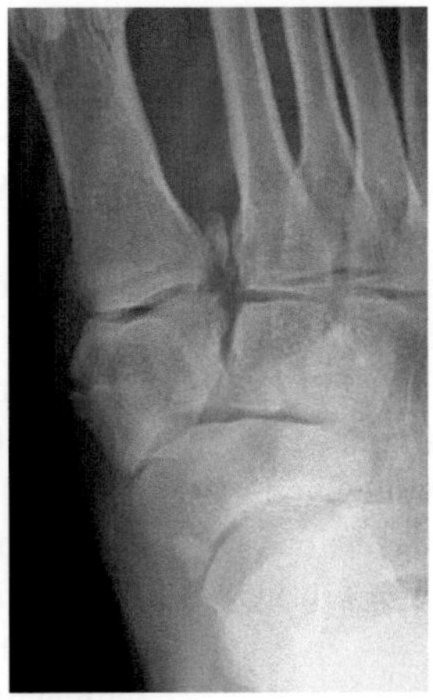

AO/OTA classification of cuneiform fracture

Type B: Comminuted fracture.
B1: Medial cuneiform fracture

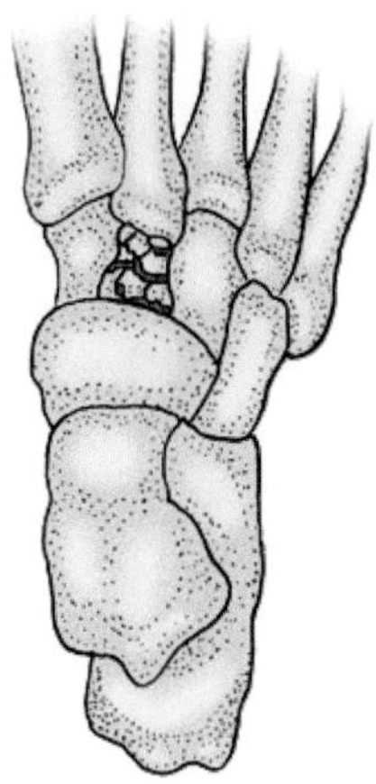

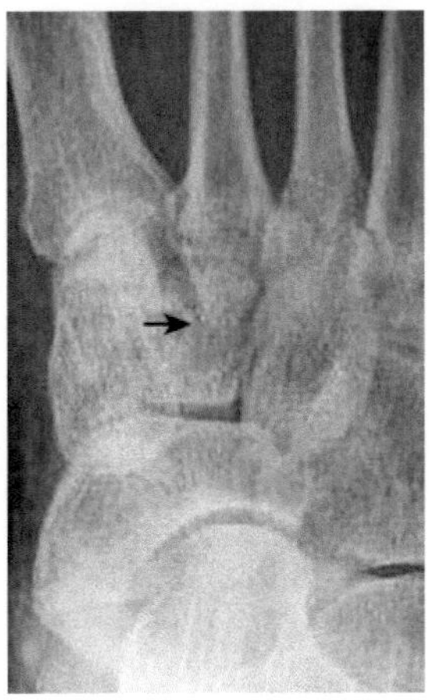

AO/OTA classification of cuneiform fracture

Type B: Comminuted fracture.
B2: Middle cuneioform fracture

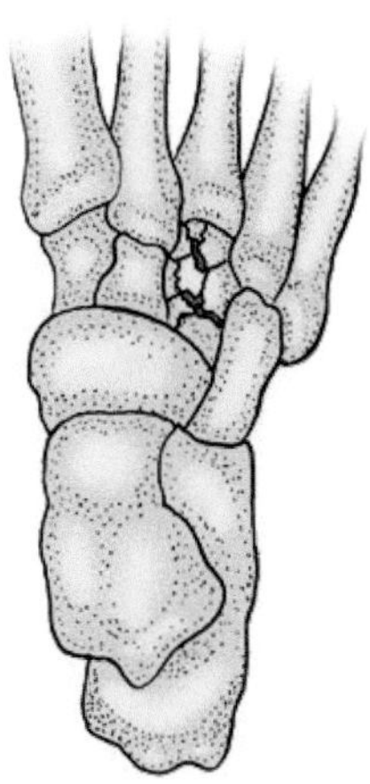

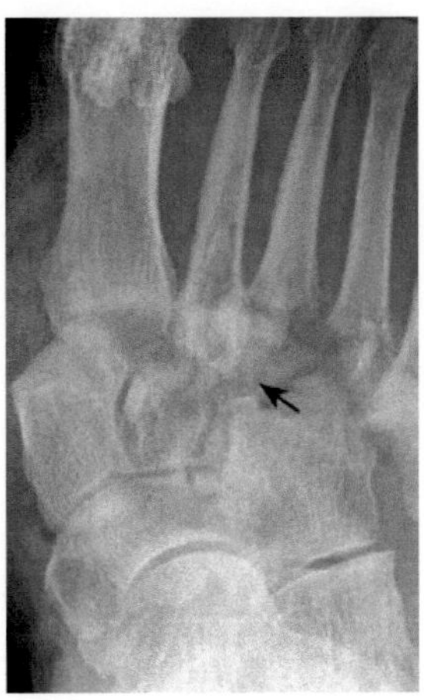

AO/OTA classification of cuneiform fracture

Type B: Comminuted fracture.
B3: Lateral cuneiform fracture

11.3.4 Midtarsal Joint (Chopart Joint) Main-Jowett Classification

1. Medial stress injury

   Midfoot adduction to the hindfoot results in varus injuries

   Chip fracture of the talus or dorsal rim of the navicular and calcaneal or lateral rim of the cuboid hints sprain injuries.

   In more severe situations, the midfoot may dislocate completely or a talonavicular joint dislocation alone may occur. A medial rotational dislocation indicates talonavicular joint dislocation and subtalar joint subluxation; however, the calcaneocuboid joint is intact.
2. Longitudinal stress injury

   A stress force transmits along the axial area of the metatarsal from the head to the proximity, leading to a compression fracture in the midfoot or between the metatarsal and talus with plantarflexion.

   A longitudinal stress force transmits through cuneiforms, leading to typical vertical navicular fractures.
3. Lateral stress injury

   A "nutcracker fracture" is a specific fracture of the cuboid joint. The abduction force stress on the forefoot causes a compressive load to the cuboid between the calcaneus and fourth and fifth metatarsal bases. The most common type is the navicular avulsion fracture combined with comminuted cuboid compression fracture. In more severe situations, a lateral subluxation of the talonavicular joint, comminuted calcaneocuboid joint fracture, and lateral column collapse may occur.
4. Plantar side stress injury

   A plantar side direct stress leads to medial tarsi sprains with avulsion fracture of the navicular, talar, or dorsal lip of the calcaneal anterior process.
5. Crush injury

11.4 Section 4 Classification of Metatarsal Fractures

11.4.1 AO/OTA Classification of Metatarsal Fractures

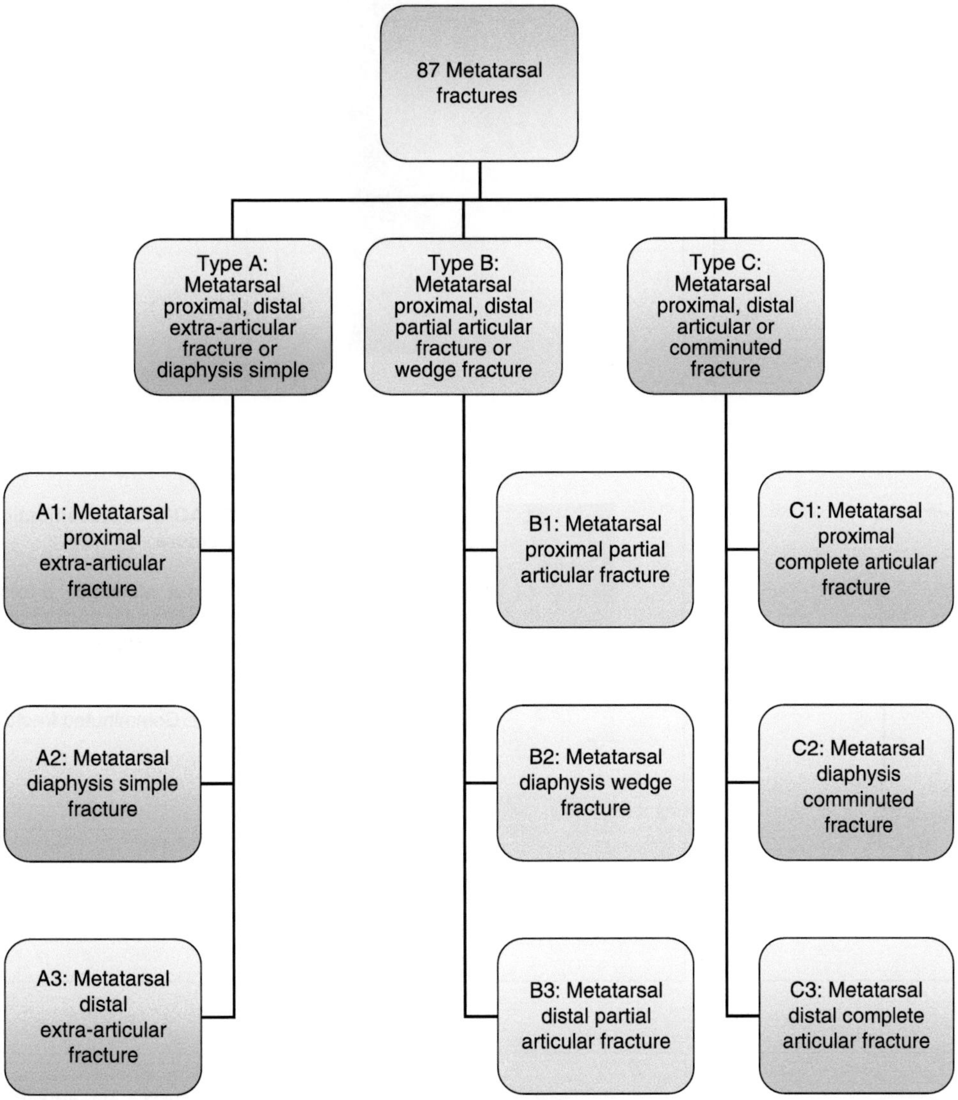

Type A: Metatarsal proximal, distal extra-articular fracture, or diaphysis simple fracture.

- Type A1: Metatarsal proximal extra-articular fracture:
  - Type A1.1: Non-comminuted fracture.
  - Type A1.2: Comminuted fracture.
- Type A2: Metatarsal diaphysis simple fracture:
  - Type A2.1: Metatarsal diaphysis simple spiral fracture, metatarsal diaphysis simple oblique fracture, and metatarsal diaphysis simple transverse fracture.
- Type A3: Metatarsal distal extra-articular fracture:
  - Type A3.1: Non-comminuted fracture.
  - Type A3.2: Comminuted fracture.

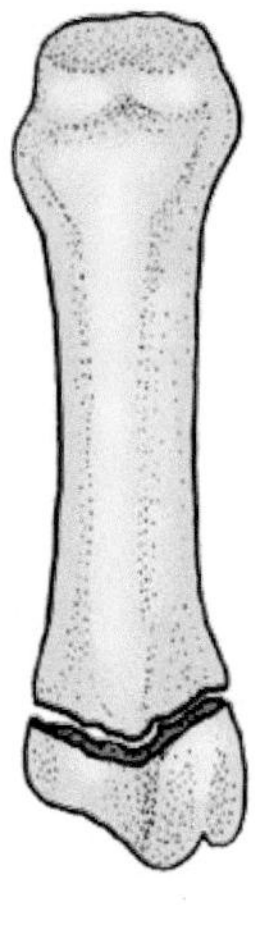

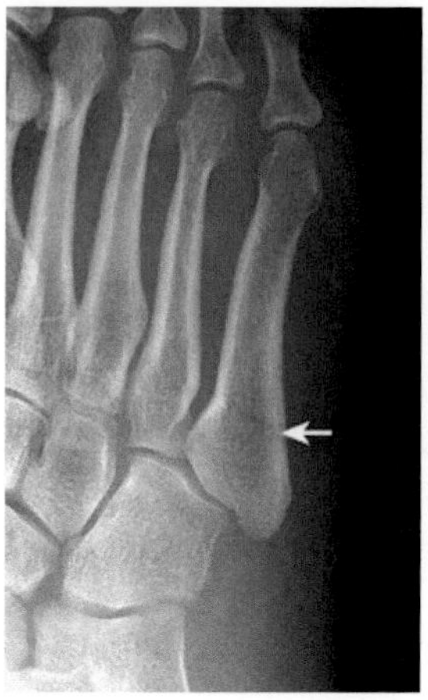

87 AO/OTA classification of Metatarsal fracture

Type A: Metatarsal proximal, distal extra-articular fracture or diaphysis simple fracture.
A1: Metatarsal proximal extra-articular fracture.
A1.1 Noncomminuted fracture

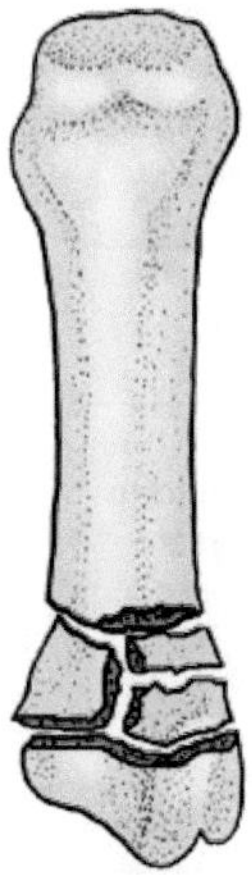

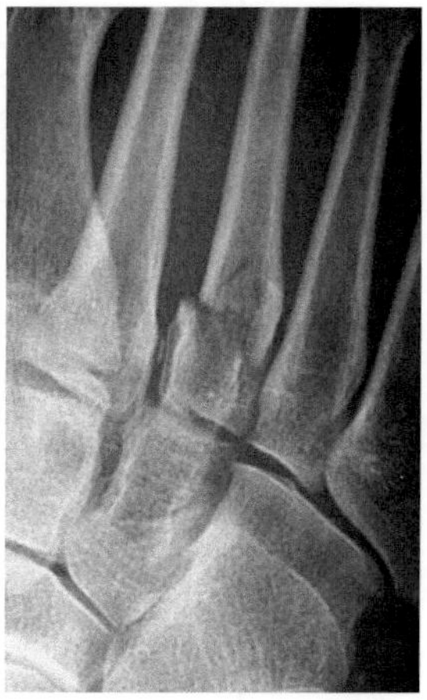

87 AO/OTA classification of Metatarsal fracture

Type A: Metatarsal proximal, distal extra-articular fracture or diaphysis simple fracture.
A1: Metatarsal proximal extra-articular fracture.
A1.2: Comminuted fracture

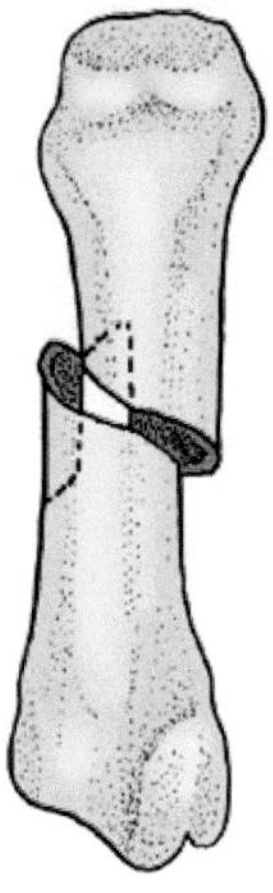

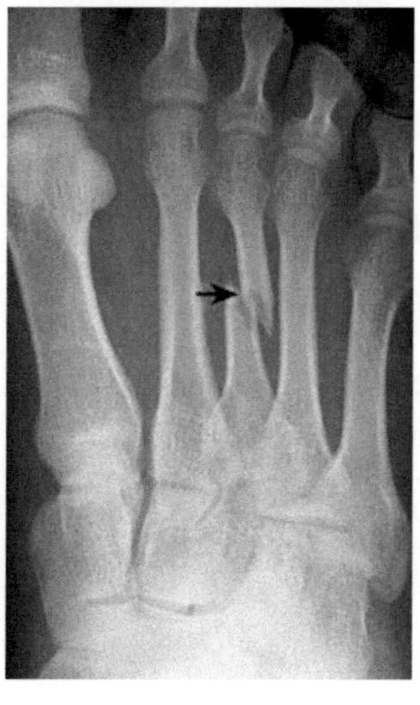

87 AO/OTA classification of Metatarsal fracture

Type A: Metatarsal proximal, distal extra-articular fracture or diaphysis simple fracture.
A2: Metatarsal diaphysis simple fracture.
A2.1: Metatarsal diaphysis simple spiral fracture

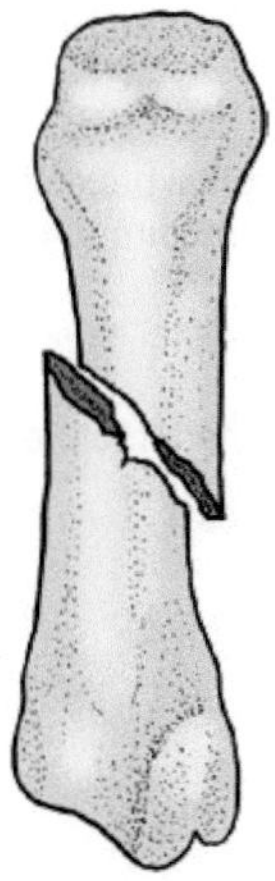

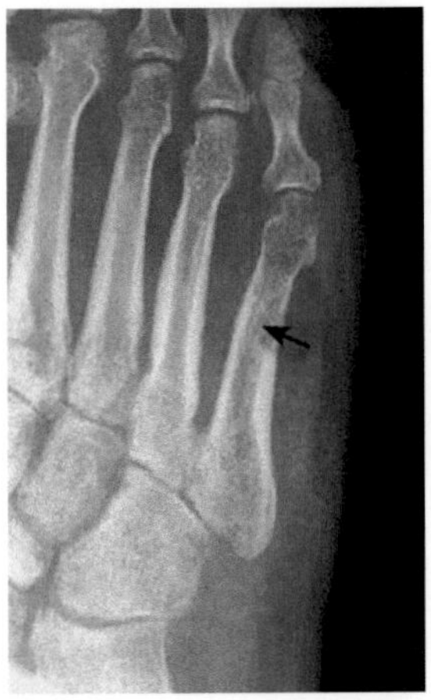

87 AO/OTA classification of Metatarsal fracture

Type A: Metatarsal proximal, distal extra-articular fracture or diaphysis simple fracture.
A2: Metatarsal diaphysis simple fracture.
A2.2: Metatarsal diaphysis simple oblique fracture

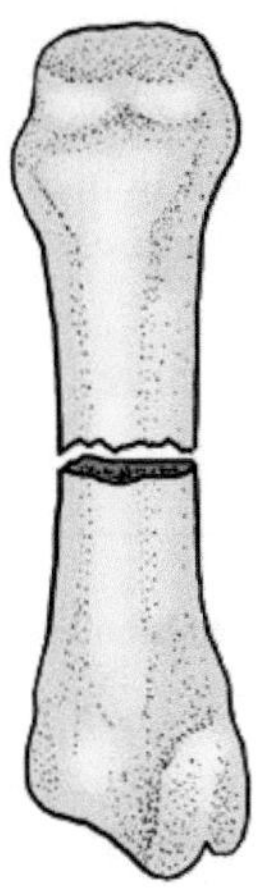

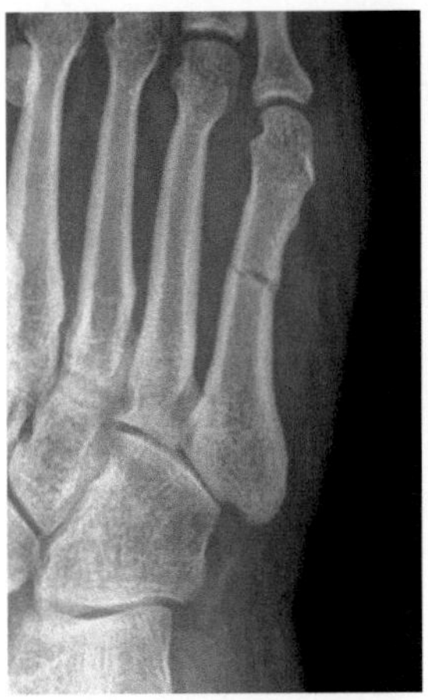

87 AO/OTA classification of Metatarsal fracture

Type A: Metatarsal proximal, distal extra-articular fracture or diaphysis simple fracture.
A2: Metatarsal diaphysis simple fracture.
A2.3: Metatarsal diaphysis simple transverse fracture

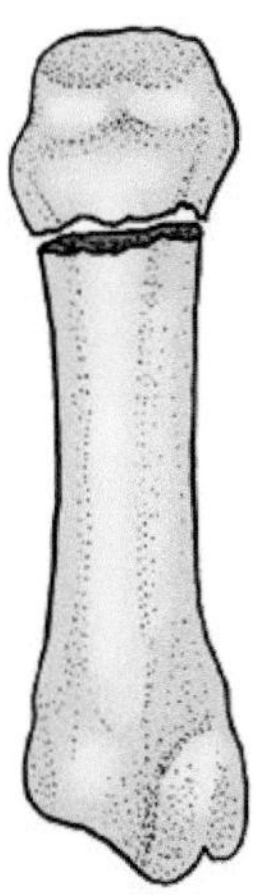

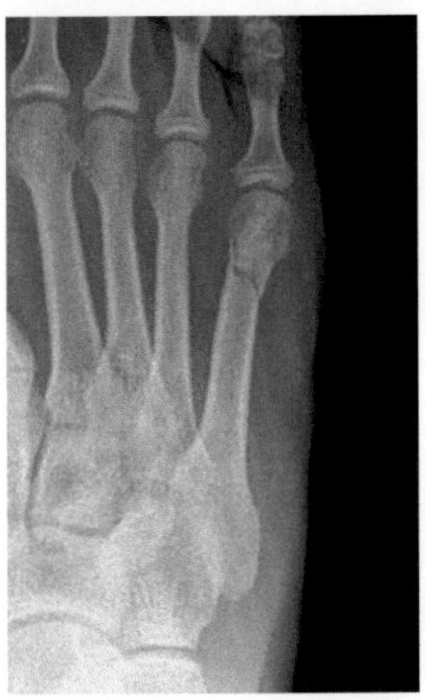

87 AO/OTA classification of Metatarsal fracture

Type A: Metatarsal proximal, distal extra-articular fracture or diaphysis simple fracture.
A3: Metatarsal distal extra-articular fracture.
A3.1: Noncomminuted fracture

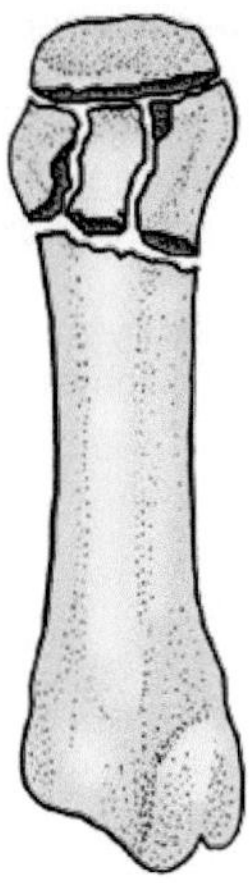

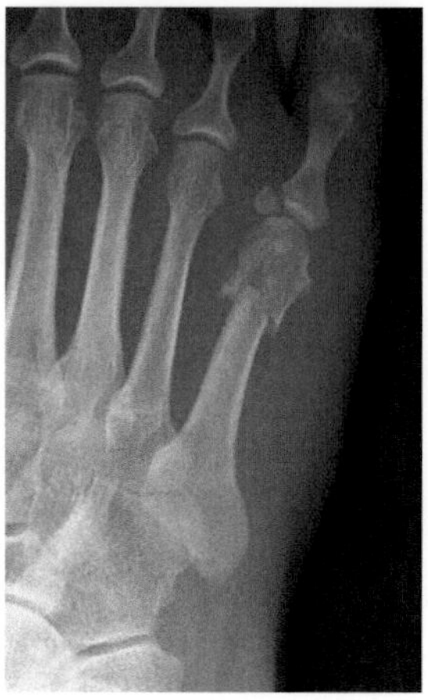

87 AO/OTA classification of Metatarsal fracture

Type A: Metatarsal proximal, distal extra-articular fracture or diaphysis simple fracture.
A3: Metatarsal distal extra-articular fracture.
A3.2: Comminuted fracture

Type B: Metatarsal proximal, distal partial articular fracture, or diaphysis wedge fracture

- Type B1: Metatarsal proximal partial articular fracture:
  - Type B1.1: Avulsion or split fracture.
  - Type B1.2: Depression fracture.
  - Type B1.3: Split-depression fracture.
- Type B2: Metatarsal diaphysis wedge fracture:
  - Type B2.1: Diaphysis spiral wedge fracture.
  - Type B2.2: Diaphysis bending wedged fracture.
  - Type B2.3: Diaphysis comminuted wedge fracture.
- Type B3: Metatarsal distal partial articular fracture:
  - Type B3.1: Avulsion or split fracture.
  - Type B3.2: Depression fracture.
  - Type B3.3: Split-depression fracture.

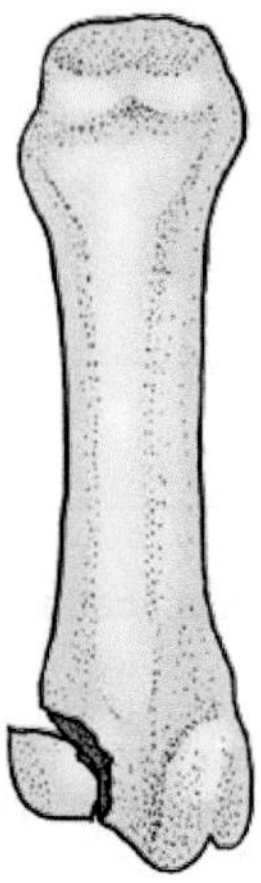

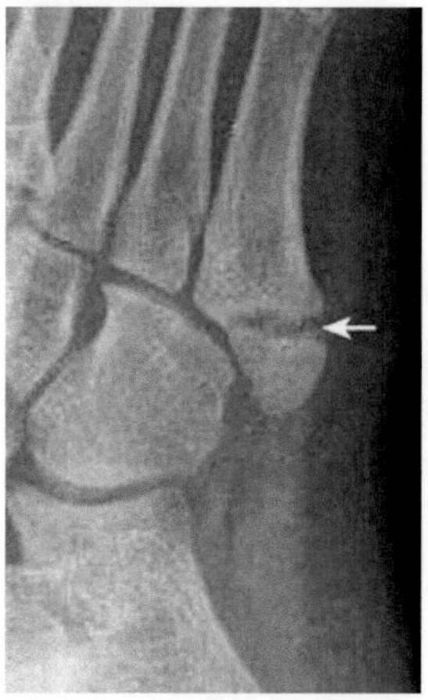

87 AO/OTA classification of Metatarsal fracture

Type B: Metatarsal proximal, distal partial articular fracture or diaphysis wedge fracture.
B1: Metatarsal proximal partial articular fracture.
B1.1: Avulsion or split fracture

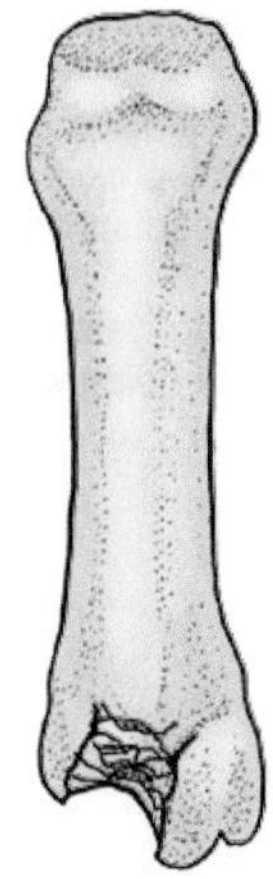

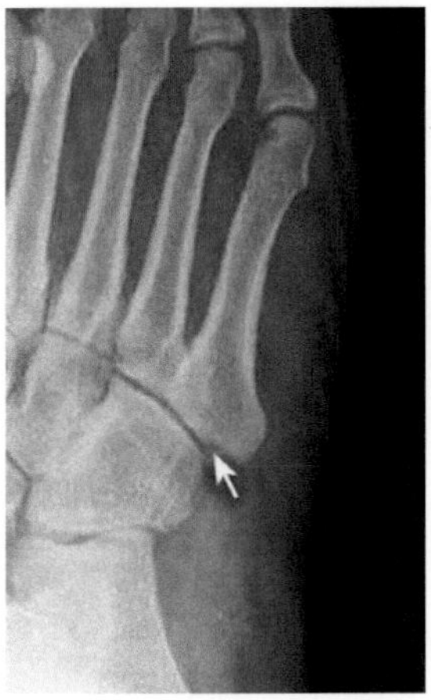

87 AO/OTA classification of Metatarsal fracture

Type B: Metatarsal proximal, distal partial articular fracture or diaphysis wedge fracture.
B1: Metatarsal proximal partial articular fracture.
B1.2: Depression fracture

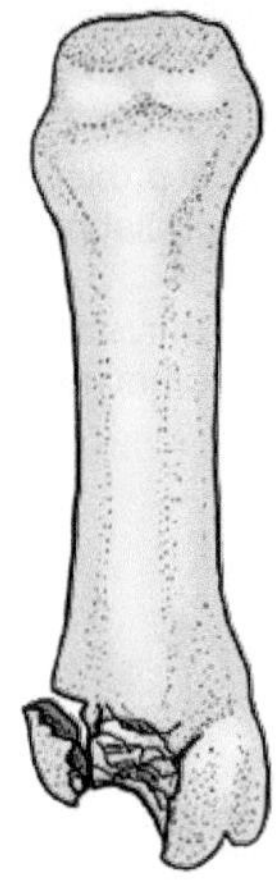

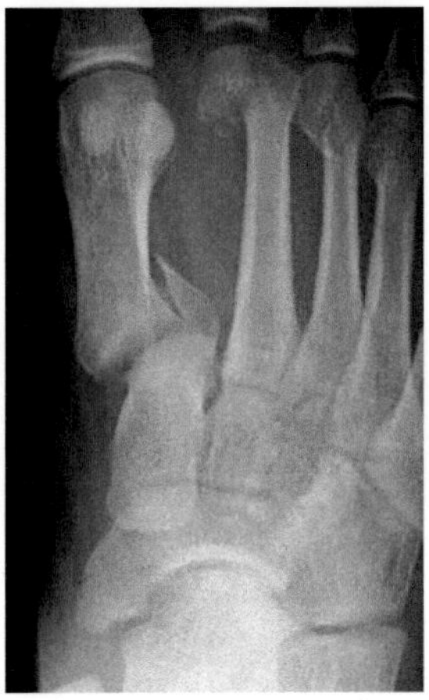

87 AO/OTA classification of Metatarsal fracture

Type B: Metatarsal proximal, distal partial articular fracture or diaphysis wedge fracture.
B1: Metatarsal proximal partial articular fracture.
B1.3: Split/depression fracture

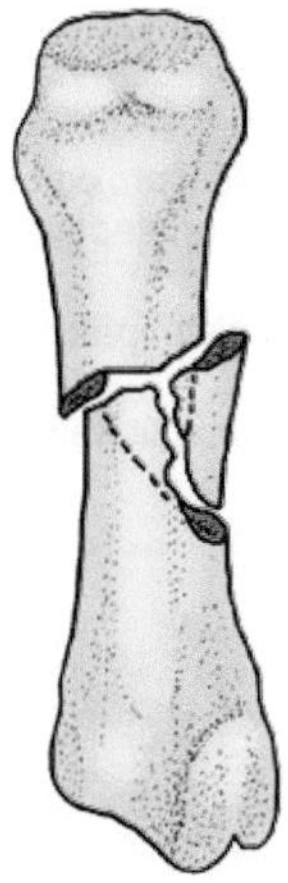

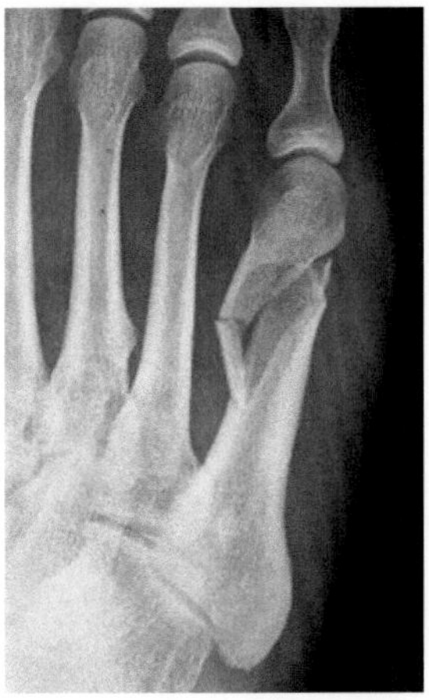

87 AO/OTA classification of Metatarsal fracture

Type B: Metatarsal proximal, distal partial articular fracture or diaphysis wedge fracture.
B2: Metatarsal diaphysis wedge fracture.
B2.1: Diaphysis spiral wedge fracture

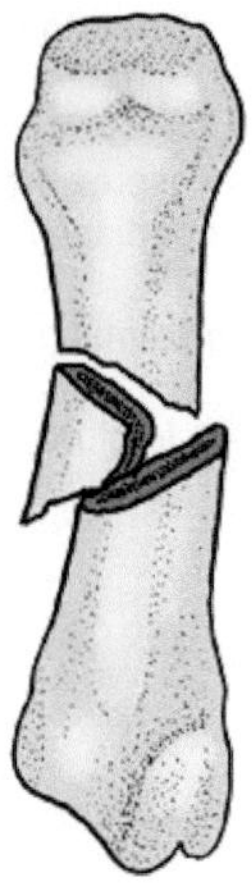

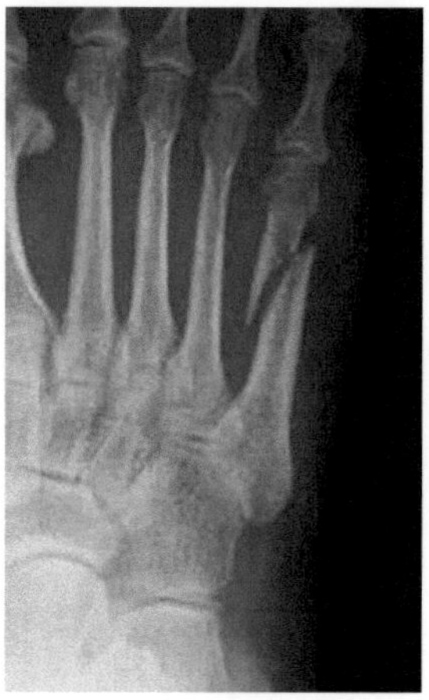

87 AO/OTA classification of Metatarsal fracture

Type B: Metatarsal proximal, distal partial articular fracture or diaphysis wedge fracture.
B2: Metatarsal diaphysis wedge fracture.
B2.2: Diaphysis bending wedged fracture

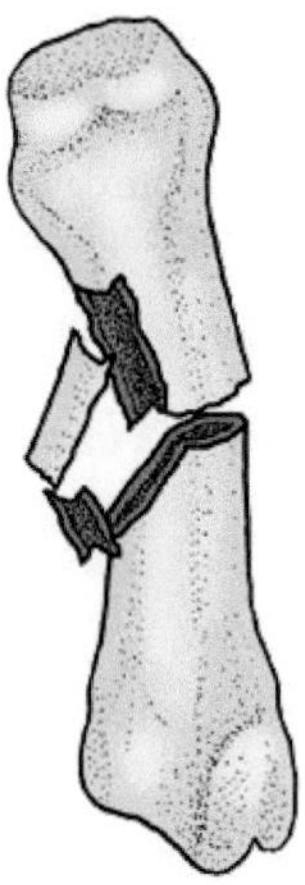

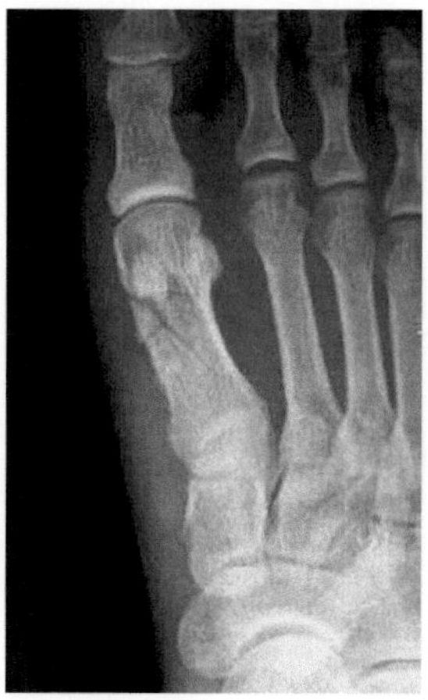

87 AO/OTA classification of Metatarsal fracture

Type B: Metatarsal proximal, distal partial articular fracture or diaphysis wedge fracture.
B2: Metatarsal diaphysis wedge fracture.
B2.3: Diaphysis comminuted wedge fracture

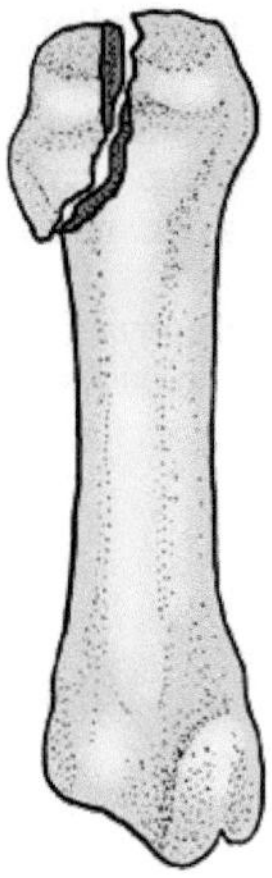

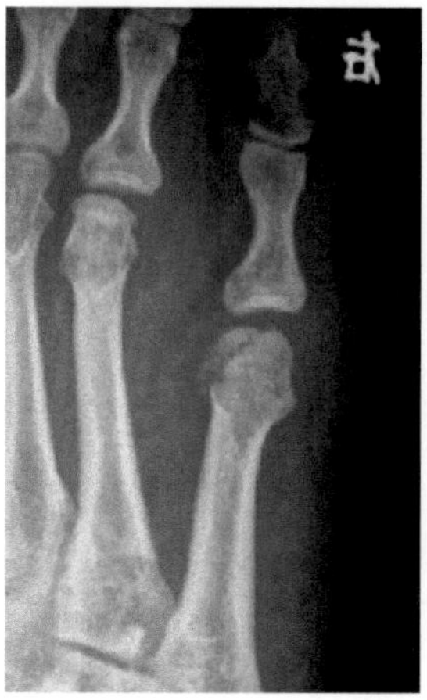

87 AO/OTA classification of Metatarsal fracture

Type B: Metatarsal proximal, distal partial articular fracture or diaphysis wedge fracture.
B3: Metatarsal distal partial articular fracture.
B3.1: Avulsion or split fracture

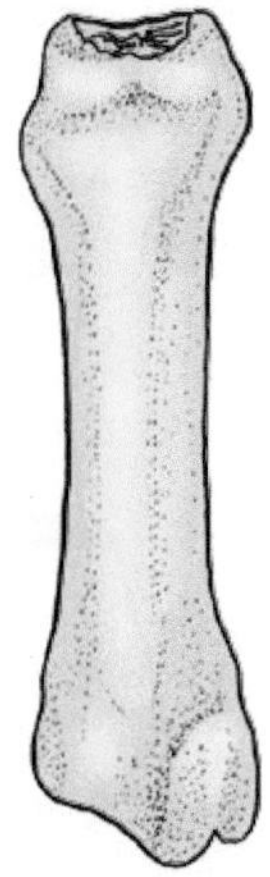

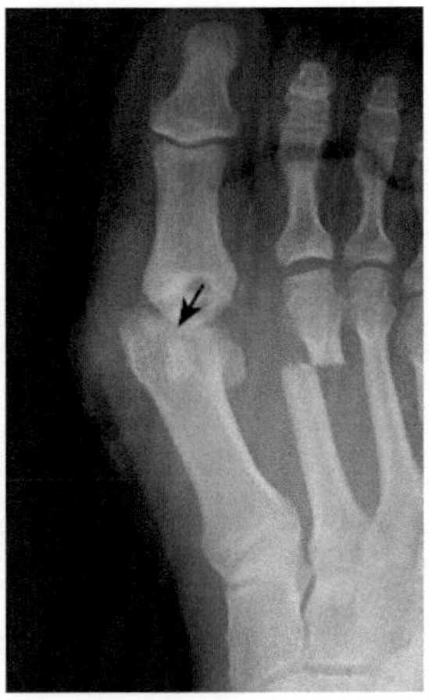

87 AO/OTA classification of Metatarsal fracture

Type B: Metatarsal proximal, distal partial articular fracture or diaphysis wedge fracture.
B3: Metatarsal distal partial articular fracture.
B3.2: Depression fracture

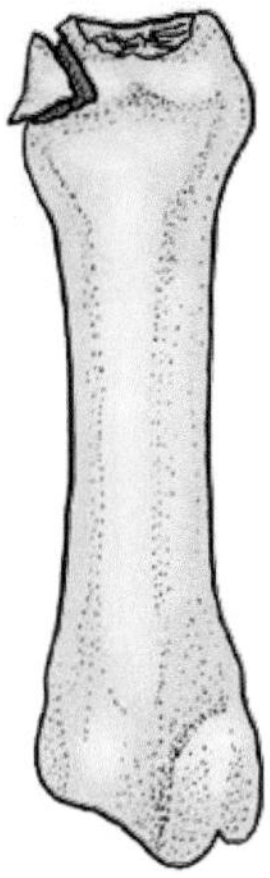

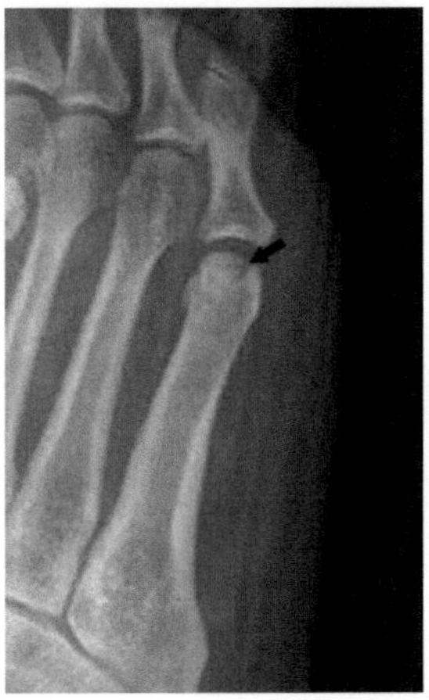

87 AO/OTA classification of Metatarsal fracture

Type B: Metatarsal proximal, distal partial articular fracture or diaphysis wedge fracture.
B3: Metatarsal distal partial articular fracture.
B3.3: Split/depression fracture

Type C: Metatarsal proximal, distal complete articular, or diaphysis comminuted fracture:
- Type C1: Metatarsal proximal complete articular fracture:
  - Type C1.1: Simple articular and metaphysis fracture.
  - Type C1.2: Simple articular, comminuted metaphysis fracture.
  - Type C1.3: Comminuted articular and metaphysis.
- Type C2: Metatarsal diaphysis comminuted fracture:
  - Type C2.1: Segmental fracture.
  - Type C2.2: Complex comminuted.

Type C3: Metatarsal distal complete articular fracture:
- Type C3.1: Simple articular and metaphysis fracture.
- Type C3.2: Simple articular, comminuted metaphysis fracture.
- Type C3.3: Comminuted articular and metaphysis.

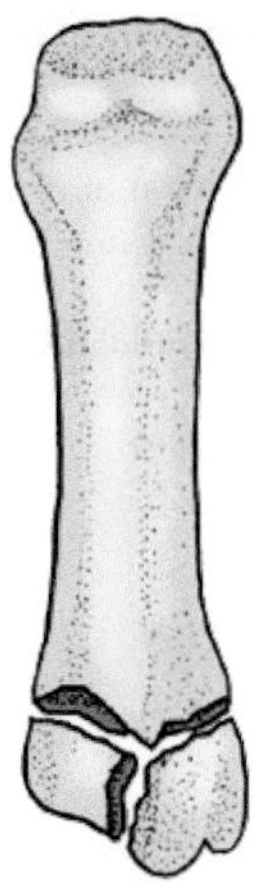

87C1.1

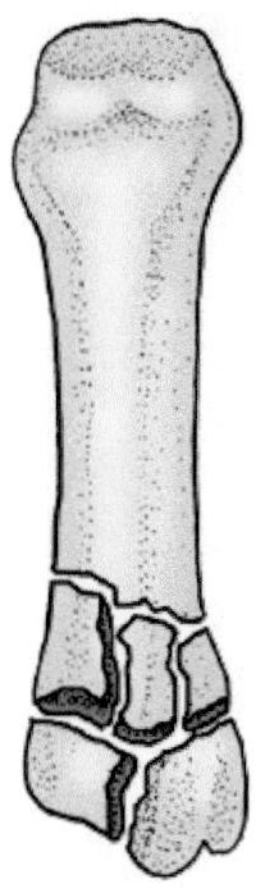

87C1.2

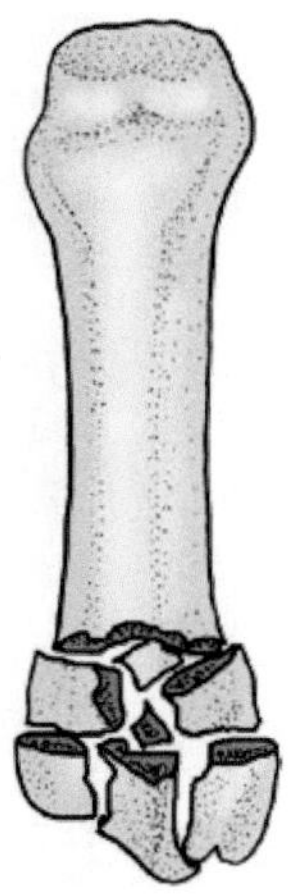

87C1.3

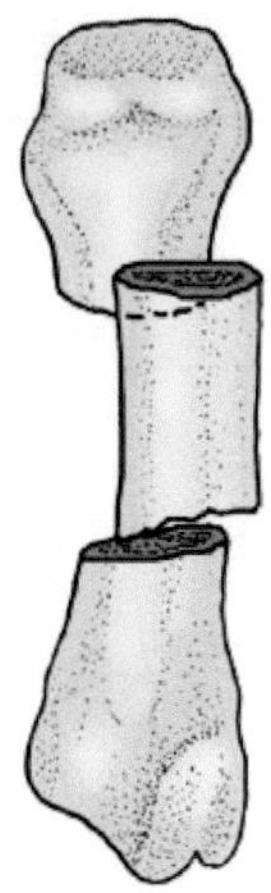

87C2.1

87C2.2

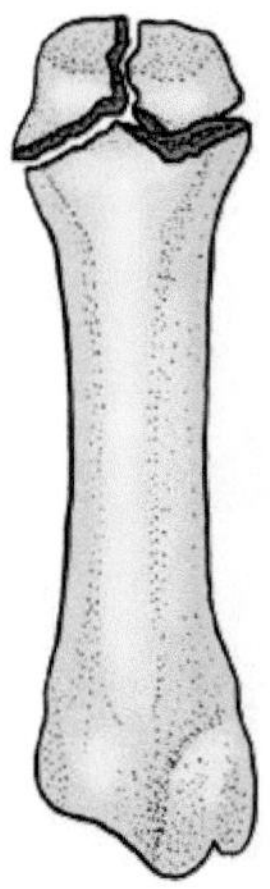

87C3.1

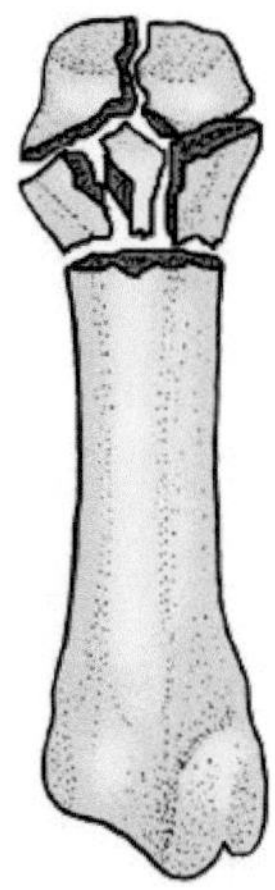

87C3.2

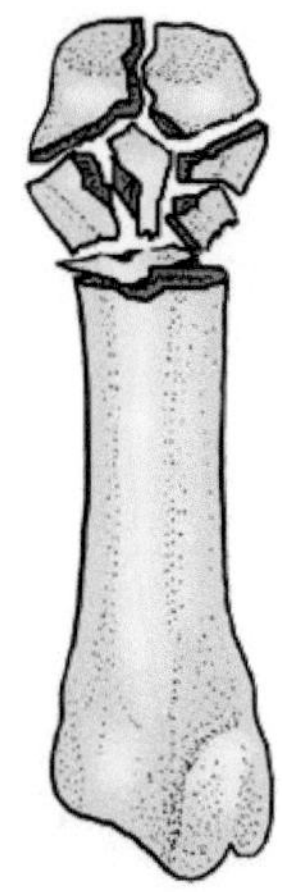

87C3.3

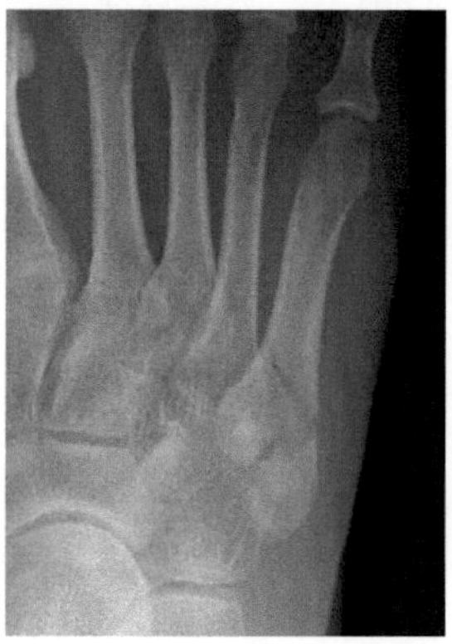

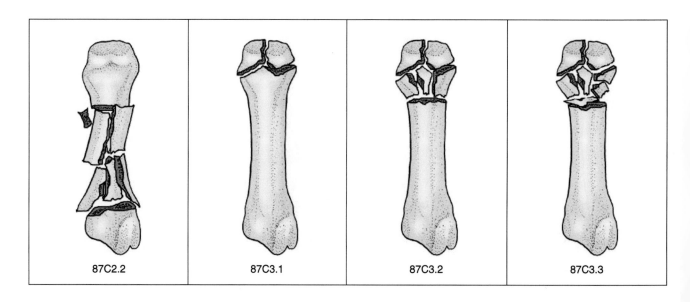

C1.1 Simple articular and metaphysis fracture

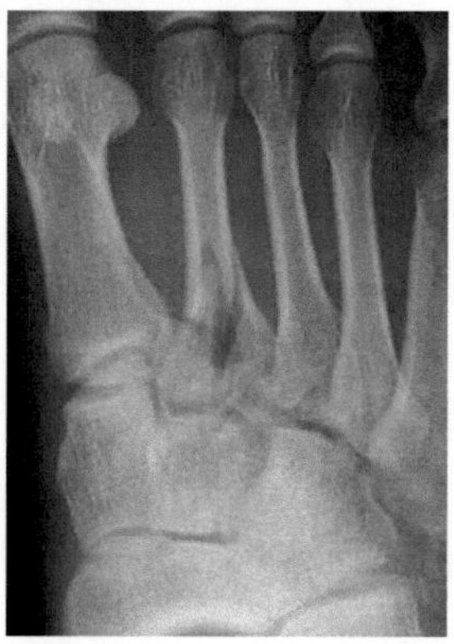

C1.2 Simple articular, comminuted metaphysis fracture

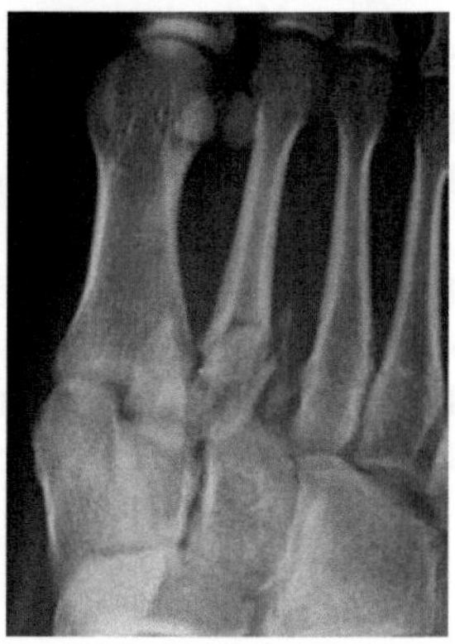

C1.3 Comminuted articular and metaphysis

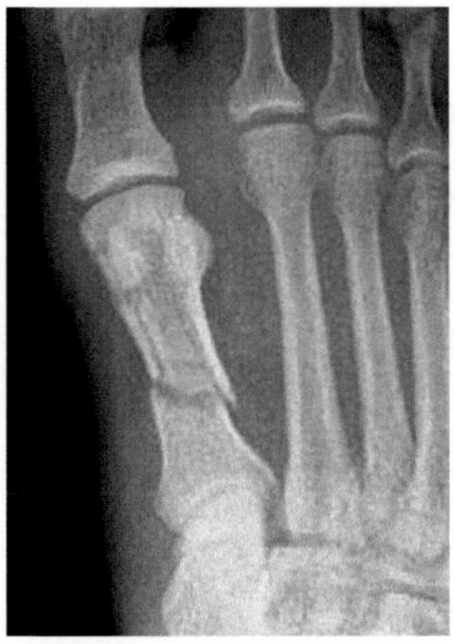

C2.1 Segmental fracture

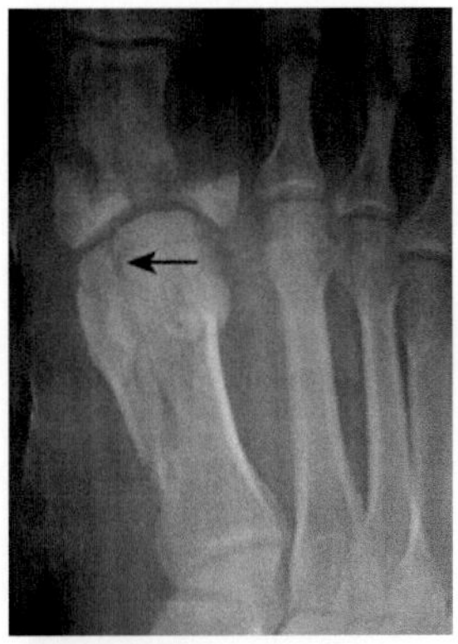

C3.1 Simple articular and metaphysis fracture

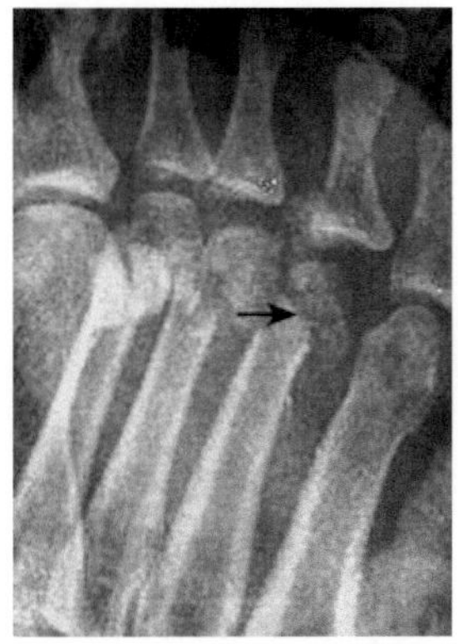

C3.3 Comminuted articular and metaphysis

11.4.2 Dameron Classification of Proximal Fifth Metatarsal Fracture

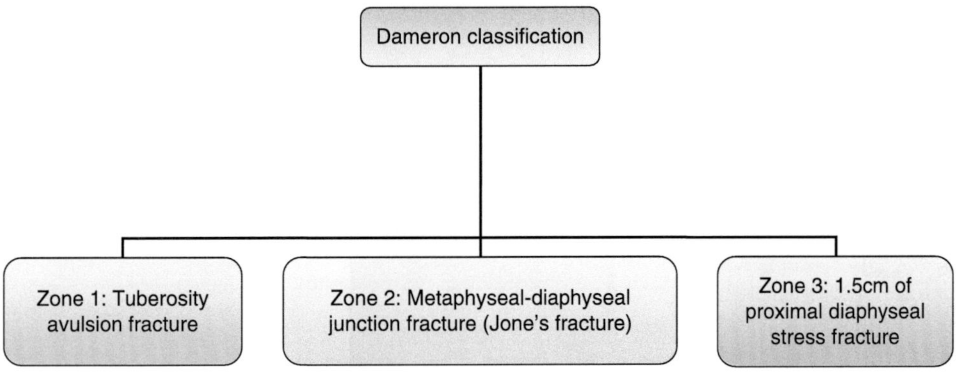

Zone 1: Tuberosity avulsion fracture.
Zone 2: Metaphyseal-diaphyseal junction fracture (Jones fracture).
Zone 3: 1.5 cm of proximal diaphyseal stress fracture.

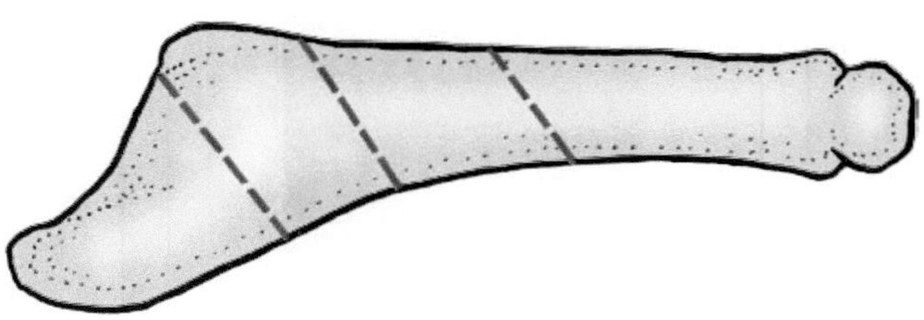

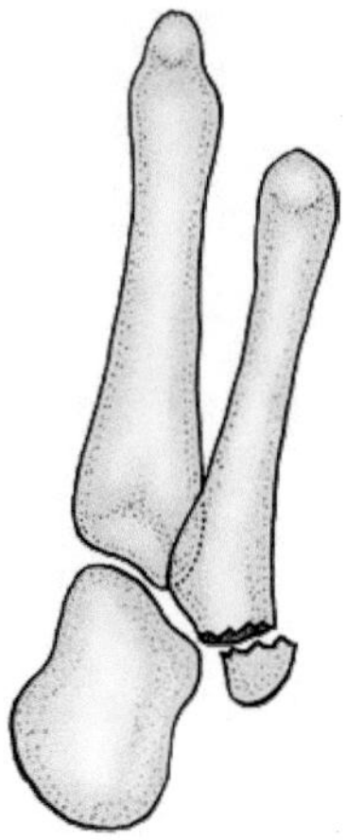

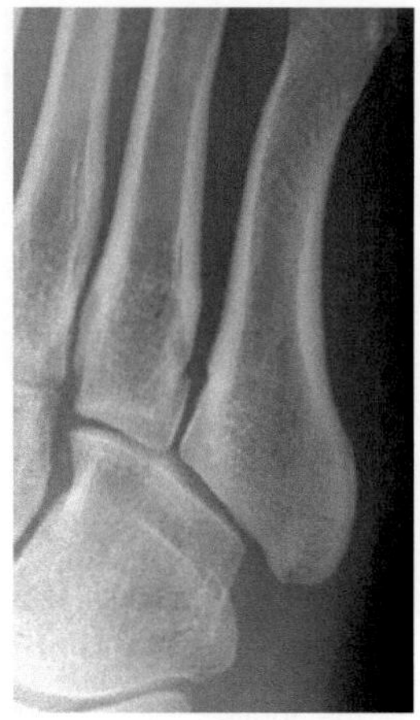

Dameron classification of proximal fifth metatarsal fracture
Zone 1: Tuberosity avulsion fracture

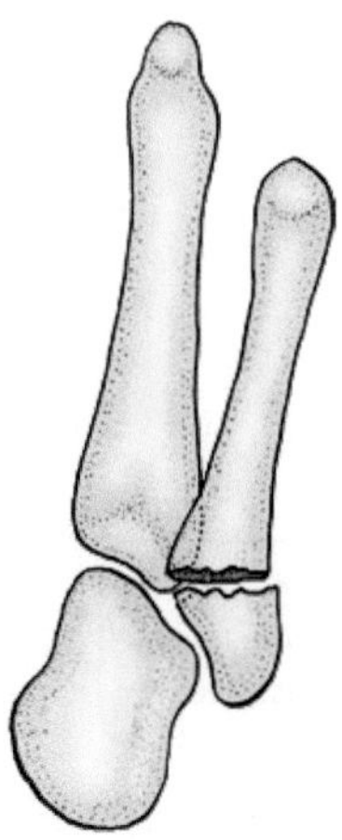

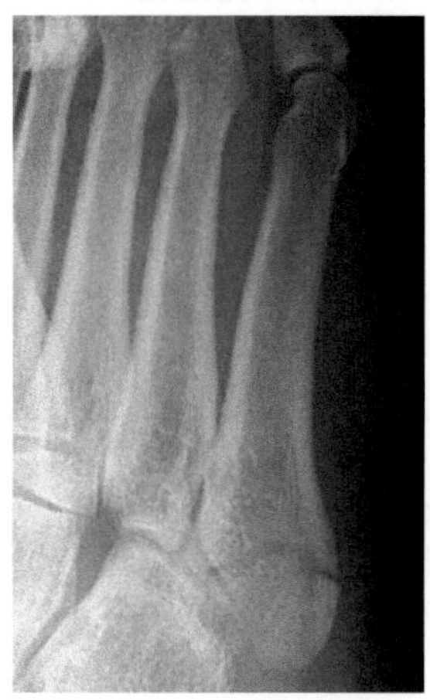

Dameron classification of proximal fifth metatarsal fracture
Zone 2: Metaphyseal-diaphyseal junction fracture (Jone's fracture)

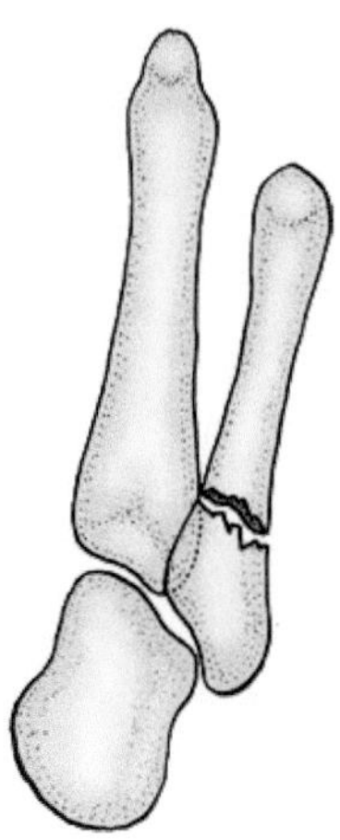

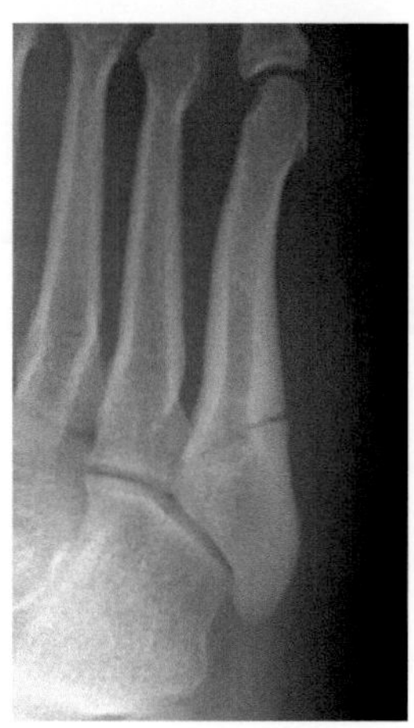

Dameron classification of proximal fifth metatarsal fracture
Zone 3: 1.5cm of proximal diaphyseal stress fracture

11.4.3 Bowers-Martin Classification of the First Metatarsophalangeal Joint Injury

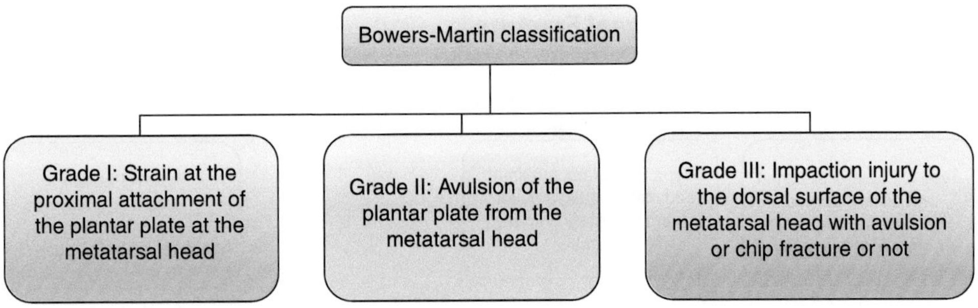

Grade I: Strain at the proximal attachment of the plantar plate at the metatarsal head.
Grade II: Avulsion of the plantar plate from the metatarsal head.
Grade III: Impaction injury to the dorsal surface of the metatarsal head with avulsion or chip fracture or not.

11.5 Section 5 Classification of Phalangeal Fracture

11.5.1 AO/OTA Classification of Phalangeal Fracture

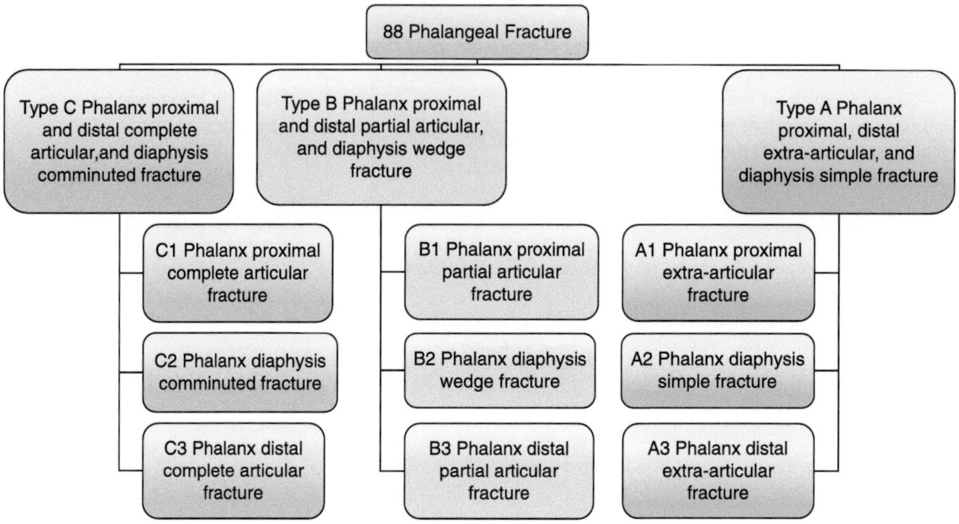

Type A: Phalanx proximal, distal extra-articular, and diaphysis simple fracture:
- Type A1: Phalanx proximal extra-articular fracture:
  - Type A1.1: Non-comminuted fracture.
  - Type A1.2: Comminuted fracture.
- Type A2: Phalanx diaphysis simple fracture:
  - Type A2.1: Simple spiral fracture.
  - Type A2.2: Simple oblique fracture.
  - Type A2.3: simple transverse fracture.
- Type A3: Phalanx distal extra-articular fracture:
  - Type A3.1: Non-comminuted fracture.
  - Type A3.2: Comminuted fracture.

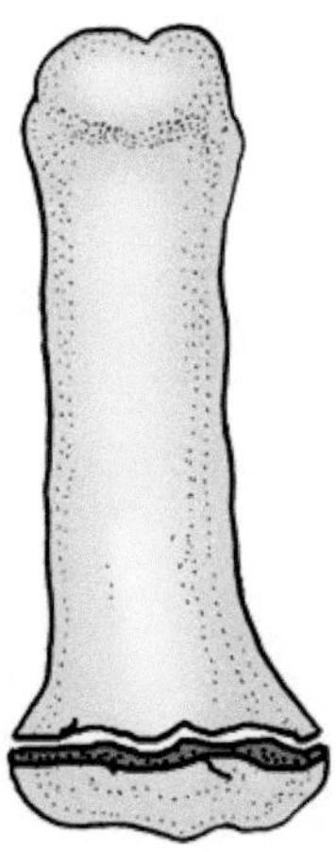

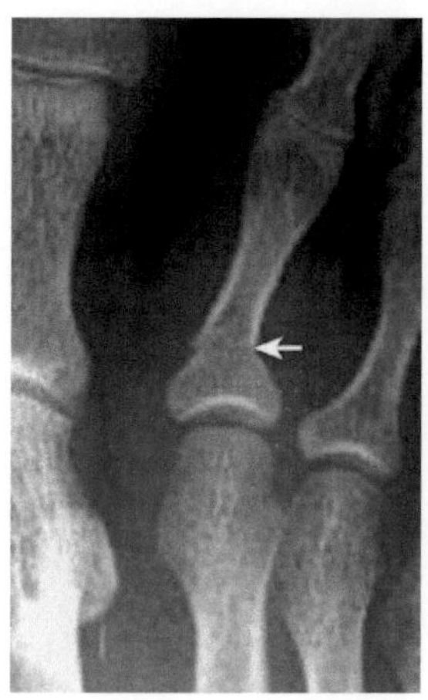

88 AO/OTA Classification of Phalangeal Fracture
Type A: Phalanx proximal, distal extra-articular, and diaphysis simple fracture.
A1: Phalanx proximal extra-articular fracture.
A1.1: Non-comminuted fracture

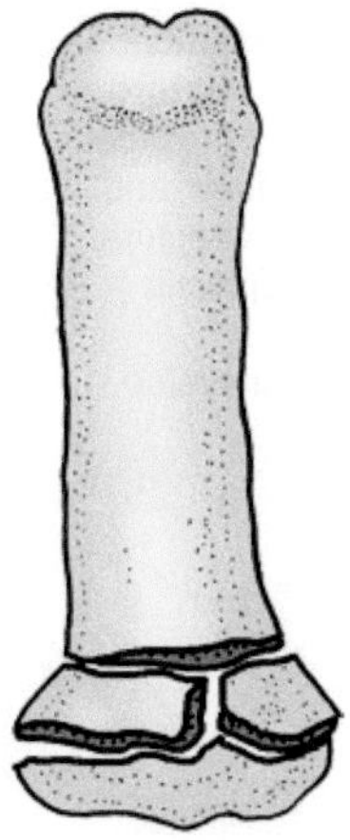

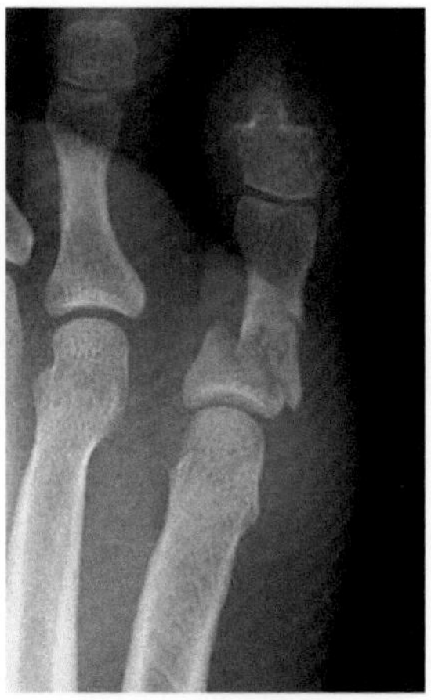

88 AO/OTA Classification of Phalangeal Fracture
Type A: Phalanx proximal, distal extra-articular, and diaphysis simple fracture.
A1: Phalanx proximal extra-articular fracture.
A1.2: Comminuted fracture

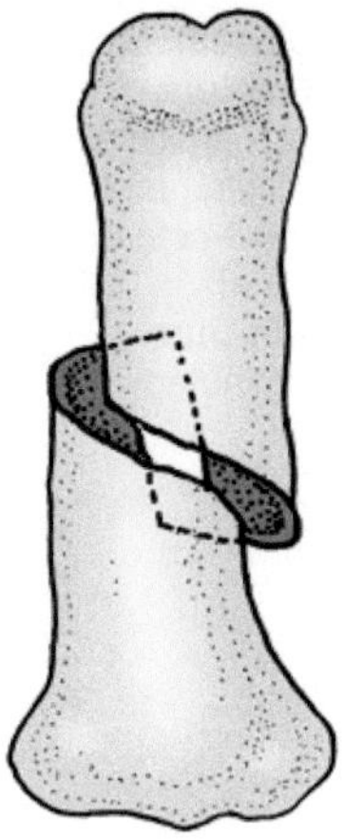

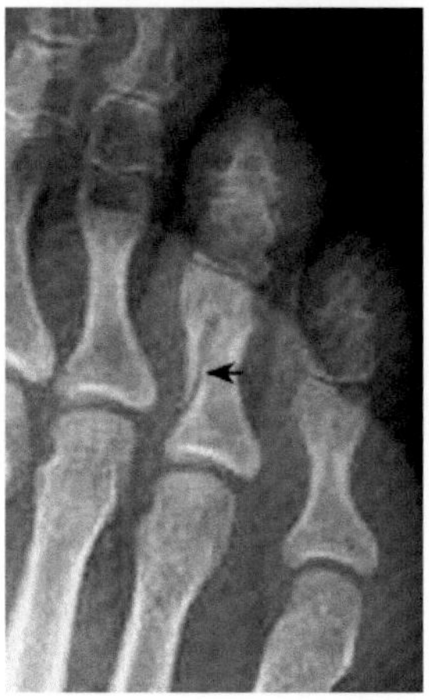

88 AO/OTA Classification of Phalangeal Fracture
Type A: Phalanx proximal, distal extra-articular, and diaphysis simple fracture.
A2: Phalanx diaphysis simple fracture.
A2.1: Simple spiral fracture

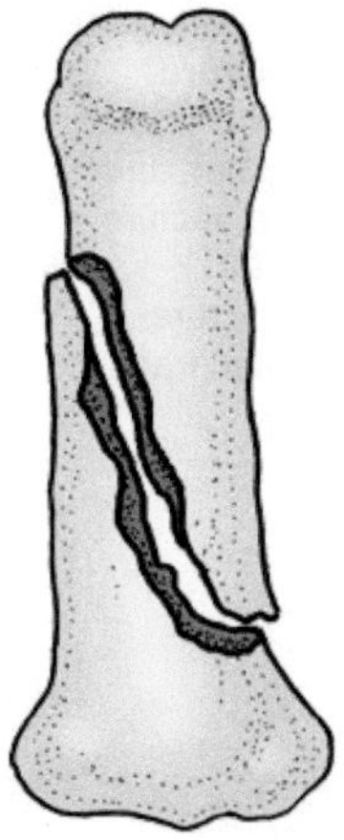

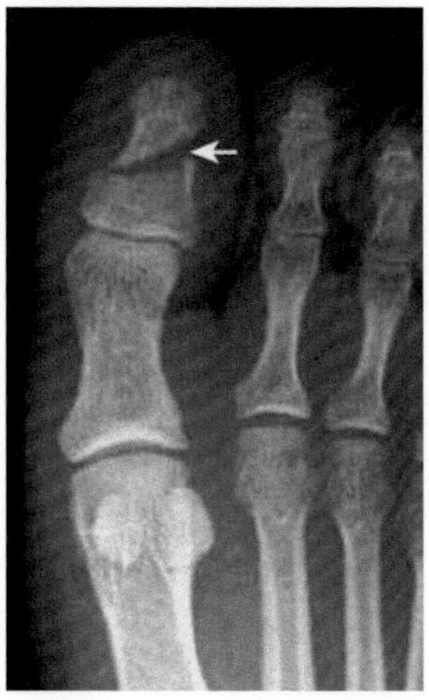

88 AO/OTA Classification of Phalangeal Fracture
Type A: Phalanx proximal, distal extra-articular, and diaphysis simple fracture.
A2: Phalanx diaphysis simple fracture.
A2.2: Simple oblique fracture

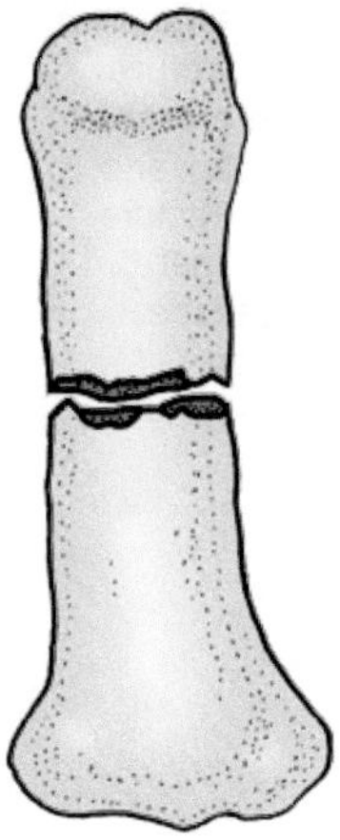

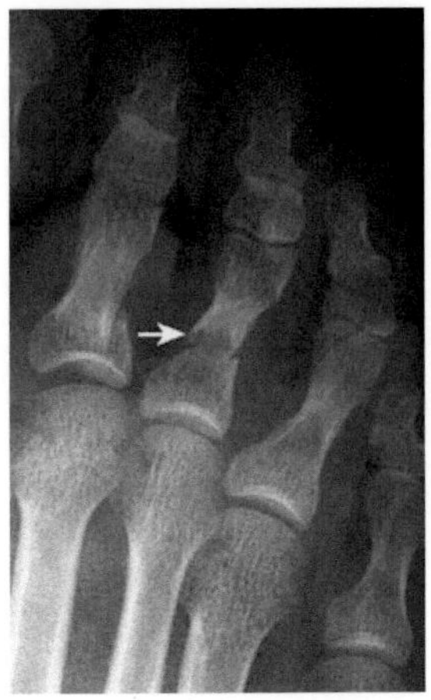

88 AO/OTA Classification of Phalangeal Fracture
Type A: Phalanx proximal, distal extra-articular, and diaphysis simple fracture.
A2: Phalanx diaphysis simple fracture.
A2.3: simple transverse fracture

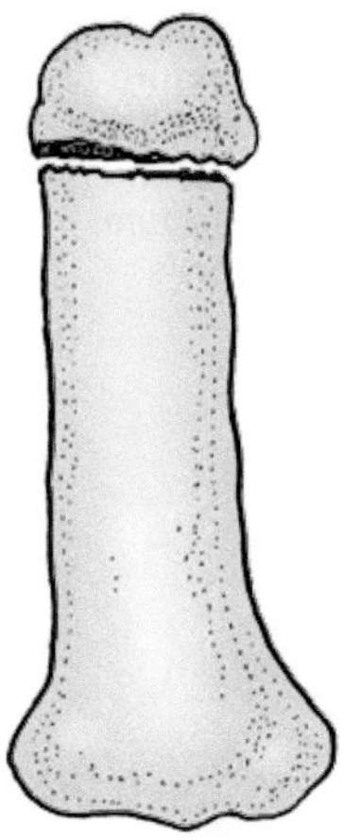

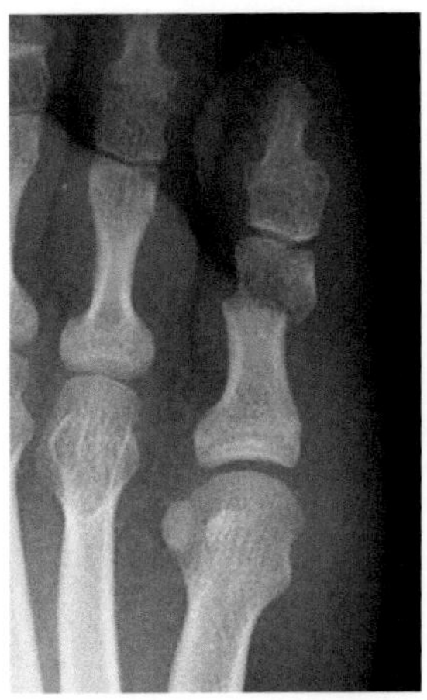

88 AO/OTA Classification of Phalangeal Fracture
Type A: Phalanx proximal, distal extra-articular, and diaphysis simple fracture.
A3: Phalanx distal extra-articular fracture.
A3.1: Noncomminuted fracture

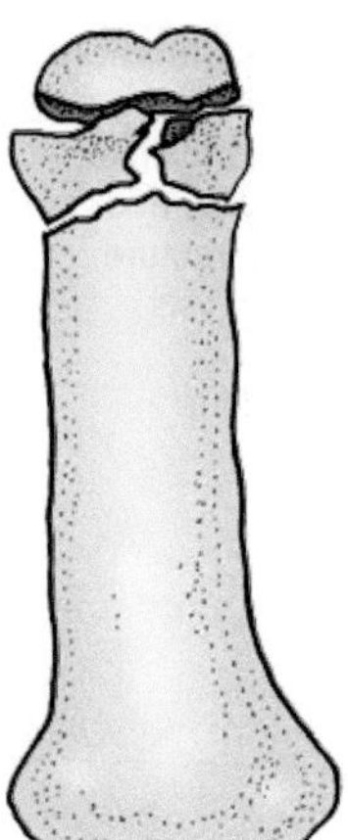

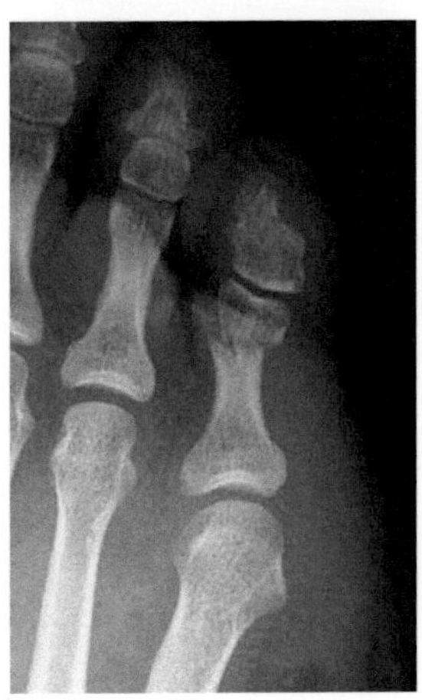

88 AO/OTA Classification of Phalangeal Fracture
Type A: Phalanx proximal, distal extra-articular, and diaphysis simple fracture.
A3: Phalanx distal extra-articular fracture.
A3.2: Comminuted fracture

Type B: Phalanx proximal and distal partial articular, and diaphysis wedge fracture:

Type B1: Phalanx proximal partial articular fracture:

Type B1.1: Avulsion or split fracture.

Type B1.2: Depression fracture.

Type B1.3: Split-depression fracture.

Type B2: Phalanx diaphysis wedge fracture:

Type B2.1: Phalanx diaphysis spiral wedge fracture.

Type B2.2: Phalanx diaphysis bending wedge fracture.

Type B2.3: Phalanx diaphysis fragmented wedge fracture.

Type B3: Phalanx distal partial articular fracture:

Type B3.1: Avulsion or split fracture.

Type B3.2: Depression fracture.

Type B3.3: Split-depression fracture.

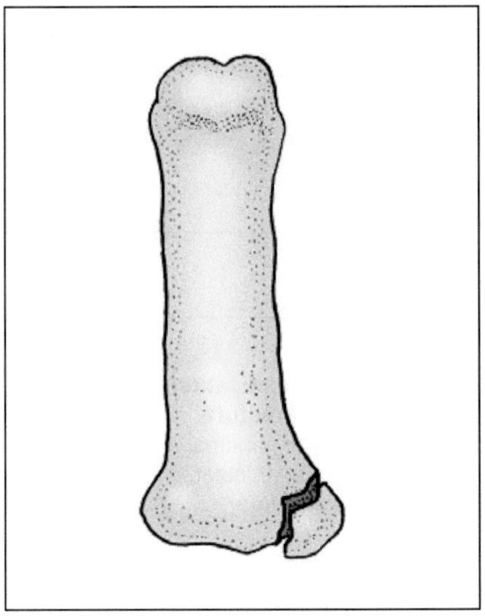

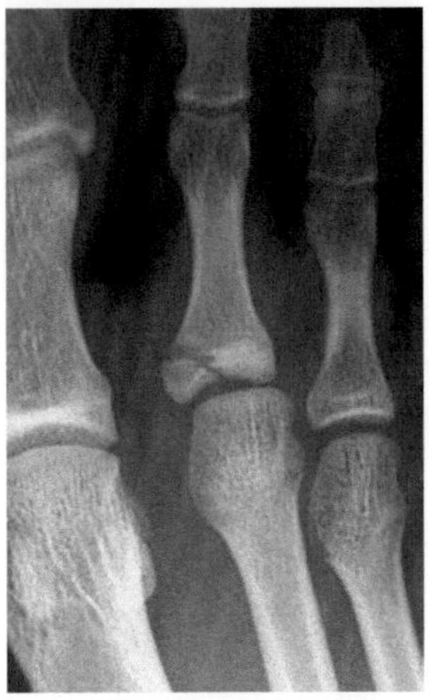

88 AO/OTA Classification of Phalangeal Fracture
Type B: Phalanx proximal and distal partial articular, and diaphysis wedge fracture.
B1: Phalanx proximal partial articular fracture.
B1.1: Avulsion or split fracture

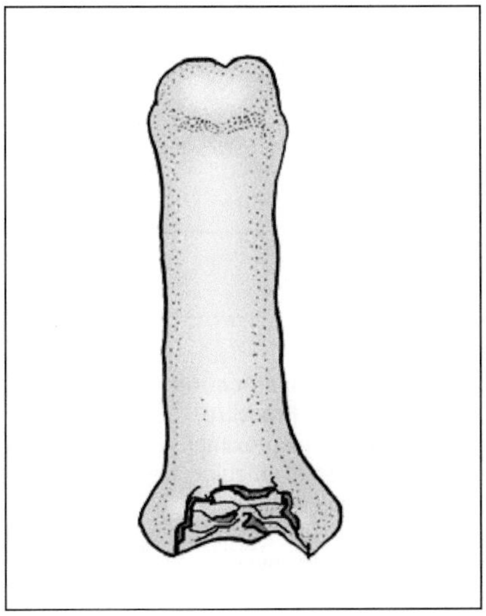

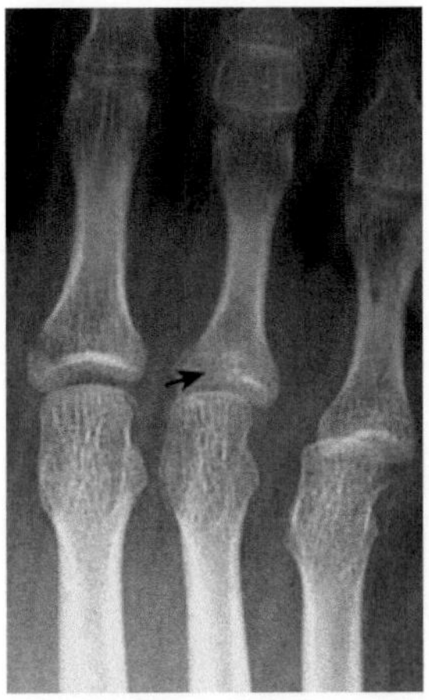

88 AO/OTA Classification of Phalangeal Fracture
Type B: Phalanx proximal and distal partial articular, and diaphysis wedge fracture.
B1: Phalanx proximal partial articular fracture.
B1.2: Depression fracture

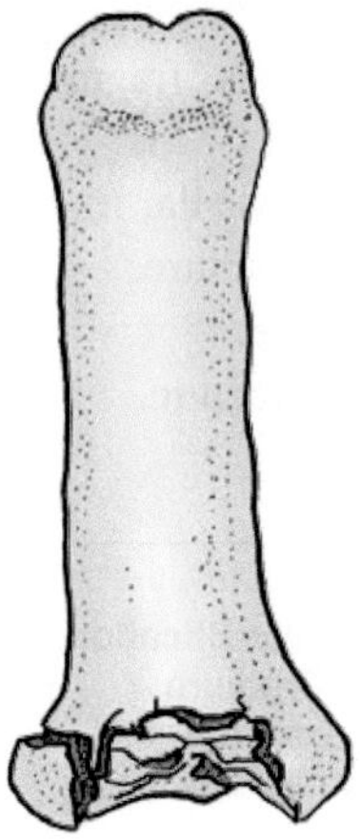

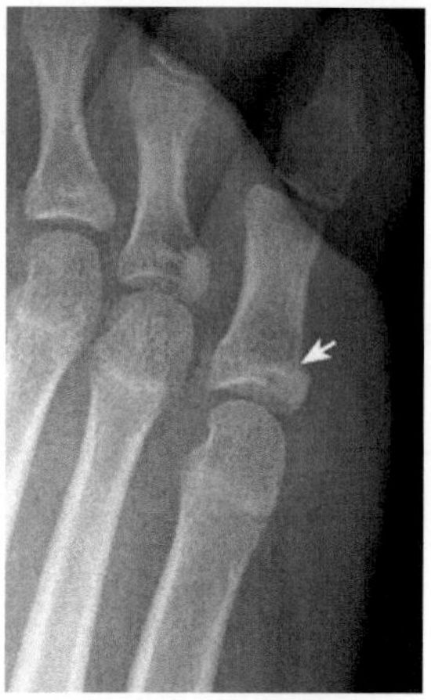

88 AO/OTA Classification of Phalangeal Fracture
Type B: Phalanx proximal and distal partial articular, and diaphysis wedge fracture.
B1: Phalanx proximal partial articular fracture.
B1.3: Split/depression fracture

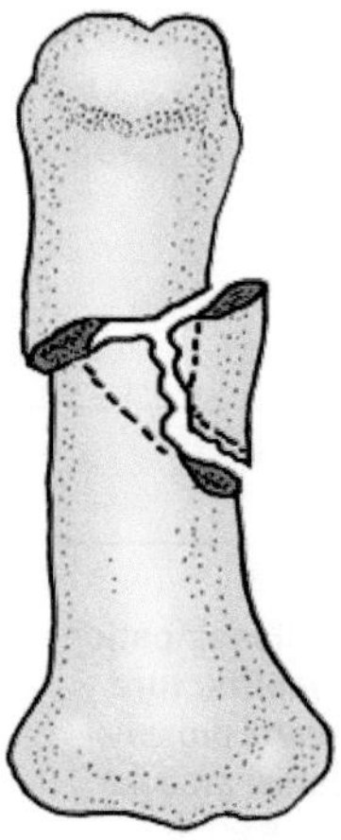

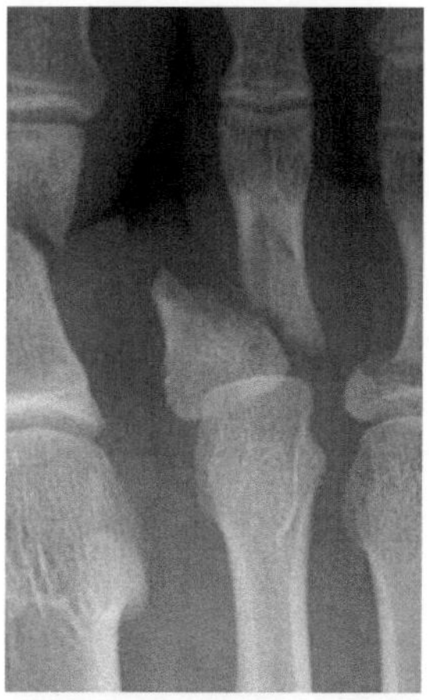

88 AO/OTA Classification of Phalangeal Fracture
Type B: Phalanx proximal and distal partial articular, and diaphysis wedge fracture.
B2: Phalanx diaphysis wedge fracture.
B2.1: Phalanx diaphysis spiral wedge fracture

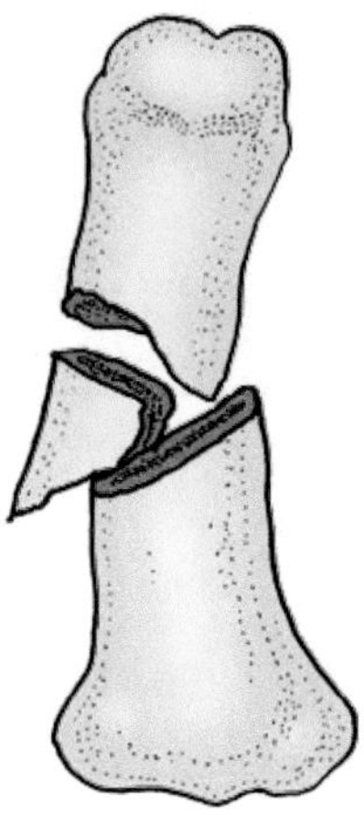

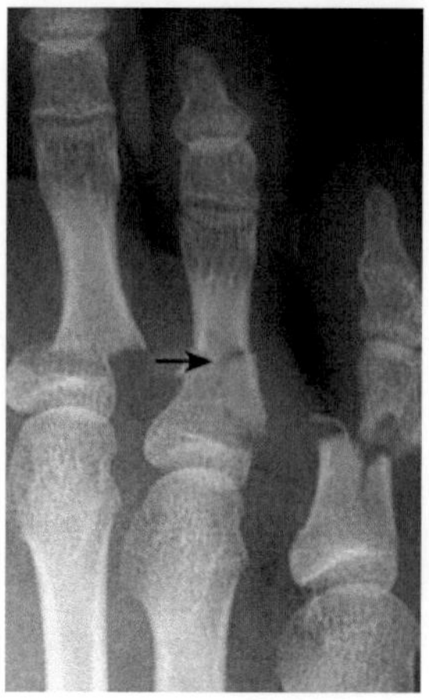

88 AO/OTA Classification of Phalangeal Fracture
Type B: Phalanx proximal and distal partial articular, and diaphysis wedge fracture.
B2: Phalanx diaphysis wedge fracture.
B2.2: Phalanx diaphysis bending wedge fracture

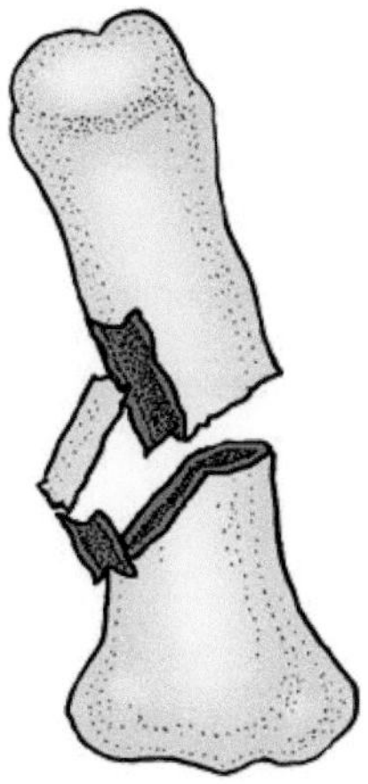

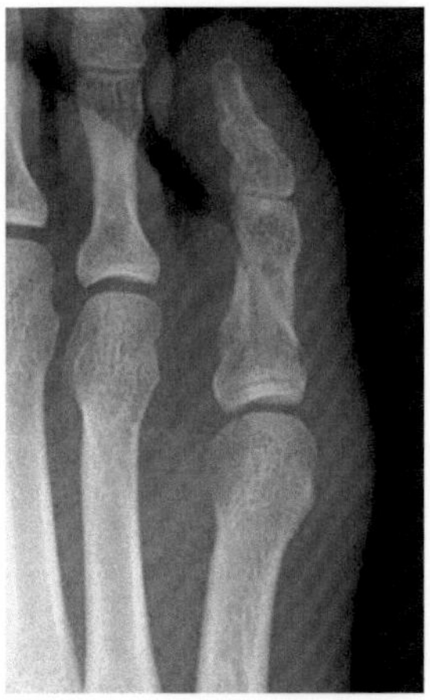

88 AO/OTA Classification of Phalangeal Fracture
Type B: Phalanx proximal and distal partial articular, and diaphysis wedge fracture.
B2: Phalanx diaphysis wedge fracture.
B2.3: Phalanx diaphysis fragmented wedge fracture

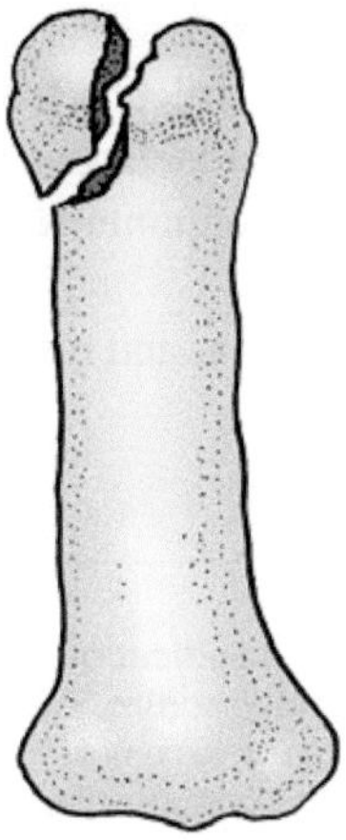

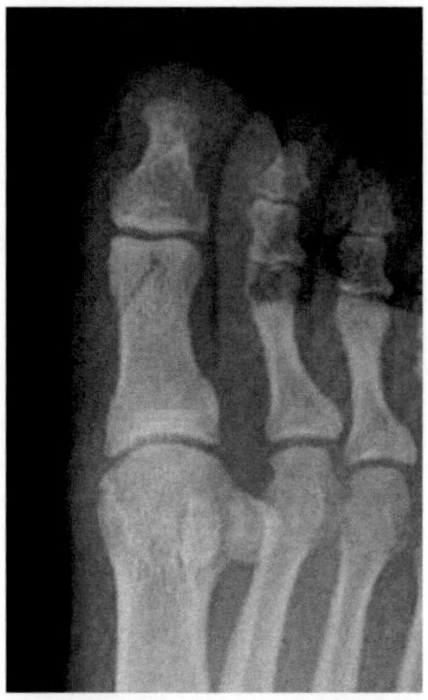

88 AO/OTA Classification of Phalangeal Fracture
Type B: Phalanx proximal and distal partial articular, and diaphysis wedge fracture.
B3: Phalanx distal partial articular fracture.
B3.1: Avulsion or split fracture

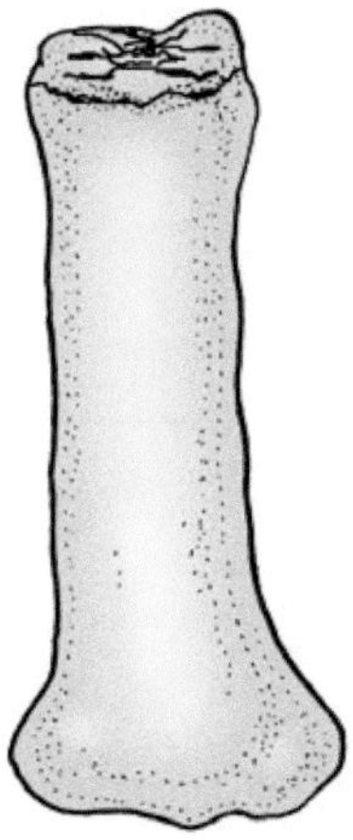

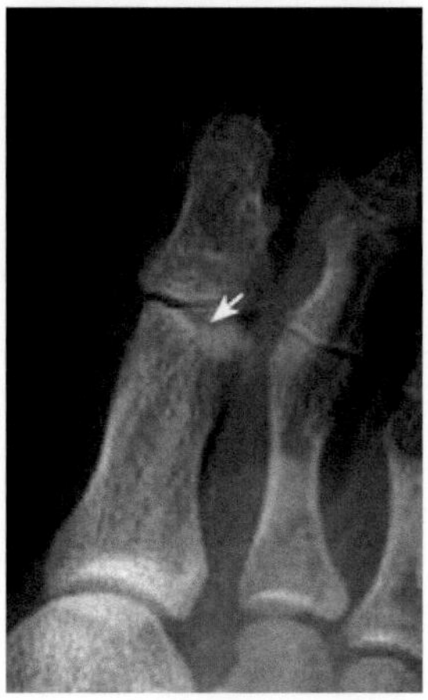

88 AO/OTA Classification of Phalangeal Fracture
Type B: Phalanx proximal and distal partial articular, and diaphysis wedge fracture.
B3: Phalanx distal partial articular fracture.
B3.2: Depression fracture

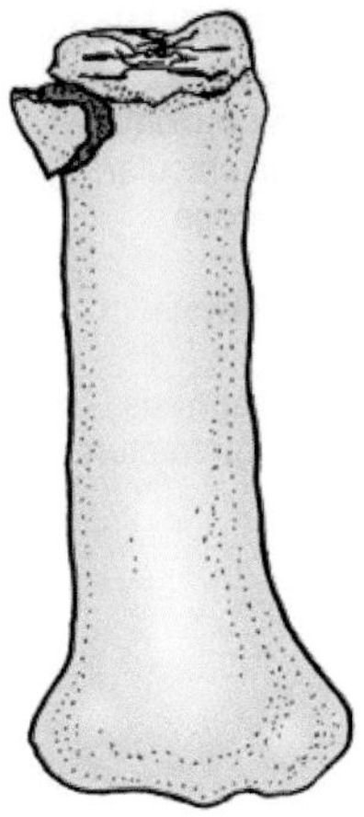

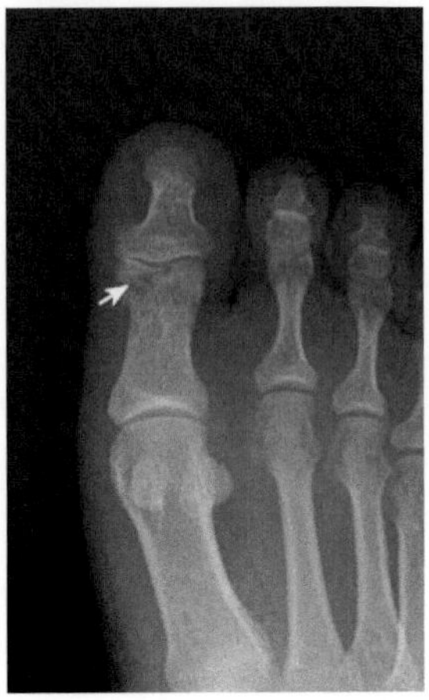

88 AO/OTA Classification of Phalangeal Fracture
Type B: Phalanx proximal and distal partial articular, and diaphysis wedge fracture.
B3: Phalanx distal partial articular fracture.
B3.3: Split/depression fracture

Type C: Phalanx proximal and distal complete articular, and diaphysis comminuted fracture:
- Type C1: Phalanx proximal complete articular fracture:
  - Type C1.1: Simple articular and metaphysis fracture.
  - Type C1.2: Simple articular, comminuted metaphysis fracture.
  - Type C1.3: Comminuted articular and metaphysis.
- Type C2: Phalanx diaphysis comminuted fracture:
  - Type C2.1: Segmental fracture.
  - Type C2.2: Complex comminuted.
- Type C3: Phalanx distal complete articular fracture:
  - Type C3.1: Simple articular and metaphysis fracture.
  - Type C3.2: Simple articular, comminuted metaphysis fracture.
  - Type C3.3: Comminuted articular and metaphysis.

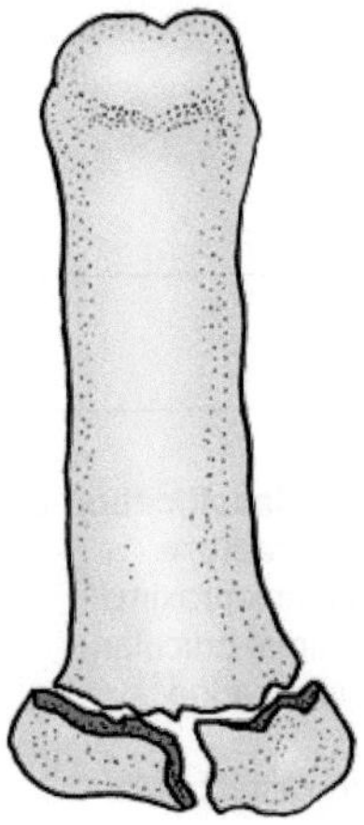

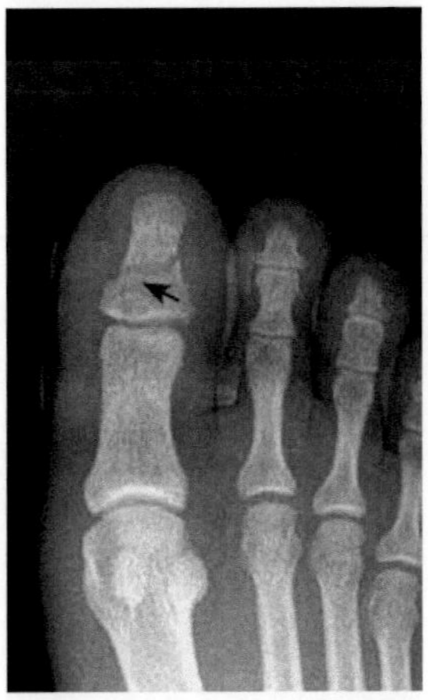

88 AO/OTA Classification of Phalangeal Fracture
Type C: Phalanx proximal and distal complete articular, and diaphysis comminuted fracture.
C1: Phalanx proximal complete articular fracture.
C1.1: Simple articular and metaphysis fracture

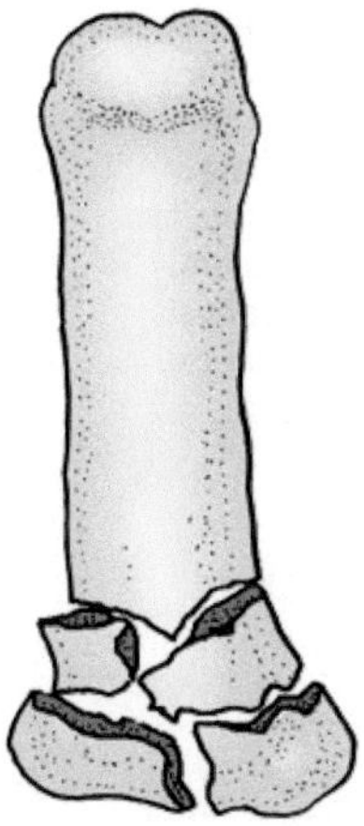

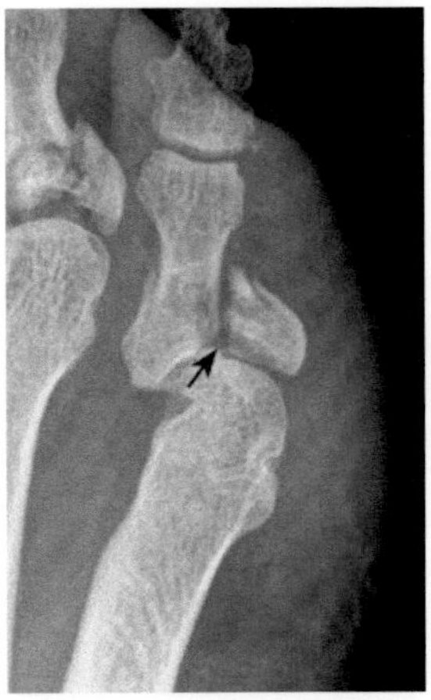

88 AO/OTA Classification of Phalangeal Fracture
Type C: Phalanx proximal and distal complete articular, and diaphysis comminuted fracture.
C1: Phalanx proximal complete articular fracture.
C1.2: Simple articular, comminuted metaphysis fracture

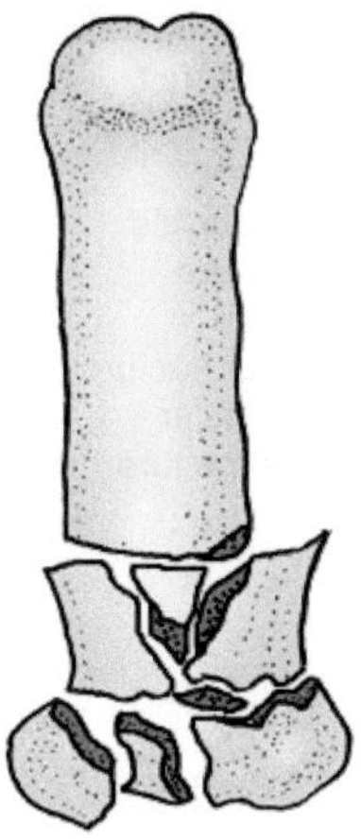

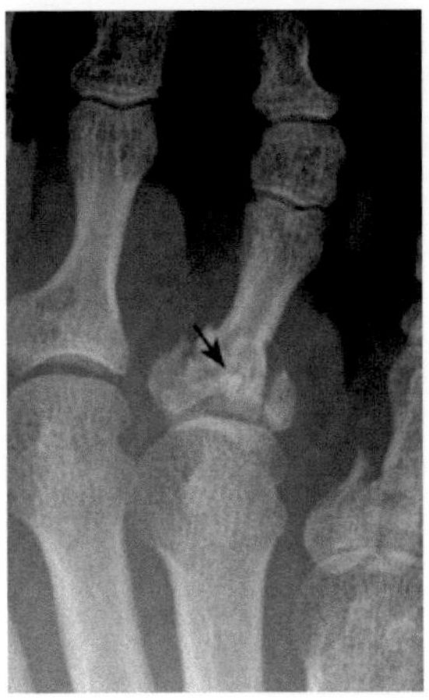

88 AO/OTA Classification of Phalangeal Fracture
Type C: Phalanx proximal and distal complete articular, and diaphysis comminuted fracture.
C1: Phalanx proximal complete articular fracture.
C1.3: Comminuted articular and metaphysis

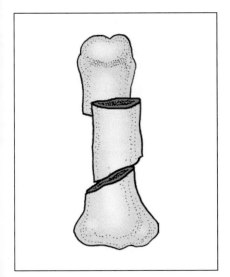

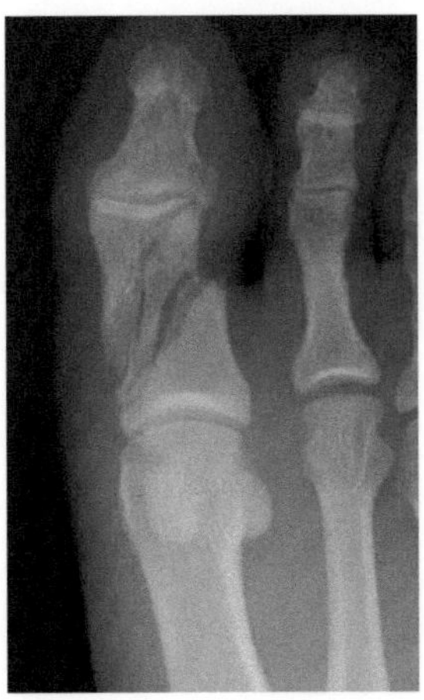

88 AO/OTA Classification of Phalangeal Fracture
Type C: Phalanx proximal and distal complete articular, and diaphysis comminuted fracture.
C2: Phalanx diaphysis comminuted fracture.
C2.1: Segmental fracture

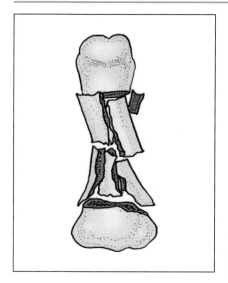

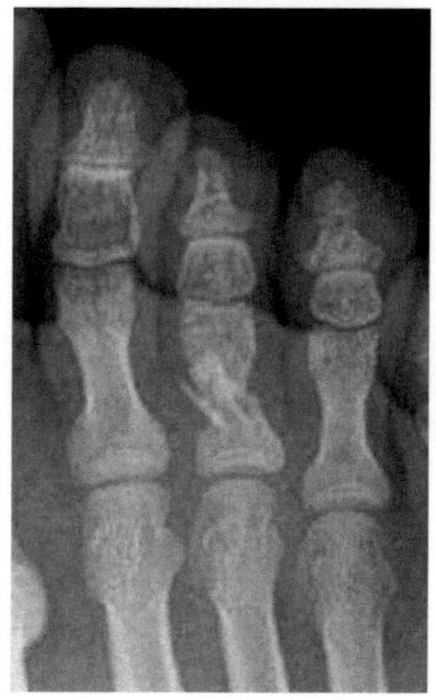

88 AO/OTA Classification of Phalangeal Fracture
Type C: Phalanx proximal and distal complete articular, and diaphysis comminuted fracture.
C2: Phalanx diaphysis comminuted fracture.
C2.2: Complex comminuted

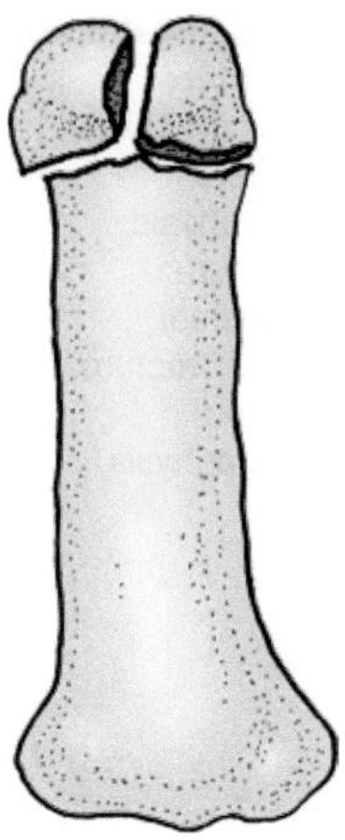

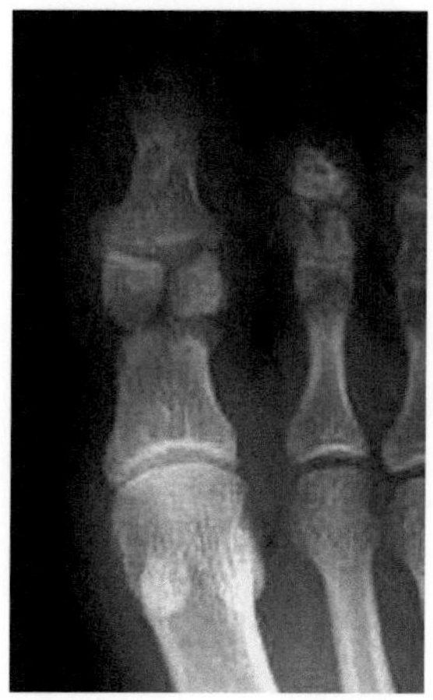

88 AO/OTA Classification of Phalangeal Fracture
Type C: Phalanx proximal and distal complete articular, and diaphysis comminuted fracture.
C3: Phalanx distal complete articular fracture.
C3.1: Simple articular and metaphysis fracture

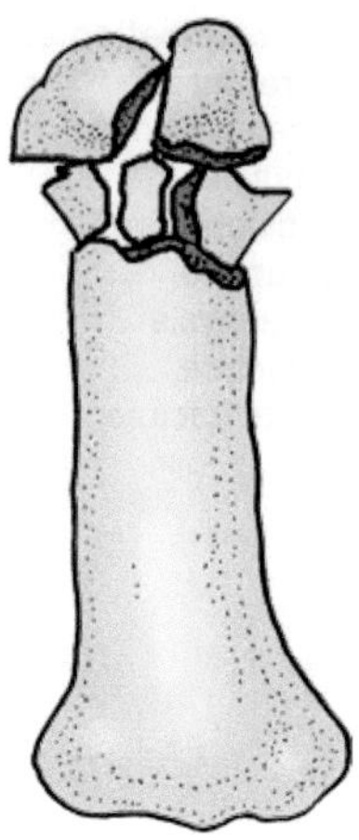

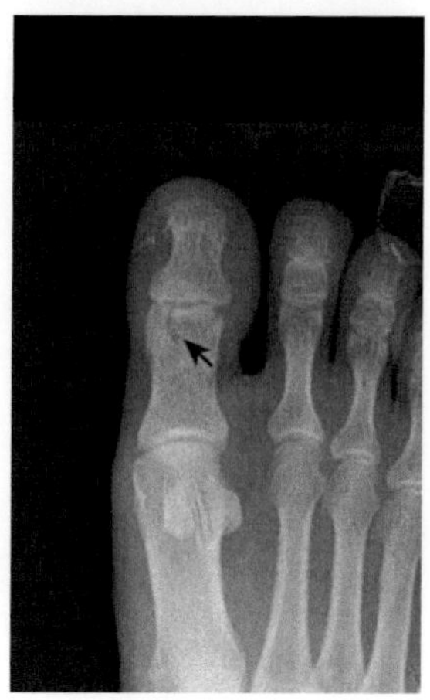

88 AO/OTA Classification of Phalangeal Fracture
Type C: Phalanx proximal and distal complete articular, and diaphysis comminuted fracture.
C3: Phalanx distal complete articular fracture.
C3.2: Simple articular, comminuted metaphysis fracture

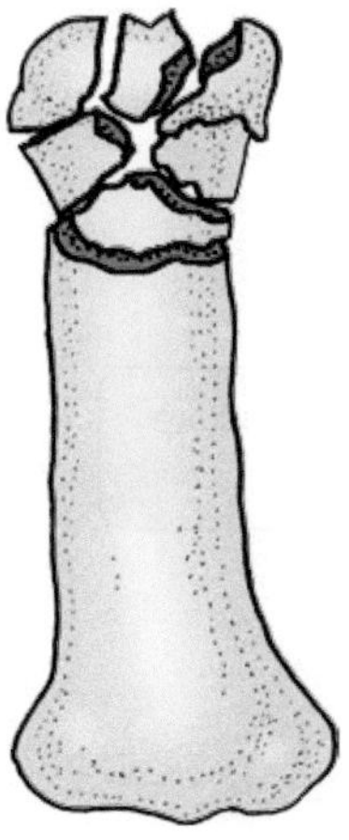

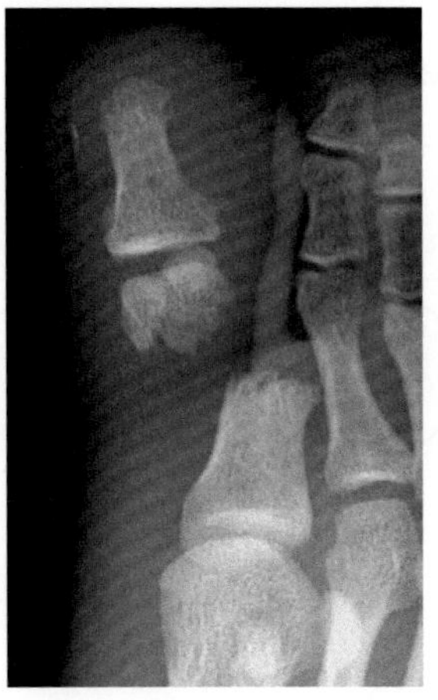

88 AO/OTA Classification of Phalangeal Fracture
Type C: Phalanx proximal and distal complete articular, and diaphysis comminuted fracture.
C3: Phalanx distal complete articular fracture.
C3.3: Comminuted articular and metaphysis

11.6 Section 5 Classification of Multiple Fracture of the Foot

11.6.1 AO/OTA Classification of Multiple Fracture of the Foot

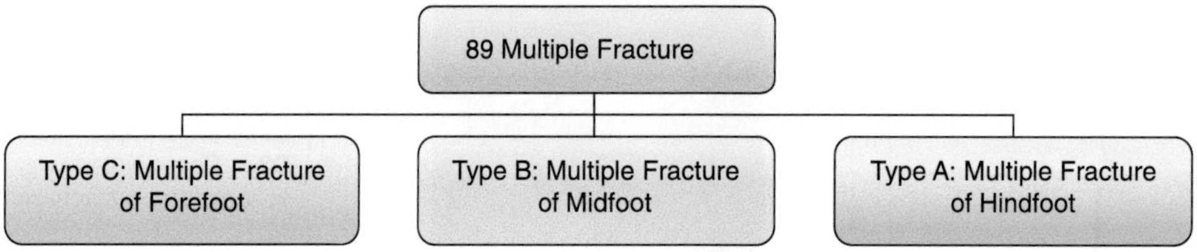

Type A: Multiple fracture of hindfoot.
Type B: Multiple fracture of midfoot.
Type C: Multiple fracture of forefoot.

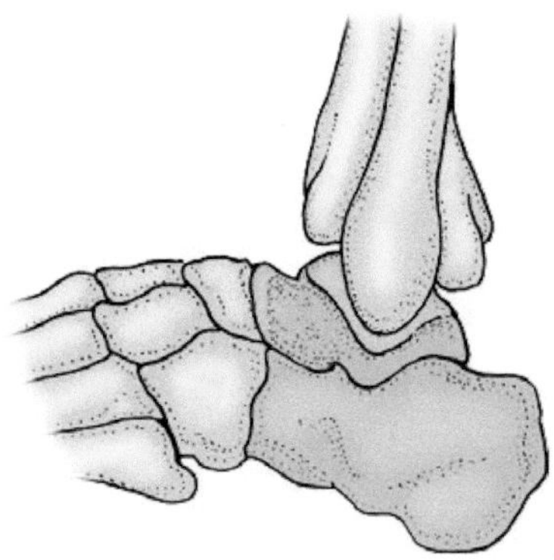

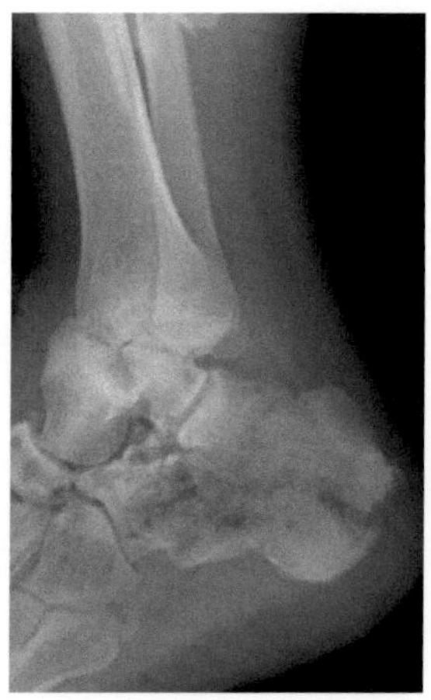

89 AO/OTA Classification of Multiple Fracture of the Foot
Type A: Multiple Fracture of Hindfoot

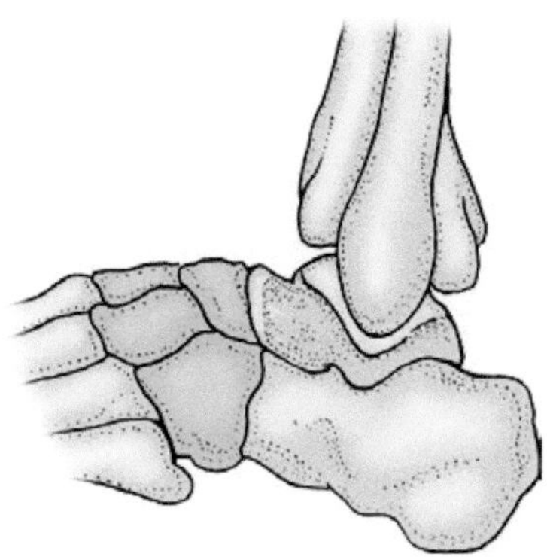

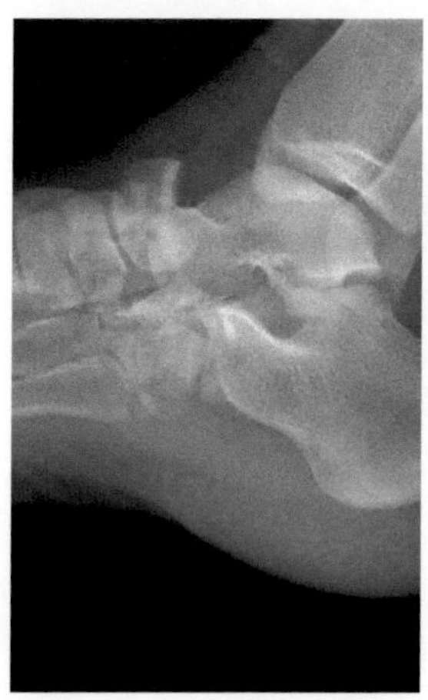

89 AO/OTA Classification of Multiple Fracture of the Foot
Type B: Multiple Fracture of Midfoot

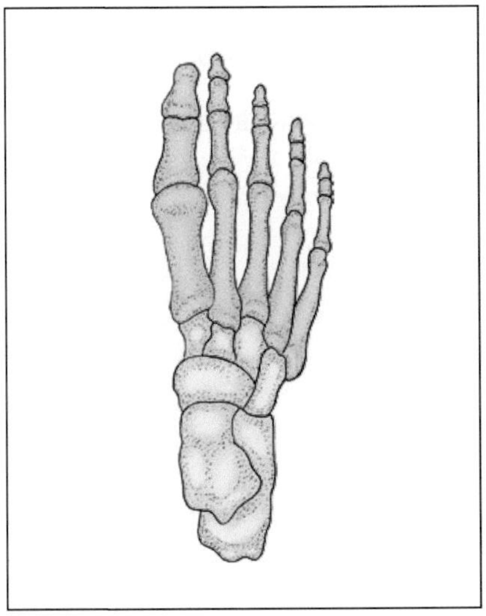

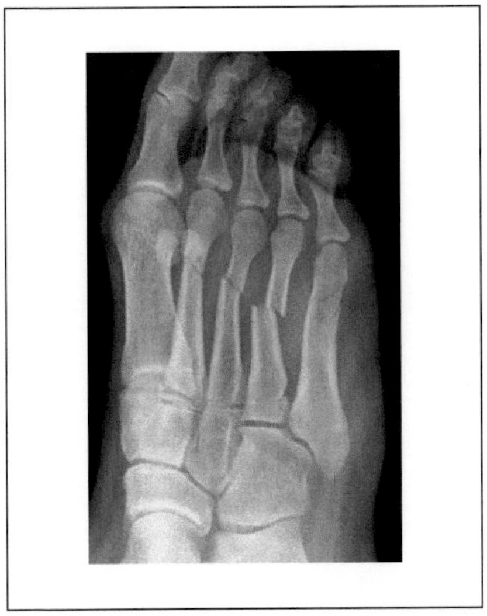

89 AO/OTA Classification of Multiple Fracture of the Foot
Type C: Multiple Fracture of Forefoot

11.6.2 Classification of Multiple Fracture of the Foot

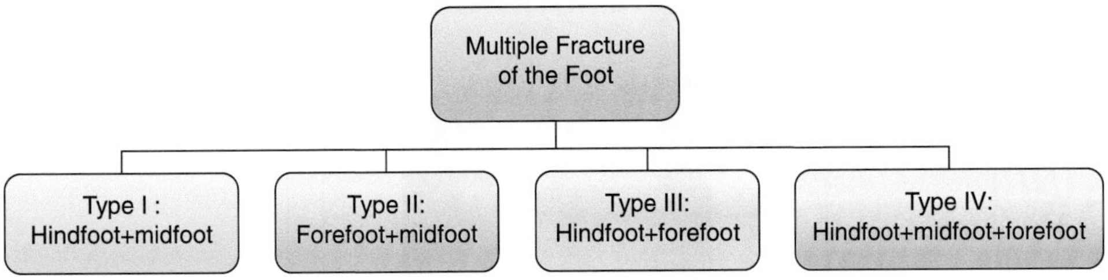

Type I: Hindfoot (single) + midfoot (single).
Type II: Forefoot (single) + midfoot (single).
Type III: Hindfoot (single) + forefoot (single).
Type IV: Hindfoot (single) + midfoot (single) + forefoot (single).

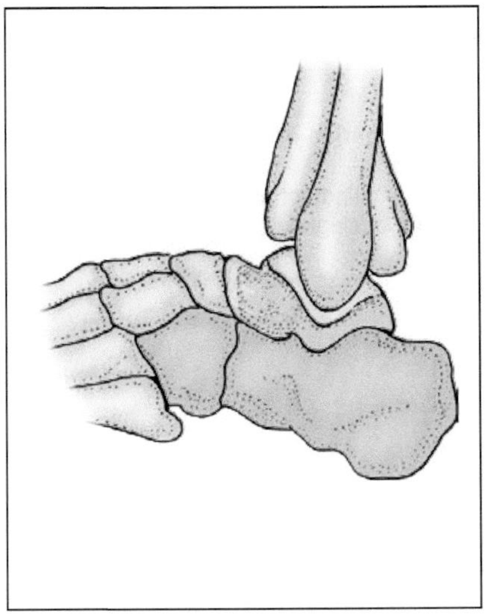

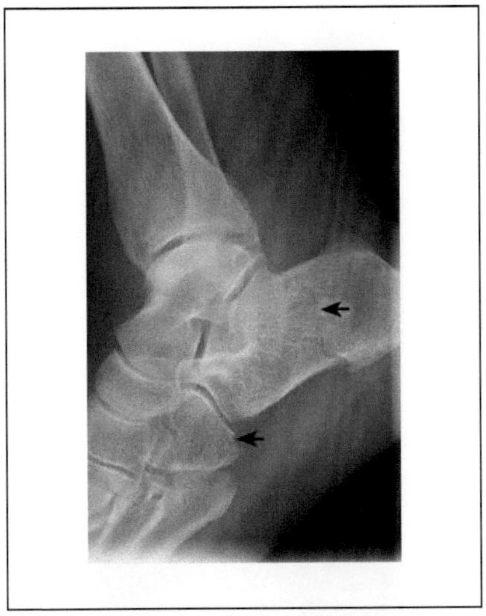

Classification of Multiple Fracture of the Foot
Type I: Hindfoot(single)+midfoot(single)

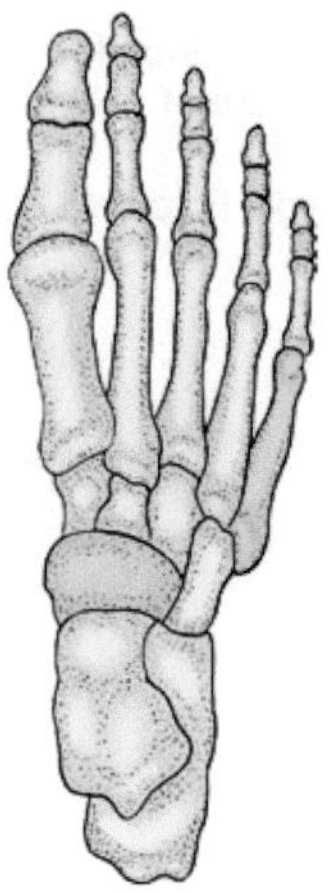

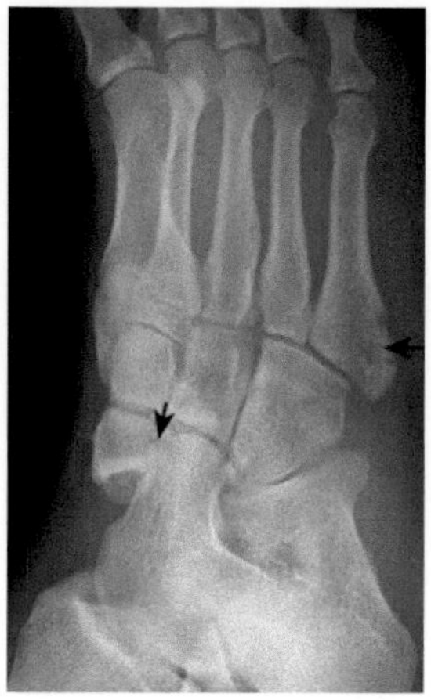

Classification of Multiple Fracture of the Foot
Type II: Forefoot(single)+midfoot(single)

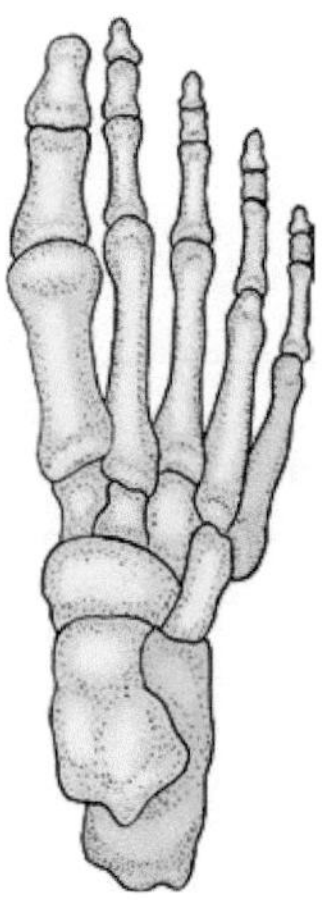

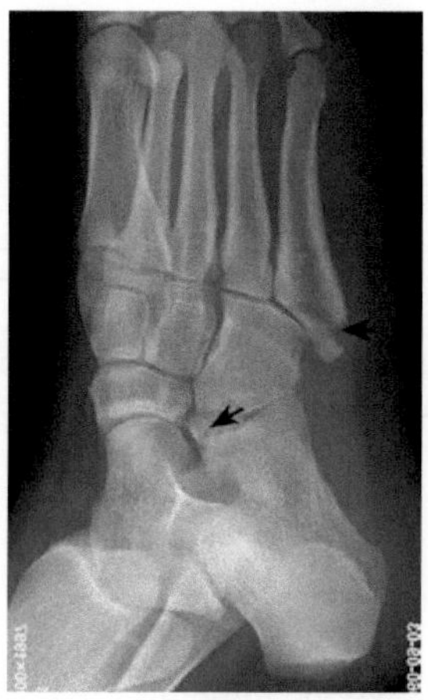

Classification of Multiple Fracture of the Foot
Type III: Hindfoot(single)+forefoot(single)

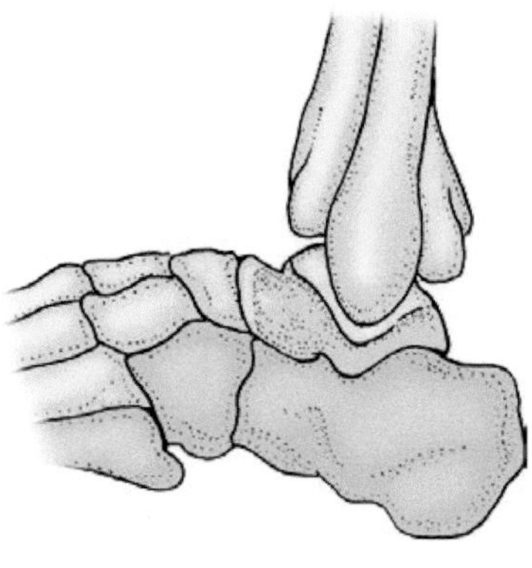

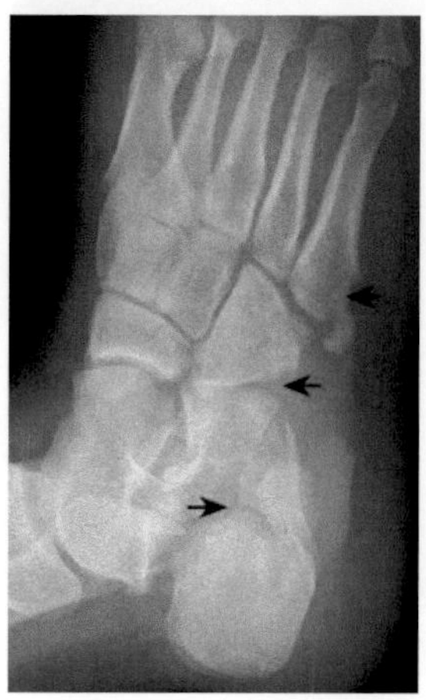

Classification of Multiple Fracture of the Foot
Type IV: Hindfoot(single)+midfoot(single)
+forefoot(single)

12 Classification of Hip Joint and Lower Extremity Dislocations

Yingze Zhang and Haotian Wu

12.1 Section 1 Classification of Hip Joint Dislocations

A classification of hip joint dislocations was first proposed by Ashley Copper in 1791, which divided them into four types; types I–III were associated with different degrees of acetabular fractures, and type IV was associated with femoral head and neck fractures.

12.1.1 Classification of Hip Joint Dislocation

12.1.1.1 **Brumback Classification** (1987, St. Louis, C V Mosby, 181–206)

Type I: Posterior hip dislocation with fracture of the femoral head involving the inferomedial portion of the femoral head (nonweight-bearing area of the femoral head).
- Type Ia: With minimum or no fracture of the acetabular rim and stable hip joint after reduction.
- Type Ib: With significant acetabular rim and unstable joint after reconstruction.

Type II: Posterior hip dislocation with fracture of the femoral head involving the supermedial portion of the femoral head (weight-bearing area of the femoral head).
- Type IIa: With minimum or no fracture of the acetabular rim and stable joint after reduction.
- Type IIb: With significant acetabular fracture and hip joint instability.

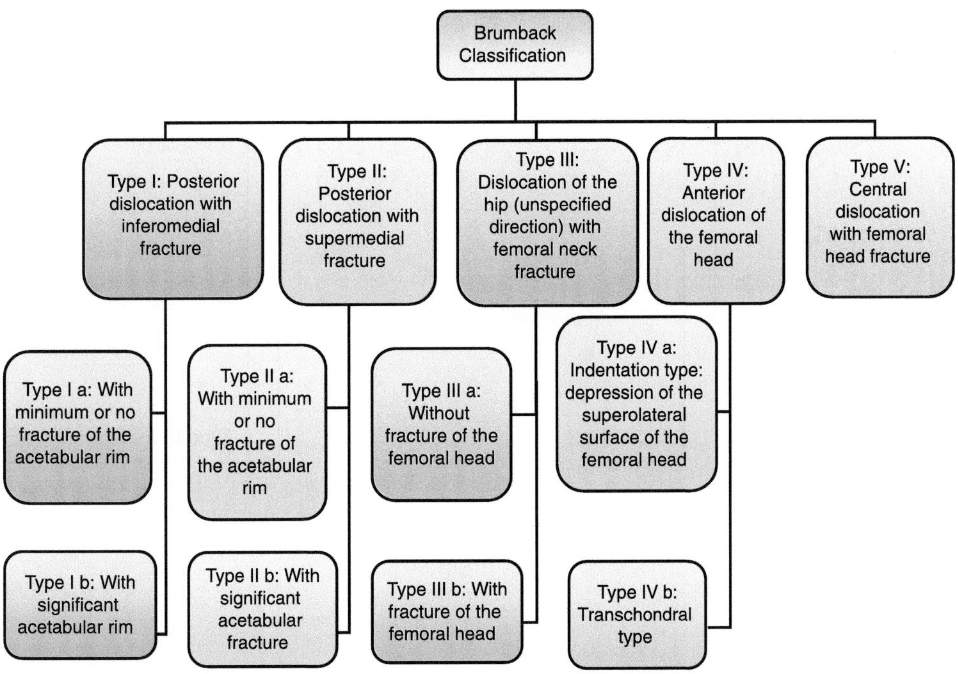

Y. Zhang (✉) • H. Wu
Department of Orthopedics,
The Third Hospital of Hebei Medical University,
Shijiazhuang, China
e-mail: yzzhangdr@126.com, yzling_liu@163.com

Y. Zhang (ed.), *Clinical Classification in Orthopaedics Trauma*, https://doi.org/10.1007/978-981-10-6044-1_12

Type III: Dislocation of the hip (unspecified direction) with femoral neck fracture.

Type IIIa: Without fracture of the femoral head.

Type IIIb: With fracture of the femoral head.

Type IV: Anterior dislocation of the femoral head.

Type IVa: Indentation type: depression of the superolateral surface of the femoral head.

Type IVb: Transchondral type; osteocartilaginous shear fracture of the weight-bearing surface of the femoral head.

Type V: Central fracture-dislocation of the hip with femoral head fracture.

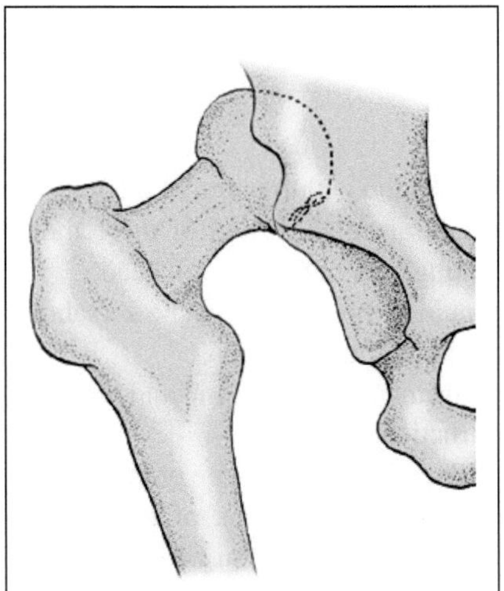
Type I a

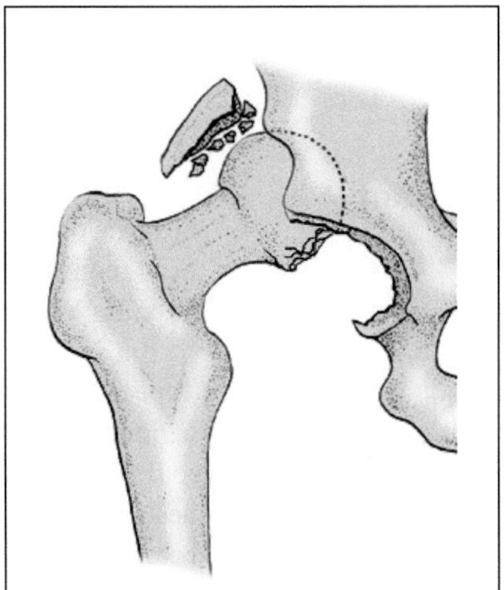
Type I b

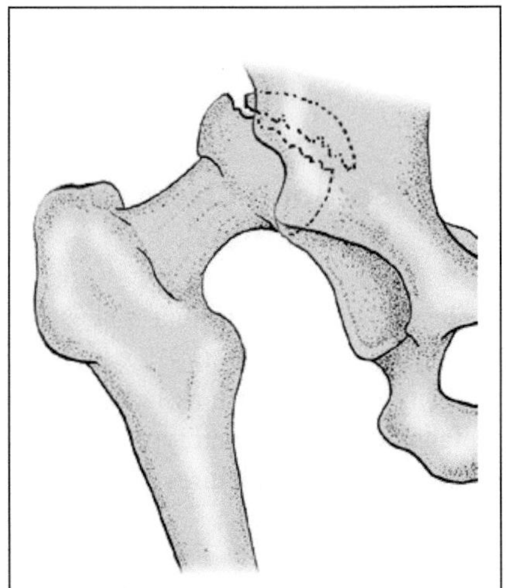
Type II b

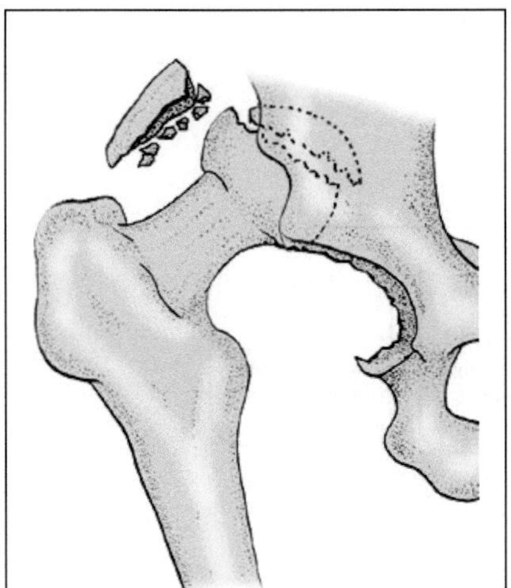
Type II b

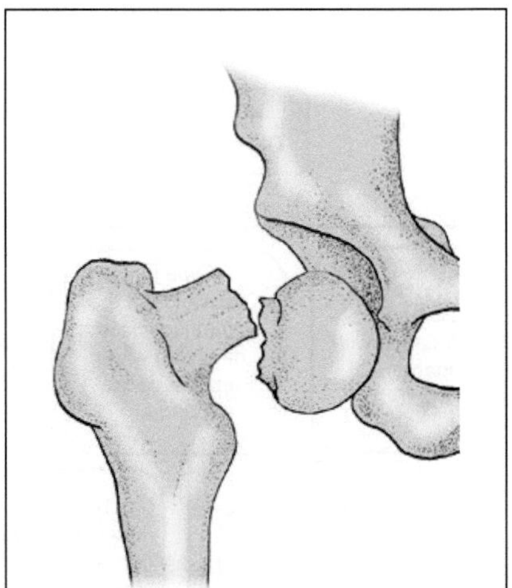
Type III a

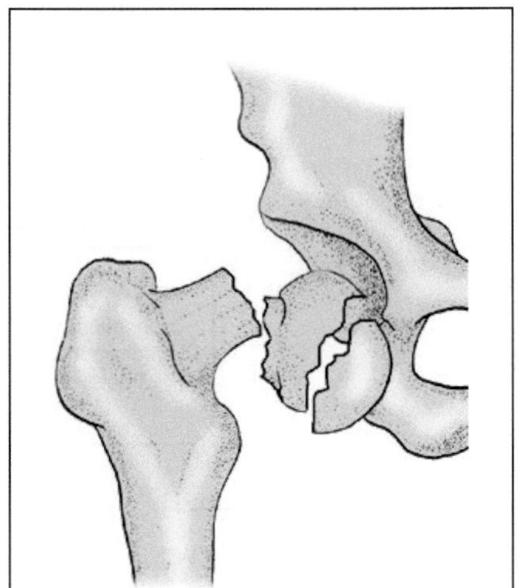
Type III b

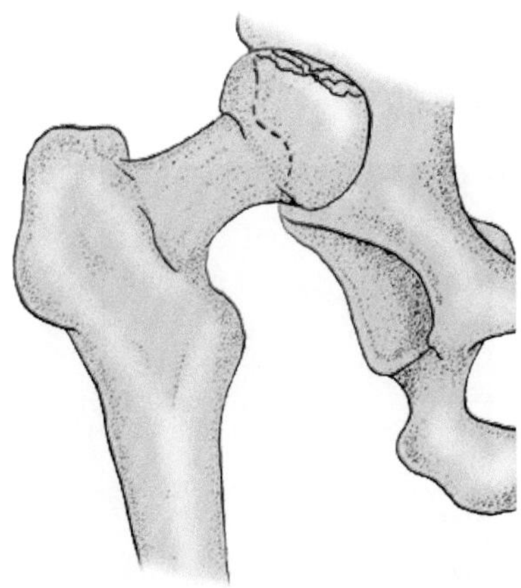
Type IV a

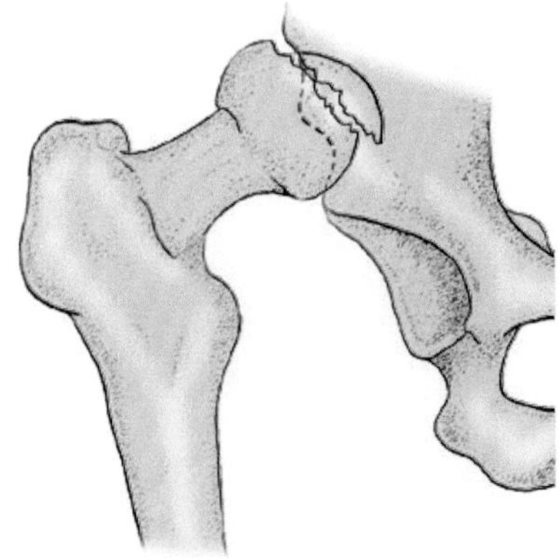
Type IV b

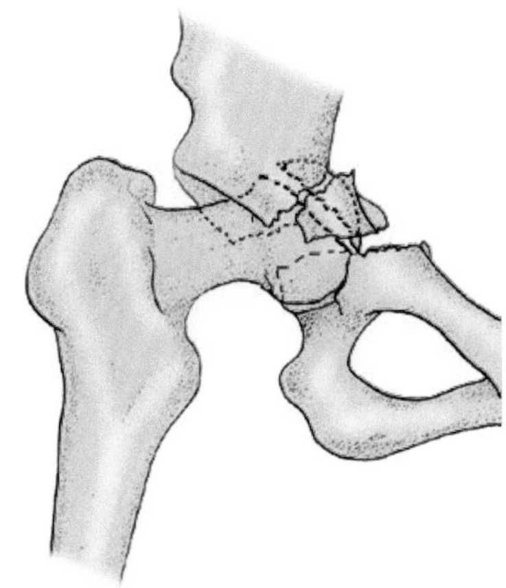
Type V

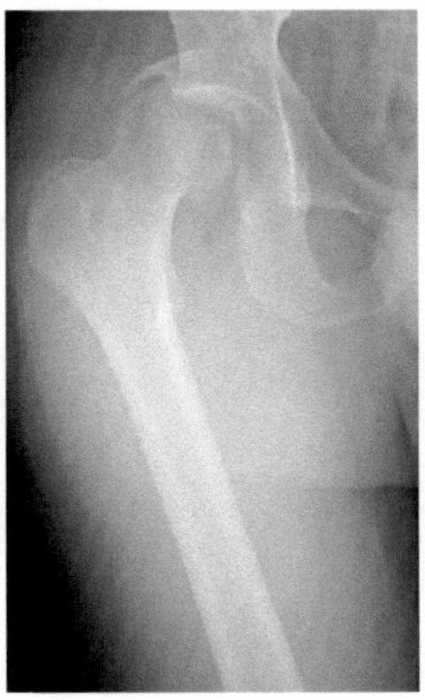
Type I b

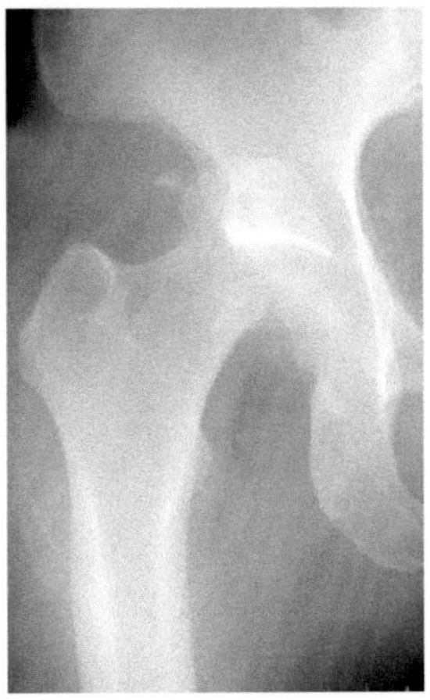
Type II a

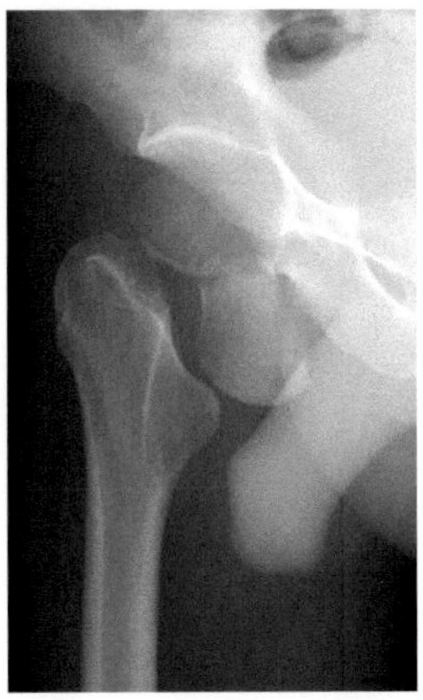
Type III b

12.1.1.2 **AO/OTA Classification** (2007, Journal of Orthopaedic Trauma. 21 supplement; Originally proposed in 80s, revised in 2007)

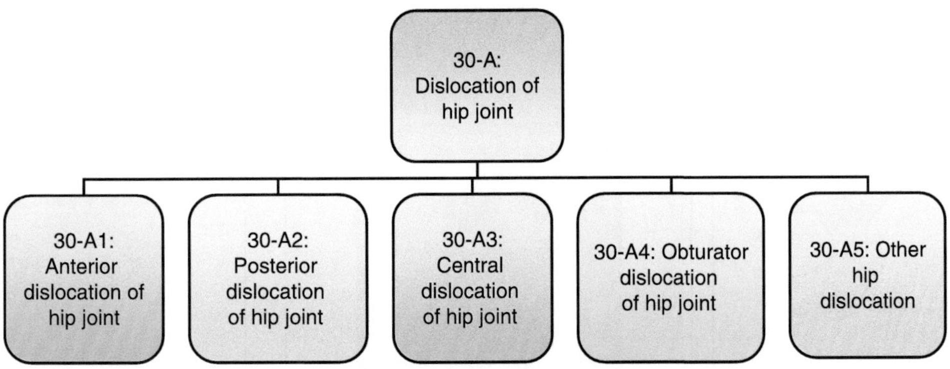

30-A1: Anterior dislocation of hip joint
30-A2: Posterior dislocation of hip joint.
30-A3: Central dislocation of hip joint.
30-A4: Obturator dislocation of hip joint.
30-A5: Other hip dislocation.

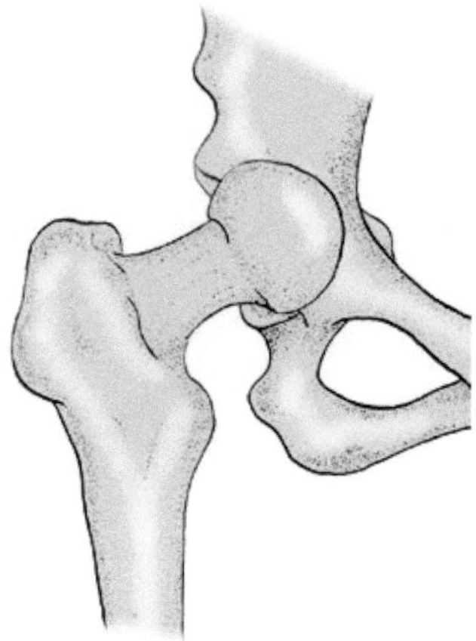

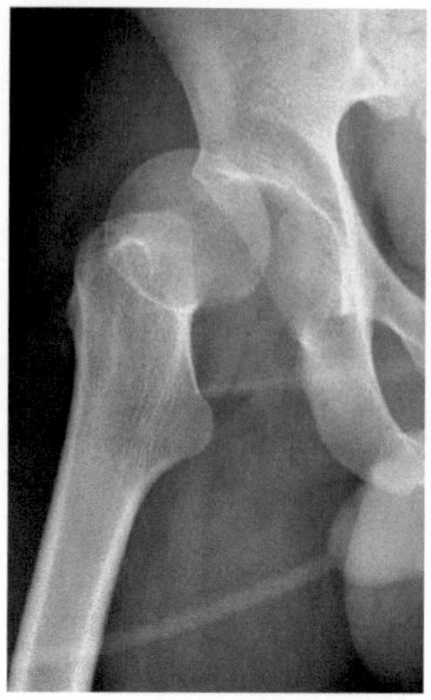

30-A AO/OTA classification of hip dislocation
A1: Anterior dislocation of hip joint)

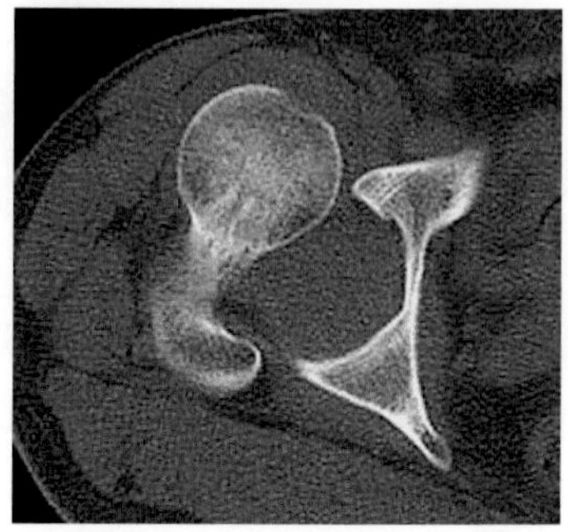

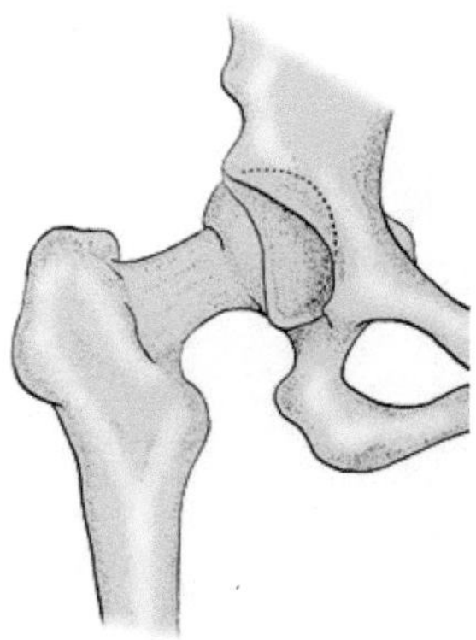

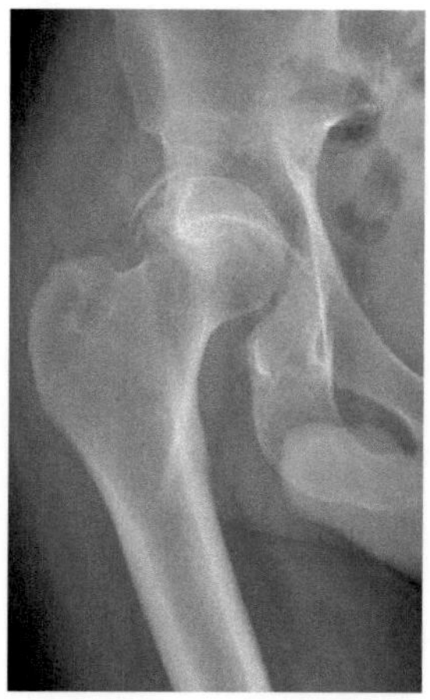

30-A AO/OTA classification of hip dislocation
A1: Anterior dislocation of hip joint)

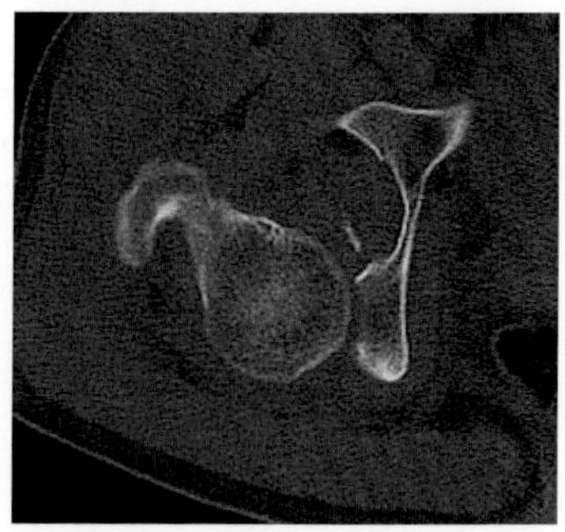

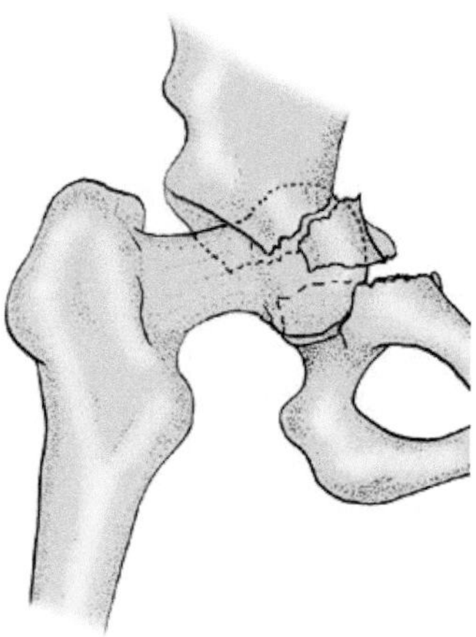

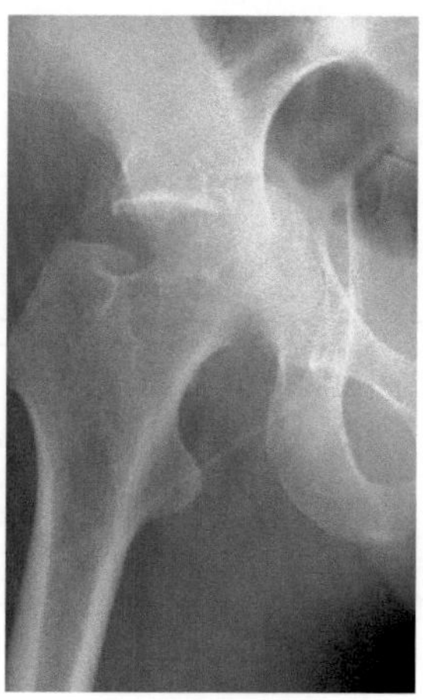

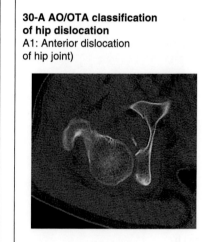

30-A AO/OTA classification of hip dislocation
A3: Central dislocation of hip joint

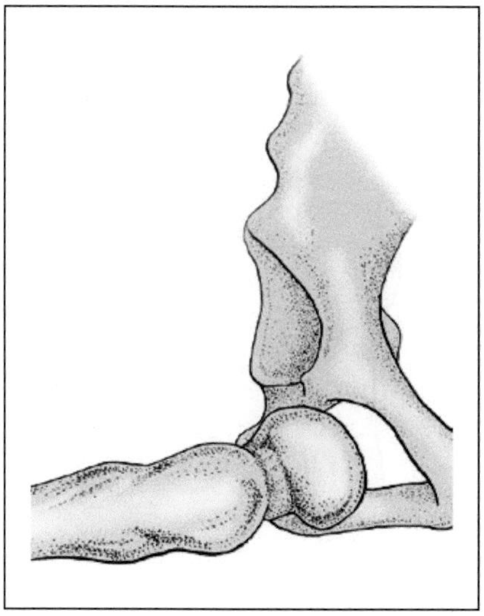

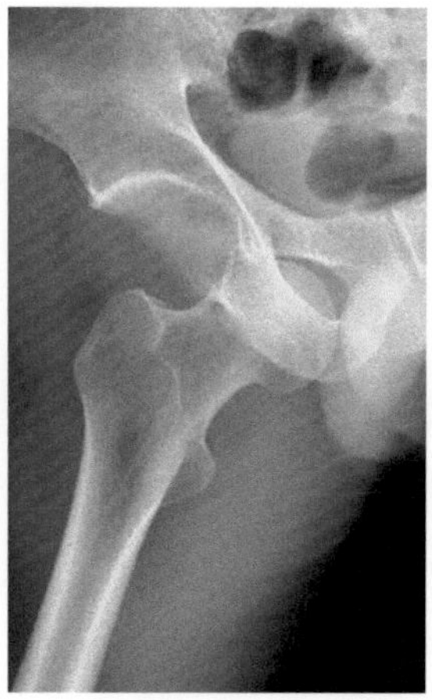

30-A AO/OTA classification of hip dislocation
A4: Obturator dislocation of hip joint

12.1.2 Classification of Anterior Hip Joint Dislocation

12.1.2.1 Epstein Classification

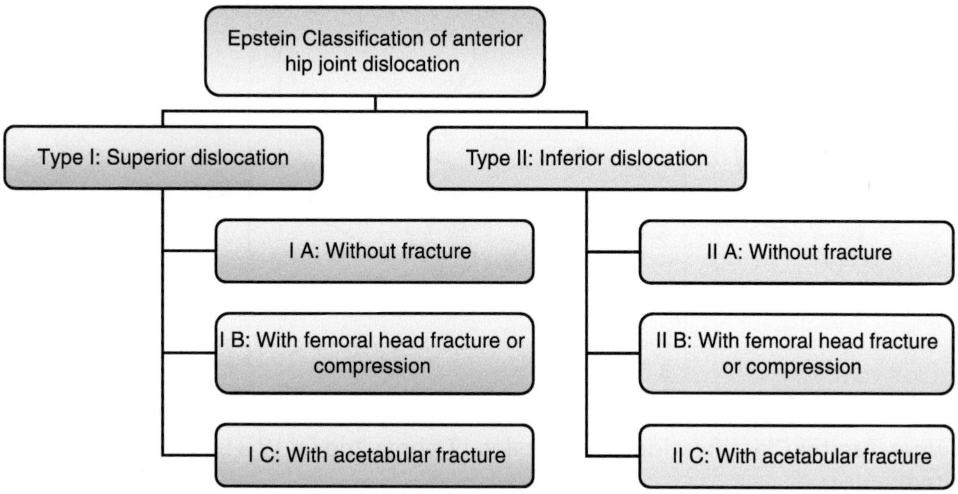

Type I: Superior dislocation of the hip.
- Type IA: Without fracture.
- Type IB: With femoral head fracture or compression.
- Type IC: With acetabular fracture.

Type II: Inferior dislocation of the hip, including obturator and perineum dislocation.
- Type IIA: Without fracture.
- Type IIB: With femoral head fracture or compression.
- Type IIC: With acetabular fracture.

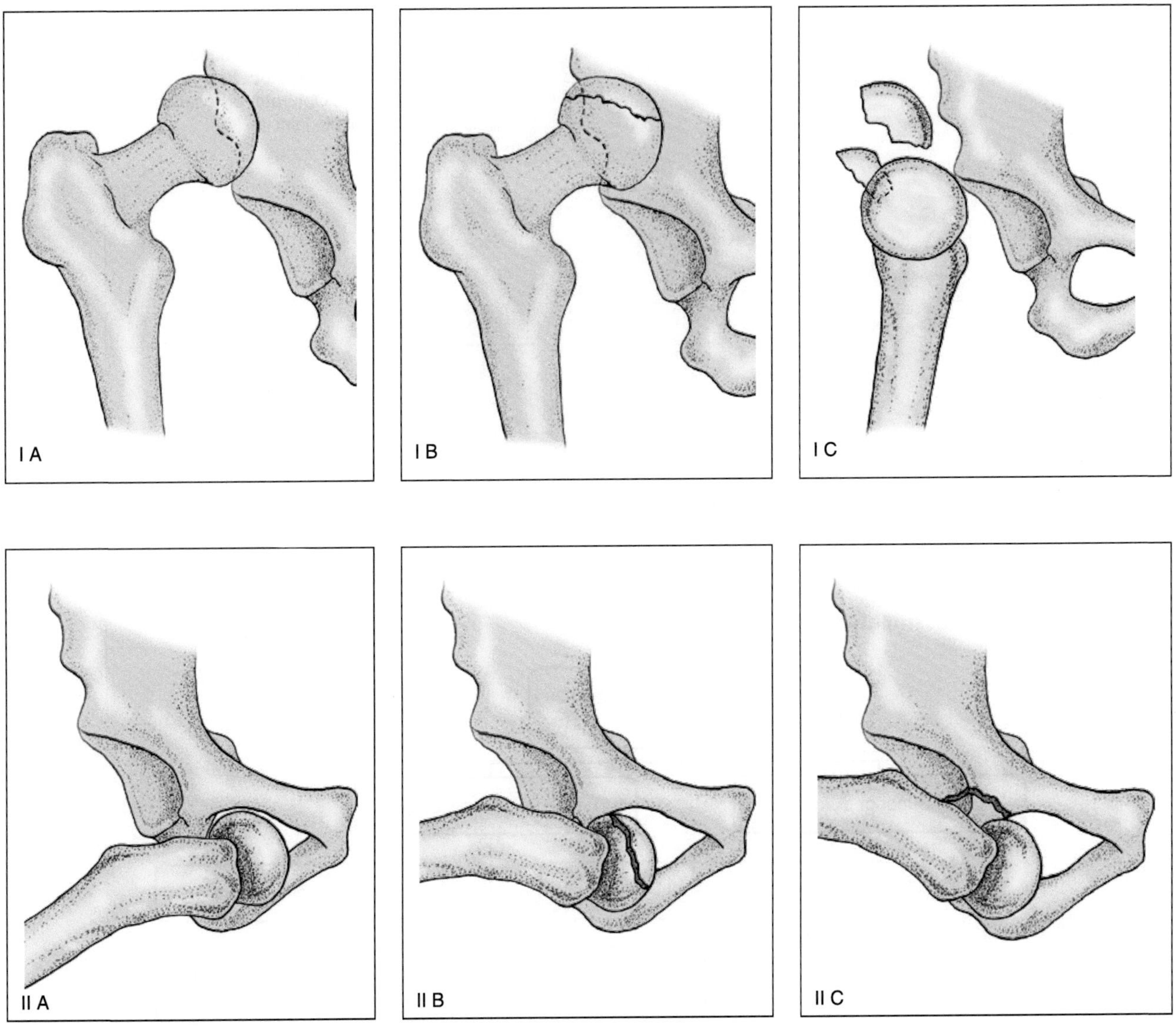

12.1.2.2 **Browner-Jupiter Classification** (1998, Skeletal Trauma 2nd Ed. W B Saunders: Harcount Publishers Limited)

Type I: No significant related to fracture, stable after axial traction.

Type II: Unreduced dislocation without femoral head and acetabulum fractures.

Type III: Unstable after traction, has potential cartilage or acetabulum labrum injury or acetabular fractures.

Type IV: Acetabulum fractures require to be rebuilt in order to obtain the stability of hip or joint symmetry.

Type V: With femoral head or neck fractures or impact.

12.1.3 Classification of Posterior Hip Joint Dislocation

12.1.3.1 Thompson-Epstein Classification (1951, J Bone Joint Surg (Am), 33:746–778)

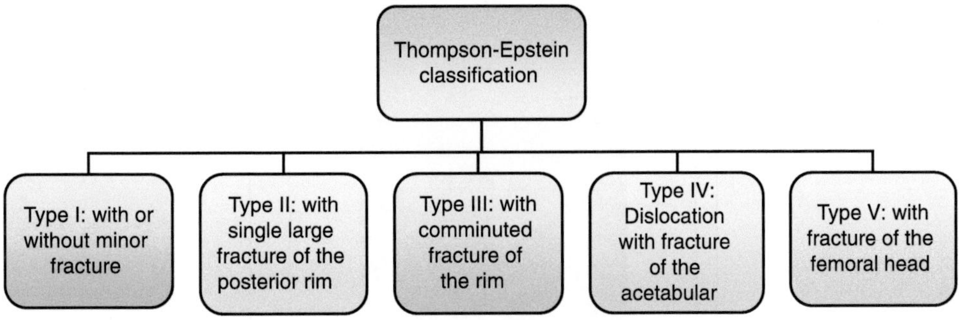

Type I: Dislocation with or without minor fracture.

Type II: Dislocation with single large fracture of the posterior rim of the acetabulum.

Type III: Dislocation with comminuted fracture of the rim, with or without a large major fragment.

Type IV: Dislocation with fracture of the acetabular floor.

Type V: Dislocation with fracture of the femoral head.

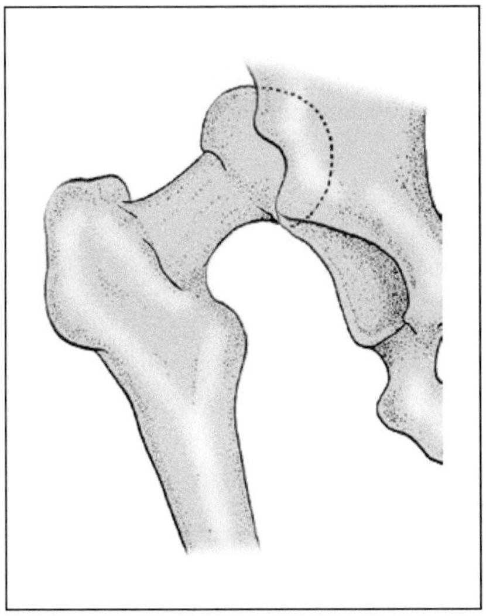

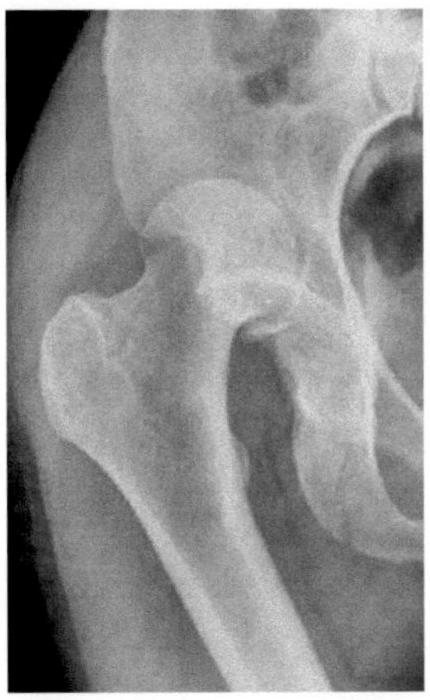

Thompson-Epstein
Classification of Posterior hip joint dislocation
Type I: Dislocation with or without minor fracture.

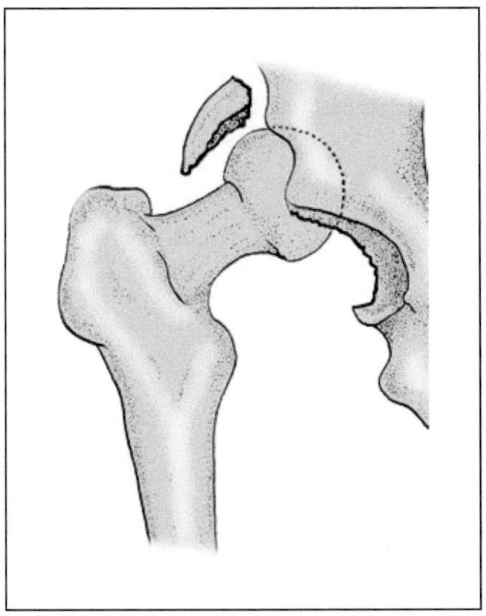

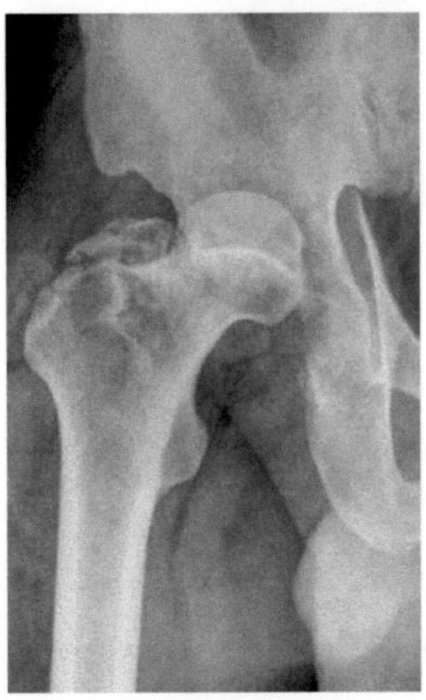

Thompson-Epstein
Classification of Posterior hip joint dislocation
Type II: Dislocation with single large fracture of the posterior rim of the acetabulum.

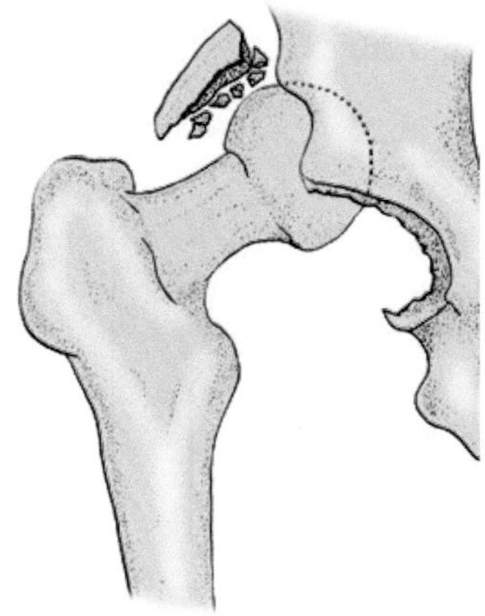

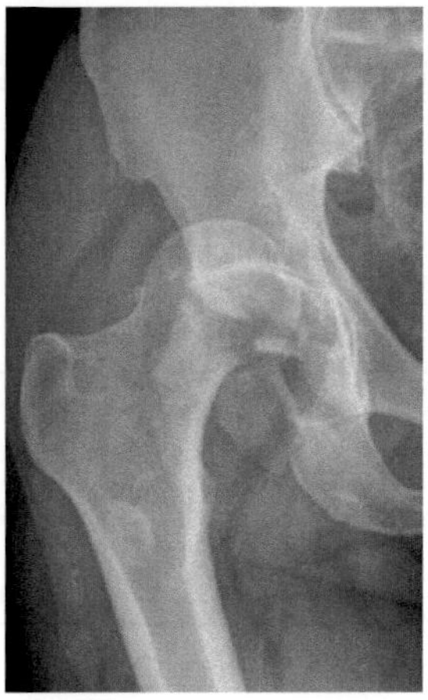

Thompson-Epstein
Classification of Posterior hip joint dislocation
Type III: Dislocation with comminuted fracture of the rim, with or without a large major fragment.

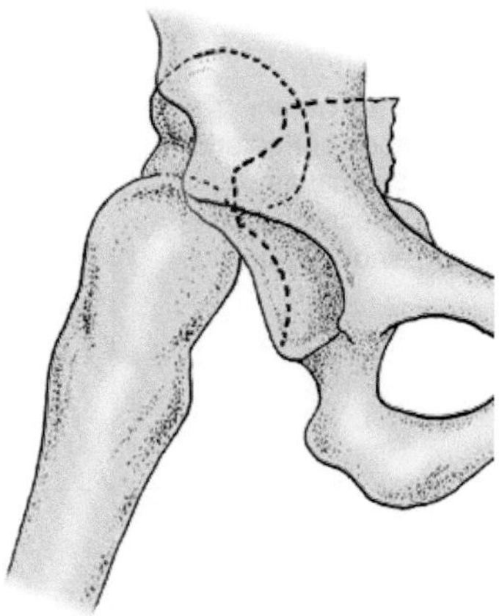

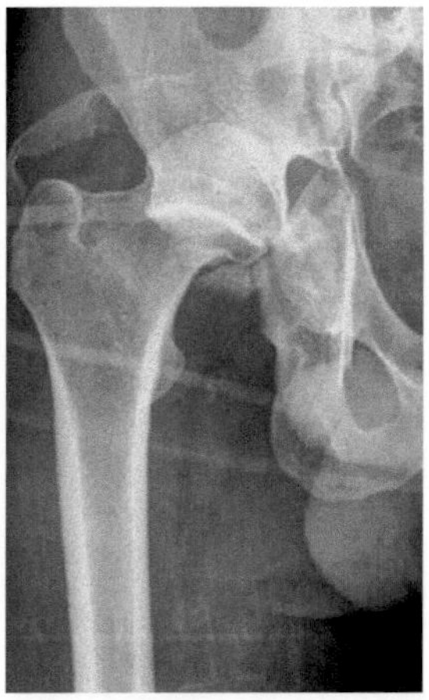

Thompson-Epstein
Classification of Posterior hip joint dislocation
Type IV: Dislocation with fracture of the acetabular floor.

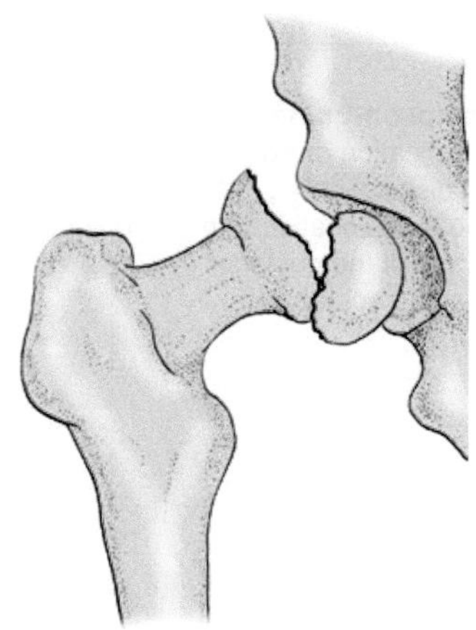

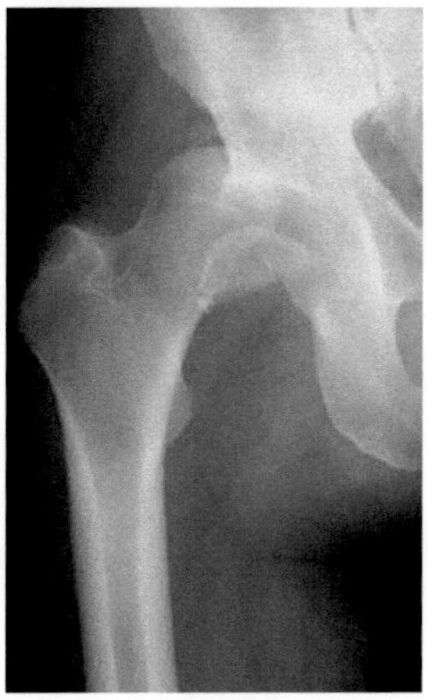

Thompson-Epstein
Classification of Posterior hip joint dislocation
Type V: Dislocation with fracture of the femoral head.

12.1.3.2 **Browner-Jupiter Classification** (1998, Skeletal Trauma 2nd Ed. W B Saunders: Harcount Publishers Limited)

Type I: No significant related to fracture, stable after axial traction.

Type II: Unreduced dislocation without femoral head and acetabulum fractures.

Type III: Unstable after traction, has potential cartilage or acetabulum labrum injury or acetabular fractures.

Type IV: Acetabulum fractures require to be rebuilt in order to obtain the stability of hip or joint symmetry.

Type V: With femoral head or neck fractures or impact.

12.2 Section 2 Classification of Knee Joint Dislocation

12.2.1 Chapman Classification of Knee Joint Dislocation (1993, Operative Orthopaedics. Ed. Philadelphia: J B Lippincott Company, 2133)

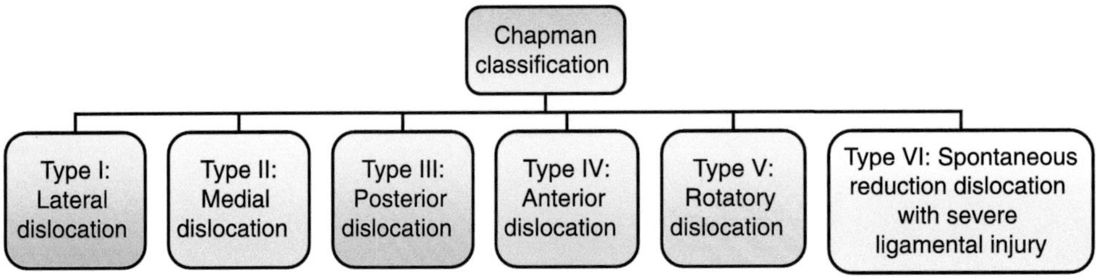

Type I: Lateral dislocation.
Type II: Medial dislocation.
Type III: Posterior dislocation.
Type IV: Anterior dislocation.
Type V: Rotatory dislocation.
Type VI: Spontaneous reduction dislocation with severe ligamental injury.

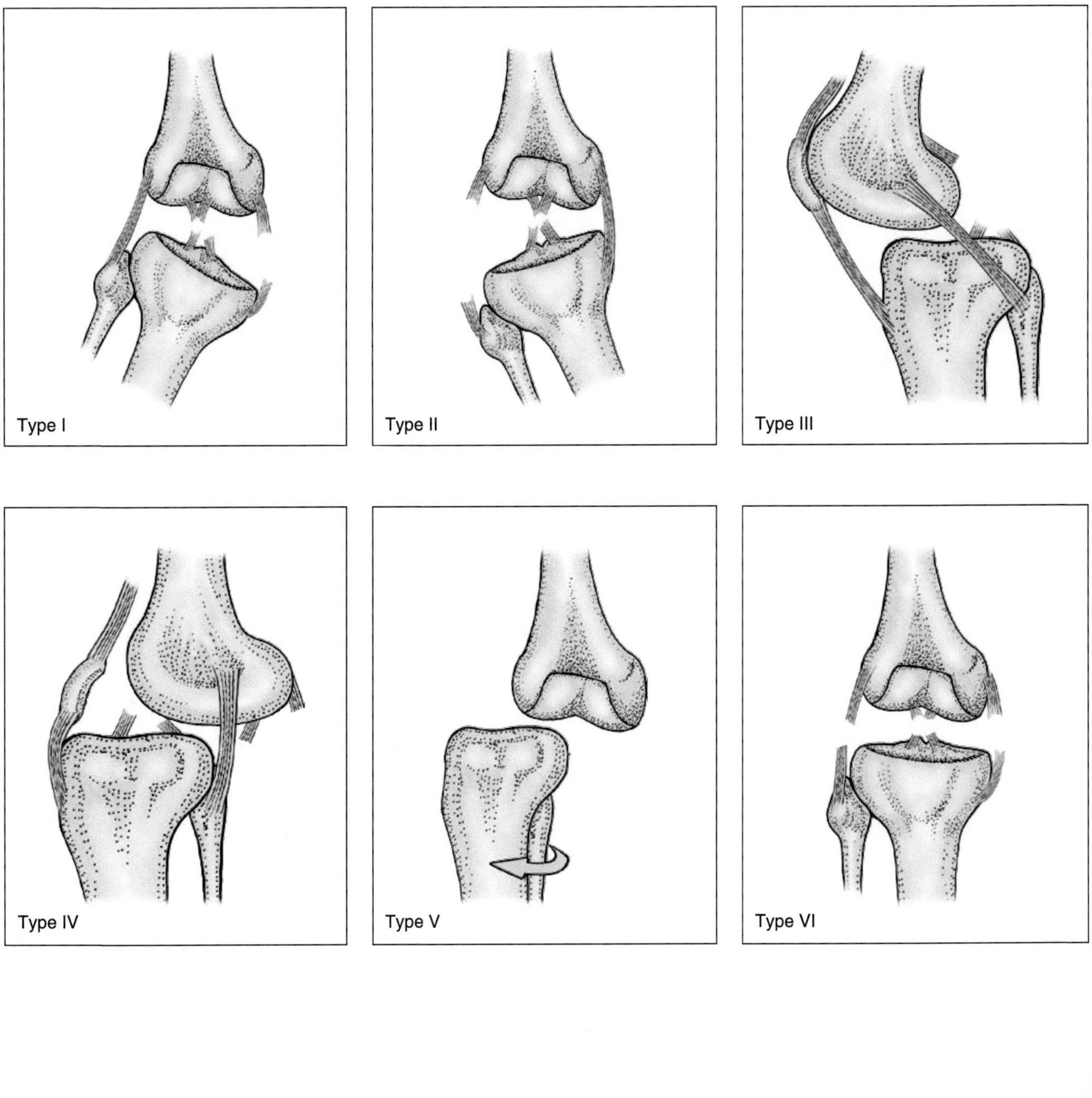

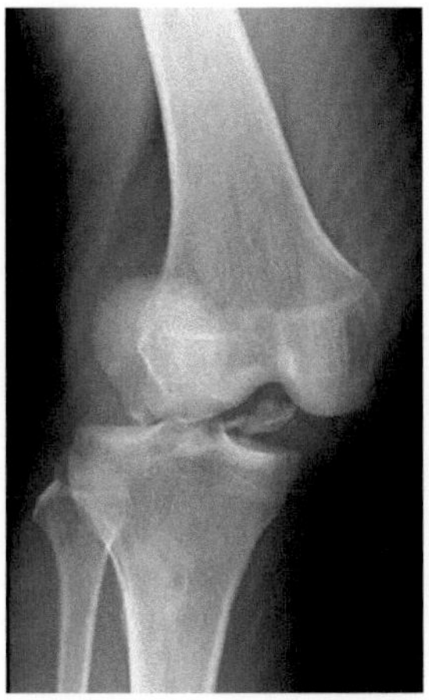
Type I

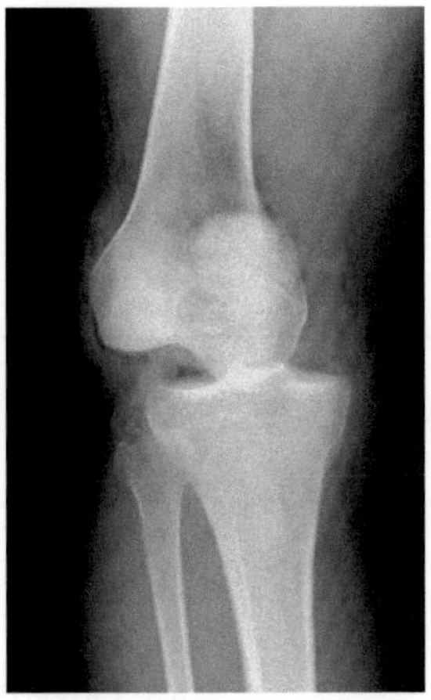
Type II

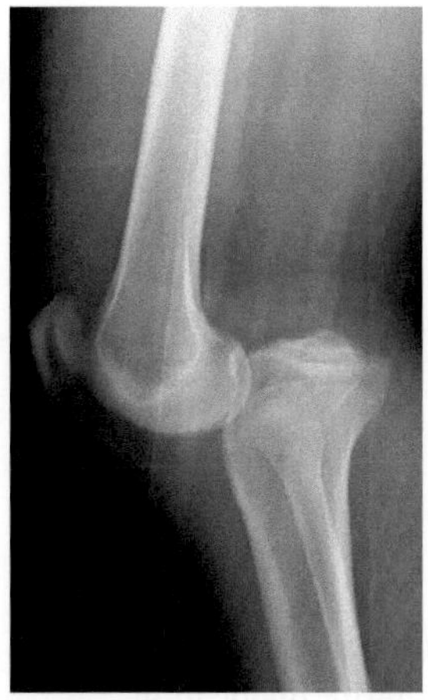
Type III

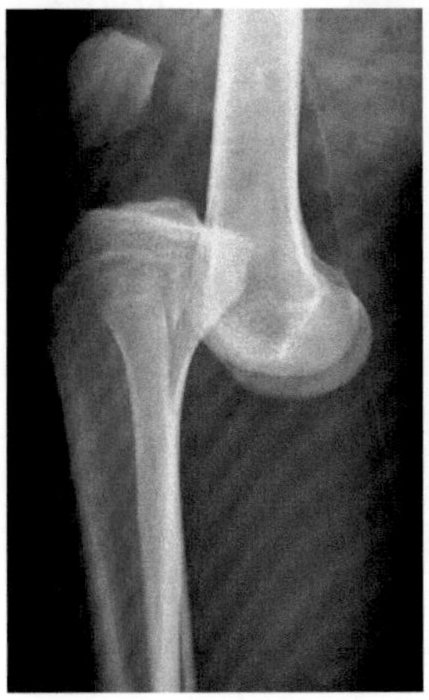
Type IV

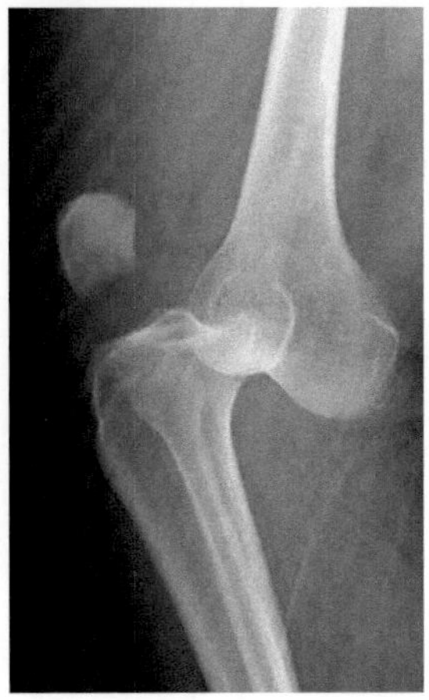
Type V

12.2.2 **Yicong Wang Classification** (2001, Bone and joint injuries. 3rd edition, Beijing: People's Health Publishing House, 1039)

Type I: Anterior dislocation: The ACL and PLC are always torn at the same time, or sometimes, only the ACL is torn. The MCL and LCL are always involved.

Type II: Posterior dislocation: The ACL and PLC are always torn at the same time, or sometimes, only the PCL is torn. The MCL and LCL are rarely involved and can be combined with a patellar tendon rupture.

Type III: Lateral dislocation: The ACL, PCL, and PCL are torn and always combined with lateral dislocation of the patella.

Type IV: Medial dislocation; rare.

Type V: Posterolateral rotational dislocation: The ACL and PCL are torn, or only the ACL is torn in an equal ratio. The herniation of the medial femoral condyle from the capsule and medial vastus muscle or retinaculum will lock the joint and make it difficult to be reduced closely.

Type VI: Fracture and dislocation; femoral or tibial condyle alone or combined, accompanied with a tibiofemoral joint dislocation.

12.2.3 AO/OTA Classification of

12.2.3.1 Tibiofemoral Joint Dislocation

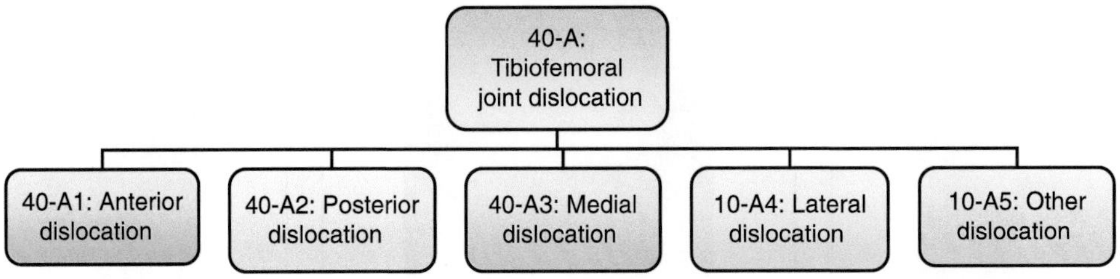

A1: Anterior dislocation
A2: Posterior dislocation
A3: Medial dislocation
A4: Lateral dislocation
A5: Other dislocation

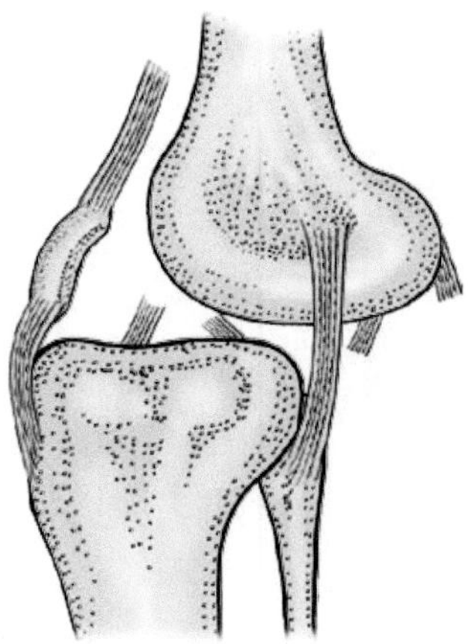

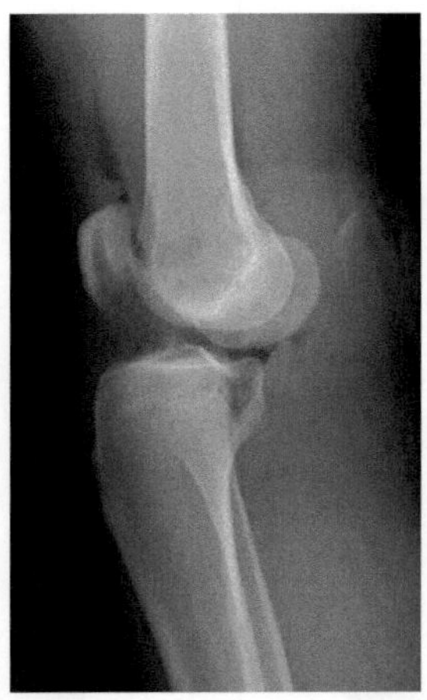

AO/OTA
40-A Tibiofemoral joint dislocation.
A1: Anterior dislocation

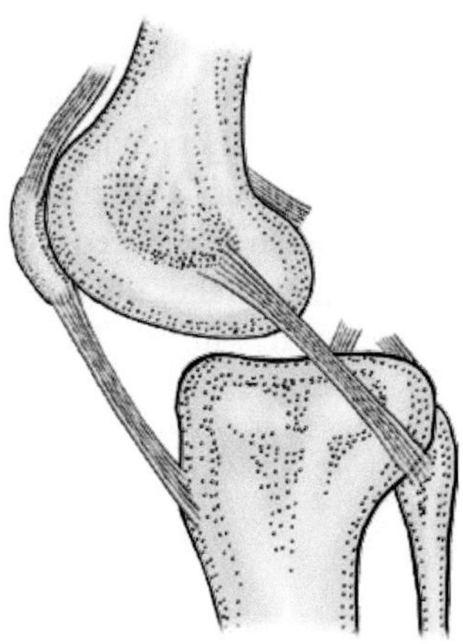

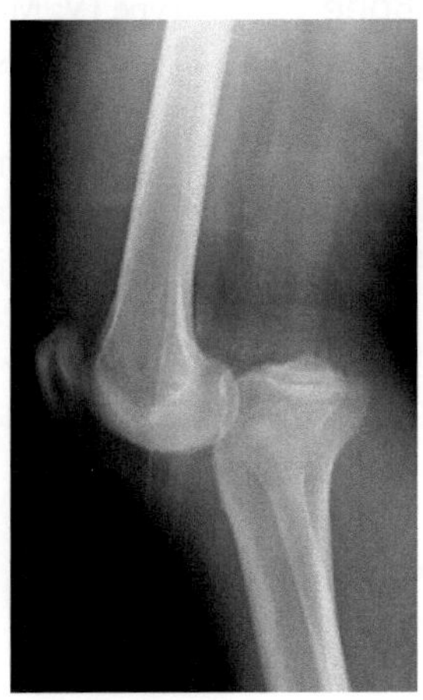

AO/OTA
40-A Tibiofemoral joint dislocation.
A1: Posterior dislocation

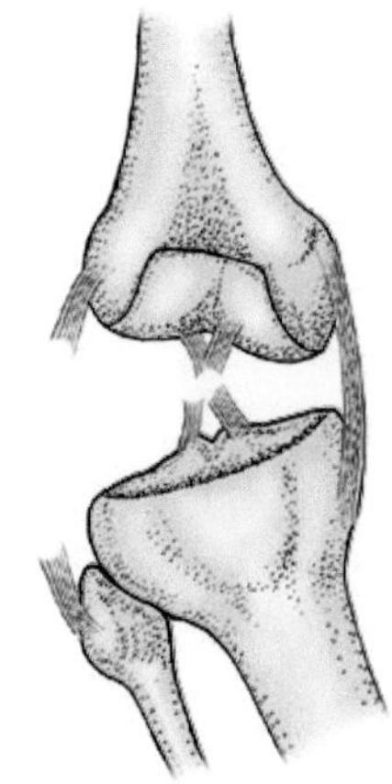

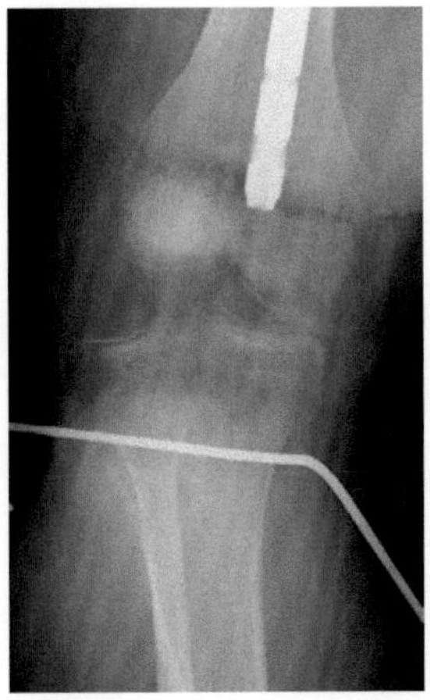

AO/OTA
40-A Tibiofemoral joint dislocation.
A1: Medial dislocation

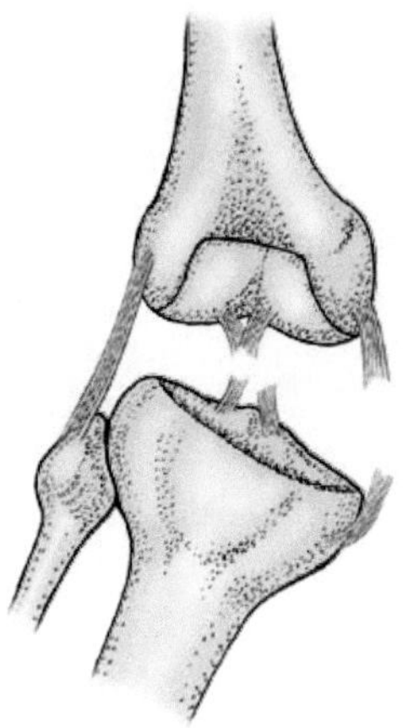

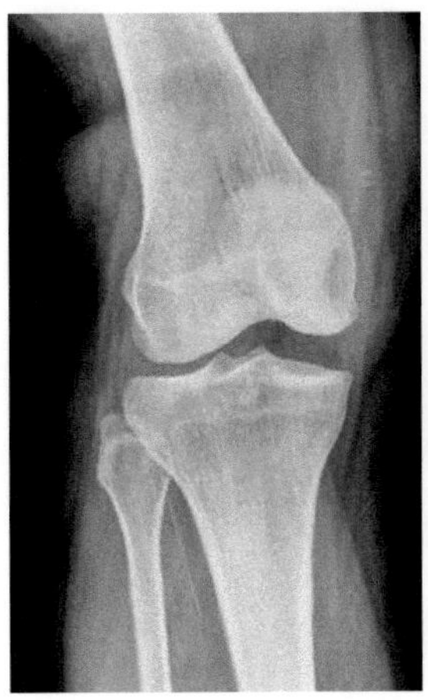

AO/OTA
40-A Tibiofemoral joint dislocation.
A1: Laterial dislocation

12.2.3.2 Patellofemoral Dislocation

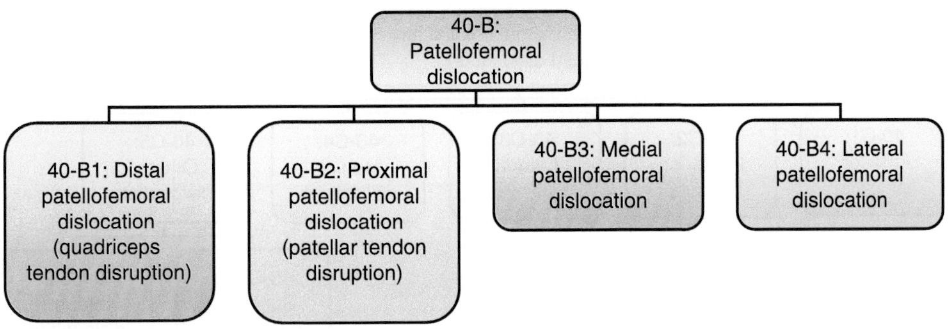

B1: Distal patellofemoral dislocation (**quadriceps tendon disruption**)
B2: Proximal patellofemoral dislocation (**patellar tendon disruption**)
B3: Medial patellofemoral dislocation
B4: Lateral patellofemoral dislocation

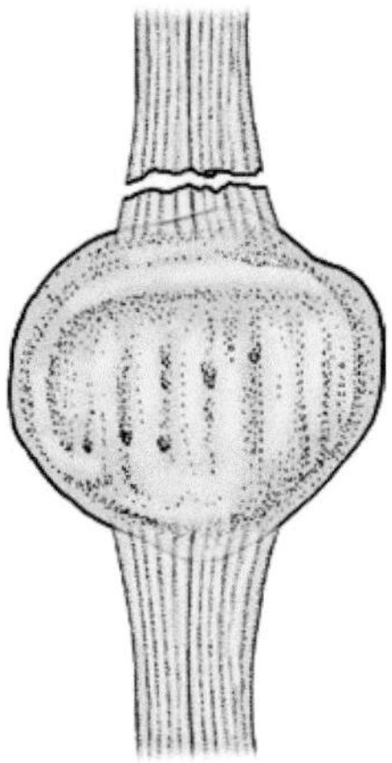
40-B1

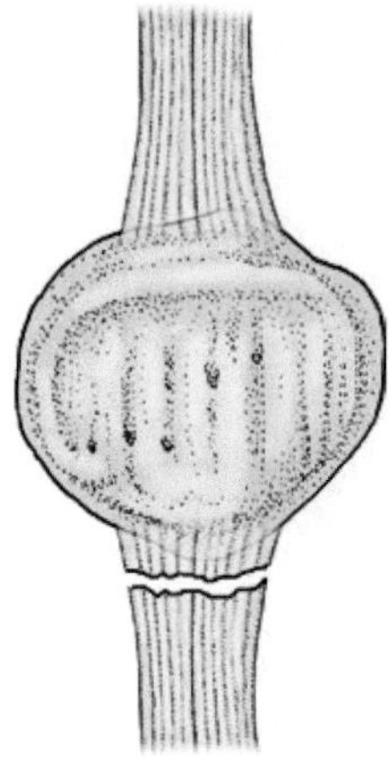
40-B2

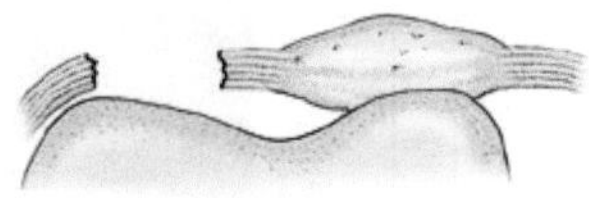
40-B3

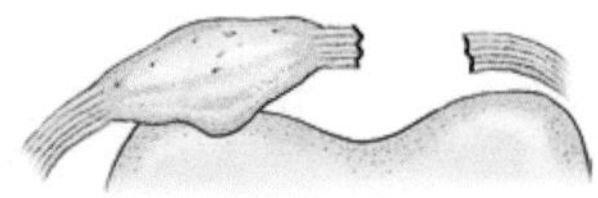
40-B4

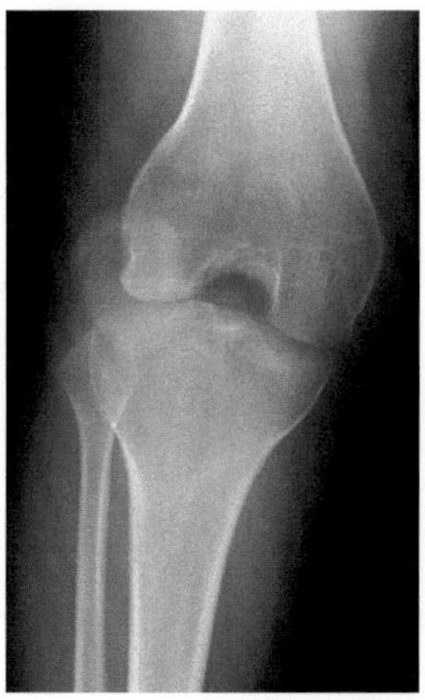
40-B1

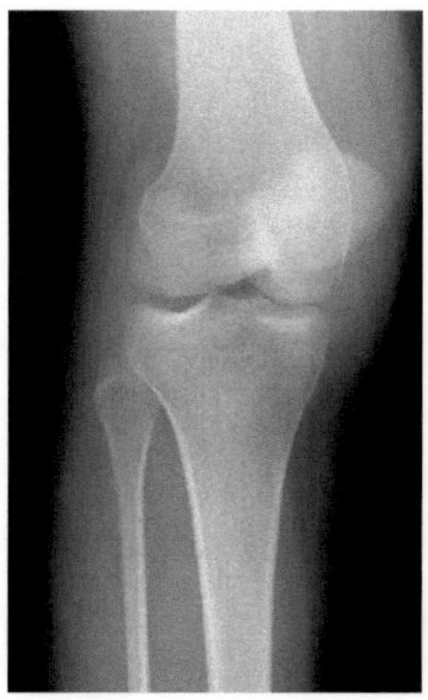
40-B3

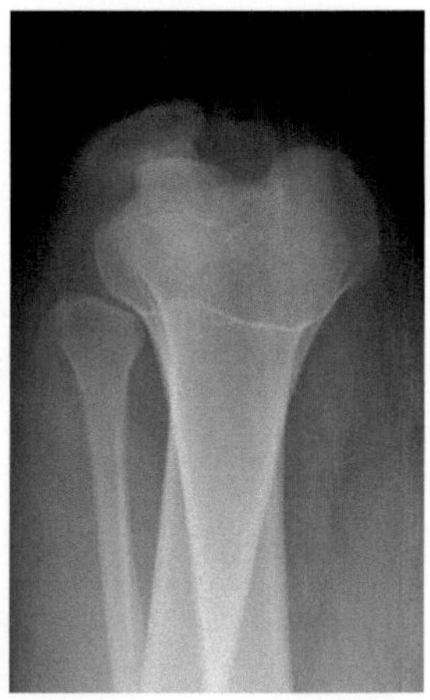
40-B4

12.2.3.3 Proximal Tibiofibular Joint Dislocation

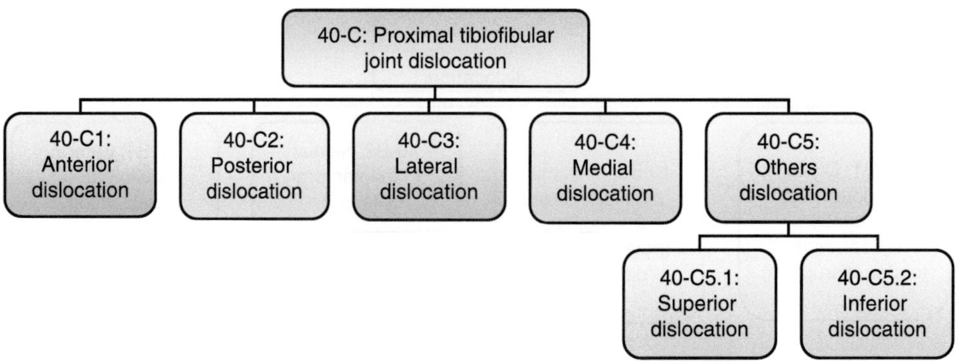

C1: Anterior dislocation of the proximal tibiofibular joint.
C2: Posterior dislocation of the proximal tibiofibular joint.
C3: Lateral dislocation of the proximal tibiofibular joint.
C4: Medial dislocation of the proximal tibiofibular joint.
C5: The other dislocations:

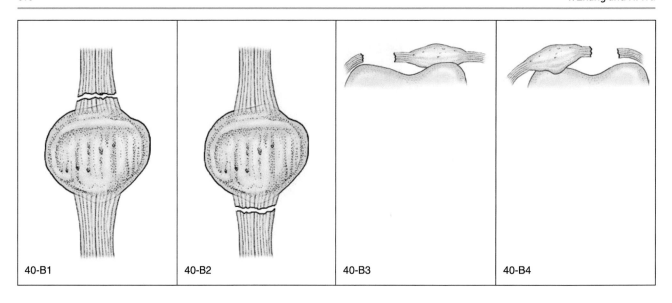

40-C5.1: Superior dislocation on the proximal tibiofibular joint

40-C5.2: Inferior dislocation on the proximal tibiofibular joint

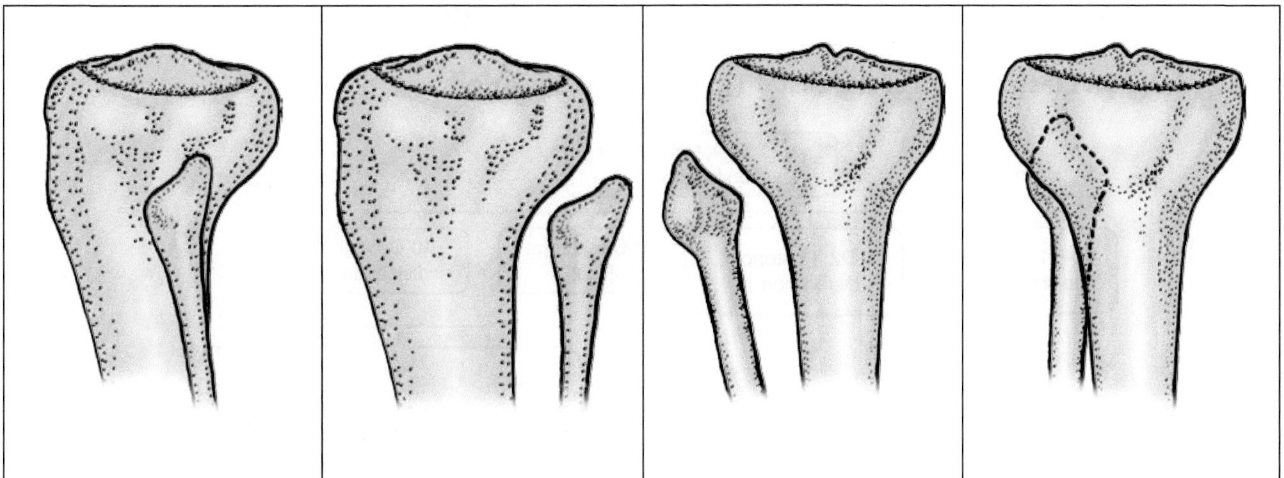

40-C1 40-C2 40-C3 40-C4

12.2.3.4 **Ogden Classification of the Proximal Tibiofibular Joint Dislocation** (1974, J Bone Joint Surg [Am], 56:145)

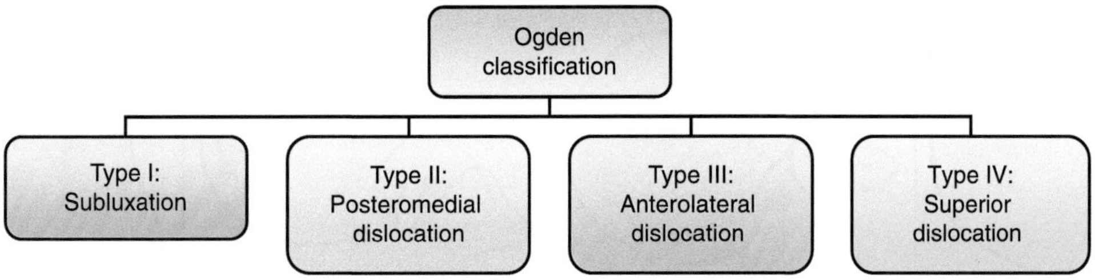

Type I: Subluxation of the proximal tibiofibular joint.
Type II: Posteromedial dislocation of the proximal tibiofibular joint.
Type III: Anterolateral dislocation of the proximal tibiofibular joint.
Type IV: Superior dislocation of the proximal tibiofibular joint.

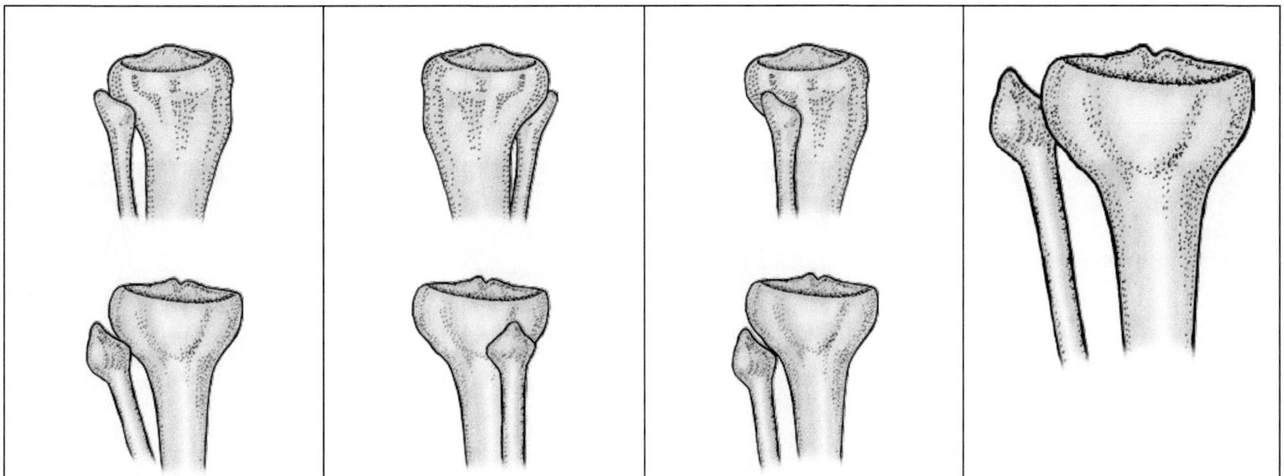

Type I Type II Type III Type IV

12.3 Section 3 Classification of Ankle Joint and Foot Dislocation

12.3.1 AO/OTA Classification of the Distal Tibiofibular Dislocation

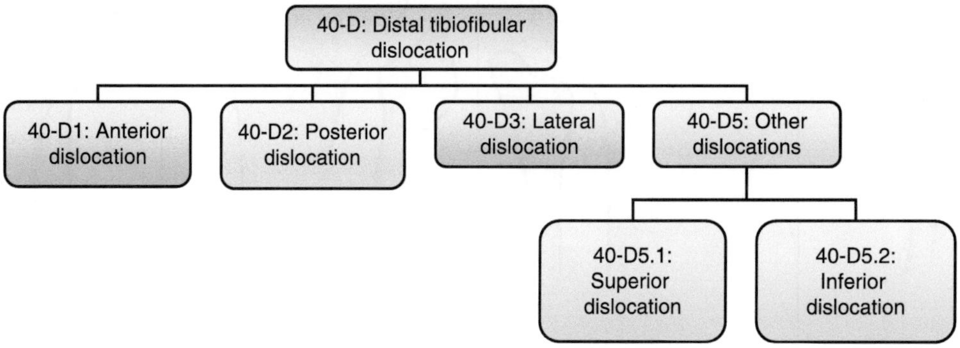

D1: Anterior dislocation of the distal tibiofibular.
D2: Posterior dislocation of the distal tibiofibular.
D3: Lateral dislocation of the distal tibiofibular.
D5: The others:
D5.1: Superior dislocation of the distal tibiofibular.
D5.2: Inferior dislocation of the distal tibiofibular.

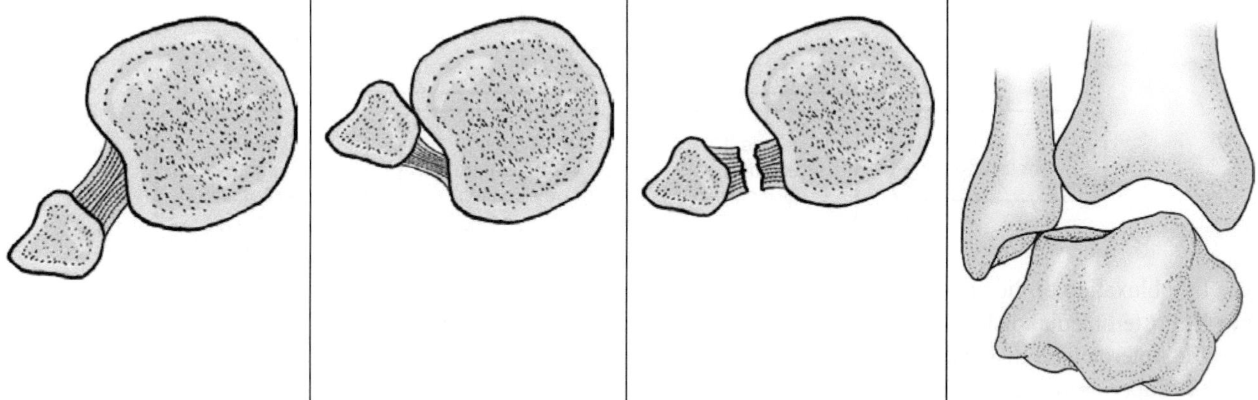

40-D1 40-D2 40-D3 40-D5.2

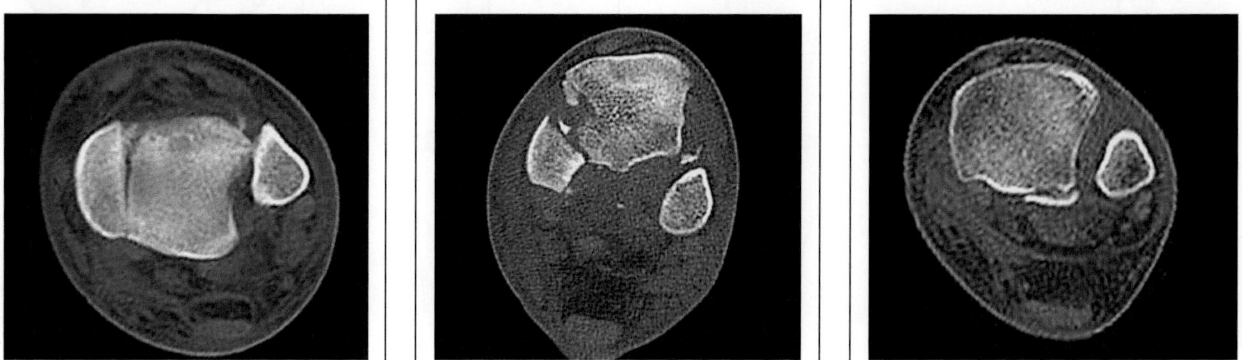

40-D1 40-D1 40-D1

12.3.2 AO/OTA Classification of the Talotibial Joint Dislocation

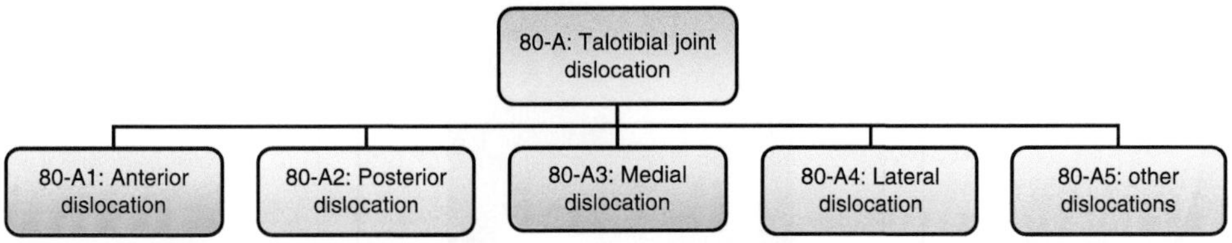

A1: Anterior dislocation of the talotibial joint.
A2: Posterior dislocation of the talotibial joint.
A3: Medial dislocation of the talotibial joint.
A4: Lateral dislocation of the talotibial joint.
A5: The others:

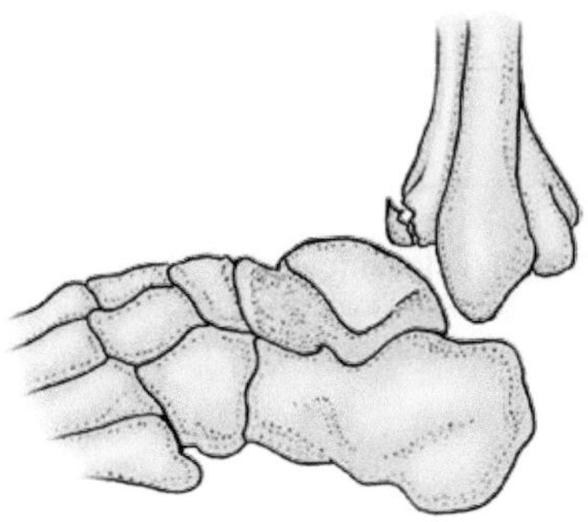

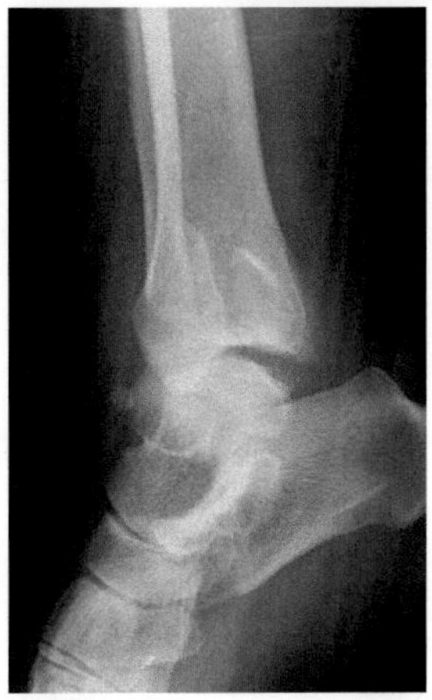

AO/OTA classification
80-A talotibial joint dislocation.
A1: Anterior dislocation

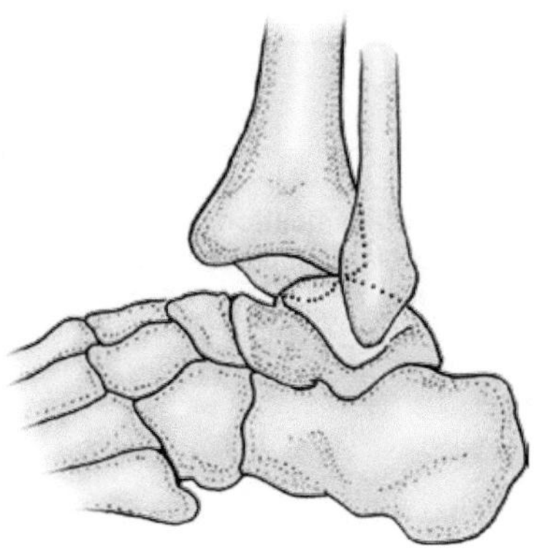

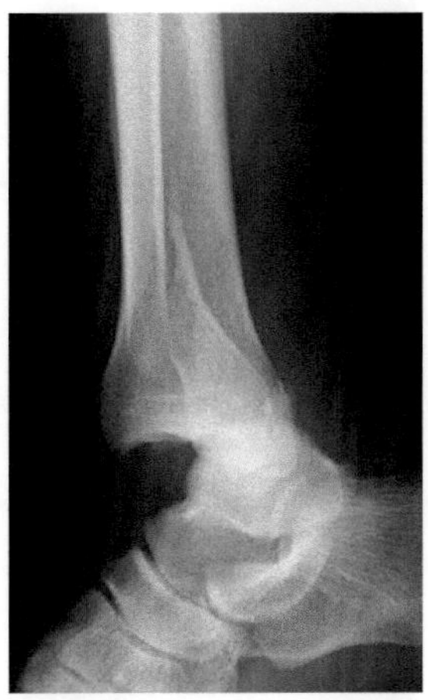

AO/OTA classification
80-A talotibial joint dislocation.
A2: Posterior dislocation

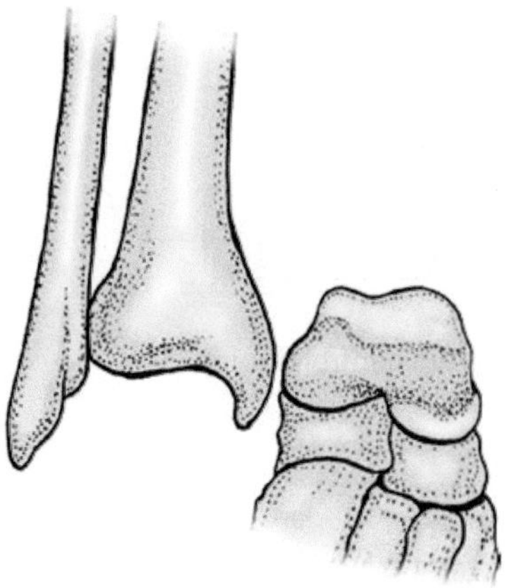

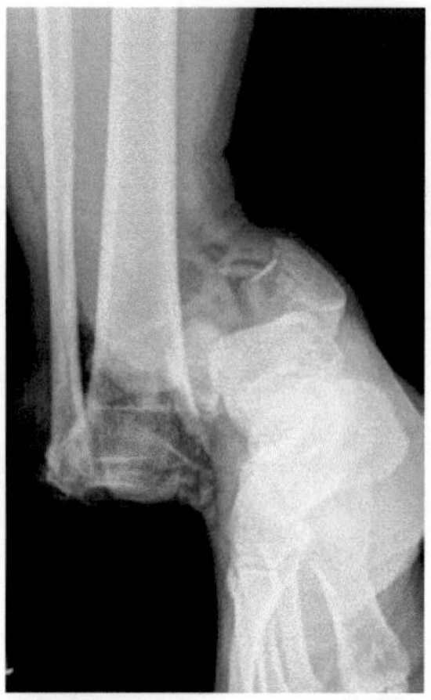

AO/OTA classification
80-A talotibial joint dislocation.
A3: Medial dislocation

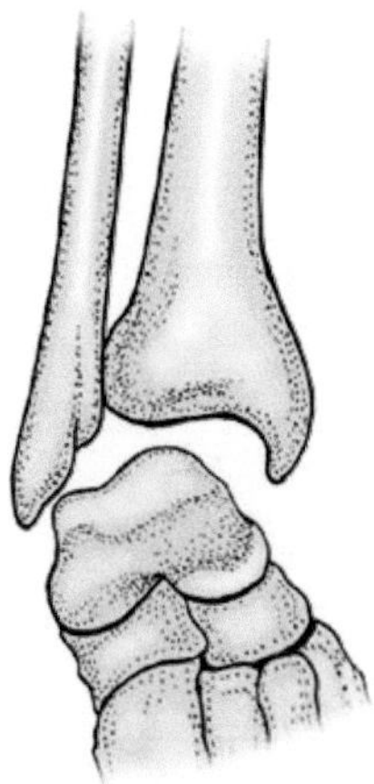

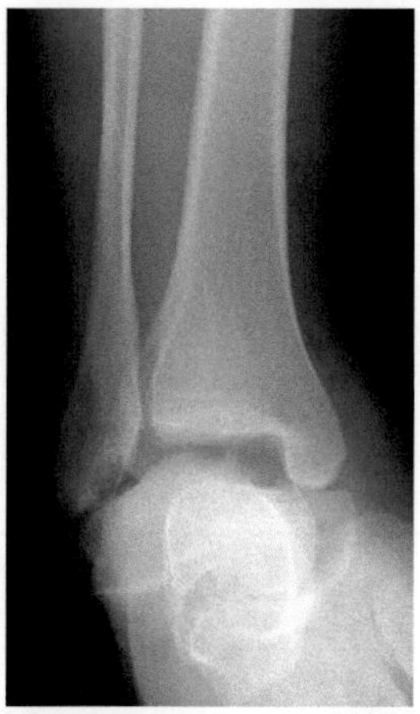

AO/OTA classification
80-A talotibial joint dislocation.
A4: Lateral dislocation

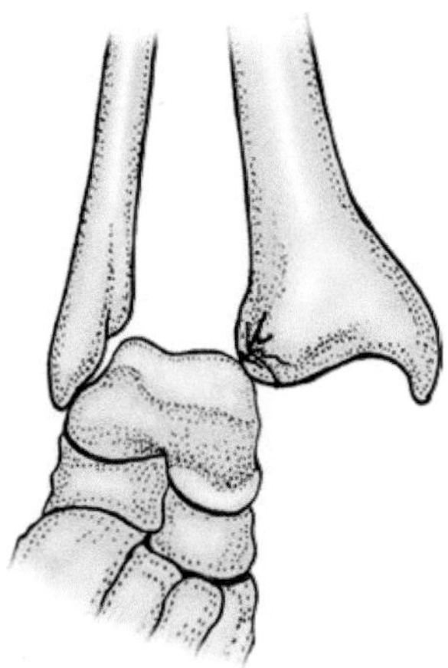

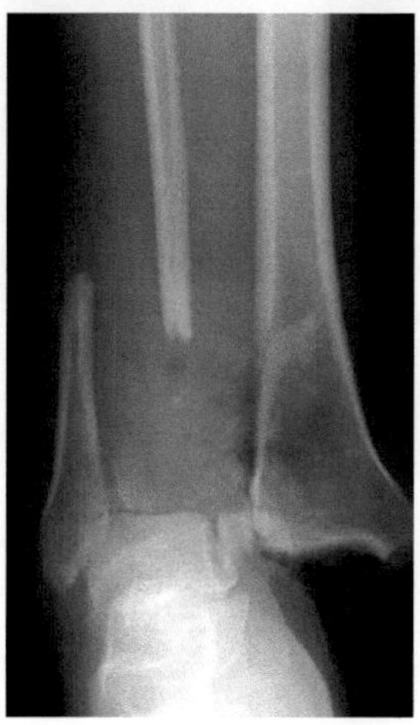

AO/OTA classification
80-A talotibial joint dislocation.
A5: the others

12.3.3 AO/OTA Classification of Subtalar Joint Dislocation

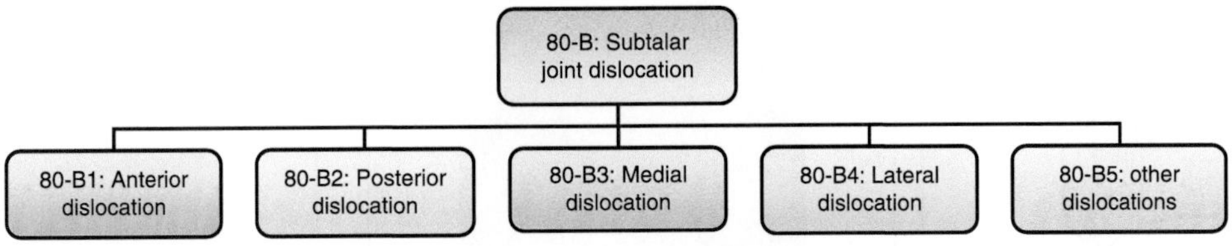

B1: Anterior dislocation
B2: Posterior dislocation
B3: Medial dislocation
B4: Lateral dislocation
B5: Other dislocation

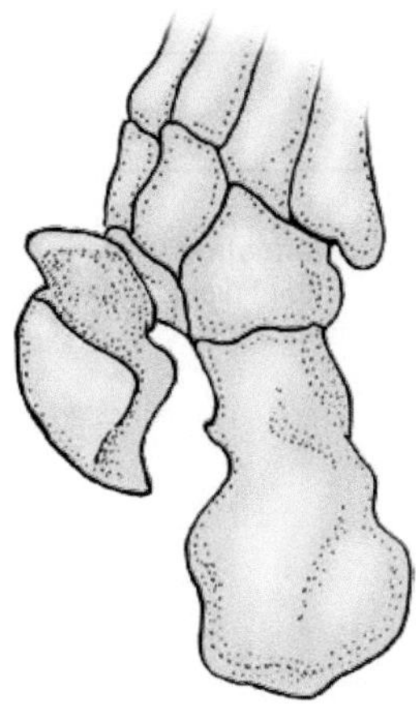

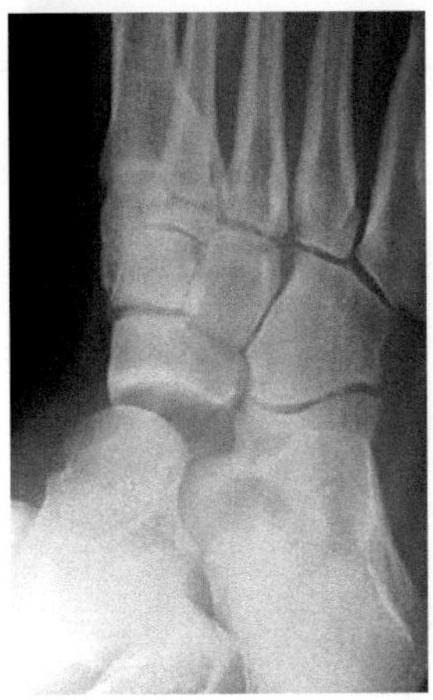

AO/OTA classification
80-B Subtalar joint dislocation.
B1: Anterior dislocation

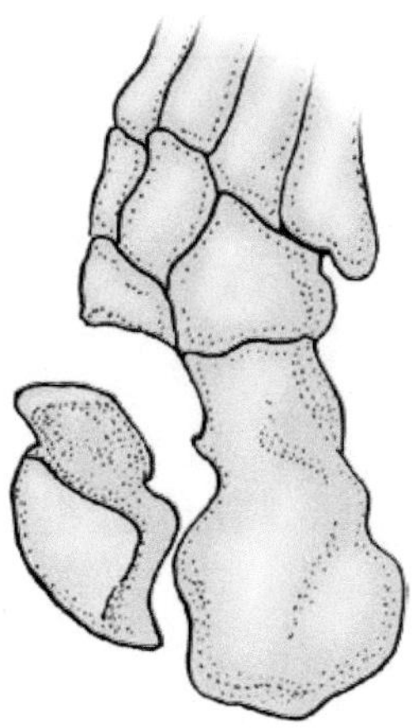

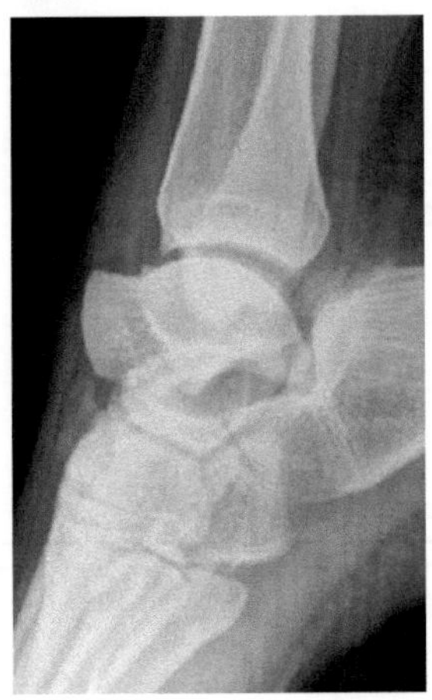

AO/OTA classification
80-B Subtalar joint dislocation.
B2: Posterior dislocation

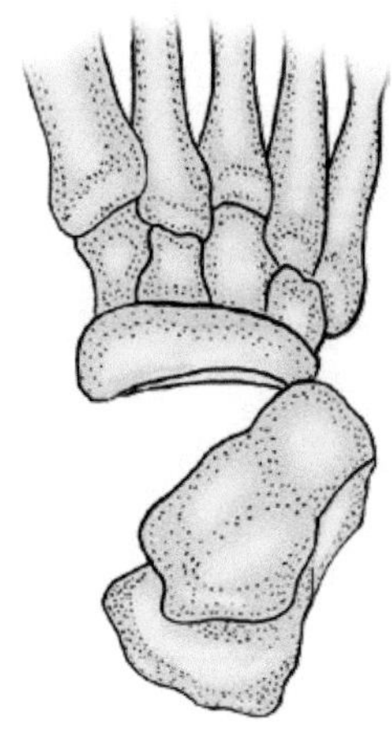

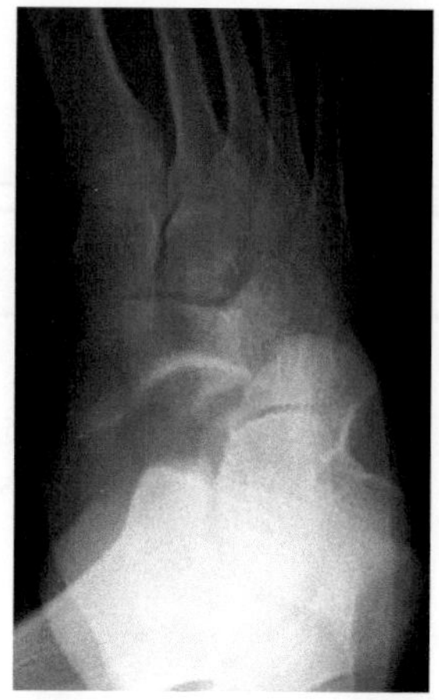

AO/OTA classification
80-B Subtalar joint dislocation.
B3: Medial dislocation

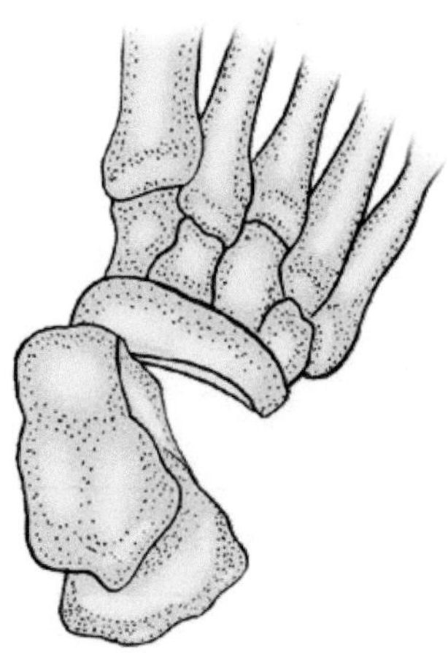

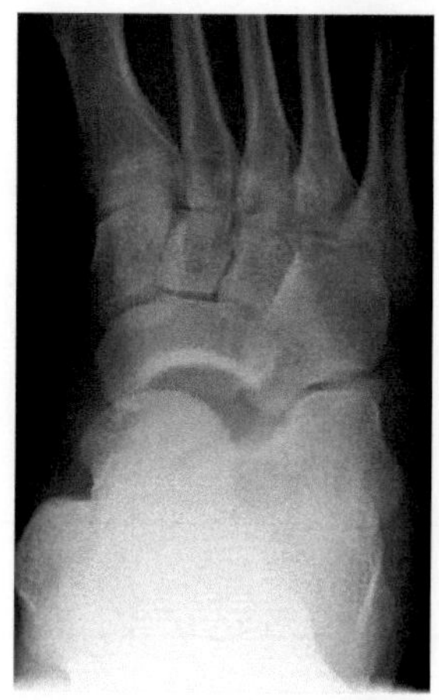

AO/OTA classification
80-B Subtalar joint dislocation.
B4: Lateral dislocation

12.3.4 Dislocation of Tarsometatarsal Joint (Lisfranc Injury)

12.3.4.1 Myerson Classification (1986, Foot Ankle, 6:228)

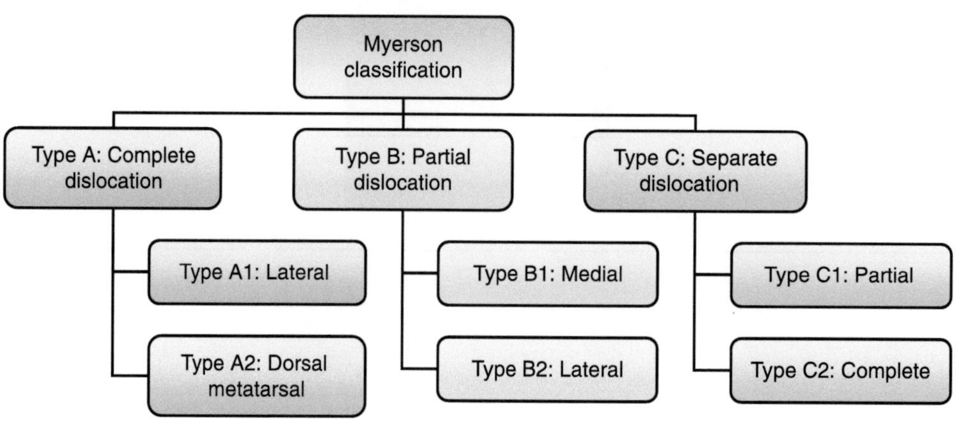

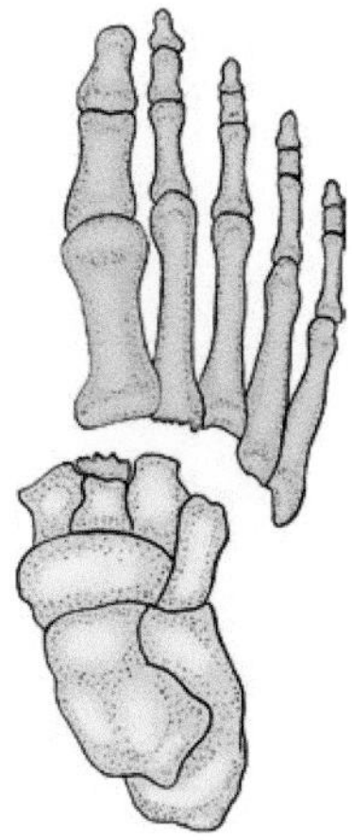

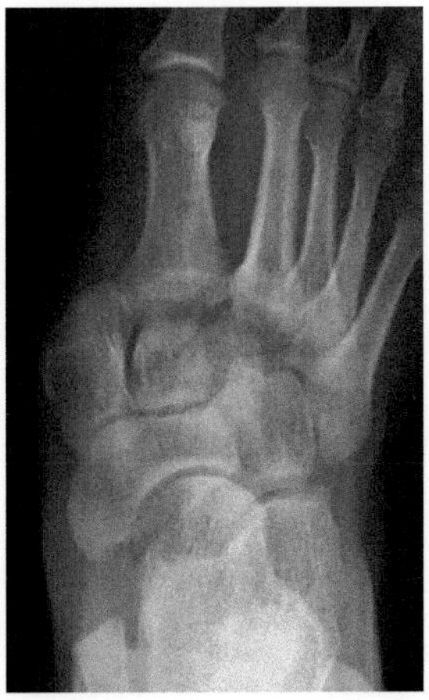

Myerson classification
Type A: Complete dislocation.
Type A1: Lateral

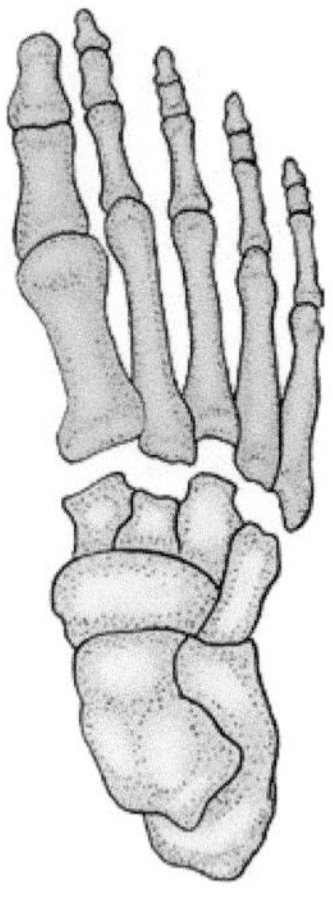

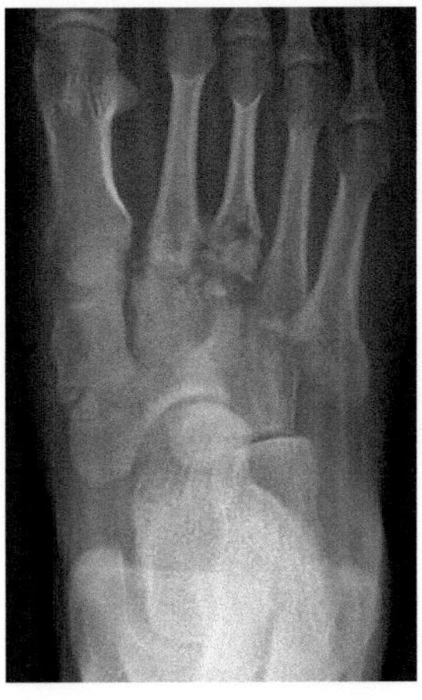

Myerson classification
Type A: Complete dislocation.
Type A2: Dorsal metatarsal

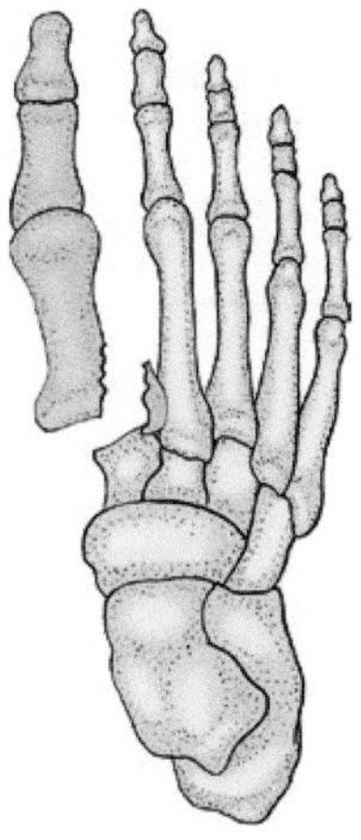

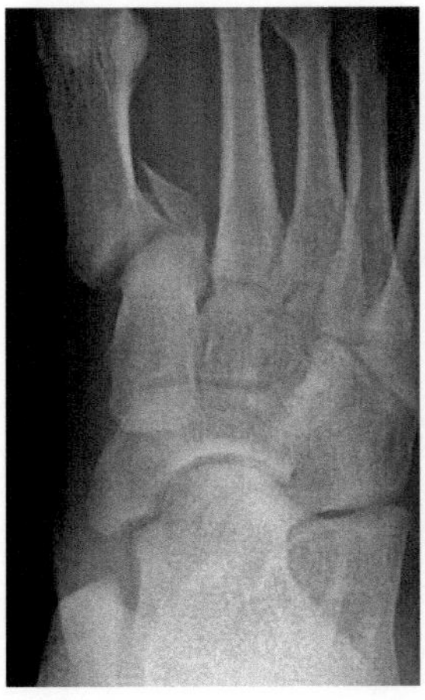

Myerson classification
Type B: Partial dislocation.
Type B1: Medial

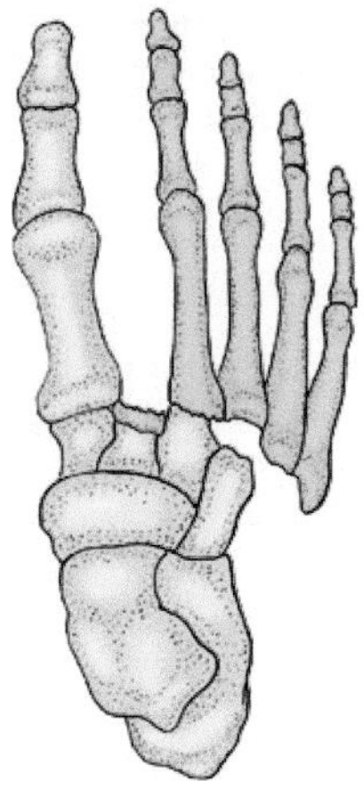

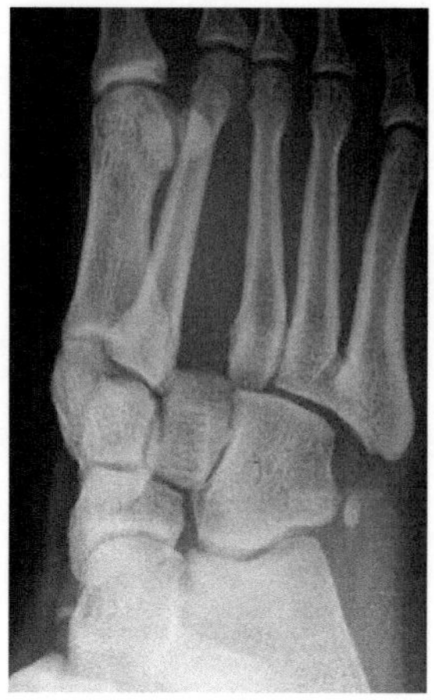

Myerson classification
Type B: Partial dislocation.
Type B2: Lateral

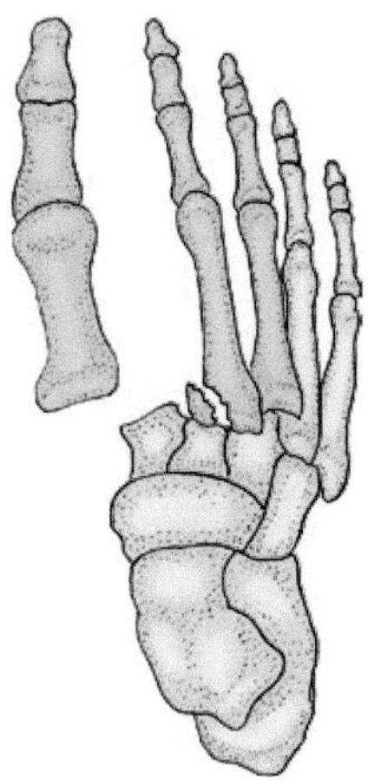

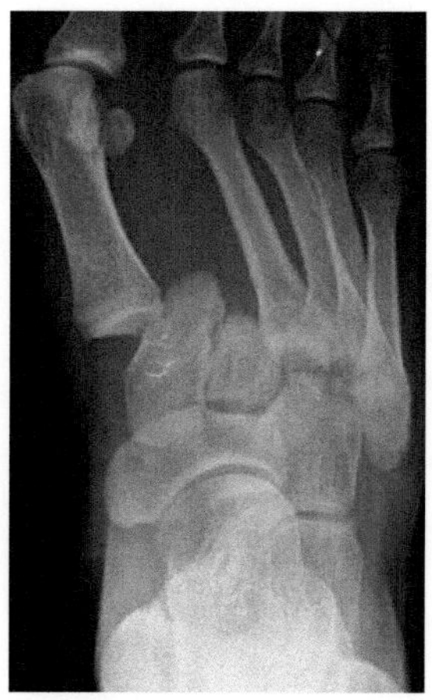

Myerson classification
Type C: Separate dislocation.
Type C1: Partial

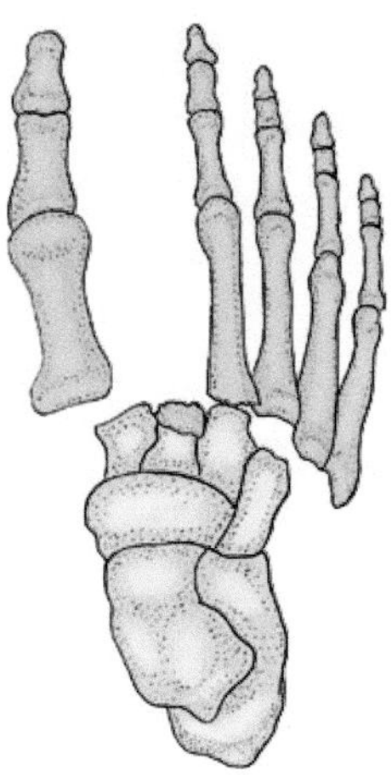

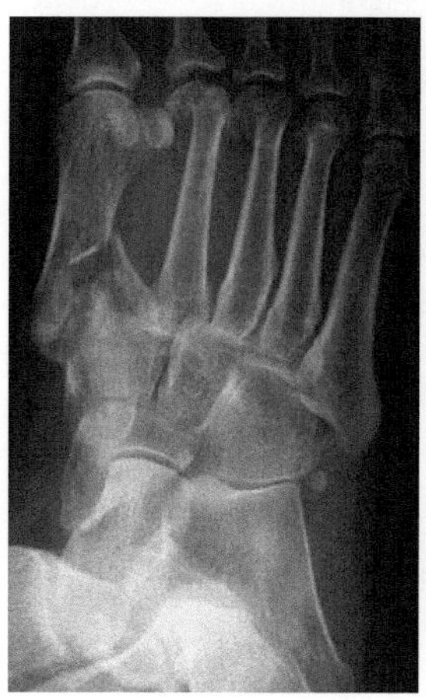

Myerson classification
Type C: Separate dislocation.
Type C2: complete

12.3.4.2 AO/OTA Classification of Midfoot Dislocation

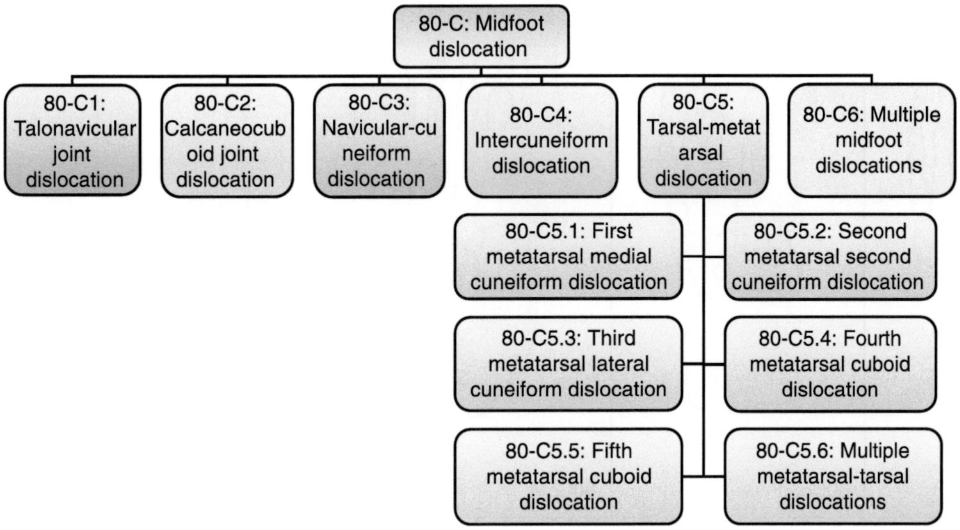

80-C: Midfoot dislocation
- 80-C1: Talonavicular joint dislocation
- 80-C2: Calcaneocuboid joint dislocation
- 80-C3: Navicular-cuneiform dislocation
- 80-C4: Intercuneiform dislocation
- 80-C5: Tarsal-metatarsal dislocation
  - C5.1: First metatarsal medial cuneiform dislocation
  - C5.2: Second metatarsal second cuneiform dislocation
  - C5.3: Third metatarsal lateral cuneiform dislocation
  - C5.4: Fourth metatarsal cuboid dislocation
  - C5.5: Fifth metatarsal cuboid dislocation
  - C5.6: Multiple metatarsal-tarsal dislocations
- 80-C6: Multiple midfoot dislocations

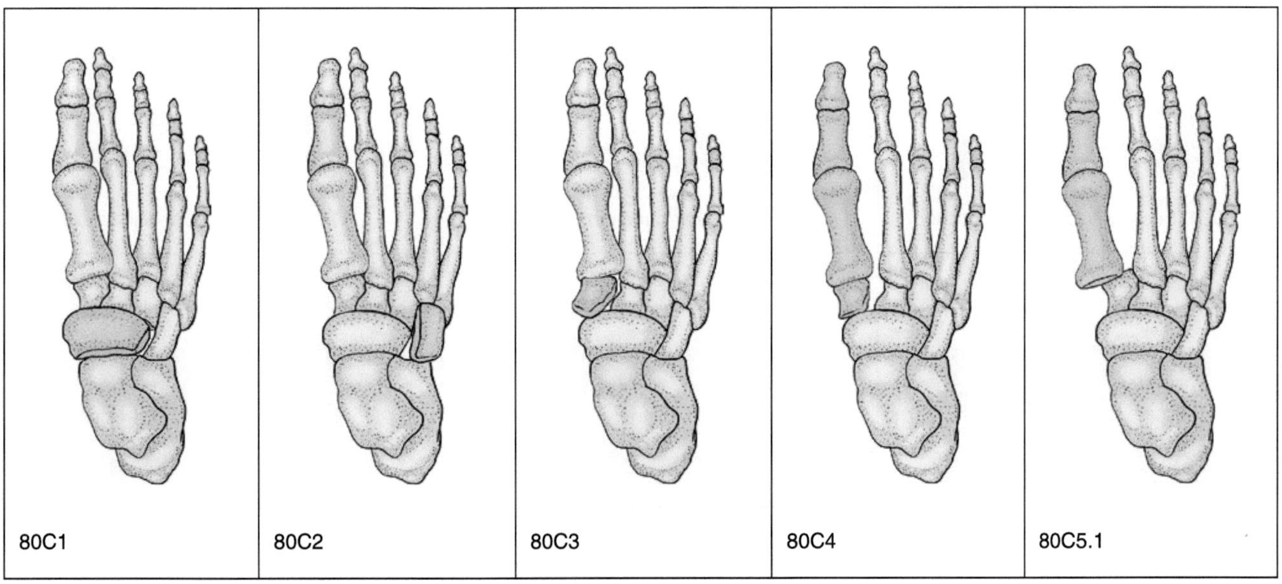

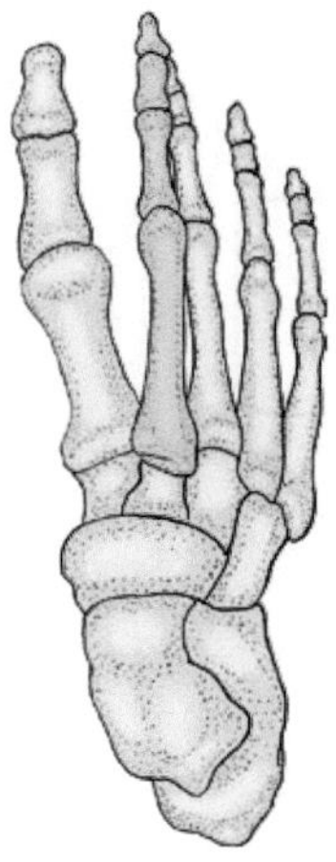
80C5.2

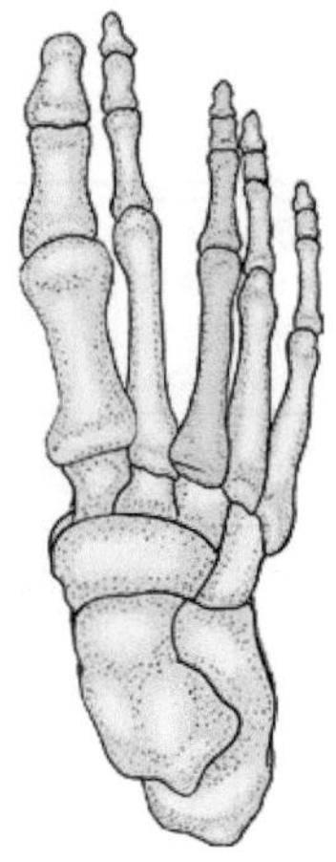
80C5.3

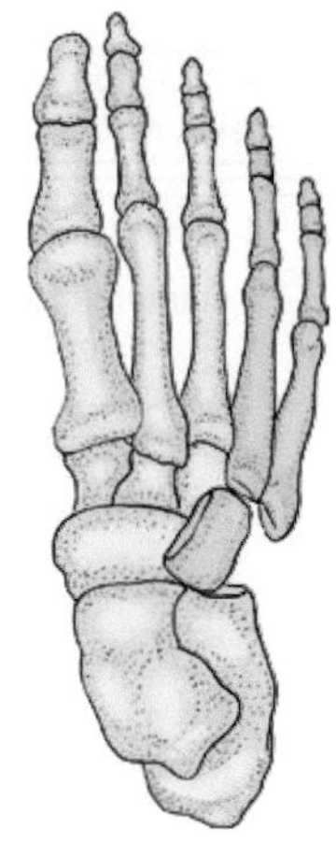
80C5.4

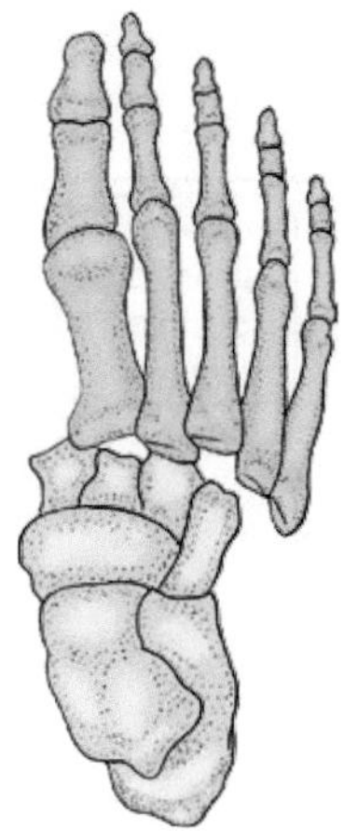
80C5.9

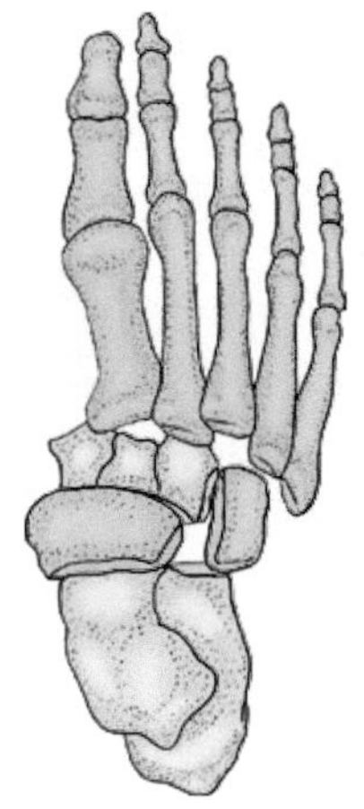
80C9

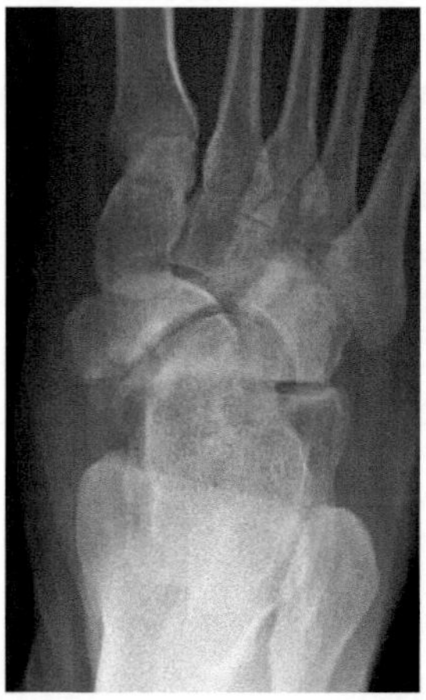
80C1 Talonavicular joint dislocation

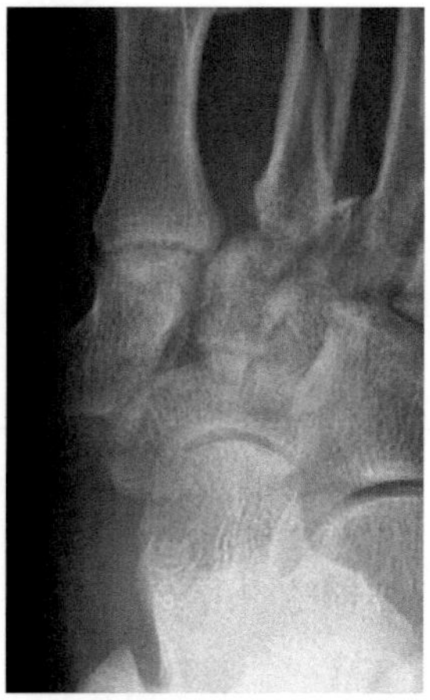
80C3 Navicular-cuneiform dislocation

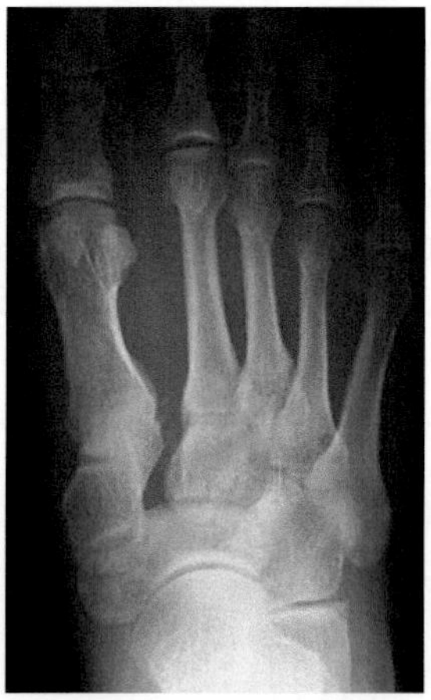
80C4 Intercuneiform dislocation

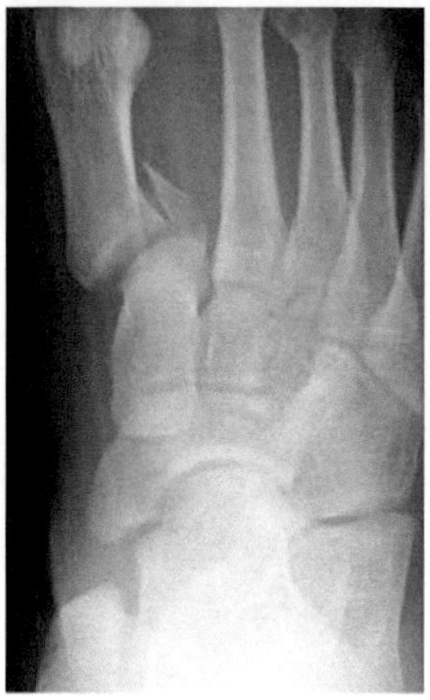
80C5.1 1st metatarsal medial cuneiform dislocation

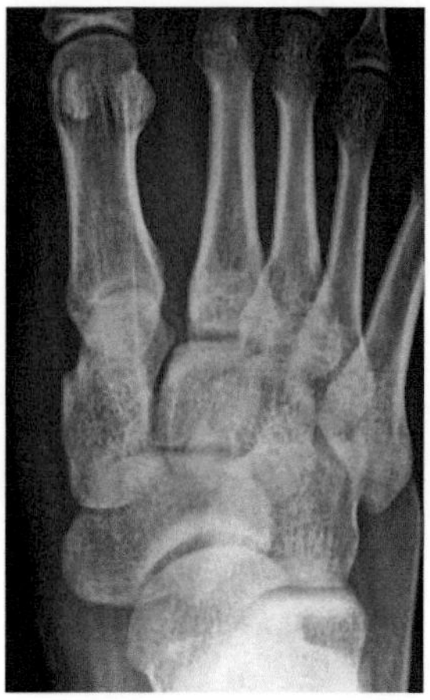
80 C5.2 2nd metatarsal second cuneiform dislocation

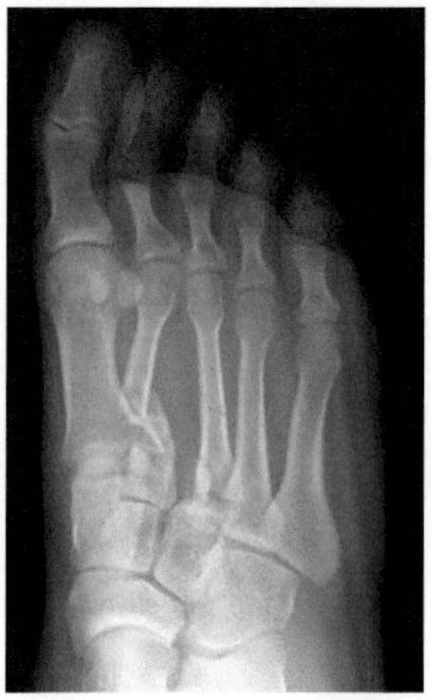
80 C5.3 3rd metatarsal lateral cuneiform dislocation

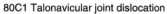

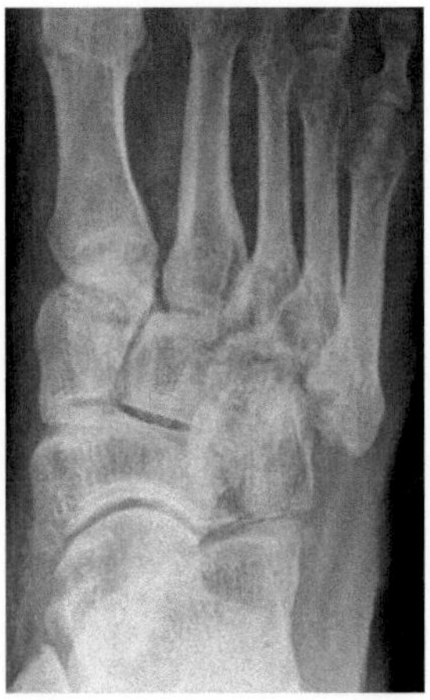

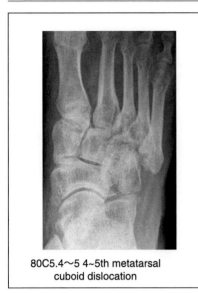

80C5.4~5 4~5th metatarsal cuboid dislocation

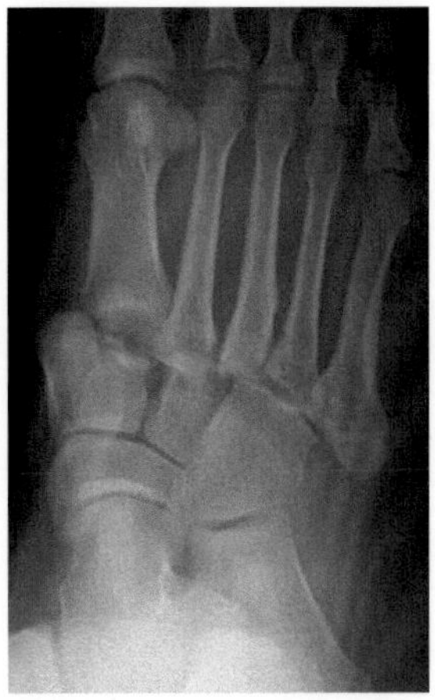

80C5.6 multiple metatarsal-tarsal dislocations

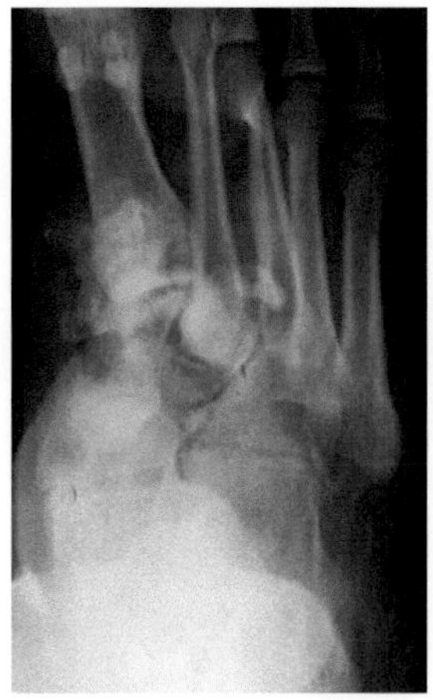

80C6 Multiple midfoot dislocations

12.3.4.3 Quenu-Kuss Classification

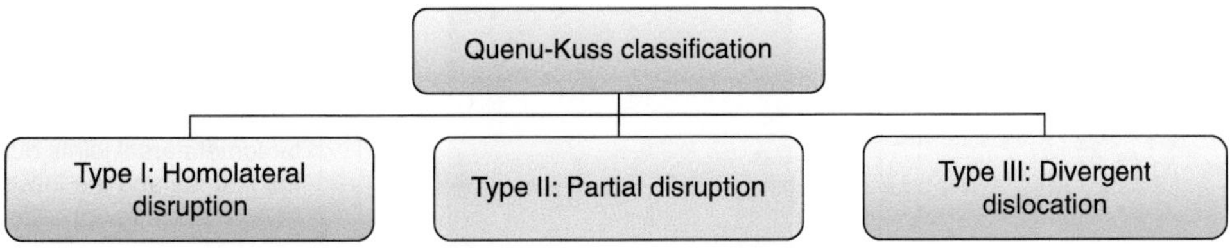

Type I: Depicts homolateral disruption where all metatarsals travel in the same direction.
Type II: Partial disruption involves only the first metatarsal or all the lesser rays.
Type III: Divergent dislocation occurs when there is complete disruption of the tarsometatarsal joints but the first ray and the lesser rays displace in opposite directions.

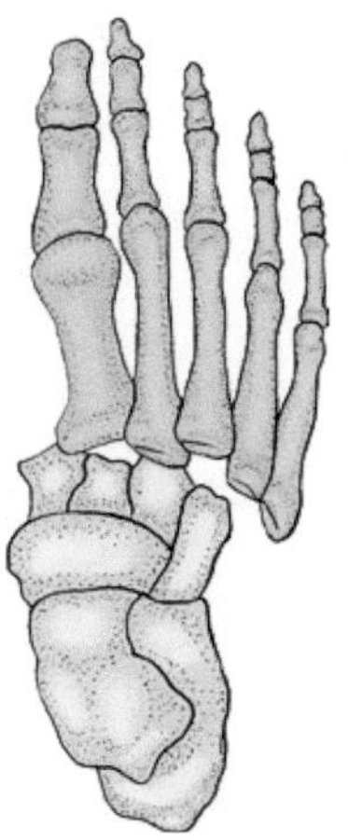

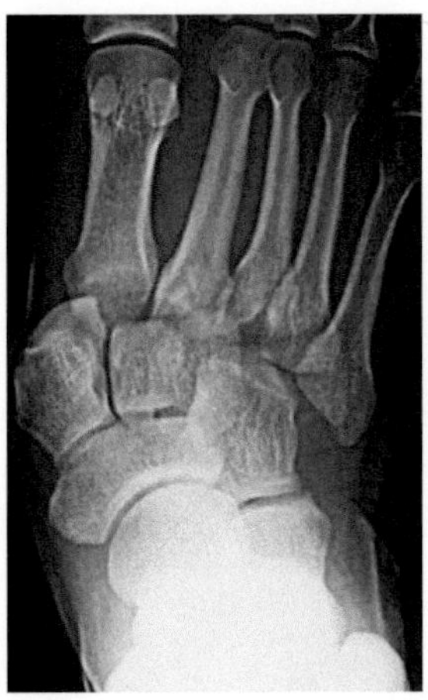

Quenu-Kuss classification
Type I: Depicts homolateral disruption where all metatarsals travel in the same direction

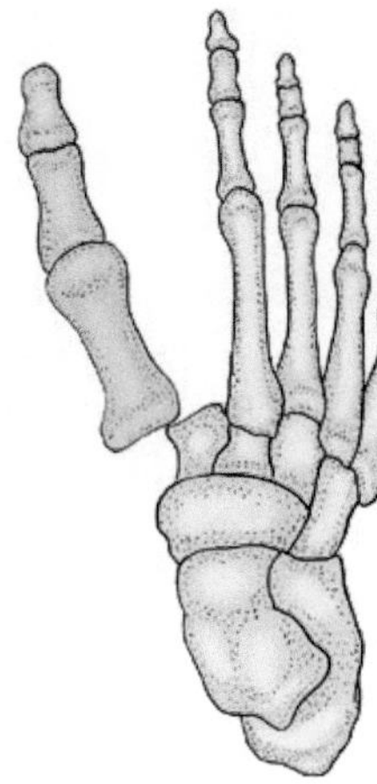

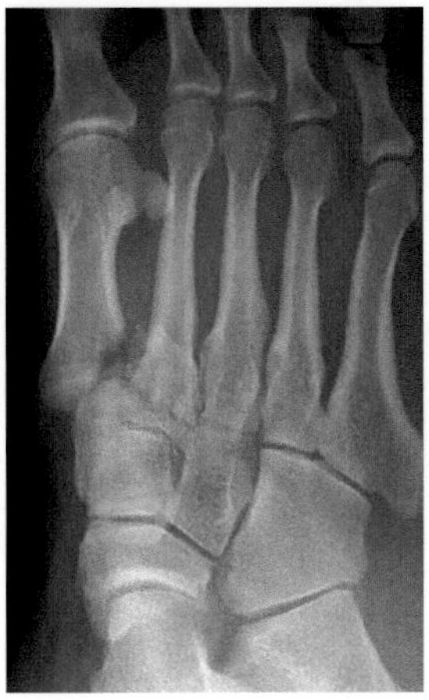

Quenu-Kuss classification
Type II: Partial disruption involves only the first metatarsal or all the lesser rays

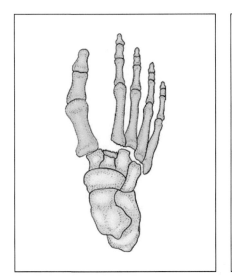

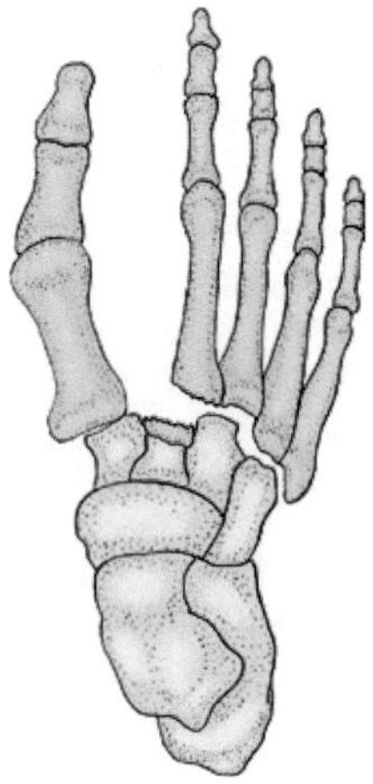

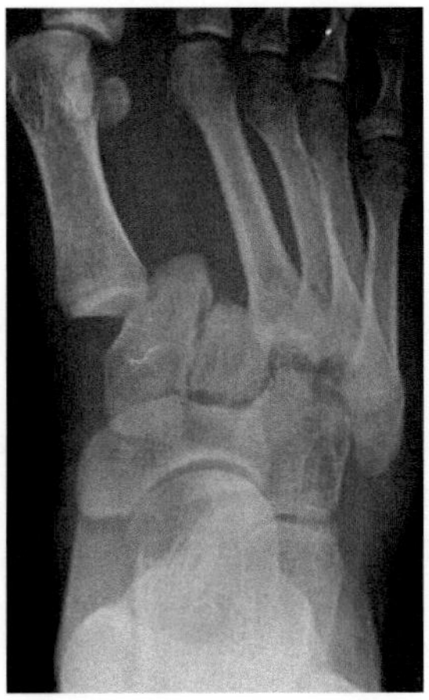

Quenu-Kuss classification
Type III: Divergent dislocation occurs when there is complete disruption of the tarsometatarsal joints but the first ray and the lesser rays displace in opposite directions

12.3.5 Forefoot Dislocation

12.3.5.1 AO/OTA Classification

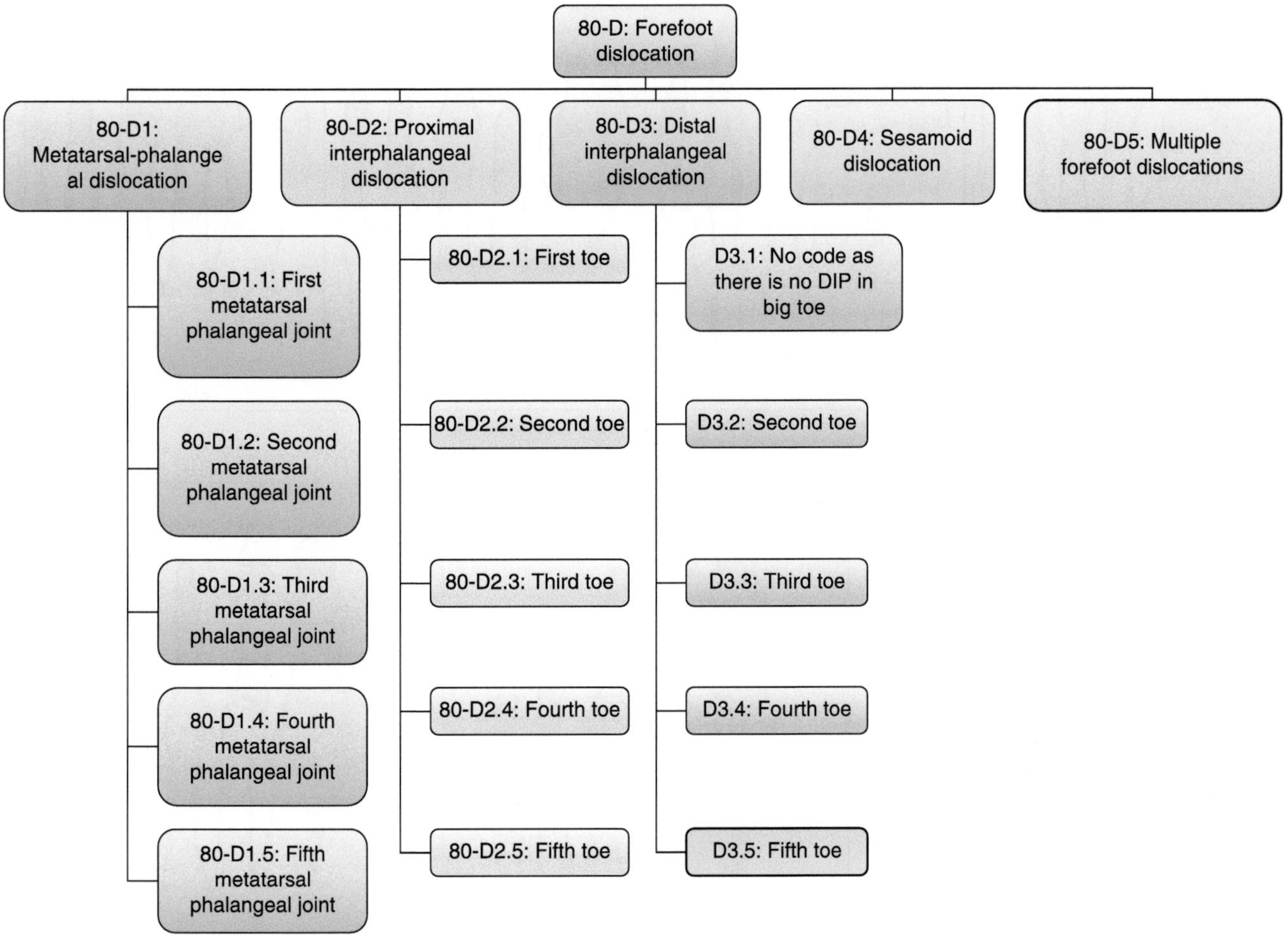

80-D: Forefoot dislocation
- 80-D1: Metatarsal-phalangeal dislocation
  - D1.1: First metatarsal phalangeal joint
  - D1.2: Second metatarsal phalangeal joint
  - D1.3: Third metatarsal phalangeal joint
  - D1.4: Fourth metatarsal phalangeal joint
  - D1.5: Fifth metatarsal phalangeal joint
- 80-D2: Proximal interphalangeal dislocation
  - D2.1: First toe
  - D2.2: Second toe
  - D2.3: Third toe
  - D2.4: Fourth toe
  - D2.5: Fifth toe
- 80-D3: Distal interphalangeal dislocation
  - D3.1: No code as there is no DIP in big toe
  - D3.2: Second toe
  - D3.3: Third toe
  - D3.4: Fourth toe
  - D3.5: Fifth toe
- 80-D4: Sesamoid dislocation
- 80-D5: Multiple forefoot dislocations

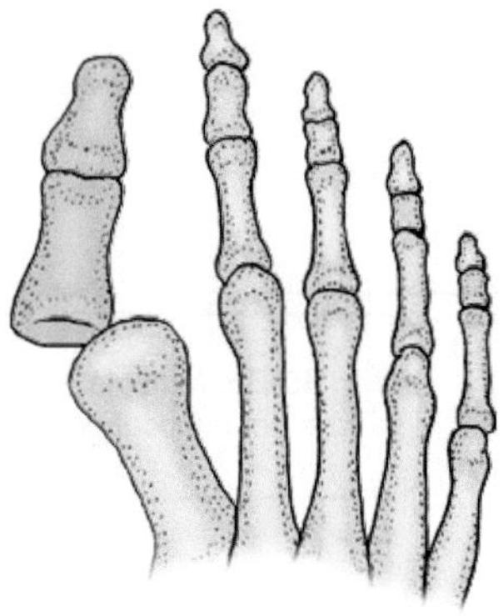
80D1.1

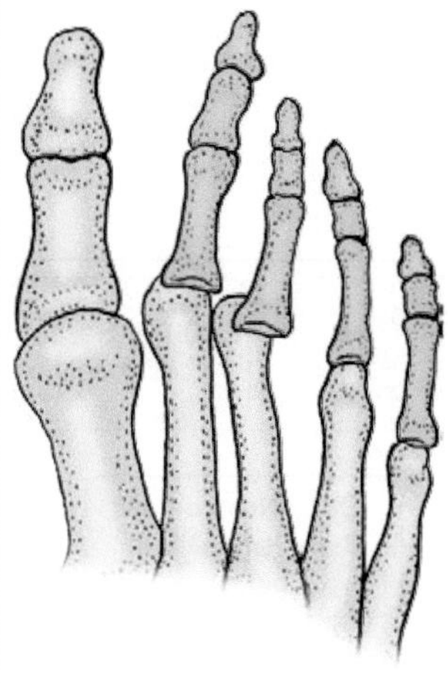
80D1.2~5

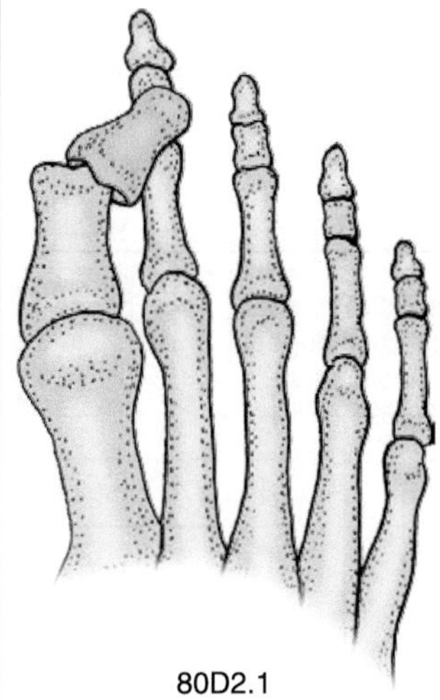
80D2.1

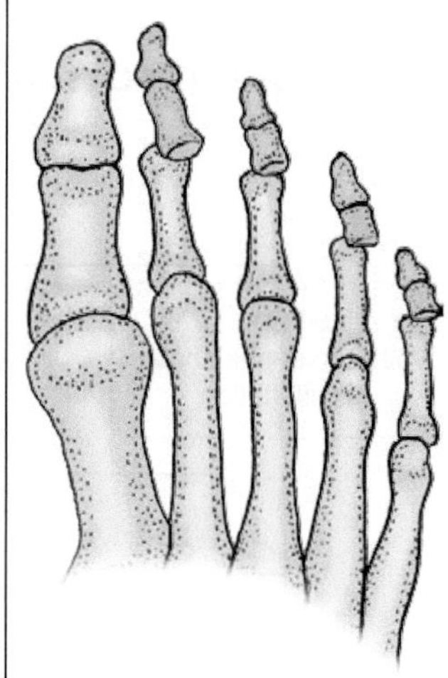
80D2.2~5

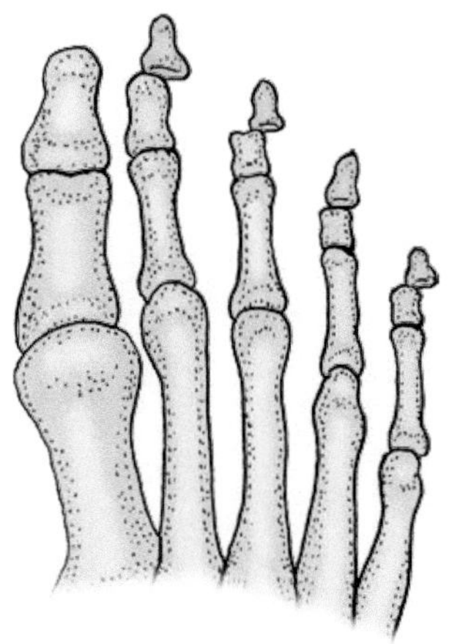
80D3.2~5

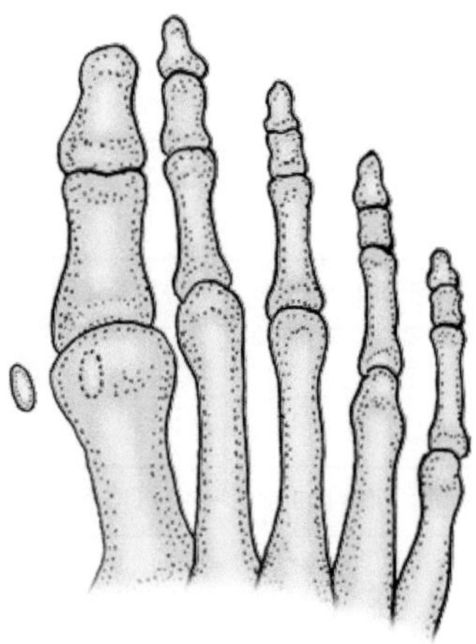
80D4

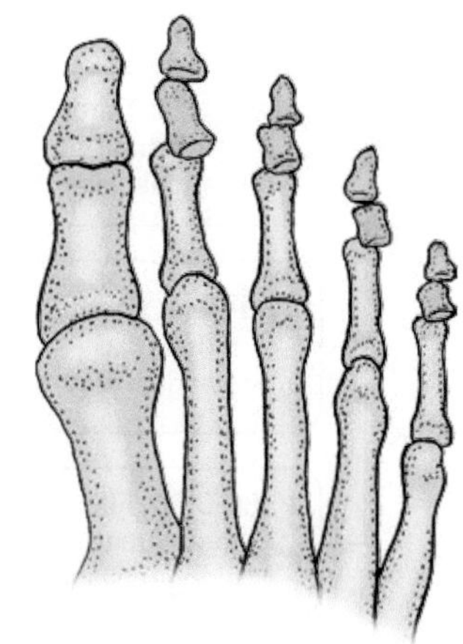
80D4

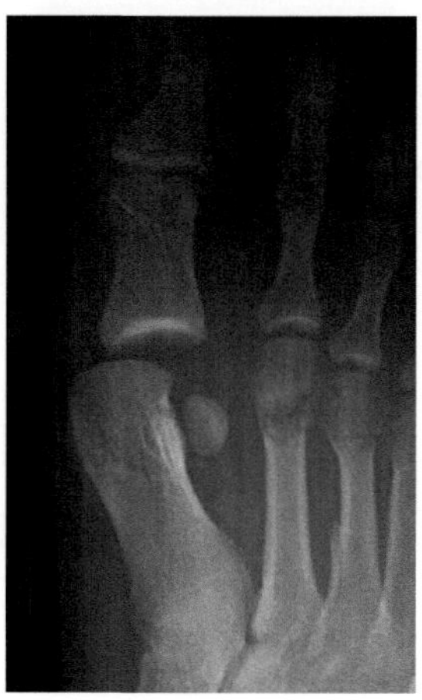
80D1.1

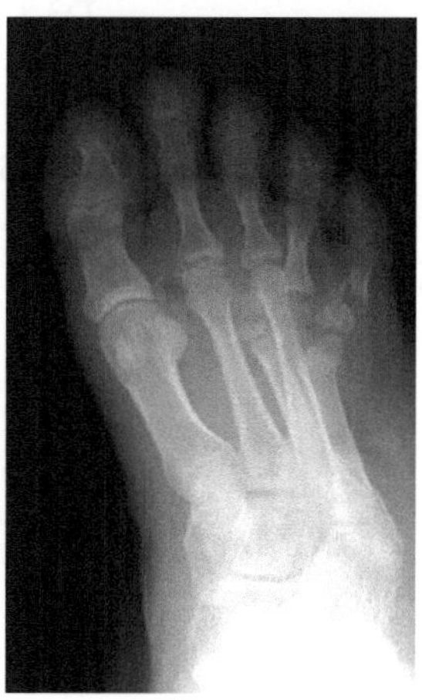
80D1.2~5

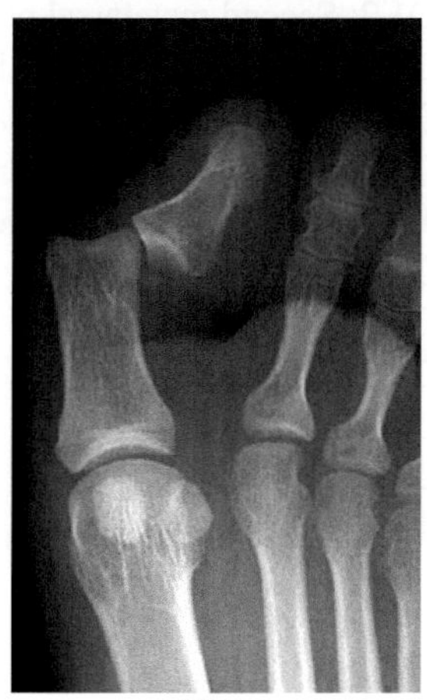
80D2.1

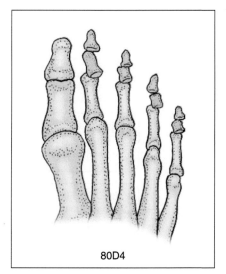

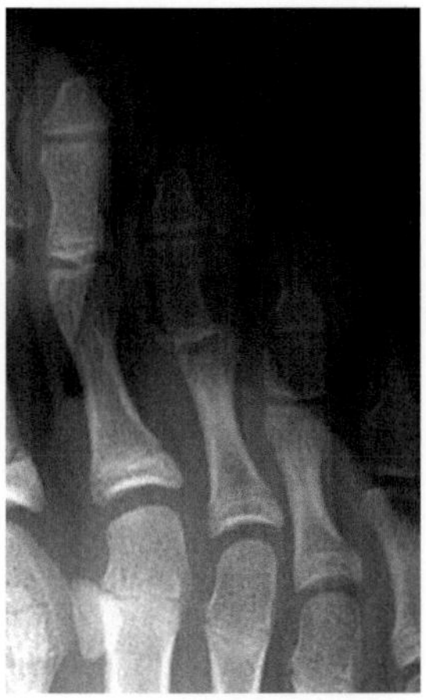

80D2.2~5

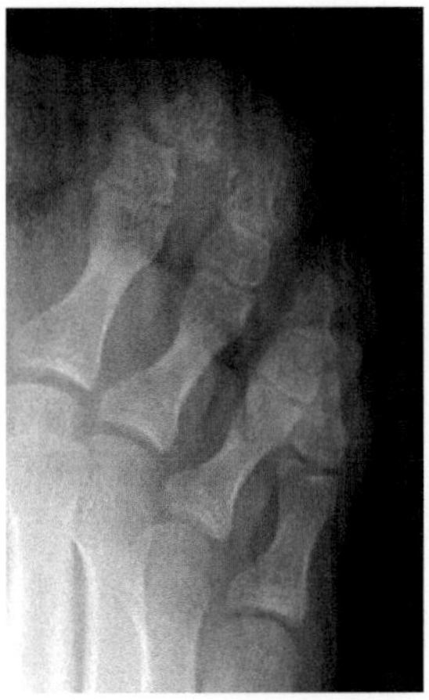

80D3.2~5

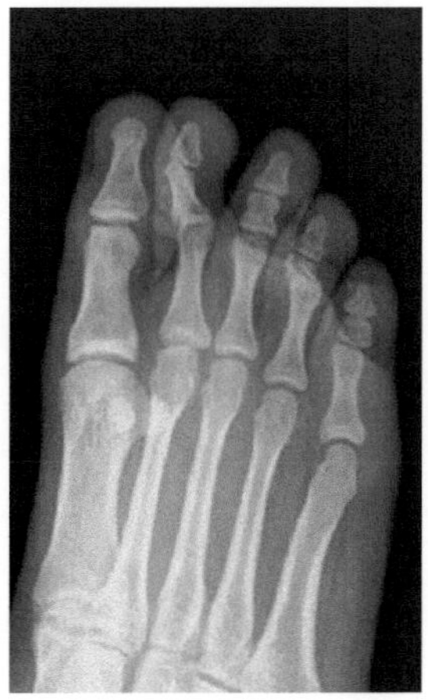

80D9

12.3.5.2 **Jahss Classification of First Metatarsophalangeal Dislocation** (1991, Disorders of the Foot and Ankle, Philadelphia: W B Saunders)

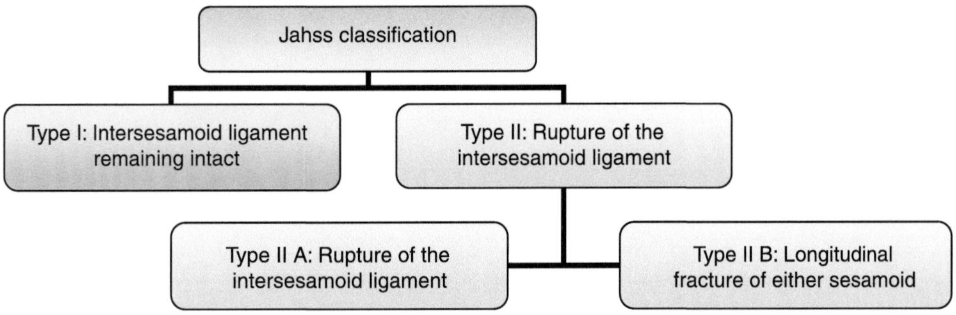

Type I: Volar plate avulsed off the first metatarsal head, proximal phalanx displaced dorsally; intersesamoid ligament remaining intact and lying over the dorsum of the metatarsal head.

Type II: Rupture of the intersesamoid ligament.

Type IIA: Rupture of the intersesamoid ligament, no fracture.

Type IIB: Longitudinal fracture of either sesamoid.

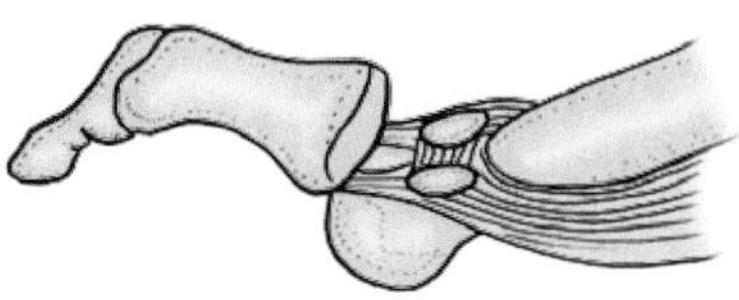

Type I

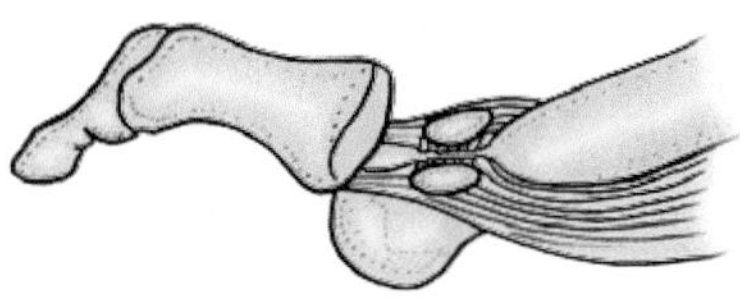

Type II A

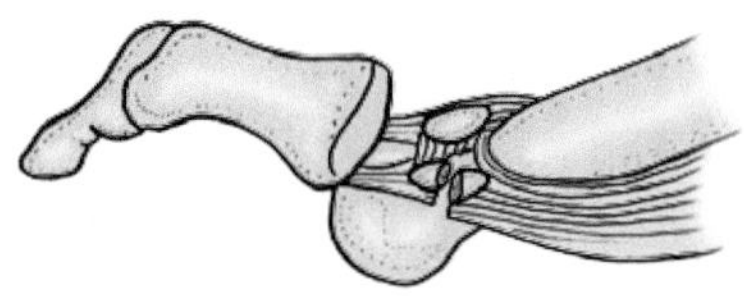

Type II B

Classifications of Soft-Tissue Injuries

13

Yingze Zhang and Xin Xing

13.1 Section 1 Classification AO of Soft-Tissue Injury

13.1.1 Classification AO of Skin Injury (IC) (Müller ME, Nazarian S, Koch P. Classification AO des fractures: Lesos longs. Berlin: Springer-Verlag, 1987)

IC1: No skin injury.
IC2: Contusion of skin, but no wound.
IC3: Limited degloving injury.
IC4: Extensive and closed degloving injury.
IC5: Contusion necrosis.

(I means cover, C means closure).

13.1.2 Classification AO of Skin Injury (IO) (Müller ME, NazarianS, Koch P. Classification AO des fractures: Lesos longs. Berlin: Springer-Verlag, 1987)

IO1: Skin from inside to outside stab.
IO2: Skin is damaged from the inside out <5 cm, the edge contusion.
IO3: Skin was damaged by >5 from inside to outside, severe contusion, and cm inactivation.
IO4: Full-thickness skin contusion, abrasions, wide-open sleeve.
IO5: Other special types of damage.

(I means cover, O means open).

13.1.3 AO Classification of Muscle and Tendon Injury (MT) (Müller ME, NazarianS, Koch P. Classification AO des fractures: Lesos longs. Berlin: Springer-Verlag, 1987)

MT1: Without muscle damage.
MT2: Limitation of muscle injury, confined to a single compartment.
MT3: Obvious muscle damage involving two compartments.
MT4: Muscle defect, tendon rupture, generalized muscle contusion.
MT5: Compartment syndrome or large-area crush syndrome.

13.1.4 AO Classification of Nerve and Vessel Injury (NV) (Müller ME, NazarianS, Koch P. Classification AO des fractures: Lesos longs. Berlin: Springer-Verlag, 1987)

NV1: Without nerve and vessel injury.
NV2: Single-nerve injury.
NV3: Local vascular injury.
NV4: Extensive segmental vascular injury.
NV5: Combined with nerve and vascular injury, including incomplete or complete disconnection.

Y. Zhang (✉) • X. Xing
Department of Orthopedics,
The Third Hospital of Hebei Medical University,
Shijiazhuang, China
e-mail: yzzhangdr@126.com, yzling_liu@163.com

Y. Zhang (ed.), *Clinical Classification in Orthopaedics Trauma*, https://doi.org/10.1007/978-981-10-6044-1_13

13.2 Section 2 Other Classification of Soft-Tissue Injuries

13.2.1 Gustilo Classification of Open Fracture (Gustilo RB, Anderson JT. Prevention of infection in the treatment of one thousand and twenty-five open fractures of long bones: Retrospective and prospective analyses. J Bone Joint Surg (Am), 1976; 58: 453–458. Gustilo RB, Mendoza RM, Williams DN. Problems in the management of type III (severe) open fractures: A new classification of type III open fractures. J Trauma. 1984; 24: 742–746)

Type I: An open fracture with a wound <1 cm in length and clean.

Type II: An open fracture with a laceration >1 cm but < 10 cm in length without extensive soft-tissue damage, flaps, or avulsions.

Type III: An open fracture with extensive soft-tissue laceration (>10 cm), damage, or loss or an open segmental fracture. This type also includes open fractures caused by farm injuries, fractures requiring vascular repair, or fractures that have been open for 8 h prior to treatment.

Type IIIA: Type III fracture with adequate periosteal coverage of the fracture bone despite the extensive soft-tissue laceration or damage.

Type IIIB: Type III fracture with extensive soft-tissue loss and periosteal stripping and bone damage. Usually associated with massive contamination. Will often need further soft-tissue coverage procedure (i.e. free or rotational flap).

Type IIIC: Type III fracture associated with an arterial injury requiring repair, irrespective of degree of soft-tissue injury.

13.2.2 Oestern and Tscherne Classification of Soft-Tissue Injury in Closed Fractures (Tscherne H, Oestern HJ. Die Klassifizierung des Weichteil-schadens bei offenen und geschlossenen. Frakturen. Unfallheilkunde, 1982, 85: 111–115)

Grade	Soft-tissue injury	Fracture pattern
0	Minimal soft-tissue damage caused by indirect injury to limb (torsion)	Simple fracture
1	Superficial abrasion or contusion	Mild fracture
2	Deep abrasion, skin or muscle contusion caused by direct trauma to limb	Severe fracture
3	Extensive skin contusion or crush injury, severe damage to underlying muscle, compartment syndrome, subcutaneous avulsion	Severe fracture

13.2.3 Classification According to the Severity of Soft-Tissue Injury

Class I: The skin is punctured from the inside to the outside.

Class II: The skin is cut or crushed, with moderate damage to the skin and muscles.

Class III: A wide range of skin, subcutaneous tissue, and muscle damage, often associated with neurovascular injury.

13.2.4 Seddon Classification of Peripheral Nerve Injury (1943)

Class	Mechanism	Pathological change	Outcome
Neurotmesis	Transection injury	Steatosis of cracked nerve fibres	Peripheral neuroma
	Traction injury	Nerve injury	
Axonotmesis	Traction injury	Steatosis of impaired nerve fibres	Regeneration
	Compression	Structure preserving	
Neuropraxia	Compression	With or without local demyelination	Recovery

Neuropraxia (Class I): It is a temporary interruption of conduction without loss of axonal continuity. In neuropraxia, there is a physiologic block of nerve conduction in the affected axons.

Other characteristics:

- It is the mildest type of peripheral nerve injury.
- There are sensory-motor problems distal to the site of injury.
- The endoneurium, perineurium, and epineurium are intact.
- There is no Wallerian degeneration.
- Conduction is intact in the distal segment and proximal segment, but no conduction occurs across the area of injury.
- Recovery of nerve conduction deficit is full, and requires days to weeks.
- EMG shows lack of fibrillation potentials (FP) and positive sharp waves.

Axonotmesis (Class II): It involves loss of the relative continuity of the axon and its covering of myelin, but preservation of the connective tissue framework of the nerve (the encapsulating tissue, the epineurium and perineurium, is preserved).

Other characteristics:

- Wallerian degeneration occurs distal to the site of injury.
- There are sensory and motor deficits distal to the site of lesion.
- There is no nerve conduction distal to the site of injury (3 to 4 days after injury).
- EMG shows fibrillation potentials (FP), and positive sharp waves (2 to 3 weeks postinjury).
- Axonal regeneration occurs and recovery is possible without surgical treatment. Sometimes surgical intervention because of scar tissue formation is required.

Neurotmesis (Class III): It is a total severance or disruption of the entire nerve fibre. A peripheral nerve fibre contains an axon (or long dendrite), myelin sheath (if existence), their Schwann cells, and the endoneurium. Neurotmesis may be partial or complete.

Other characteristics:

- Wallerian degeneration occurs distal to the site of injury.
- There is connective tissue lesion that may be partial or complete.
- Sensory-motor problems and autonomic function defect are severe.
- There is no nerve conduction distal to the site of injury (3 to 4 days after lesion).
- EMG and NCV findings are as axonotmesis.
- Because of lack of nerve repair, surgical intervention is necessary.

13.2.5 Sunderland Classification of Peripheral Nerve Injury. (Sunderland S. Nerves and Nerve Injuries. Edinburgh and London: Livingstone, 1968)

First-degree (Class I): Seddon's neurapraxia and first-degree are the same.

Second-degree (Class II): Seddon's axonotmesis and second-degree are the same.

Third-degree (Class III): Third-degree is included within Seddon's neurotmesis. It's a nerve fibre interruption. There is a lesion of the endoneurium, but the epineurium and perineurium remain intact. Recovery from a third-degree injury is possible, but surgical intervention may be required.

Fourth-degree (Class III): Fourth-degree is included within Seddon's neurotmesis. Only the epineurium remains intact. In this case, surgical repair is required.

Fifth-degree (Class III): Fifth-degree is included within Seddon's neurotmesis. A complete transection of the nerve. Recovery is not possible without an appropriate surgical treatment.

13.2.6 Cervicular Vascular Injury Scale (Moore EE, Malangoni MA, Cogbill TH, et al. Organ injury scaling VII: Cervical vascular, peripheral vascular, adrenal, penis, testis, and scrotum. J Trauma, 1996, 41:523–524)

Grade	Description of injury	AIS-90
I	Vena thyreoidea, common facial vein, external jugular vein, non-named arterial/venous branches	1–3
II	External carotid branches (ascending pharyngeal artery, superior thyroid artery, lingual artery, etc.)	1–3
	Thyrocervical trunk and its first-level branches	1–3
	Internal jugular vein	1–3
III	External jugular vein	2–3
	Subclavian vein	3–4
	Vertebral artery	2–4
IV	Common carotid artery	3–5
	Subclavian artery	3–4
V	Internal carotid (extracranial)	3–5

Increase one grade for multiple grade III or IV injuries involving >50% vessel circumference. Decrease one grade for <25% vessel circumference disruption for grades IV or V

13.2.7 Peripheral Vascular Organ Injury Scale (Moore EE, Malangoni MA, Cogbill TH, et al. Organ injury scaling VII: Cervical vascular, peripheral vascular, adrenal, penis, testis, and scrotum. J Trauma, 1996, 41:523–524)

Grade	Description of injury	AIS-90
I	Digital artery/vein, palmar artery/vein, deep palmar artery/vein, dorsalis pedis artery, planter artery/vein, non-named arterial/venous branches	1 ~ 3
II	Basilic/cephalic vein, saphenous vein, radial artery, ulnar artery	1 ~ 3
III	Axillary vein, superficial/deep femoral vein, popliteal vein, brachial artery	2 ~ 3
	Anterior tibial artery, posterior tibial artery, peroneal artery	1 ~ 3
	Tibioperoneal trunk	2 ~ 3
IV	Superficial/deep femoral artery	3 ~ 4
	Popliteal artery	2 ~ 3
V	Axillary artery	2 ~ 3
	Common femoral artery	3 ~ 4

13.2.8 Zhang Yingze Classification of Cruciate Ligament Injury of the Knee Joint

Class I: No loosening of the knee joint by the KT-1000 test; no difference in the tibial displacement between the affected side and the contralateral side.

Class II: Ligament fibre bundle fracture ≤1/3; no knee joint relaxation by the KT-1000 test; knee displacement difference of <2 mm.

Class III:

Class IIIA: Ligament fibre bundle fracture 1/3–2/3; mild knee laxity by the KT-1000 test; knee displacement difference of 2–3 mm

Class IIIB: Avulsion fracture of the intercondylar eminence (no displacement or avulsion <2 mm).

Class IV:

Class IVA: Ligament rupture >2/3; moderate knee laxity by the KT-1000 test; knee displacement difference of ≥3 mm

Class IVB: Avulsion fracture of the intercondylar eminence (avulsion ≥2 mm).

Class V:

Class VA: Complete rupture of the ligament; severe knee laxity by the KT-1000 test; knee displacement difference of ≥5 mm

Class VB: Avulsion fracture of the intercondylar eminence (complete avulsion).

14 Fracture and Dislocation Classification for Children

Yingze Zhang and Liang Shi

14.1 Section 1 Epiphyseal Injury/Fracture in Children

Poland first proposed the classification of epiphyseal injuries in children in 1898. In 1863, Salter-Harris divided epiphyseal injuries in children into five types, which has been widely accepted. Mercer Rang added type VI based on the classification of Salter-Harris.

14.1.1 Salter-Harris Classification (1963, J Bone Joint Surg (Am), 45:587–622)

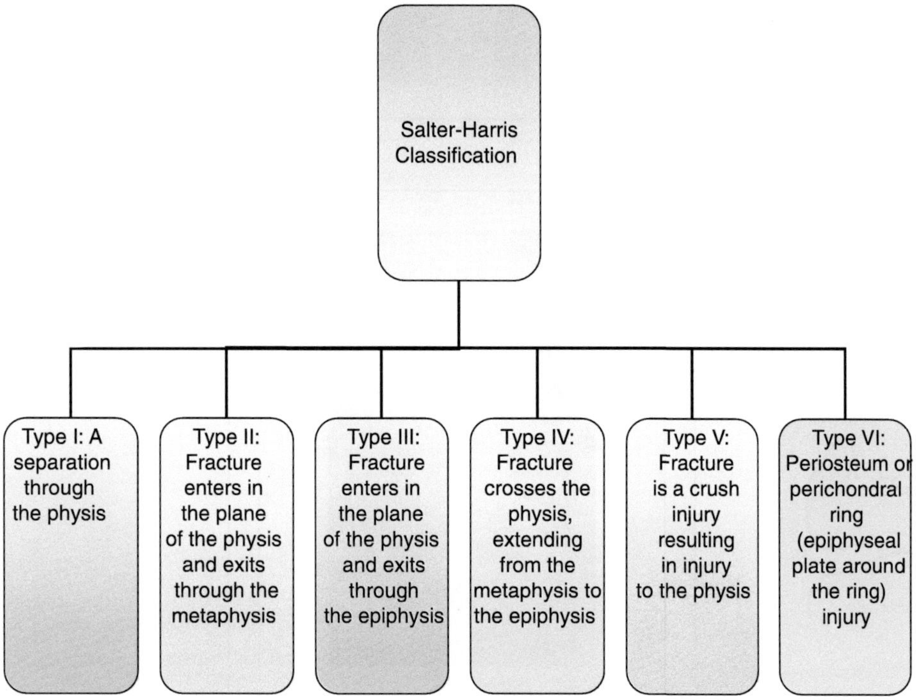

Y. Zhang (✉) • L. Shi
Department of Orthopedics,
The Third Hospital of Hebei Medical University,
Shijiazhuang, China
e-mail: yzzhangdr@126.com, yzling_liu@163.com

Y. Zhang (ed.), *Clinical Classification in Orthopaedics Trauma*, https://doi.org/10.1007/978-981-10-6044-1_14

Type I: A separation through the physis.

Type II: Fracture enters in the plane of the physis and exits through the metaphysis.

Type III: Fracture enters in the plane of the physis and exits through the epiphysis.

Type IV: Fracture crosses the physis, extending from the metaphysis to the epiphysis.

Type V: Fracture is a crush injury resulting in injury to the physis.

Type VI: Periosteum or perichondral ring (epiphyseal plate around the ring) injury, less common.

In types I and II injuries, the fracture line does not pass through the epiphysis and does not usually cause growth retardation; types III and IV injuries in the epiphysis can cause growth retardation and progressive deformity.

Mercer Rang (1994, J Pediatr Orthop, 14:439) adds type VI to this classification.

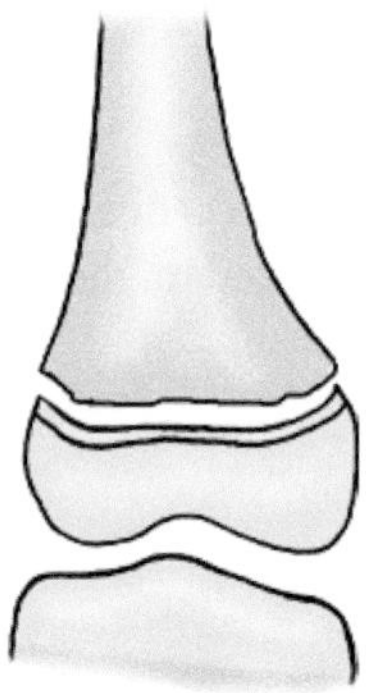

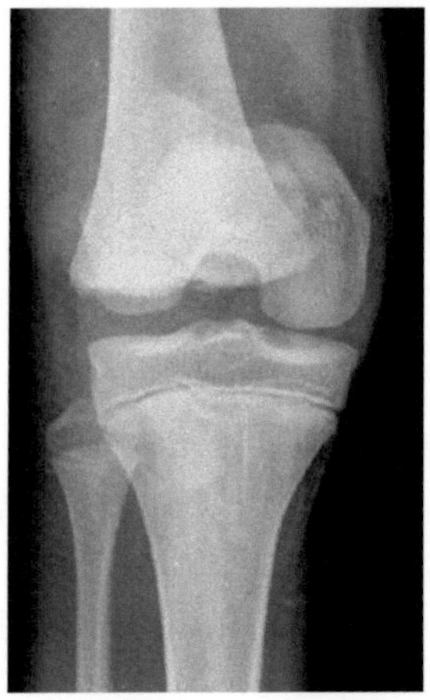

Salter-Harris classification of pediatric physeal fractures
Type I: A separation through the physis

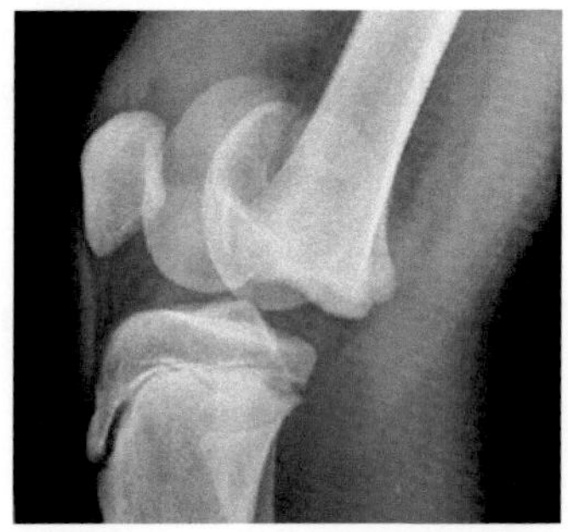

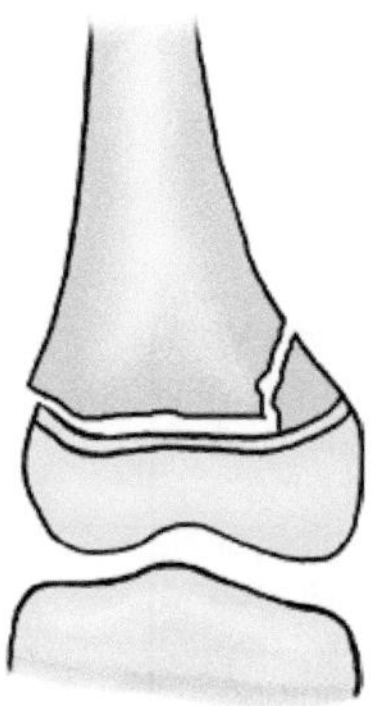

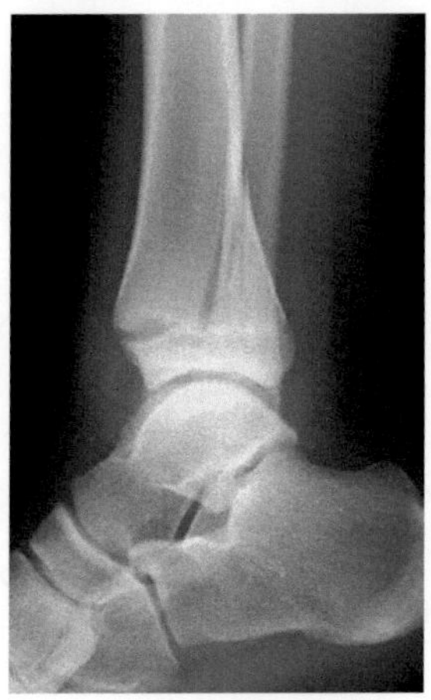

Salter-Harris classification of pediatric physeal fractures
Type II: Fracture enters in the plane of the physis and exits through the metaphysis

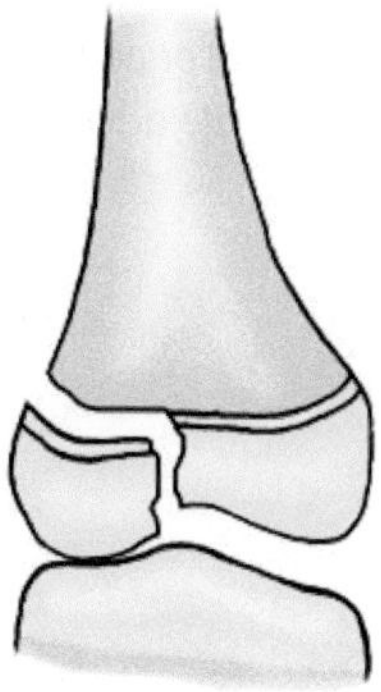

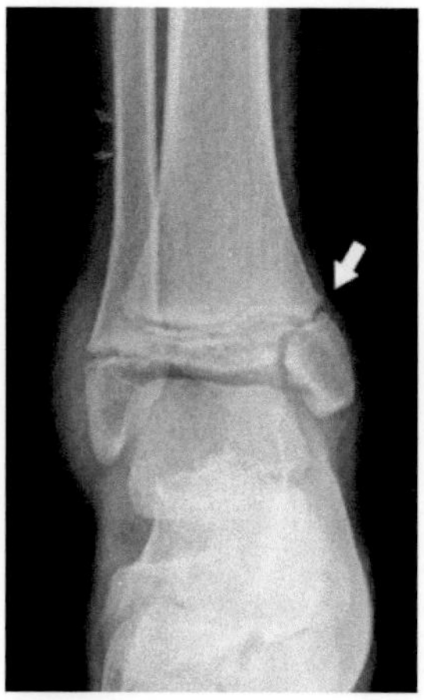

Salter-Harris classification of pediatric physeal fractures
Type III: Fracture enters in the plane of the physis and exits through the epiphysis

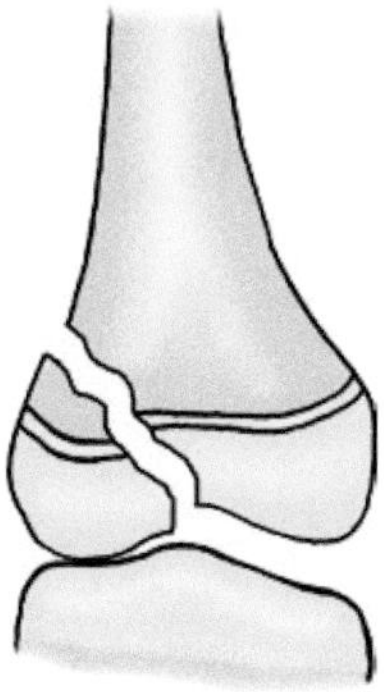

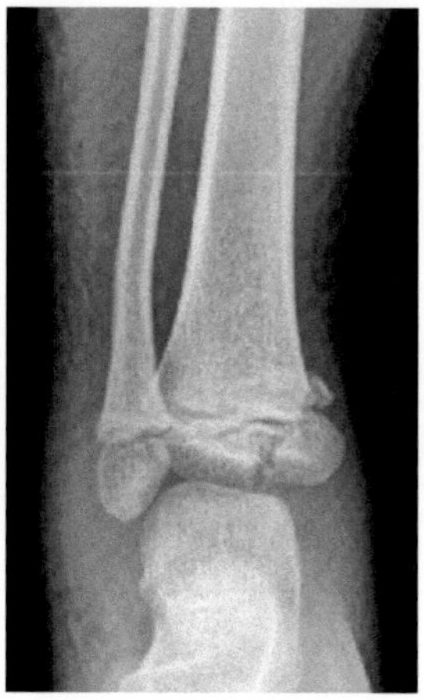

Salter-Harris classification of pediatric physeal fractures
Type IV: Fracture crosses the physis, extending from the metaphysis to the epiphysis

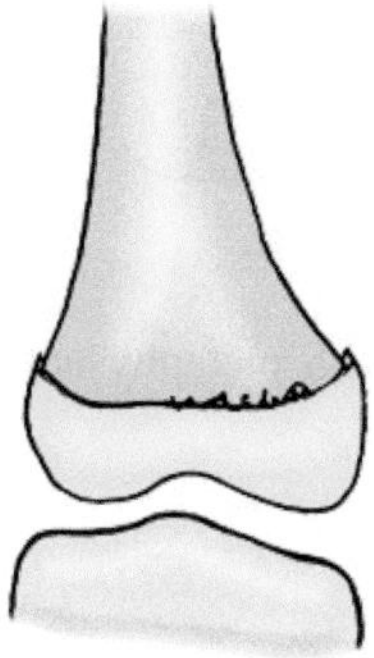

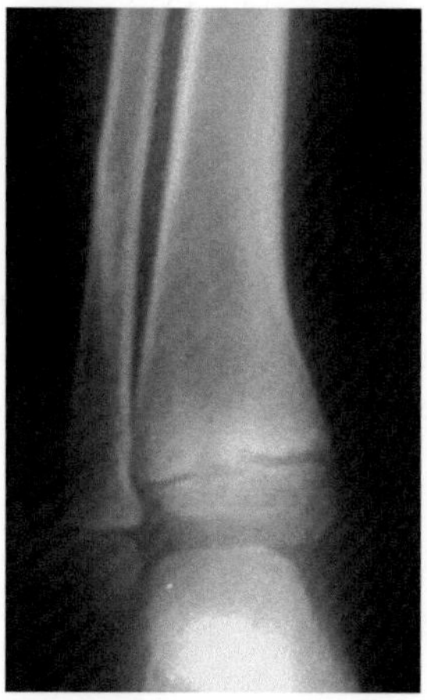

Salter-Harris classification of pediatric physeal fractures
Type V: Fracture is a crush injury resulting in injury to the physis

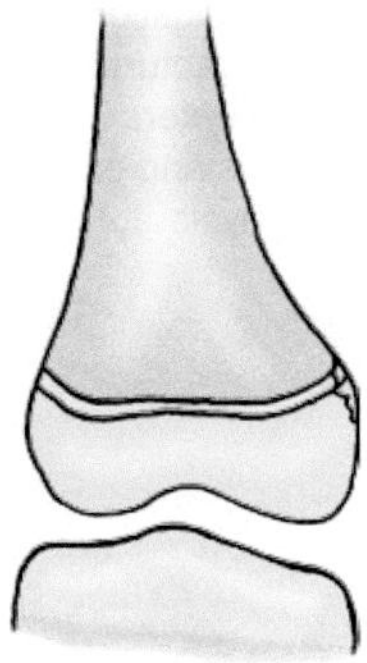

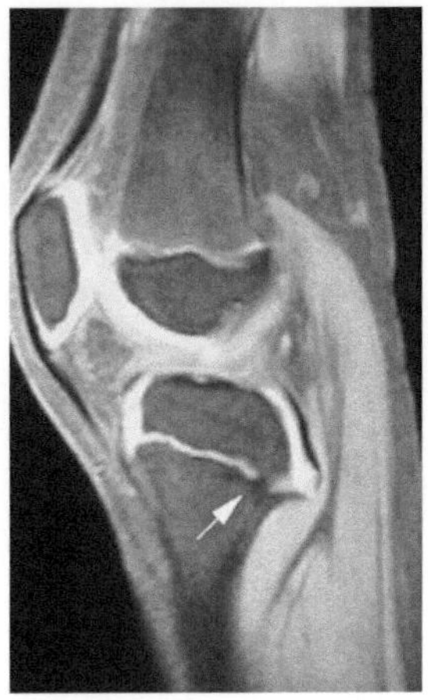

Salter-Harris classification of pediatric physeal fractures
Type VI: Periosteum or perichondral ring (epiphyseal plate around the ring) injury

14.1.2 **Poland Classification** (1898, Traumatic Separation of the Epiphyses. London: Smith, Elder & Company)

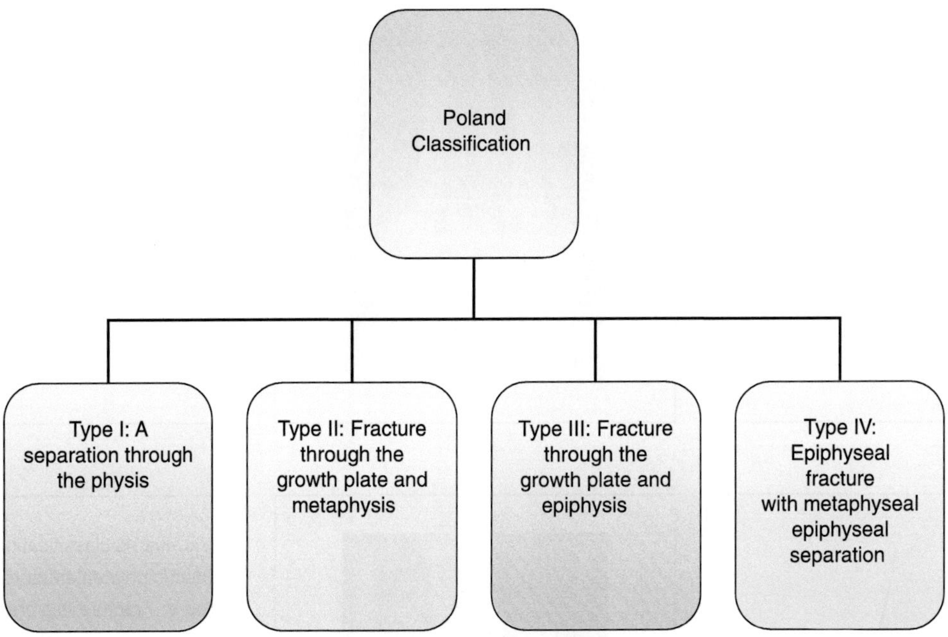

Type I: A separation through the physis.
Type II: Fracture through the growth plate and metaphysis.
Type III: Fracture through the growth plate and epiphysis.
Type IV: Epiphyseal fracture with metaphyseal epiphyseal separation.

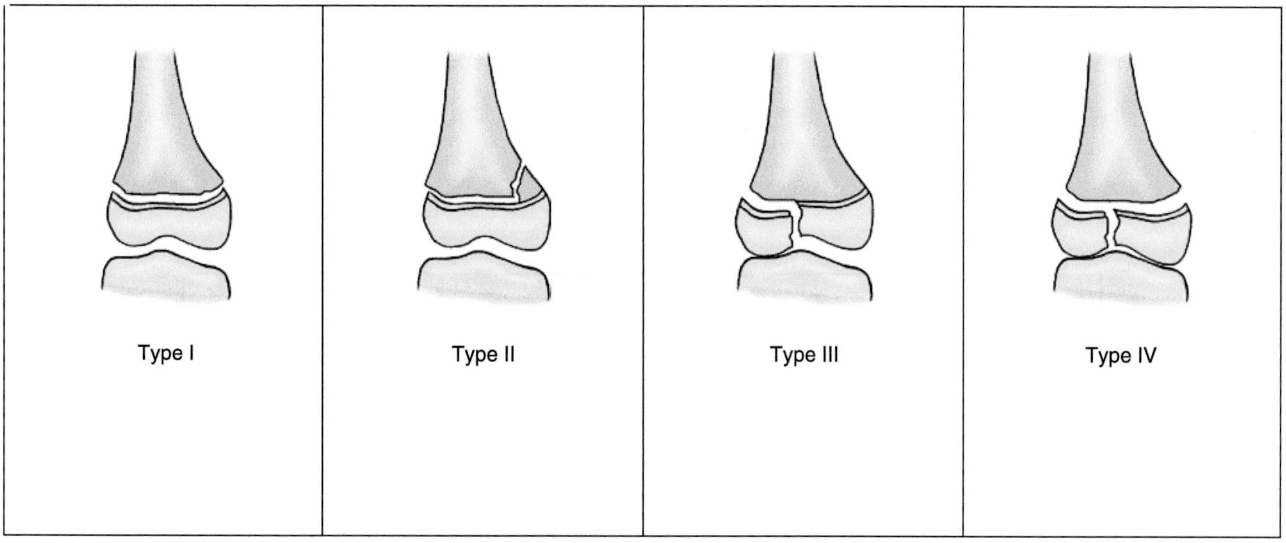

14.1.3 Aitken Classification (1936, J Bone Joint Surg, 18:685–691)

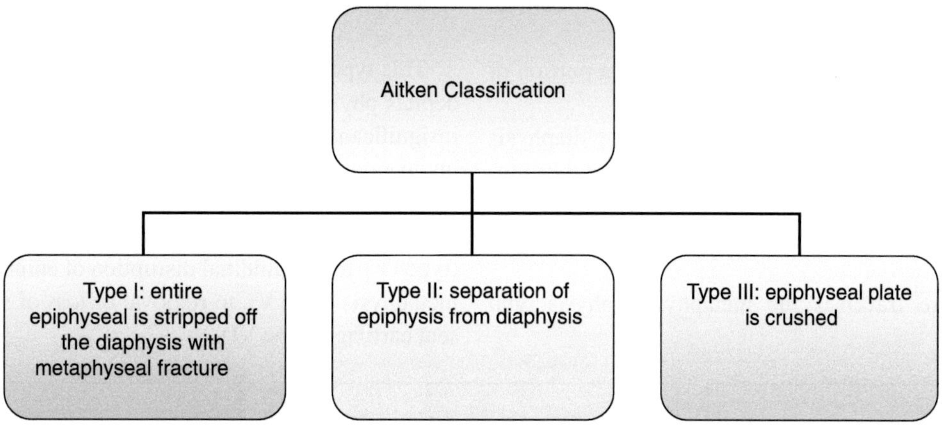

Type I: Avulsion fracture, entire epiphyseal is stripped off the diaphysis with metaphyseal fracture.

Type II: Compression fracture, separation of epiphysis from diaphysis.

Type III: Compression fracture, epiphyseal plate is crushed, deformity in this type is common.

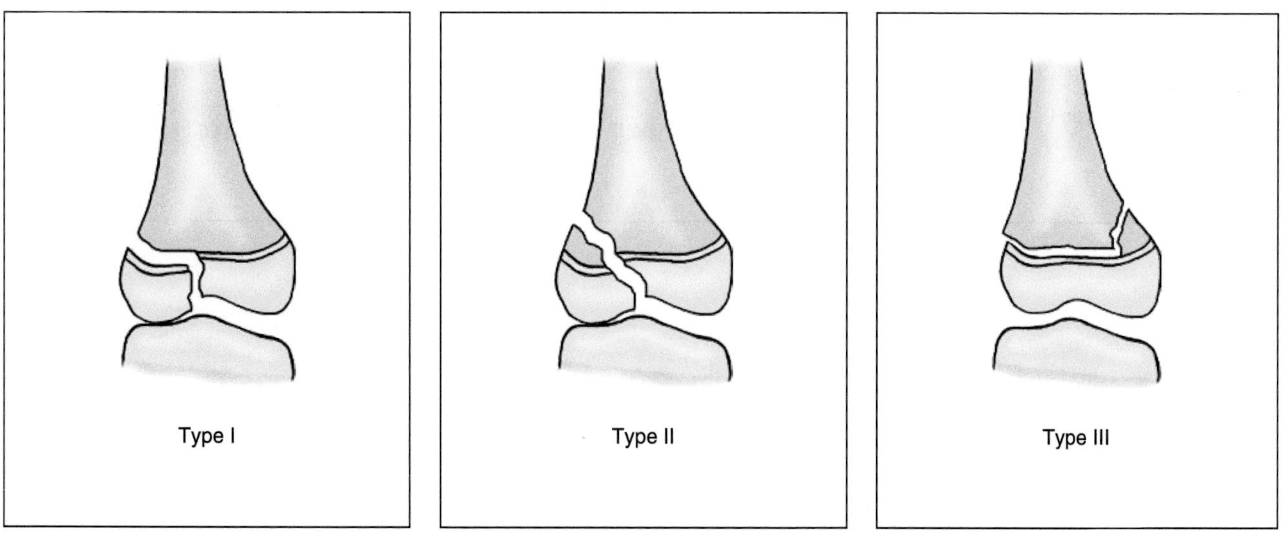

14.1.4 Peterson Classification (1994, J Pediatr Orthop, 14:431–448)

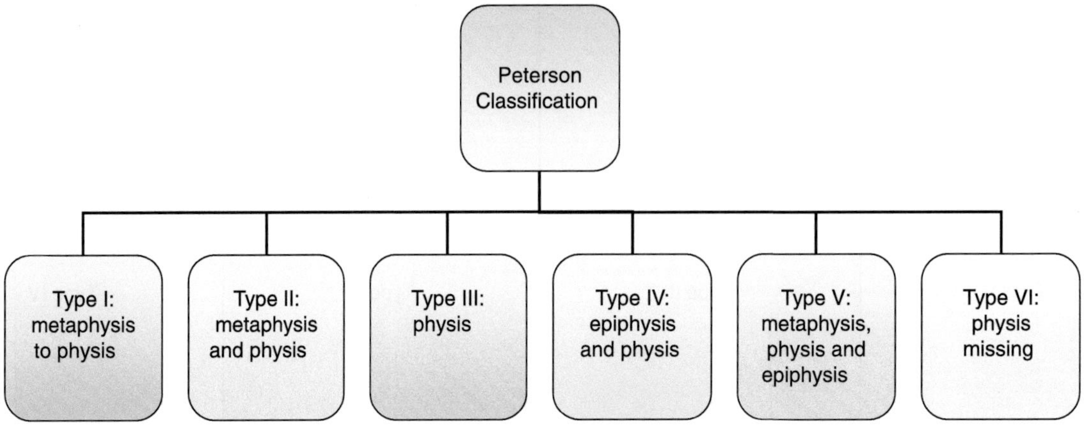

Type I: Transverse fracture of the metaphysis with extension to the physis. There may be a small eccentric cortical fragment not attached to either epiphysis or cortical fragment.

Type II: Separation of a part of the physis, with a portion of the metaphysis attached to the epiphysis.

Type III: Separation of the epiphysis from the diaphysis through any of the layer of the physis disrupting the complete physis.

Type IV: Fracture of the epiphysis extending to and along the physis.

Type V: Fracture traverses the metaphysis, physis, and epiphysis.

Type VI: The fracture in which a portion of the physis has been removed or is missing and typically is described as an open "lawnmower" type of injury.

This type of classification has a sound anatomic basis; it depicts physeal tissue injury as a continuum from relatively insignificant involvement (type I), to progressively more involvement (type II), to complete transphyseal disruption (type III), to transphyseal disruption with epiphyseal fracture, which ensures damage to the germinal layer of cells (type IV), to longitudinal disruption of epiphysis, physis, and metaphysis (type V), to removal or loss of some of the physeal cartilage (type VI).

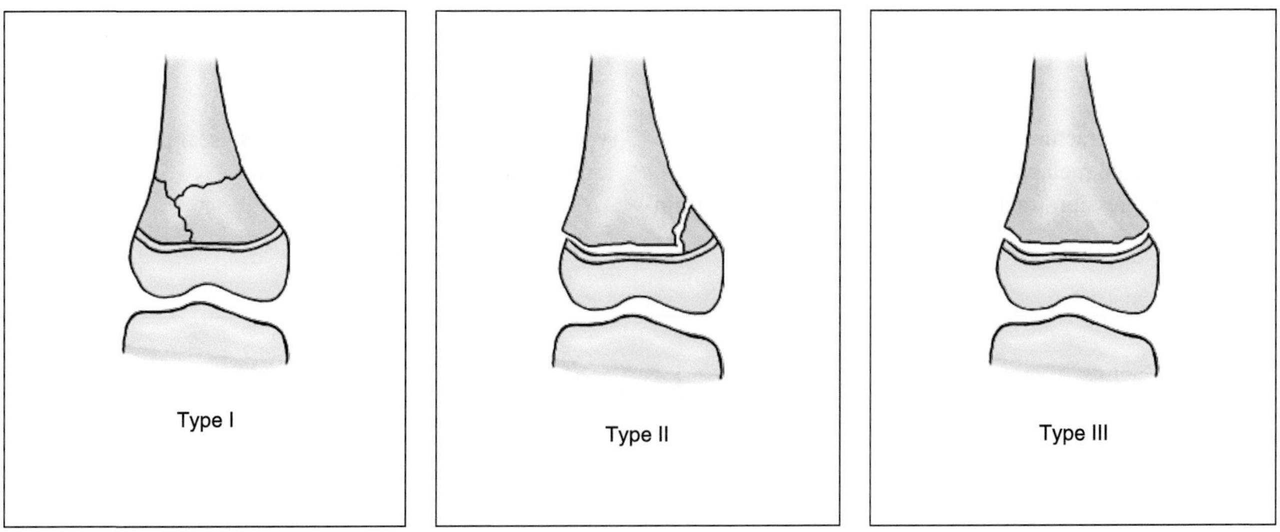

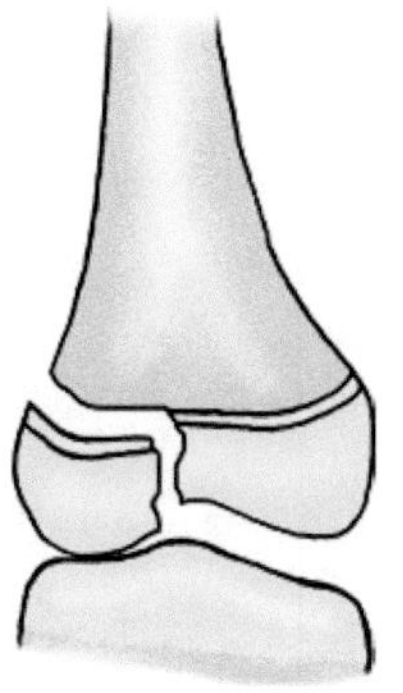

Type V

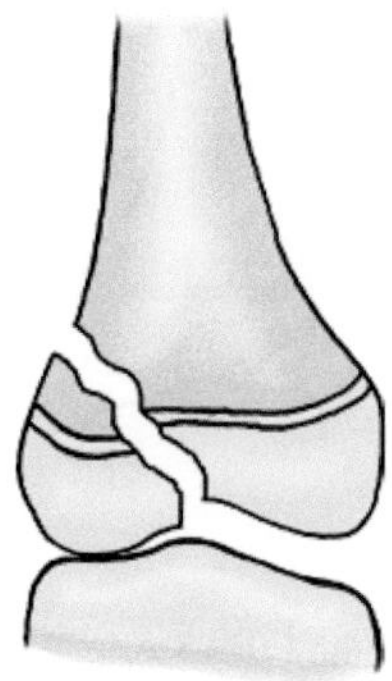

Type IV

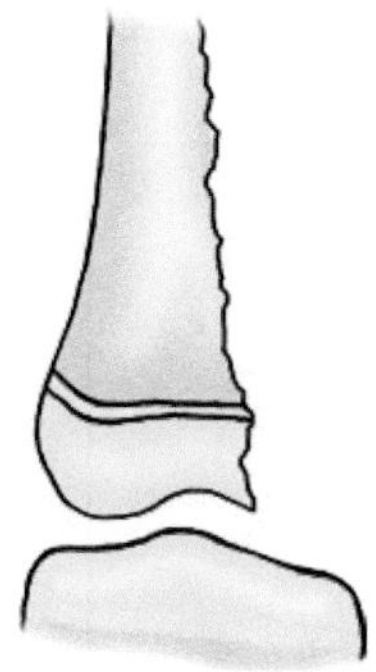

Type VI

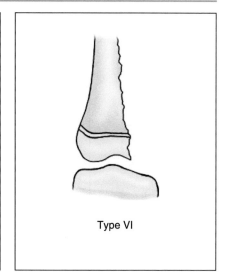

14.1.5 Weber and Brunner Classification

Type A: Equivalent to Salter-Harris classification of type 1 and type 2.

Type B: Equivalent to Salter-Harris classification of type 3 and type 4.

14.1.6 Ogden Classification

Ogden in 1981 proposed a classification of 9 types with 11 subtypes, thus producing 20 types.

The first five types are those of Salter and Harris.

Type VI: Periosteum or perichondral ring injury described by Rang.

Type VII: Epiphyseal fracture (tibial ridge, internal and external condylar avulsion fracture).

Type VIII: Metaphyseal structure damage.

Type IX: Diaphysis → periosteum → growth-shaping disorder.

Though this classification and author's depictions of growth arrest with each type are valid, it has not gained widespread use, probably because the multiple subtypes are too difficult to remember and because types VII, VIII, and IX are common nonphyseal fractures that rarely result in growth arrest.

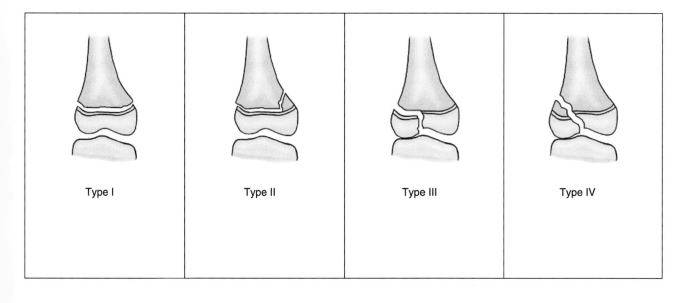

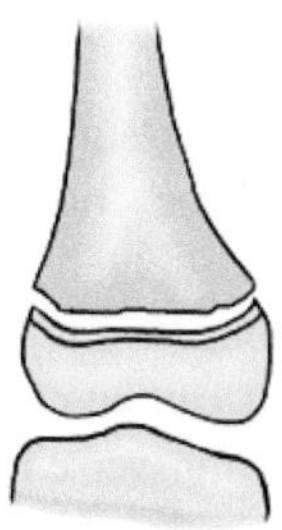

Type I

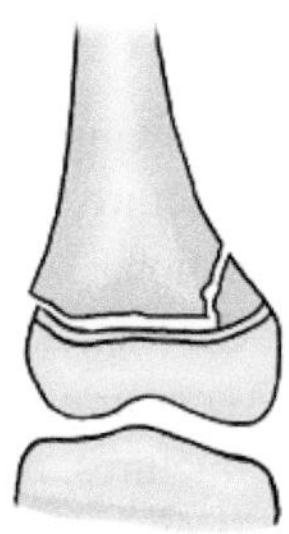

Type II

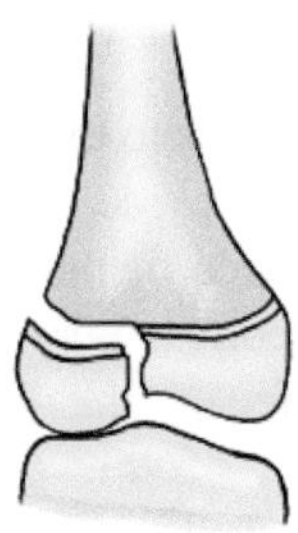

Type III

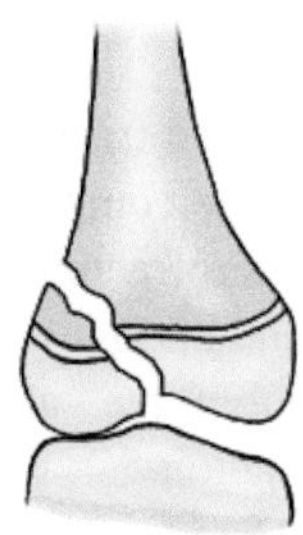

Type IV

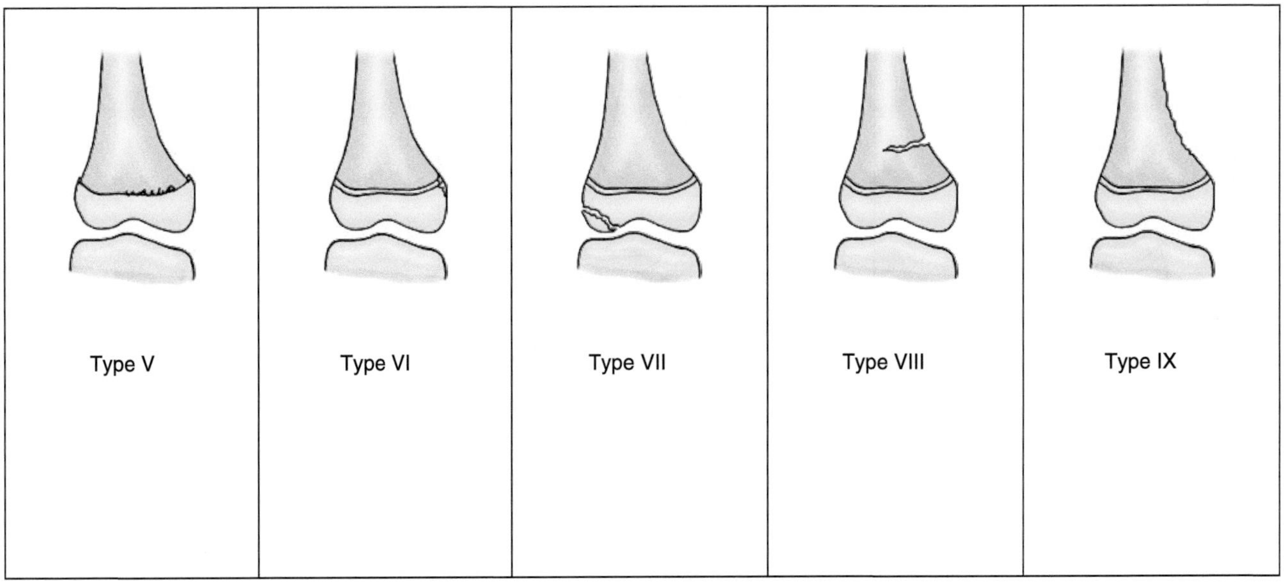

14.1.7 Children with Long Tubular Bone Fracture Jones Classification (1998)

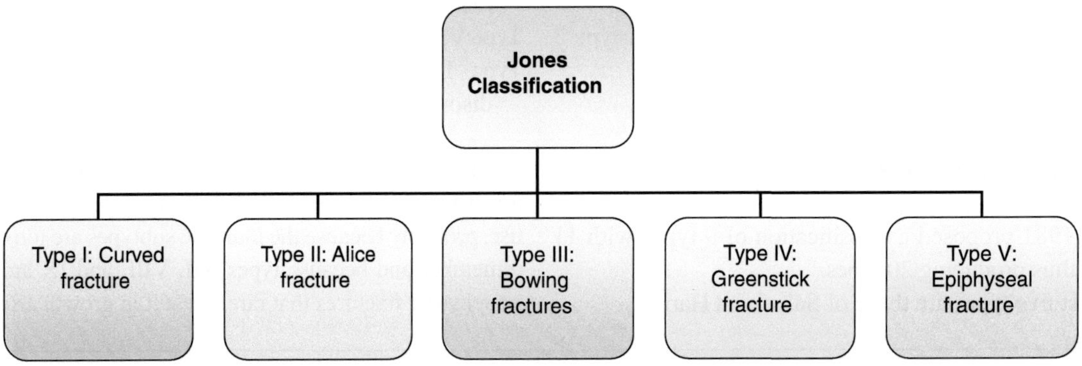

Type I: Curved fracture. Bending stress leads to the concave side of the compression side and convex side of the tension microfracture. But the tension side of the fracture line limitations, not spread to the cortex, removes the external force after the backbone of the bending deformation.

Type II: Alice fracture. Mostly for the metaphyseal and bone at the angle of compression fractures.

Type III: Bowing fractures. Bone-bending stress, tension-side fracture, concave side of the bone-bending deformation.

Type IV: Greenstick fracture. Cortical bone is completely broken. According to the fracture line it can be divided into spiral fractures, oblique fracture, and transverse fracture.

Type V: Epiphyseal fracture. Epiphyseal fractures often affect the epiphyseal plate.

14.2 Section 2 Children Humeral Fractures

14.2.1 AO/OTA Classification

14.2.1.1 Proximal Humerus Epiphyseal Fractures (11-E)

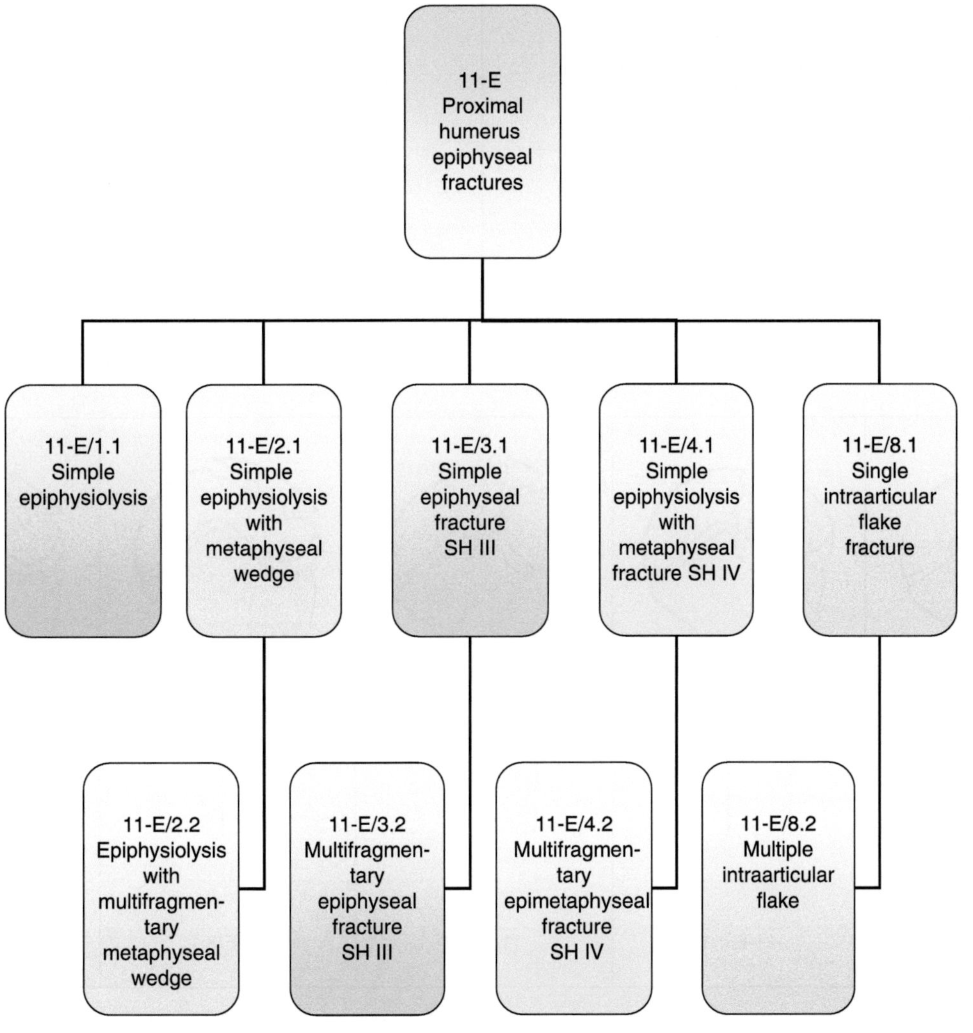

11-E: Proximal humeral epiphyseal fractures:

1.1: Simple epiphysiolysis.
2.1: Simple epiphysiolysis with metaphyseal wedge.
2.2: Epiphysiolysis with multifragmentary metaphyseal wedge.
3.1: Simple epiphyseal fracture SH III.
3.2: Multifragmentary epiphyseal fracture SH III.
4.1: Simple epiphysiolysis with metaphyseal fracture SH IV.
4.2: Multifragmentary epimetaphyseal fracture SH IV.
8.1: Single intra-articular flake fracture.
8.2: Multiple intra-articular flake.

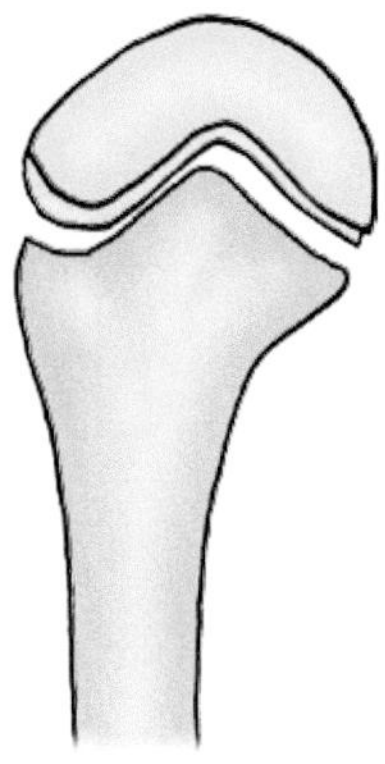
11-E/1.1

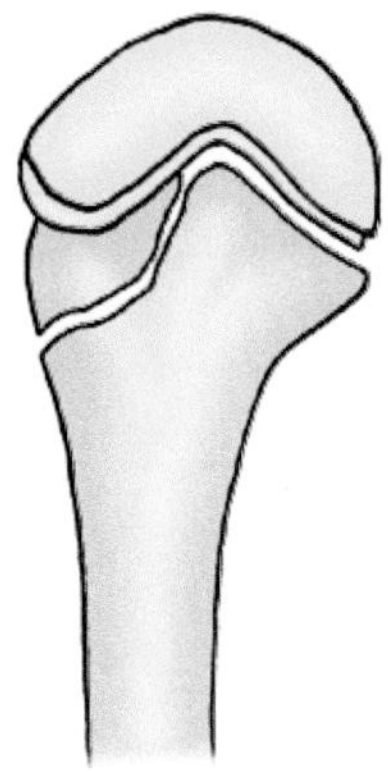
11-E/2.1

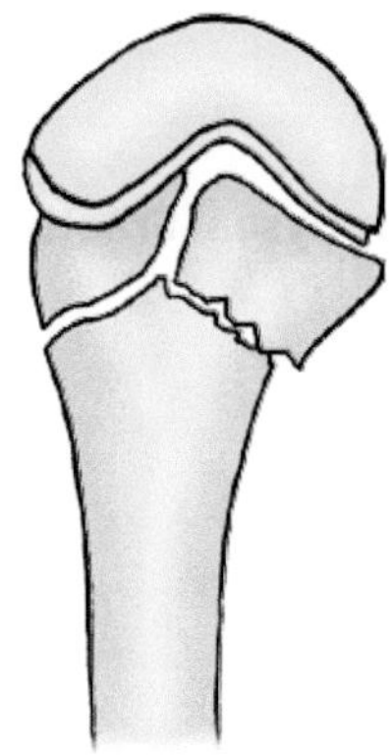
11-E/2.2

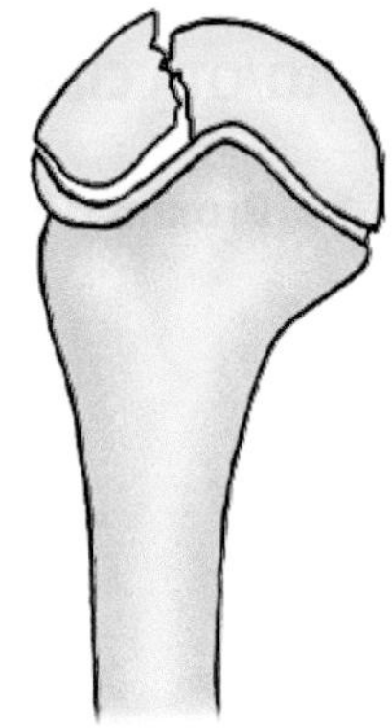
11-E/3.1

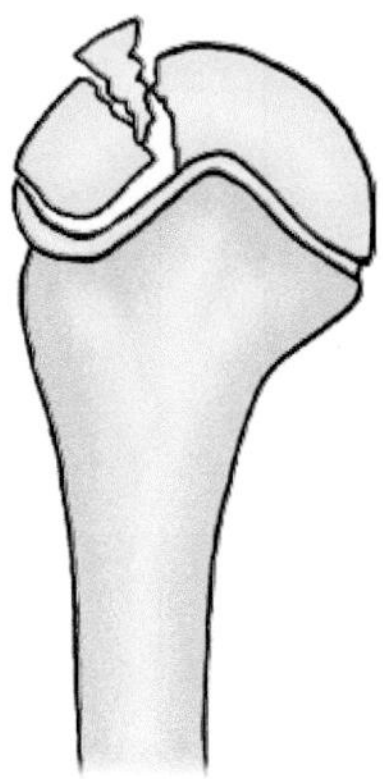
11-E/3.2

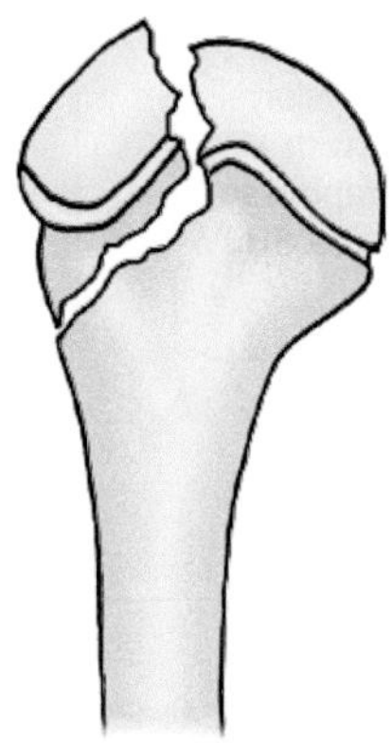
11-E/4.1

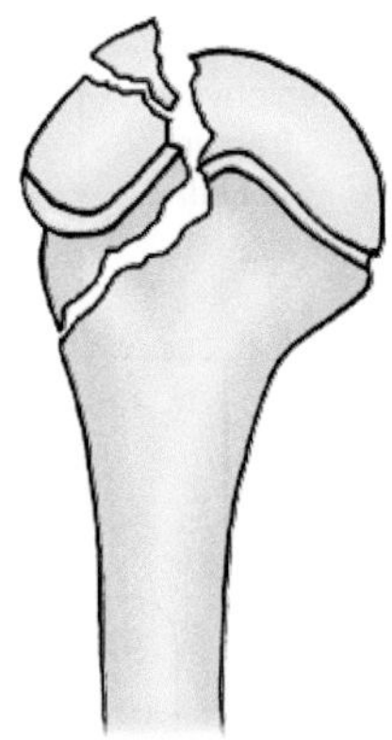
11-E/4.2

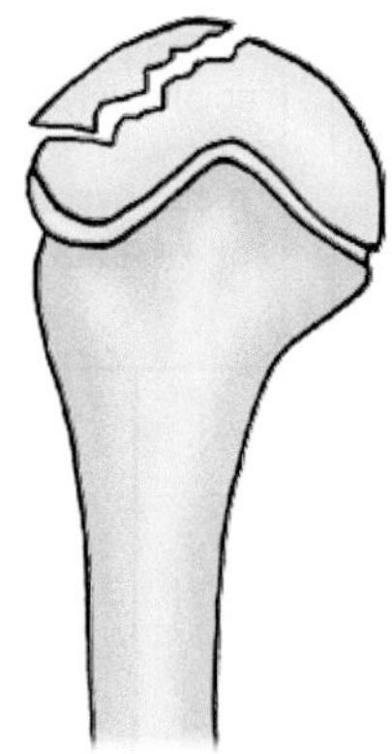
11-E/8.1

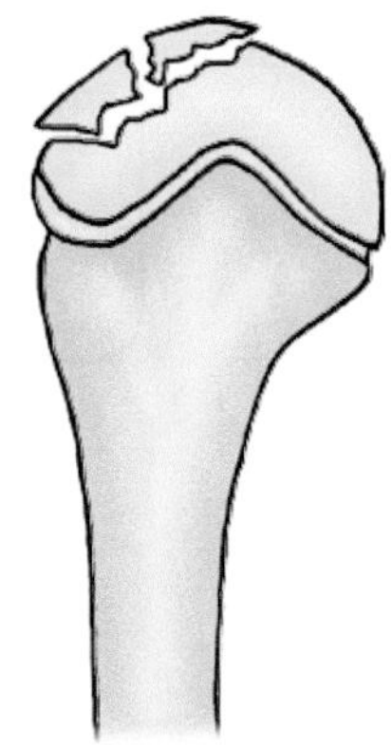
11-E/8.2

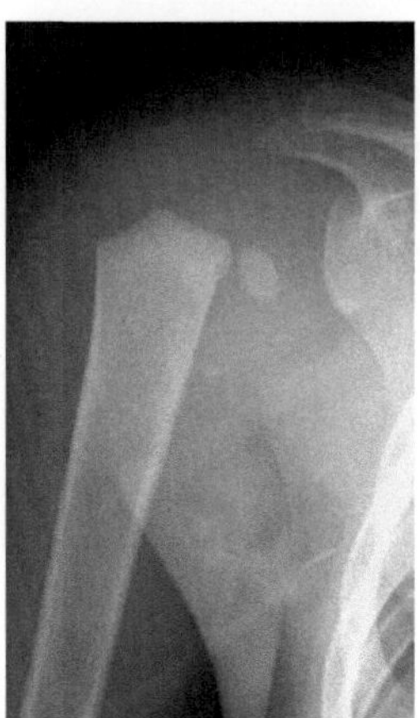
11-E/1.1

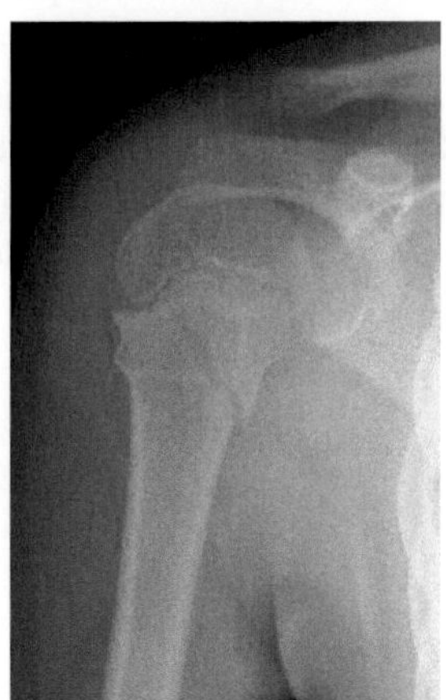
11-E/2.2

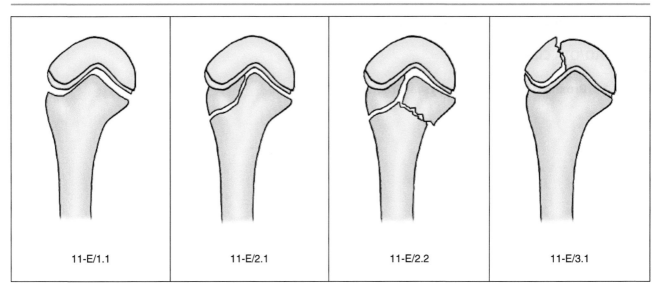

14.2.1.2 Proximal Metaphyseal Fracture of the Humerus (11-M)

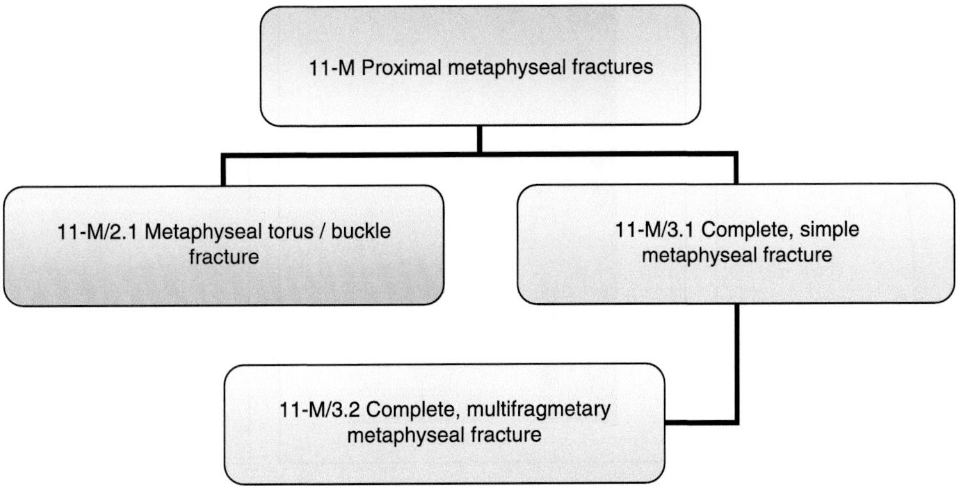

11-M: Proximal metaphyseal fractures of the humerus:

2.1: Metaphyseal torus/ buckle fracture.
3.1: Complete, simple metaphyseal fracture.
3.2: Complete, multifragmentary metaphyseal fracture.

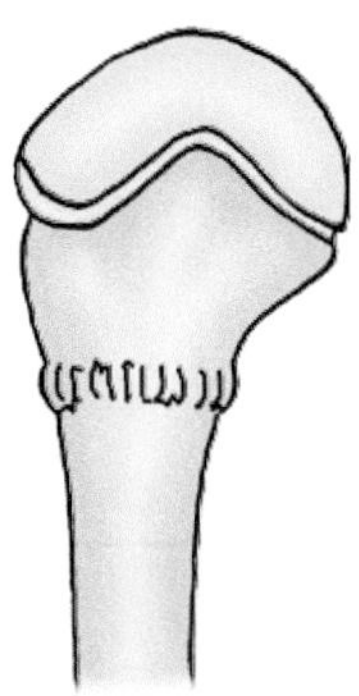

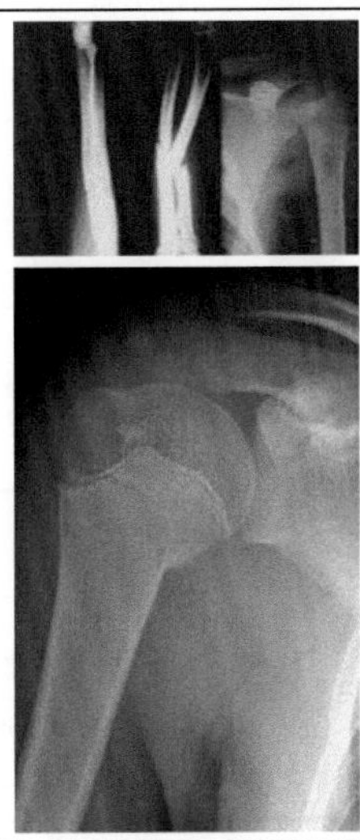

Proximal metaphyseal fracture of the humerus, AO/OTA classification
11-M Proximal metaphyseal fractures:
2.1 Metaphyseal torus / buckle fracture

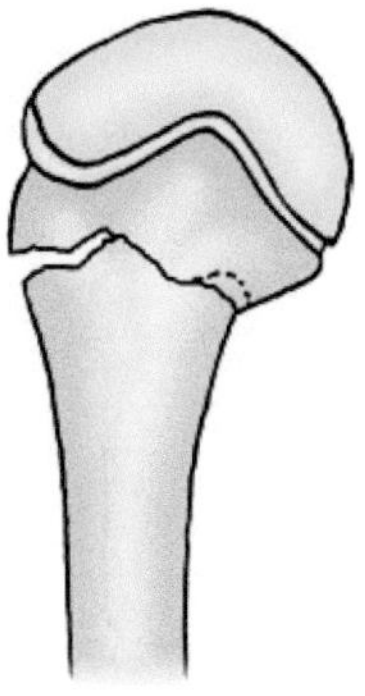

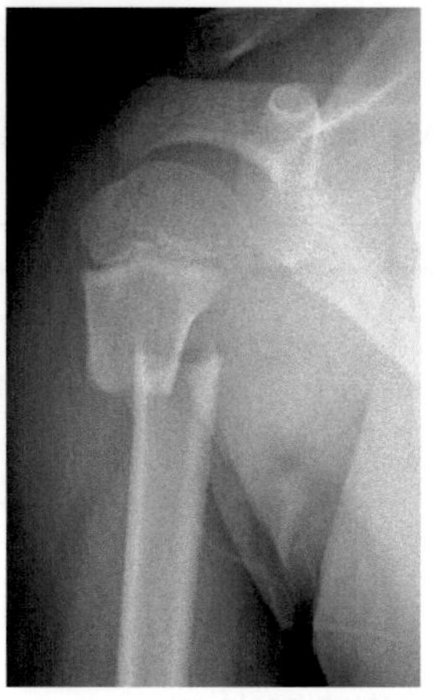

Proximal metaphyseal fracture of the humerus, AO/OTA classification
11-M Proximal metaphyseal fractures:
3.1 Complete, simple metaphyseal fracture

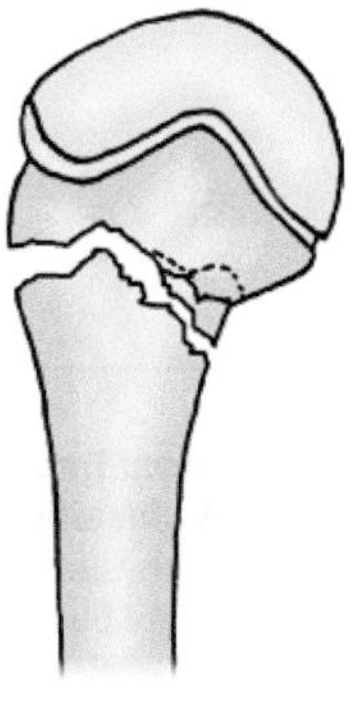

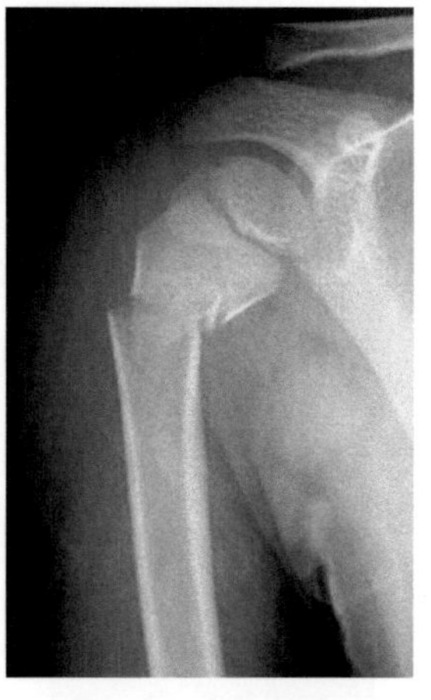

Proximal metaphyseal fracture of the humerus, AO/OTA classification
11-M Proximal metaphyseal fractures:
3.2 Complete, multifragmetary metaphyseal fracture

14.2.1.3 Fracture of the Humeral Shaft (12-D)

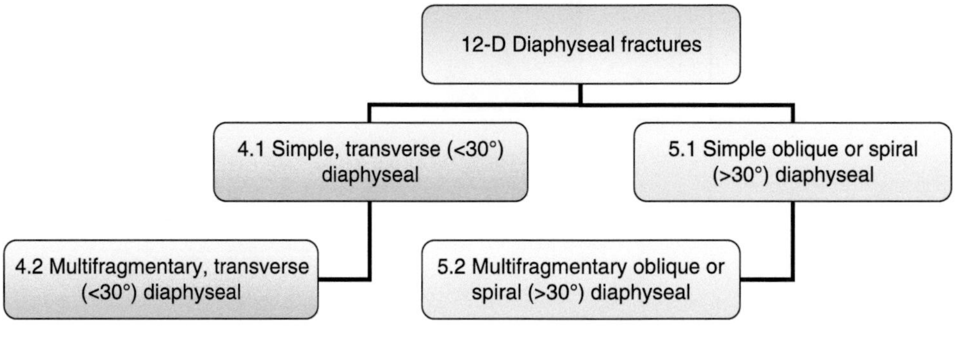

12-D: Humeral shaft fracture:

4.1: Simple, transverse (<30°) diaphyseal fracture.
4.2: Multifragmentary, transverse (<30°) diaphyseal fracture.
5.1: Simple oblique or spiral (>30°) diaphyseal fracture.
5.2: Multifragmentary oblique or spiral (>30°) diaphyseal fracture.

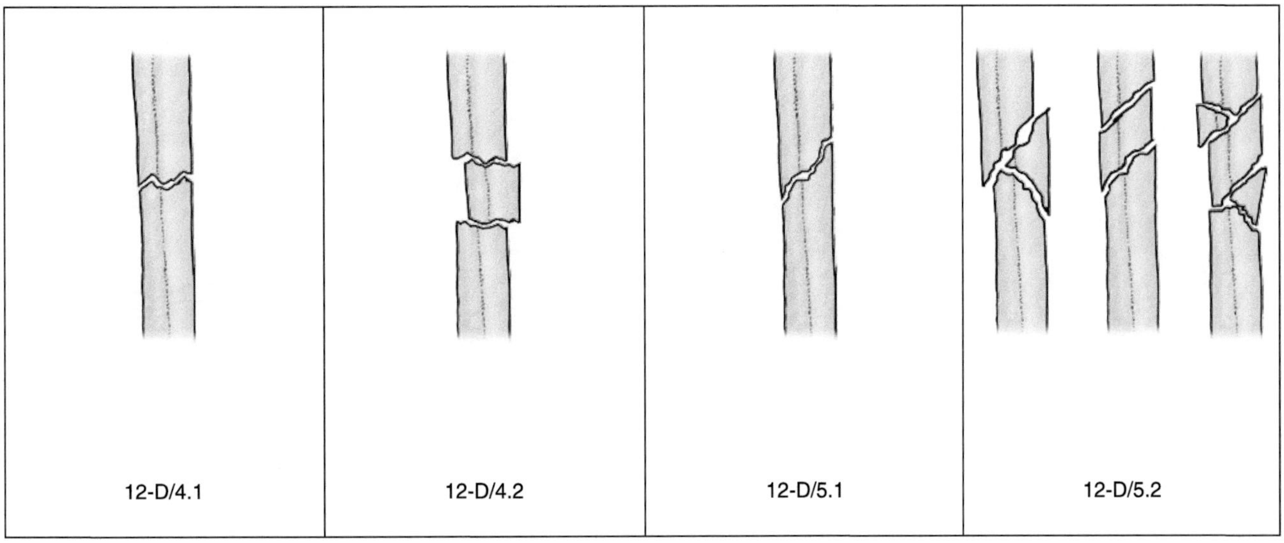

14.2.1.4 Distal Metaphyseal Fracture of the Humerus (13-M)

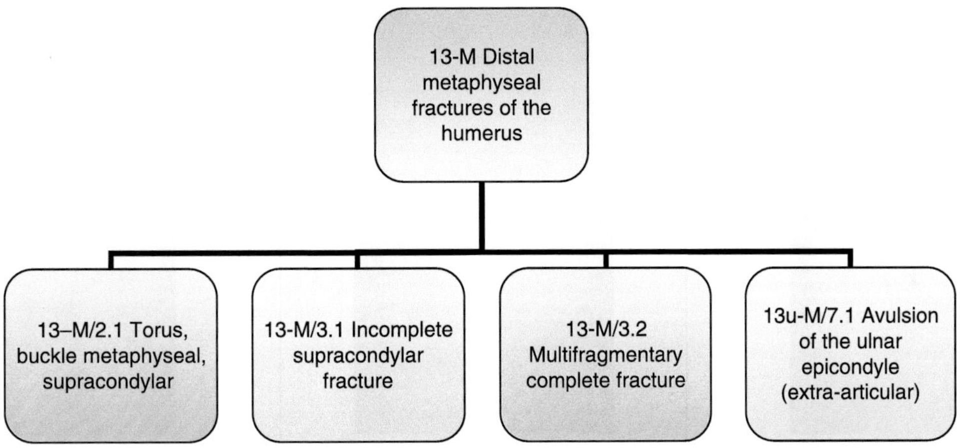

13-M: Distal metaphyseal fractures of the humerus:

2.1: Torus, buckle metaphyseal, supracondylar fracture.
3.1: Incomplete supracondylar fracture.
3.2: Multifragmentary complete fracture.
7.1: Avulsion of the ulnar epicondyle (extra-articular).

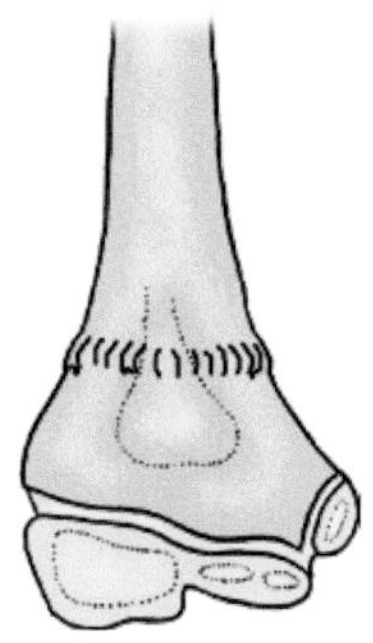

13–M/2.1

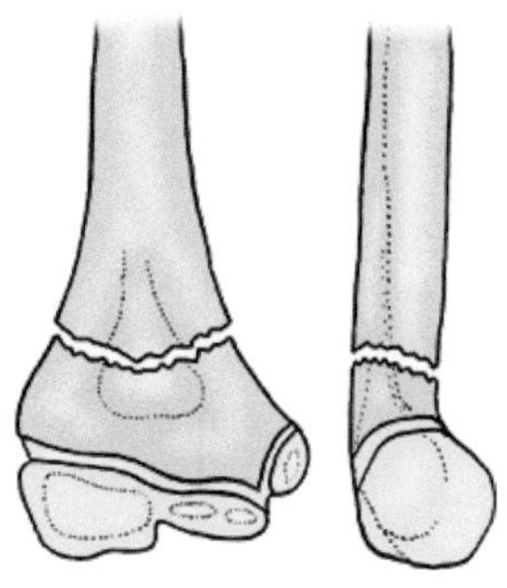

13–M/3.1

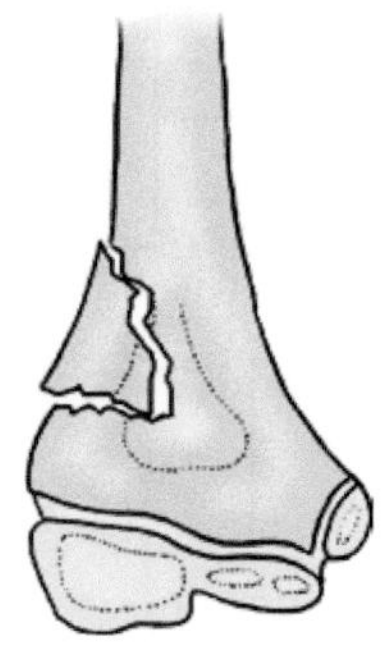

13–M/3.2

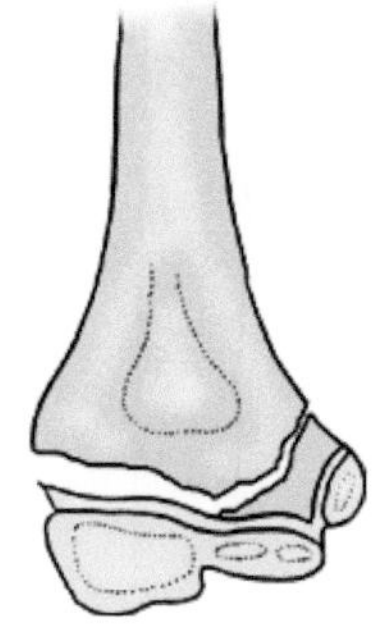

13–M/7.1

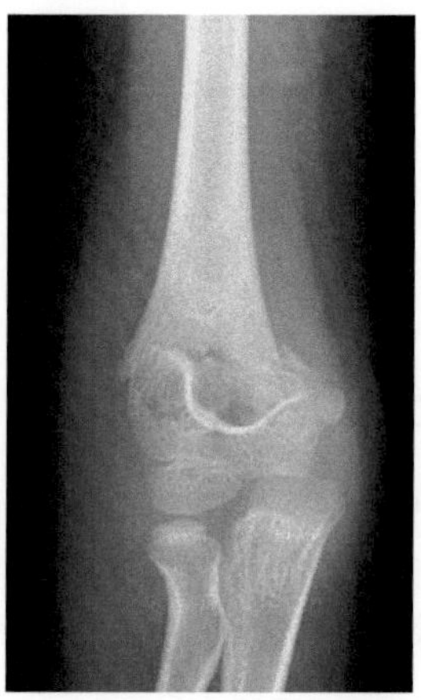

13–M/3.1

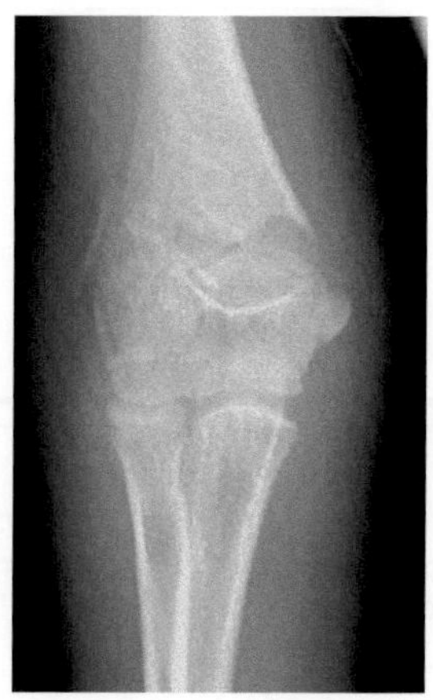

13–M/3.2

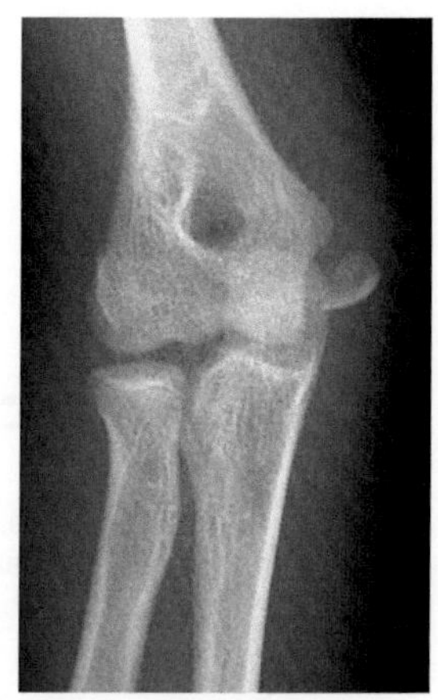

13–M/7.1

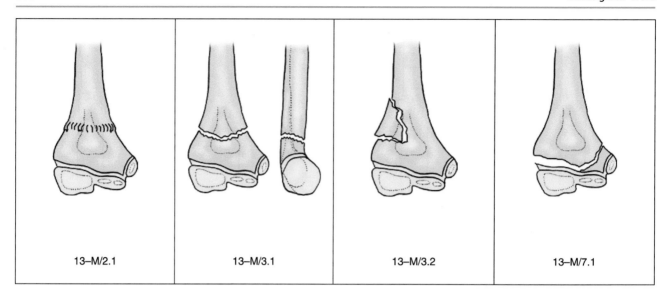

14.2.1.5 Distal Epiphyseal Fractures of the Humerus (13-E)

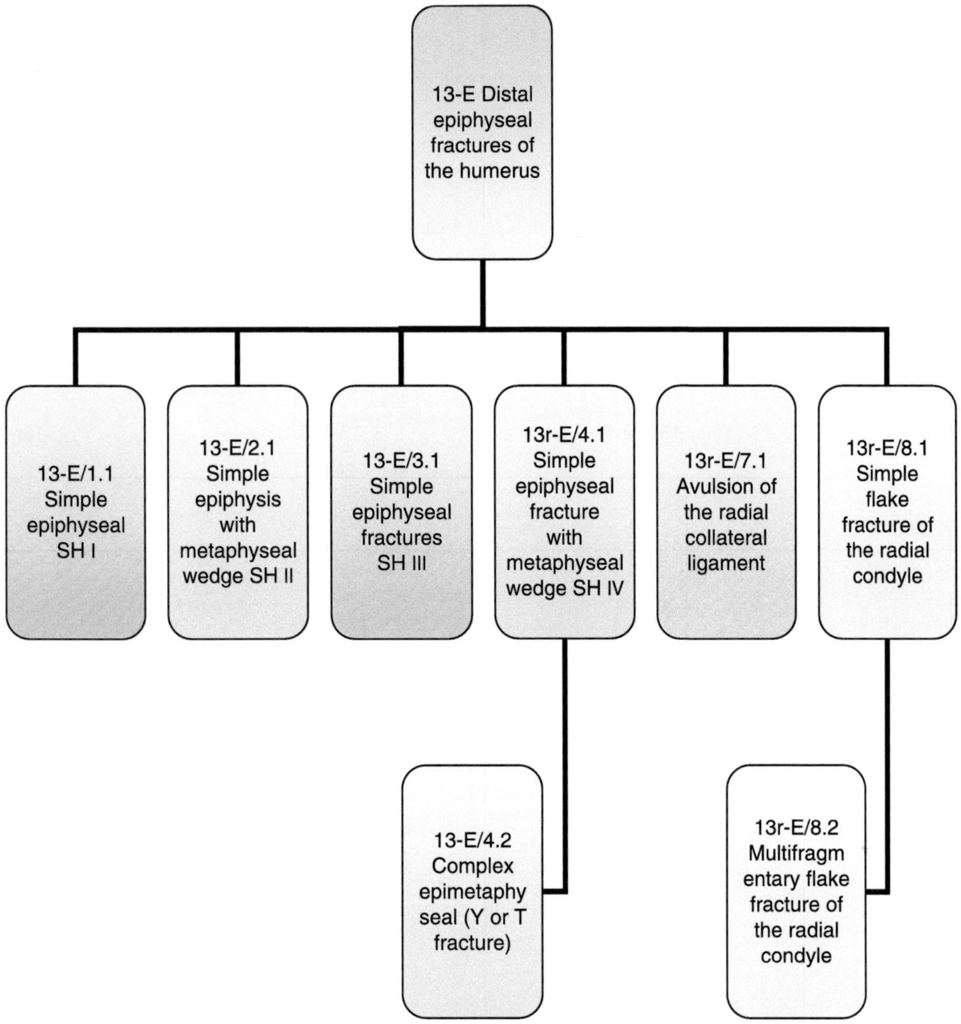

13-E: Distal epiphyseal fractures of the humerus:

1.1: Simple epiphyseal SH I.
2.1: Simple epiphysis with metaphyseal wedge SH II.
3.1: Simple epiphyseal fractures SH III.

13r-E: Distal epiphyseal fractures of the humerus:

4.1: Simple epiphyseal fracture with metaphyseal wedge SH IV.
4.2: Complex epimetaphyseal (Y or T fracture).
7.1: Avulsion of the radial collateral ligament.
8.1: Simple flake fracture of the radial condyle.
8.2: Multifragmentary flake fracture of the radial condyle.

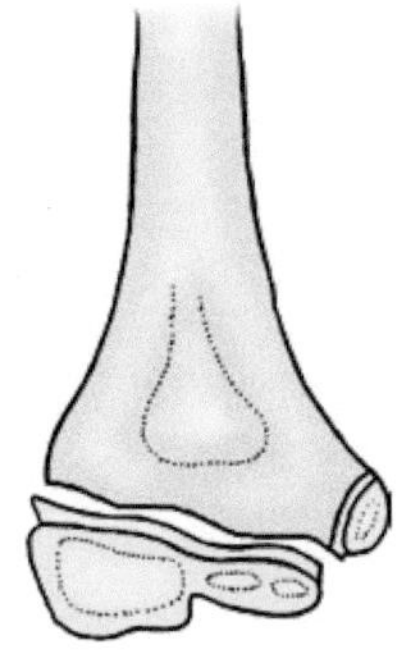

13-E/1.1

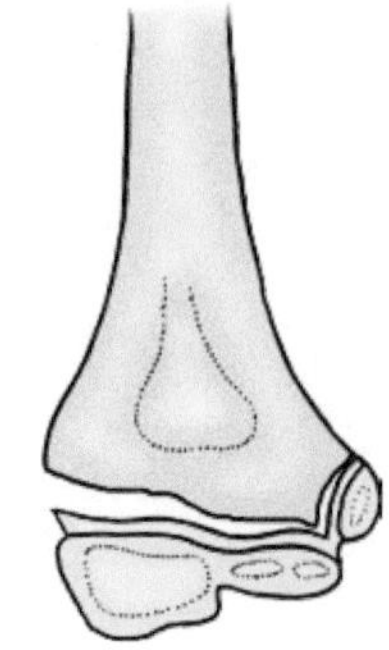

13-E/2.1

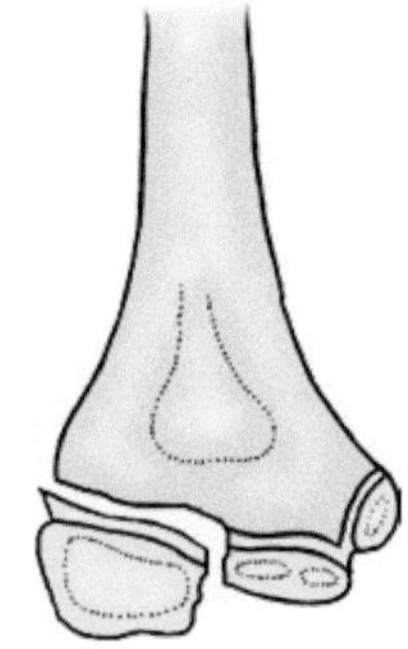

13-E/3.1

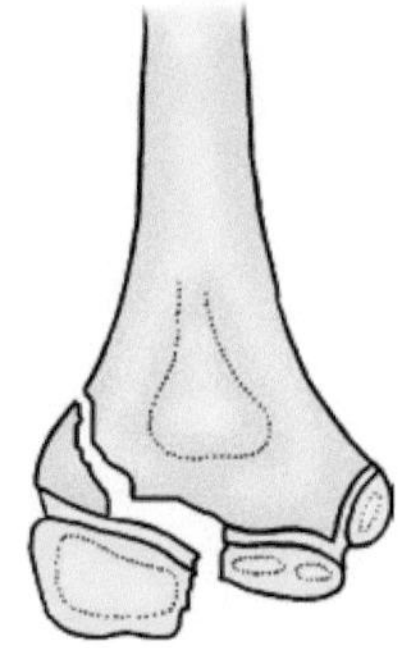

13r-E/4.1

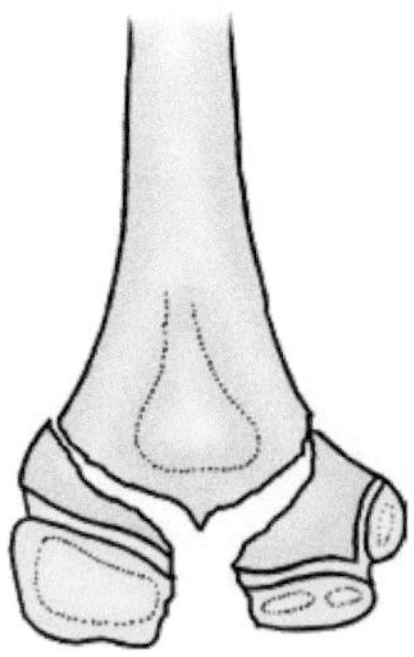

13r-E/4.2

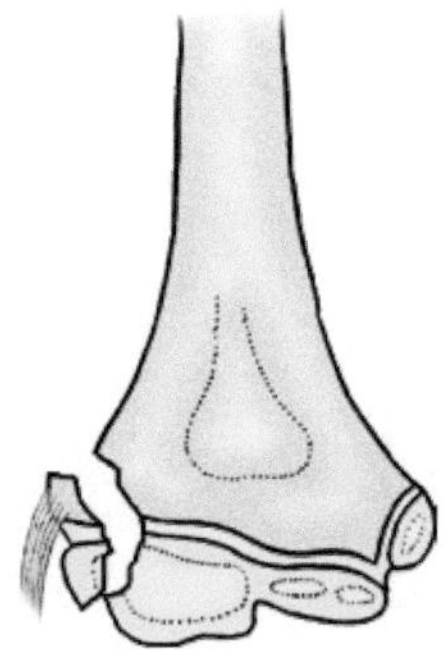

13r-E/7.1

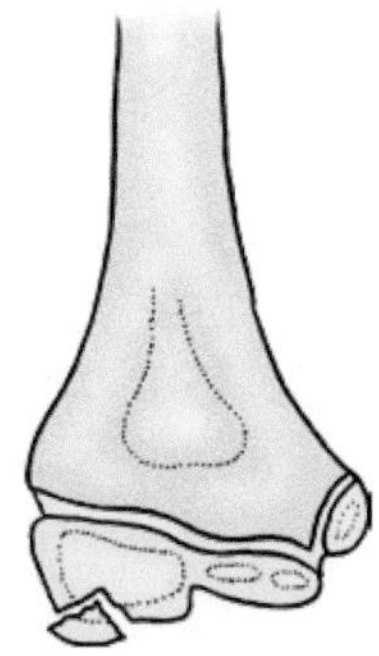

13r-E/8.1

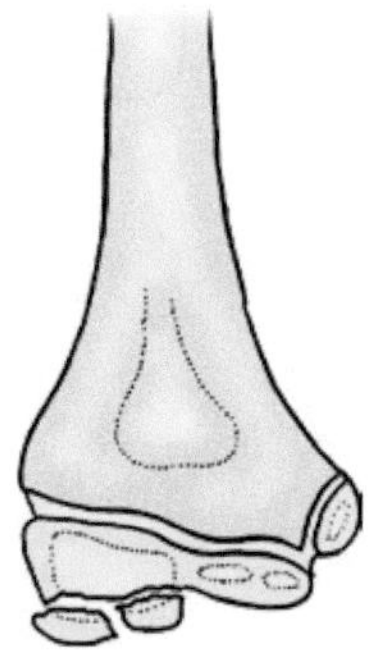

13r-E/8.2

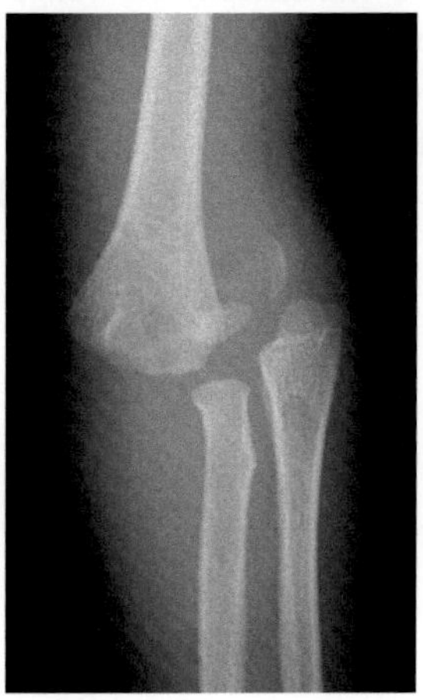

13-E/1.1 SH I

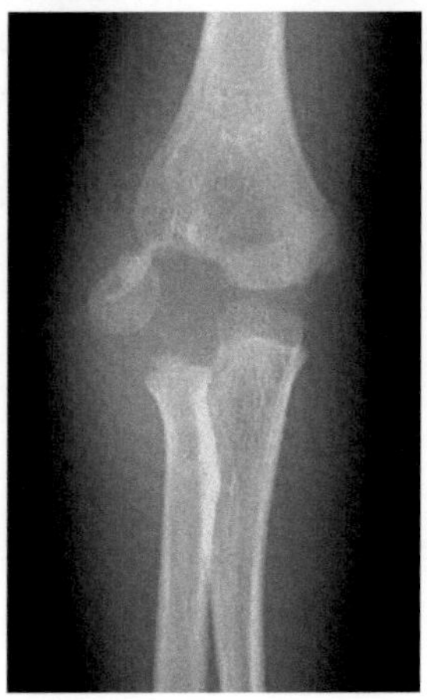

13-E/2.1 SH II

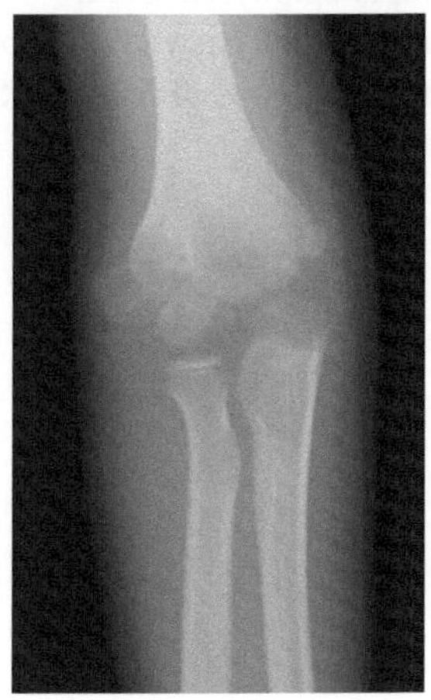

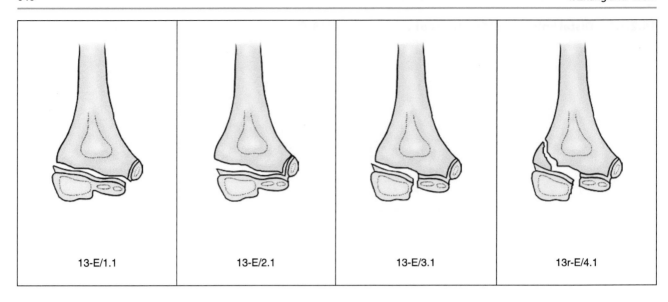

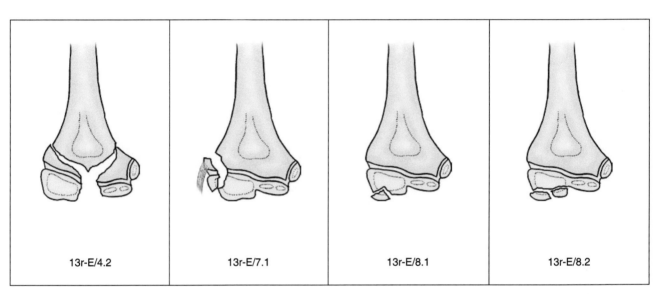

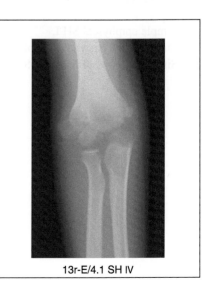

13r-E/4.1 SH IV

14.2.2 **Injuries of the Capitular** (Lateral Humeral Condylar) Epiphysis, Wadsworth Classification (1972, Clin Orthop 85:127–142)

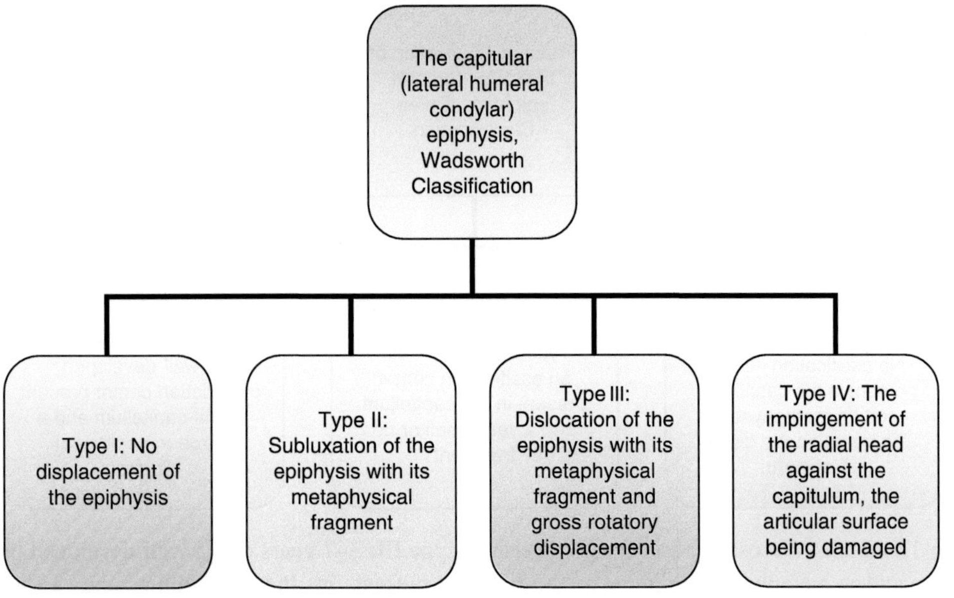

Type I: Frequently the metaphysical fragment is a rim of bone and no displacement of the epiphysis.

Type II: There is subluxation of the epiphysis with its metaphysical fragment and consequent instability of the elbow joint.

Type III: There is dislocation of the epiphysis with its metaphysical fragment and gross rotatory displacement so that the articular surface may be in contact with the fracture surface and the lower end of the humerus.

Type IV: The impingement of the radial head against the capitulum, the articular surface being damaged.

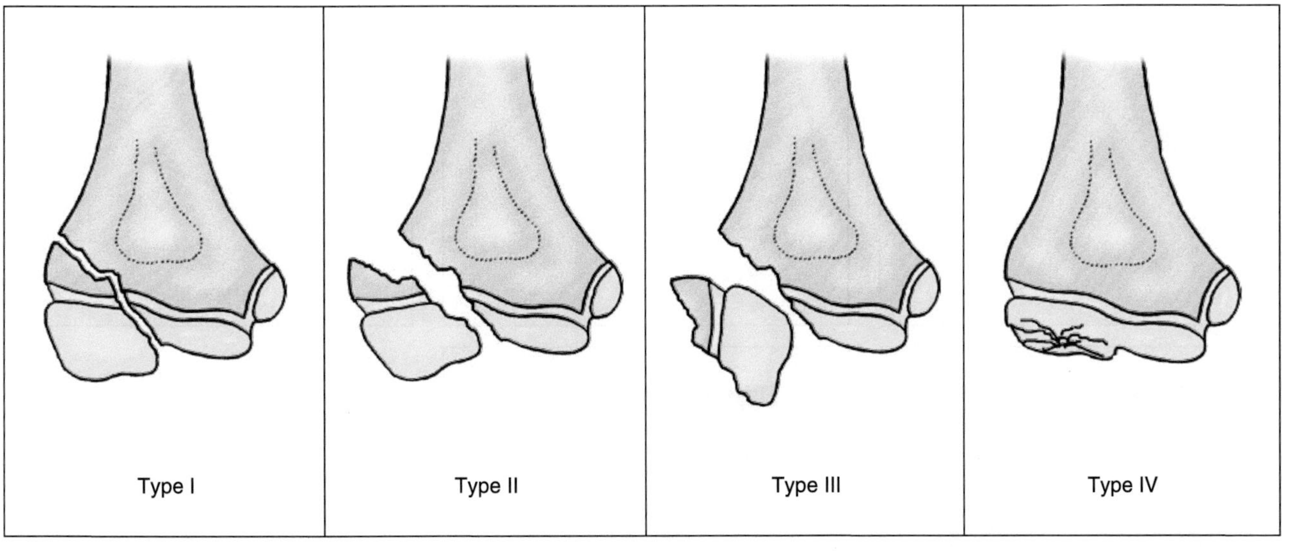

14.2.3 Delee Classification, Fracture-Separation of the Distal Humeral Epiphysis
(1980, JBJS (Am), 62:46–51)

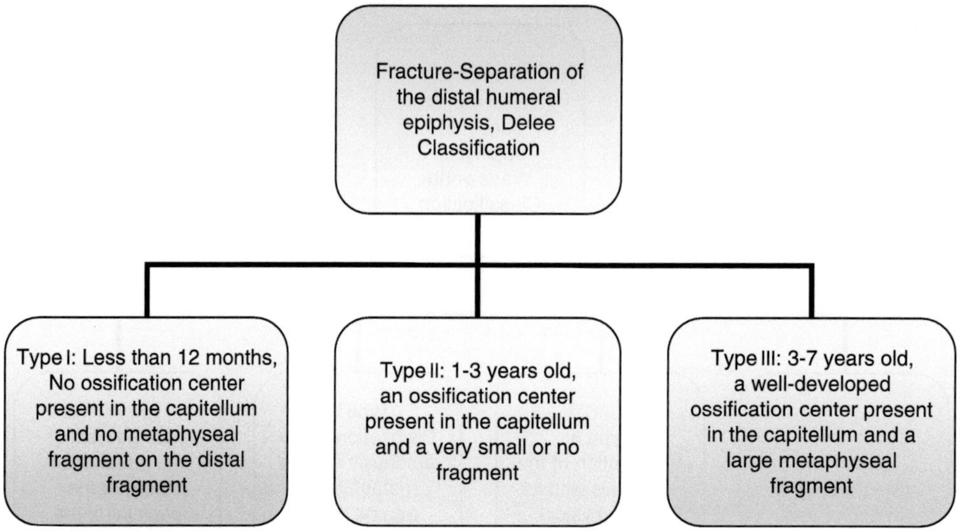
Fracture-Separation of the distal humeral epiphysis, Delee Classification
Type I: Less than 12 months, No ossification center present in the capitellum and no metaphyseal fragment on the distal fragment
Type II: 1-3 years old, an ossification center present in the capitellum and a very small or no fragment
Type III: 3-7 years old, a well-developed ossification center present in the capitellum and a large metaphyseal fragment

Type I: Less than 12 months. No ossification centre present in the capitellum and no metaphyseal fragment on the distal fragment.

Type II: 1–3 years old, an ossification centre present in the capitellum and a very small or no fragment.

Type III: 3–7 years old, a well-developed ossification centre present in the capitellum and a large metaphyseal fragment.

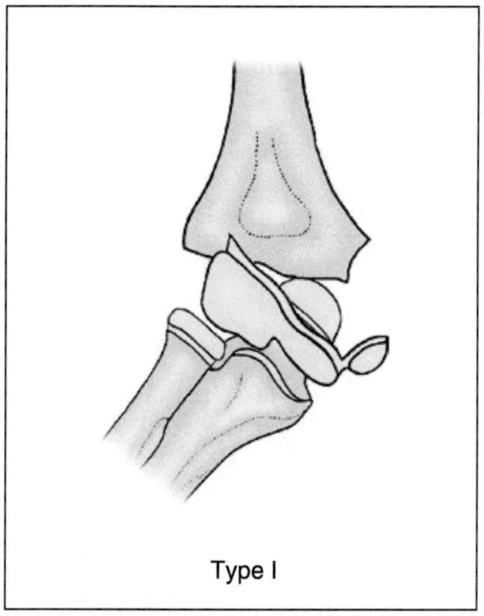
Type I

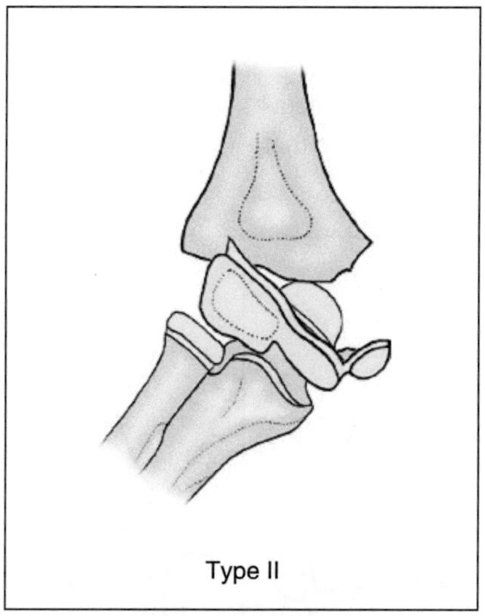
Type II

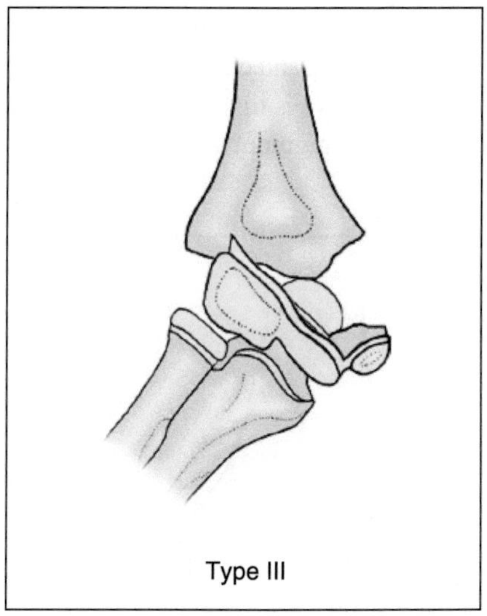
Type III

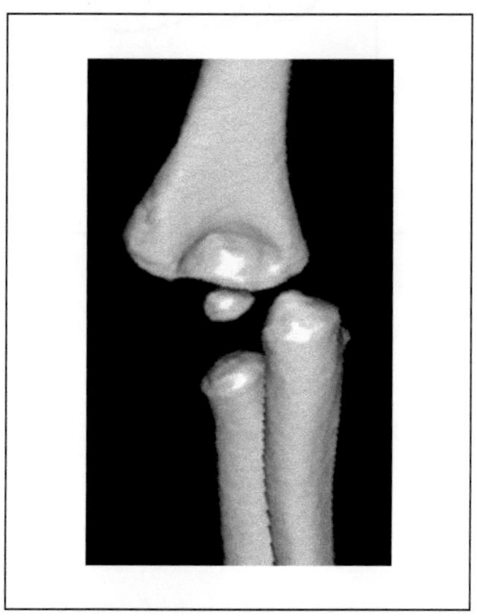

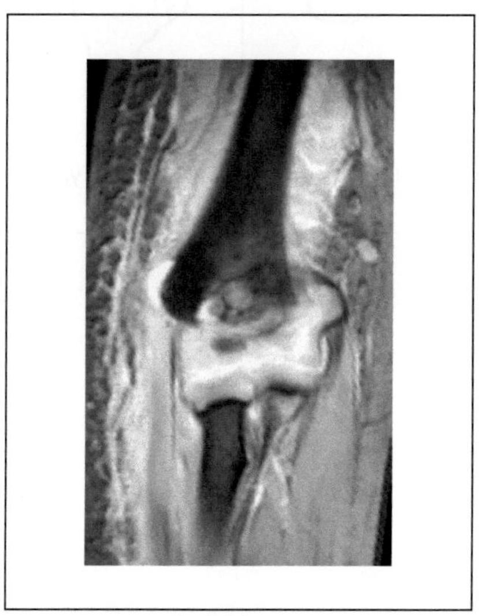

14.3 Section 3 Children Ulnar Radius Fractures

14.3.1 AO/OTA Classification

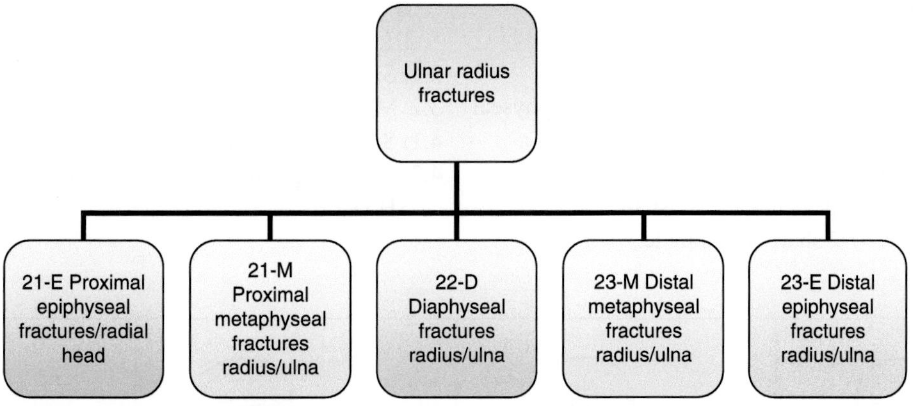

14.3.1.1 Proximal Epiphyseal Fractures/Radial Head (21-E)

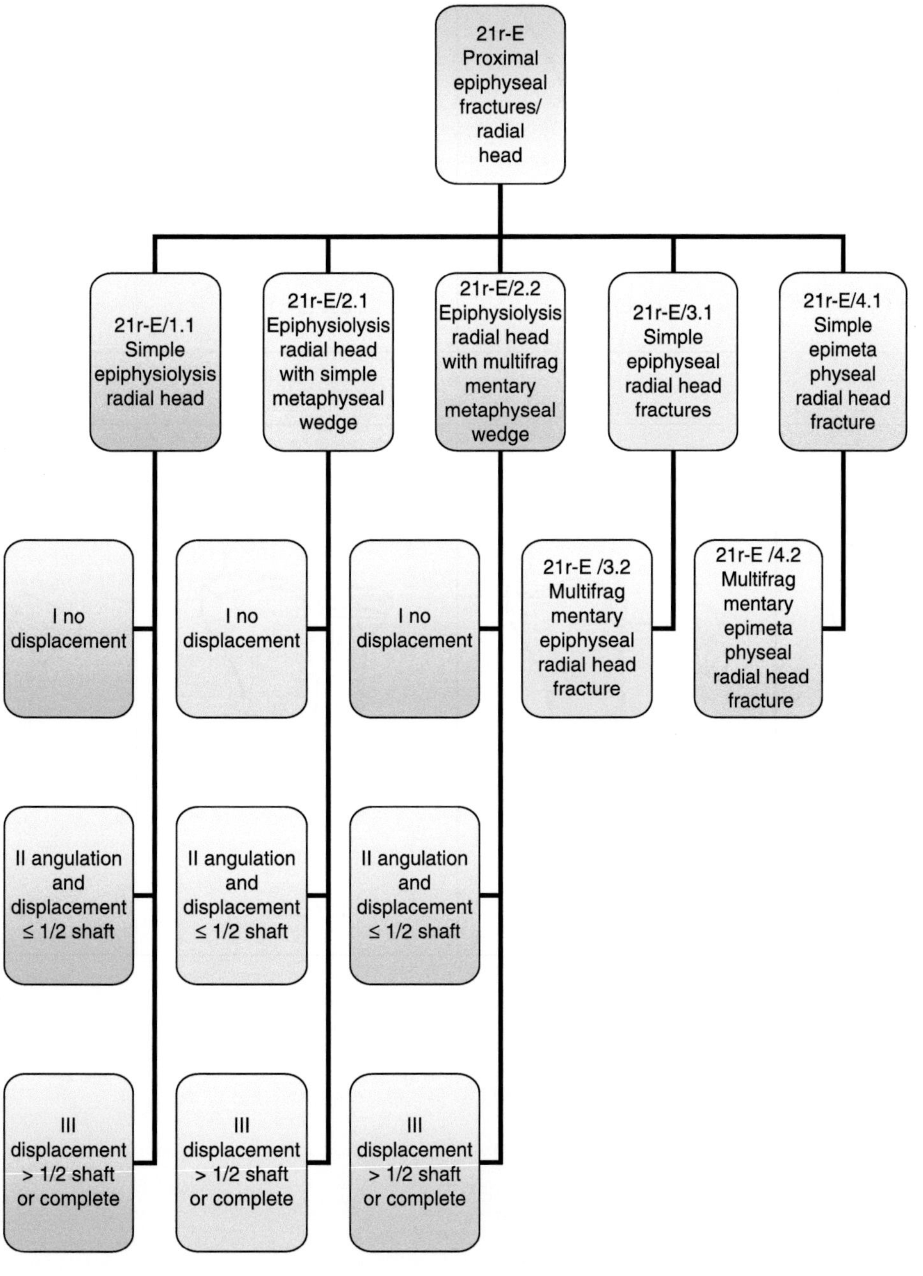

Proximal epiphyseal fractures/radial head (21r-E):

1.1: Simple epiphysiolysis radial head (SHI).
  I: No displacement.
  II: Angulation and displacement ≤1/2 shaft.
  III: Displacement >1/2 shaft or complete.

2.1: Epiphysiolysis radial head with simple metaphyseal wedge (SH II):
  I: No displacement.
  II: Angulation and displacement ≤1/2 shaft.
  III: Displacement >1/2 shaft or complete.

2.2: Epiphysiolysis radial head with multifragmentary metaphyseal wedge (SH II):
  I: No displacement.
  II: Angulation and displacement ≤1/2 shaft.
  III: Displacement >1/2 shaft or complete.

3.1: Simple epiphyseal radial head fractures SH III.

3.2: Multifragmentary epiphyseal radial head fracture SH III.

4.1: Simple epimetaphyseal radial head fracture SH IV.

4.2: Multifragmentary epimetaphyseal radial head fracture SH IV.

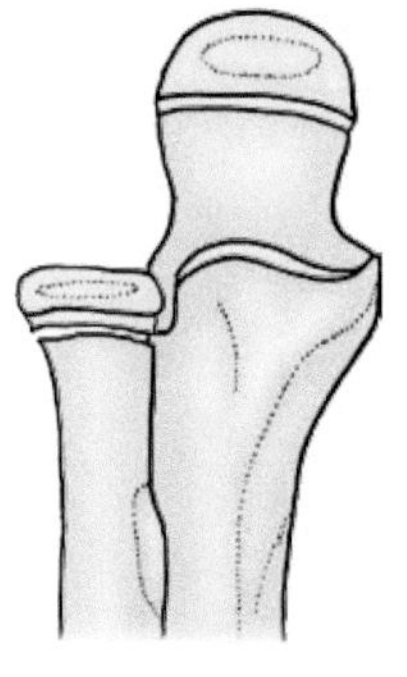
21r-E/1.1 I

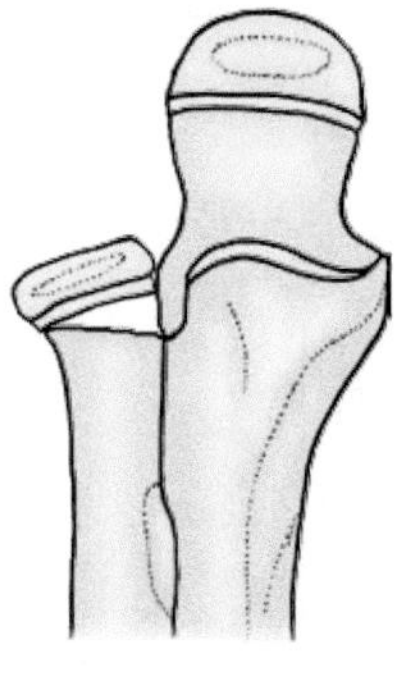
21r-E/1.1 II

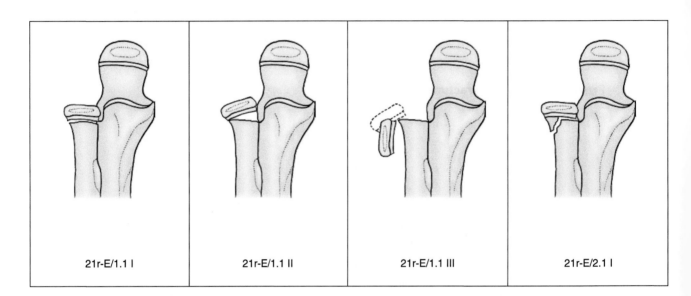

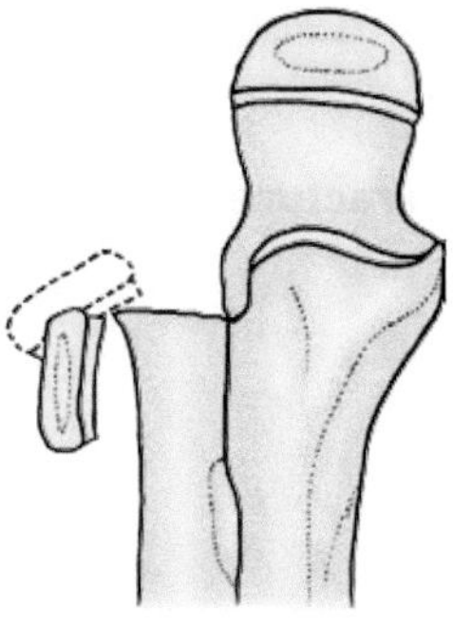
21r-E/1.1 III

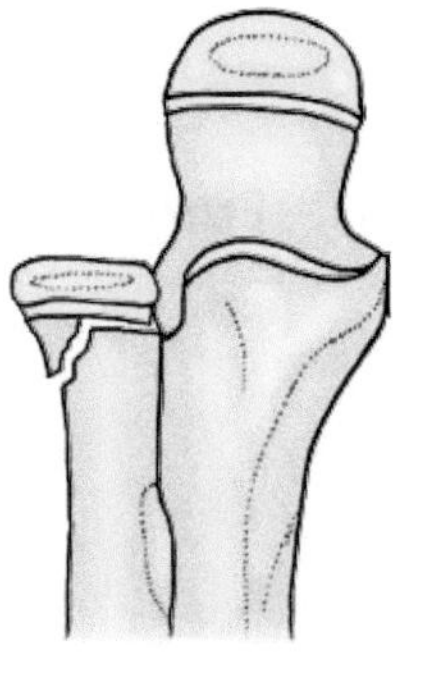
21r-E/2.1 I

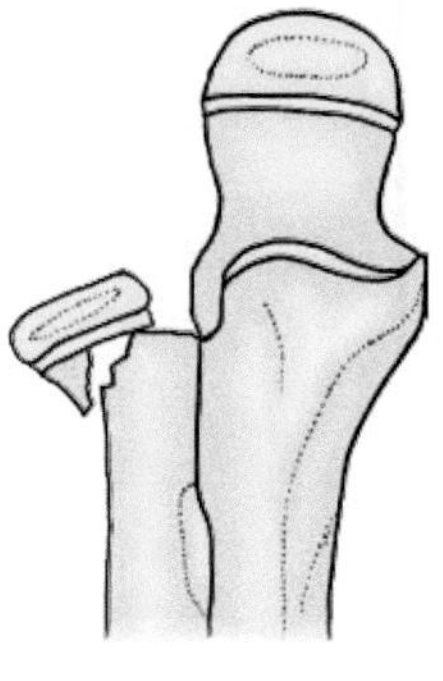
21r-E/2.1 II

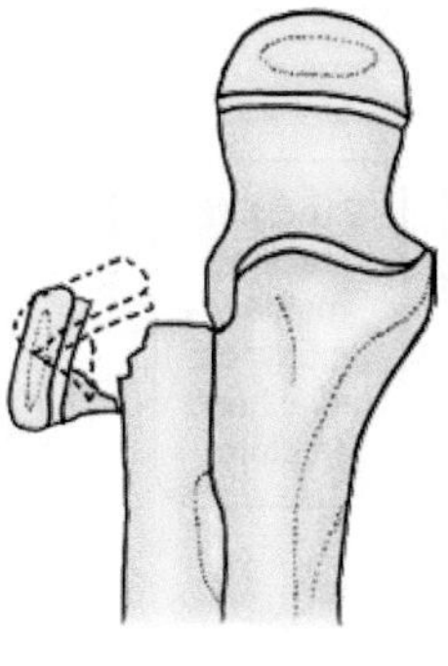
21r-E/2.1 III

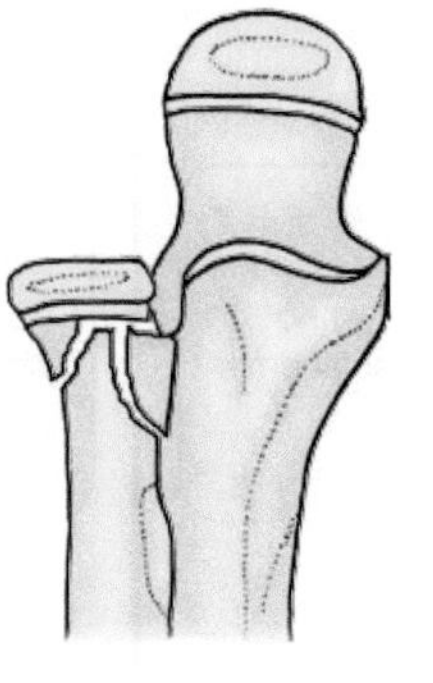
21r-E/2.2 I

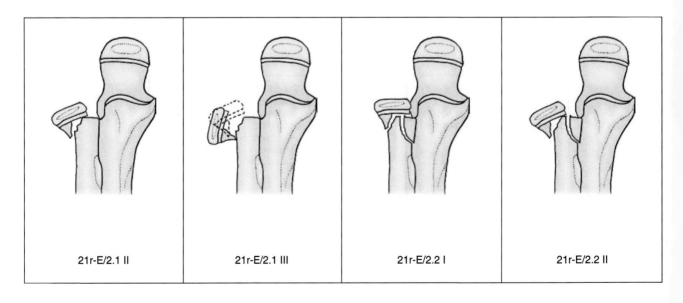

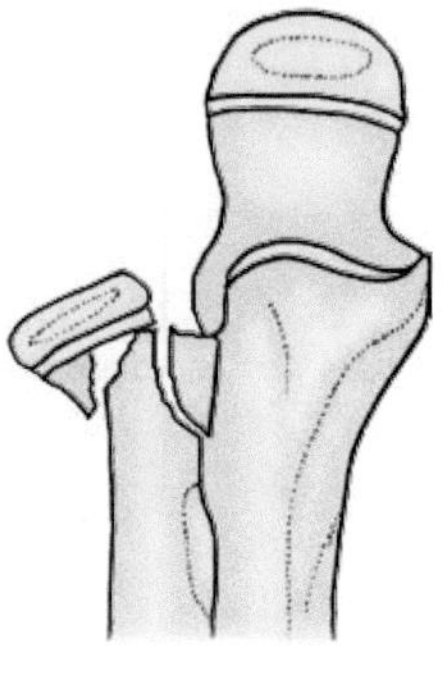
21r-E/2.2 II

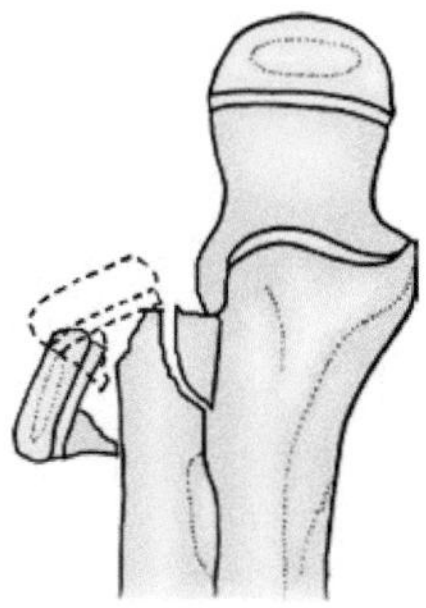

21r-E/2.2 III

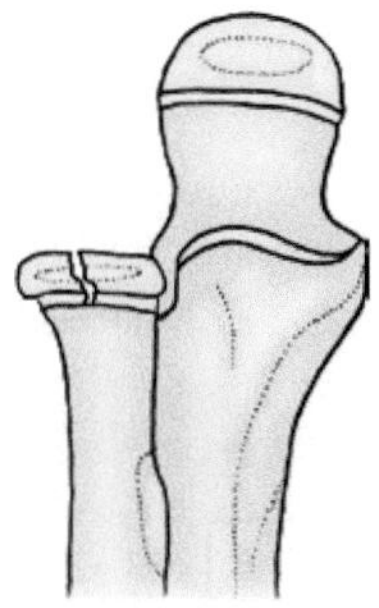

21r-E/3.1

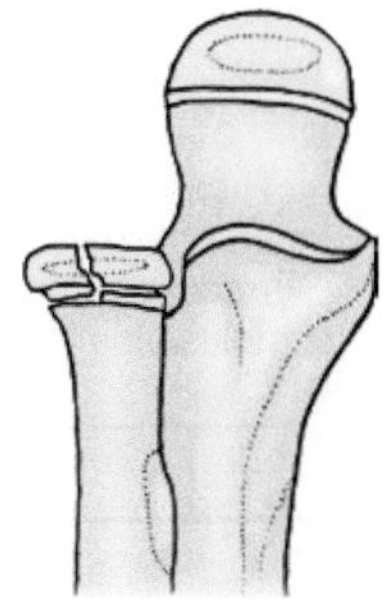

21r-E/3.2

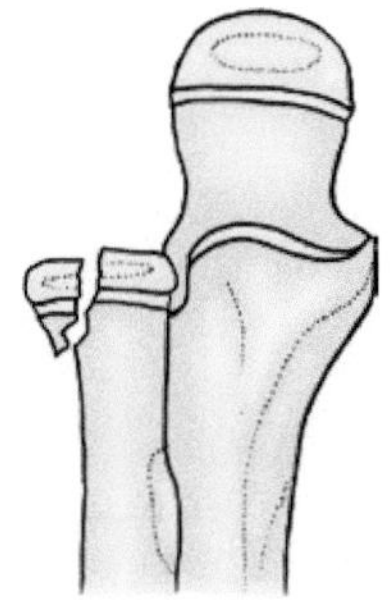

21r-E/4.1

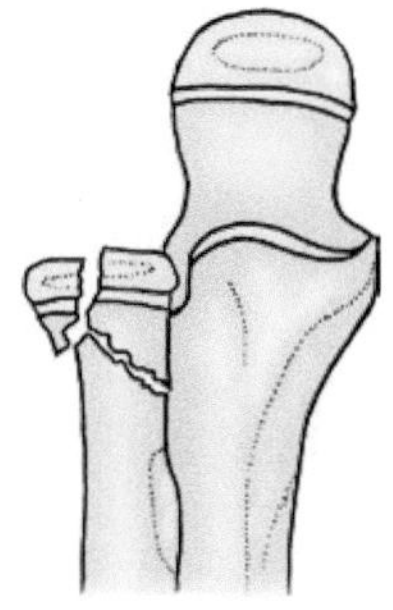

21r-E/4.2

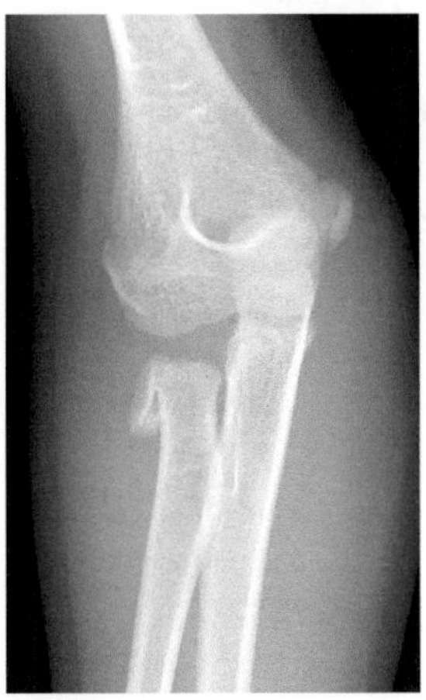

21r-E/1.1 III

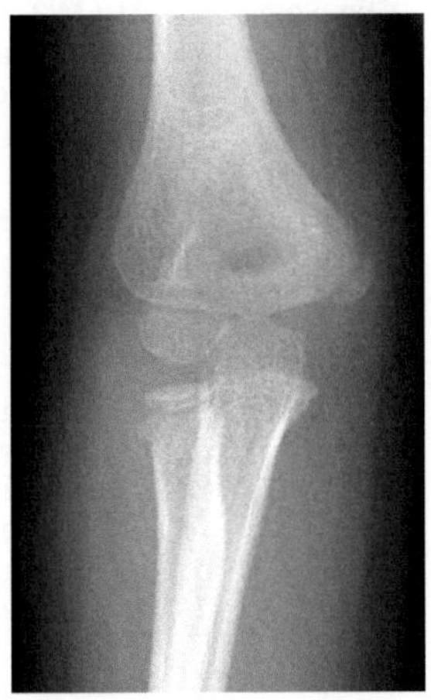

21r-E/2.1 I

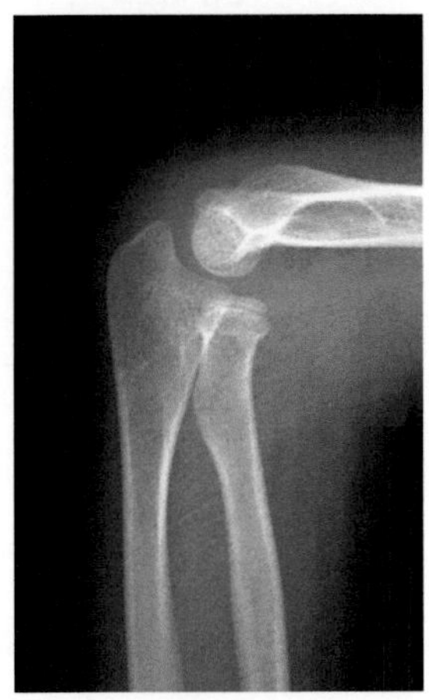

21r-E/4.1

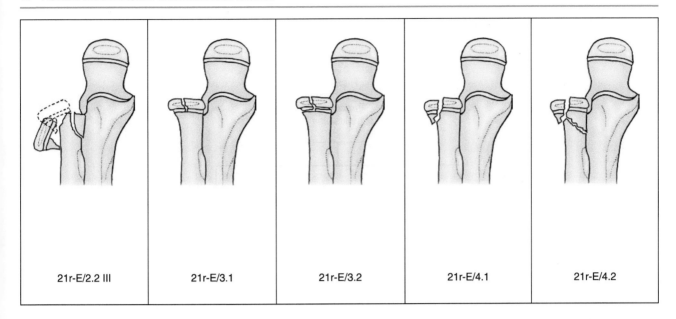

14.3.1.2 Proximal Metaphyseal Fractures Radius/Ulna (21-M)

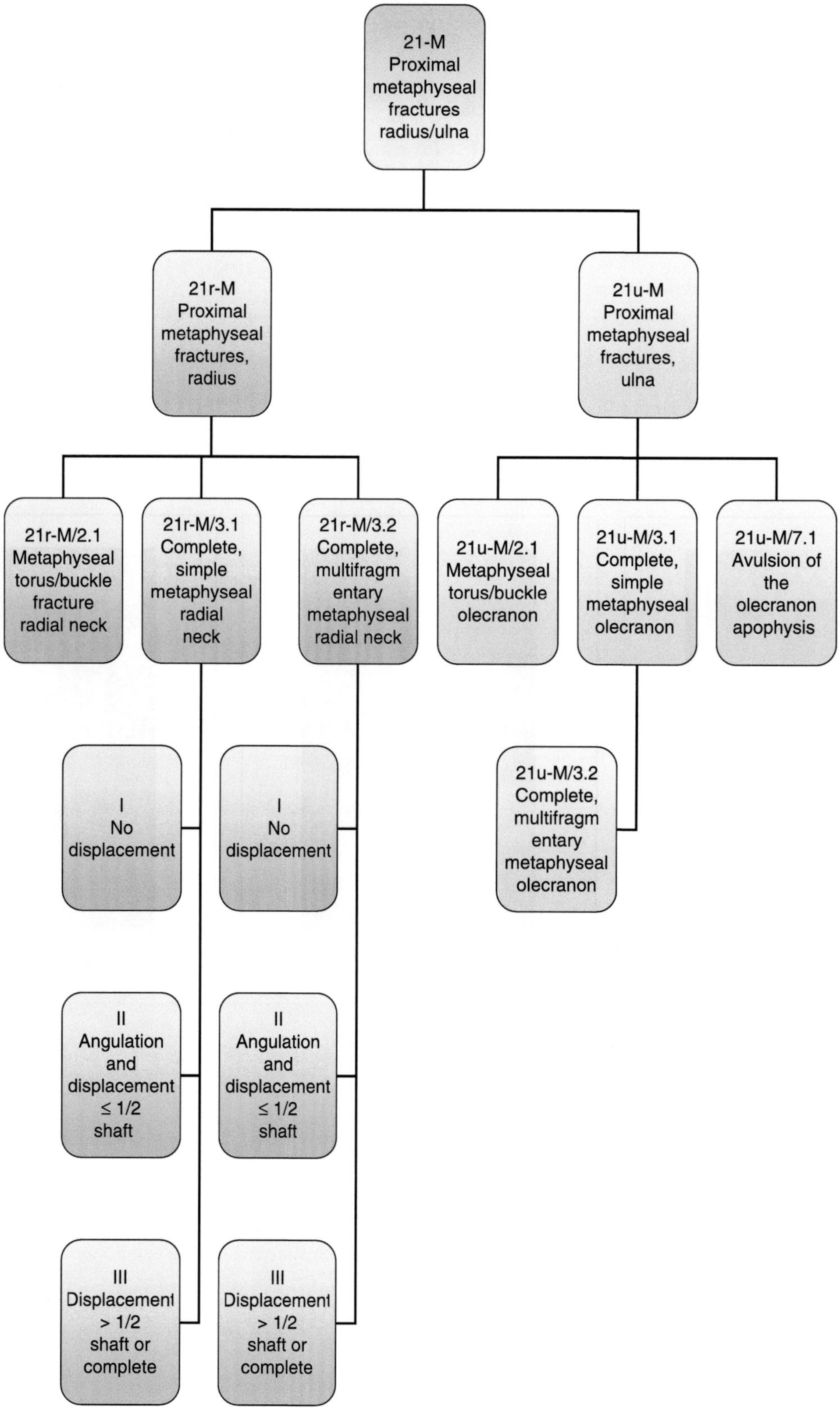

21r-M: Proximal metaphyseal fractures, radius.

2.1: Metaphyseal torus/buckle fracture radial neck.
3.1: Complete, simple metaphyseal radial neck:
  I: No displacement.
  II: Angulation and displacement ≤1/2 shaft.
  III: Displacement >1/2 shaft or complete.
3.2: Complete, multifragmentary metaphyseal radial neck:
  I: No displacement.
  II: Angulation and displacement ≤1/2 shaft.
  III: Displacement >1/2 shaft or complete.

21u-M: Proximal metaphyseal fractures, ulna:

2.1: Metaphyseal torus/buckle olecranon.
3.1: Complete, simple metaphyseal olecranon.
3.2: Complete, multifragmentary metaphyseal olecranon.
7.1: Avulsion of the olecranon apophysis.

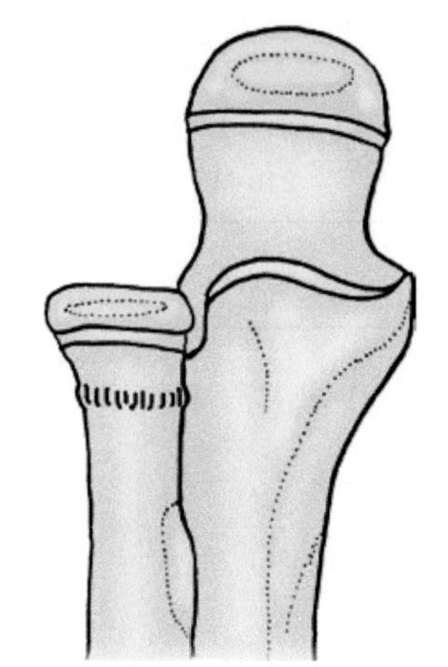
21r-M/2.1

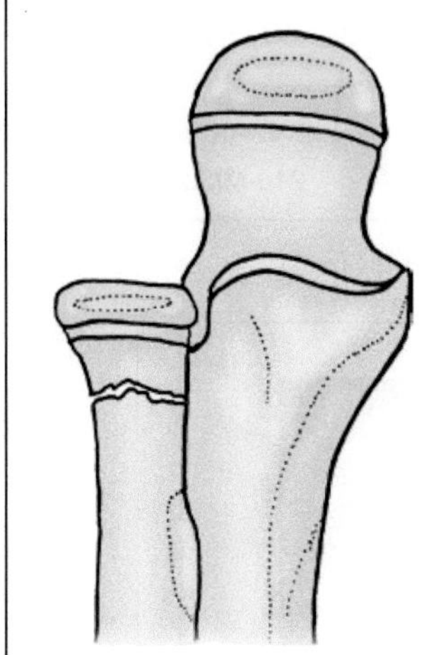
21r-M/3.1 I

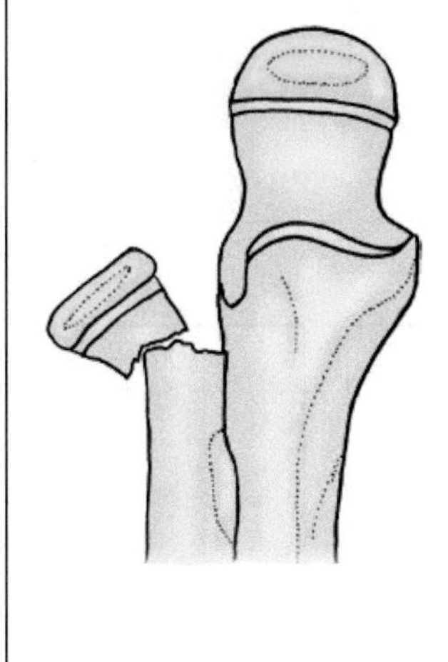
21r-M/3.1 II

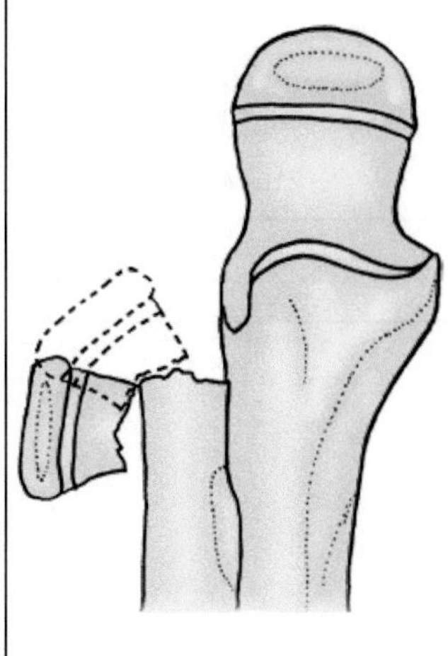
21r-M/3.1 III

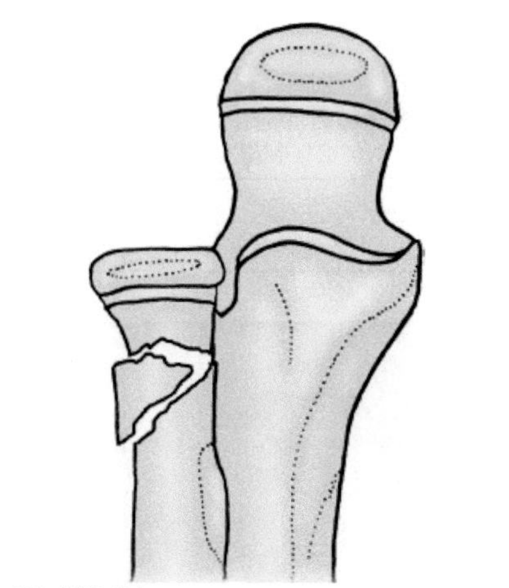
21r-M/3.2 I

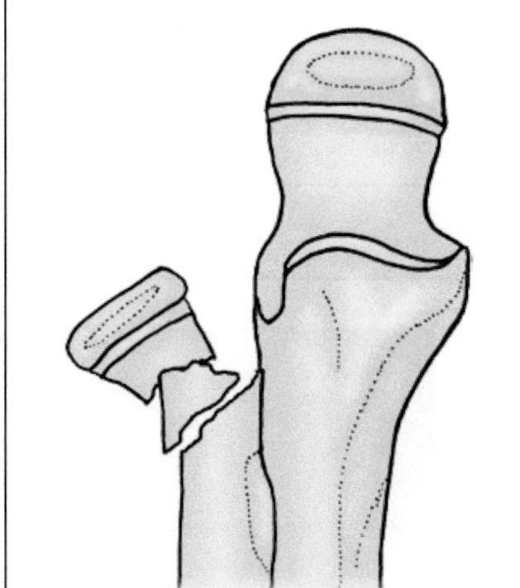
21r-M/3.2 II

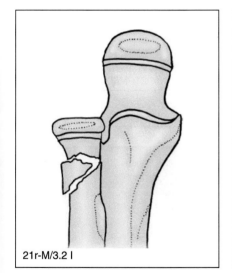

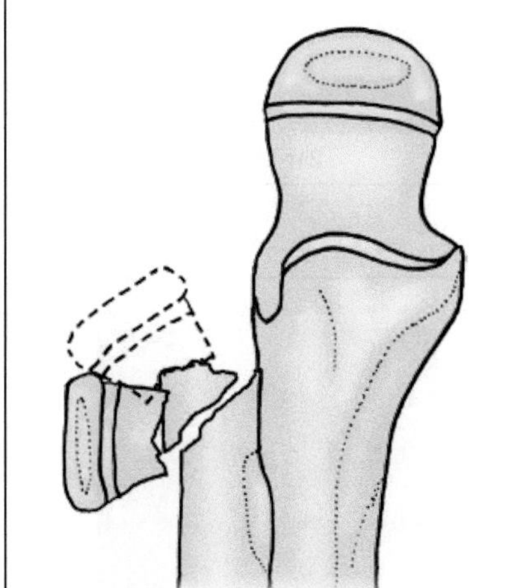
21r-M/3.2 III

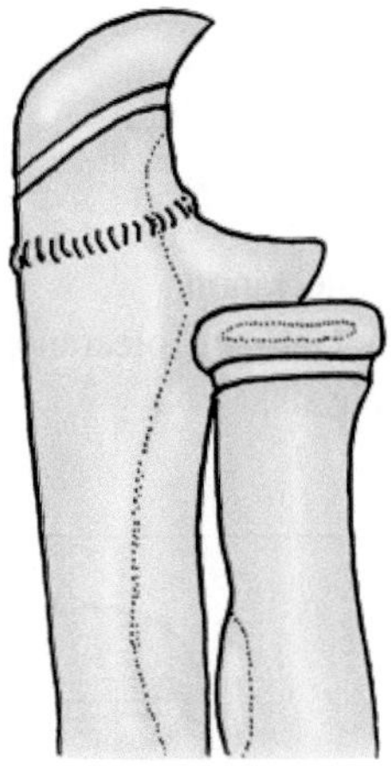
21u-M/2.1

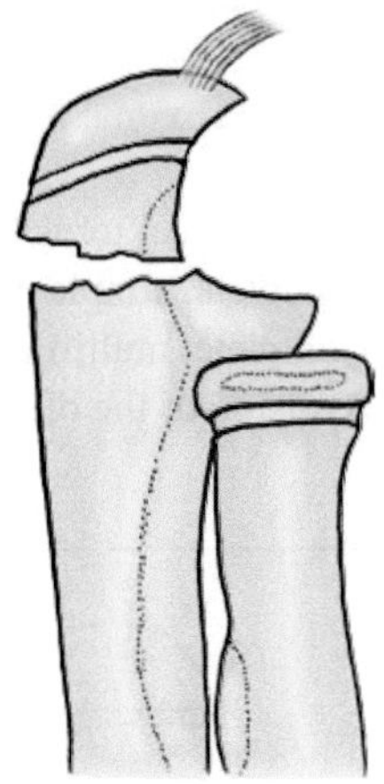
21u-M/3.1

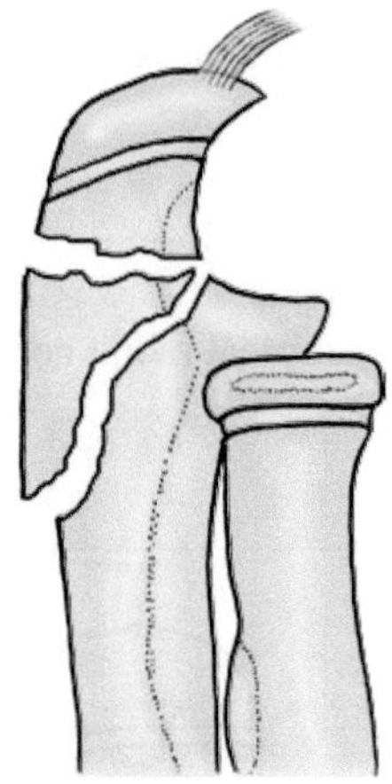
21u-M/3.2

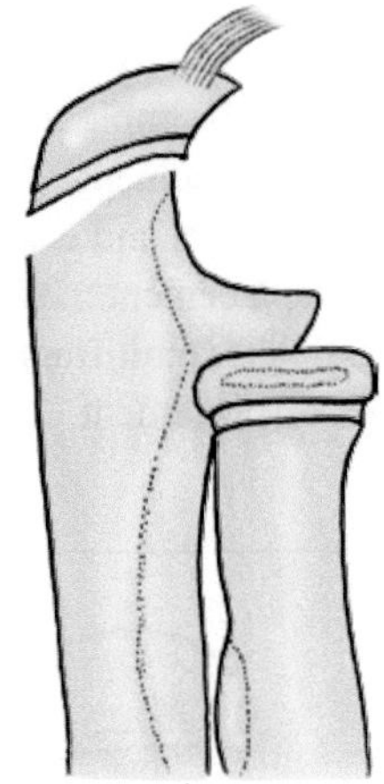
21u-M/7.1

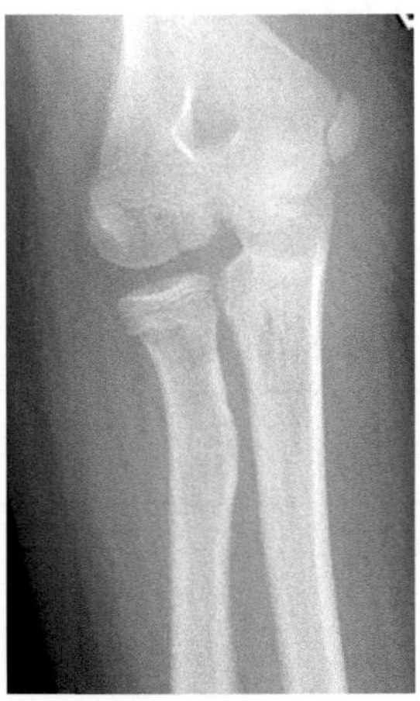
21r-M/2.1

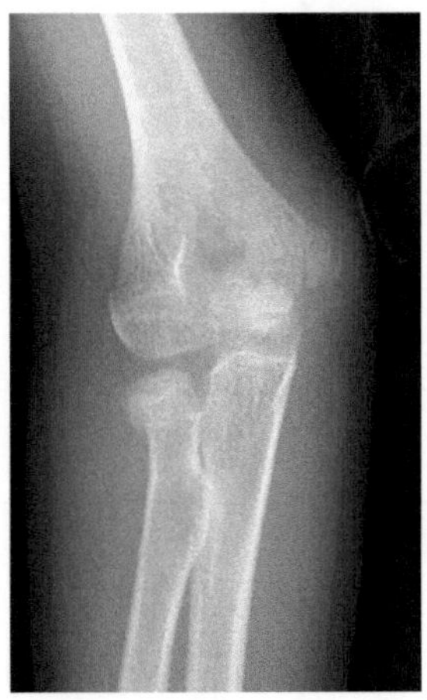
21r-M/3.1 II

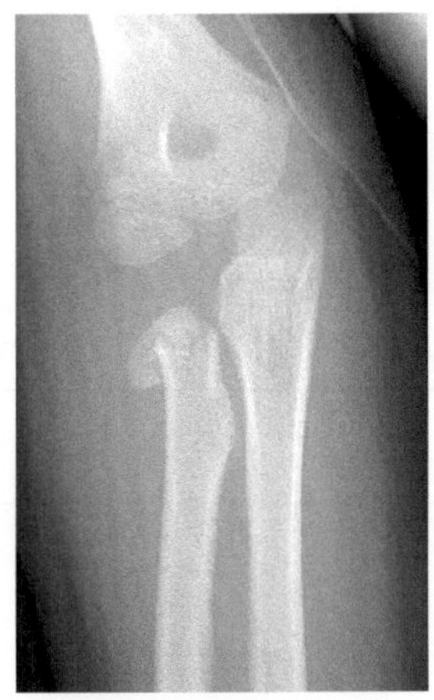
21r-M/2.1 III

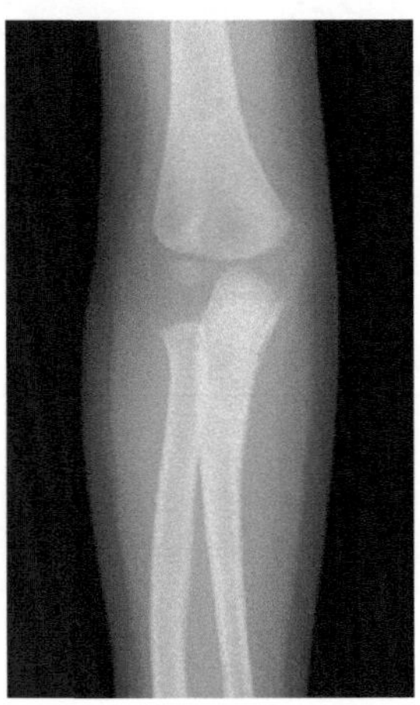
21u-M/3.1

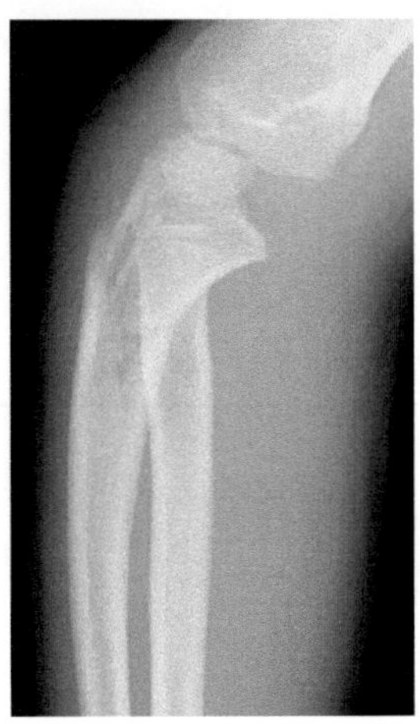
21u-M/3.2

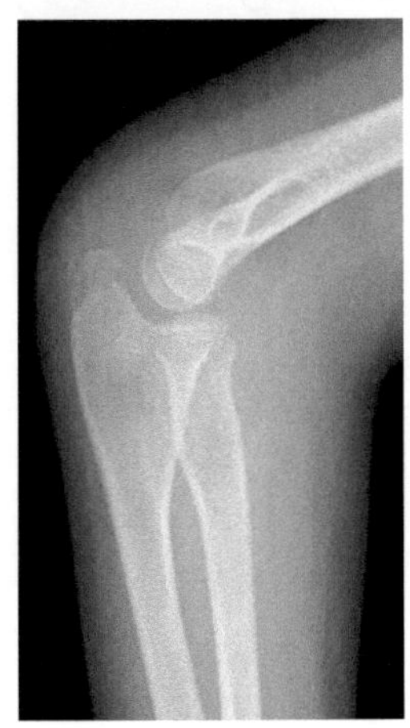
21u-M/7.1

14.3.1.3 Diaphyseal Fractures Radius/Ulna (22-D)

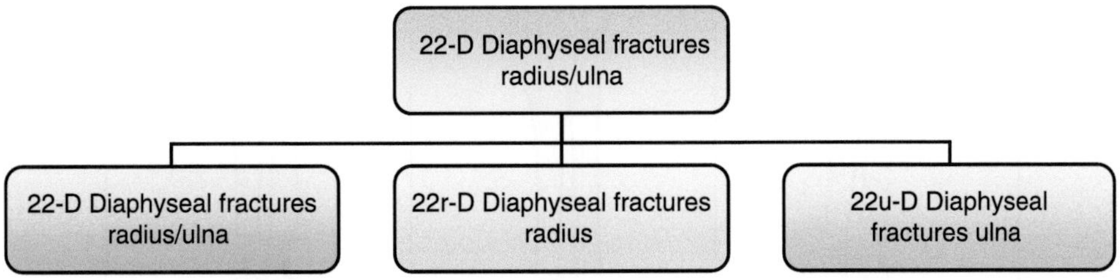

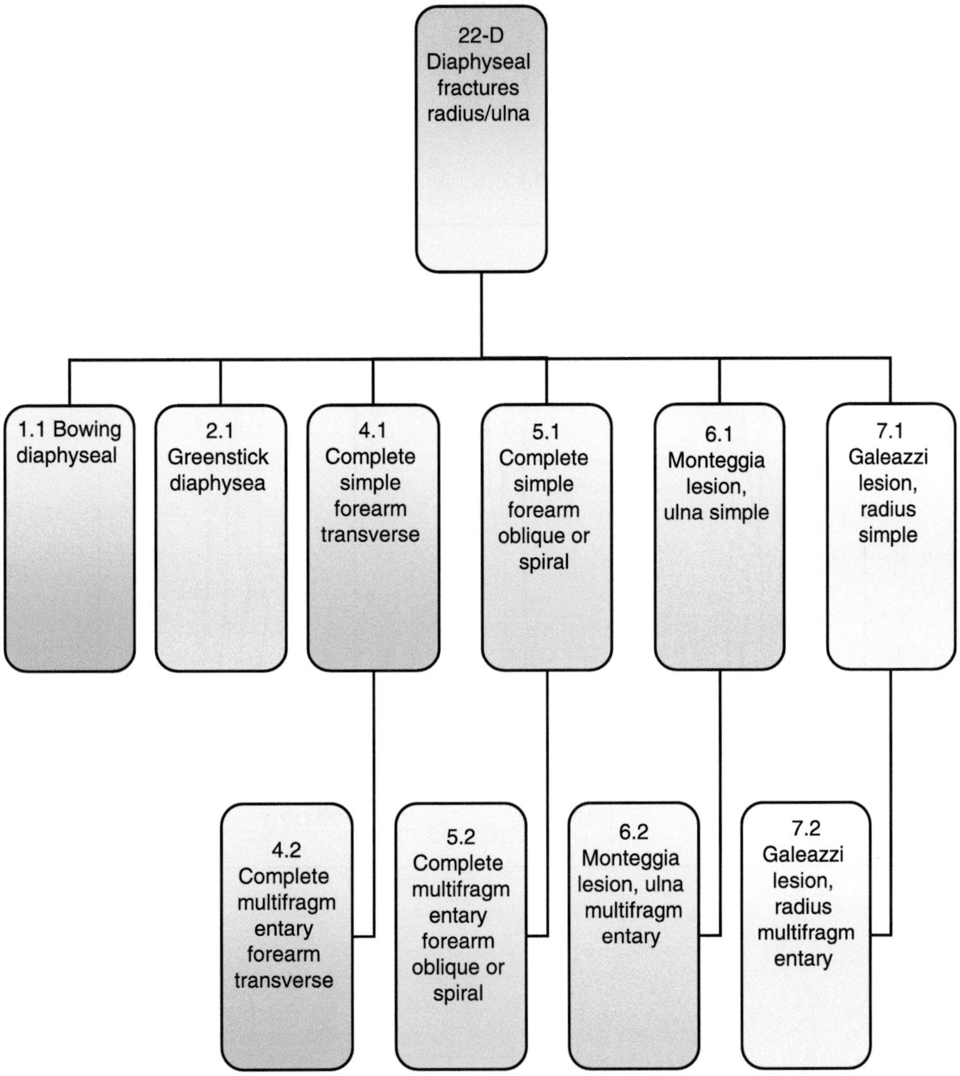

22-D: Diaphyseal fractures radius/ulna:

1.1: Bowing diaphyseal.
2.1: Greenstick diaphyseal.
4.1: Complete simple forearm transverse.
4.2: Complete multifragmentary forearm transverse.
5.1: Complete simple forearm oblique or spiral.
5.2: Complete multifragmentary forearm oblique or spiral.
6.1: Monteggia lesion, ulna simple.
6.2: Monteggia lesion, ulna multifragmentary.
7.1: Galeazzi lesion, radius simple.
7.2: Galeazzi lesion, radius multifragmentary.

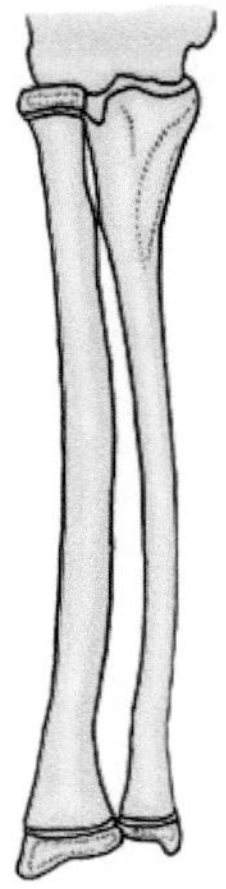
22-D/1.1

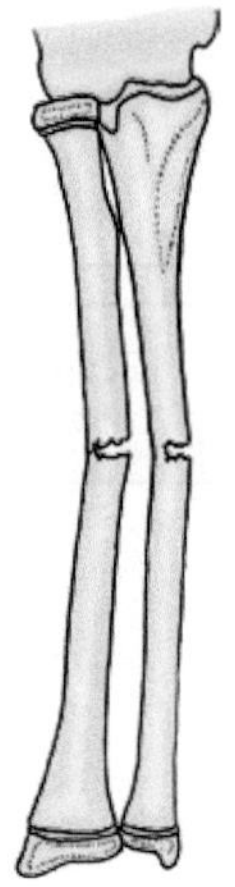
22-D/2.1

22-D/4.1

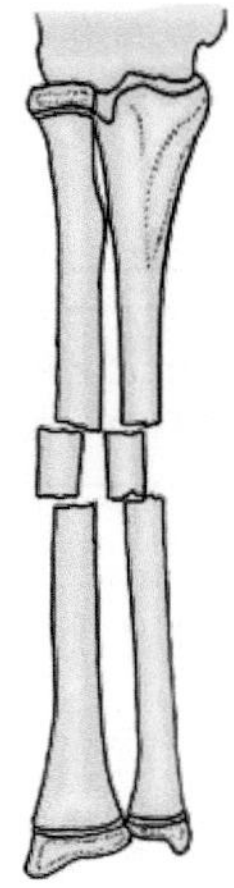
22-D/4.2

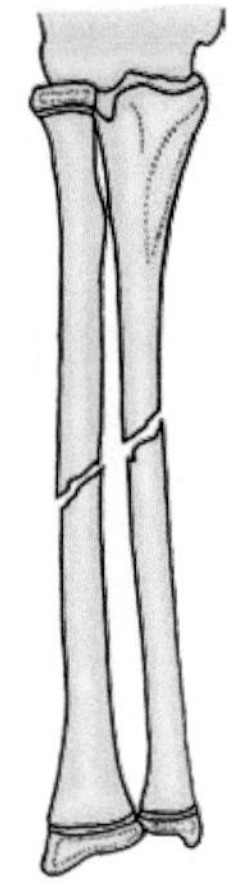
22-D/5.1

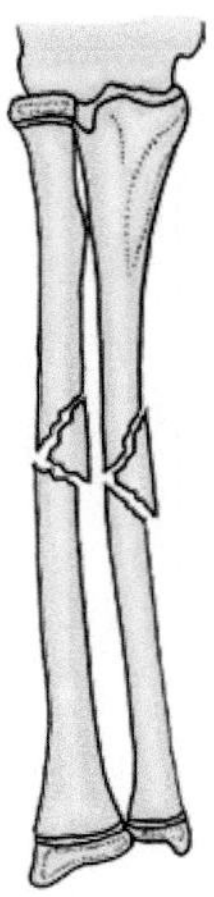
22-D/5.2

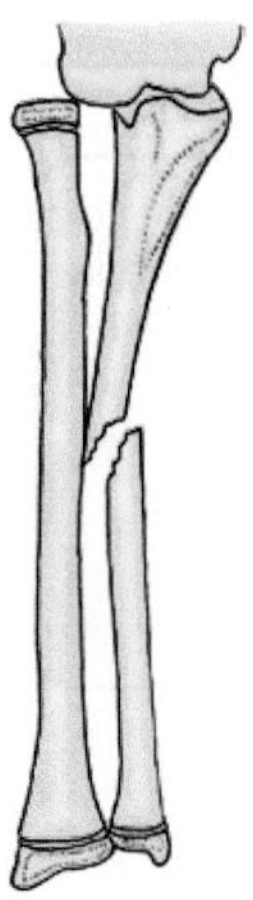
22-D/6.1

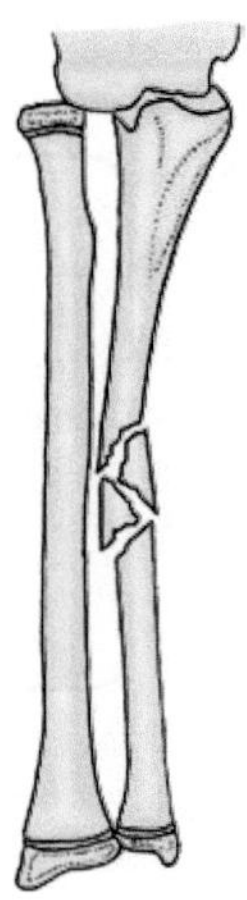
22-D/6.2

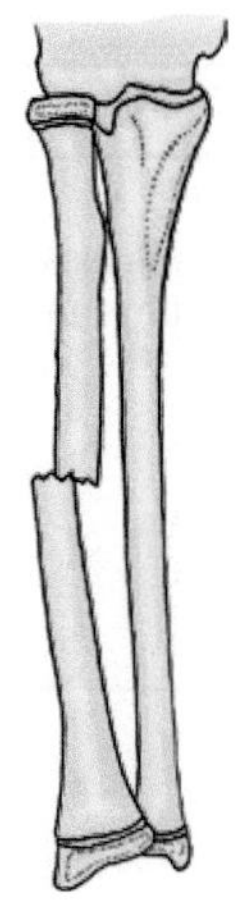
22-D/7.1

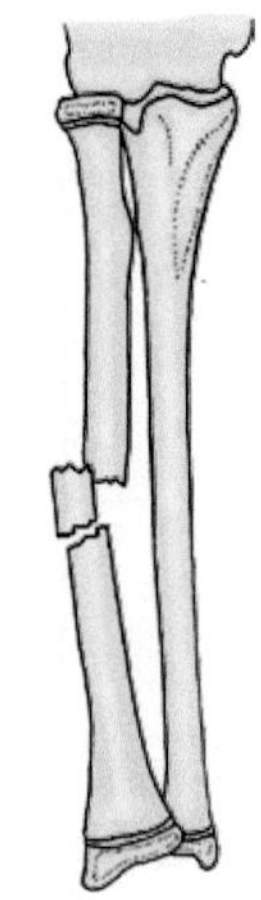
22-D/7.2

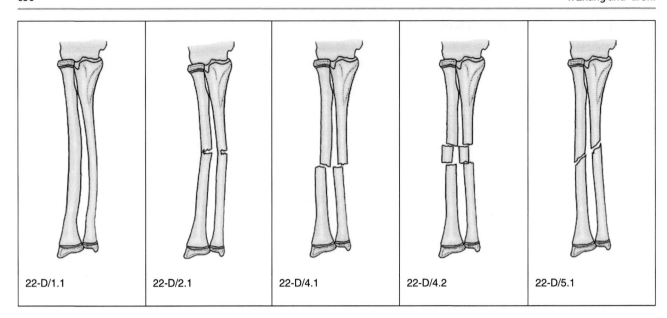

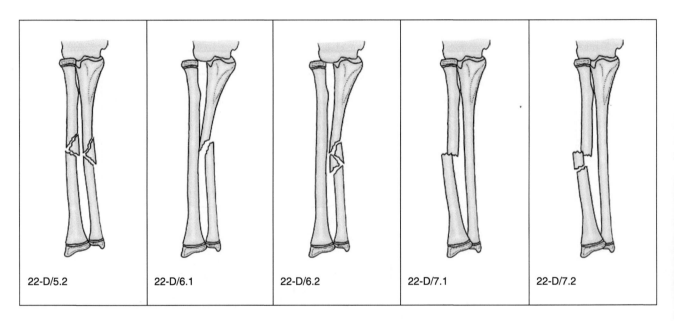

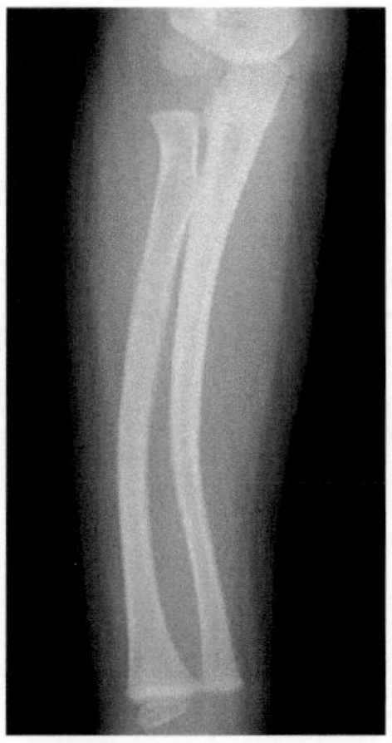

22-D/1.1

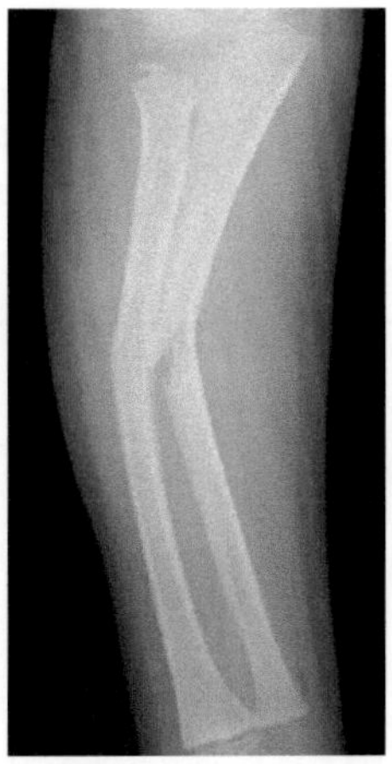

22-D/2.1

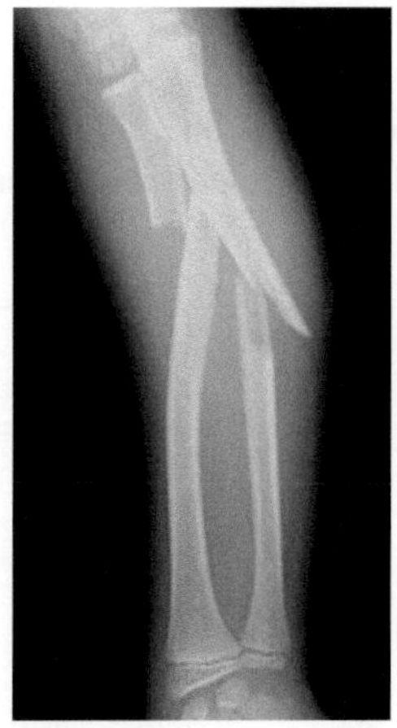

22-D/5.1

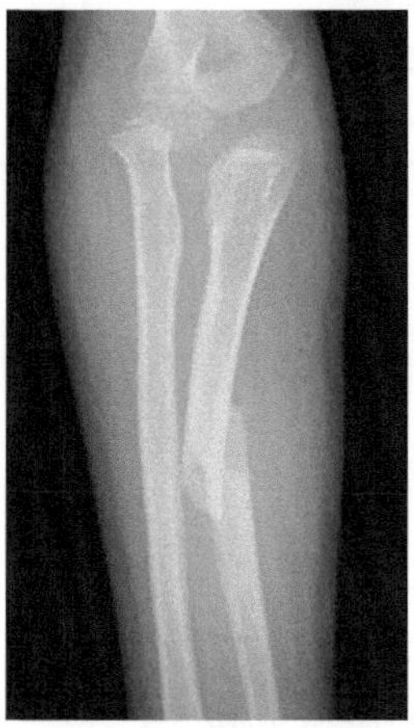

22-D/6.1

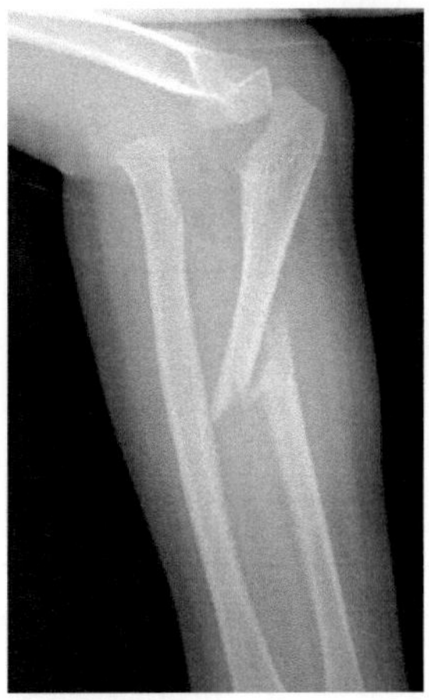

22-D/6.2

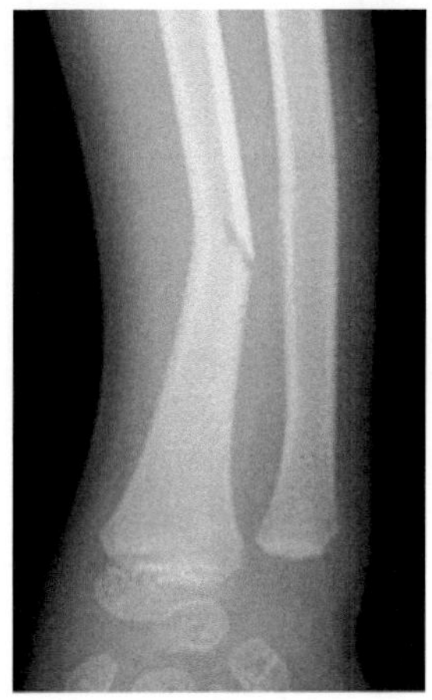

22-D/7.1

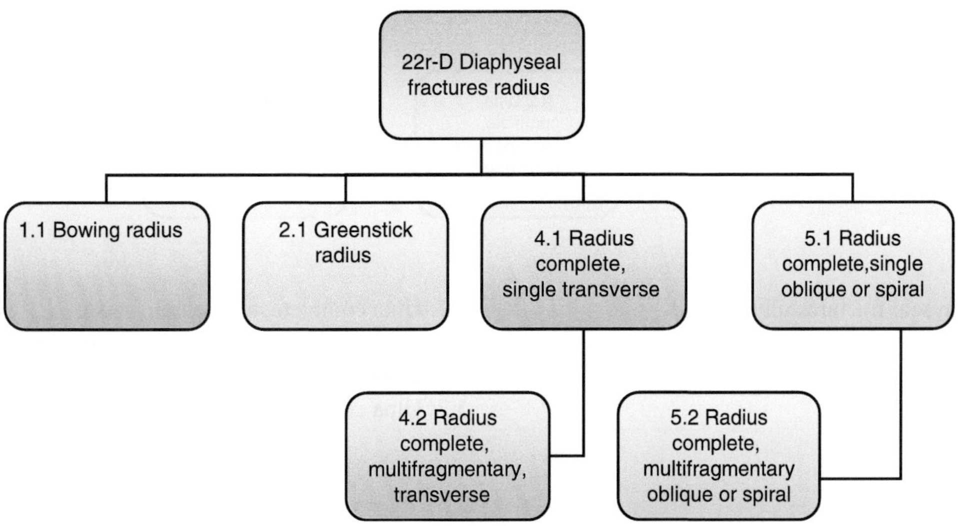

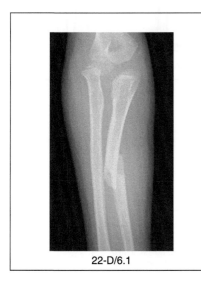

22r-D: Diaphyseal fractures radius:

1.1: Bowing radius.
2.1: Greenstick radius.
4.1: Radius complete, single transverse.
4.2: Radius complete, multifragmentary transverse.
5.1: Radius complete, single oblique or spiral.
5.2: Radius complete, multifragmentary oblique or spiral.

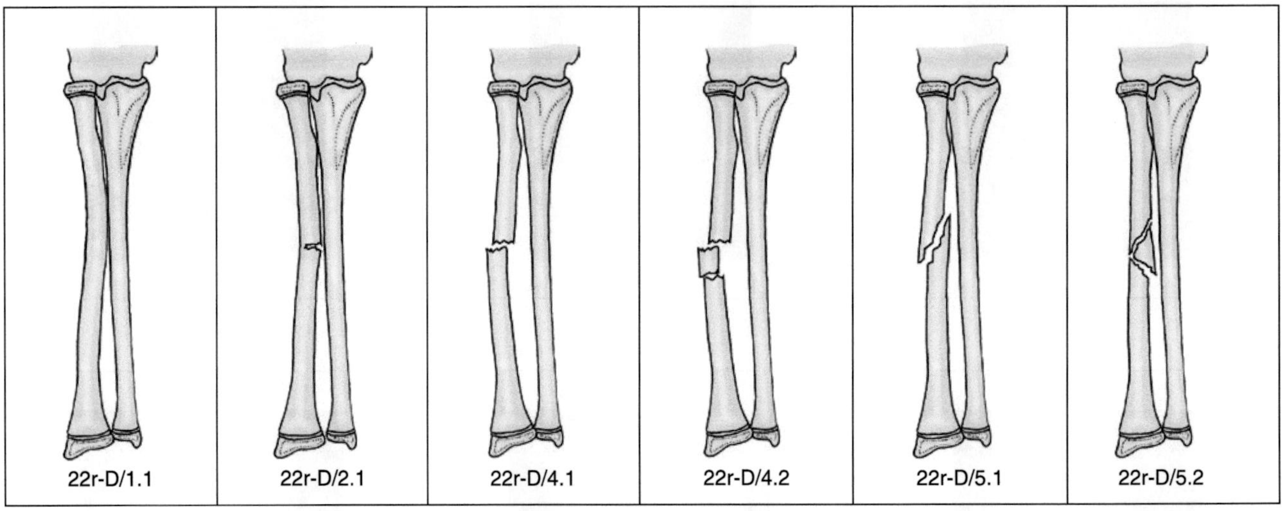

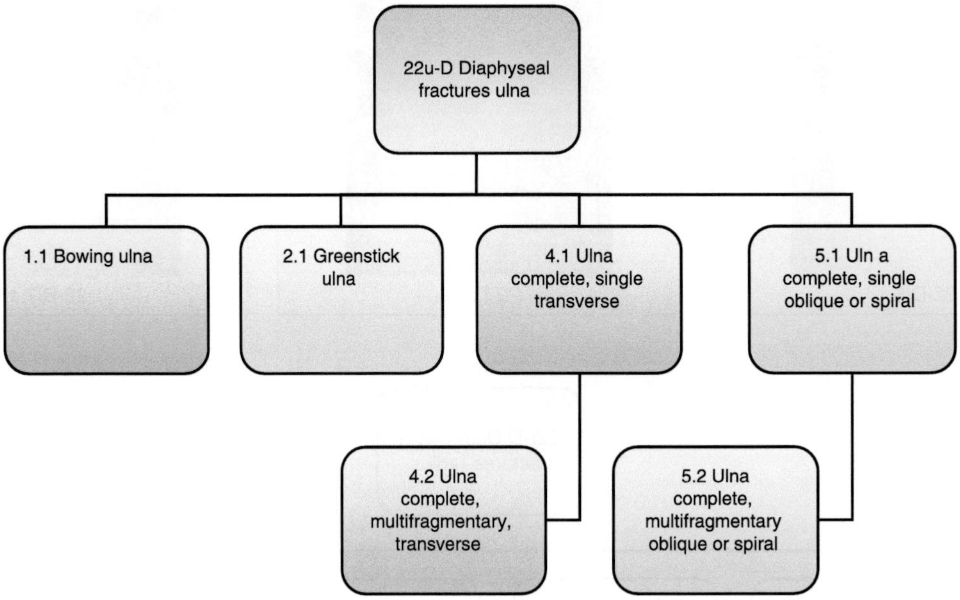

22u-D: Diaphyseal fractures ulna:

1.1: Bowing ulna.
2.1: Greenstick ulna.
4.1: Ulna complete, single transverse.
4.2: Ulna complete, multifragmentary, transverse.
5.1: Ulna complete, single oblique or spiral.
5.2: Ulna complete, multifragmentary oblique or spiral.

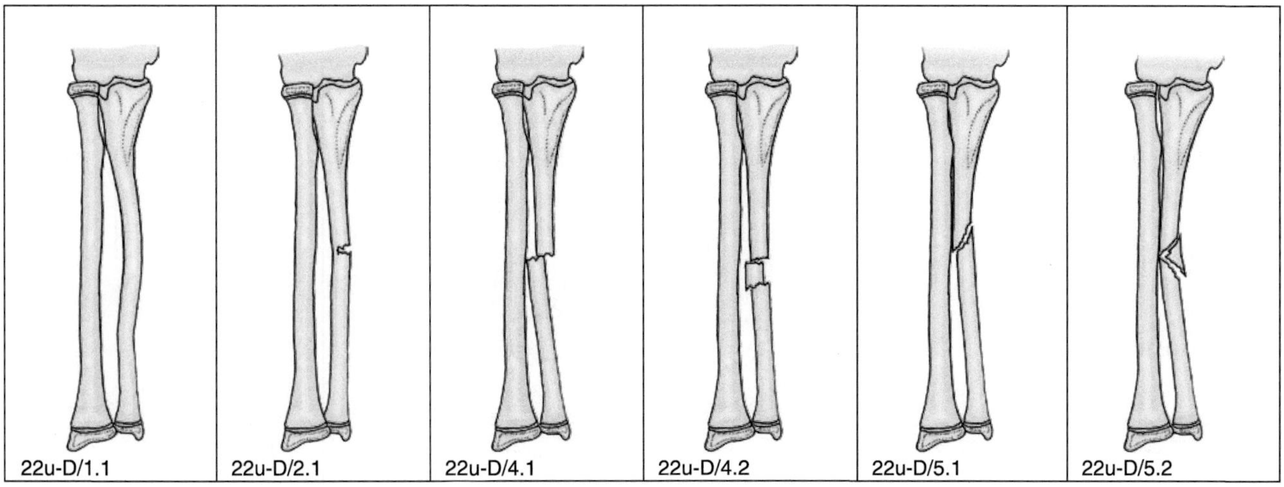

14.3.1.4 Distal Metaphyseal Fractures Radius/Ulna (23-M)

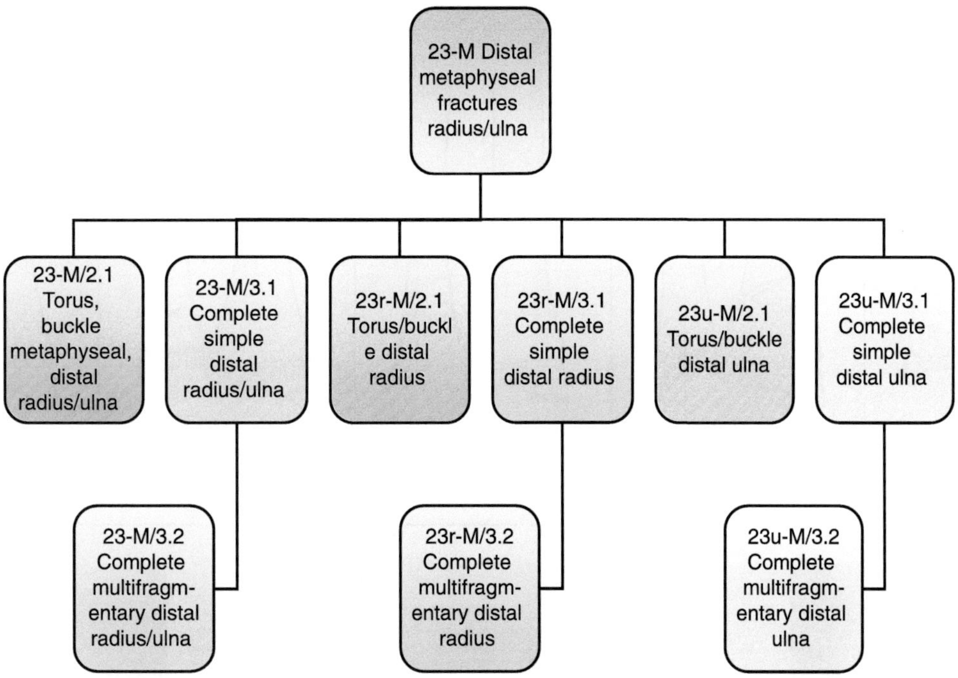

23-M: Distal metaphyseal fractures radius/ulna:

2.1: Torus, buckle metaphyseal, distal radius/ulna.
3.1: Complete simple distal radius/ulna.
3.2: Complete multifragmentary distal radius/ulna.

23r-M: Distal metaphyseal fractures radius:

2.1: Torus/buckle distal radius.
3.1: Complete simple distal radius.
3.2: Complete multifragmentary distal radius.

23u-M: Distal metaphyseal fractures ulna:

2.1: Torus/buckle distal ulna.
3.1: Complete simple distal ulna.
3.2: Complete multifragmentary distal ulna.

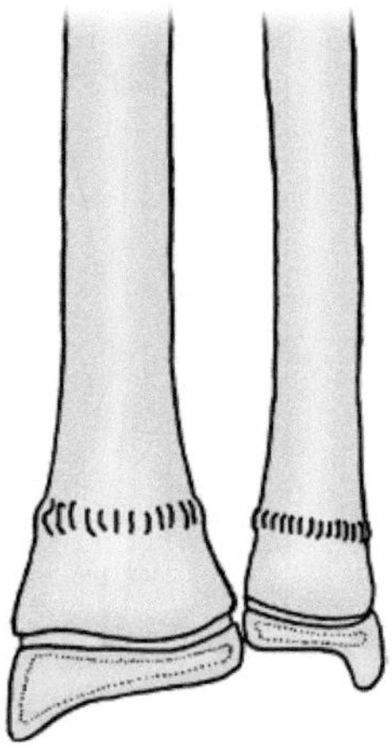
23-M/2.1

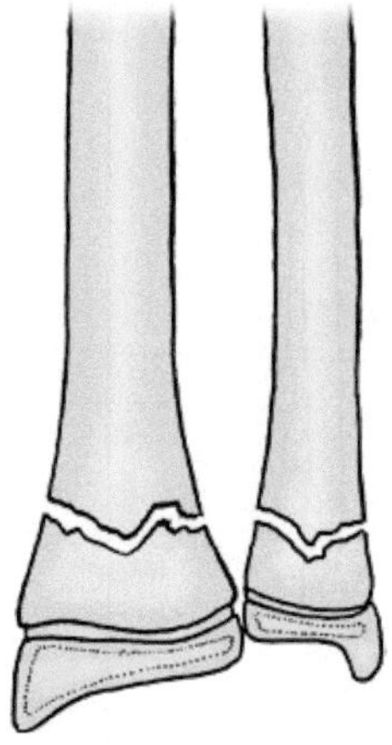
23-M/3.1

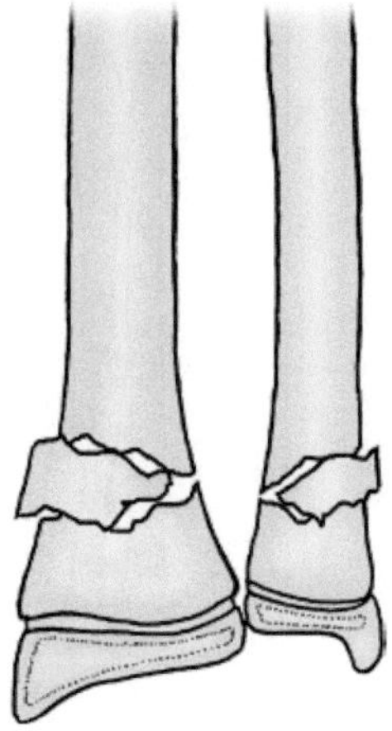
23-M/3.2

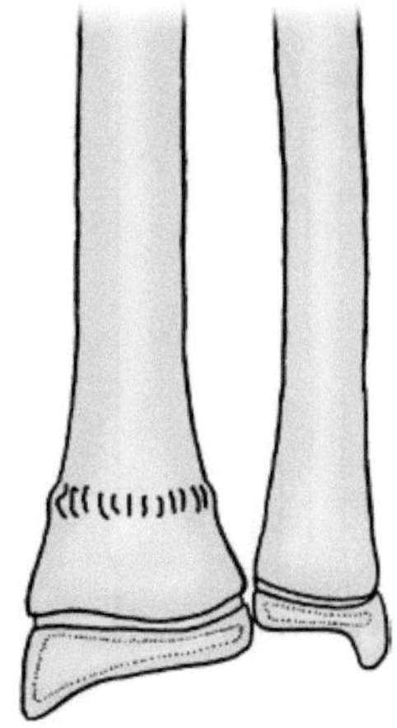
23r-M/2.1

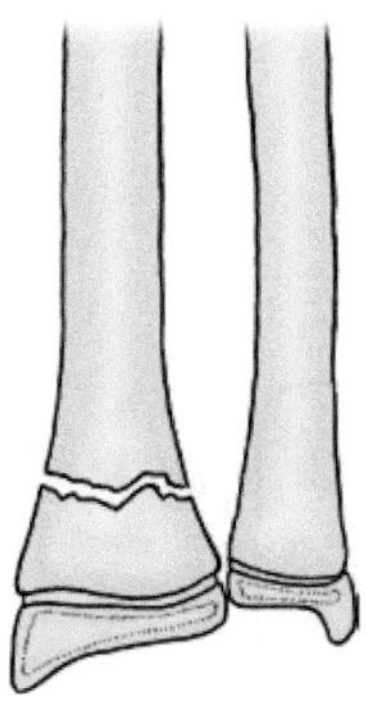
23r-M/3.1

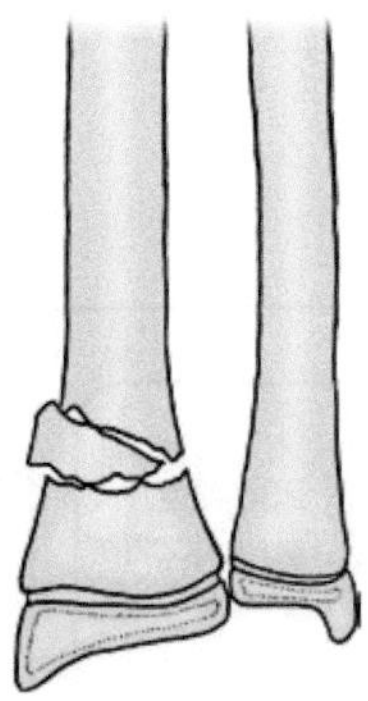
23r-M/3.2

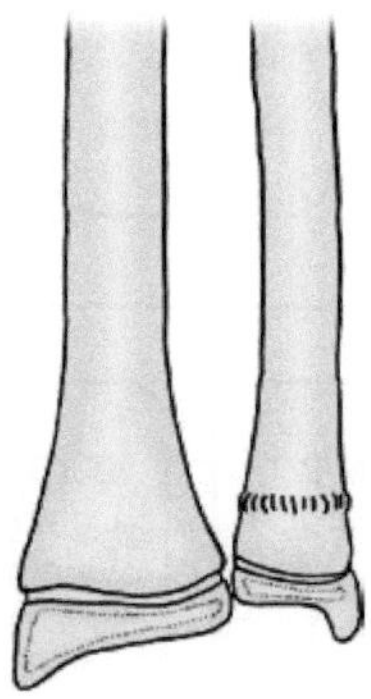
23u-M/2.1

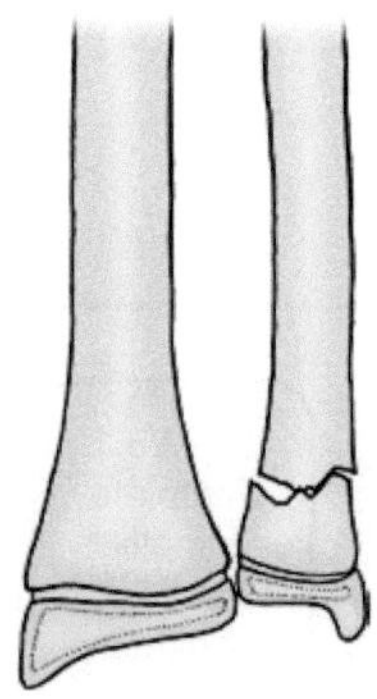
23u-M/3.1

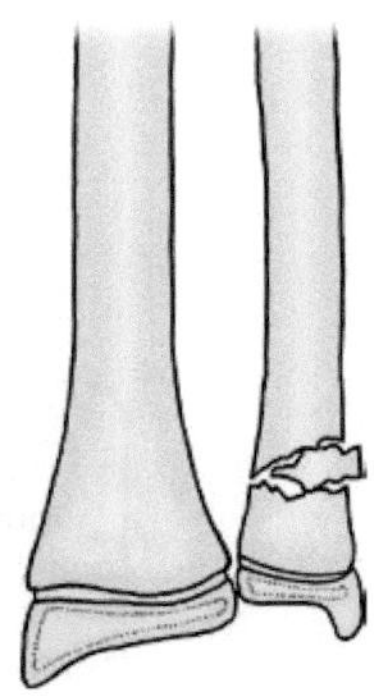
23u-M/3.2

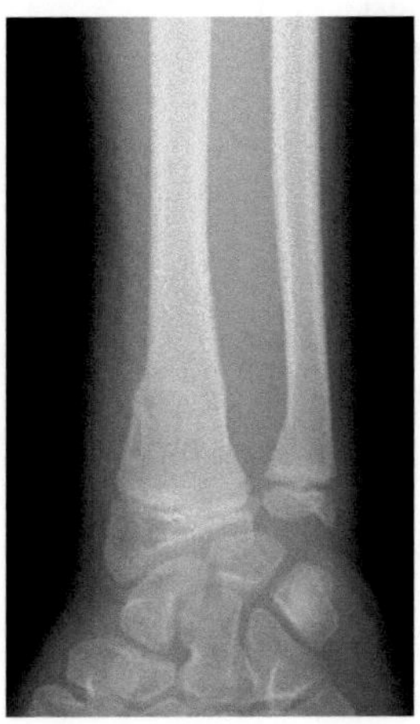
23-M/2.1

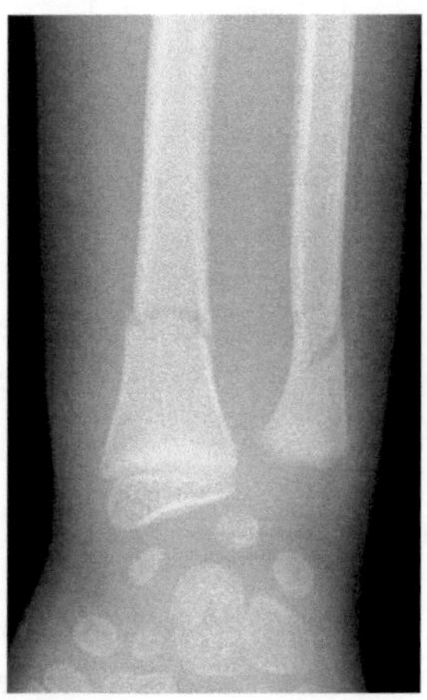
23-M/3.1

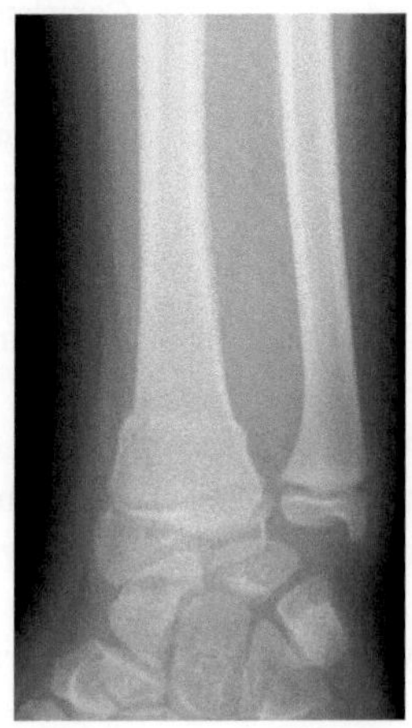
23r-M/2.1

14.3.1.5 Distal Epiphyseal Fractures Radius/Ulna (23-E)

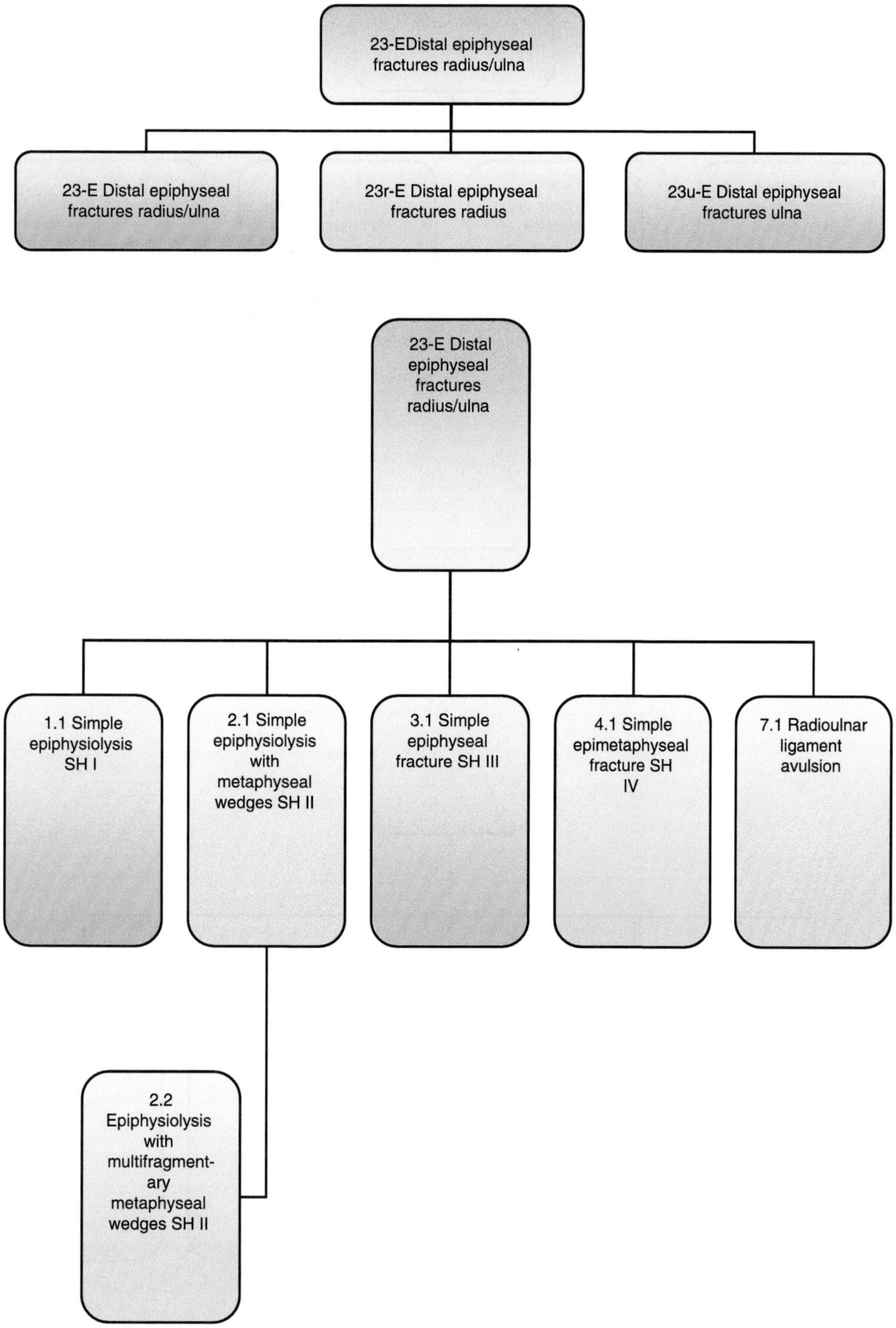

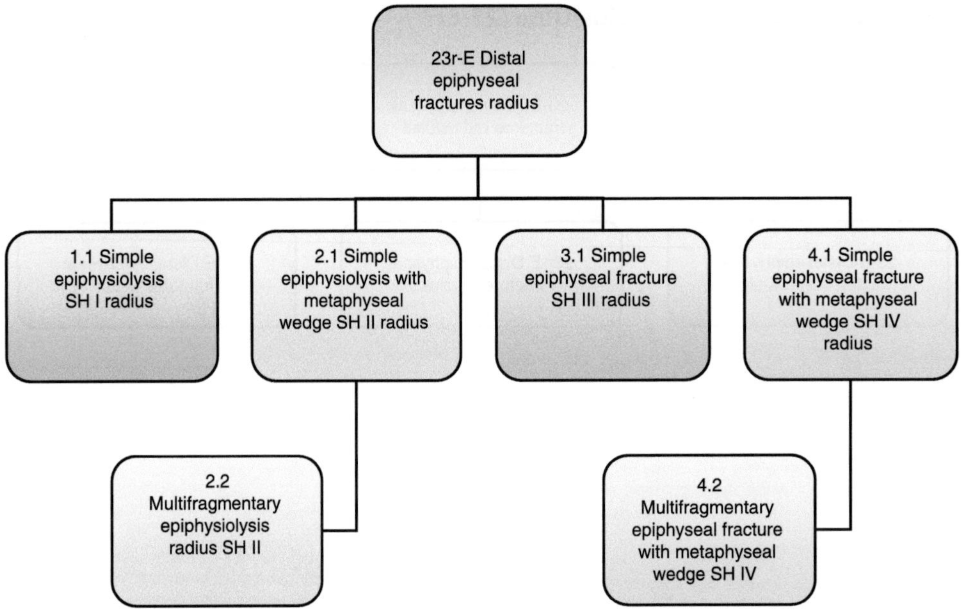
23r-E Distal epiphyseal fractures radius
1.1 Simple epiphysiolysis SH I radius
2.1 Simple epiphysiolysis with metaphyseal wedge SH II radius
3.1 Simple epiphyseal fracture SH III radius
4.1 Simple epiphyseal fracture with metaphyseal wedge SH IV radius
2.2 Multifragmentary epiphysiolysis radius SH II
4.2 Multifragmentary epiphyseal fracture with metaphyseal wedge SH IV

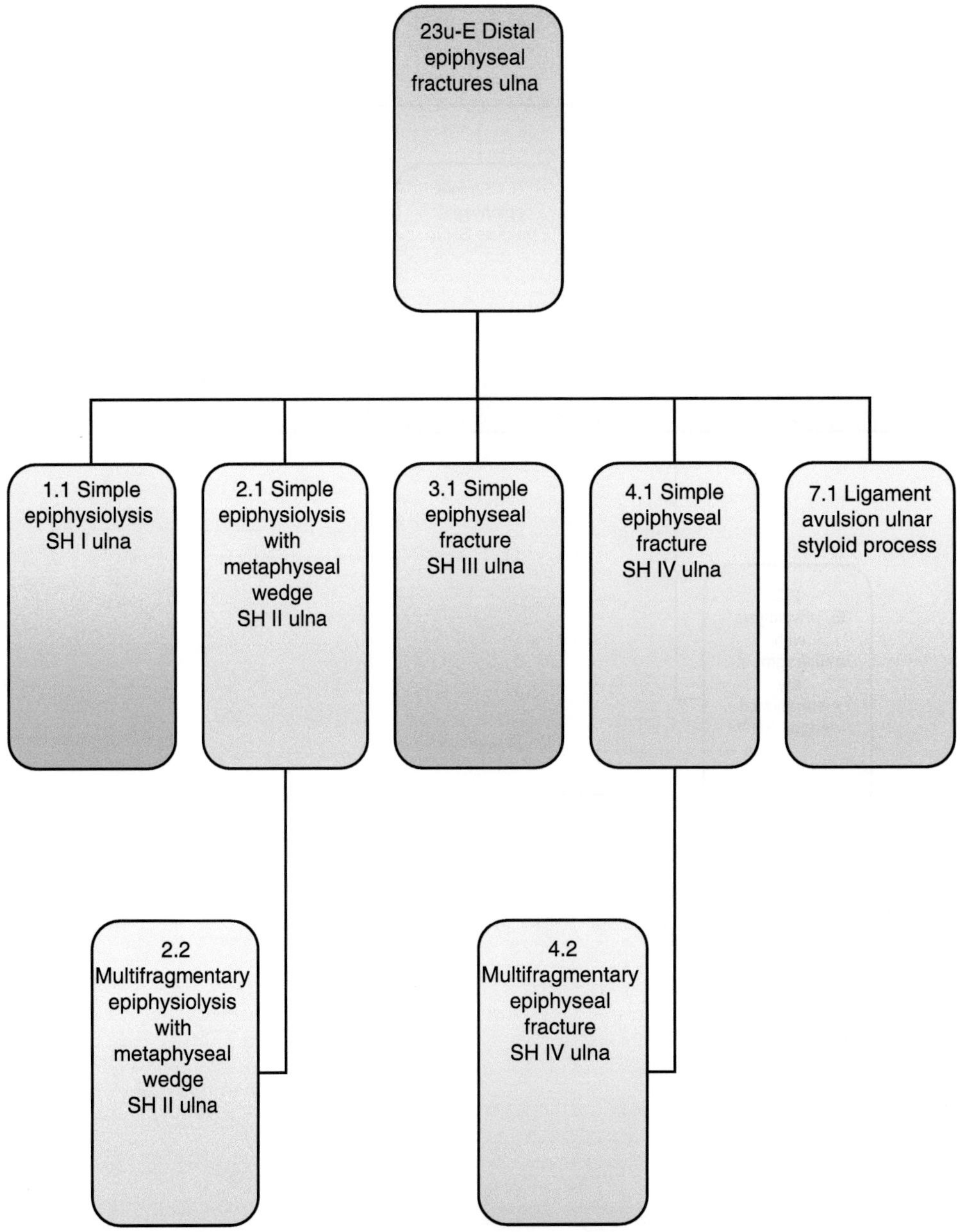
23u-E Distal epiphyseal fractures ulna
1.1 Simple epiphysiolysis SH I ulna
2.1 Simple epiphysiolysis with metaphyseal wedge SH II ulna
3.1 Simple epiphyseal fracture SH III ulna
4.1 Simple epiphyseal fracture SH IV ulna
7.1 Ligament avulsion ulnar styloid process
2.2 Multifragmentary epiphysiolysis with metaphyseal wedge SH II ulna
4.2 Multifragmentary epiphyseal fracture SH IV ulna

23-E: Distal epiphyseal fractures radius/ulna:

1.1: Simple epiphysiolysis SH I.
2.1: Simple epiphysiolysis with metaphyseal wedges SH II.
2.2: Epiphysiolysis with multifragmentary metaphyseal wedges SH II.
3.1: Simple epiphyseal fracture SH III.
4.1: Simple epimetaphyseal fracture SH IV.
7.1: Radioulnar ligament avulsion.

23r-E: Distal epiphyseal fractures radius:

1.1: Simple epiphysiolysis SH I radius.
2.1: Simple epiphysiolysis with metaphyseal wedge SH II radius.
2.2: Multifragmentary epiphysiolysis radius SH II.
3.1: Simple epiphyseal fracture SH III radius.
4.1: Simple epiphyseal fracture with metaphyseal wedge SH IV radius.
4.2: Multifragmentary epiphyseal fracture with metaphyseal wedge SH IV radius.

23u-E: Distal epiphyseal fractures ulna:

1.1: Simple epiphysiolysis SH I ulna.
2.1: Simple epiphysiolysis with metaphyseal wedge SH II ulna.
2.2: Multifragmentary epiphysiolysis with metaphyseal wedge SH II ulna.
3.1: Simple epiphyseal fracture SH III ulna.
4.1: Simple epiphyseal fracture SH IV ulna.
4.2: Multifragmentary epiphyseal fracture SH IV ulna.
7.1: Ligament avulsion ulnar styloid process.

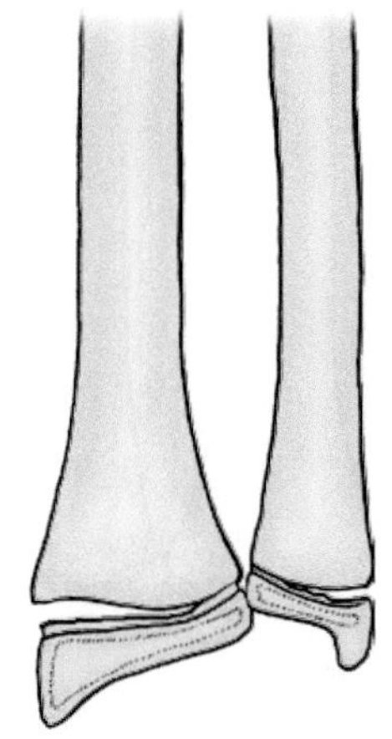
23-E/1.1

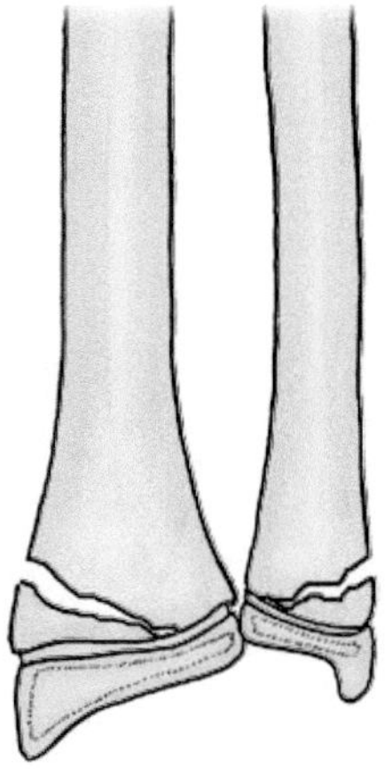
23-E/2.1

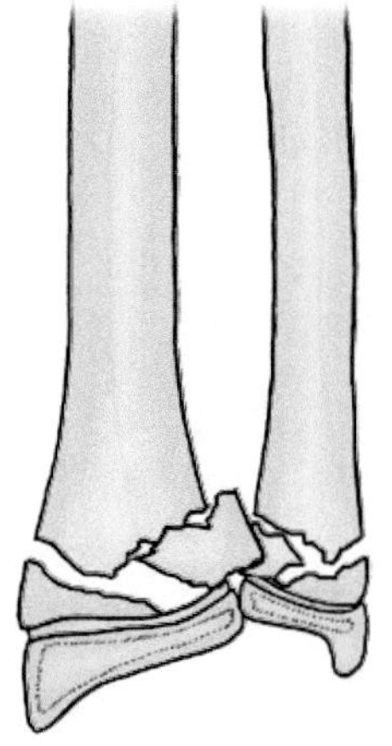
23-E/2.2

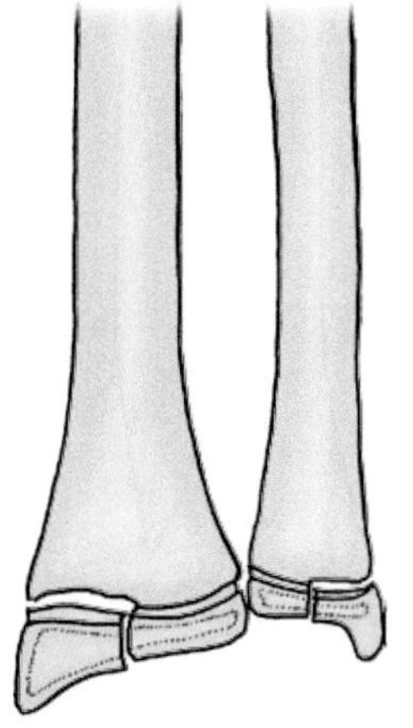
23-E/3.1

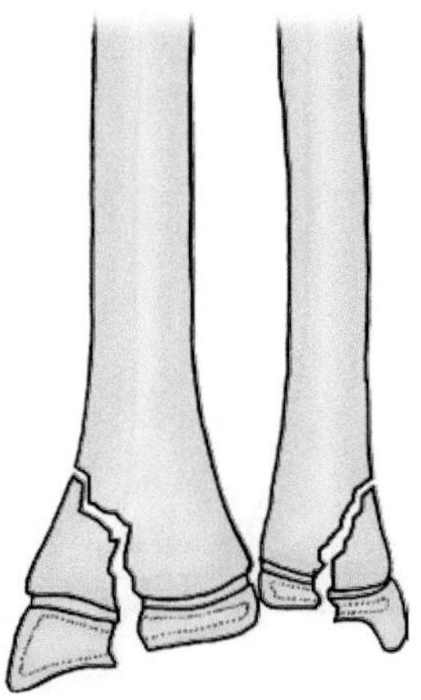
23-E/4.1

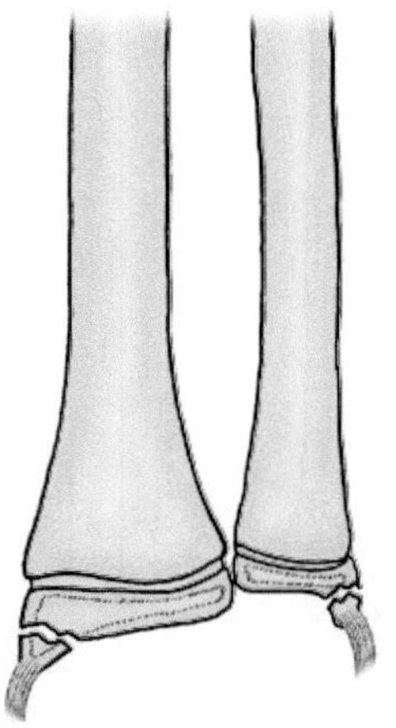
23-E/7.1

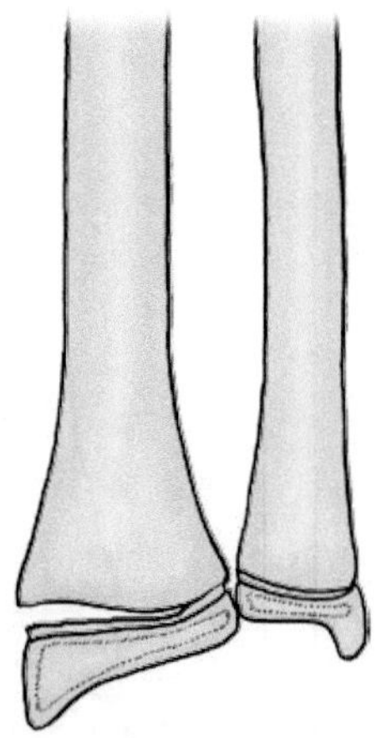
23r-E/1.1

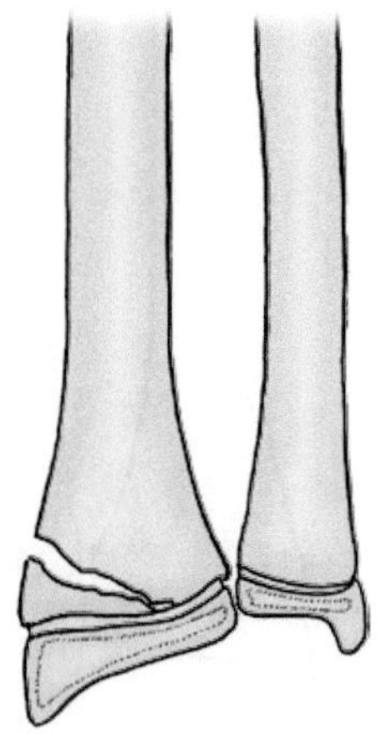
23r-E/2.1

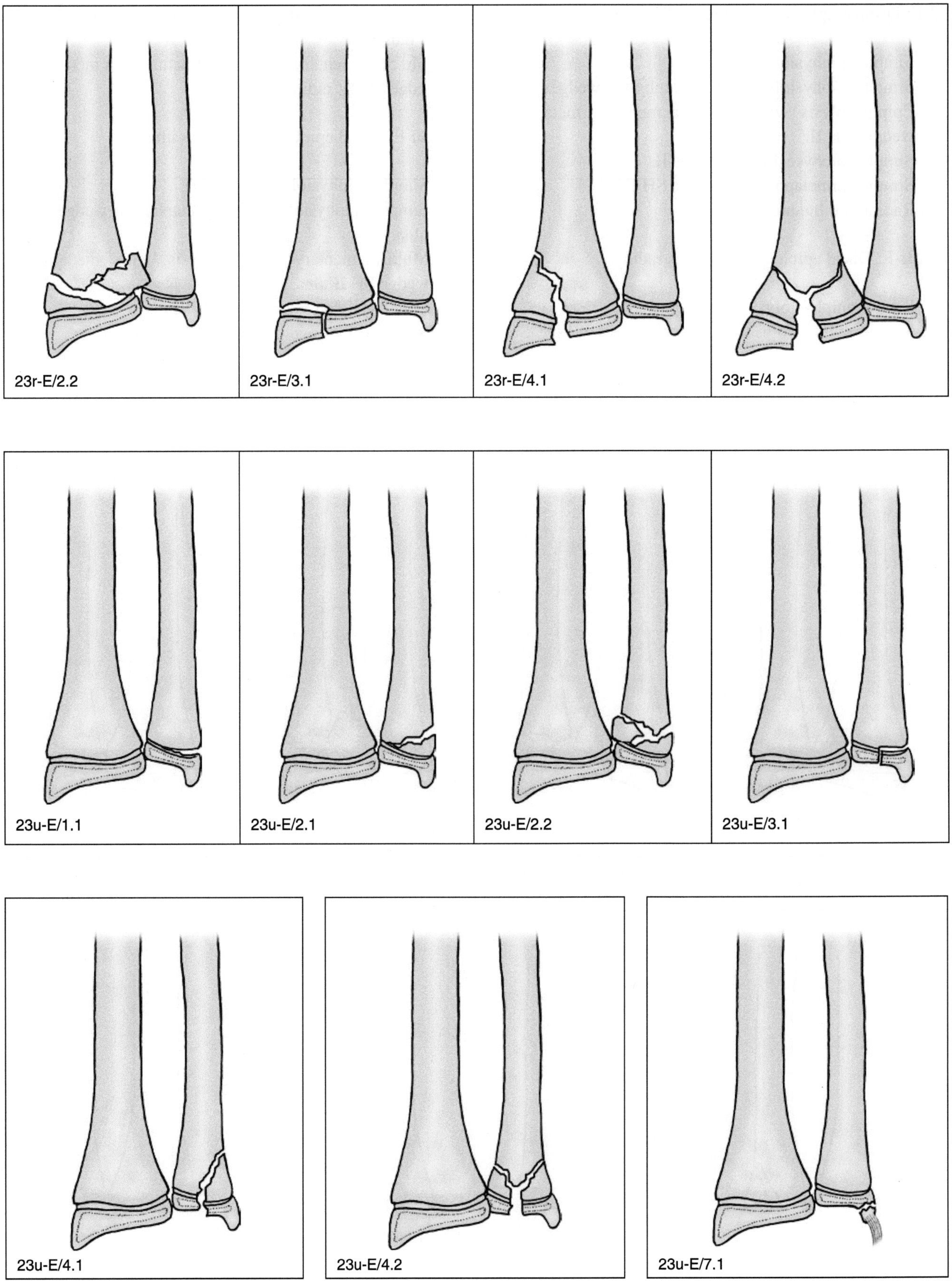
23r-E/2.2
23r-E/3.1
23r-E/4.1
23r-E/4.2
23u-E/1.1
23u-E/2.1
23u-E/2.2
23u-E/3.1
23u-E/4.1
23u-E/4.2
23u-E/7.1

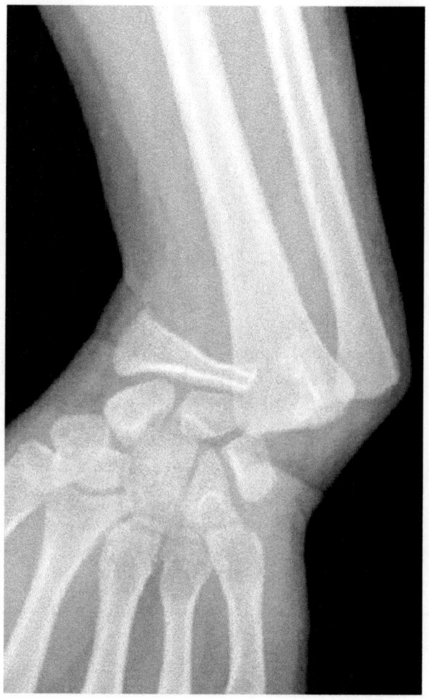

23-E/1.1 SH I

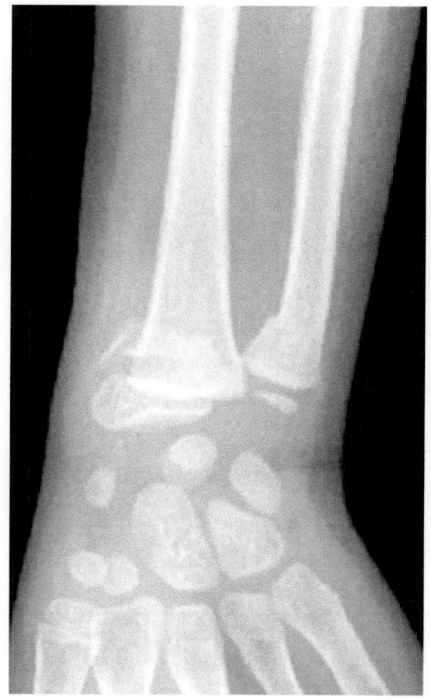

23r-E/2.2 SH II

14.3.1.6 Frequent Fracture Combinations in Paired Bones

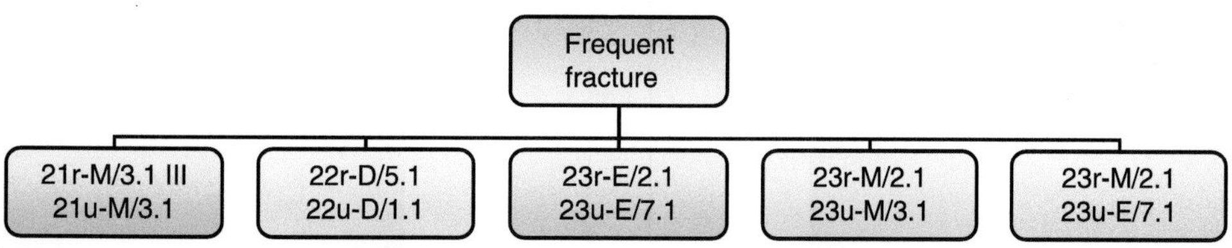

1. 21r–M/3.1III
   21u–M/3.1
   Complete radial neck type III and olecranon fracture.
2. 22r–D/5.1
   22u–D/1.1
   Simple oblique or spiral complete radius and bowing of the ulna.
3. 23r–E/2.1
   23u–E/7.1
   Radial SH II and fracture of the ulnar styloid.
4. 23r–M/2.1
   23u–M/3.1
   Torus/buckle of the radius and complete metaphyseal ulna.
5. 23r–M/2.1
   23u–E/7.1
   Torus/buckle of the radius and fracture of the ulnar styloid.

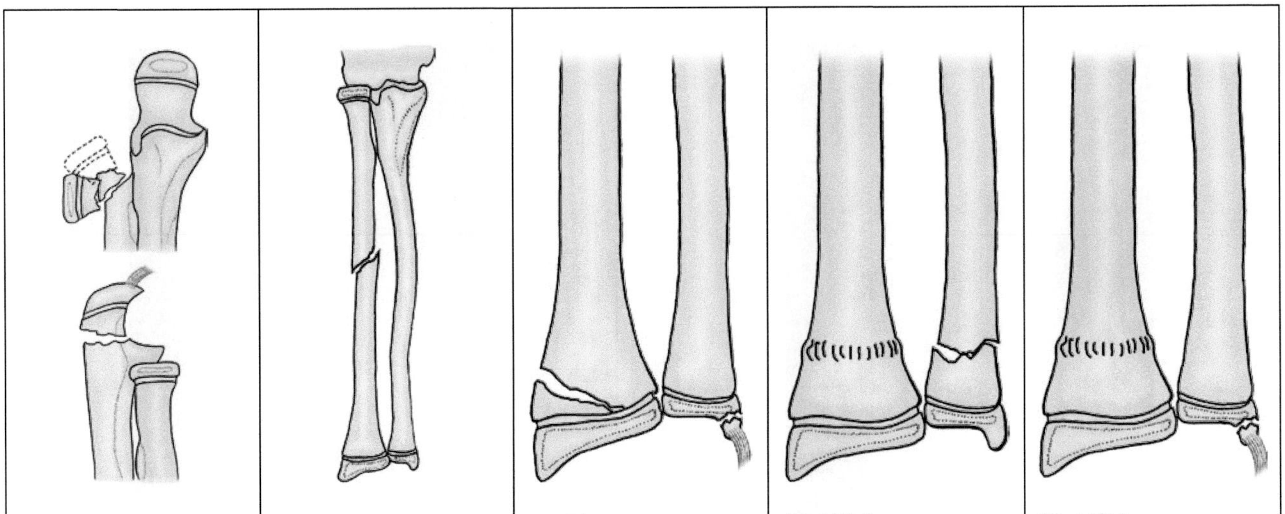

21r-M/3.1 III 21u-M/3.1	22r-D/5.1 22u-D/1.1	23r-E/2.1 23u-E/7.1	23r-M/2.1 23u-M/3.1	23r-M/2.1 23u-E/7.1

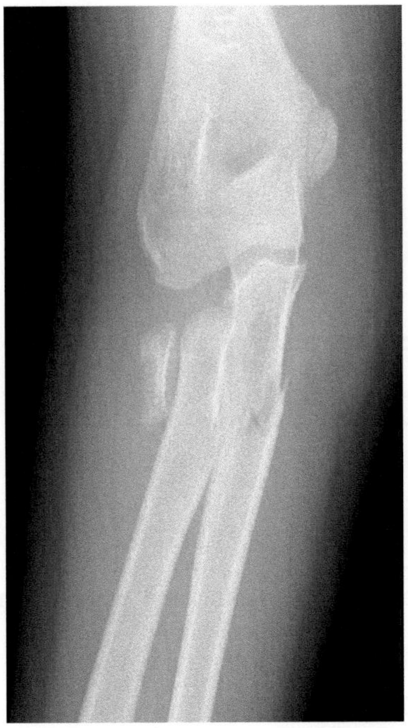

21r-M/3.1III
21u-M/3.1

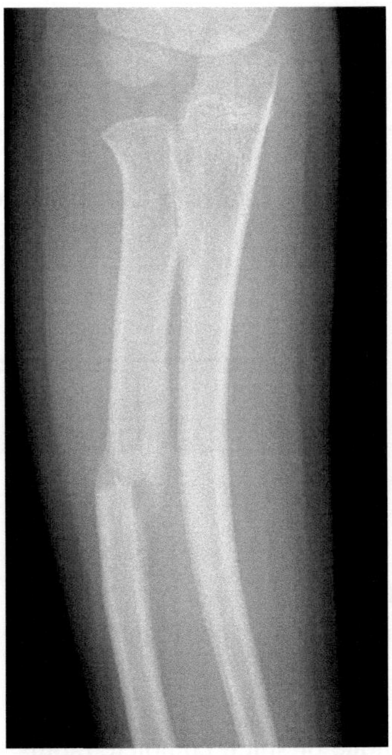

22r-D/5.1
22u-D/1.1

14.3.2 Xu Yijing Classification of Children Ulnar Coronoid Fracture

Type I: Small pieces of coronal processes of avulsion fracture.

Type II: Single or multiple crushed bones, fractures do not exceed 50% of the coronal processes.

Type III: Single or multiple crushed bones, fractures more than 50% of coronal processes.

14.4 Section 4 Children Pelvic Fracture

14.4.1 Torode-Zie Classification

Type I: Avulsion fracture, mainly avulsion of cartilage plate, like sports injury.

Type II: Iliac wing fracture. Mainly caused by direct violence, probably iliac crest or iliac wing fracture caused by lateral forces.

Type III: Single ring fracture. Including pubic branch fracture or pubic symphysis separation. For the children pelvic elasticity, generally partial laceration of anterior sacroiliac ligament does not have sacroiliac joint instability.

Type IV: Pelvic ring fracture. Instability of pelvic ring produced by fracture or joint separation.

- Type IVa: Bilateral pubic ramus fractures (straddle injury).
- Type IVb: One side of pubic rami fractures or pubic symphysis separation involves posterior pelvic fracture or sacroiliac joint separation.
- Type IVc: Fracture involving anterior ring and acetabulum.

14.4.2 **Tile Classification** (1988, J Bone Joint Surg (Br), 70:1–12)

Similar to adult pelvic fracture classification.

14.4.2.1 Stable Fracture

1. The secondary ossification centre avulsion; common in adolescent athletes, occurs in any secondary ossification centre. It is more common in:
   (a) Anterior superior iliac spine, the start of sartorius muscle avulsion.
   (b) Anterior inferior iliac spine, the start of rectus femoris avulsion.
   (c) Sciatic tuberosity, the start of hamstring avulsion.
2. Pelvic ring stable fracture: Pelvic posterior tension band stability of this fracture, that is, posterior ligament of posterior pelvic bearing surface not broken.
   (a) Anterior-posterior compression (open book): Pubic symphysis fractures were more common than ramus pubis.
   (b) Lateral compression ("Y"-shaped cartilage injury): Lateral crush injuries can involve "Y"-shaped cartilage, which has potential early closure of the epiphyseal plate, can lead to acetabular dysplasia.

14.4.2.2 Unstable Fracture

Unstable pelvic fractures (double-longitudinal fractures) similar to adults, the anterior injury can be pubic symphysis separation, pubic branch fracture or the both, the posterior injury is often the sacroiliac joint dislocation, occasionally the sacrum or iliac fracture. More severe posterior injuries were bilateral. Bilateral sacroiliac joint dislocation without anterior injury, children are more common than adults, this damage is mostly caused by extrusion or ahead violence.

14.4.3 Young-Burgess Classification

Pelvic fractures are more common in adults, and children with pelvic fractures are also cited in the literature.

1. Anterior-posterior compression (APC)
2. Lateral compression
3. Vertical shear
4. Complex pattern

14.4.4 Kane Classification

Type I: Fractures not involving the ring.
Type II: Single fracture of the ring.
Type III: Two fractures of the ring.
Type IV: Fractures of the acetabulum.

14.4.5 Trunkey Classification

Type I: Crushing, more than three fractures of anterior and posterior pelvic ring.

Type II: Unstable, anterior and posterior pelvic ring fracture and dislocation.

Type III: Stable, isolated fracture or pubic branch fracture.

14.4.6 Other Classifications

In addition to Trunkey classification, there were also Orden classification and Maull classification, but few references in the literature.

14.5 Section 4 Children Femur Fractures

14.5.1 AO/OTA Classification

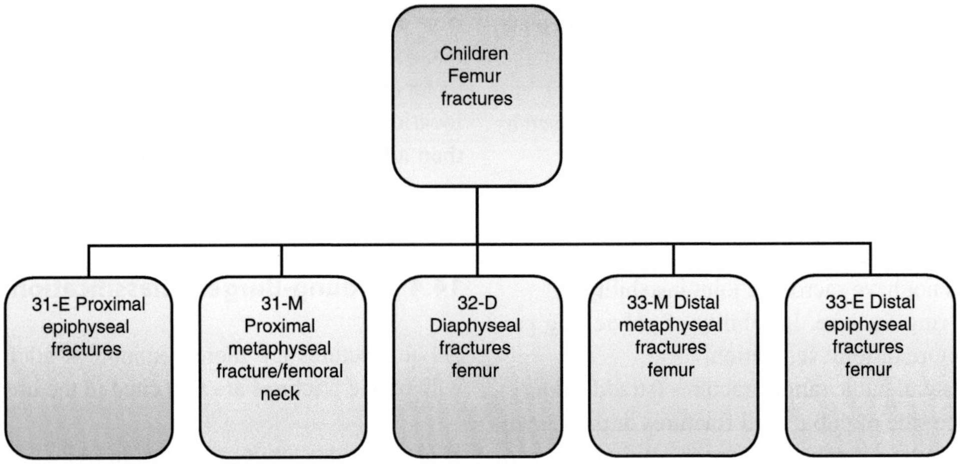

14.5.1.1 Proximal Epiphyseal Fractures (31-E)

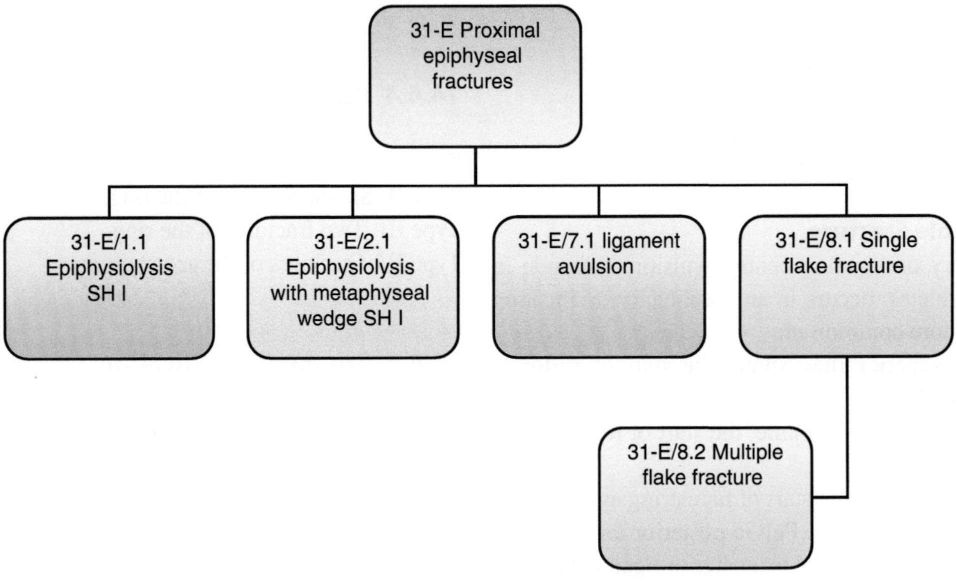

31-E: Proximal epiphyseal fractures.

1.1: Epiphysiolysis (SUFE/SCFE) SH I.
2.1: Epiphysiolysis (SUFE/SCFE) with metaphyseal wedge SH I.
7.1: Ligament avulsion (ligamentum capitis femoris).
8.1: Single flake fracture.
8.2: Multiple flake fracture.

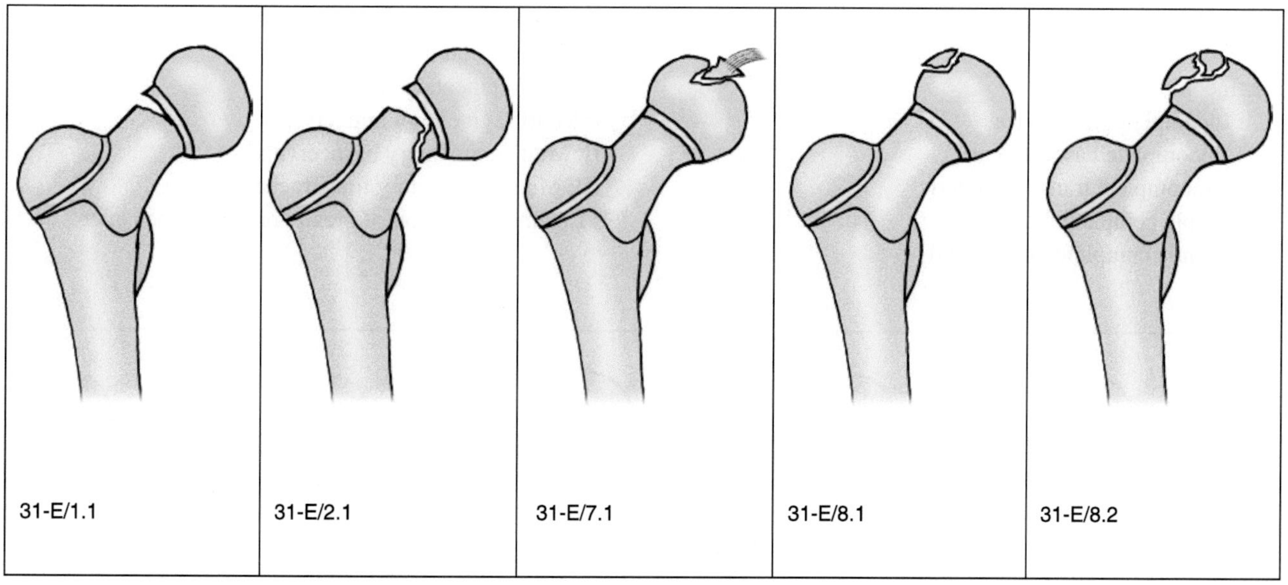

14.5.1.2 Proximal Metaphyseal Fracture/Femoral Neck (31-M)

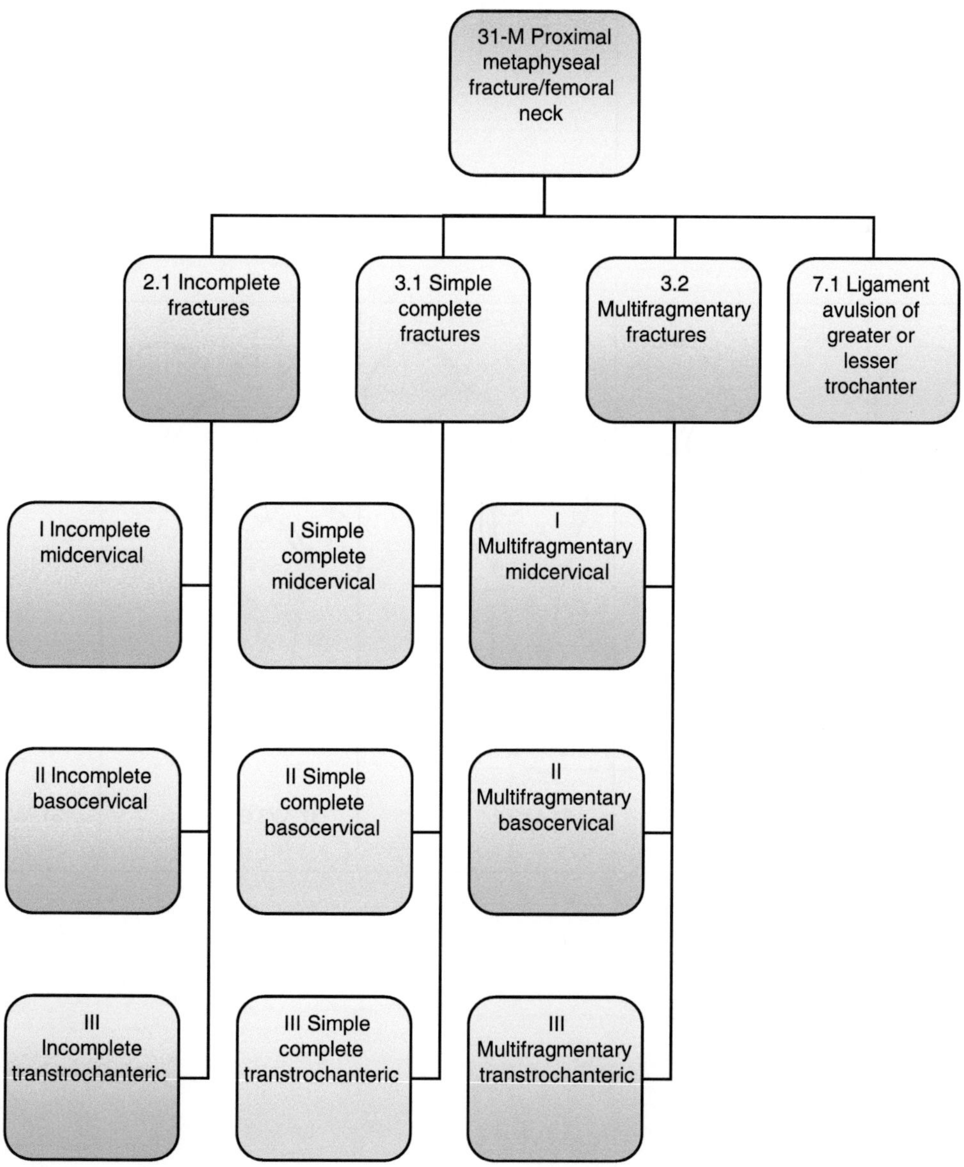

31-M: **Proximal metaphyseal fracture/femoral.**

2.1: Incomplete fractures:
- I: Incomplete midcervical
- II: Incomplete basocervical
- III: Incomplete transtrochanteric

3.1: Simple complete fractures:
- I: Simple complete midcervical
- II: Simple complete basocervical
- III: Simple complete transtrochanteric

3.2: Multifragmentary fractures:
- I: Multifragmentary midcervical
- II: Multifragmentary basocervical
- III: Multifragmentary transtrochanteric

7.1: Ligament avulsion of greater or lesser trochanter

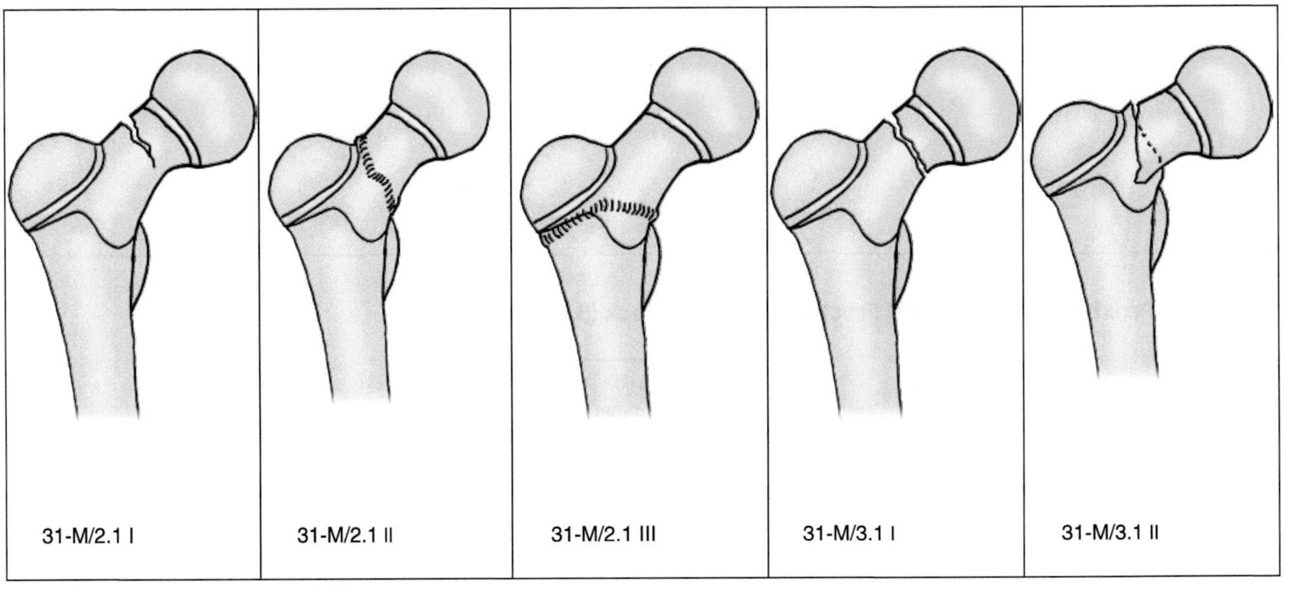

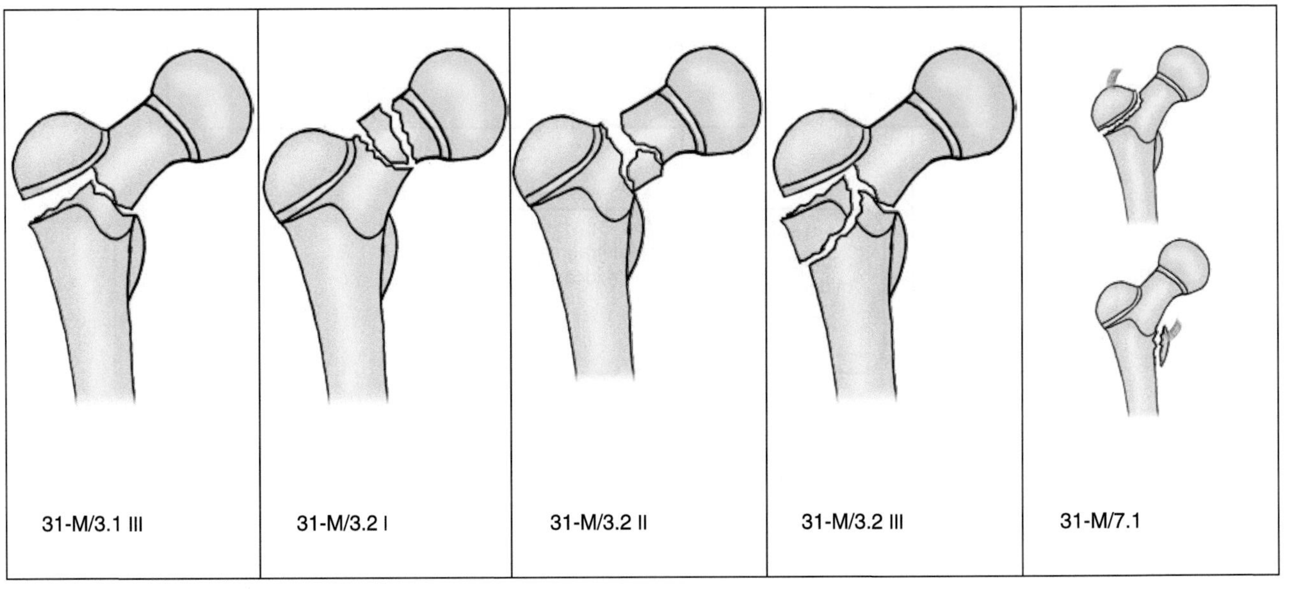

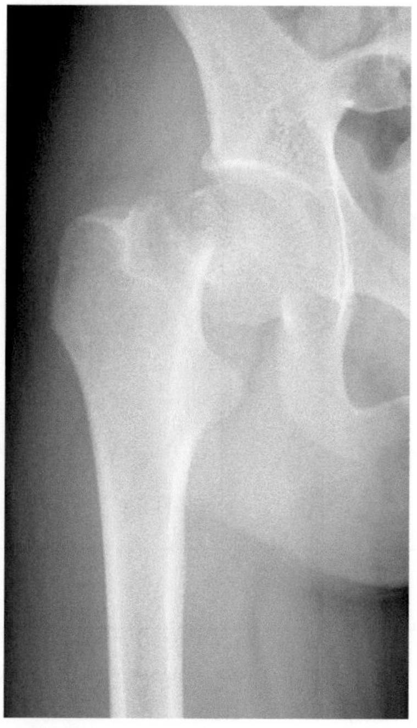

31-M/3.1 I

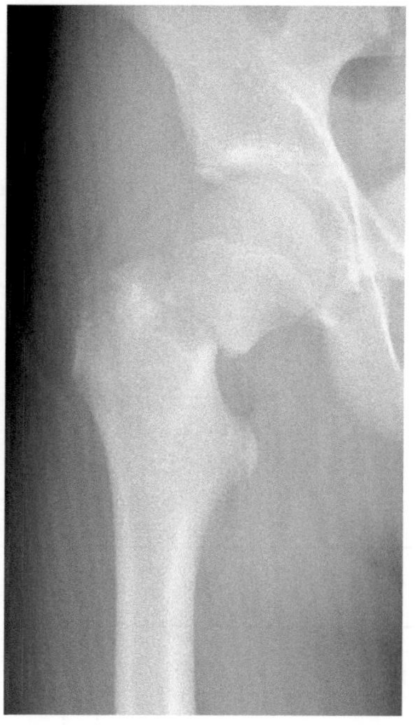

31-M/3.1 II

14.5.1.3 Diaphyseal Fractures Femur (32-D)

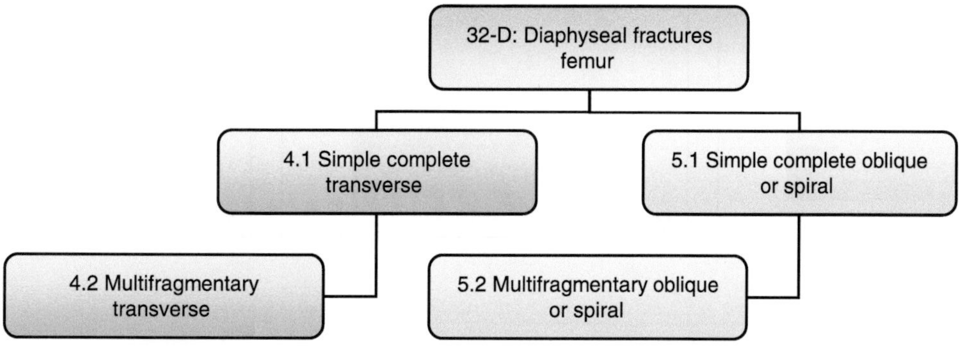

32-D: Diaphyseal fractures femur.

4.1: Simple complete transverse (≤30°).
4.2: Multifragmentary transverse (≤30°).
5.1: Simple complete oblique or spiral (>30°).
5.2: Multifragmentary oblique or spiral (>30°).

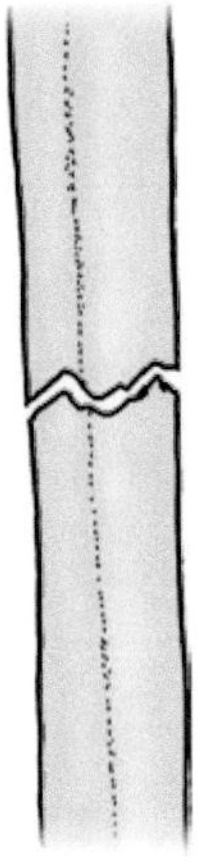
32-D/4.1

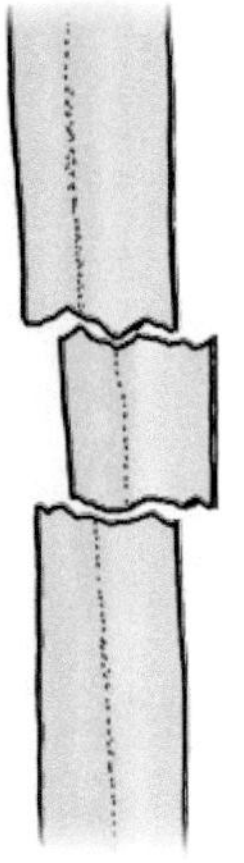
32-D/4.2

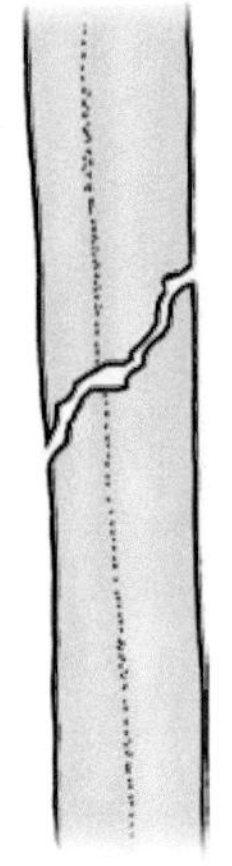
32-D/5.1

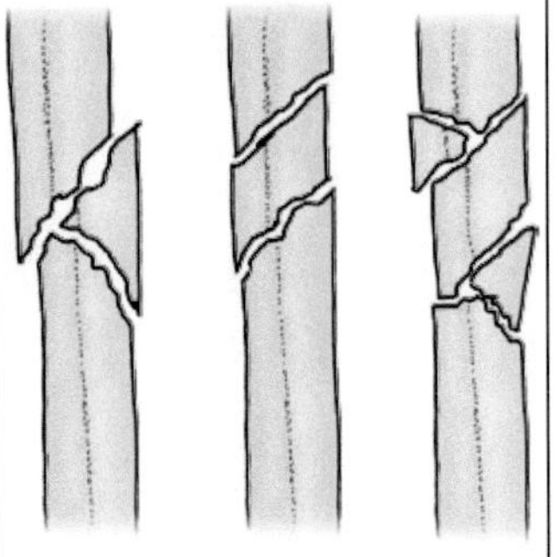
32-D/5.2

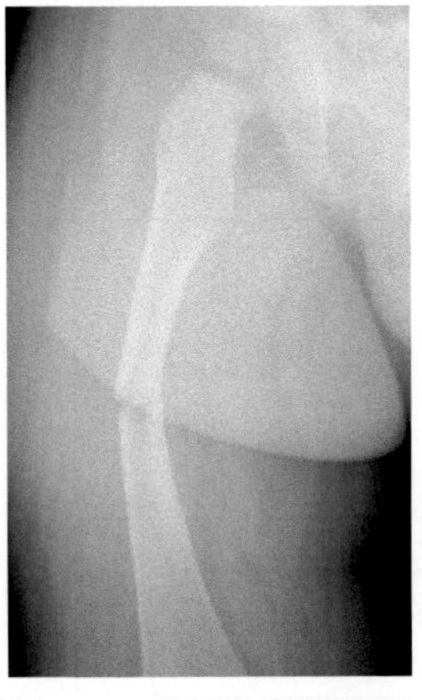
32-D/4.1

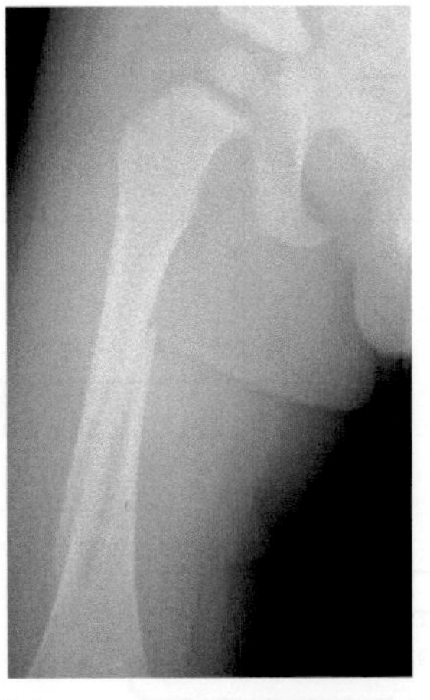
32-D/5.1

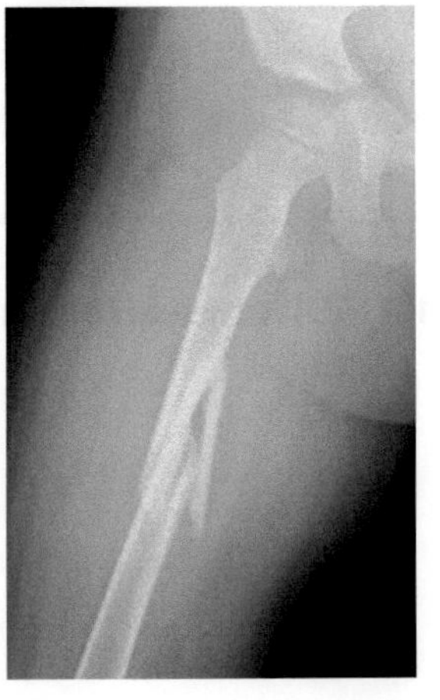
32-D/5.2

14.5.1.4 Distal Metaphyseal Fractures Femur (33-M)

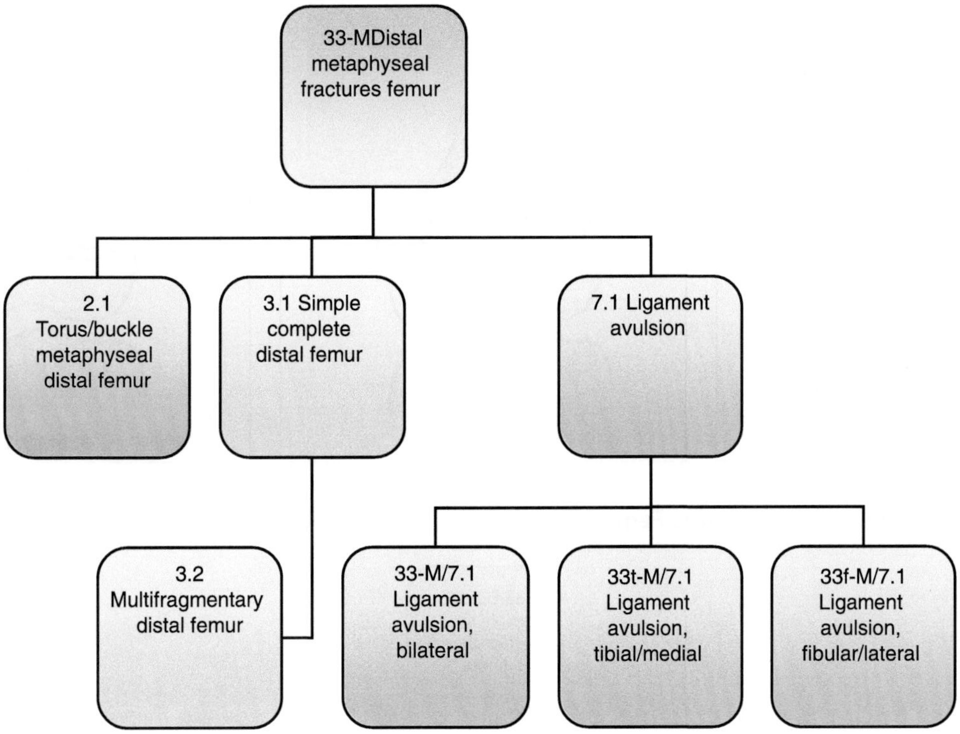

33-M: Distal metaphyseal fractures femur.

2.1: Torus/buckle metaphyseal distal femur.
3.1: Simple complete distal femur.
3.2: Multifragmentary distal femur.

33-M/7.1: Ligament avulsion, bilateral.
33t-M/7.1: Ligament avulsion, tibial/medial.
33f-M/7.1: Ligament avulsion, fibular/lateral.

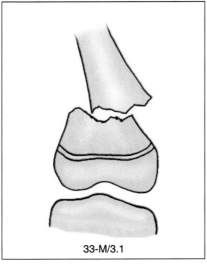

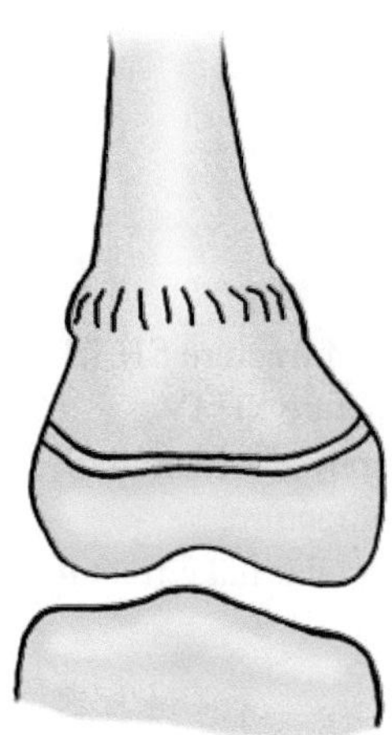

33-M/2.1

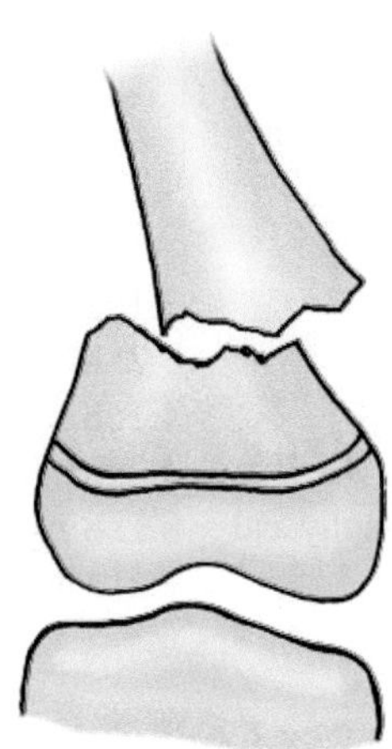

33-M/3.1

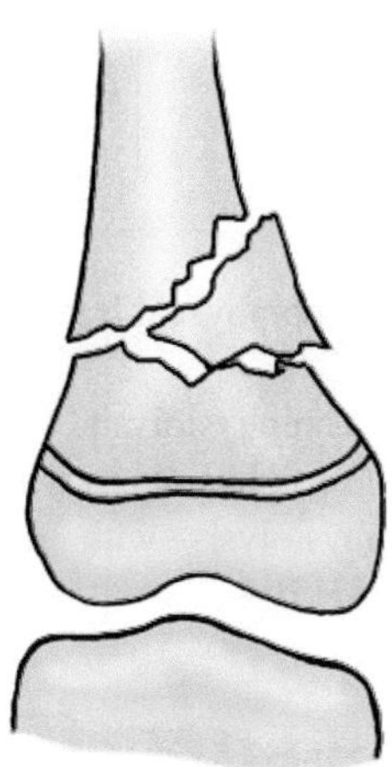

33-M/3.2

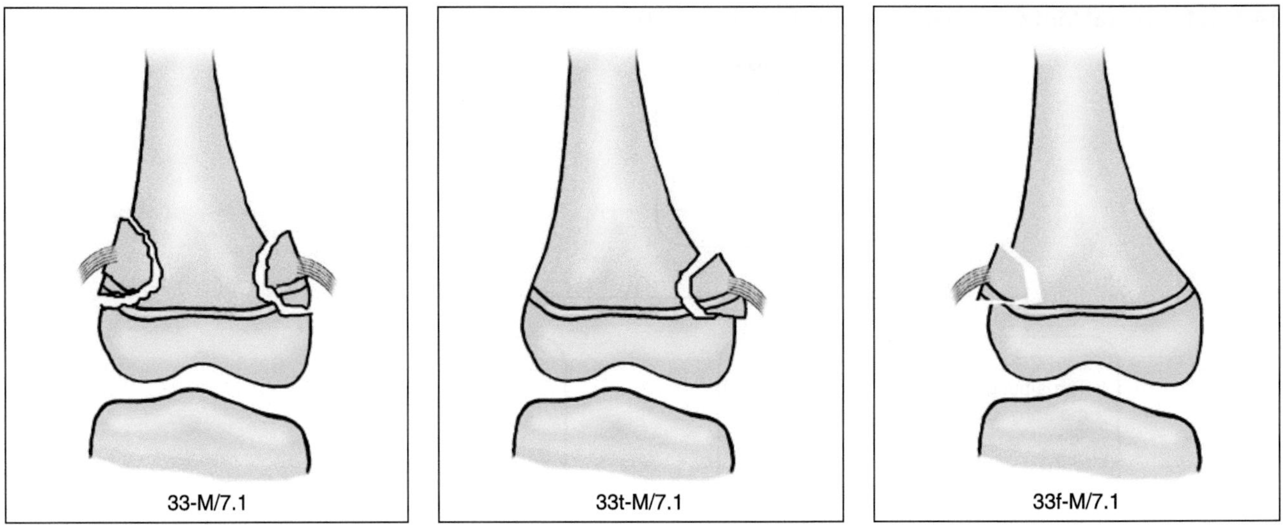

14.5.1.5 Distal Epiphyseal Fractures Femur (33-E)

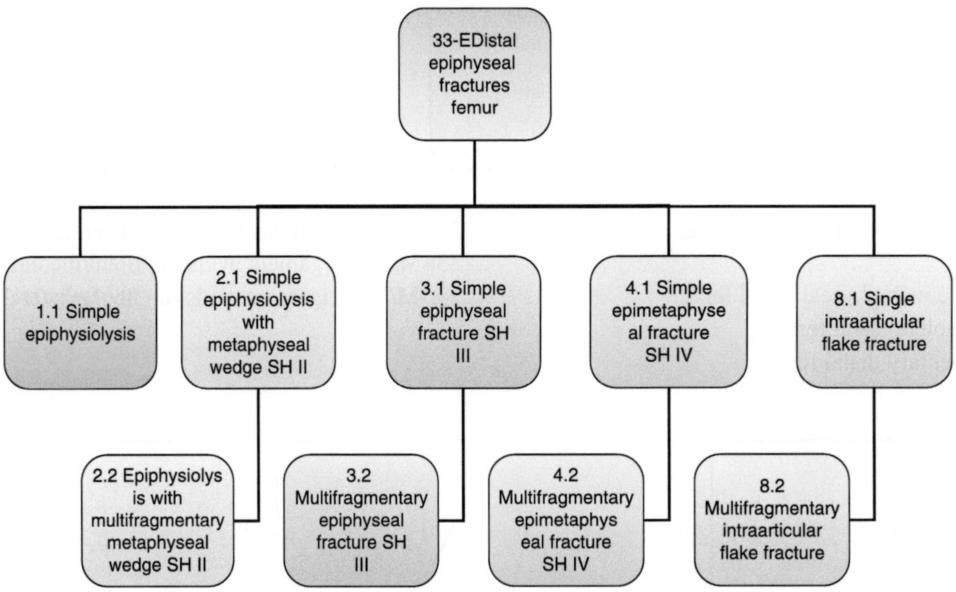

33-E: Distal epiphyseal fractures femur.

1.1: Simple epiphysiolysis.
2.1: Simple epiphysiolysis with metaphyseal wedge SH II.
2.2: Epiphysiolysis with multifragmentary metaphyseal wedge SH II.
3.1: Simple epiphyseal fracture SH III.
3.2: Multifragmentary epiphyseal fracture SH III.
4.1: Simple epimetaphyseal fracture SH IV.
4.2: Multifragmentary epimetaphyseal fracture SH IV.
8.1: Single intra-articular flake fracture.
8.2: Multifragmentary intra-articular flake fracture.

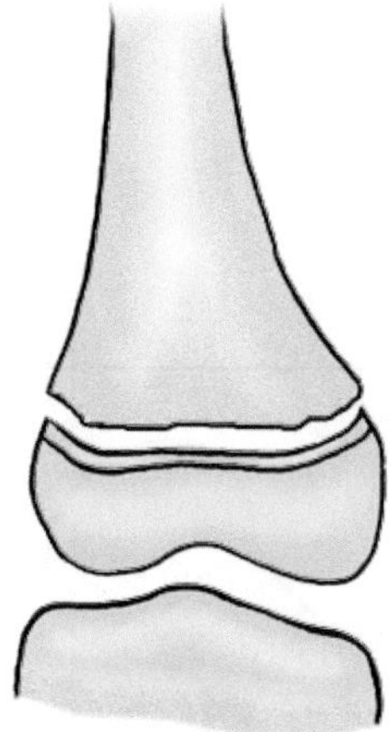
33-E/1.1

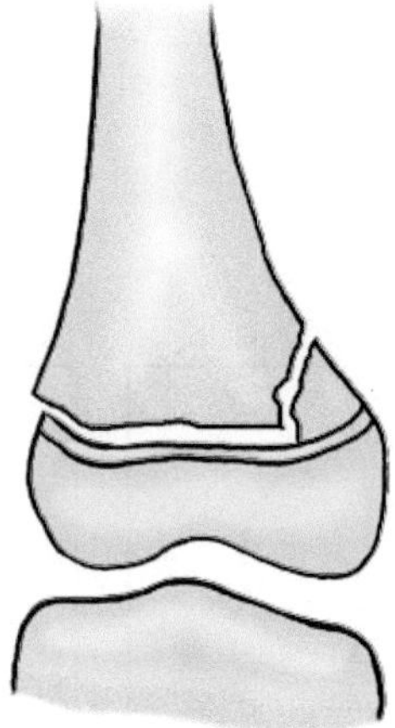
33-E/2.1

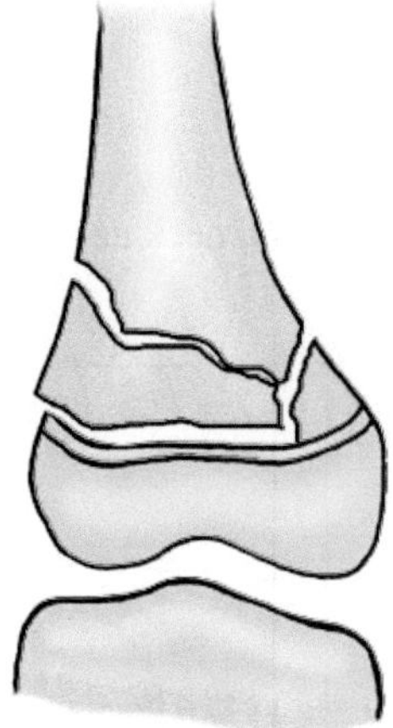
33-E/2.2

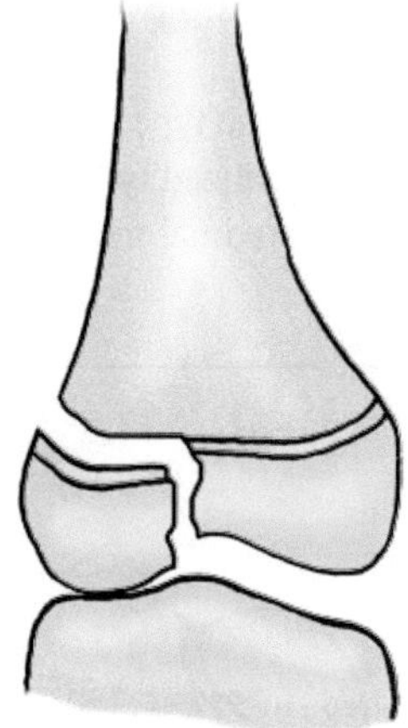
33-E/3.1

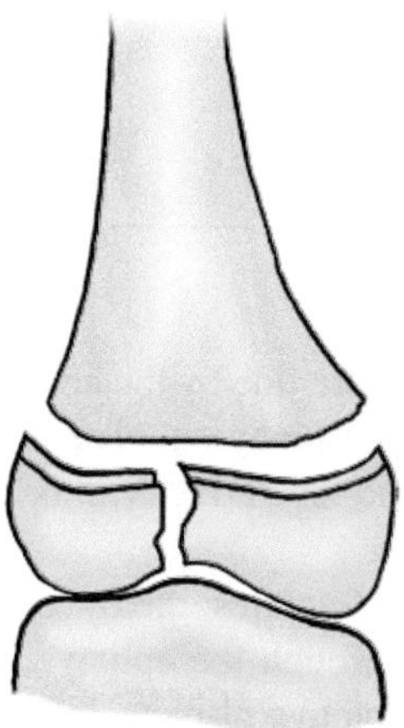
33-E/3.2

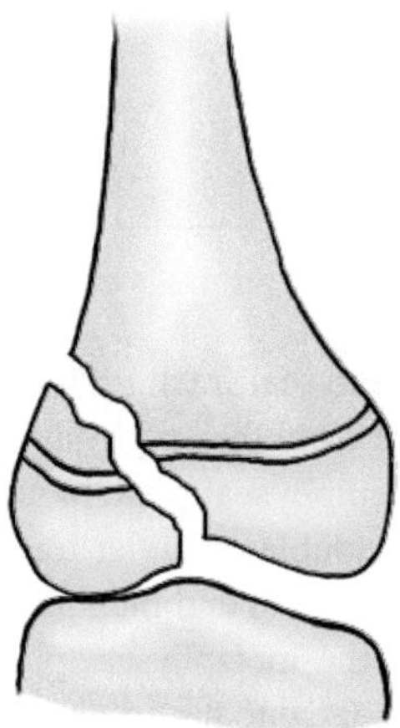
33-E/4.1

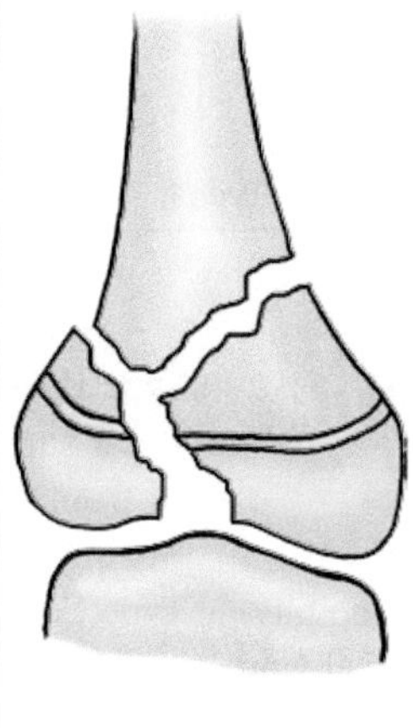
33-E/4.2

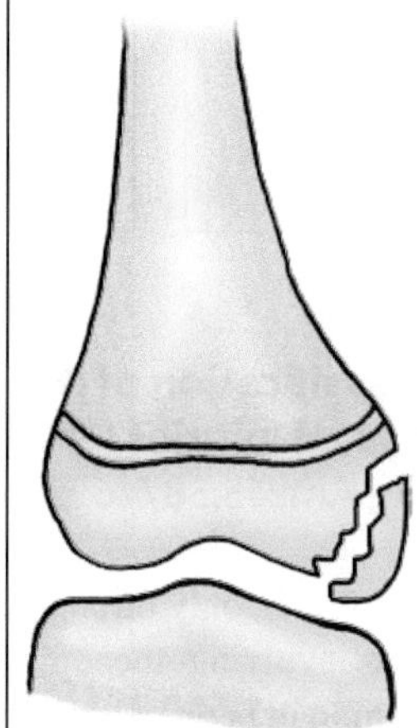
33-E/8.1

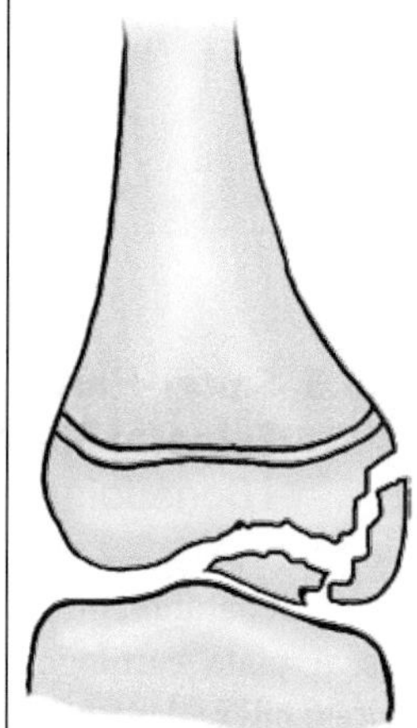
33-E/8.2

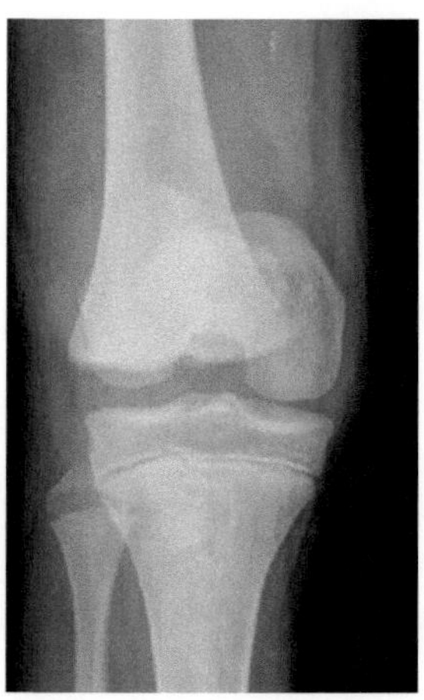
33-E/1.1

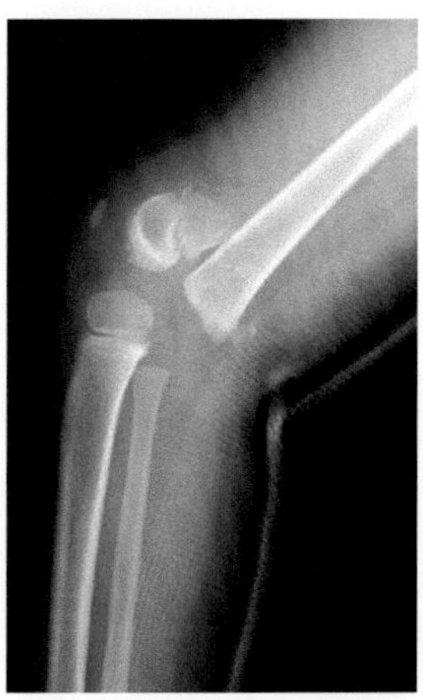
33-E/2.1 SH II

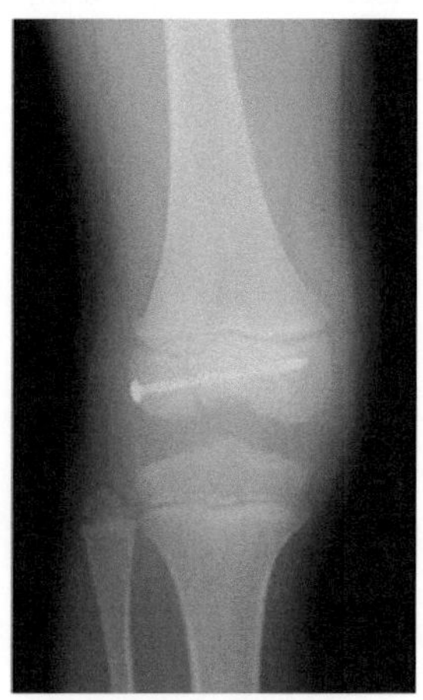
33-E/3.1 SH III

14.5.2 Proximal Metaphyseal Fracture/Femoral Neck and Aseptic Necrosis (1962, J Bone Joint Surg (Br), 44:528–542)

Type I: Diffuse type
Type II: Localized type
Type III: Proximal metaphyseal and femoral neck necrosis

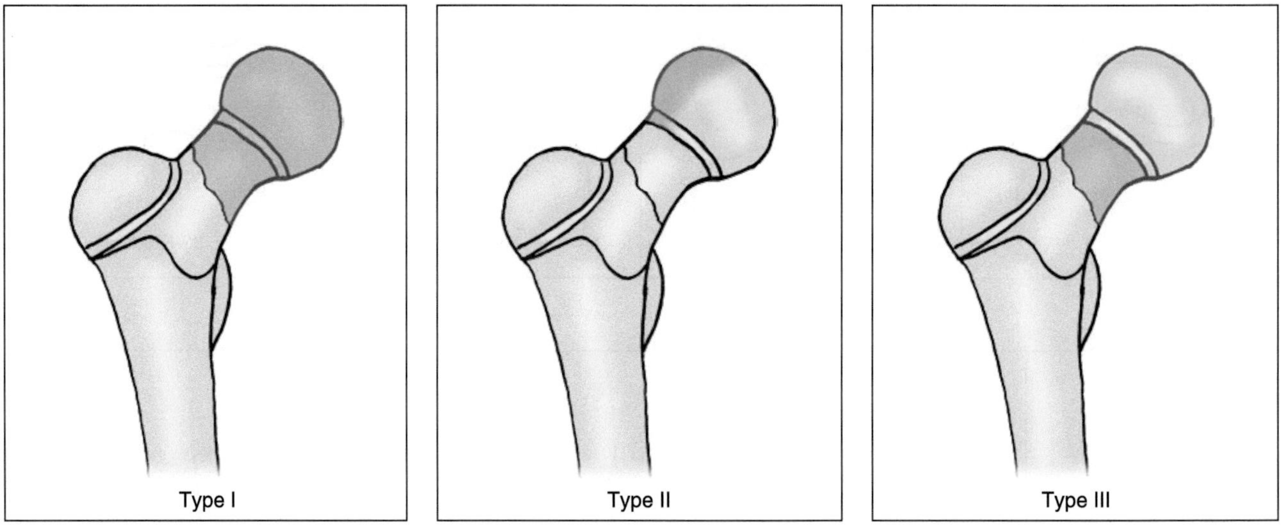

14.5.3 Salter-Harris Classification of Distal Femoral Epiphyseal Injuries (1963, J Bone Joint Surg Am, 45:587–622)

Type I: Separation of the epiphysis; only through the epiphyseal plate cartilage, not involving the epiphyseal and metaphyseal plates; common in neonatal epiphyseal separation and juvenile undisplaced epiphyseal separation.

Type II: Separation of the epiphysis with metaphyseal fractures; fracture line through the epiphyseal plate extending to the metaphyseal plate. The separation of the epiphyseal and metaphyseal bones from the triangular piece bone is the most common type of injury.

Type III: Epiphyseal fracture; the fracture line by the articular surface from the epiphysis to the epiphyseal plate and from the epiphyseal plate to around the surface can be a single- or double-condylar fracture.

Type IV: Epiphyseal and metaphyseal fractures; the fracture line from the metaphyseal plate through the epiphyseal plate cartilage into the epiphysis (epiphyseal-metaphyseal fractures) involves the articular surface.

Type V: Epiphyseal plate compression injury; epiphyseal plate compression fracture; very rare, only accounting for 1%. The vertical compression injury easily leads to early closure of the epiphyseal plate.

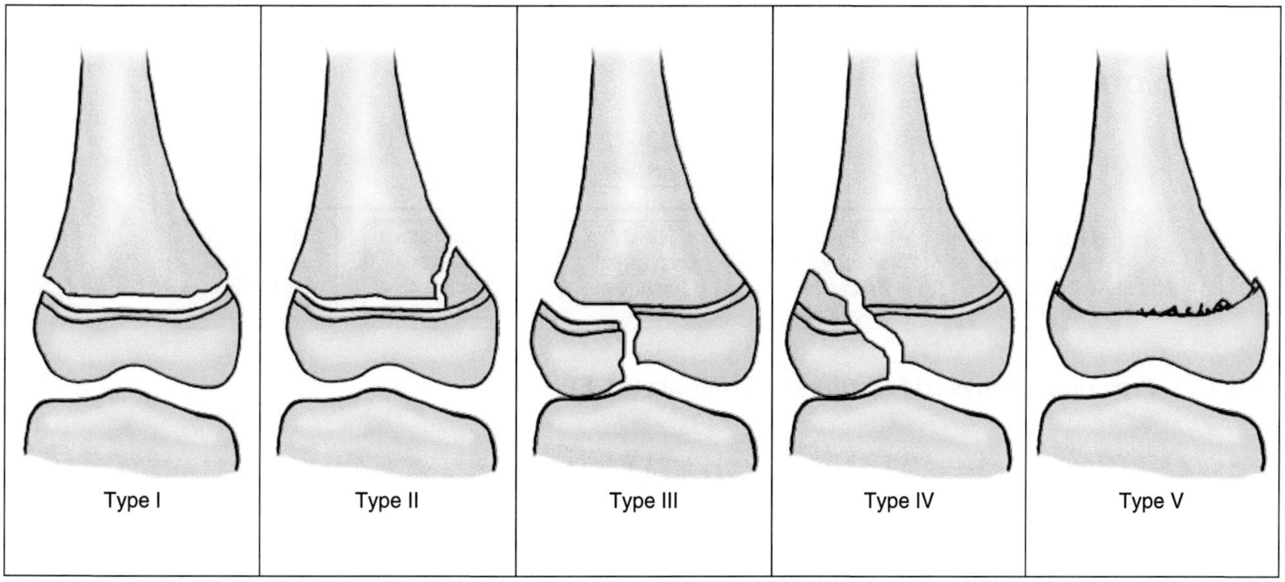

14.5.4 Delbe Classification of Femoral Neck Fracture in Children

Type I: Epiphyseal separation.
Type II: Neck type.
Type III: Base type.
Type IV: Femoral neck–interbody type.

14.5.5 The Rockwood Classification of Epiphyseal Plate Growth (1984, Fractures in Children. Philadelphia: J B Lippincott, 146)

Type I: Peripheral type; bone bridge is involved in the perichondrium ring, can be confined to the edge of the epiphyseal plate or half of the epiphyseal plate, this type of bone bridge is the most common.
Type II: Central type; bone bridge located in the central or partial side of the epiphyseal plate, does not involve the radial membrane ring area.
Type III: Mixed type; bone bridge involving the epiphyseal plate around the centre, section was linear.

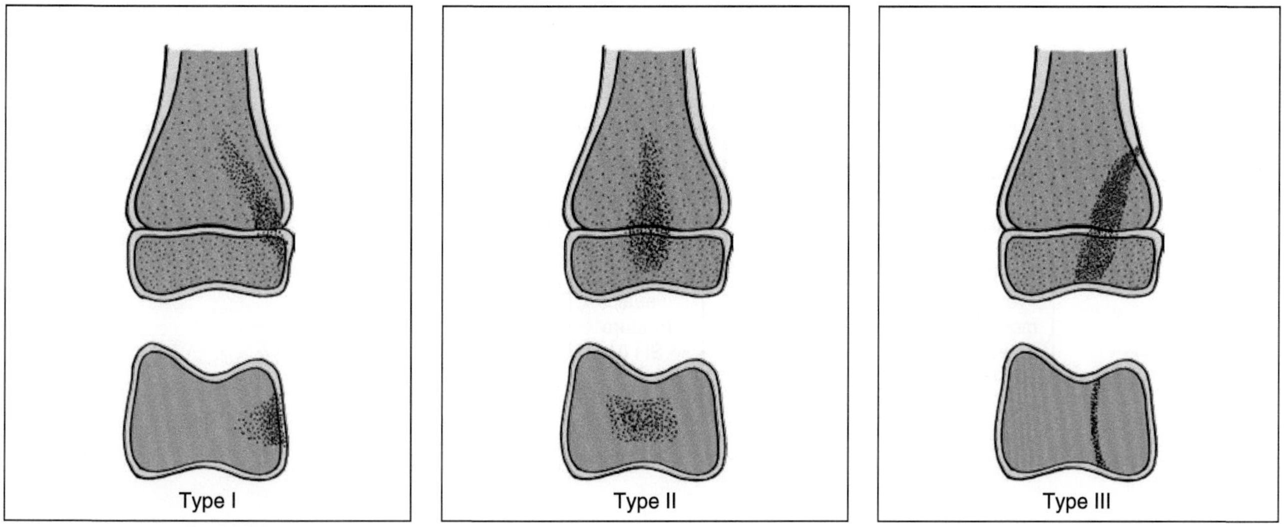

14.6 Section 4 Children Tibia/Fibula Fractures

14.6.1 AO/OTA Classification

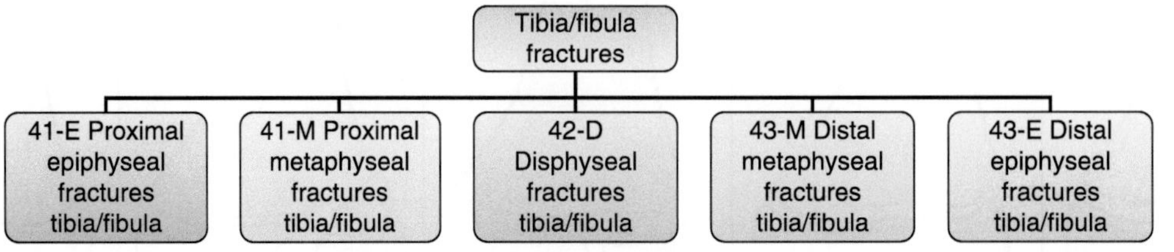

14.6.1.1 Proximal Epiphyseal Fractures Tibia/Fibula (41-E)

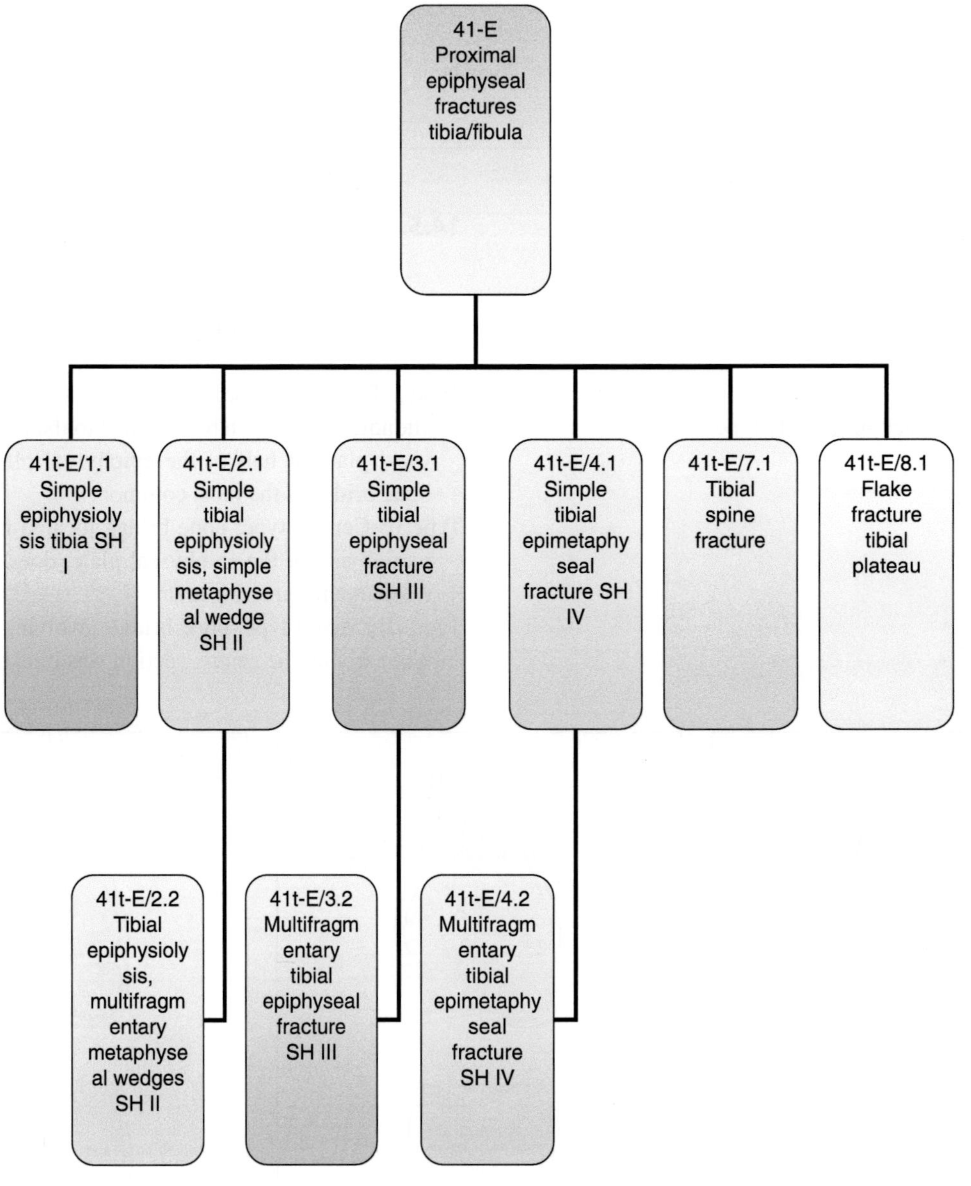

41t–E: Proximal epiphyseal fractures tibia/fibula (41-E):

1.1: Simple epiphysiolysis tibia SH I.
2.1: Simple tibial epiphysiolysis, simple metaphyseal wedge SH II.
2.2: Tibial epiphysiolysis, multifragmentary metaphyseal wedges SH II.
3.1: Simple tibial epiphyseal fracture SH III.
3.2: Multifragmentary tibial epiphyseal fracture SH III.
4.1: Simple tibial epimetaphyseal fracture SH IV.
4.2: Multifragmentary tibial epimetaphyseal fracture SH IV.
7.1: Tibial spine fracture.
8.1: Flake fracture tibial plateau.

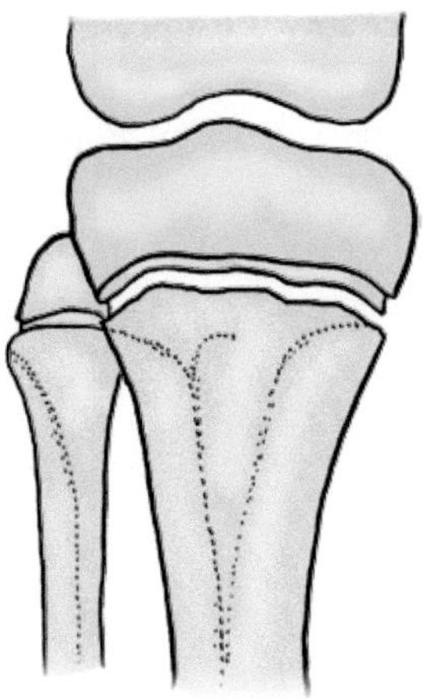
41t-E/1.1 SH I

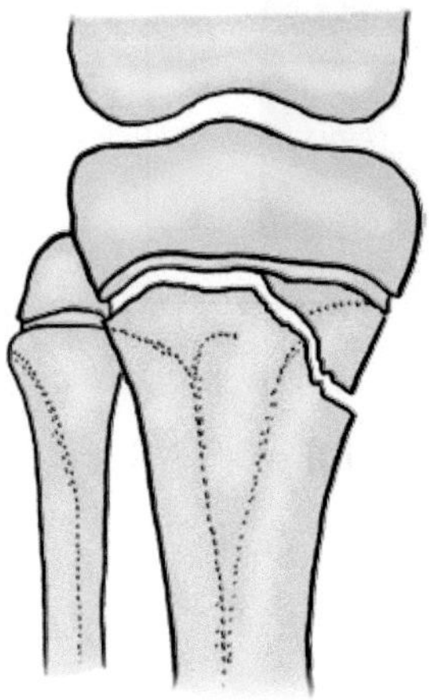
41t-E/2.1 SH II

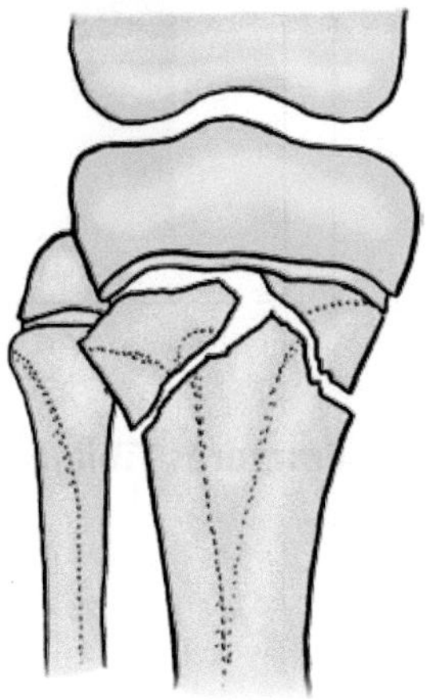
41t-E/2.2 SH II

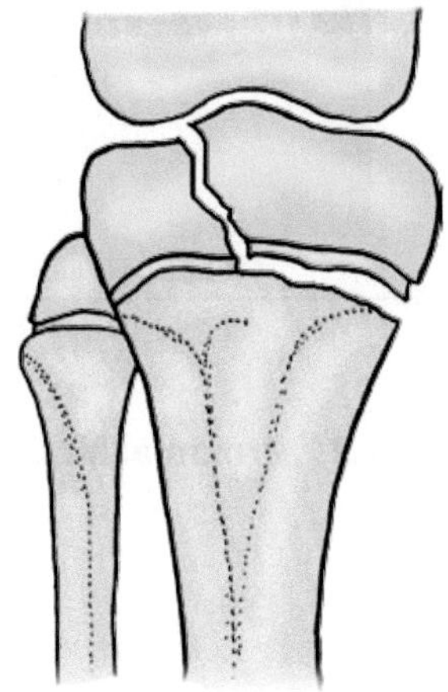
41t-E/3.1 SH III

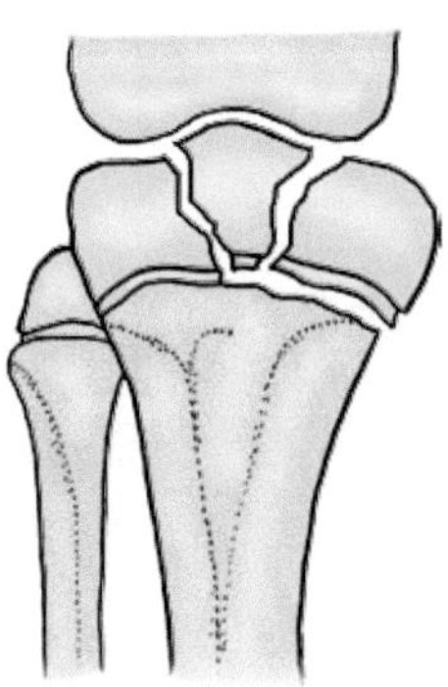
41t-E/3.2

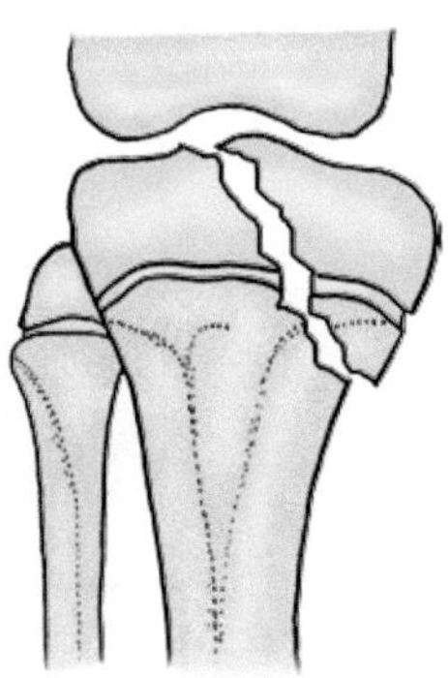
41t-E/4.1

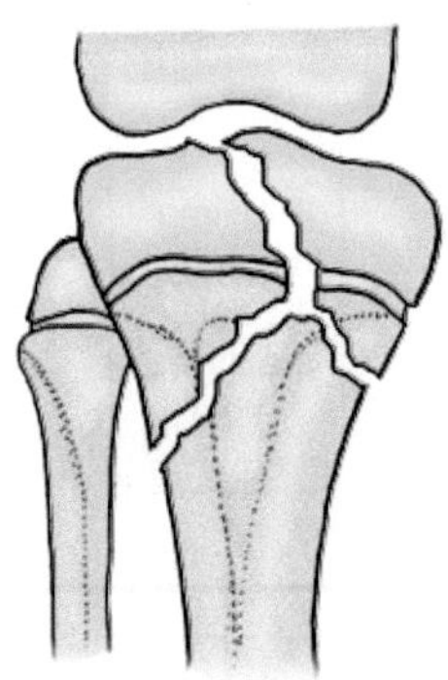
41t-E/4.2

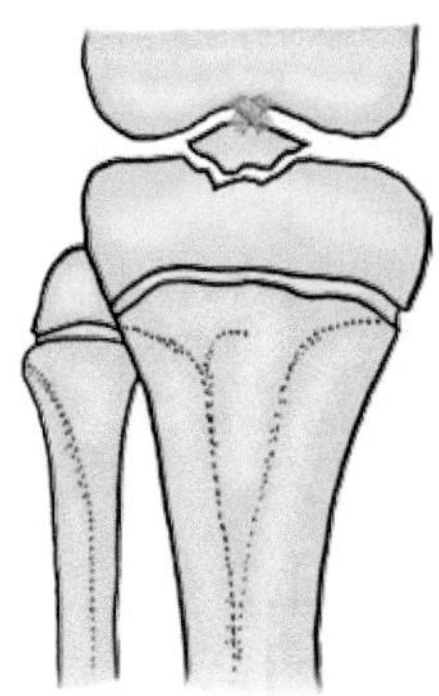
41t-E/7.1

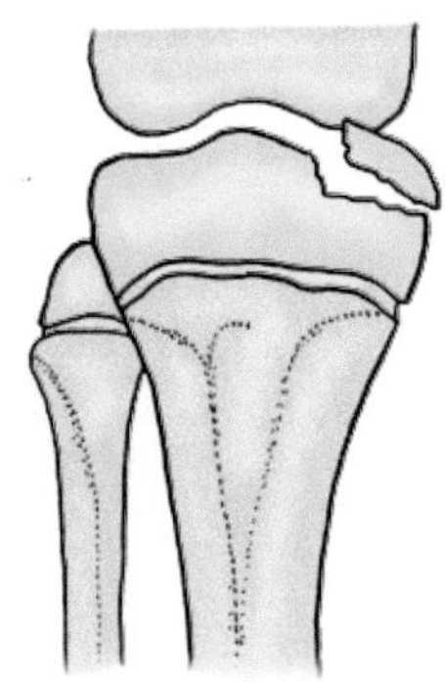
41t-E/8.1

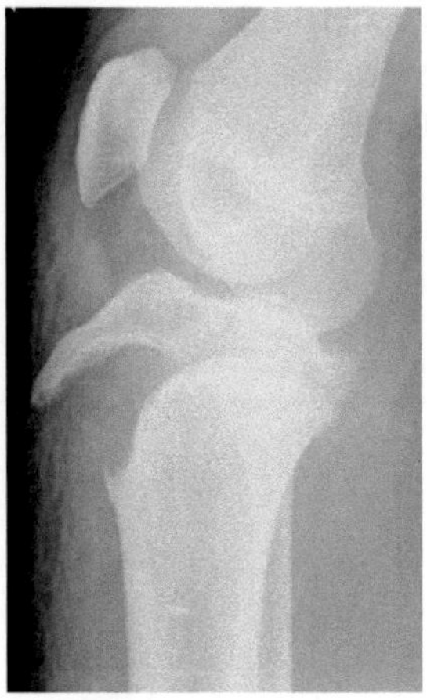

41t-E/3.1 SH III

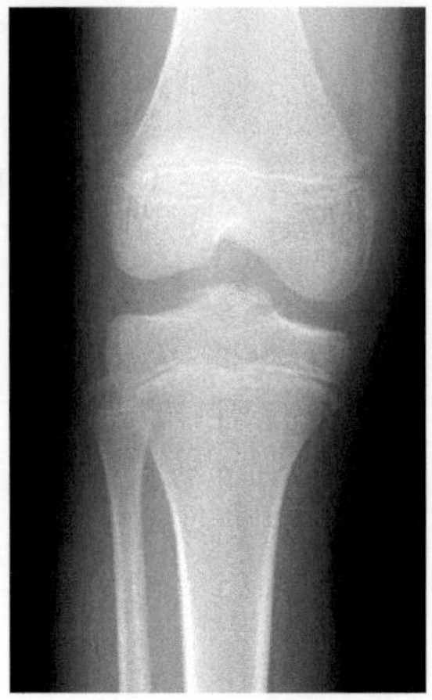

41t-E/3.1 SH III

14.6.1.2 Proximal Metaphyseal Fractures Tibia/Fibula (41-M)

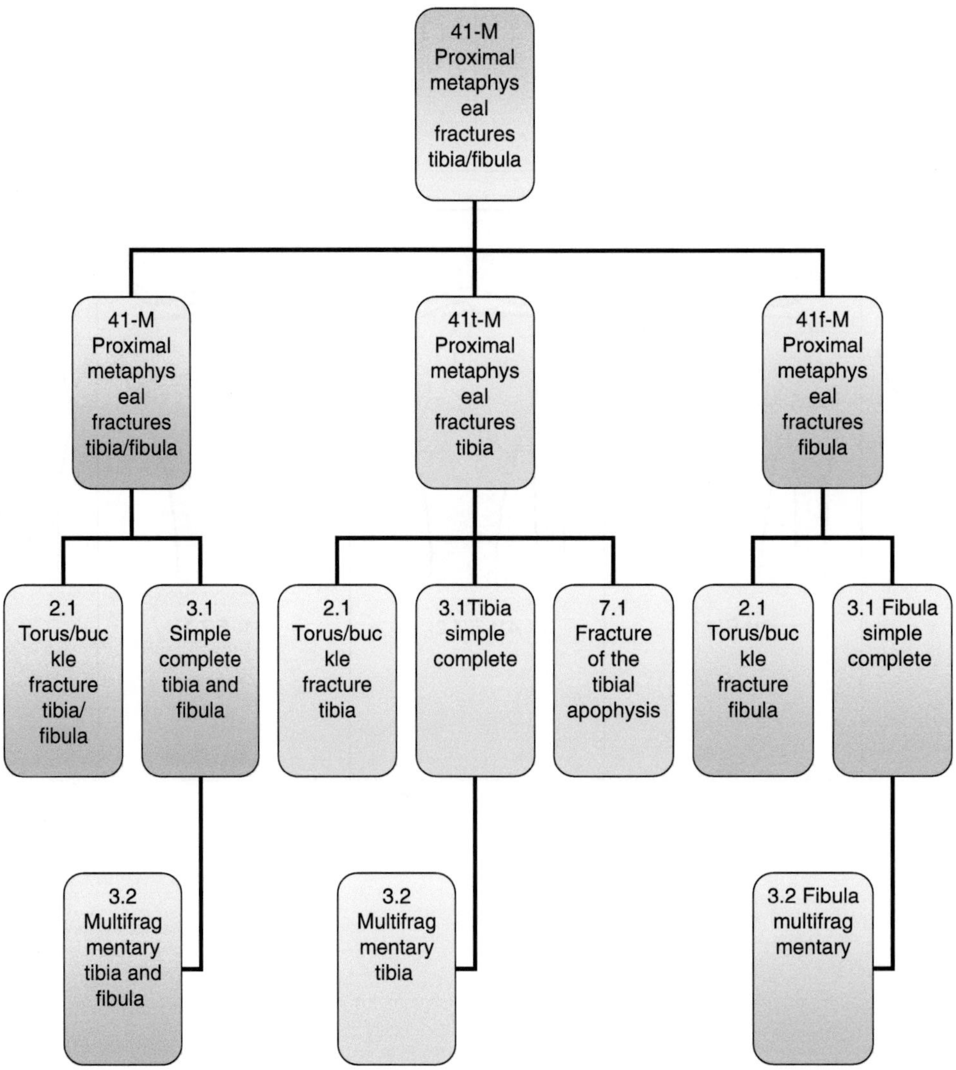

41-M: Proximal metaphyseal fractures tibia/fibula:

2.1: Torus/buckle fracture tibia/fibula.
3.1: Simple complete tibia and fibula.
3.2: Multifragmentary tibia and fibula.

41t-M: Proximal metaphyseal fractures tibia:

2.1: Torus/buckle fracture tibia.
3.1: Tibia simple complete.
3.2: Multifragmentary tibia.
7.1: Fracture of the tibial apophysis.

41f-M: Proximal metaphyseal fractures fibula:

2.1: Torus/buckle fracture fibula.
3.1: Fibula simple complete.
3.2: Fibula multifragmentary.

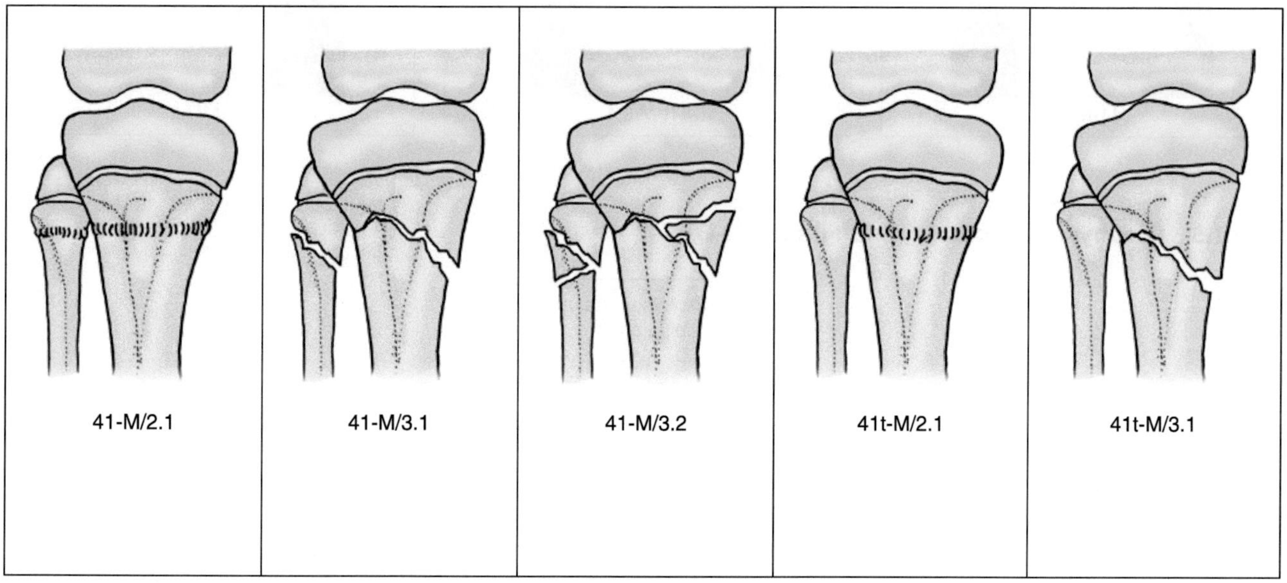

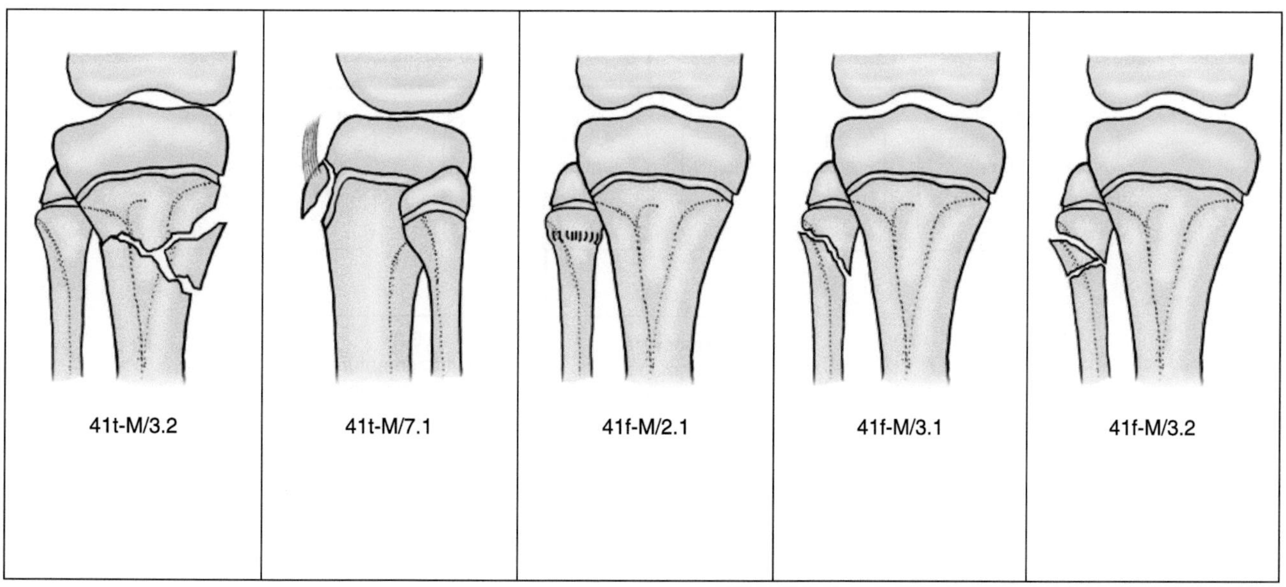

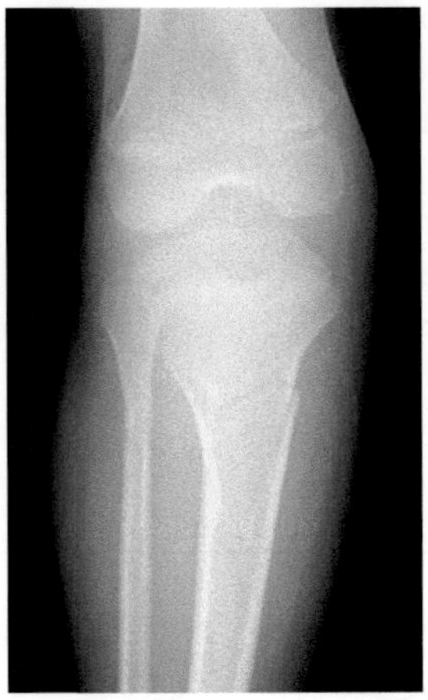
41-M/3.1

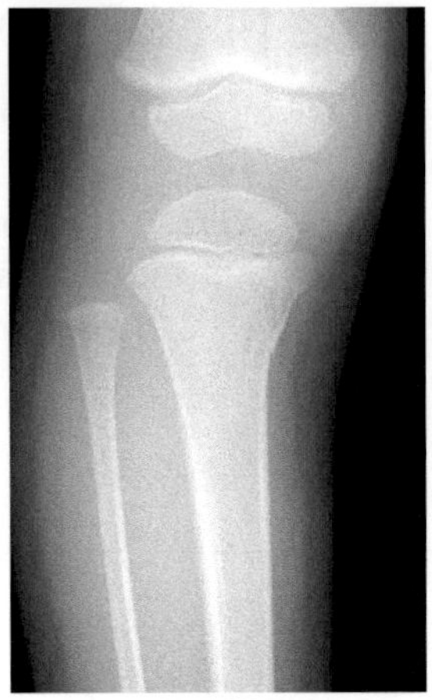
41t-M/2.1

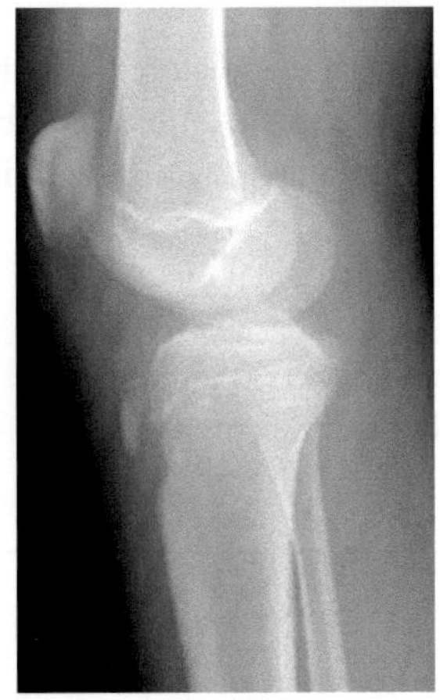
41t-M/7.1

14.6.1.3 Diaphyseal Fractures Tibia/Fibula (42-D)

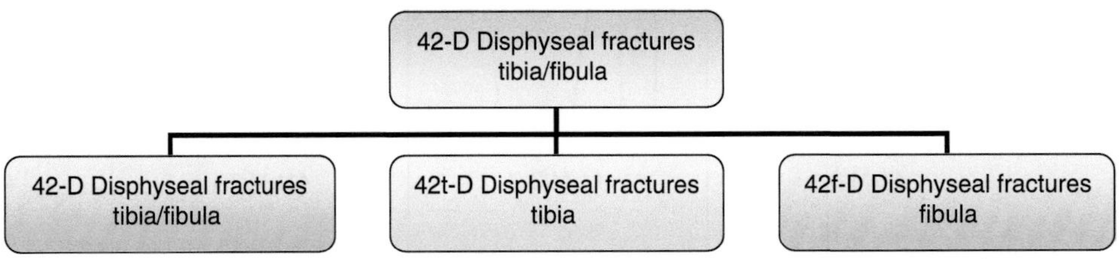

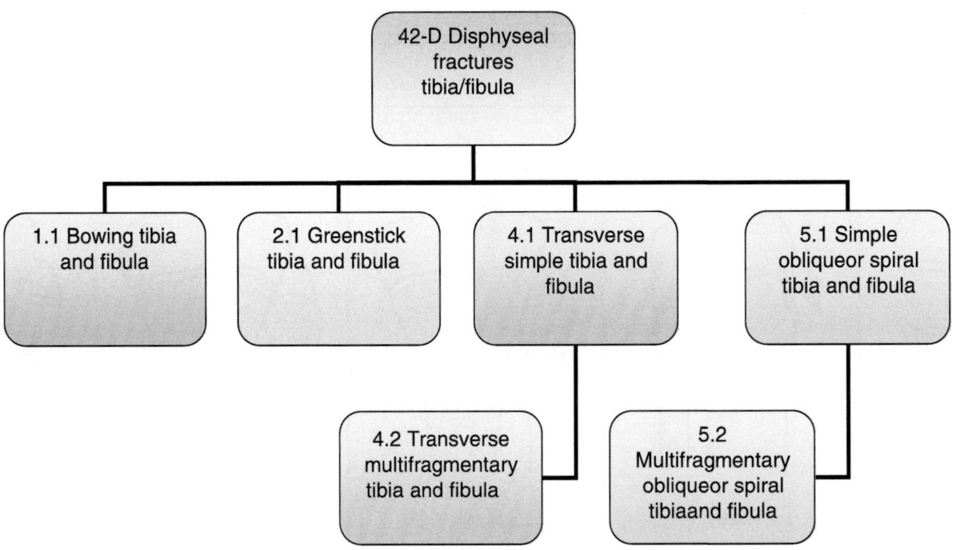

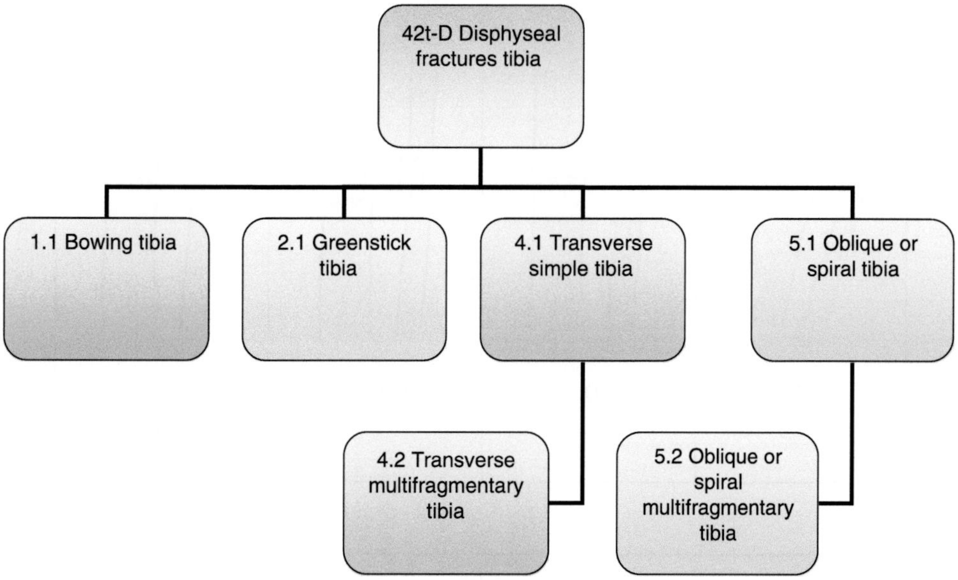

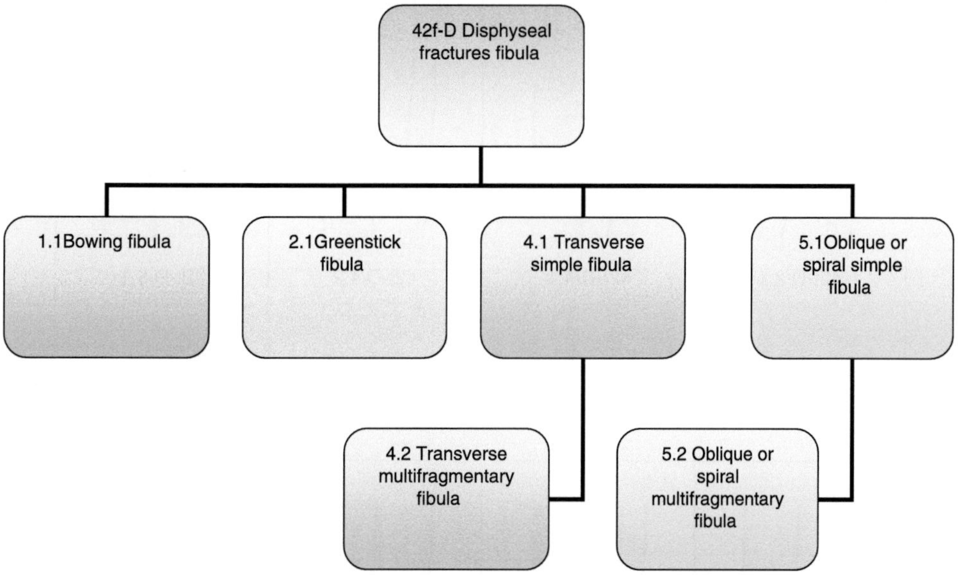

42-D: Diaphyseal fractures tibia/fibula.

1.1: Bowing tibia and fibula.
2.1: Greenstick tibia and fibula.
4.1: Transverse simple tibia and fibula (≤30°).
4.2: Transverse multifragmentary tibia and fibula (≤30°).
5.1: Simple oblique or spiral tibia and fibula (>30°).
5.2: Multifragmentary oblique or spiral tibia and fibula (>30°).

42t-D: Diaphyseal fractures tibia:

1.1: Bowing tibia.
2.1: Greenstick tibia.
4.1: Transverse simple tibia (≤30°).
4.2: Transverse multifragmentary tibia (≤30°).
5.1: Oblique or spiral tibia (>30°).
5.2: Oblique or spiral multifragmentary tibia (>30°).

42f-D: Diaphyseal fractures fibula:

1.1: Bowing fibula;
2.1: Greenstick fibula;
4.1: Transverse simple fibula (≤30°);
4.2: Transverse multifragmentary fibula (≤30°);
5.1: Oblique or spiral simple fibula (>30°);
5.2: Oblique or spiral multifragmentary fibula (>30°).

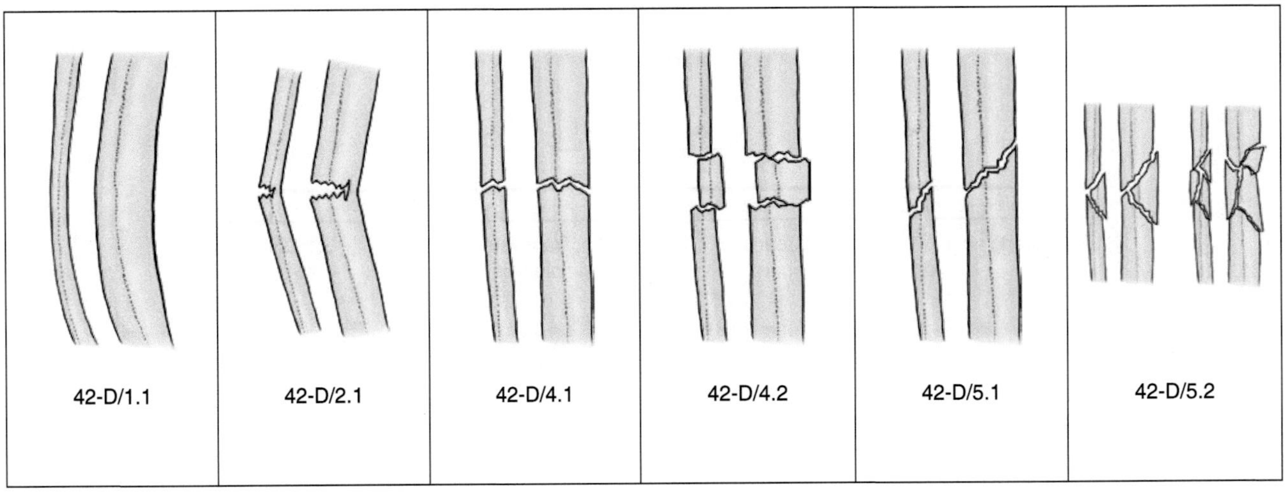
42-D/1.1
42-D/2.1
42-D/4.1
42-D/4.2
42-D/5.1
42-D/5.2

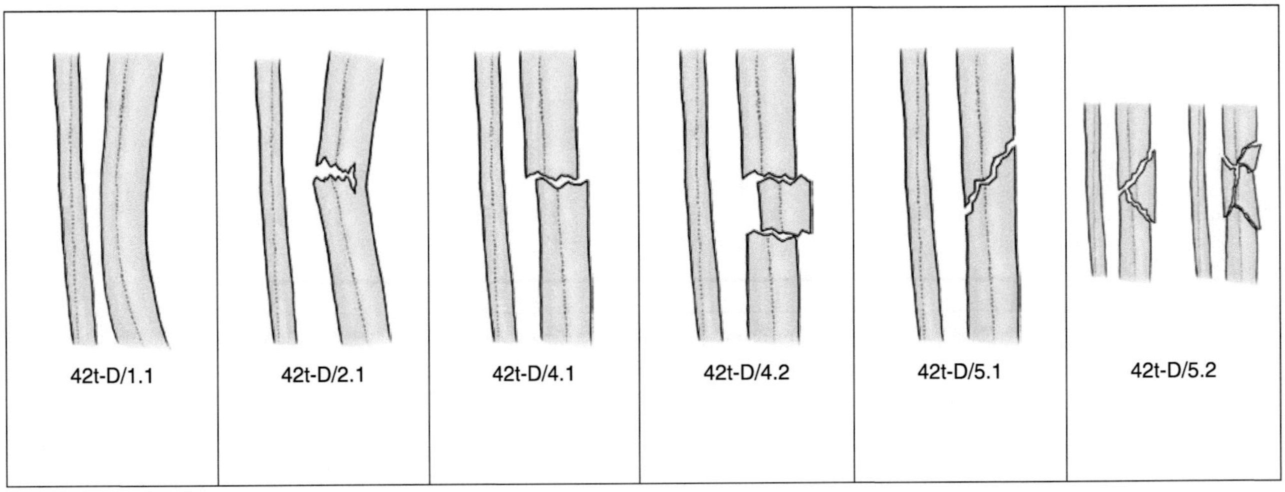
42t-D/1.1
42t-D/2.1
42t-D/4.1
42t-D/4.2
42t-D/5.1
42t-D/5.2

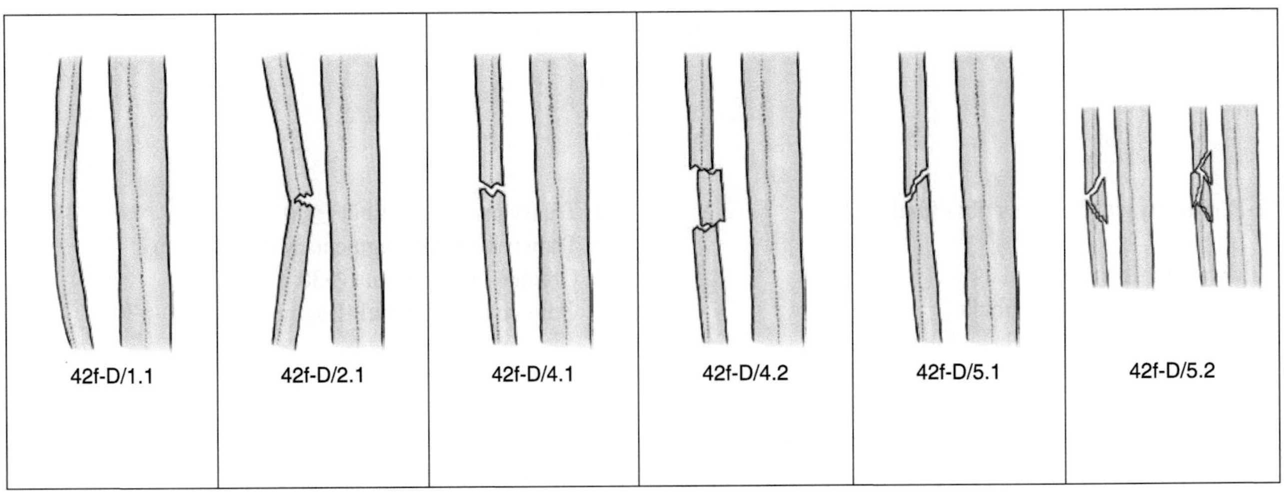
42f-D/1.1
42f-D/2.1
42f-D/4.1
42f-D/4.2
42f-D/5.1
42f-D/5.2

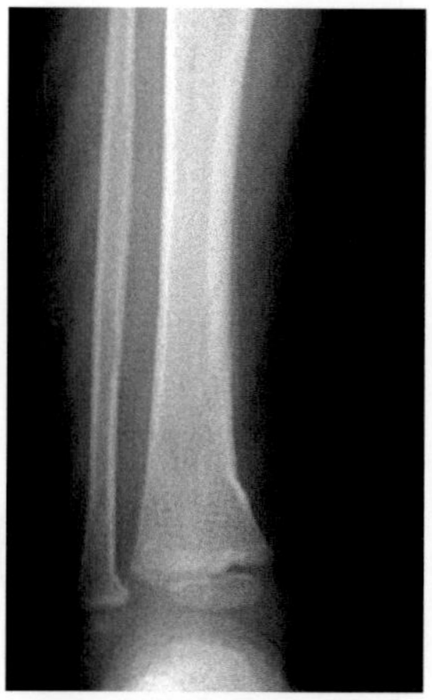

42t-D/2.1

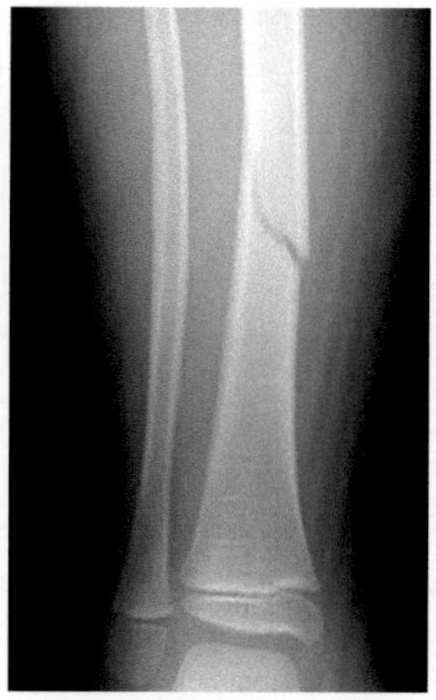

42t-D/4.1

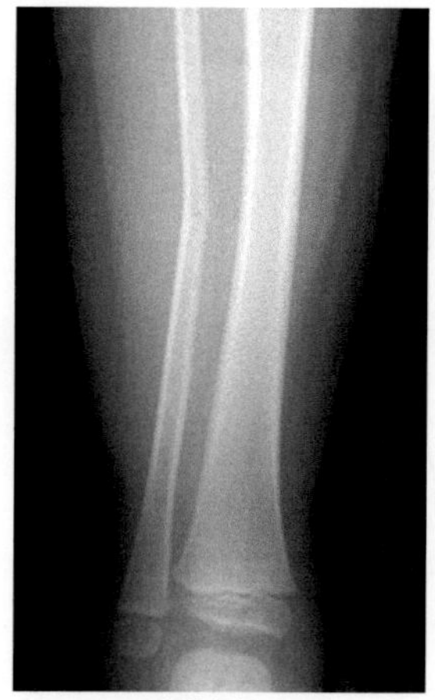

42f-D/1.1

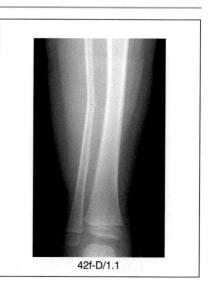

14.6.1.4 Distal Metaphyseal Fractures Tibia/Fibula (43-M)

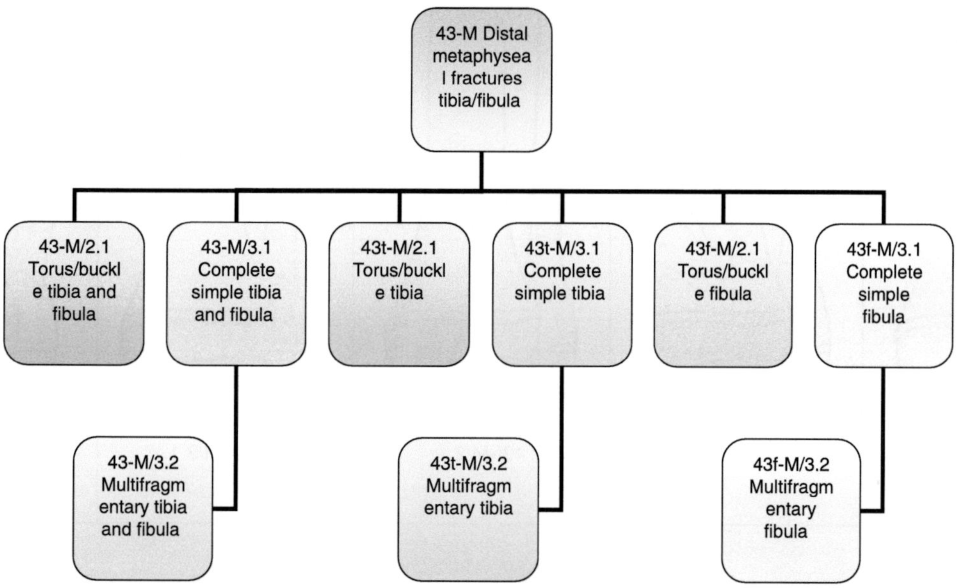

43-M: Distal metaphyseal fractures tibia/fibula:

2.1: Torus/buckle tibia and fibula.
3.1: Complete simple tibia and fibula.
3.2: Multifragmentary tibia and fibula.

43t-M: Distal metaphyseal fractures tibia:

2.1: Torus/buckle tibia.
3.1: Complete simple tibia.
3.2: Multifragmentary tibia.

43f-M: Distal metaphyseal fractures fibula:

2.1: Torus/buckle fibula.
3.1: Complete simple fibula.
3.2: Multifragmentary fibula.

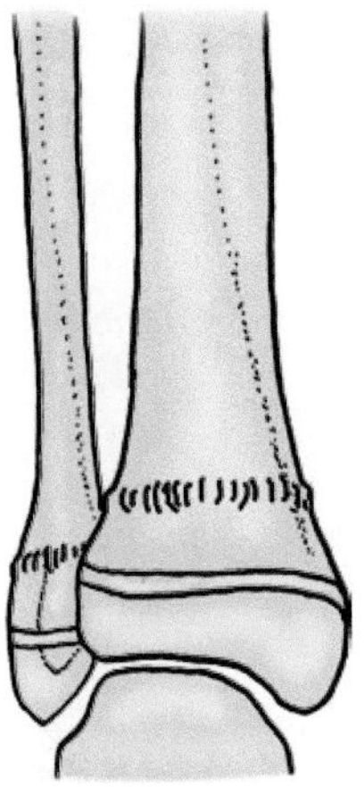
43-M/2.1

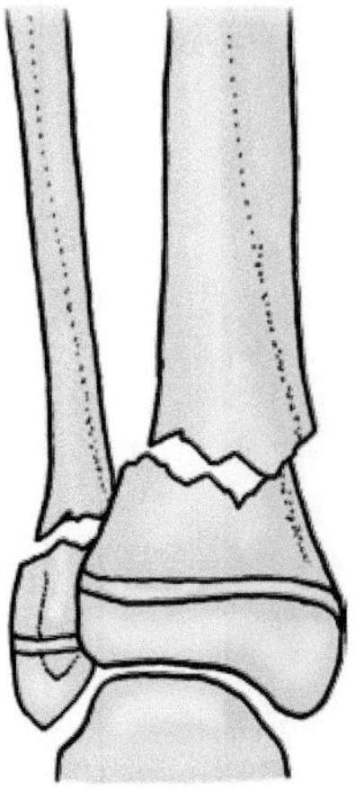
43-M/3.1

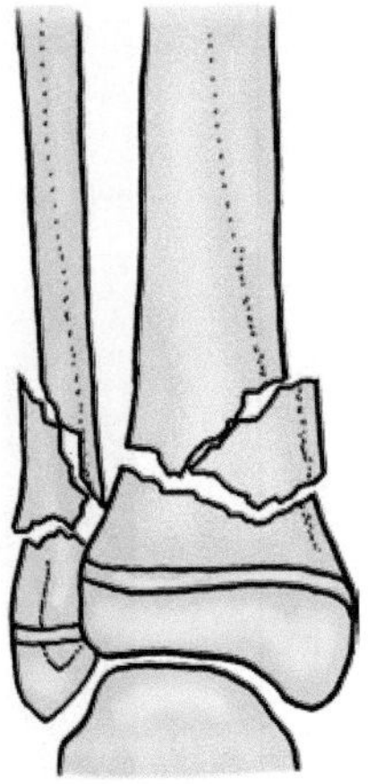
43-M/3.2

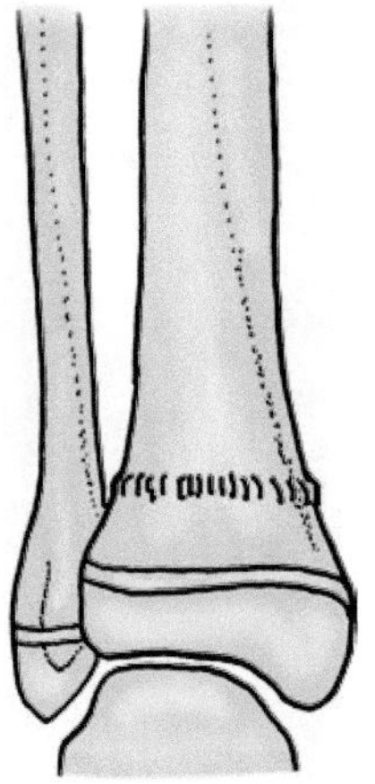
43t-M/2.1

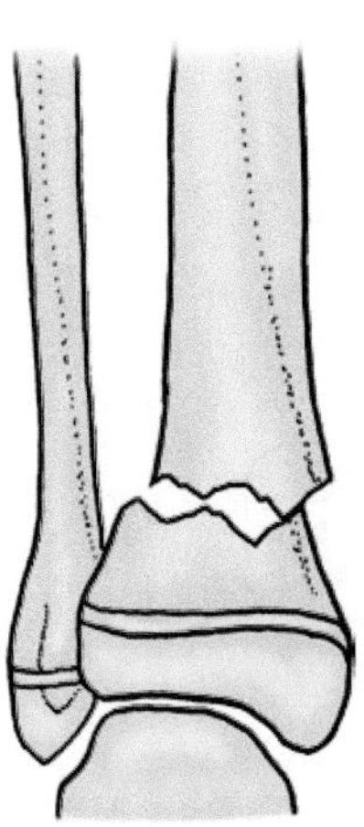
43t-M/3.1

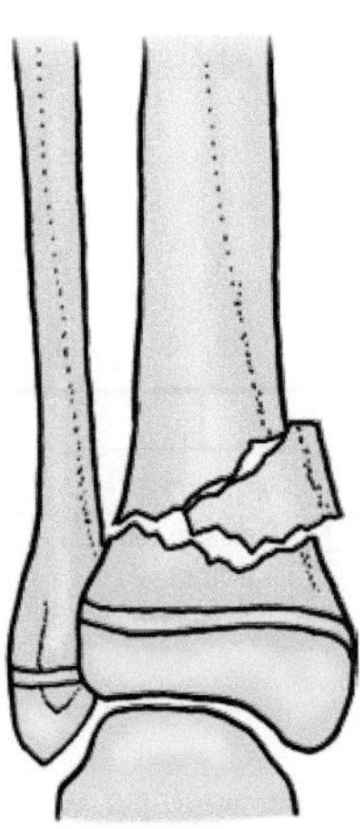
43t-M/3.2

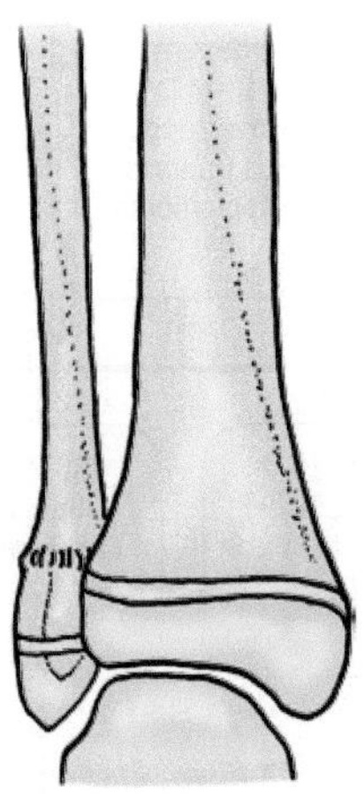
43f-M/2.1

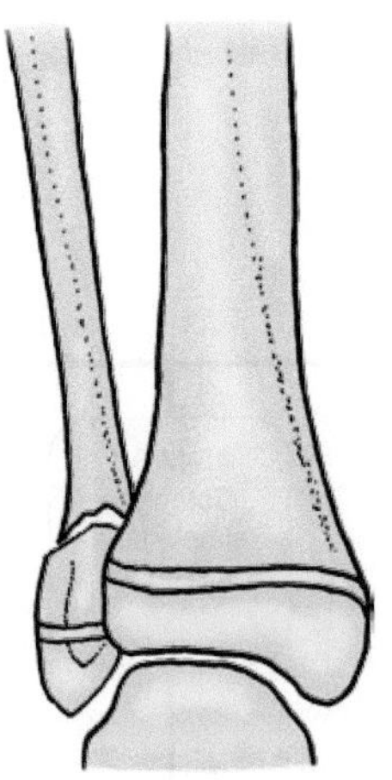
43f-M/3.1

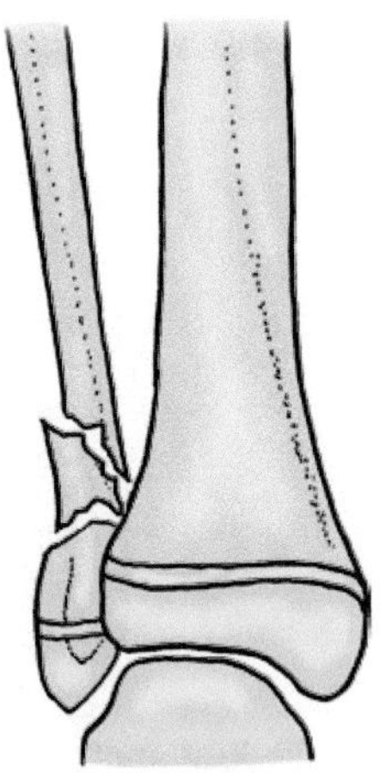
43f-M/3.2

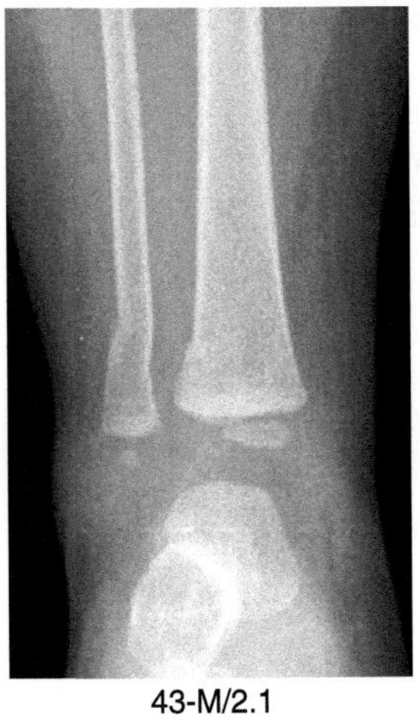
43-M/2.1

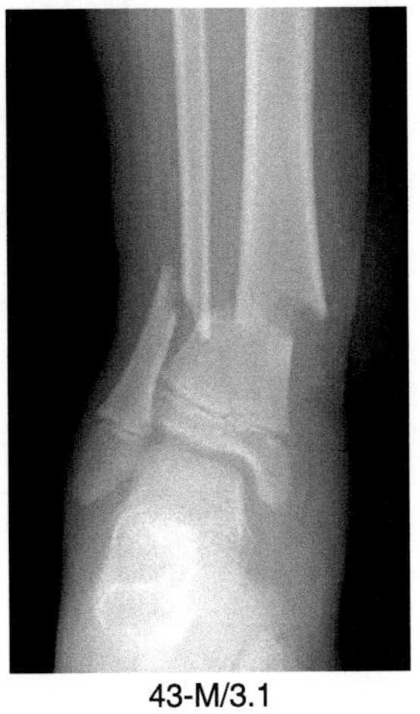
43-M/3.1

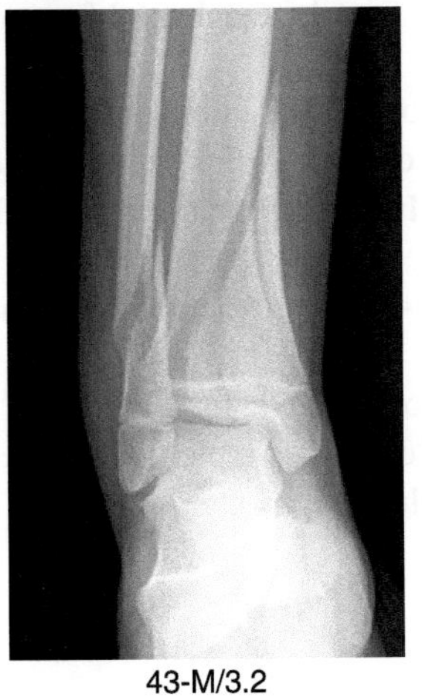
43-M/3.2

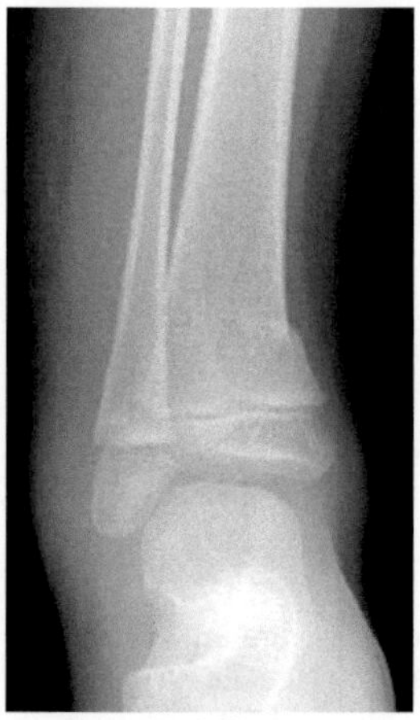

43t-M/2.1

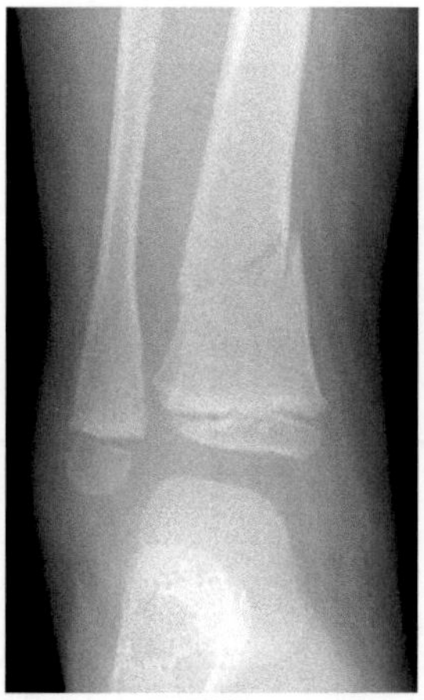

43t-M/3.1

14.6.1.5 Distal Epiphyseal Fractures Tibia/Fibula (43-E)

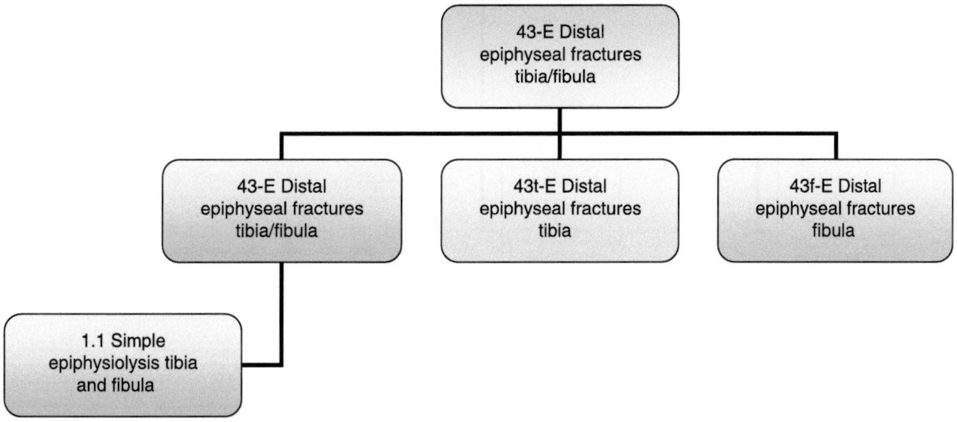

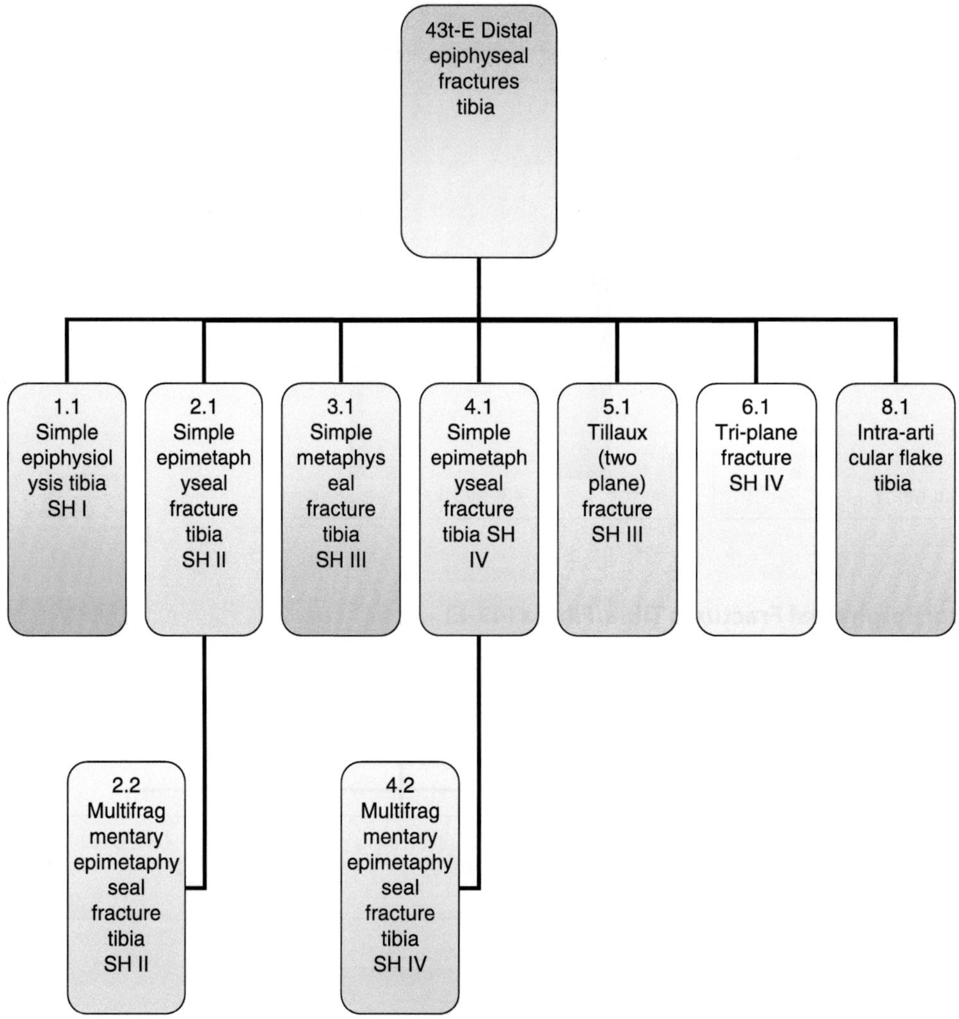
43t-E Distal epiphyseal fractures tibia
1.1 Simple epiphysiolysis tibia SH I
2.1 Simple epimetaphyseal fracture tibia SH II
3.1 Simple metaphyseal fracture tibia SH III
4.1 Simple epimetaphyseal fracture tibia SH IV
5.1 Tillaux (two plane) fracture SH III
6.1 Tri-plane fracture SH IV
8.1 Intra-articular flake tibia
2.2 Multifragmentary epimetaphyseal fracture tibia SH II
4.2 Multifragmentary epimetaphyseal fracture tibia SH IV

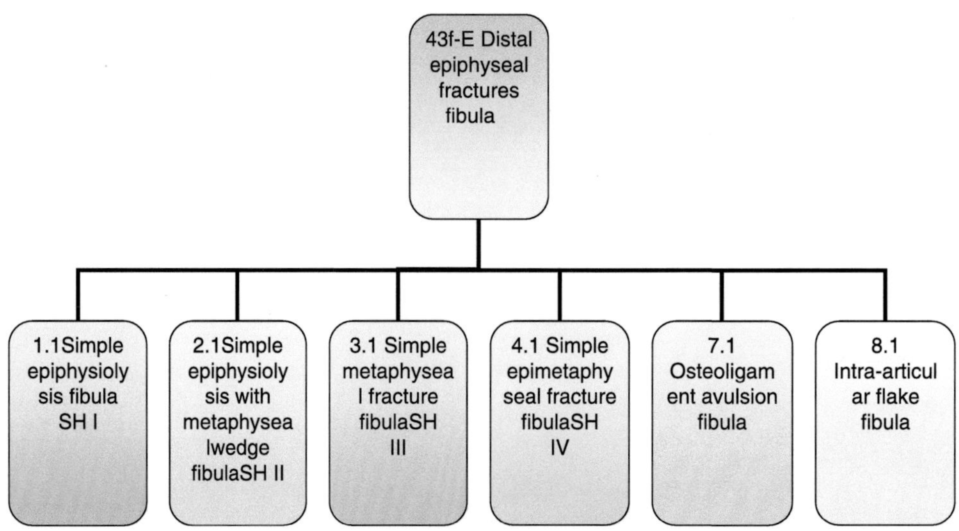
43f-E Distal epiphyseal fractures fibula
1.1Simple epiphysiolysis fibula SH I
2.1Simple epiphysiolysis with metaphysealwedge fibulaSH II
3.1 Simple metaphyseal fracture fibulaSH III
4.1 Simple epimetaphyseal fracture fibulaSH IV
7.1 Osteoligament avulsion fibula
8.1 Intra-articular flake fibula

43-E: Distal epiphyseal fractures tibia/fibula:

1.1: Simple epiphysiolysis tibia and fibula.

43t-E: Distal epiphyseal fractures tibia:

1.1: Simple epiphysiolysis tibia SH I.
2.1: Simple epimetaphyseal fracture tibia SH II.
2.2: Multifragmentary epimetaphyseal fracture tibia SH II.
3.1: Simple metaphyseal fracture tibia SH III.
4.1: Simple epimetaphyseal fracture tibia SH IV.
4.2: Multifragmentary epimetaphyseal fracture tibia SH IV.
5.1: Tillaux (two plane) fracture SH III.
6.1: Tri-plane fracture SH IV.
8.1: Intra-articular flake tibia.

43f-E: Distal epiphyseal fractures fibula:

1.1: Simple epiphysiolysis fibula SH I.
2.1: Simple epiphysiolysis with metaphyseal wedge fibula SH II.
3.1: Simple metaphyseal fracture fibula SH III.
4.1: Simple epimetaphyseal fracture fibula SH IV.
7.1: Osteoligament avulsion fibula.
8.1: Intra-articular flake fibula.

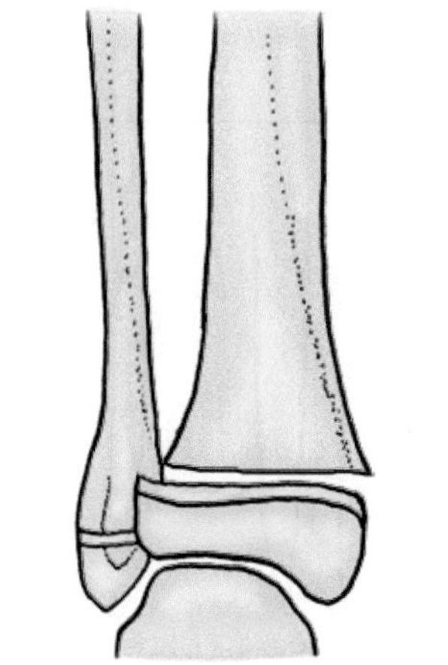
43-E/1.1

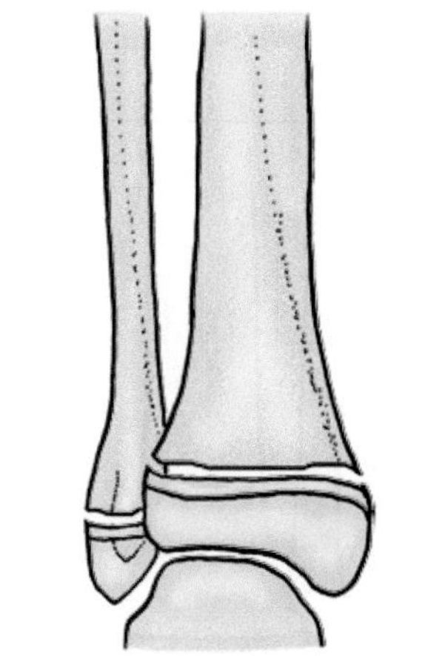
43t-E/1.1

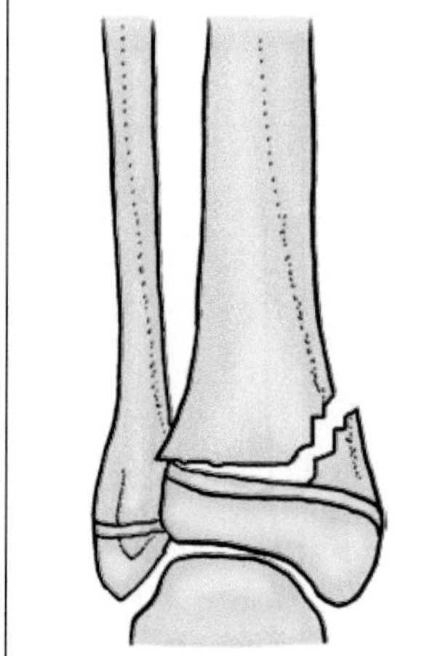
43t-E/2.1

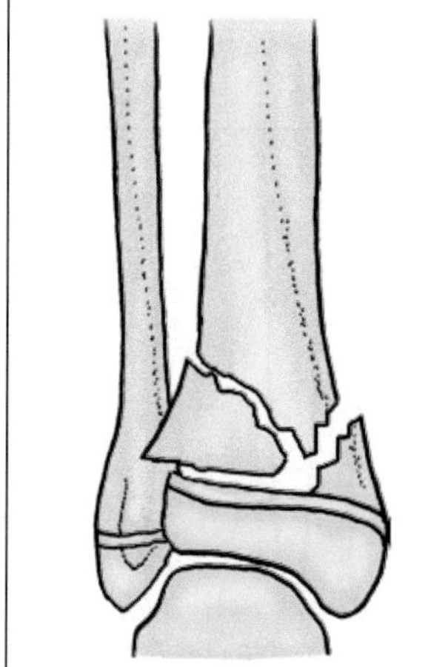
43t-E/2.2

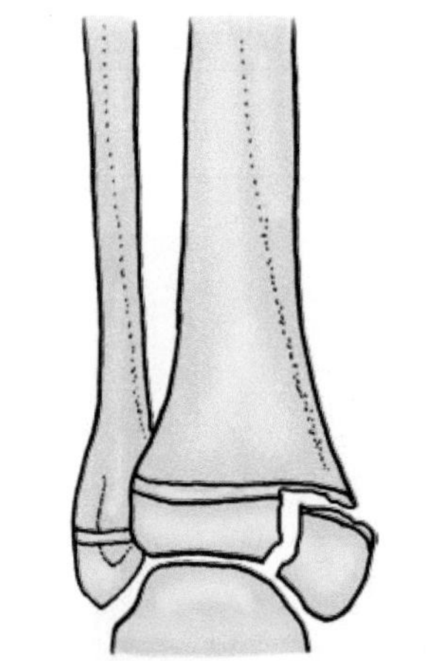
43t-E/3.1

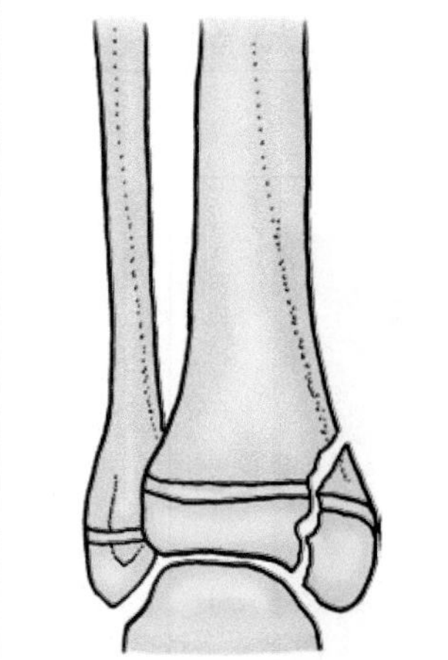
43t-E/4.1

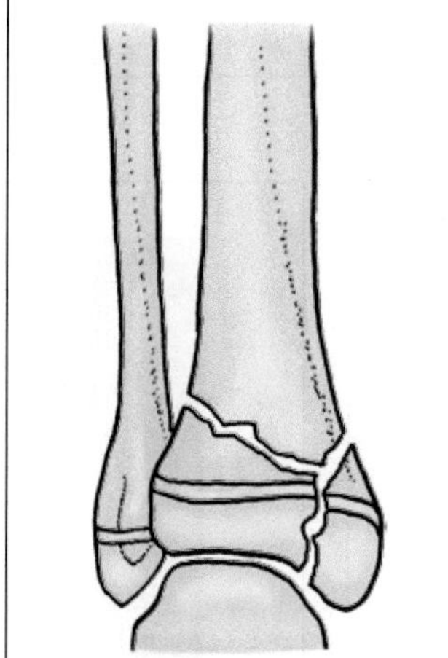
43t-E/4.2

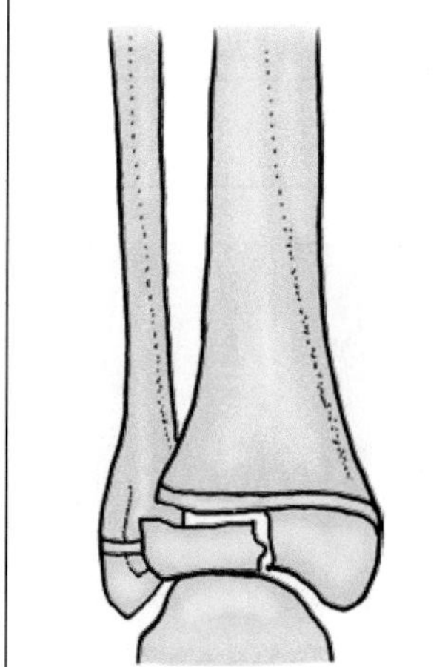
43t-E/5.1

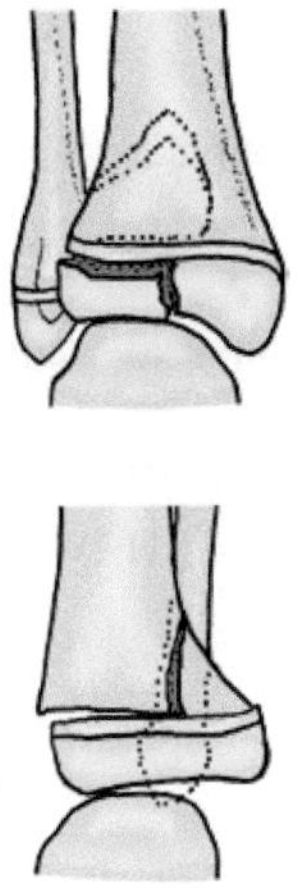
43t-E/6.1

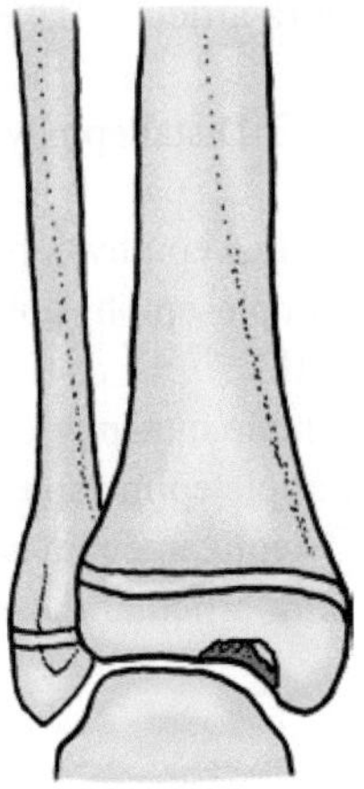
43t-E/8.1

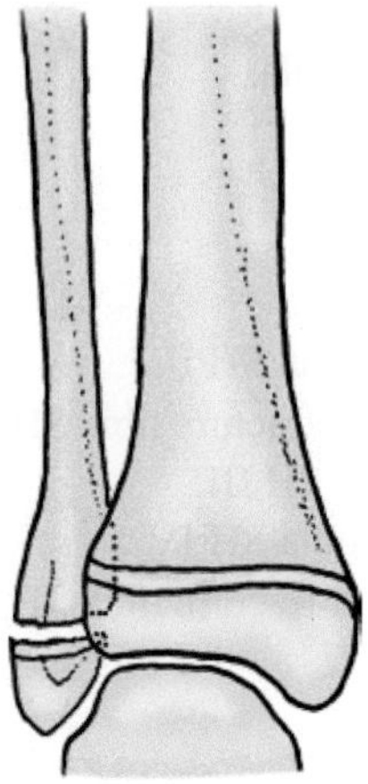
43f-E/1.1

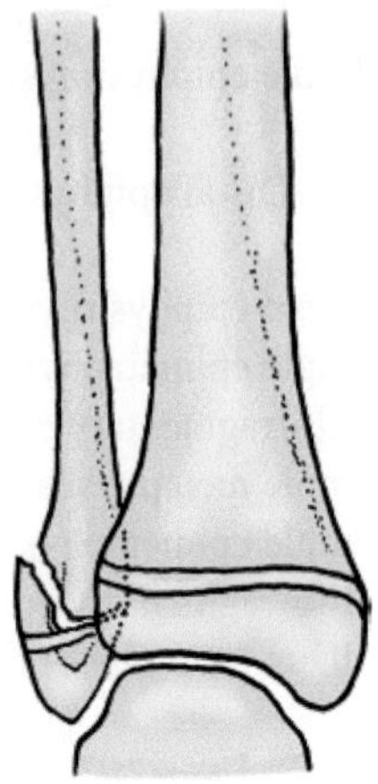
43f-E/2.1

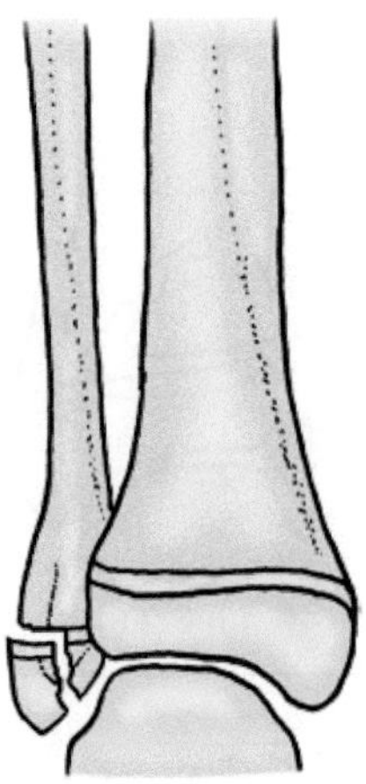
43f-E/3.1

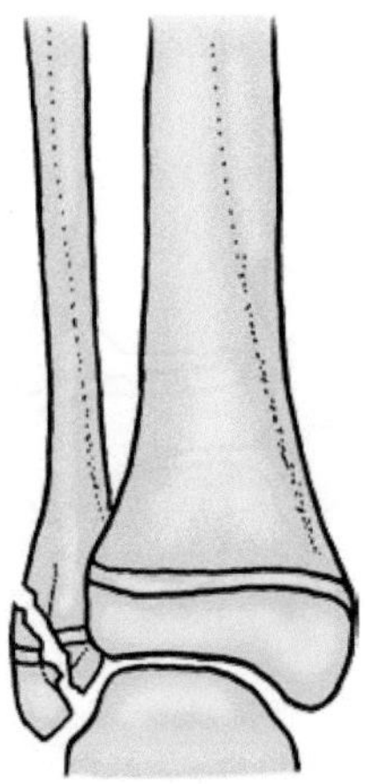
43f-E/4.1

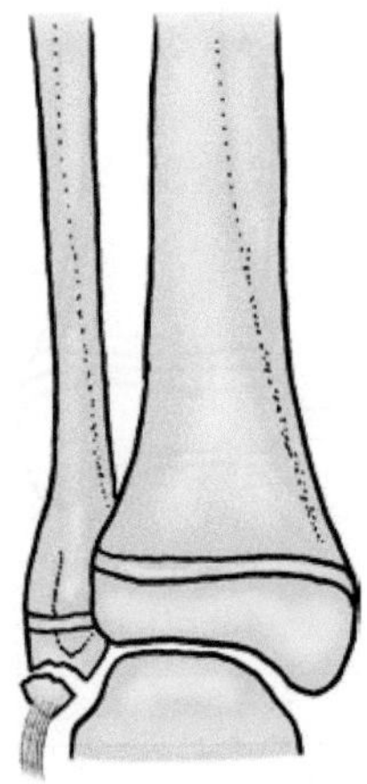
43f-E/7.1

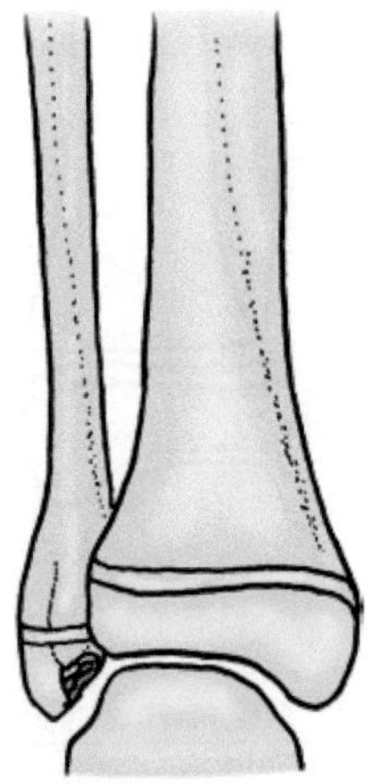
43f-E/8.1

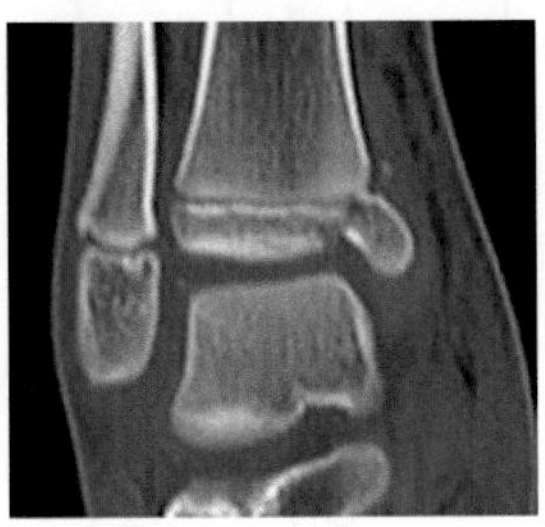
43t-E/3.1 SH III

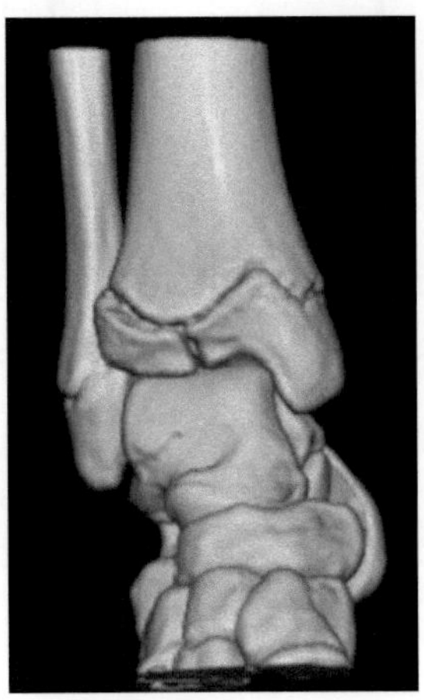
43t-E/5.1 SH III

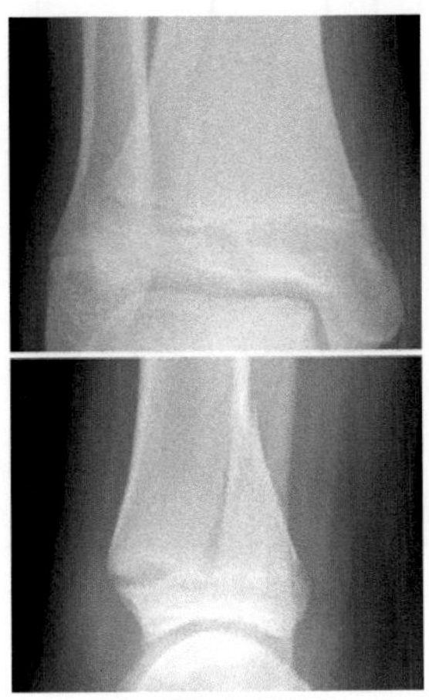
43t-E/6.1 SH IV

14.6.1.6 Frequent Fracture Combinations in Paired Bones

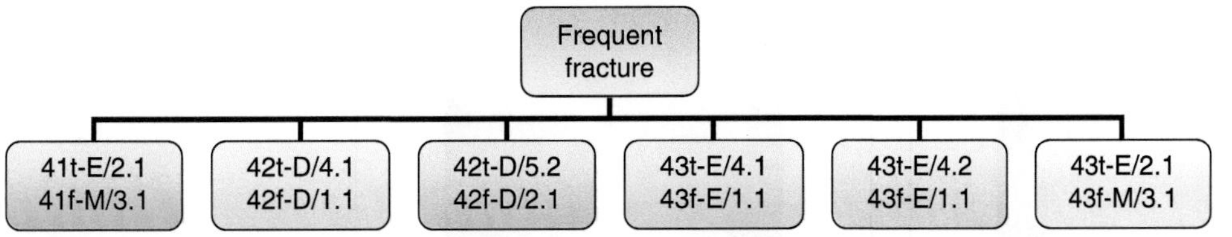

1. 41 t-E/2.1
   41f-M/3.1
   SH II tibia and complete metaphyseal fibula.
2. 42 t-D/4.1
   42f-D/1.1
   Complete diaphyseal tibia and bowing of the fibula.
3. 42 t-D/5.2
   42f-D/2.1
   Multifragmentary diaphyseal tibia and greenstick fibula.
4. 43 t-E/4.1
   43f-E/1.1
   Combined fracture SH III tibia and SH I fibula.
5. 43 t-E/4.2
   43f-E/1.1
   Multifragmentary epiphyseal fracture tibia SH III and SH I fibula.
6. 43 t-E/2.1
   43f-M/3.1
   Distal lower leg SH II tibia and complete metaphyseal fibula.

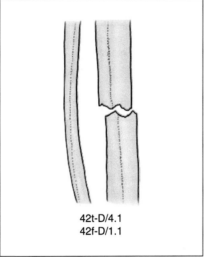

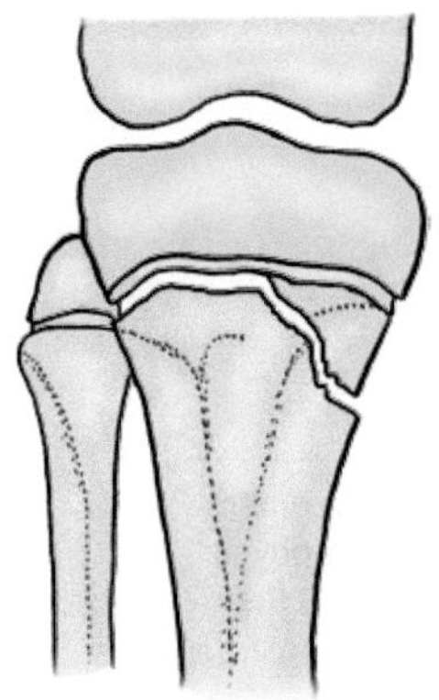
41t-E/2.1
41f-M/3.1

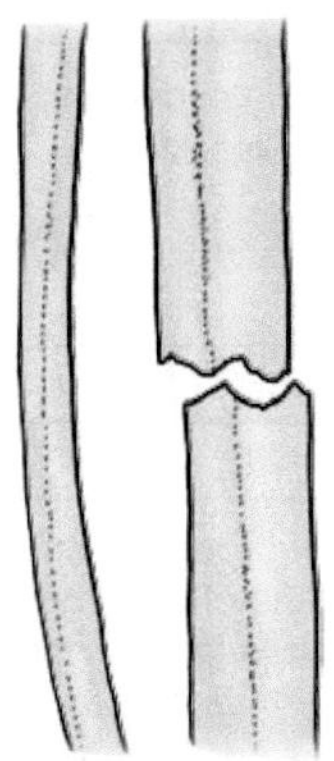
42t-D/4.1
42f-D/1.1

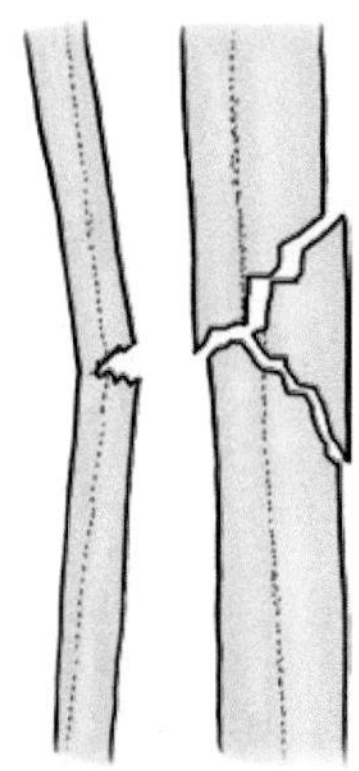
42t-D/5.2
42f-D/2.1

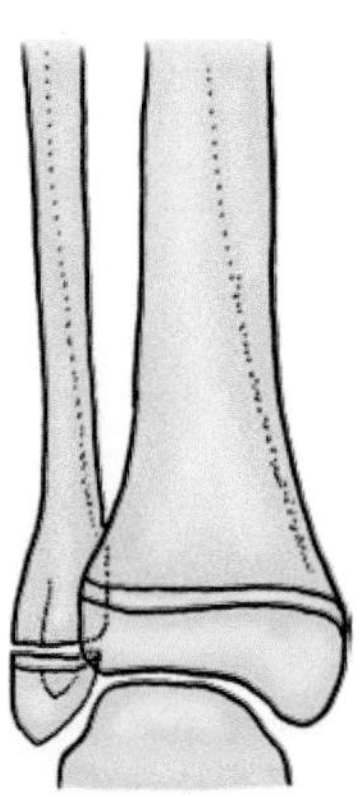
43t-E/4.1
43f-E/1.1

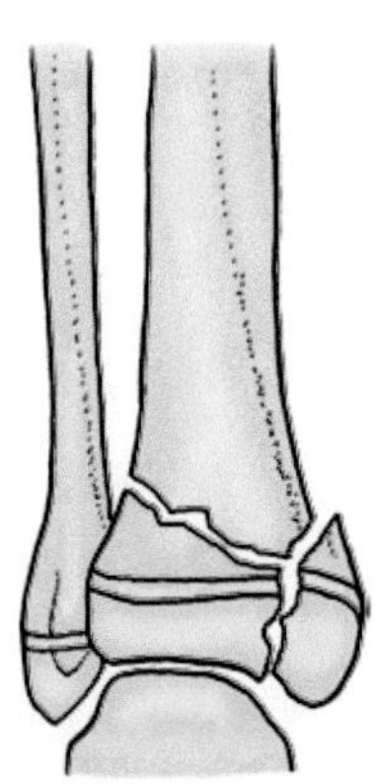
43t-E/4.2
43f-E/1.1

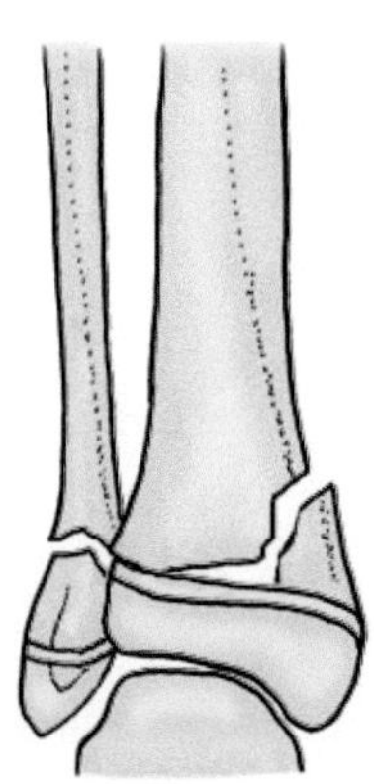
43t-E/2.1
43f-M/3.1

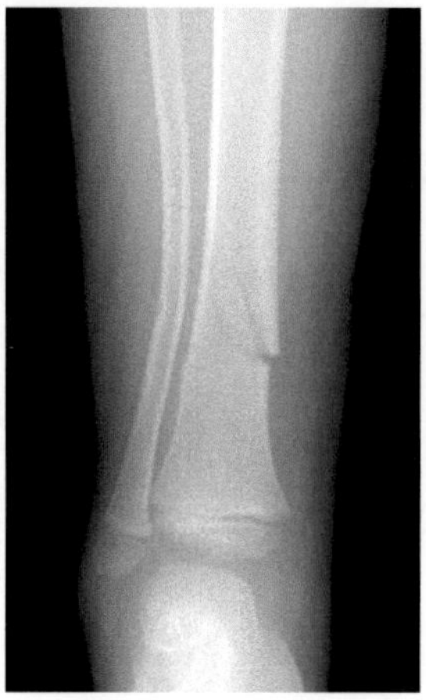
42t-D/4.1； 42f-D/1.1

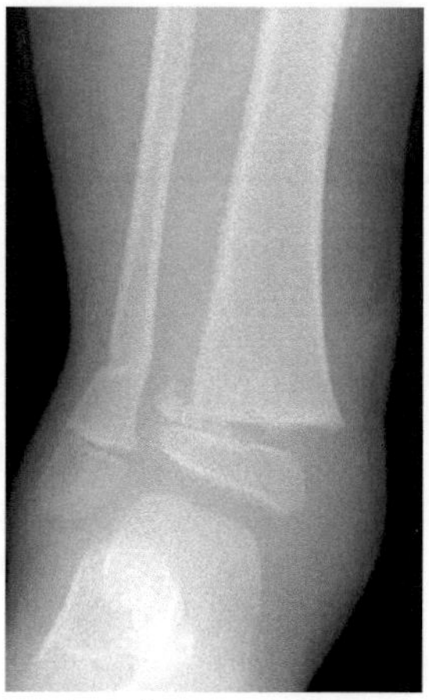
43t-E/2.1； 43f-M/3.1

14.6.2 Classification of Tibial Tubercle Avulsion Fractures

14.6.2.1 Watson-Jones Classification (Fractures and Joint Injures. ed. by J U Wilson. 5th Ed. Churchill Livingstone Edinburgh. London & New York, 1976, 1047–1050)

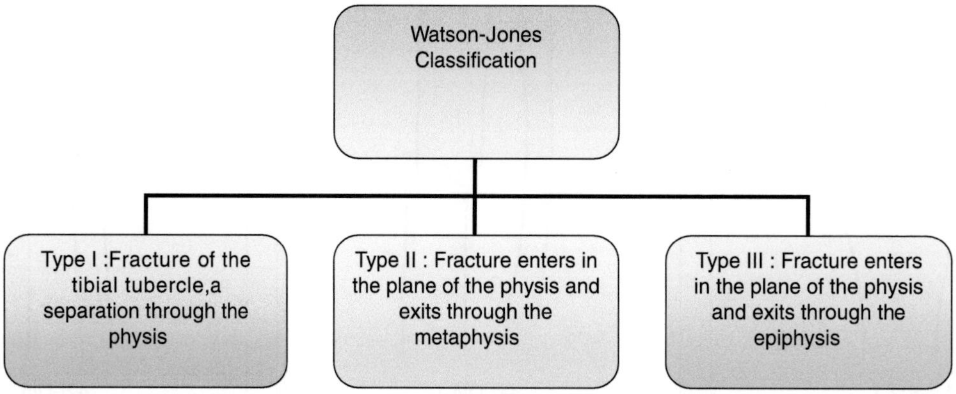

Type I: Fracture of the tibial tubercle, a separation through the physis.

Type II: Fracture enters in the plane of the physis and exits through the metaphysis.

Type III: Fracture enters in the plane of the physis and exits through the epiphysis.

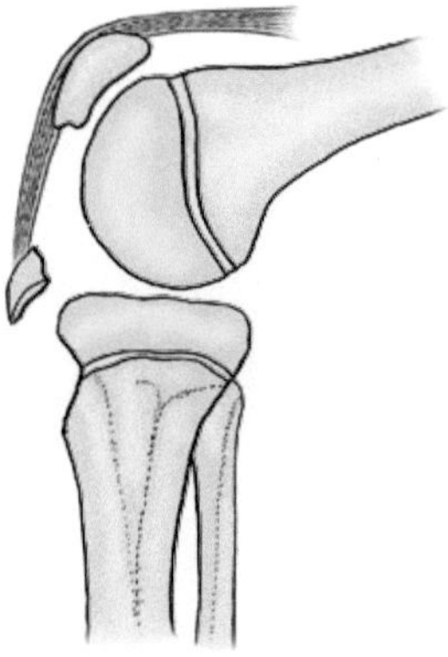

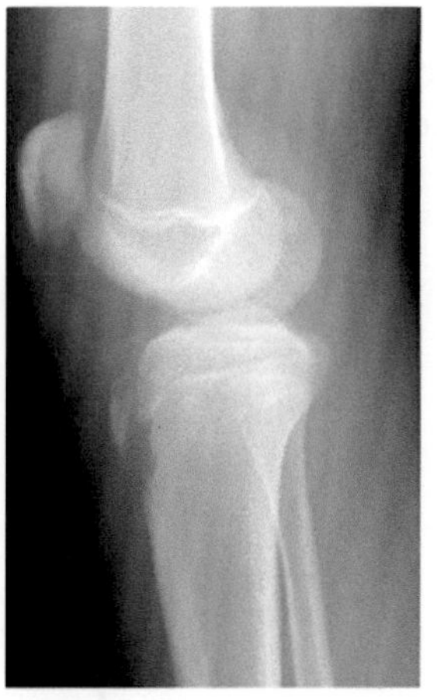

Tibial tubercle avulsion fractures, Watson-Jones Classification
Type I: Fracture of the tibial tubercle, a separation through the physis

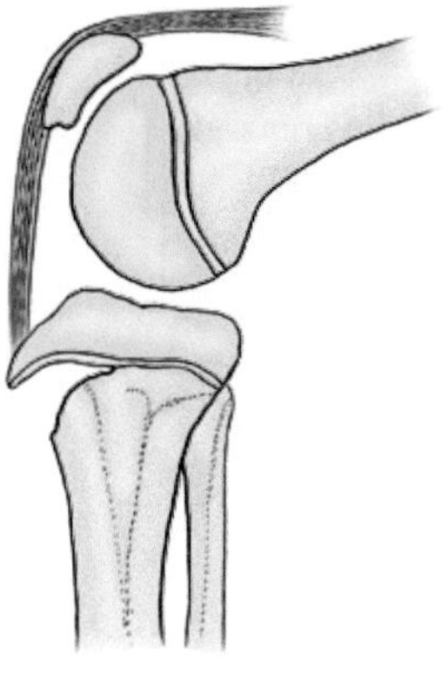

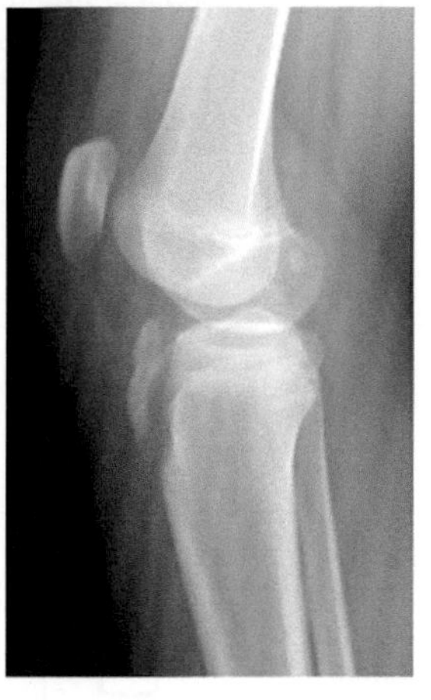

Tibial tubercle avulsion fractures, Watson-Jones Classification
Type II: Fracture enters in the plane of the physis and exits through the metaphysis

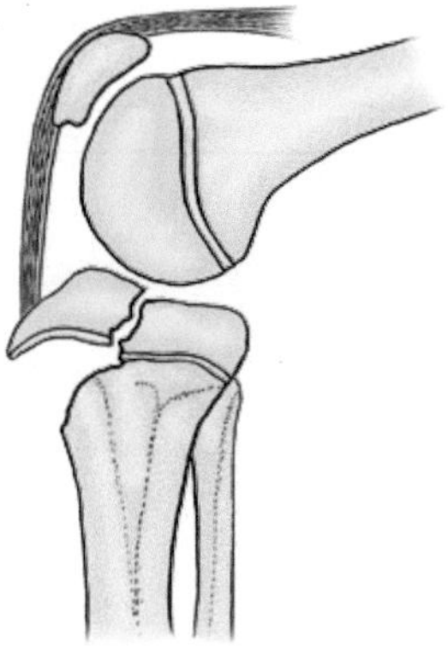

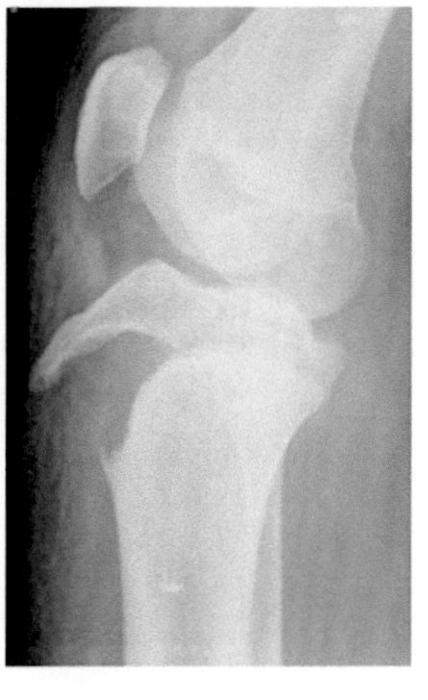

Tibial tubercle avulsion fractures, Watson-Jones Classification
Type III : Fracture enters in the plane of the physis and exits through the epiphysis

14.6.2.2 Watson-Jones and Ogden Classification

Ogden also divides each type of tibial tuberosity fractures into a and b types according to their displacement and comminution based on the Watson-Jones classification.

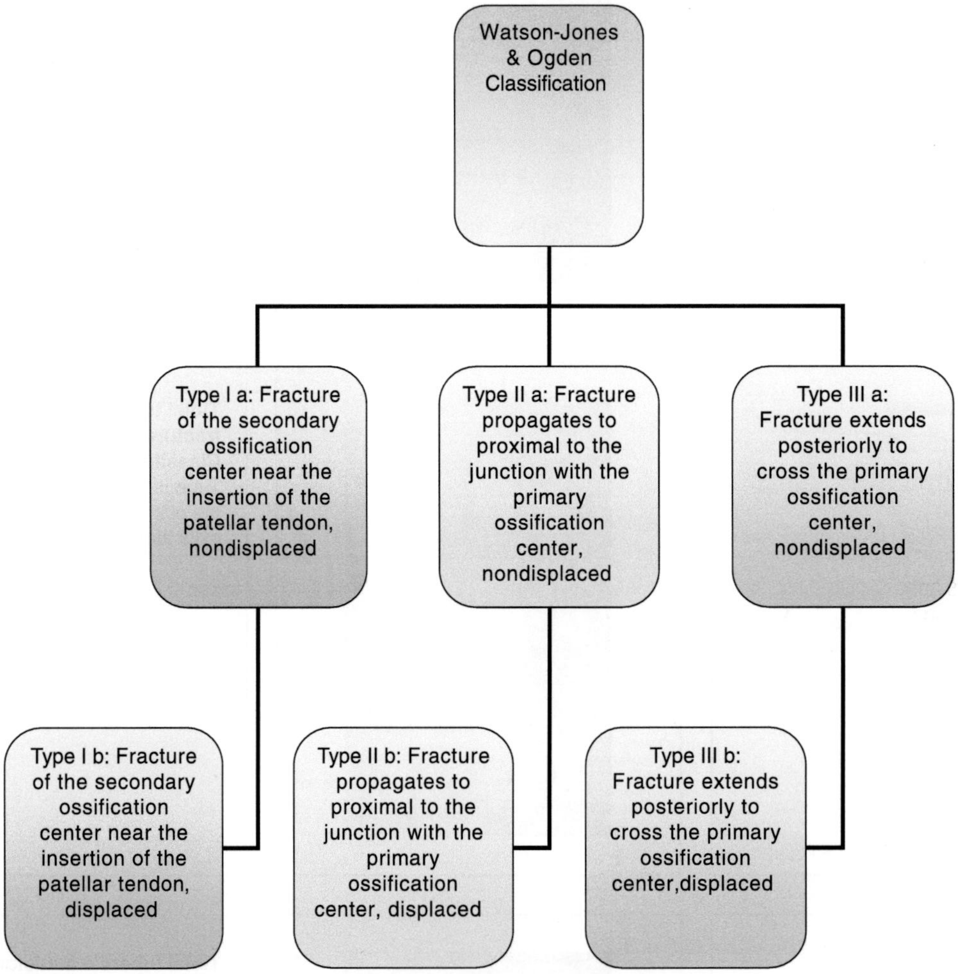

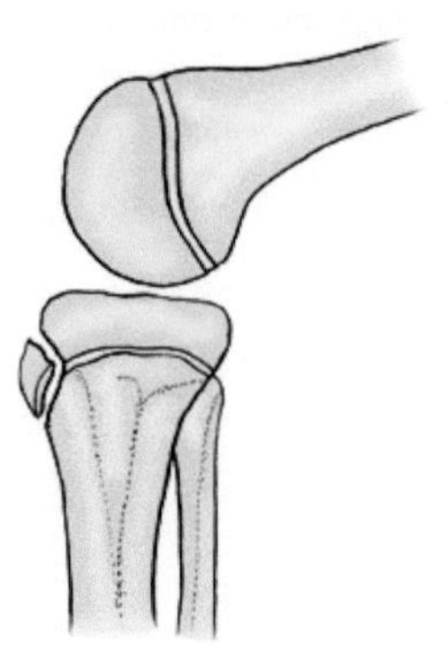

Type I a: Fracture of the secondary ossificationcenter near the insertion of the patellar tendon, nondisplaced

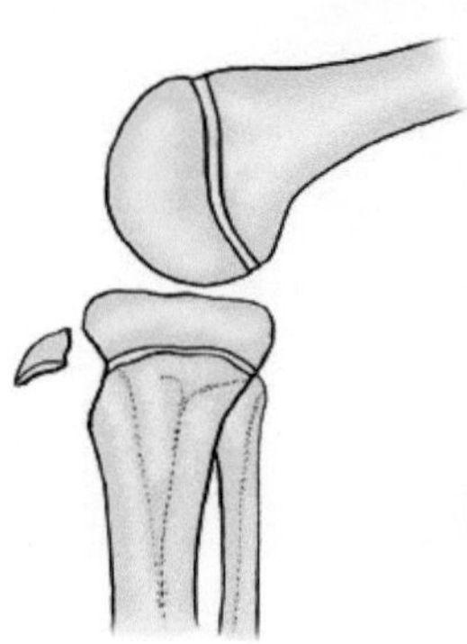

Type I b: Fracture of the secondary ossification center near the insertion of the patellar tendon, displaced

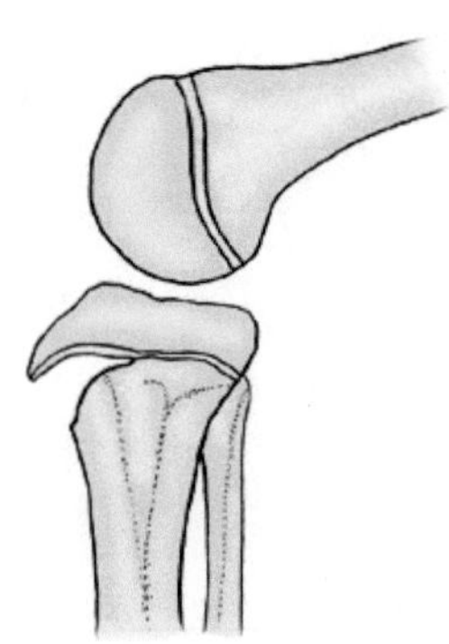

Type II a: Fracture propagates to proximal to the junction with the primary ossification center, nondisplaced

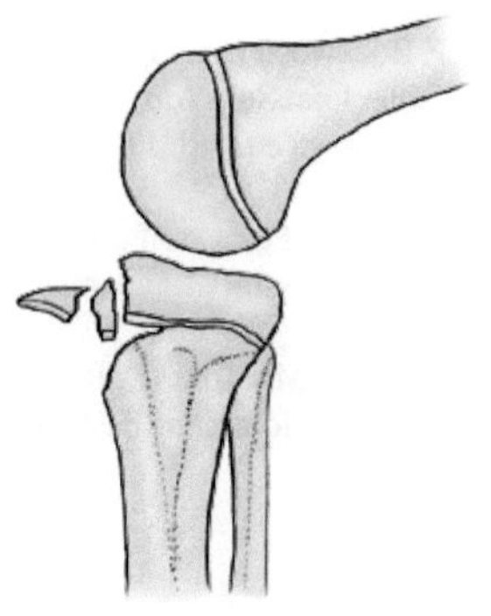

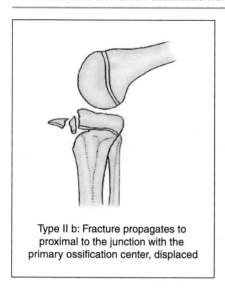

Type II b: Fracture propagates to proximal to the junction with the primary ossification center, displaced

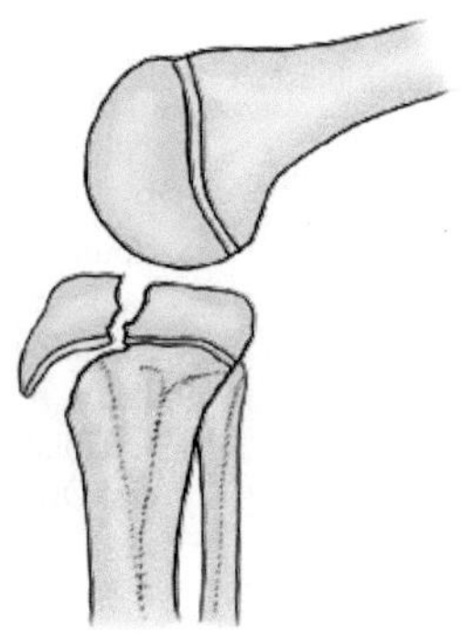

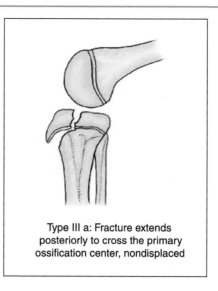

Type III a: Fracture extends posteriorly to cross the primary ossification center, nondisplaced

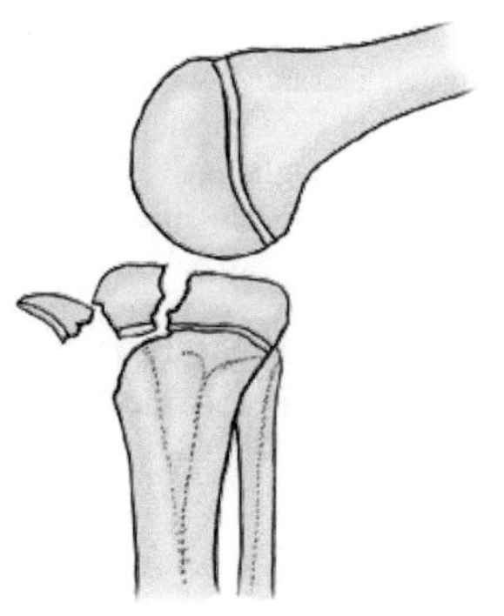

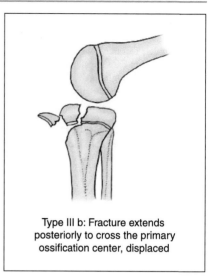

Type III b: Fracture extends posteriorly to cross the primary ossification center, displaced

14.6.3 Classification of a Special Type of Epiphyseal Injury

Type I: Juvenile Tillaux fracture (1964, J Bone Joint Surg (Am), 46:25–32).

The distal tibial epiphyseal line closure starts from the age of 12 to 13 years and occurs first at the central area, followed by at the medial bone, and finally at the outside in a total of 18 months. Before the lateral closure, strong external rotation of the foot due to tibiofibular anterior ligament traction may occur, which could consequently lead to development of this fracture.

Type II: Three-plane tibial distal epiphyseal fractures (1972, Clin Orthop, 86: 187–190).

Type IIa: Three-plane three-fracture fracture:

1. Distal tibial anterolateral.
2. Tibial metaphyseal spiral fracture with residual distal tibia.
3. Distal tibial bone.

Type IIb: Three-plane two-fracture fracture.

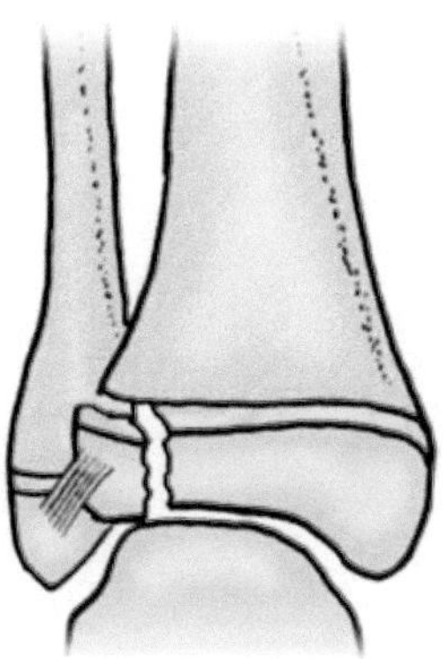

I 型

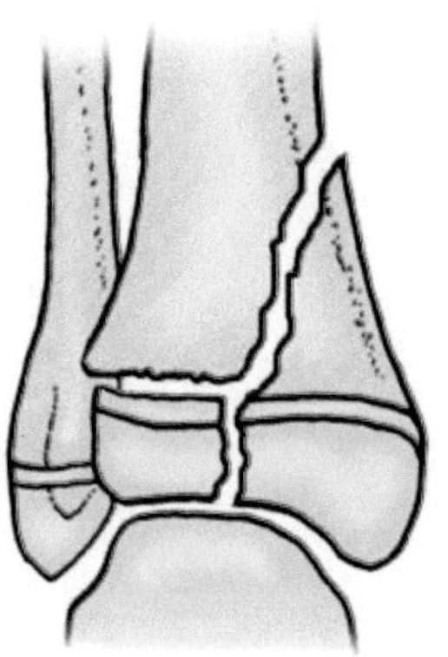

II a

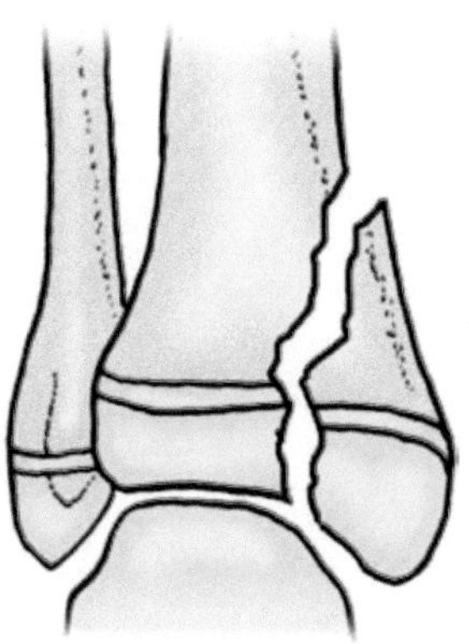

II b

References

1. Brown JH, DeLuca SA. Growth plate injuries: salter-Harris classification. Am Fam Physician. 1992;46:1180–4.
2. Cepela DJ, Tartaglione JP, Dooley TP, Patel PN. Classifications in brief: Salter-Harris classification of pediatric physeal fractures. Clin Orthop Relat Res. 2016;474:2531–7.
3. Aitken AP. Fractures of the proximal tibial epiphysial cartilage. Clin Orthop Relat Res. 1965;41:92–7.
4. Peterson HA. Physeal fractures: Part 3. Classification. J Pediatr Orthop. 1994;14:439–48.
5. Wadsworth TG. Injuries of the capitular (lateral humeral condylar) epiphysis. Clin Orthop Relat Res. 1972;85:127–42.
6. DeLee JC, Wilkins KE, Rogers LF, Rockwood CA. Fracture-separation of the distal humeral epiphysis. J Bone Joint Surg Am. 1980;62:46–51.
7. Tile M. Pelvic ring fractures: should they be fixed. J Bone Joint Surg Br. 1988;70:1–12.
8. Young JW, Burgess AR, Brumback RJ, Poka A. Pelvic fractures: value of plain radiography in early assessment and management. Radiology. 1986;160:445–51.
9. Jakoi A, Freidl M, Old A, Javandel M, Tom J, Realyvasquez J. Tibial tubercle avulsion fractures in adolescent basketball players. Orthopedics. 2012;35:692–6.